QZ 17

Library
1st Floor, Education Centre
Queen Elizabeth Hospital Birmingham
Mindelsohn Way
Birmingham B15 2WB

D1325310

Atlas of
Diagnostic Oncology

Dana-Farber Cancer Institute
Atlas of Diagnostic Oncology

FOURTH EDITION

Edited by

Arthur T. Skarin, MD, FACP, FCCP

Associate Professor of Medicine
Harvard Medical School
Senior Attending Physician
Lowe Center for Thoracic Oncology
Dana-Farber Cancer Institute
Department of Medicine,
Brigham and Women's Hospital

Associate Editors

Kitt Shaffer, MD, PhD

Radiology Department, Harvard Medical School
Dana-Farber Cancer Institute
Brigham and Women's Hospital

Tad Wieczorek, MD

Pathology Department
Harvard Medical School
Brigham and Women's Hospital

Janina Longtine, MD

Pathology Department
Harvard Medical School
Brigham and Women's Hospital

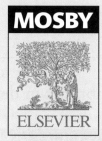

MOSBY

ELSEVIER

An Imprint of Elsevier

To my wife, for her patience, encouragement, and devotion during the preparation for this atlas;
To William C. Moloney, M.D., and Emil Frei III, M.D., who stimulated my interest in
hematology and oncology
and
To all our patients who have contributed so much to medical education

MOSBY
ELSEVIER

1600 John F. Kennedy Blvd,
Ste 1800
Philadelphia, PA 19103-2899

ATLAS OF DIAGNOSTIC ONCOLOGY   ISBN: 978-0-323-05905-3
© 2010 by Mosby, Inc., an affiliate of Elsevier Inc. All rights reserved.

No part of this publication may be reproduced or transmitted in any form or by any means, electronic or
mechanical, including photocopying, recording, or any information storage and retrieval system, without
permission in writing from the Publisher. Details on how to seek permission, further information about
the Publisher's permissions policies and our arrangements with organizations such as the Copyright
Clearance Center and the Copyright Licensing Agency, can be found at our website: www.elsevier.com/
permissions.

This book and the individual contributions contained in it are protected under copyright by the Publisher
(other than as may be noted herein).

Notices

Knowledge and best practice in this field are constantly changing. As new research and experience
broaden our understanding, changes in research methods, professional practices, or medical
treatment may become necessary.

Practitioners and researchers must always rely on their own experience and knowledge in
evaluating and using any information, methods, compounds, or experiments described herein. In
using such information or methods they should be mindful of their own safety and the safety of others, including parties for whom they have a professional responsibility.

With respect to any drug or pharmaceutical products identified, readers are advised to check the
most current information provided (i) on procedures featured or (ii) by the manufacturer of each
product to be administered, to verify the recommended dose or formula, the method and duration
of administration, and contraindications. It is the responsibility of practitioners, relying on their own
experience and knowledge of their patients, to make diagnoses, to determine dosages and the best
treatment for each individual patient, and to take all appropriate safety precautions.

To the fullest extent of the law, neither the Publisher nor the authors, contributors, or editors
assume any liability for any injury and/or damage to persons or property as a matter of products liability, negligence or otherwise, or from any use or operation of any methods, products, instructions,
or ideas contained in the material herein.

Previous editions copyrighted 1996, 2003

Library of Congress Cataloging-in-Publication Data

Atlas of diagnostic oncology / [edited by] Arthur T. Skarin ... [et al.]. — 4th ed.
    p. ; cm.
  At head of title: Dana-Farber Cancer Institute.
  Includes bibliographical references and index.
  ISBN 978-0-323-05905-3
1. Cancer–Atlases.   I. Skarin, Arthur T., 1935–   II. Dana-Farber Cancer Institute.
  [DNLM: 1. Neoplasms–diagnosis–Atlases. QZ 17 A8809 2009]
  RC254.6.A75 2009
  616.99'4075--dc22   2009035668

Acquisitions Editor: Dolores Meloni
Developmental Editor: Jessica Pritchard
Design Direction: Ellen Zandle
Project Manager: Mary B. Stermel
Marketing Manager: Helena Mutak

Working together to grow
libraries in developing countries

www.elsevier.com | www.bookaid.org | www.sabre.org

ELSEVIER   BOOK AID International   Sabre Foundation

Printed in Canada

Last digit is the print number: 9 8 7 6 5 4 3 2 1

Contents

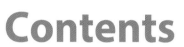

Foreword

As the field of clinical oncology moves forward, so must the published reference literature. The rate of new knowledge has accelerated and resulted in new diagnostic and therapeutic modalities. Understanding the unique biology of tumors that were previously included in major disease groups has resulted in their separation as distinct entities in the *Atlas of Diagnostic Oncology* – entities such as mesothelioma, gastrointestinal stromal tumors, and neuroendocrine gastrointestinal neoplasms. The updates, graphics, and comprehensive summaries have made this a classic in the past and assure its status in the near future. Nuclear radiology is an emerging field that has brought imaging into a new era. Imaging technology has improved the accuracy of staging and the evaluation of response. There is a new section that has brought this field forward and up to date.

Dr. Arthur Skarin brings to this volume his commitment to visual and graphic aspects of medical oncology. He is a talented photographer and outstanding medical oncologist. He brings these talents together as editor of the *Atlas of Diagnostic Oncology*. In recognition of his talents, he has been a long-serving editor of "Images in Oncology" in the *Journal of Clinical Oncology*. I am particularly proud to write this foreword as 16 of the 21 chapters have authors who trained at the Dana-Farber Cancer Institute. This edition includes writers who are now on staffs of the Massachusetts General Hospital and Brigham and Women's Hospital. This edition will offer the clinician a ready reference to all the important issues in the daily practice of clinical oncology. The clinician will also be able to use the accompanying ExpertConsult web site to download teaching illustrations. This is indeed a multidisciplinary text with contributors from the related areas of surgery, pathology, radiology, and dermatology. The *Atlas of Diagnostic Oncology* continues an important tradition in the oncologic literature. It is renowned for its unique combination of talents. The fourth edition enhances this reputation further. I am very proud of my professional relationships with the editors and contributors. The honor is mine to write this foreword.

George P. Canellos, MD
William Rosenberg Professor of Medicine,
Harvard Medical School
Senior Physician, Dana-Farber Cancer Institute

Preface

Considerable progress has occurred in the fields of oncology and hematologic malignancies during the 7 years since the third edition of the *Atlas of Diagnostic Oncology* was published. As a result, it was felt that a fourth edition of this teaching textbook was justified. All chapters from the previous edition have been updated, many with new co-authors, and several chapters have been extensively revised to include new knowledge and data in molecular biology, genetic studies, and staging procedures. Two new topics have been added, the first to Chapter 7: "Cancer of the Gastrointestinal Tract" (Neuroendocrine Tumors by Dr. Matthew Kulke) and the second to Chapter 12: "Sarcomas of Soft Tissue and Bone" (Gastrointestinal Stromal Tumor by Drs. Suzanne George, Jason Hornick, and George Demetri). With the rapid progress in technology, specialization, and staging studies in the field of radiology, the topic of nuclear medicine has been expanded into a new and separate chapter organized by Drs. Annick van den Abbeele and Steven Burrell. Likewise, a new chapter, titled "Malignant Mesothelioma," has been developed by Drs. Pasi Jänne, David Wu, and Lucian Chirieac, experts in this challenging and aggressive disease now seen with increased frequency worldwide. Malignant mesothelioma was previously covered in the Lung Cancer chapter, after initial discussion in the Sarcoma chapter. One other new chapter has been added to this Atlas—Chapter 20, "Complications of Cancer," by Dr. Nadine A. Jackson and myself—to complement Chapter 21, "Systemic and Mucocutaneous Reactions to Chemotherapy". Thus, the fourth edition of *Atlas of Diagnostic Oncology* has five new chapters and topics with a total of 24 new authors and coauthors, all with academic positions at Harvard Medical School and cancer experts at the Dana-Farber Cancer Institute, Massachusetts General Hospital, and the Brigham and Women's Hospital.

The chapter format has remained the same: a general review of the cancer including incidence, epidemiology, etiology, and histopathology with molecular biology when relevant, and clinical features, which is followed by diagnostic studies and current clinical and pathologic staging. Most of the chapters use staging nomenclature from the sixth edition (2002) of the American Joint Committee on Cancer (AJCC). The seventh edition of the AJCC staging system will be published in late 2009. A new TNM staging system has been developed by the International Association for the Study of Lung Cancer (IASLC) in collaboration with the International Union Against Cancer (IUAC) and the AJCC and is included in Chapter 5. Detailed charts are used for histopathologic classification, diagnostic studies, and prognostic factors when important. Generous illustrations with detailed figure legends are utilized for examples of histopathology, staging, radiographs, CT, MRI, and PET images and differential diagnosis, along with examples of various clinical manifestations and relevant up-to-date references. As with previous editions, detailed treatment recommendations are not included since these are outside the goals of this book. The reader is referred to standard oncology textbooks and current review articles for details concerning management of cancer and hematologic malignancy patients.

Of note, previous editions of this Atlas had 35-mm slide sets included for teaching purposes. With advances in computer technology it was possible to provide a CD-ROM with the second and third editions. With the fourth edition, a website will be available to download images of choice. These images have proven to be of great value for teaching medical and nursing students, house staff, and fellows. These images will also increase the scope of this Atlas by allowing for use in tumor boards, lectures, and other teaching applications. This fulfills our original goals of preparing a unique and illustrative educational *Atlas of Diagnostic Oncology*.

Arthur T. Skarin, MD
September, 2009

Contributors

Annick D. van den Abbeele, MD
Associate Professor of Radiology, Harvard Medical School;
Chief, Department of Radiology and Founding Director,
Center for Biomedical Imaging in Oncology,
Dana-Farber Cancer Institute, Boston, Massachusetts

Jeremy S. Abramson, MD
Instructor, Department of Medicine,
Harvard Medical School; Clinical Director,
Lymphoma Program, Cancer Center,
Massachusetts General Hospital,
Boston, Massachusetts

Kenneth C. Anderson, MD
Kraft Family Professor of Medicine, Harvard Medical School;
Chief, Division of Hematologic Neoplasia,
Dana-Farber Cancer Institute, Department of Medicine,
Brigham and Women's Hospital,
Boston, Massachusetts

Karen H. Antman, MD
Provost of Medical Campus; Dean, School of Medicine;
Professor of Medicine, Boston University School of Medicine,
Boston, Massachusetts
Formerly
Associate Professor of Medicine, Harvard Medical School;
Director, Solid Tumor Autologous Marrow Program,
Dana-Farber Cancer Institute, Boston, Massachusetts

Ramon Blanco, MD
Department of Pathology, Falmouth Hospital,
Falmouth, Massachusetts
Formerly
Fellow in Surgical Pathology, Department of Pathology,
Brigham and Women's Hospital, Boston, Massachusetts

Steven Burrell, MD, FRCPC
Center for Biomedical Imaging in Oncology,
Dana-Farber Cancer Institute, Harvard
Medical School, Boston, Massachusetts
Formerly
Assistant Professor of Radiology, Dalhousie University;
Department of Diagnostic Imaging, Queen Elizabeth II Health
Sciences Centre,
Halifax, Nova Scotia, Canada

Susana M. Campos, MD, MPH
Assistant Professor of Medicine, Harvard Medical School,
Dana-Farber Cancer Institute, Boston, Massachusetts

Wendy Y. Chen, MD, MPH
Assistant Professor in Medicine, Harvard Medical School;
Attending Physician, Dana-Farber Cancer Institute,
Brigham and Women's Hospital,
Boston, Massachusetts

Lucian R. Chirieac, MD
Assistant Professor, Department of Pathology,
Harvard Medical School; Associate Pathologist,
Pathology, Brigham and Women's Hospital,
Boston, Massachusetts

Toni K. Choueiri, MD
Instructor in Medicine, Harvard Medical School;
Attending Physician, Dana-Farber Cancer Institute,
Boston, Massachusetts

John R. Clark, MD
Clinical Director, Center for Head and Neck Cancers,
Massachusetts General Hospital Cancer Center,
Boston, Massachusetts
Formerly
Instructor in Medicine, Harvard Medical School;
Attending Physician, Head and Neck Tumor Clinic,
Adult Oncology Division, Dana-Farber Cancer Institute,
Department of Medicine, Brigham and Women's Hospital,
Boston, Massachusetts

A. Dimitros Colevas, MD
Associate Professor of Medicine, Stanford University,
Stanford, California
Formerly
Instructor in Medicine, Harvard Medical School;
Attending Physician, Head and Neck Tumor Center,
Adult Oncology Division, Dana-Farber Cancer Institute,
Brigham and Women's Hospital,
Boston, Massachusetts

Christopher Corless, MD, PhD
Assistant Professor of Pathology, Department of Pathology,
Oregon Health and Sciences University,
Portland, Oregon

Formerly
Instructor of Pathology, Harvard Medical School,
Department of Pathology, Brigham and Women's Hospital,
Boston, Massachusetts

George D. Demetri, MD
Associate Professor of Medicine, Harvard Medical School;
Director, Ludwig Center at Dana-Farber/Harvard Cancer
Center; Director, Center for Sarcoma and Bone Oncology,
Dana-Farber Cancer Institute, Boston, Massachusetts

David M. Dorfman, MD, PhD
Assistant Professor of Pathology, Harvard Medical School;
Medical Director, Hematology Laboratory;
Associate Pathologist, Department of Pathology,
Brigham and Women's Hospital,
Boston, Massachusetts

Joseph P. Eder, MD
Associate Professor, Department of Medicine,
Harvard Medical School; Clinical Director,
Experimental Therapeutics Program,
Dana-Farber Cancer Institute; Associate Physician,
Medicine, Beth Israel Deaconess Medical Center,
Boston, Massachusetts

Philip Friedlander, MD, PhD
Instructor of Medicine, Harvard Medical School;
Instructor of Medicine, Dana-Farber Cancer Institute;
Instructor of Medicine, Brigham and Women's Hospital,
Boston, Massachusetts

Suzanne George, MD
Instructor in Medicine, Harvard Medical School;
Clinical Director, Center for Sarcoma and Bone Oncology,
Dana-Farber Cancer Institute,
Boston, Massachusetts

Holcombe E. Grier, MD
Professor of Pediatrics, Harvard Medical School;
Associate Chief, Pediatric Clinical Oncology,
Dana-Farber Cancer Institute,
Boston, Massachusetts

Robert Haddad, MD
Assistant Professor of Medicine, Harvard Medical School;
Clinical Director, Head and Neck Oncology Program,
Dana-Farber Cancer Institute,
Boston, Massachusetts

Daniel F. Hayes, MD
Professor, Internal Medicine, Hematology, and
Oncology, University of Michigan Comprehensive
Cancer Center, Ann Arbor, Michigan
Formerly
Assistant Professor of Medicine, Harvard Medical School;
Gillette Center for Women's Cancer's, Adult Oncology
Division, Dana-Farber Cancer Institute,
Boston, Massachusetts

Michelle S. Hirsch, MD, PhD
Assistant Professor of Pathology, Harvard Medical School;
Associate Pathologist, Department of Surgical Pathology,
Division of Women's and Perinatal Pathology,
Brigham and Women's Hospital,
Boston, Massachusetts

F. Stephen Hodi, MD
Instructor in Medicine, Harvard Medical School;
Department of Medical Oncology/Solid Tumor Oncology,
Dana-Farber Cancer Institute; Department of Medicine,
Brigham and Women's Hospital, Boston, Massachusetts

Fredric A. Hoffer, MD
Professor of Radiology, University of Washington
Medical Center; Department of Radiology,
Seattle Children's Hospital, Seattle, Washington
Formerly
Associate Professor of Radiology, Harvard
Medical School; Radiologist, Children's
Hospital, Boston, Massachusetts

Jason L. Hornick, MD, PhD
Assistant Professor, Department of Pathology,
Harvard Medical School; Consultant in Pathology, Pathology,
Dana-Farber Cancer Institute; Consultant, Pathology,
Children's Hospital Boston; Staff Pathologist, Pathology,
Brigham and Women's Hospital,
Boston, Massachusetts

Eric Jacobsen, MD
Instructor in Medicine, Harvard Medical School;
Attending Physician, Dana-Farber Cancer Institute,
Boston, Massachusetts

Pasi A. Jänne, MD, PhD
Associate Professor of Medicine, Harvard Medical School;
Attending Physician, Lowe Center for Thoracic Oncology,
Dana-Farber Cancer Institute; Department of Medicine,
Brigham and Women's Hospital, Boston, Massachusetts
Formerly
Assistant Professor of Medicine, Harvard Medical School;
Dana-Farber Cancer Institute, Department of Medicine,
Brigham and Women's Hospital, Boston, Massachusetts

Nancy E. Joste, MD
Professor of Pathology, University of New Mexico
School of Medicine; Head of Surgical Pathology,
University of New Mexico Hospitals,
Albuquerque, New Mexico
Formerly
Instructor of Pathology, Harvard Medical School;
Department of Pathology, Brigham and
Women's Hospital,
Boston, Massachusetts

Philip W. Kantoff, MD
Chief Clinical Research Officer;
Chief, Division of Solid Tumor Oncology;
Director, Lank Center for Genitourinary Oncology,

Dana-Farber Cancer Institute; Professor of Medicine,
Harvard Medical School; Department of Medicine,
Brigham and Women's Hospital,
Boston, Massachusetts

Karen J. Krag, MD
Department of Medical Oncology, North Shore Cancer
Center, Danvers, Massachusetts
Formerly
Clinical Instructor in Medicine, Harvard Medical School;
Adult Oncology Division, Dana-Farber Cancer Institute;
Department of Medicine, Brigham and Women's Hospital,
Boston, Massachusetts

Matthew H. Kulke, MD
Assistant Professor, Department of Medicine,
Harvard Medical School; Associate Physician,
Brigham and Women's Hospital,
Dana-Farber Cancer Institute,
Boston, Massachusetts

Janina A. Longtine, MD
Associate Professor of Pathology, Harvard Medical School;
Co-Director, Center for Advanced Molecular Diagnostics;
Director, Molecular Diagnostics, Department of Pathology,
Brigham and Women's Hospital, Boston, Massachusetts

Elizabeth A. Maher, MD, PhD
Associate Professor of Internal Medicine and Neurology,
Theodore H. Strauss Professor of Neuro-Oncology,
Simmons Cancer Center, University of Texas Southwestern
Medical Center, Dallas, Texas
Formerly
Instructor in Medicine, Harvard Medical School;
Neuro-Oncology Program, Adult Oncology Division,
Dana-Farber Cancer Institute; Department of Medicine,
Brigham and Women's Hospital,
Boston, Massachusetts

Ursula A. Matulonis, MD
Assistant Professor of Medicine, Harvard Medical School;
Department Medical Oncology/Solid Tumor Oncology,
Gynecologic Oncology Program, Dana-Farber Cancer Institute;
Department of Medicine, Brigham and Women's Hospital,
Boston, Massachusetts

Nadine Jackson McCleary, MD, MPH
Instructor in Medicine, Harvard Medical School;
Dana-Farber Cancer Institute,
Boston, Massachusetts

Ann C. McKee, MD
Director, VISN-1 Neuropathology, New England
Veterans Administration Medical Centers;
Associate Professor of Neurology and Pathology,
Boston University School of Medicine;
Director, Brain Banks, Framingham Heart Study,
Centenarian Study Center for the Study of Traumatic
Encephalopathy, Boston, Massachusetts
Formerly

Instructor of Pathology, Harvard Medical School;
Division of Neuropathology, Massachusetts General
Hospital, Boston, Massachusetts

Jeffrey A. Meyerhardt, MD, MPH
Assistant Professor of Medicine, Harvard Medical School;
Associate Physician, Gastrointestinal Cancer Center,
Dana-Farber Cancer Institute,
Boston, Massachusetts

Francis D. Moore, Jr., MD
Professor of Surgery, Harvard Medical School;
Chief, Division of General and Gastrointestinal Surgery;
Senior Surgeon; Chief, Endocrine Surgery Unit,
Brigham and Women's Hospital,
Boston, Massachusetts

William K. Oh, MD
Associate Director for Clinical Research, The Tisch Cancer Institute;
Chief, Division of Hematology-Medical Oncology;
Professor of Medicine and Urology; Ezra M. Greenspan, MD,
Professor in Clinical Cancer Therapeutics, The Mount Sinai
Hospital, New York, New York
Formerly
Associate Professor of Medicine, Harvard Medical School;
Clinical Director, Lank Center for Genitourinary Oncology,
Adult Oncology Division, Dana-Farber Cancer Institute;
Department of Medicine, Boston, Massachusetts

Antonio Perez-Atayde, MD, PhD
Associate Professor of Pathology, Harvard Medical School;
Department of Pathology, Children's Hospital,
Boston, Massachusetts

Marshall Posner, MD
Associate Professor in Medicine, Harvard Medical School;
Medical Director, Head and Neck Oncology Program,
Dana-Farber Cancer Institute,
Boston, Massachusetts

Noopur Raje, MD
Assistant Professor of Medicine, Harvard Medical School;
Director, Center for Multiple Myeloma, Massachusetts
General Hospital, Boston, Massachusetts
Formerly
Dana-Farber Cancer Institute; Department of Medicine,
Brigham and Women's Hospital,
Boston, Massachusetts

Robert Ross, MD
Instructor in Medicine, Harvard Medical School;
Medical Oncologist, Dana-Farber Cancer Institute;
Department of Medicine, Brigham and Women's Hospital,
Boston, Massachusetts

Peter M. Sadow, MD, PhD
Instructor of Pathology, Harvard Medical School;
Staff Pathologist, Massachusetts General Hospital,
Boston, Massachusetts

Ravi Salgia, MD, PhD
Professor of Medicine, Pathology, and Dermatology;
Director, Thoracic Oncology Research Program, Center for
Advanced Medicine, University of Chicago Medical Center;
Head of the Aerodigestive Tract Program Translational Research
Laboratories, University of Chicago,
Chicago, Illinois
Formerly
Assistant Professor of Medicine, Harvard Medical School;
Lowe Center for Thoracic Oncology, Adult Oncology
Division, Dana-Farber Cancer Institute; Department of
Medicine, Brigham and Women's Hospital,
Boston, Massachusetts

David T. Scadden, MD
Gerald and Darlene Jordan Professor of Medicine; Professor
and Co-Chair, Department of Stem Cell and Regenerative
Biology, Harvard University; Co-Director, Harvard Stem Cell
Institute; Director, Hematologic Malignancies and Center
for Regenerative Medicine, Massachusetts General Hospital,
Boston, Massachusetts

Kitt Shaffer, MD, PhD
Associate Professor of Radiology,
Boston University School of Medicine;
Vice-Chair of Radiology, Boston Medical Center,
Boston, Massachusetts
Formerly
Associate Professor, Department of Radiology,
Harvard Medical School; Clinical Director, Radiology,
Dana-Farber Cancer Institute, Brigham and Women's Hospital,
Boston, Massachusetts

Arthur T. Skarin, MD, FACP, FCCP
Associate Professor of Medicine, Harvard Medical School;
Senior Attending Physician, Lowe Center for Thoracic
Oncology, Dana-Farber Cancer Institute;
Department of Medicine, Brigham and Women's Hospital,
Boston, Massachusetts

Mark A. Socinski, MD
Professor of Medicine Hematology/Oncology, University of
North Carolina at Chapel Hill, Lineberger Comprehensive
Cancer Center, Chapel Hill, North Carolina
Formerly
Medical Oncology Fellow, Harvard Medical School;
Adult Oncology Division, Dana-Farber Cancer Institute;
Department of Medicine, Brigham and Women's Hospital,
Boston, Massachusetts

James N. Suojanen, MD
Department of Radiology, South Shore Hospital,
South Weymouth, Massachusetts
Formerly

Instructor of Radiology, Harvard Medical School;
Director of Neuroradiology, Deaconess Hospital,
Boston, Massachusetts

Jerrold R. Turner, MD, PhD
Professor and Associate Chair, Department of Pathology,
The University of Chicago, Chicago, Illinois
Formerly
Instructor of Pathology, Harvard Medical School;
Staff Pathologist, Department of Pathology,
Brigham and Women's Hospital,
Boston, Massachusetts

Elsa F. Velazquez, MD
Assistant Professor of Pathology, Harvard Medical School;
Associate Dermatopathologist, Brigham and Women's
Hospital, Boston, Massachusetts

Stephan D. Voss, MD, PhD
Assistant Professor of Radiology; Staff Radiologist,
Department of Radiology, Children's Hospital Boston,
Boston, Massachusetts

Martha Wadleigh, MD
Instructor in Medicine, Harvard Medical School;
Dana-Farber Cancer Institute, Department of Medical
Oncology; Hematologic Oncology, Brigham and Women's
Hospital, Boston, Massachusetts

Michael M. Wick, MD, PhD
Chairman, Chief Executive Officer and President, Telik, Inc.,
Palo Alto, California
Formerly
Associate Professor of Dermatology,
Harvard Medical School; Laboratory of Molecular
Dermatologic Oncology,
Dana-Farber Cancer Institute; Department of Medicine,
Brigham and Women's Hospital,
Boston, Massachusetts

Tad Wieczorek, MD
Instructor in Pathology, Harvard Medical School;
Pathologist, Brigham and Women's/Faulkner Hospitals,
Boston, Massachusetts

David Wu, MD, PhD
Assistant Professor, University of Washington Medical School,
Department of Laboratory Medicine,
University of Washington, Seattle, Washington
Formerly
Clinical Fellow in Pathology, Harvard Medical School;
Department of Pathology, Brigham and Women's Hospital,
Boston, Massachusetts

Acknowledgments

I would like to acknowledge the associate editors of the first edition, Dr. Maxine Jochelson (currently Director of Oncologic Radiology and Women's Imaging, Cedars-Sinai Medical Center, Los Angeles, CA) and Dr. Robert Penny (currently Director of Hematopathology, Community and St. Vincent's Hospital of Indianapolis, IN). Their immense help in organizing and evaluating the radiographic and pathology material for the chapters contributed significantly to the success of the Atlas. In the extensive revision and update for the third and fourth editions, I deeply appreciate the work of the current associate editors, Dr. Kitt Shaffer, former Clinical Director of Radiology at Dana-Farber Cancer Institute and Drs. Tad Wieczorek, and Nina Longtime of the Pathology Department at Brigham and Women's Hospital. Their expertise was invaluable in emphasizing the illustrative and teaching aspects of these editions. I also appreciate the work of the editorial staff at Elsevier, including Dolores Meloni, Elena Pushaw, Jessica Pritchard, and Ellen Sklar, in preparing the revised layouts and keeping all of the chapters on schedule.

Introduction

The likelihood of developing cancer during one's lifetime is one in two for males and one in three for females, based on the 1998–2000 Surveillance, Epidemiology and End Results (SEER) database (Gloeckler et al., 2003; Hayat et al., 2007). The median age at cancer diagnosis is 68 years for men and 65 years for women. The overall 5-year relative survival rate for all patients is 62.7%, with considerable variation by cancer site and stage at diagnosis. The variation in cancer statistics over recent years in the United States is depicted in Figures 1 and 2 (Hayat et al., 2007). The American Cancer Society estimates that in 2009 the total number of new cases will be 1,479,350 with 562,340 deaths (see Fig. 3 for the percent distribution of the more common cancer types) (Jemal et al., 2006, 2008, 2009). The death rate from all cancers combined has decreased by 1.5% per year since 1993 among men and by 0.8% per year since 1992 for women. The mortality rate in men has also continued to decrease for the three most common sites (lung/bronchus, colorectal, and prostate), as has the rate for breast and colorectal cancers in women. Of interest, since 1999, cancer has surpassed heart disease as the leading cause of death for those under 85 years of age (Jemal et al., 2006). The reverse exists for those over age 85. This latest update on cancer statistics was recently published and confirms a decrease in deaths, particularly from lung, prostate, and colorectal cancer in men and breast and colorectal cancer in women (Jemal et al., 2009).

Worldwide, an estimated 11 million new cases and 7 million cancer deaths occurred in 2002, while nearly 25 million people were living with cancer (Kamangar et al., 2006). Global disparities in cancer incidence, mortality, and prevalence relate to genetic susceptibility and aging, but also to modifiable risk factors such as tobacco abuse, infectious agents, certain dietary factors, and physical activity. Other modifiable factors include overweight/obesity, urban air pollution, indoor smoke from household fires, unsafe sex, and contaminated injections in health-care settings (Ezzati et al., 2005). At least one third of world cancer deaths are believed to be preventable. The associations of established causes of human cancers have been categorized as chemicals and naturally occurring compounds, medicines and hormones, infectious agents, and mixtures (Neugent and Li, 2007). Lung cancer, for example, is the most common cancer in the world and the leading cause of cancer-related mortality, with about 1,179,000 deaths per year. A recent report from China estimated 673,000 deaths in 2005 attributable to smoking with 538,200 among men and 134,800 among women. The leading causes of these smoking-related deaths were cancer (40%), cardiovascular disease (22%), and respiratory disease (10%) (Gu et al., 2009). To counter the tobacco epidemic, the World Health Organization Framework Convention on Tobacco

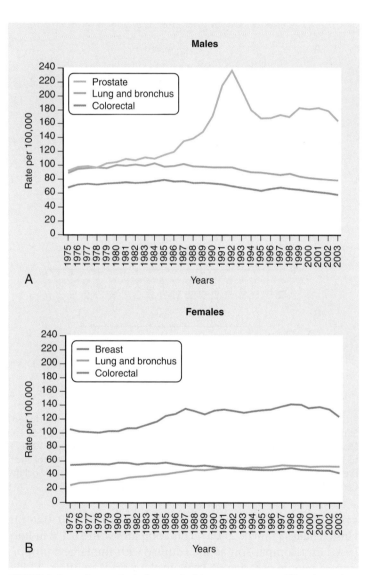

FIGURE 1 Annual age-adjusted cancer incidence rates among **(A)** males and **(B)** females for selected cancers in the United States, 1975–2003. (Data from Surveillance, Epidemiology and End Results [SEER] program [http://seer.cancer.gov] SEER*Stat Database: Incidence-SEER 9 Regs Public-Use, Nov 2005 [Sub 1973–2003], National Cancer Institute, DCCPS, Surveillance Research Program, Cancer Statistics Branch, released April 2006, based on the 25 November 2005 submission.)

Control, organized in 2003, has proposed restrictions on advertising, established clean indoor air controls, and strengthened legislation against tobacco smuggling (Roemer et al. 2005).

Because of the improvements in health care and other factors, there is an increasing aging population in the United States and many other countries in the world. It has been estimated that the proportion of people over age 65 years will increase

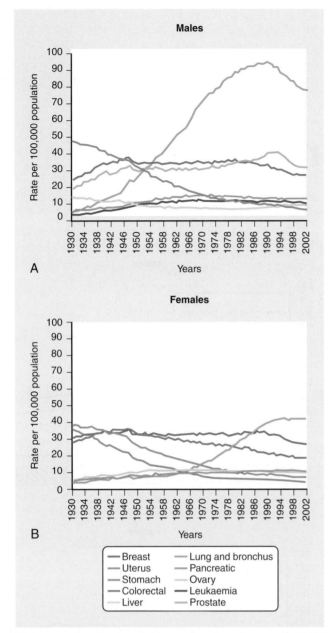

FIGURE 2   Age-adjusted cancer death rates for selected cancers in the United States between 1930 and 2002 for **(A)** males and **(B)** females. (Source: U.S. Mortality Public Use Data Tapes, 1960 to 2002; U.S. Mortality Volumes, 1930 to 1959, National Center for Health Statistics, Centers for Disease Control and Prevention, 2005. Reproduced with permission from American Cancer Society. Cancer Facts and Figures 2006. Atlanta: American Cancer Society, Inc.)

from 12.6% in 2000 to 14.7% in 2015 and 20% in 2030 in the United States (Yancik, 2005). This compares with 18.1% in Italy (used as a comparison as the country with the largest proportion of people over age 65 years in the world) in 2000, 22.2% in 2015, and 28.1% in 2030. Since the incidence of cancer increases with age, a rising number of cancer cases and deaths is predicted. Screening for cancer is therefore extremely important for early detection and subsequent cure. The annual screening recommendations by the American Cancer Society have been published (Neugent and Li, 2007; Smith et al., 2009).

Winning the war against cancer will include not only a multidisciplinary therapeutic plan but also a strong public health approach. The latter includes primary prevention through reduction in risk factors and changes to the environment that reduce human exposure to widely consumed cancer-promoting agents, as well as vaccination against virus-associated cancers, and secondary prevention by effective screening and early treatment (Frieden et al., 2008).

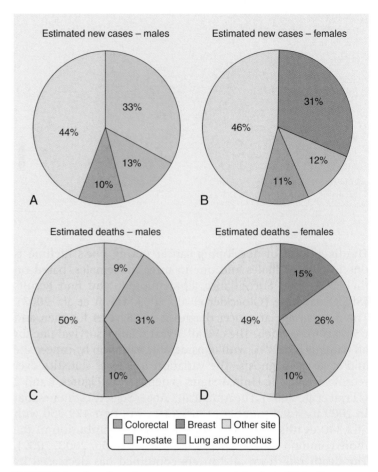

FIGURE 3   Leading sites of new cancer cases and deaths—2006 estimates. **(A)** Estimated new cases—males. **(B)** Estimated new cases—females. **(C)** Estimated deaths—males. **(D)** Estimated deaths—females. (Source: American Cancer Society, Inc., Surveillance Research. Estimates of new cases are based on incidence rates from 1979 to 2002, National Cancer Institute's Surveillance, Epidemiology, and End Results program, nine oldest registries. Estimates of deaths are based on data from U.S. Mortality Public Use Data Tapes, 1969 to 2003. National Center for Health Statistics, Centers for Disease Control and Prevention, 2006.)

Cancer prevention is extremely important, and the progress in information technology has been recently reviewed (Jimbo et al., 2006). Important characteristics of neoplasms and the associated molecular targets that may be adversely affected by chemoprevention or definitive treatment programs are noted in Table 1 (Hanahan and Weinberg, 2000).

With completion of the Human Genome Project, new knowledge has become available about genetic variations that can aid in understanding the family history as a risk factor for most cancer types. Identification of mutations in genes (*BRCA1*, *BRCA2*, *TP53*, *PTEN*, and others) may identify individuals at high risk for certain cancers, allowing for early detection, as well as an increased understanding of the etiologic subtypes of cancer and inherited alterations in drug metabolism. This exciting field of molecular epidemiology may thus impact favorably on cancer prognosis (Chen and Hunter, 2005). The importance of the above underscores the need for collection and storage of adequate tumor tissue for study.

The new information explosion in molecular biology has led to important discoveries in unique patterns of gene expression characteristic of certain malignancies (Cam et al., 2008). This genetic expression profiling will be important not only for accurate diagnosis but also for determining prognosis and candidates for certain therapies (Quackenbush, 2006). In addition, exciting work in identification and characterization of cancer stem cells is underway (Boman et al., 2008).

Table 1

Molecular Biomarkers Associated with Neoplasia Characteristics

Evading Apoptosis
BCL-2, BAX, caspases, FAS, TNF receptor, DRS, IGF/PI3K/AKT, mTOR, p53, PTEN, *RAS* IL-3, NF-κB

Insensitivity to Antigrowth Signals
SMADs, pRb, cyclin-dependent kinases, MYC

Limitless Replicative Potential
hTERT, pRb, p53

Self-sufficiency in Cell Growth
Epidermal growth factor, platelet-derived growth factor, MAPK, PI3K

Sustained Angiogenesis
VEGF, basic fibroblast growth factor, α, β thrombospondin-1, hypoxia-inducible factor 1α

Tissue Invasion and Metastasis
Matrix metalloproteinases, MAPK, E-cadherin

BAX, BCL-2 associated X protein; BCL-2, B-cell lymphoma 2; DR5, death receptor 5; FAS, fatty acid synthase; hTERT, human telomerase reverse transcriptase; IGF, insulin-like growth factor; IL, interleukin; MAPK, mitogen-activated protein kinase; mTOR, mammalian target of rapamycin; NF, nuclear factor; PI3K, phosphatidylinositol 3-kinase; pRb, retinoblastoma protein; PTEN, phosphatase and tensin homolog deleted on chromosome 10; TNF, tumor necrosis factor; VEGF, vascular endothelial growth factor.

Another new blossoming area of research is cancer proteomics (Geho et al., 2004). In this field, as the result of carcinogenesis, abnormalities in protein networks extend outside the cancer cell to the tissue microenvironment in which exchange of cytokines, enzymes, and other proteins occurs to the advantages of the malignant cell. These molecules can be identified and become the target for new diagnostic and/or therapeutic targets. Major progress is occurring in the proteomics field in the discovery of biomarkers that may be useful in predicting the clinical response to anticancer therapy (Smith et al., 2006). New discoveries in cancer genetics have begun to be integrated into clinical care (Senter and Chun, 2008). Inherited susceptibility to common malignancies such as lung, breast, colorectal, prostate, and pancreatic cancers can now be used for screening and early detection when cures can be achieved (Foulkes, 2008; NCCN Clinical Practice Guidelines in Oncology, 2008). In less common cancers, such as patients with the Li-Fraumeni syndrome, surveillance strategy using modern studies may detect asymptomatic resectable lesions (Masciari et al., 2008). Major research advances have occurred not only during the past few years in cancer biology, genetics, prevention, and screening, but also in cancer treatment (Gralow et al., 2008; Huang and Ratain, 2009). In this *Atlas of Diagnostic Oncology* general treatment guidelines are often mentioned, but for specific management details readers are referred to readily available publications and textbooks.

Arthur T. Skarin

References and Suggested Readings

Boman BM, Graham HF, Wacha MS: Cancer stem cells: a step toward the cure, J Clin Oncol 26:2795–2799, 2008.

Cam RL, Neumeister V, Rimm DL: A decade of tissue microarrays: progress in the discovery and validation of cancer biomarkers, J Clin Oncol 26:5630–5637, 2008.

Chen Y, Hunter DJ: Molecular epidemiology of cancer, Cancer J Clin 55(1):45–54, 2005.

Ezzati M, Henley SJ, Lopez AD, Thun MJ: Role of smoking in global and regional cancer epidemiology: current patterns and data needs, Int J Cancer 116:963–971, 2005.

Foulkes W: Inherited susceptibility to common cancers, N Engl J Med 359:2143–2153, 2008.

Frieden TR, Myers JE, Krauskopf MS, et al: A Public Health approach to winning the war against cancer, Oncologist 13:1306–1313, 2008.

Geho DH, Petricoin EF, Liotta LA: Blasting into the microworld of tissue proteomics: a new window on cancer, Clin Cancer Res 10:825–827, 2004.

Gloeckler LA, Reichman MR, Riedel Lewis D, et al: Cancer survival and incidence from the Surveillance, Epidemiology, and End Results (SEER) program, Oncologist 8:541–552, 2003.

Gralow J, Ozols RF, Bajorin DF, et al: Clinical Cancer Advances 2007: major research advances in cancer treatment, prevention, and screening—A Report from the American Society of Clinical Oncology, J Clin Oncol 26:313–325, 2008.

Gu D, Kelly TN, Wu X, et al: Mortality attributable to smoking in China, N Engl J Med 360:150–159, 2009.

Hanahan D, Weinberg RA: The hallmarks of cancer, Cell 100:57–70, 2000.

Hayat MJ, Howladerl N, et al: Cancer statistics, trends and multiple primary cancer analyses from the surveillance, epidemiology, and end results (SEER) program, Oncologist 12:20–37, 2007.

Huang RS, Ratain MJ: Pharmacogenetics and Pharmacogenomics of Anticancer Agents, CA Cancer J Clin 59:42–55, 2009.

Jemal A, Siegel R, Ward E, et al: Cancer statistics, 2006, CA Cancer J Clin 56:106–130, 2006.

Jemal A, Siegel R, Ward E, et al: Cancer statistics, 2008, CA Cancer J Clin 58:71–96, 2008.

Jemal A, Siegel R, Ward E, et al: Cancer statistics, 2009, CA Cancer J Clin 59:225–249, 2009.

Jimbo M, Nease DE, Ruffin MT, et al: Information technology and cancer prevention, CA Cancer J Clin 56:26–36, 2006.

Kamangar F, Dores GM, Andreson WF: Patterns of cancer incidence, mortality, and prevalence across five continents: defining priorities to reduce cancer disparities in different geographic regions of the world, J Clin Oncol 24(14):2137–2150, 2006.

Masciari S, van den Abbeele AD, Diller LR, et al: ^{18}F-Fluorodeoxyglucose-Positron emission tomography/computed tomography screening in Li-Fraumeni syndrome, JAMA 299:1315–1319, 2008.

Neugent AI, Li FP: Cancer epidemiology and prevention, Sci Am 12:2–12, 2007.

Quackenbush J: Microarray analysis and tumor classification, N Engl J Med 354:2463–2472, 2006.

Roemer R, Taylor A, Lariviere J: Origins of the WHO framework convention on tobacco control, Am J Public Health 95:936–938, 2005.

Senter L, Chun N: Cancer genetic testing: applying scientific discovery to clinical practice, Commun Oncol 5:660–664, 2008.

Smith L, Lind MJ, Welham KJ, et al: Cancer proteomics and its application to discovery of therapy response markers in human cancer, Cancer 107(2):232–241, 2006.

Smith RA, Cokkinides V, Brawley OW: Cancer screening in the United States, 2009: a review of current American Cancer Society Guidelines and Issues in Cancer Screening, CA Cancer J Clin 59:27–41, 2009.

Yancik R: Population aging and cancer: a cross-national concern, Cancer J 11:437–441, 2005.

Zon RT, Gross E, Vogel VG, et al: American Society of Clinical Oncology Policy Statement: the role of the oncologist in cancer prevention and risk assessment, J Clin Oncol 27:986–993, 2008.

The Role of Molecular Probes and Other Markers in the Diagnosis of Malignancy

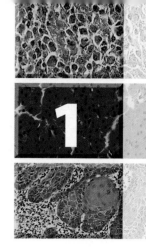

TAD WIECZOREK • JANINA A. LONGTINE

Histopathologic assessment is still the cornerstone in the diagnosis, classification, and grading of malignancies. Light microscopic evaluation augmented by histochemical stains is sufficient in the majority of cases to provide adequate information for diagnosis and prognostication. However, it is limited by subjectivity and imprecision in the evaluation of poorly differentiated malignancies, tumors of unknown primary origin, and unusual neoplasms. In an era of increasingly sophisticated therapeutic protocols (which sometimes target the molecular events leading to cancer) and the need to maximize information gained from minimally invasive samples (such as core biopsy or fine-needle aspiration), ancillary techniques have been developed to increase the specificity and reproducibility of diagnosis. These rely on cell-specific antigen expression and, more importantly, tumor-specific genetic changes that provide diagnostic, prognostic, and/or therapeutic information.

In most instances the advent of monoclonal antibodies directed against cellular proteins, coupled with the immunoperoxidase technique, has superseded direct ultrastructural evaluation in allowing more accurate designation of the epithelial, mesenchymal, hematolymphoid, neuroendocrine, or glial origin of neoplasms. A cardinal example is immunolocalization of cytoskeletal intermediate filaments, which are differentially expressed in different cell types. Table 1.1 lists the intermediate filaments most useful in determining the cell lineage of tumors. The cytokeratins are a complex family of polypeptides that are expressed in various combinations in different epithelial cell types. Antibodies to cytokeratin subtypes can sometimes be used to identify the epithelial origin of a metastatic carcinoma of unknown primary site. For example, the pattern of reactivity for cytokeratin 7 (54 kDa), which is expressed in most glandular and ductal epithelium and transitional epithelium of the urinary tract, and for cytokeratin 20 (46 kDa), which is more restricted in its expression, has been helpful in this regard (Chu et al., 2000).

In addition to the intermediate filaments, other monoclonal antibodies to cellular or tumor antigens are available. In the past decade, advances in the technique of immunohistochemistry have allowed consistent, reliable application in routinely processed surgical pathology specimens (Chan, 2000). Antigen retrieval techniques (including proteolytic digestion and heat-induced antigen retrieval), sensitive detection systems, automation, and a broad range of antibodies have all contributed to this advance. Table 1.2 lists a panel of antibodies that can be used in routine formalin-fixed paraffin-embedded tissue to diagnose poorly differentiated neoplasms. A differential diagnosis is generated by clinical and morphologic features, which can then be further refined by the use of immunohistochemistry. It is important to realize that the majority of antibodies are not entirely specific in lineage determination, and "aberrant" staining patterns are observed. In addition, there is biologic variation in poorly differentiated neoplasms resulting in variation in protein expression. Therefore, accuracy is enhanced by using a panel of antisera to determine lineage or primary site. One application of this principle is distinguishing between poorly differentiated adenocarcinoma and mesothelioma in pleural tumors. Table 1.3 demonstrates the differential immunoprofile.

Although a panel of monoclonal markers greatly aids in the diagnosis of a particular cancer, three malignancies can be confirmed solely by demonstrating the presence of a highly specific protein. Papillary and follicular thyroid carcinomas are characterized by immunoreactivity to thyroglobulin, prostate carcinoma by detection of prostate-specific antigen, and breast carcinoma by a positive reaction for gross cystic disease fluid protein, which is present in approximately 50% to 70% of cases. It is noteworthy that the latter protein is also present in the rare apocrine gland carcinoma. Other antibodies that are not tissue-specific markers but are useful in antibody panels include TIF-l for pulmonary adenocarcinoma, RCC antigen for renal cell carcinoma, CD117 (c-kit) for gastrointestinal stromal tumors, and CD31 (platelet endothelial cell adhesion molecule) for vascular endothelial neoplasms. Immunostains are also helpful in the delineation of normal tissue architecture and its abrogation in neoplasia. For example, immunostaining for p63 (a nuclear antigen expressed in myoepithelial cells of the breast and basal cells of the prostate) aids in the detection of ductal/glandular structures without the normal myoepithelial framework, the hallmark of invasive neoplasia.

Although the cellular proteins expressed in particular types of neoplasia are fundamental to their diagnostic characterization, somatic mutations (i.e., mutations that occur in the genes of nongermline tissues) are central to the development of cancer. A series of different mutations in critical genes is probably necessary for malignant transformation to occur. The mutations may be deletions, duplications, point mutations, and/or chromosomal translocations in the DNA of the tumor precursor cell. The mutations affect regulation of the cell cycle, differentiation, apoptosis, or cell-cell and cell-matrix interactions. Different neoplasms have different combinations of genetic alterations, which lead to clonal proliferations of cells. These genetic alterations, though fundamental in tumor biology, can also be used

Table 1.1

Cytoskeletal Intermediate Filaments

Cell Type	Intermediate Filaments	Molecular Weight or Subtype	Presence in Tumor
Epithelial	Cytokeratins	40–67	Keratinizing and nonkeratinizing carcinomas
Mesenchymal	Vimentin	58	Wide distribution: sarcomas, melanomas, many lymphomas, some carcinomas
Muscle	Desmin	53	Leiomyosarcomas, rhabdomyosarcomas
Glial astrocytes	Glial fibrillary acidic protein	57	Gliomas (including astrocytomas), ependymomas
Neurons	Neurofilament proteins	68, 160, 200	Neural tumors, neuroblastomas

Table 1.2

Immunocytochemistry in the Differential Diagnosis of Malignancies

Malignancy	Keratin	Chromogranin Synaptophysin	S100	MART-1	LCA	OCT 3/4	SMA/ Desmin
Carcinoma	+	–	–/+	–	–	–	–
Germ cell	+/–*	–	–	–	–	+/–	–
Lymphoma	–	–	–	–	+	–	–
Melanoma	–	–	+	+/–	–	–	–
Neuroendocrine	+/–	+	–	–	–	–	–
Sarcoma†	–/+	–	–/+	–/+	–	–	+/–

LCA, leukocyte common antigen; MART-1, melanoma antigen recognized by T cells 1; OCT 3/4, organic cation transporter 3/4; SMA, smooth muscle actin.
+ positive; – negative; +/– mainly positive, occasionally negative; –/+ mainly negative, occasionally positive.
*Keratin is usually negative in seminomas but positive in nonseminomatous germ cell tumors.
†Sarcomas are a heterogeneous family of neoplasms, and immunohistochemical staining patterns depend on the specific histologic subtype.

as diagnostic or prognostic markers for malignancies. This is best characterized in lymphomas and leukemias wherein specific genetic translocations result in the production of chimeric messenger RNA (mRNA) and novel proteins. These translocations are the sine qua non for the classification of some leukemias, such as the Philadelphia chromosome t(9;22)(q34;q11) for chronic myelogenous leukemia and t(15;17)(q22;q11–21) for acute promyelocytic leukemia. Single-nucleotide mutations may also be important in hematopoietic neoplasia; for example, the *JAK2* V617F mutation is frequently present in chronic myeloproliferative disorders (Percy and McMullin, 2005; Swerdlow et al., 2008). Although genetic alterations in carcinomas are more complex than single point mutations or chromosome translocations, simple chromosomal translocations also commonly occur in (and characterize) soft tissue tumors (Antonescu, 2006; Sandberg, 2002).

A global assessment of structural cytogenetic changes in a neoplasm is provided by full karyotypic analysis, which requires fresh, viable tumor. By contrast, fluorescence in situ hybridization (FISH) is a more targeted approach that can be performed on interphase nuclei obtained from frozen or fixed

Table 1.3

Antibody Panel in the Differential Diagnosis of Adenocarcinoma and Mesothelioma

Malignancy	Keratin*	WT-1	CD15 (Leu-M1)	CEA
Adenocarcinoma	+	–	+	+
Mesothelioma	+	+	–	–

CEA, carcinoembryonic antigen.
+ positive; – negative.
*Keratin positivity in the appropriate clinicopathologic setting limits the differential diagnosis to adenocarcinoma and mesothelioma.

paraffin-embedded tissue and can identify specific characteristic cytogenetic abnormalities as an adjunct to tumor diagnosis. For example, FISH probes that flank the *EWS* gene region show a "split apart" signal when an *EWS* rearrangement is present, as in Ewing's sarcoma (see Fig. 1.1). In addition, many of the characteristic cytogenetic abnormalities of neoplasms have been cloned and sequenced, allowing for the utilization of molecular biology techniques such as Southern blot hybridization or, more commonly, the polymerase chain reaction (PCR). These techniques use fresh or frozen tumor, or even fixed, embedded tissue (with PCR), and improve diagnoses by identifying the characteristic chromosomal translocations of malignancies at the molecular level. With PCR a specific translocation can be detected in as few as 1 in 100,000 or 1 in 1,000,000 cells as compared with 1 in 100 cells for FISH analysis. Thus, PCR provides a sensitive method for diagnosis and for monitoring response to therapy. For example, the t(9;22)(q34;q11) of chronic myelogenous leukemia juxtaposes the *BCR* and *ABL1* genes, resulting in a unique chimeric mRNA that can be detected by a quantitative real-time reverse transcription (RT)-PCR technique. Peripheral blood cell RNA is converted to complementary DNA by RT. The resultant *BCR-ABL1* complementary DNA is quantified by monitoring fluorescently labeled oligonucleotide probes that specifically hybridized with the target during each cycle of PCR amplification (see Fig. 1.2). Clinical trials with the tyrosine kinase inhibitor imatinib defined a target of a minimal residual level of *BCR-ABL1* RNA transcripts that is associated with progression-free survival (see Fig. 1.3) (O'Brien et al., 2003; Hughes et al., 2003). Rising levels of BCR-ABL1 mRNA in patients taking tyrosine kinase inhibitors or status post-transplantation are indicative of a molecular relapse and the need for alternate or additional therapy. Southern blot hybridization or PCR can also identify clonal rearrangements of the immunoglobulin or T-cell receptor genes as an adjunct to the diagnosis of lymphoma or lymphoid leukemias (see Fig. 1.4).

Genetic analysis of neoplasms may also provide prognostic information, such as identifying the *BCR-ABL1* rearrangement in Philadelphia chromosome–positive acute lymphoblastic leukemia or *N-MYC* amplification in neuroblastoma. In addition, genetic analysis is playing an increasing role in therapeutic planning, as therapies tailored to specific genetic "lesions" are developed. Examples of such lesions include *HER2* amplification in breast cancer and the epidermal growth factor receptor gene (*EGFR*) mutation in lung cancer (Lauren-Puig, 2009; Lynch et al., 2004; Paez et al., 2004). These genetic lesions may be detected either by evaluation of aberrant protein expression (as in immunohistochemical detection of membranous overexpression of HER2 oncoprotein in breast cancer), by gene amplification (as in FISH analysis of *HER2*), or by molecular testing (as in *EGFR* point or small-deletion mutation analysis in lung cancer, see Fig. 1.5). Quantification of the expression levels of large numbers of genes in specific types of neoplasia by oligonucleotide chips or cDNA microarrays, "expression profiling," has led to the identification of subsets of genes that provide prognostic information, such as in diffuse large B-cell lymphoma (see Fig. 1.6) (Shipp et al., 2002). It has even become feasible to measure the expression level of multiple

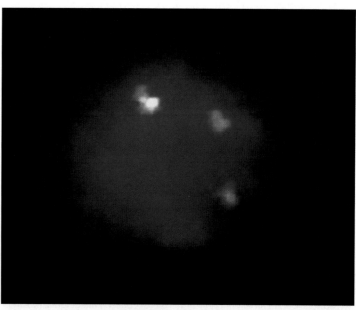

FIGURE 1.1 Fluorescence in situ hybridization (FISH) on a sample obtained by fine-needle aspiration shows an interphase nucleus with red and green probes flanking each of two copies of the *EWS* gene, demonstrating one fused and one split signal. The split signal indicates rearrangement of the *EWS* gene region. (Courtesy of Dr. Paola Dal Cin, Cytogenetics Laboratory, Brigham and Women's Hospital.)

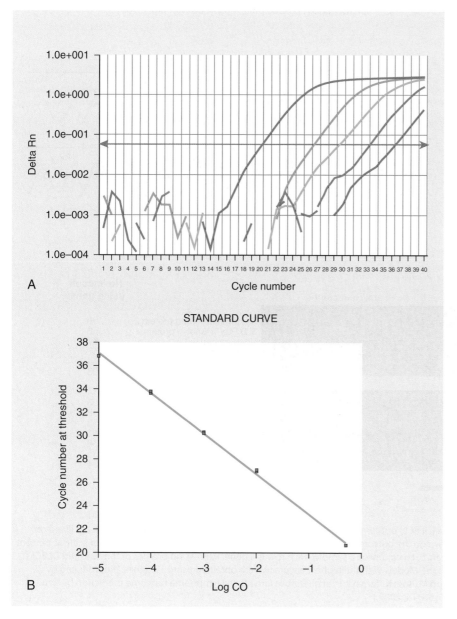

A

STANDARD CURVE

B

FIGURE 1.2 **(A)** "Taq-Man'Y" (Applied Biosystems) quantitative RT-PCR results for dilutions (1:1, 10^{-2}, 10^{-3}, 10^{-4}, 10^{-5}) of K562 cell line RNA, which express chimeric *BCR-ABL1* mRNA. After approximately 15 cycles of PCR, the sample with the most *BCR-ABL1* mRNA (1:1) enters the linear phase of exponential amplification as measured by fluorescence accumulation monitored in real time. Samples with less target require more PCR cycles to reach the exponential phase. **(B)** For quantitation a standard curve is generated plotting the PCR cycle number at threshold (red line in middle of exponential phase) against log concentration of target. Unknown samples can be quantified by plotting against the standard curve. (From Chen WY, Wardley A, Skarin AT, editors: *Dana-Farber Cancer Institute: Breast Cancer*, Philadelphia, Mosby, Elsevier Ltd, p 14.)

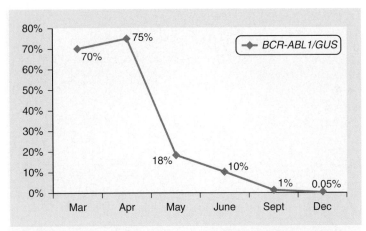

FIGURE 1.3 Timeline of response to the tyrosine kinase inhibitor imatinib as monitored by real-time RT-PCR analysis of *BCR-ABL1* mRNA expressed as a ratio to the normalizing gene, *GUS*. Patients who achieve a 3-log reduction of transcript level by 12 months of therapy have a negligible risk of disease progression in the following 12 months. (From Chen WY, Wardley A, Skarin AT, editors: *Dana-Farber Cancer Institute: Breast Cancer*, Philadelphia, Mosby, Elsevier Ltd, p 15.)

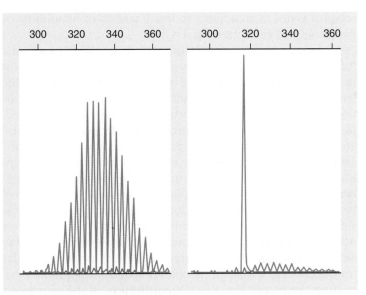

FIGURE 1.4 PCR amplification of the immunoglobulin heavy chain (IgH) gene with primers to the variable and joining regions that flank the unique IgH gene rearrangement of B cells. B-cell IgH rearrangements differ by size and sequence. Fluorescent primers are incorporated into the PCR product, which are then analyzed by capillary gel electrophoresis. **(A)** The Gaussian distribution of a polyclonal population of B cells. **(B)** A dominant peak of 318 base pairs representing a monoclonal population in a B-cell lymphoma. (From Chen WY, Wardley A, Skarin AT, editors: *Dana-Farber Cancer Institute: Breast Cancer*, Philadelphia, Mosby, Elsevier Ltd, p 16.)

FIGURE 1.5 Lung adenocarcinoma DNA sequence analysis of exon 21 of the *EGFR* gene. The top row shows the normal or wild-type exon sequence. The bottom row shows the heterozygous T→C point mutation, which characterizes the L858R mutation, a common mutation in carcinomas responsive to tyrosine kinase inhibitors. (From Chen WY, Wardley A, Skarin AT, editors: *Dana-Farber Cancer Institute: Breast Cancer*, Philadelphia, Mosby, Elsevier Ltd, p 17.)

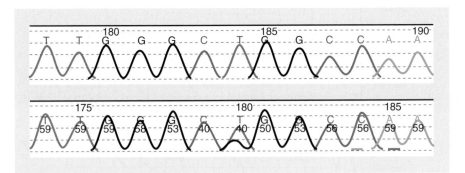

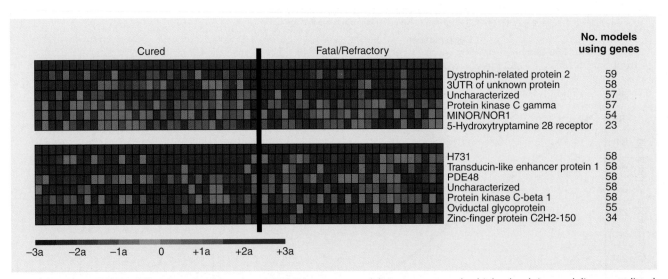

FIGURE 1.6 Genes included in the diffuse large B cell lymphoma (DLBCL) outcome model. Genes expressed at higher levels in cured disease are listed on top, and those that were more abundant in fatal disease are shown on the bottom. Red indicates high expression; blue, low expression. Color scale at bottom indicates relative expression in standard deviations from the mean. Each column is a sample; each row is a gene. Expression profiles of the 32 cured DLBCLs are on the left; profiles of the fatal/refractory tumors are on the right. Models with the highest accuracy were obtained using 13 genes. (Reproduced by permission from Macmillan Publishers Ltd. Nature Medicine. Shipp M, Ross K, Tamayo P, et al: Diffuse large B-cell lymphoma outcome prediction by gene expression profiling and supervised machine learning, *Nat Med* 8: 68–74, 2002.)

genes (by RT-PCR) in routinely prepared, paraffin-embedded tumor samples, as in the multigene assay to predict recurrence of tamoxifen-treated, node-negative breast cancer (Paik et al., 2004). This assay measures the expression level of genes involved in key aspects of tumor biology such as proliferation, invasion, and estrogen response, and its quantitative result has potential application in therapeutic planning (Sorlie, 2009). Because key genes (and hence proteins) are identified by expression profiling, expression can be assayed by routine immunohistochemistry. An important and practical example of this strategy was the development of a specific antibody to P504S (AMACR/racemase), a protein product strongly expressed in prostatic adenocarcinoma and prostatic intraepithelial neoplasia, but typically not in benign prostatic epithelium (Beach et al., 2002). This immunostain is therefore useful in supporting a diagnosis of prostatic adenocarcinoma in cases wherein the morphologic findings are subtle—as in the diagnosis of minimal adenocarcinoma on needle biopsy.

The genetics of cancer also extends to inherited predisposition to neoplasms described in a number of families (Scriver et al., 2001). These syndromes include germline mutations of tumor suppressor genes, such as familial retinoblastoma, and mutations of DNA repair genes as in ataxia telangiectasia or hereditary nonpolyposis colon cancer. Some of these are listed in Table 1.4.

Table 1.4

Examples of Inherited Syndromes Predisposing to Cancer

Syndrome	Chromosome Locus	Gene
Ataxia-telangiectasia	11q22	ATM
Hereditary breast/ovarian cancer	17q21	BRCA1
	13q12	BRCA2
Familial adenomatous polyposis	5q21–q22	APC
Familial retinoblastoma	13q14	RB1
Hereditary nonpolyposis colorectal cancer (Lynch syndrome)	2q22–p21	MSH2
	3p21	MLH1
	2q31–q33	PMS1
	7p22	PMS2
Li-Fraumeni	17p13	TP53
Multiple endocrine neoplasia, type 1	11q13	MEN1
Multiple endocrine neoplasia, type 2	10q11.2	RET
Neurofibromatosis, type 1	12q11	NF1
Neurofibromatosis, type 2	22q12	NF2
von Hippel–Lindau disease	3p26–p25	VHL

References and Suggested Readings

Antonescu CR: The role of genetic testing in soft tissue sarcoma, *Histopathology* 48:13–21, 2006.

Beach R, Gown AM, De Peralta-Venturina MN, et al: P504S immunohistochemical detection in 405 prostatic specimens including 376 18-gauge needle biopsies, *Am J Surg Pathol* 26:1588–1596, 2002.

Camp RL, Neumeister V, Rimm DL: A decade of tissue microarrays: progress in the discovery and validation of cancer biomarkers, *J Clin Oncol* 26:5630–5637, 2008.

Chan JKC: Advances in immunohistochemistry: impact on surgical pathology practice, *Semin Diagn Pathol* 17:170–177, 2000.

Chiang AC, Massagué J: Molecular origins of cancer: molecular basis of metastasis, *N Engl J Med* 359:2814–2828, 2008.

Chu P, Wu E, Weiss LM: Cytokeratin 7 and cytokeratin 20 expression in epithelial neoplasms: a survey of 435 cases, *Mod Pathol* 13(9):962–971, 2000.

Hughes TP, Kaeda J, Branford S, et al: Frequency of major molecular responses to imatinib or interferon alfa plus cytarabine in newly diagnosed chronic myeloid leukemia, *N Engl J Med* 349:1423–1432, 2003.

Lauren-Puig P, Lievre A, Blons H: Mutations and response to epidermal growth factor receptor inhibitors. *Clin Cancer Res* 15:1133–1139, 2009.

Lynch TJ, Bell DW, Sordella R, et al: Activating mutations in the epidermal growth factor receptor underlying responsiveness of non-small-cell lung cancer to gefitinib, *N Engl J Med* 350:2129–2139, 2004.

O'Brien SG, Guilhot F, Larson RA, et al: Imatinib compared with interferon and low-dose cytarabine for newly diagnosed chronic-phase chronic myeloid leukemia, *N Engl J Med* 348:994–1004, 2003.

Paez JG, Janne PA, Lee JC, et al: EGFR mutations in lung cancer: correlation with clinical response to gefitinib therapy, *Science* 304:1497–1500, 2004.

Paik S, Shak S, Tang G, et al: A multigene assay to predict recurrence of tamoxifen-treated, node-negative breast cancer, *N Engl J Med* 351:2817–2826, 2004.

Percy MJ, McMullin MF: The V617F *JAK2* mutation and the myeloproliferative disorders, *Hematol Oncol* 23:91–93, 2005.

Sandberg AA: Cytogenetics and molecular genetics of bone and soft-tissue tumors, *Am J Med Genet* 115:189–193, 2002.

Scriver CR, Beaudet AL, Sly WS, Valle D, editors: *Metabolic and Molecular Bases of Inherited Disease*, ed 3, New York, 2001, McGraw-Hill.

Shipp M, Ross K, Tamayo P, et al: Diffuse large B-cell lymphoma outcome prediction by gene expression profiling and supervised machine learning, *Nat Med* 8:68–74, 2002.

Slamon DJ, Leyland-Jones B, Shak S, et al: Use of chemotherapy plus a monoclonal antibody against HER2 for metastatic breast cancer that overexpresses HER2, *N Engl J Med* 344:783–792, 2001.

Sorlie T: Introducing molecular subtyping of breast cancer into the clinic, *J Clin Oncol* 27(8):1153–1154, 2009.

Swerdlow SH, Campo E, Harris NL, editors: *World Health Organization Classification of Tumours, Pathology and Genetics of Tumours Haematopoietic and Lymphoid Tissues*, Lyon, 2008, IARC Press.

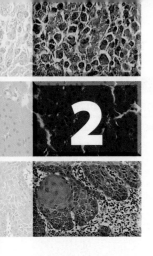

2

Radiographic Evaluation of Cancer

KITT SHAFFER

Imaging Goals

Goals of radiographic imaging vary in patients with malignancies depending upon whether the specific malignant diagnosis is already known and whether the imaging is performed to stage disease or to follow disease. Each type of malignancy has its own spectrum of findings on imaging studies, which will be covered in detail in subsequent chapters. In this chapter, generalized imaging principles will be reviewed, with some attention to new imaging techniques that may have greater application in diagnosis and follow-up of malignancies in the future. Nuclear medicine will be covered in a separate chapter. Lymphangiography, angiography, and myelography will not be covered specifically in this chapter, because they are used less frequently in current practice. Detailed information regarding these types of studies may be obtained in a variety of oncoradiologic texts (Vanel and Stark, 1993; Stomper, 1993).

Imaging findings in cancer patients may be very nonspecific or very specific (see Fig. 2.1). In choosing a particular method for imaging cancer patients, the specificity and sensitivity of the imaging modality must be considered with particular reference to the type of malignancy suspected. The risk to the patient for the imaging modality must also be weighed, along with the actual cost of the study. The strengths and weaknesses of many common studies will be considered individually, with a discussion of imaging assistance for biopsy, which is often the final path to conclusive diagnosis of malignancy.

It is important even in cancer patients, who may have already received large doses of radiation as part of their treatment and who are considered to have life-threatening conditions, to keep in mind the principle of ALARA (as low as reasonably achievable), which guides efforts to minimize radiation exposure in imaging of all patients. Recent evidence suggests that overuse of medical imaging can lead to an increase in cancer risk, particularly in women and in young patients (Einstein et al., 2007). As treatments for cancer become more successful and patients live longer, the cumulative risk of follow-up imaging, particularly multidetector computed tomographic (CT) scans, must be considered in planning appropriate management.

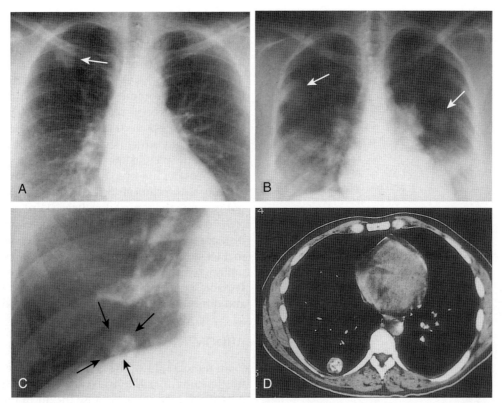

FIGURE 2.1 Although the chest radiograph is very sensitive for detection of lung abnormalities, findings may or may not be specific. **(A)** Frontal view of the chest in the PA projection in an asymptomatic 42-year-old female shows a slightly lobular 2-cm mass in the right upper lobe, projecting behind the right clavicle. At surgery *a noncalcified granuloma* was removed. This lesion radiographically could not be distinguished from other solitary pulmonary nodules, such as lung carcinoma, pulmonary amyloid, or a rheumatoid nodule. **(B)** Frontal view of the chest in the PA projection in a 39-year-old female with a cough shows bilateral ill-defined lung nodules (*arrows*), with bilateral hilar enlargement. At open-lung biopsy *alveolar sarcoidosis* was found. Many other processes could have caused a similar appearance on the chest radiograph, such as bilateral pneumonia, lung metastases, pulmonary lymphoma, or bronchoalveolar carcinoma. **(C)** Close-up from a frontal view of the chest in the PA projection in an asymptomatic 33-year-old male obtained as part of a pre-employment physical examination shows a 1-cm smoothly rounded nodule at the right lung base (*arrows*). Calcification is present in a characteristic chunky, curved distribution indicating a specific benign diagnosis. **(D)** CT image at the right lung base in the same patient as in **C**, displayed with mediastinal windows, shows this calcification more clearly, resembling "popcorn," diagnostic of a *pulmonary hamartoma*. In this case the chest radiograph (and CT) were both sensitive and specific in making the correct diagnosis.

Plain Radiography

Digital radiographic imaging has replaced analog (film-screen) imaging for most plain radiography. In computed radiography a phosphor-coated plate is substituted for the photographic film used in analog radiography. This plate is exposed using standard x-ray equipment and is then read out electronically in the form of digital imaging data. The plate can be erased and reused. The digital imaging data can be used to print images on transparent film or paper or displayed on a monitor. Digital imaging has many advantages over film-screen radiography, including fewer under- or overpenetrated films, ability to change contrast and brightness of the image after acquisition, existence of edge-enhancing algorithms for image processing, and digital storage, allowing electronic transfer of imaging information (Cowen et al., 1993). Drawbacks include slightly lower spatial resolution (not noticeable without special testing methods) and initial expense of installation. Combination of digital imaging systems with radiology scheduling and reporting systems allows progression to a "film-less" radiology department, using a totally integrated "picture archiving and communication system" or PACS (Choplin et al., 1992). Particularly with newer, faster computer systems and improvements in rate of data transfer, PACS systems have proliferated at most academic centers and have become the standard for large institutions throughout the country.

Plain radiographs are often the most cost-effective method to begin a diagnostic search for malignancy or to follow effects of treatment. Table 2.1 compares cost, radiation dose, and practical limitations for various plain radiographic examinations. Cost estimates are for a large U.S. tertiary-care teaching institution in New England and will vary in other types of institutions and other parts of the country. Dose information is given as skin entry dose, which is at best a crude estimate of actual absorbed dose. Specific absorbed doses to particularly sensitive organs should also be considered and will vary depending on the specific views obtained. For example, the breast glandular dose from an anteroposterior (AP) chest radiograph (wherein the beam enters the front of the patient) is about 70 times greater than the breast glandular dose from a posterior-anterior (PA) chest radiograph. Overall, approximately 50% of the average radiation dose to the general public is from radon gas and only about 15% from medical imaging, including nuclear medicine (Broadbent and Hubbard, 1992).

CHEST RADIOGRAPHS

The chest radiograph provides an excellent survey of the lungs, mediastinum, bony thorax, and pleura in a very short exam time and at a relatively low radiation dose. Because of the natural contrast between air in the lungs and soft tissue in other parts of the chest, the chest radiograph is particularly sensitive for diagnosis of many pulmonary malignancies, though usually not very specific. Chest radiographs may also provide useful staging information for lung tumors in some cases, because bone metastases and mediastinal adenopathy may be demonstrated along with the primary tumor. Chest radiographs are also useful in detection of

Table 2.1

A Comparison of Cost and Dose of Common Radiographic Studies

Exam	Cost	Radiation Dose[†]
PA/lat CXR	1 cost unit*	0.007–0.01 cG (PA) 0.02–0.03 cG (lat)
Portable AP CXR	1.25	0.01–0.02 cG
KUB	0.5	0.06–0.1 cG
Decubitus abdomen	0.5	0.06–0.1 cG
AP & lat C-spine	1	0.06 cG (AP) 0.05 cG (lat)
AP & lat T-spine	1	0.2 cG (AP) 0.3–0.6 cG (lat)
AP & lat L-spine	1	0.07–0.1 cG (AP) 0.2–0.3 cG (lat)
Femur, humerus	0.75	0.08–0.2 cG each view
Pelvis	0.85	0.05–0.06 cG
Ribs	0.75	0.15 cG (two views)
Knee, shoulder, hip	1	0.07–0.1 cG each view
AP & lat skull	1	0.1–0.3 cG (AP) 0.1–0.3 cG (lat)
Barium swallow	1.4	3–5 cG
UGI (air-contrast)	2.25	8–15 cG
UGI/SBFT	2.75	10–25 cG
SBFT	2.25	3–5 cG
Enteroclysis	3	10–15 cG
BE (air-contrast)	3.1	15–30 cG
Mammogram	2	3 mG or less film-screen, per view ~2 mG or less digital, per view
Head CT	3.25 (1–) 3.75 (1+) 4 (1–/1+)	4–6 cG
Chest or abdomen CT	3.6 (1–) 3.9 (1+) 4.25 (1–/1+)	1–3 cG
Pelvis CT	3.25 (1–) 3.75 (1+) 4 (1–/1+)	1–3 cG

AP, anterior-posterior; BE, barium enema; C, cervical; cG, centiGray; CT, computed tomography; CXR, chest radiograph; KUB, plain radiograph of kidney urinary bladder; L, lumbar: lat, lateral; PA, posterior-anterior: SBFT, small bowel follow-through; T, thoracic; UGI, upper gastrointestinal series; 1–, without intravenous contrast infusion; 1–/1+, without intravenous contrast followed by images with intravenous contrast infusion; 1+, with intravenous contrast infusion.

*One cost unit, for comparison purposes, is defined as the cost for a PA and lateral CXR, including both technical and professional fees.

[†]Doses are given as skin entry doses; actual absorbed dose will vary considerably depending on radiographic technique, body habitus, and site examined. These doses also assume use of state-of-the-art image receptors and optimal radiographic technique.

many treatment-related problems, such as infections, drug toxicities, fluid overload, and misplaced support lines. Problems with support lines are one of the most common abnormalities detected on portable radiographs. Even a subtle abnormality may have clinical importance. A finding of an abnormally placed line on a chest radiograph may require additional studies, such as CT or digital subtraction angiography, to determine the exact line position and whether it can be used for infusion of chemotherapy.

Chest radiographs in obese patients will show decreased contrast, but even in patients in excess of 160 kg (352 lb), diagnostically useful radiographs can usually still be obtained. There is an overall decrease in diagnostic quality of many types of imaging studies in obese patients, but in the cancer setting this is less

of a problem than in the general population. For solving specific problems in the chest, special views may be useful, such as oblique views (helpful for detection of rib, pleural, or chest wall lesions and for confirming the presence of questionable lung nodules), decubitus views (for demonstrating loculation of pleural fluid and for improving visualization of the lung base in the presence of large nonloculated pleural effusions), apical lordotic views (for projection of the apical portion of the lung free of overlying bony structures), or apical kyphotic views (for examination of the pleural apex). Chest radiography can be performed at the bedside; however, the quality of these exams is limited by certain fixed technical factors. The portable x-ray machine does not generate the same kilovoltage (kVp) as a standard chest unit (60–90 kVp vs 120 kVp for standard chest radiography). Also, the distance from the tube to the receptor is shorter than for departmental radiographs (0.9–1.2 m vs 1.8 m for standard chest radiography), which increases distortion and geometric indistinctness. Portable radiography may also be limited by patient condition and difficulty in properly positioning the receptor and x-ray tube.

ABDOMINAL RADIOGRAPHS

Plain radiographs of the abdomen provide a less sensitive diagnostic study for abdominal organs than the chest radiograph provides for the lung, because the air in the bowel provides the only natural contrast among the abdominal contents. Detection of retroperitoneal and solid-organ abnormalities is limited, unless calcification is present. Fat planes within the abdomen may provide enough contrast to allow delineation of some solid-organ contours but is variable among patients. Fat planes may be particularly diminished in cancer patients, because of weight loss related to their disease or their treatment. However, for detection of abnormalities of the bowel, plain abdominal radiographs can be very helpful and again, are inexpensive, can be obtained at a relatively low radiation dose, can be performed at the bedside, and require only minimal patient cooperation. Special views that may be helpful include decubitus views (left side down for detection of minimal pneumoperitoneum outlined by the liver), prone views (to move gas into the rectum and rule out distal colonic obstruction), and upright views (to detect air-fluid levels, which are only normal in the stomach and duodenal bulb, but can be seen in the colon in patients with diarrhea or in the small bowel in cases of ileus or obstruction). Upright abdominal radiographs can also be used to detect pneumoperitoneum, but the upright chest radiograph is preferable because the x-ray beam is centered closer to the dome of the diaphragm and therefore will more clearly demonstrate very small collections of air. Abdominal fluoroscopy is not usually performed without contrast administration.

BONE RADIOGRAPHS

Bone plain radiographs are moderately sensitive in detection of many primary and metastatic malignancies but are most useful when interpreted in conjunction with results of nuclear medicine bone scans. Interpretation of bone radiographs can be confounded by a variety of normal variants and benign lesions and experience in interpretation of bone radiographs is essential. In surveying the body for bone metastases, nuclear medicine scanning is preferred to skeletal surveys, because the bone scan is more sensitive, less expensive, and gives a lower radiation dose. The exception to this rule is in multiple myeloma or in very aggressive purely lytic bone metastases, wherein bone scanning may be negative (Woolfenden et al., 1980). In these cases, skeletal surveys or plain radiographs of long bones, skull, spine, and pelvis are preferred. Consultation with a radiologist may often be helpful in limiting any bone examination to the most appropriate radiographs. For certain bones, such as the sacrum, scapula, and sternum, CT or tomography is required for best visualization of the entire bone. The particular views included in a standard study of any bone or joint will vary from department to department. Therefore, if a specific question is to be answered regarding a bone or joint, adequate clinical information must be given to the radiologist to decide if additional views must be obtained to supplement the standard views.

Gastrointestinal Contrast Studies

The role of gastrointestinal (GI) contrast studies has become progressively more limited, with many of the indications for theses studies being replaced by CT or magnetic resonance imaging (MRI). However, for direct examination of dynamic peristaltic function or for detection of perforation, these studies still can have a role. Care must be taken in planning the sequence of GI studies when staging a cancer patient, particularly if contrast studies are needed. If a barium enema, bone scan, upper GI series, and CT are all planned, the CT or bone scan should usually be done first (in that barium from the other two studies will severely limit the ability to perform the CT or nuclear medicine studies for varying lengths of time, up to a week). The barium enema should then be performed before the upper GI series, because residual contrast will hamper either study, and contrast from a barium enema is usually eliminated more rapidly than that from an upper GI study. When in doubt about how best to schedule a series of different types of radiologic studies, consultation with a radiologist or nuclear medicine physician is often helpful.

Intravenous Contrast Studies

Intravenous (IV) contrast agents used in radiology are now almost entirely iso-osmolar to blood (non-ionic agents), having replaced older ionic agents that were less expensive but more toxic. The incidence of fatal contrast reactions with either type of agent is approximately 1/100,000 uses (Caro et al., 1991). The nephrotoxic effect of non-ionic agents is probably less than with older ionic agents, and the incidence of minor contrast reactions (nausea, vomiting, hives) is definitely much lower with non-ionic agents, which leads to much better patient acceptance. All contrast agents must be used with caution in patients with multiple myeloma, diabetes, sickle cell disease, or chronic renal insufficiency.

In patients with a history of serious reactions to IV contrast material, a premedication protocol using steroids and histamine blockers is often used before a planned contrast administration (Kelly et al., 1978). Whenever possible, IV contrast should be administered after the patient has taken nothing by mouth for several hours, because food or liquids in the stomach may increase the risk of vomiting. Because venous access is often a problem in cancer patients, placement of an IV catheter before a planned study is often helpful to prevent delays or cancellation of the study. In CT, optimal examinations require rapid bolus contrast administration. Therefore, the largest-caliber catheter

that can be easily inserted should usually be used. Contrast material that leaks from a small-caliber catheter into the surrounding tissues (infiltration) can lead to considerable pain, swelling, and even tissue necrosis. With newer multidetector CT (MDCT) equipment, which is capable of completing the scan of a region such as the liver in a very short time, it is now possible to reliably obtain image sequences at various phases after injection to optimize visualization of lesions such as metastases (Silverman, 2006).

INTRAVENOUS AND RETROGRADE UROGRAPHY

The advent of CT and ultrasound has markedly decreased indications for IV and retrograde urography. In an IV pyelogram, after injection of a bolus of IV contrast material, radiographs and tomograms are obtained rapidly to demonstrate the enhancement of the renal parenchyma, followed by more delayed radiographs to show the contour of the collecting systems, ureters, and bladder. Filling of the collecting systems is highly variable, and it is not uncommon for small segments of the ureters to be poorly visualized. If small mucosal lesions of the collecting system are suspected, retrograde studies may be preferable. Cystography involves filling the bladder with contrast via catheter, usually under fluoroscopic guidance. To visualize the urethra, the catheter can be withdrawn after filling of the bladder and radiographs obtained during urination in a voiding cystourethrogram (VCUG). In conjunction with cystoscopy, the ureters can also be cannulated and retrograde injections may be performed into the collecting systems under fluoroscopic guidance. This provides the best visualization of the entire collecting system. The cost for an IV pyelogram is approximately 3.25 cost units, and the radiation dose is 3–6 cG. The cost of a cystogram is approximately 1.5 cost units, a VCUG is 2.25 cost units, and a retrograde CUG is 2.5–3 cost units. The radiation dose is 3–6 cG, with particularly high gonadal doses for the VCUG.

Mammography

The quality of imaging in mammography has improved rapidly in recent years. The two goals of maximizing spatial and contrast resolution and minimizing patient dose have led to many technical innovations. Early mammography was performed with standard radiographic equipment and one view of each breast. Current mammographic standards require dedicated mammographic equipment, strict quality control standards, and two views of each breast, in the craniocaudal and mediolateral oblique projections. Specialized views may also be obtained, such as spot compression (to search for nodules or architectural distortion), rolled or rotated (to help localize a lesion within the breast), or magnification views (to detect and characterize microcalcifications). When a mass is present that may represent a cyst, breast ultrasound may be useful. In recent years most large centers have switched from film-screen to digital mammography (Fig. 2.2). Mammography was the last radiographic imaging modality to convert to a digital format because of the extremely high spatial resolution required for diagnostic images. New receptors had to be developed as well as a new generation of high-resolution high-brightness viewing monitors before digital mammography became a practical reality. Most studies have shown similar sensitivity and specificity of digital and film-screen mammography except in the setting of dense breast tissue, where digital mammography is probably slightly more sensitive (Knutson and Steiner, 2007). Another advantage of digital mammography is the ability to apply sophisticated computer-aided diagnostic techniques to the images to improve sensitivity and specificity. The overall breast radiation dose for digital mammography is slightly lower than for conventional film-screen imaging if imaging parameters are optimized (Chevalier et al., 2004).

There are a number of interesting new technical adaptations of mammography on the horizon that may greatly increase our ability to detect small early breast tumors. These include breast tomosynthesis (which creates a three-dimensional [3D] view of the breast) and contrast-enhanced mammography (which may image neovascularity in tumors) (Singletary, 2007; Diekmann and Bick, 2007). The mean glandular dose from modern film-screen or digital mammography is under 0.3 cG for each view, which would yield approximately 10/1,000,000 excess cases of breast cancer in 50-year-old patients due to the radiation from a standard four-view examination (Gofman and O'Connor, 1985). This produces a risk of dying from a radiation-induced breast carcinoma comparable to the risk of dying due to smoking 14 cigarettes, breathing the air of an industrialized city in the U.S. Northeast for a month, or living in Denver for 2 years (Wilson, 1979). Mammographic dose varies with breast size, density, degree of compression, and type of x-ray target used, and radiation risk from mammography decreases with increasing patient age.

It is very important when ordering a mammogram that any prior mammograms be available to the radiologist at the time of the examination. Having prior mammographic reports is not sufficient, and actual images are needed to optimize the search for subtle changes in density and architecture. Comparison with prior studies greatly decreases the need for extra views and other workup, such as ultrasound, also greatly decreasing patient anxiety. Findings on mammography generally can be grouped into categories based on the likelihood of malignancy, with vary-

ing follow-up recommendations based on this classification (Table 2.2). A normal mammogram does not exclude malignancy, because the false-negative rate of mammography ranges from 10% to 20% (Holland et al., 1983; Bird et al., 1992). Mammography may be uncomfortable for the patient, because firm compression of the breast is needed for best diagnostic image quality (Feig, 1987). Patients are instructed not to use deodorant on the day of their exam, because it may be visible on the images and can mimic pathology (microcalcifications). If patients experience cyclic changes in sensitivity of their breasts, it is helpful to schedule their mammogram at a time when they anticipate the least sensitivity. Mammograms are not generally recommended for women under the age of 30, but with newer equipment, adequate studies may be obtained even in young women if the clinical situation is sufficiently worrisome. For example, in patients who received mediastinal radiation at a young age for treatment of Hodgkin's lymphoma, routine yearly mammography should generally begin approximately 10–15 years after completion of the radiation, which in many patients will be at an age well under 30 (Diller et al., 2003).

If the clinician feels a palpable lesion that is to be evaluated, the exact location of that lesion should be clearly communicated to the radiologist and may ideally be marked on the skin to further help in planning the examination. Mammography in people with breast implants is more complicated and requires a total of four views of each breast in most cases (Eklund et al., 1988). Breast size does not alter the technical ability to perform an adequate mammogram, and high-quality images can be obtained in small-breasted women as well as in most men. Patient immobility can compromise the examination, because this may limit the ability of the technologist to bring the entire breast into the x-ray field. Other features of oncologic patients that may compromise mammography include massive ascites; recent breast, axillary, or chest wall surgery; and implanted reservoir catheters overlying the upper breast.

Table 2.2			
Classification of Common Mammographic Findings			
Finding	**Significance (BI-RADS* category)**	**Follow-up**	**Additional Procedures**
Vascular calcification	Benign (BI-RADS 2)	Routine[†]	None
Skin calcification	Benign (BI-RADS 2)	Routine	Tangential radiographs
Simple cysts	Benign (BI-RADS 2)	Routine	Aspirate, if painful
Intramammary lymph nodes	Benign (BI-RADS 2)	Routine	Ultrasound, to rule out cyst, detect fatty hilum of node
Complex cyst	Indeterminate (BI-RADS 4)	Depends on results of aspiration	Aspirate or excise
Multiple bilateral clusters of microcalcifications	Indeterminate (BI-RADS 3 or 4)	6-month f/up	Needle localization, if any one group is more worrisome in morphology
Solid, smoothly marginated nodule on initial study	Indeterminate (BI-RADS 3 or 4)	6-month f/up	Consider core biopsy or excision; ultrasound to rule out cyst
Multiple nodules	Indeterminate (BI-RADS 3)	6-month f/up	Consider core biopsy or excision if any are irregular in outline
Asymmetrical parenchymal densities	Indeterminate (BI-RADS 3)	6-month f/up	Spot compression radiographs to exclude underlying architectural distortion
Single cluster of microcalcifications	Possibly malignant (BI-RADS 4)	Depends on results of biopsy	Biopsy, with needle localization
New solid nodule	Possibly malignant (BI-RADS 4)	Depends on results of biopsy	Biopsy, with needle localization if not palpable
Architectural distortion	Possibly malignant (BI-RADS 4 or 5)	Depends on results of biopsy	Biopsy, with needle localization if not palpable
Spiculated mass	Probably malignant (BI-RADS 5)	Depends on results of biopsy	Biopsy, with needle localization if not palpable

f/up, follow-up.

*BI-RADS (Breast Imaging-Reporting and Data System) categories based on American College of Radiology quality assurance program for breast imaging.

†Routine mammographic follow-up, as recommended by the American College of Radiology, consists of yearly or biennial mammography for women between the ages of 40 and 49 and yearly mammography for women aged 50 or older (Smart CR: Mammographic screening: efficacy and guidelines, *Curr Opin Radiol* 4:108–117, 1992.).

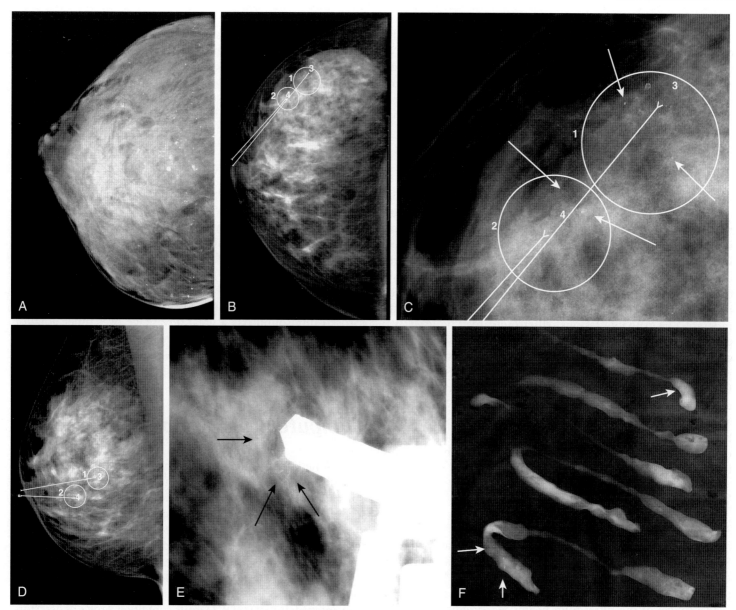

FIGURE 2.2 **DIGITAL MAMMOGRAPHY AND WORKUP OF BREAST CALCIFICATIONS.** **(A)** Craniocaudal (CC) view in a 43-year-old woman for routine screening. Digital mammography penetrates dense breast tissue better than film-screen mammography, clearly showing diffuse benign pattern of large and small calcifications throughout the breast. **(B)** CC view in a 46-year-old woman for routine screening. Digital mammography shows two areas of very faint calcification in the outer breast that require further workup. **(C)** Close-up view of the image from **B**, showing the calcifications (*arrows*) to be variable in size and shape, which is worrisome for malignancy, particularly ductal carcinoma in situ. Such tiny calcifications in a background of dense breast stroma are easier to see on digital than on film-screen mammography. Computer-assisted diagnosis programs also help the radiologist to locate even tiny groups of faint calcifications such as these. **(D)** Mediolateral view in the same patient as in image **B**, showing that the calcifications are in the lower breast. **(E)** Image from stereo core biopsy procedure in the same patient as in image **B**, showing the core needle immediately proximal to one of the groups of calcifications. Stereo core biopsy allows histologic sampling of tiny groups of calcifications, which can be very helpful in planning surgical approach. This interventional procedure can decrease the total number of surgeries that a patient must undergo to achieve definitive treatment. **(F)** Radiograph of specimen from stereo core biopsy procedure on the same patient as in image **B**, showing that there are several tiny calcifications (*arrows*) within some of the core samples. Pathologic analysis of the core biopsy revealed ductal carcinoma in situ, high grade, with comedo features.

Ultrasound

Ultrasound offers many advantages as an imaging modality for the cancer patient. The study is generally painless and can be performed rapidly at the bedside. Ultrasound does not involve ionizing radiation, and no oral or IV contrast materials are generally needed. The study is particularly attractive for frequent follow-up examinations for these reasons. Ultrasound can be used as a guide for biopsy or for drainage of pleural, pericardial, or peritoneal fluid. Using intracavity probes, very detailed images of pelvic organs can be obtained, as well as biopsies. Ultrasound can be combined with endoscopy for examination of the heart or esophagus (Botet et al., 1991) and can also be performed intraoperatively to assist in accurate tumor localization (Clarke et al., 1989). With color flow and Doppler capability, venous thrombosis can be detected noninvasively. Vascular imaging of the upper extremity with ultrasound is more difficult than the lower extremity because of the sound-dampening qualities of the bony thorax and clavicle. In any ultrasound examination, an acoustic "window" is needed to allow the sound beam to pass into the area to be examined. Bone and air do not transmit sound waves, and therefore ultrasound of the chest is limited to the heart (which can be approached through the mediastinal tissues just lateral to the sternum for evaluation of cardiac chamber size, wall motion, and pericardial fluid) and pleural fluid collections that touch the inner chest wall. The cost of ultrasound examinations ranges from 1.75 cost units for a breast ultrasound to 3.25 cost units for bilateral lower extremity venous ultrasounds.

BREAST ULTRASOUND

Breast ultrasound may be a helpful adjunct to mammography but is not useful as a screening tool (Jackson, 1990). Ultrasound can demonstrate the cystic quality of some breast lesions, eliminating the need for further workup. The exam is very operator-dependent, and images may be difficult to reproduce because of variable transducer position and settings from one exam to the next. Therefore, breast ultrasound is best used in evaluating specific lesions, such as nodules visible on mammography or palpable lesions. Ultrasound may be used as a guide for cyst aspiration, which can be both diagnostic and therapeutic. Ultrasound-guided core biopsy of the breast has greatly improved our ability to quickly assess for possible recurrences in breast cancer patients, and may even be able to locate and diagnose sentinel nodes before definitive surgery (Nathanson et al., 2007). Ultrasound is also useful in detection of rupture of breast implants. Future directions for breast ultrasound include detailed Doppler analysis of blood flow in the region of possible tumors as an indicator of neovascularity (Chang et al., 2007).

ABDOMINAL ULTRASOUND

Abdominal ultrasound in the cancer patient may detect liver metastases, dilated bile ducts, hydronephrosis, and masses. Some liver metastases may be better seen with ultrasound than with CT. Measurement of liver and spleen size can be obtained but may be difficult to reproduce because of the relatively small field of view of the ultrasound beam. Measurements are particularly difficult in patients with marked organomegaly, which moves the borders of the organ beyond the range of the transducer, requiring multiple images to encompass the entire organ. Ultrasound is very sensitive in detection of ascites and may be useful in guiding paracentesis. It can also be used to guide percutaneous biopsies of abdominal lesions and for placement of nephrostomy tubes. Evaluation of the pancreas can be limited in some patients by gas in the stomach and duodenum, which blocks sound waves. Ultrasound of the abdomen may also be limited in very obese patients, because the transducers have fixed depths of penetration and fat is relatively attenuating to the sound beam. The presence of barium in the GI tract can severely limit abdominal ultrasound, because the barium blocks sound. Only minimum patient cooperation is required for most abdominal ultrasound examinations, which can be performed at the bedside.

PELVIC ULTRASOUND

Pelvic ultrasound is generally useful to detect small amounts of ascites or to detect tumors of the pelvic organs. For examination of the uterus and ovaries, either a transabdominal or transvaginal approach may be used. Many patients prefer the transvaginal approach, because the transabdominal approach requires pressing the transducer against a full bladder to provide an acoustic "window" onto the pelvis. For prostate examination, similarly, a transabdominal or transrectal approach may be used. More patient cooperation is required for transvaginal or transrectal ultrasound than for the abdominal approach, which can be performed at the bedside. Biopsies can be performed using special needle guides on the rectal and vaginal probes. As in the abdomen, obesity can limit imaging using the transabdominal approach.

ULTRASOUND ABLATION

The ultrasound beam can be focused into a small area with special electronics to produce tissue heating at a single point or plane, called high-intensity focused ultrasound. Any lesion that can be visualized with routine ultrasound is a potential target for ultrasound ablation, which has been performed in the prostate (Rouviere et al., 2007), for uterine fibroids (Stewart et al., 2007), and in many other solid-organ tumors such as liver, kidney, and pancreas (Haar and Coussios, 2007). High-intensity focused ultrasound has a great advantage over other ablation techniques in that it does not require insertion of a catheter into the organ to be treated, because probes can be placed on the skin surface and treatments may require only light sedation.

Computed Tomography

CT scanners have undergone a technical revolution since the introduction of the first helical scanners. Helical scanning, with continuous rotation of the radiation source and continuous feeding of the patient through the scanning gantry, offers much shorter scan times than older single-slice units. The most recent technical development in CT is the development of MDCT scanners, which are units containing several rows of detectors that can simultaneously detect photons while the patient passes through the imaging field, generating much more data in an even shorter time interval. Initial (MDCT) units contained 8 rows of detectors, but current units contain 64 and even more will be available in the future. CT offers many advantages over other imaging methods, including accurate, reproducible measurement of tumors, detection of bone metastases, and detection of enlarged lymph nodes (Ueda et al., 2006). MDCT, with its vast amount of data, allows sophisticated 3D applications to become a practical reality. In CT colonography, even quite small mucosal lesions can be seen (Fig. 2.3), and automated volumetric measurements are now possible for even small lung nodules, which should allow greatly improved assessment of treatment response (Marten and Engelke, 2007). CT is relatively expensive, with many examinations costing over 3.5 cost units. Examinations of contiguous portions of the body require separate exams, so that the bill for a head, chest, abdomen, and pelvis study can total over 15 times the cost of a PA and lateral chest exam. The cost is even higher if IV contrast is used. However, for many areas of the body, such as the abdomen or mediastinum, no other imaging modality offers such complete information.

In the past, helical or spiral CT scanning required several minutes to complete for a study encompassing the chest, abdomen, and pelvis. This limited the thickness of slices that could reasonably be obtained without patient movement, and prevented routine multiplanar reconstruction of data. However, with the introduction of MDCT scanners, which are capable of scanning extremely quickly over large areas of the body, it is now routine to obtain slices thinner than 1 mm, which can easily be reconstructed in sagittal and coronal planes, as well as in 3D volumetric reconstructions (Fig. 2.4). Such sophisticated multiplanar methods allow much more accurate determination of tumor volumes and response rates to be routinely calculated.

The downside of these technical developments is the increase in total numbers of images that must be interpreted in each CT study, but application of computer-assisted diagnostic methods will provide assistance with these image management issues in the future (Bielen and Kiss, 2007).

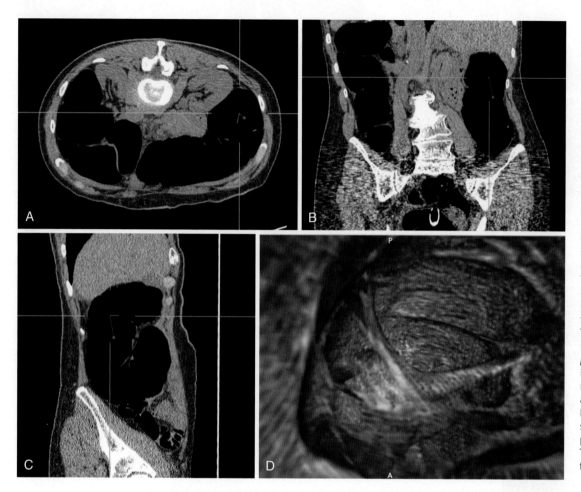

FIGURE 2.3 CT COLONOGRAPHY AND 3D SURFACE RENDERINGS IN CANCER DIAGNOSIS. (A) Axial image in the prone position from CT colonography showing point of view for endoluminal surface rendering within the lumen of colon (*purple dot*). For this study, air is insufflated into the colon after the patient has undergone routine colonoscopy preparation, and the patient is scanned in the prone and then in the supine position. **(B)** Coronally reconstructed image from the same patient as in **A**, showing point of view (*purple*) within the ascending colon, viewed from behind. There is scoliosis and degenerative change in the spine. The rectal tube used to insufflate air is visible at the bottom of the image. **(C)** Sagittally reconstructed image from the same patient as in **A**. The point of view for endoluminal reconstructions is again shown in *purple*. The liver is at the top of the image. **(D)** Endoluminal surface rendered image, simulating the appearance of actual colonoscopy. Polyps may be visible down to the size of several millimeters if the patient preparation is adequate. This view shows normal colonic folds and strands of mucus.

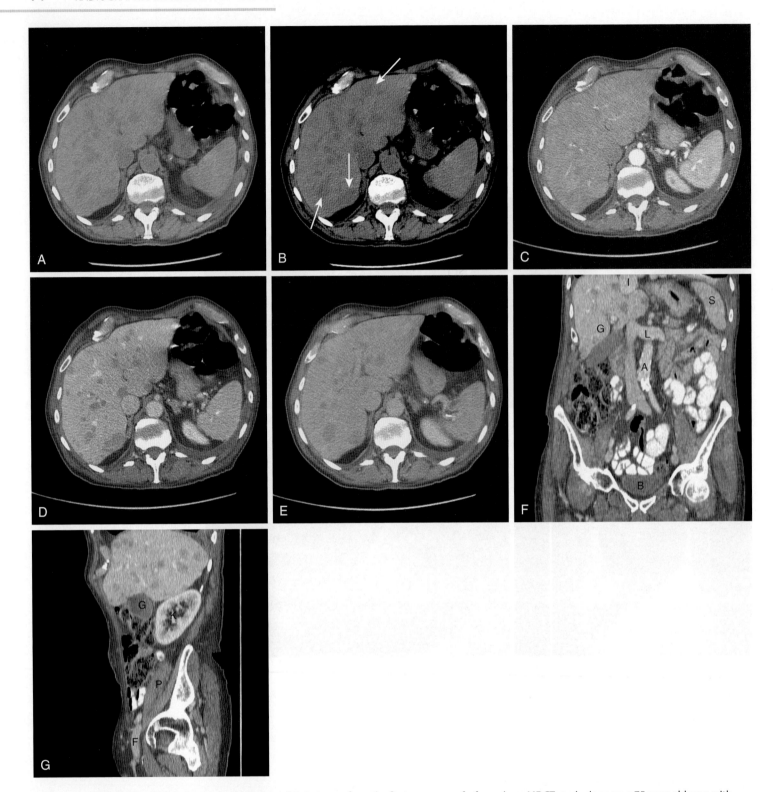

FIGURE 2.4 MDCT AND MULTIPLANAR RECONSTRUCTIONS. (A) An image from the first sequence of a four-phase MDCT study done on a 75-year-old man with unexplained weight loss. On this image before administration of IV contrast, the liver appears slightly heterogeneous but does not show definite focal abnormalities. **(B)** Same image as in **A**, displayed with liver windows. These particular brightness and contrast settings can be useful in detection of subtle abnormalities in the liver and in this case demonstrate several questionable areas of decreased attenuation (*arrows*) that are suspicious for metastatic disease. **(C)** Second sequence in the same patient as in **A**, showing the appearance of the liver during the arterial phase of imaging, with a delay of less than a minute after injection. There is enhancement of the liver, spleen, and top of the left kidney. No definite liver lesions are evident. **(D)** Third sequence in the same patient as in **A**, showing the appearance of the liver during the portal phase of imaging, with a delay of just over 1 minute after injection. Multiple rounded low-attenuation lesions are now clearly evident, representing metastatic disease from an unknown primary site. **(E)** Final phase of the same MDCT sequence, showing appearance of the liver on delayed imaging, approximately 5 minutes after contrast injection. The largest liver lesions are still visible but are less distinct than in image **D**, and many of the smaller lesions are not well seen. The appearance of liver lesions varies considerably between images **C, D,** and **E**, showing the importance of consistency in imaging when assessing tumors for response. Using liver windows as in image **B** might allow measurement of lesions without use of IV contrast, which would remove variables such as injection rate, timing, patient blood volume, and cardiac output, which can all alter the appearance of liver lesions as shown in this image sequence. **(F)** Coronal reconstruction from MDCT on the same patient as in **A**, showing anatomic structures adjacent to the liver. A, aorta; B, bladder; G, gallbladder; I, inferior vena cava; L, left renal vein; S, spleen. Because of the very thin sections possible with MDCT, the quality of coronal and sagittal reconstructions is greatly improved over standard helical scanning. **(G)** Sagittal reconstruction from MDCT on the same patient as in **A**, showing anatomic structures adjacent to the liver. F, femoral vein; G, gallbladder; K, right kidney; P, psoas muscle. In planning surgery or radiation therapy, use of multiplanar reconstructions can be extremely valuable in determining the 3D relationships of adjacent organs.

USE OF INTRAVENOUS CONTRAST

Administration of IV contrast for CT scanning is useful in most studies in cancer patients but is not required for all imaging. Lung lesions can be detected without IV contrast because of the inherent contrast provided by air in the alveoli. For specific problems in the chest, such as detection of hilar masses, vascular dissection, or thrombi, bolus contrast administration is needed. In the brain, increased doses of contrast and delayed imaging may increase detection of metastases (Davis et al., 1991). CT imaging of the neck generally requires IV contrast, because it is difficult to discriminate between vessels and nodes without vascular enhancement as a result of the frequency of anatomic variations in the veins of the neck. Although there have been no new IV contrast agents developed in recent years, research has focused on optimizing delivery of existing agents using automated injection systems and sequential injection of contrast followed by saline (Rutten and Prokop, 2007).

In the liver, the appearance and size of metastatic lesions may vary considerably when comparing studies performed after IV contrast injection to studies not enhanced by contrast (Fig. 2.5). Comparison between two studies both performed with IV contrast can also be limited by unavoidable variations, such as differences in size of catheter used to inject the contrast, location of vein used for injection, amount of contrast administered, cardiac output of the patient at the time of contrast administration, patient blood volume, and any delays between completion of injection and initiation of scanning (technical problems, emesis). Therefore, in following cancer patients with liver metastases, noncontrast scans (for those lesions visible without IV contrast) may provide a more reproducible method of tumor measurement. In some very vascular tumors, the exact timing of imaging after contrast administration may be particularly crucial, because some relatively vascular lesions in the liver may actually become less conspicuous after contrast administration, either transiently or for prolonged periods (Bressler et al., 1987). Use of MDCT may obviate some of these problems through more accurate control of the timing of contrast delivery for more reproducible imaging, but certain patient factors may be beyond the control of the imaging process. For this reason, a two-phase approach to liver metastasis imaging may be optimal, including images both before and after IV contrast administration.

IV contrast administration can also obscure tiny areas of hemorrhage or calcifications, such as might be present in the kidneys or in certain types of metastases. Patients who have received chemotherapy often have poor venous access, and insertion of a peripheral catheter of sufficient caliber for safe contrast administration may be difficult. Therefore, in cancer patients it is often helpful to begin any CT examination without IV contrast and then to assess the need for contrast injection on a case-by-case basis.

FIGURE 2.5 **DETECTION OF LIVER AND SPLEEN ABNORMALITIES WITH CT AND MRI: USE OF IV CONTRAST.** **(A)** CT image through the liver, without IV contrast, obtained for staging in a 35-year-old patient with breast cancer. Two small, low-attenuation lesions are visible in the liver periphery (*arrows*), consistent with metastases. **(B)** CT image in the same patient as Figure 2.2A, obtained at a similar level in the liver on the same day, after IV contrast administration. The liver lesions are no longer visible. Good opacification of hepatic vessels is evident, indicating adequate injection rate and prompt imaging. This study demonstrates that occasionally relatively vascular metastases in the liver may be better seen without IV contrast. **(C)** CT image in the same patient as in Figure 2.2A, obtained at a similar level in the liver several months later, confirming growth of the two lesions initially detected (*arrows*), as well as documenting the appearance of new lesions. **(D)** CT image through the liver in a 70-year-old male with carcinoid tumor of the cecum, after IV contrast administration. Good opacification of hepatic vessels and aorta is evident. No liver lesions are visible. **(E)** CT image in the same patient as in Figure 2.2D, at a similar level in the liver obtained 45 minutes after the previous image. Two low-attenuation liver lesions are now evident (*arrows*), consistent with metastases. This study demonstrates that timing of imaging after IV contrast administration can be crucial in detection of liver metastases, with some metastases less visible immediately after contrast administration. **(F)** CT images through the upper abdomen without IV contrast in a 45-year-old patient with lymphoma and new left upper quadrant pain. An irregular low-attenuation lesion is evident in the spleen and contains central areas of faint higher attenuation (*arrow*) consistent with hemorrhage. This faint density was not visible after IV contrast administration. This study demonstrates the usefulness of noncontrast scanning for detection of subtle high-attenuation abnormalities, such as blood or calcification. **(G)** CT image through the liver in a 35-year-old woman with breast cancer, obtained after IV contrast administration. Adequate opacification of hepatic vessels is evident. No discrete liver lesions are seen, although contrast enhancement is somewhat heterogeneous throughout the liver. **(H)** Axial T_2-weighted MR image through the liver in the same patient as in Figure 2.2G obtained 5 days later. Many discrete, rounded liver lesions are evident, consistent with metastases. This study demonstrates that MRI may sometimes demonstrate lesions that are not visible on CT.

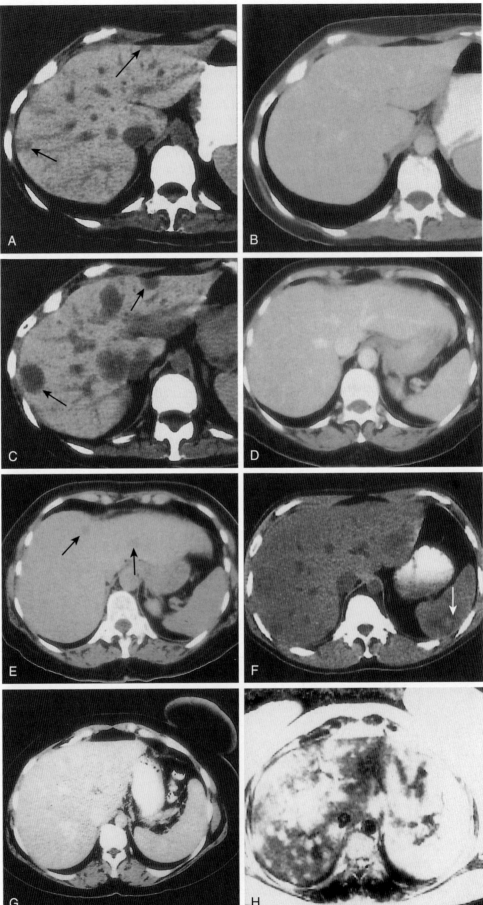

ORAL CONTRAST

For most CT examinations of the abdomen and pelvis in cancer patients, oral contrast is essential. Dilute barium or water-soluble material must be administered beginning several hours before the planned examination to allow complete transit through the bowel. In cancer patients, who may have nausea, offering several different oral preparation options is ideal, because the CT study will be of limited value if the patient does not drink enough contrast material. In particular, when cystic tumor collections or abscesses are suspected, meticulous care must be taken in adequately filling the GI tract with contrast, since fluid-filled bowel loops may mimic other cystic collections. This process takes 1–4 hours in most cases, and overnight preparation may sometimes be required. In detection of masses near the pancreatic head, additional imaging after further oral contrast administration may sometimes be needed to allow separation of pancreas from duodenum. If esophageal abnormalities are suspected, a thicker barium paste may be given orally, which remains in the lumen of the esophagus long enough to provide contrast for imaging. When pelvic masses are evaluated, rectal contrast administration is often useful and is usually well tolerated, in that much less contrast is needed than for a barium enema. Insertion of a tampon into the vagina may be useful in evaluation of uterine or vaginal masses, because the air within the tampon is clearly visible on CT. Placement of external markers may be useful when CT is used for radiation therapy planning.

RADIATION DOSE

Calculation of radiation dose from CT scans is a complex task. The dose of a single slice cannot be simply multiplied by the number of slices to obtain the total dose, because there is some radiation delivered outside the imaging section and radiation is also scattered within the patient (Rothenberg and Pentlow, 1992). Table 2.3 gives dose information for various types of CT examinations. Dose varies among CT machines, based on types of detectors used and other technical parameters. Dose on a given machine can also vary from day to day and from patient to patient. Dose will obviously be much higher if the patient is scanned multiple times, as in protocols to assess different vascular phases within suspected tumors. Such elaborate imaging is generally not needed in follow-up scans to assess response to treatment. In those circumstances it is most important to be consistent in the imaging methodology, so that comparable

images can be obtained that will allow accurate measurement of tumor volumes.

TECHNICAL FACTORS IN COMPUTED TOMOGRAPHY

The radiologist controls many technical parameters in planning a CT scan, which can alter duration of exam, radiation dose, and quality of images. Most imaging parameters that increase the quality of the image do so at the expense of increasing the patient dose (Rothenberg and Pentlow, 1992). The reconstruction algorithm and brightness/contrast settings ("windows") of the image can be changed without effect on dose and may alter conspicuity of lesions (Fig. 2.6). For detection of interstitial lung processes, high-resolution imaging is recommended, consisting of thin sections (1-mm thickness or less) and reconstruction with a high-resolution algorithm (Swensen et al., 1992). MDCT is particularly useful in rapid imaging of moving areas (heart, lungs) or vascular areas (kidneys, carotids) after bolus IV contrast. Disadvantages of MDCT scanning include increased equipment cost and some blurring of the image, with slight resultant decrease in spatial resolution. Ultrafast CT uses a specially designed machine with no moving parts and allows scans to be obtained in milliseconds. This provides the most detailed examination of rapidly moving structures, such as the heart (Stanford et al., 1991). However, ultrafast CT is not routinely available and has no advantages in oncologic imaging.

Most CT examinations require only minimal patient cooperation. Breath holding is needed for optimal chest examination, but an adequate study can usually be obtained during quiet breathing, particularly with MDCT. In searching for adenopathy it must be remembered that lymphadenopathy is diagnosed on CT scans based only on nodal size, which is at best a crude method for detection of metastases (Stomper et al., 1987). Even normal-sized nodes may contain micrometastatic deposits. CT is generally not reliable for detection of invasion of the mediastinum or body wall, unless clear-cut bony erosion or growth into vascular structures is present (Pennes et al., 1985). Invasion may be suspected but not proven when a tumor has a wide area of contact with an adjacent structure (Fig. 2.7).MRI may provide more specific information in questions of invasion (see Magnetic Resonance Imaging). Dense barium from prior fluoroscopic contrast studies or metallic hardware, such as hip replacements or spinal rods, will seriously degrade CT images. Most CT tables have a patient weight limit of 135–160 kg (297–352 lb). Agitated patients must be sedated, because no useful imaging can be obtained in a moving patient. In patients with pain, consideration must be made of the length of time the patient will be required to lie still for the examination, particularly if a multiphase study is planned. A chest CT scan on an MDCT scanner takes under 5 seconds for data acquisition. Most of the time spent in the scan suite is in positioning the patient and arranging for contrast injection, if contrast is to be used. A scan of the chest, abdomen, and pelvis takes under 20 seconds for data acquisition, with delays of several minutes between sequences if a multiphase protocol is planned. In the era of MDCT, almost any patient, even a patient in considerable pain, can hold still long enough for at least one data acquisition.

Table 2.3

Organ-Specific Radiation Doses from CT Examinations*

Site	Head CT	Chest CT	Abdomen CT	Pelvic CT
Bone marrow	0.3–0.4 cG	0.4–0.6 cG	0.6–1.0 cG	0.5–0.8 cG
Lens of the eye	3.2–3.8 cG	–	–	–
Thyroid	0.05–0.12 cG	0.2–0.3 cG	–	–
Breast	–	2.3–2.7 cG	–	–
Lungs	–	1.9–2.5 cG	–	–
Average total skin entry	2.2–6.8 cG	2.0–2.5 cG	2.0–2.5 cG	2.0–2.5 cG

cG, centiGray; CT, computed tomography.
From Wagner LK: Absorbed dose in imaging: why measure it? *Radiology* 178: 622–623, 1991.

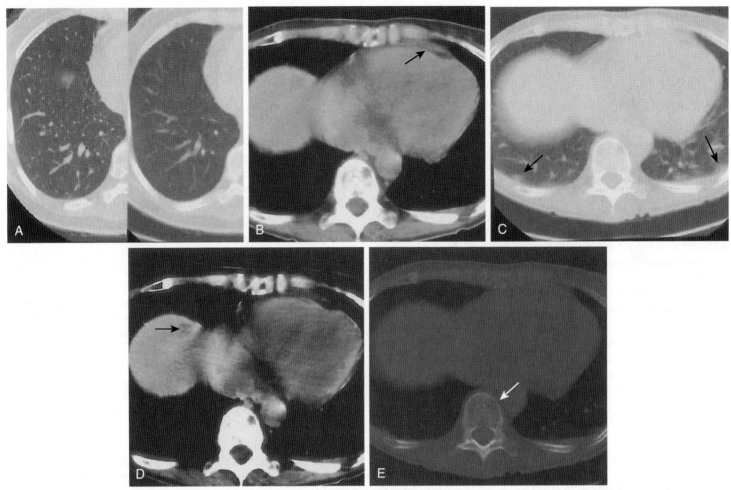

FIGURE 2.6 **TECHNICAL PARAMETERS IN CT: SLICE THICKNESS, RECONSTRUCTION ALGORITHM, AND WINDOWS. (A)** Two CT images through the same portion of the right lung base in a 40-year-old female with a history of thyroid carcinoma. The image on the left was obtained using 1.5-mm slice thickness and high-resolution reconstruction algorithm and is preferable for detection of interstitial processes in the lung, such as lymphangitic carcinomatosis. Image on the right was obtained using 10-mm slice thickness and standard reconstruction algorithm and is preferable for detection of nodular processes in the lung, such as hematogenous metastasis. No metastases or interstitial abnormalities are evident on these images. **(B)** CT image through the lung base in a 45-year-old female patient, performed for staging of breast cancer, and viewed with contrast and brightness settings optimum for mediastinal structures (mediastinal windows). A small amount of pericardial fluid is seen on this image (*arrow*). **(C)** Same CT image as in **B**, viewed with brightness and contrast settings optimum for lung (lung windows). Several ill-defined peripheral lung nodules are now visible (*arrows*), consistent with metastases. **(D)** Same CT image as in **B**, viewed with brightness and contrast settings optimum for the liver (liver windows). A single liver metastasis is now visible (*arrow*). **(E)** Same CT image as in **B**, viewed with brightness and contrast settings optimum for bony structures (bone windows). A lytic metastasis in the vertebral body is now visible (*arrow*). It is likely that viewing of the CT image with only one or two windows would have missed at least some of these abnormalities.

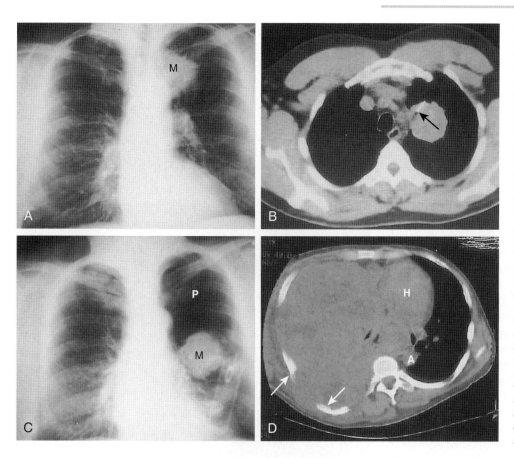

FIGURE 2.7 CT is generally not specific in detection of invasion of adjacent structures by tumor, unless destruction, erosion, or replacement of structures is seen. **(A)** Frontal chest radiograph in the PA projection in a 53-year-old male with hemoptysis showing a large left upper lobe mass (M) abutting the upper left mediastinum in the region of the aortic arch. Emphysema is noted in both upper lobes. **(B)** CT image in the same patient as in Figure 2.5A obtained during a percutaneous needle biopsy shows the biopsy needle tip within the mass (*arrow*) and possible infiltration of the adjacent mediastinal fat by the mass. Detection of such invasion is important, because it may alter surgical therapy. **(C)** Frontal chest radiograph in the PA projection after completion of the biopsy in the same patient shows a large left pneumothorax (P), with the mass (M) freely falling away from the mediastinum, proving that the mass does not invade the mediastinum. Risk of pneumothorax after percutaneous needle biopsy of the lung is increased in patients with adjacent emphysema. **(D)** CT can only conclusively diagnose invasion of adjacent structures by tumor in advanced disease, such as this CT image through the lower chest in a 25-year-old male with a large, recurrent malignant schwannoma. Tumor fills the right hemithorax and displaces the heart (H) to the left. The tumor is destroying ribs posteriorly (*arrows*), which is definitive evidence of chest wall invasion. The patient clinically had chest wall pain and compromised cardiac output due to compression of the right atrium by tumor. A, descending aorta.

Computed Tomography as a Screening Tool

In the era of MDCT scanning, allowing the entire chest to be imaged in a matter of seconds, the role of CT as a screening tool for lung tumors must be reconsidered (Petersen and Harpole, 2006). Special techniques can be used to decrease radiation dose (which also decreases image quality), but this method may become more widespread in the future. Careful cost-benefit analyses are needed, and several large trials are continuing to determine if early detection with CT actually has an impact on survival (Henschke et al., 2007; Sone et al., 2001). The problem of false-positive findings of small nonspecific nodules can be significant, particularly in parts of the country where histoplasmosis or coccidioidomycosis is endemic. In these regions most patients screened may have nodules, requiring difficult management decisions.

Positron Emission Tomography– Computed Tomography

Positron emission tomography (PET) is a noninvasive diagnostic imaging modality that provides whole-body functional imaging capability and holds great promise for cancer patients. It uses positron-emitting isotopes of elements such as carbon (^{11}C), nitrogen (^{13}N), oxygen (^{15}O), and fluorine (^{18}F) to label compounds that are similar to naturally occurring substances in the body. These radiopharmaceuticals can be used as tracers for physiologic and pathophysiologic processes that correlate with various disease states.

2-[^{18}F]-Fluoro-2-deoxy-D-glucose (^{18}F-FDG) is a U.S. Food and Drug Administration–approved positron-emitting glucose analog, which is transported into tumor cells, phosphorylated by hexokinase into FDG-6-phosphate, but does not go further along the glycolytic pathway and remains trapped within the cell. This "metabolic trapping" leads to progressive intracellular accumulation of ^{18}F-FDG over time, with preferential accumulation in tissues with higher glucose metabolism (Fig. 2.8).

Tumor cells show an increased expression of glucose transporter messenger RNA and glucose transporter molecules (GLUT-1 and GLUT-3), as well as an increased activity of hexokinase II (the isoenzyme associated with anaerobic glycolysis) and downregulation of glucose-6-phosphatase enzymes. This increased glycolytic activity is the rationale for the use of ^{18}F-FDG in the functional imaging of cancer.

The positron emitted by the radionuclide travels a short distance (~1 mm) in human tissue, combines with an electron in an annihilation reaction. This reaction results in the production of two 511-keV photons that are emitted very close to 180 degrees from each other. These high-energy photons can be detected at the same time (in "coincidence"), defining a line of response along which lies the site of the annihilation reaction. The resulting information can be reconstructed to produce a 3D map of the tracer concentration throughout the body. There are a variety of cameras able to perform PET, ranging from modified traditional nuclear medicine cameras to systems dedicated solely to coincidence imaging. The image quality and performance of the latter tend to be much better than that of the former.

Details of PET technique will be discussed in a separate chapter. The normal distribution of ^{18}F-FDG 1 hour after injection of the tracer includes the brain, the blood pool, urinary activity within the renal collecting system, and the bladder, as well as uptake in smooth and striated muscles. Myocardial uptake is highly dependent on the fasting state and is enhanced in the presence of insulin, as is the uptake in skeletal muscle (Fig. 2.9). These normal areas of activity limit the utility of PET in certain regions of the body for detection of tumors. The inherent low spatial resolution of PET images can lead to difficulties in localizing areas of activity within organs. PET-CT is a method by which rapidly sequential PET and CT images are obtained that allow correlation of anatomic (CT) with functional (PET) imaging and better localization of sites of disease (Fig. 2.10). As previously discussed, CT is exquisitely sensitive for detection and demonstration of anatomy and structure within the body, but the findings of CT alone are very nonspecific. In imaging adenopathy, for example, CT can easily detect minimally enlarged nodes but cannot determine whether they contain active tumor. PET produces images of limited resolution and clarity, but with exquisite specificity for metabolically active tumor. In PET-CT a single piece of equipment is capable of imaging a patient with both CT and PET in rapid sequence (Wong et al., 2007). Because the imaging is done in close temporal relationship there is little opportunity for movement, and images can be fused to allow optimal localization in terms of both anatomy and function.

It is important to keep in mind, however, that the quality of the CT scan obtained in PET-CT imaging is generally not the same as in a dedicated CT study. With the rapid development of new CT equipment, it is not practical for PET-CT units to all contain the latest CT methodology. Therefore, although the CT portion of the PET-CT study is very helpful in localizing the metabolic activity seen on PET, it may not be detailed enough to capture sophisticated data routinely possible with MDCT, such as multiple-phase vascular imaging and 3D reconstructions (Kuehl et al., 2007).

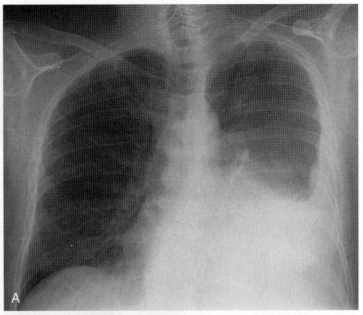

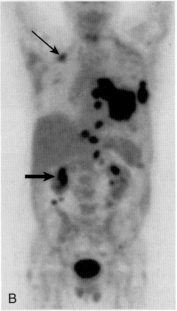

FIGURE 2.8 PET imaging depends on accumulation of ^{18}F-FDG in tissues with high rates of glucose metabolism and often demonstrates disease sites not suspected on routine imaging. **(A)** Chest radiograph in a 77-year-old man with known poorly differentiated lung cancer and new shortness of breath. A large left pleural effusion obscures most of the left chest. **(B)** The projection image from the patient's PET scan shows extensive abnormal uptake in the left lower lobe in a masslike configuration not typical for malignant effusion. This large lung mass was obscured by the pleural effusion on the chest radiograph. Areas of abnormal uptake near the midline are consistent with metastases to mediastinal nodes, and there is also left lateral chest wall uptake suspicious for skeletal invasion. A focal area of uptake on the right (*small black arrow*) indicates unsuspected contralateral supraclavicular spread. Uptake in the renal collecting systems (*large black arrow*) is normal.

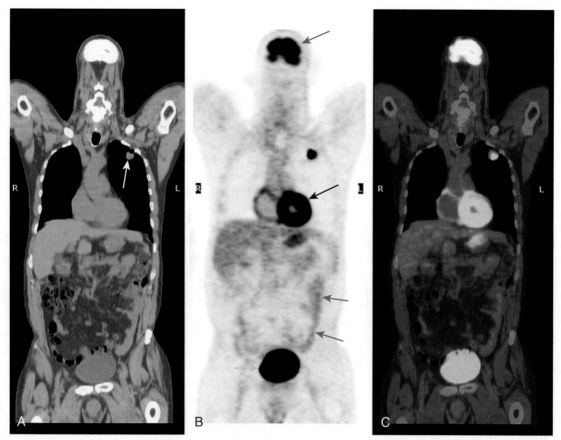

FIGURE 2.9 **PET-CT** WITH FUSION OF DATA TO DEMONSTRATE BOTH ANATOMIC AND FUNCTIONAL PATHOLOGY. **(A)** Coronally reformatted CT data on a 50-year-old smoker with cough and a solitary pulmonary nodule noted on chest radiography. A nodule is evident in the left upper lung (*arrow*). No other nodules or enlarged nodes were seen. **(B)** PET image from the same patient as in **A**, showing abnormal uptake in the left upper lobe nodule, indicating high metabolic activity and highly suggestive of lung cancer. Other areas of normal PET activity are shown including brain (*red arrow*), bladder (*yellow arrow*), and faint uptake in the colon (*blue arrows*). If the patient has not fasted before the study, the myocardium also will also show marked uptake, as in this case (*black arrow*). **(C)** Fusion image with PET and CT data overlaid to confirm correspondence of areas of normal and abnormal uptake. Because the CT and PET are acquired with the same equipment and within a short time frame, there is generally good registration of data, as shown in this case.

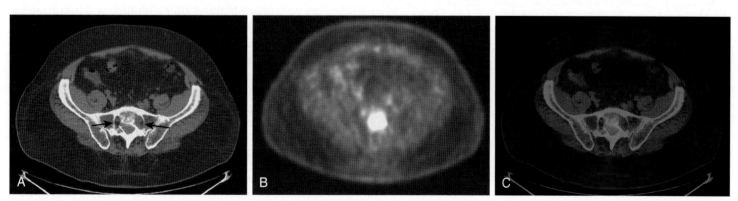

FIGURE 2.10 VALUE OF COMBINING **PET** AND **CT** DATA TO ACCURATELY LOCALIZE SITES OF DISEASE. **(A)** Axial CT image in a 49-year-old man with a known diagnosis of non-Hodgkin's lymphoma and new low back pain. There is subtle asymmetry of the sacral neural foramina (*arrows*) but no other obvious abnormality. **(B)** Axial PET image in the same patient as in **A**, showing a focus of abnormal uptake in the pelvis. On PET alone, this would be difficult to localize and could lie within bone, nodes, or possibly bowel. **(C)** Fusion image using data from **A** and **B**, showing that the abnormal PET activity is located within the sacrum and probably accounts for the subtle sacral foramen asymmetry noted on the CT scan. This was confirmed on biopsy to represent involvement of the bone with lymphoma.

IHB TRUST LIBRARY
ꓛЕН

Magnetic Resonance Imaging

Use of MRI in cancer patients is becoming more common as equipment becomes more sophisticated and new pulse sequences and specialized detection apparatus are developed. Imaging in MRI depends on electromagnetic properties of nuclei, which vary depending on their bonding to other atoms and their local electromagnetic environment (Smith and McCarthy, 1992). The patient is placed in a high-field-strength magnet (0.3–3.0 tesla) and radiofrequency energy is introduced, which is absorbed by the patient. As time passes this energy is lost and radiofrequency energy is emitted by the patient as a signal, which is detected by receivers called "coils." Imaging signal can be obtained from a variety of nuclei, but hydrogen is most often used because it is so abundant, producing a strong signal at a relatively low field strength. MRI is particularly useful in evaluation of the brain and spinal cord and has replaced CT and myelography in most instances.

Much research in MRI focuses on methods to image function rather than simple anatomy. Use of macromolecular contrast media may allow direct assessment of microvascularity, which may have important implications for treatment with antitumor agents that act on angiogenesis (Barrett et al., 2006). Imaging at 3 tesla offers faster scan times, better image resolution, and greater potential for use of MR spectroscopy (Tanenbaum, 2006). More sophisticated use of MR spectroscopy may allow analysis of in vivo metabolic changes of apoptosis and other signs of tumor response to therapy (Cao et al., 2006). More detailed analysis of vascular patterns in tumors with MR, using either existing contrast agents or novel new agents tagged to tumor markers or cellular processes, may allow better diagnosis of viable tumor within masses and more precise measurement of response to therapy (Strijkers et al., 2007). Several new MR techniques show promise for imaging of the oxygen status of tissues, which is important in many pathologic states and may have particular implications for radiation therapy (Krishna et al., 2001). Diffusion-weighted MRI, which detects changes in the ability of water to diffuse through tissues, may allow more accurate assessment of effects of ablation, chemoembolization, and standard chemotherapy upon tumor deposits throughout the body (Vossen et al., 2006).

MAGNETIC RESONANCE PHYSICS

Two properties of nuclei combine to produce MR signal: T_1 and T_2, which are relaxation times or decay times for nuclei to return to their baseline state after excitation by a radiofrequency pulse. Two operator-determined variables are altered in basic MR examinations to change the contribution of T_1 and T_2 to the imaging data: TR (repetition time between cycles of radiofrequency excitations) and TE (time to echo). Therefore, most MR imaging includes at least two types of pulse sequences: those designed to most clearly demonstrate contrast due to differences in T_1 (T_1-weighted images) and those demonstrating contrast due to differences in T_2 (T_2-weighted images). T_1-weighted sequences have short TR and short TE, whereas T_2-weighted sequences have long TR and long TE. Other sequences may also be obtained, including those that are most dependent on actual quantity of hydrogen present (rather than on T_1 or T_2), called proton density images. Varying of other parameters, such as flip angle or adding pulses to saturate certain specific types of nuclei, can also alter image appearance. In general, T_1-weighted images display more fine anatomic detail, and water (cerebrospinal fluid, edema, effusions, ascites) appears low in signal (black) in the image. T_2-weighted images display more contrast between normal and pathologic tissues, and water appears high in signal (white) in the image (Fig. 2.11).

Objects that move into and out of the section plane during the time of the scan, such as flowing blood, appear low in signal (black) in T_1- and T_2-weighted sequences. Special sequences may be used, such as gradient echo imaging, time-of-flight, or phase-contrast imaging, which will cause flowing blood to appear high in signal (white) in the image, without requiring administration of IV contrast material (see Table 2.3). Such imaging is sometimes called MR angiography and may yield information regarding flow velocity and direction as well as delineating the anatomy of vascular structures, thrombi, and caliber of vessels (Atlas, 1994). MR data, which are generated by electrically modifying a magnetic field, can be obtained in any plane. Coronal, sagittal, or oblique imaging can be particularly advantageous in certain parts of the body, such as at the lung apex or diaphragm. True volumetric acquisitions are possible, which can be useful in surgical and radiation therapy planning. Unlike CT contrast material, which contains iodine, most MR contrast agents contain gadolinium. Gadolinium alters the T_1 of nearby tissues, so only T_1-weighted images are generally obtained after gadolinium administration (Hendrick and Haacke, 1993). Gadolinium is particularly useful in detection of lesions in the brain, spinal canal, and breast (Fig. 2.12). Intravenous gadolinium agents were formerly administered to patients regardless of renal function, but recent case reports indicate that there is a low risk of development of a severe skin and multisystem reaction (nephrogenic systemic fibrosis) to gadolinium in patients with severe renal dysfunction (Khurana et al., 2007). Because of this risk, IV gadolinium is no longer administered to patients with lowered creatinine clearance.

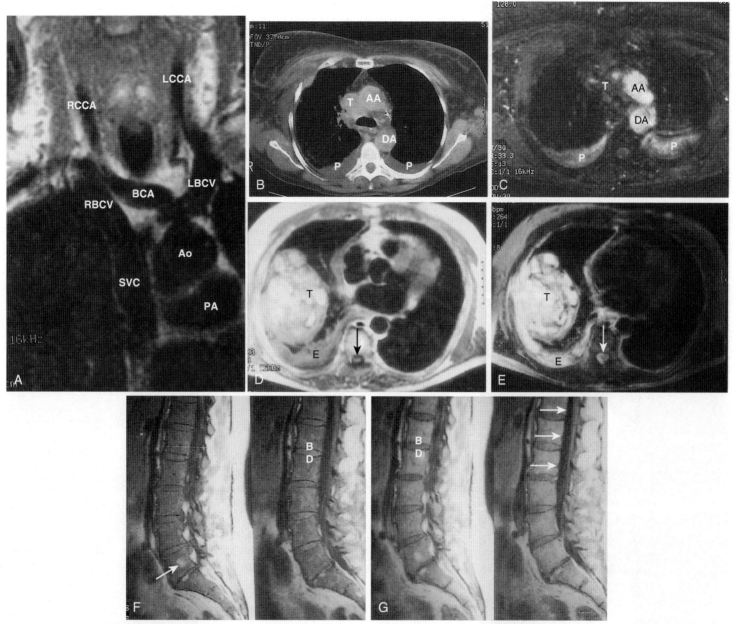

FIGURE 2.11 TECHNICAL FACTORS IN MRI. (A) Coronal T_1-weighted image through a normal mediastinum, demonstrating vascular structures, without the use of IV contrast. On this pulse sequence, flowing blood appears low in signal (*black*). Ao, aorta; BCA, brachiocephalic artery; LBCV, left brachiocephalic vein; LCCA, left common carotid artery; PA, main pulmonary artery; RBCV, right brachiocephalic vein; RCCA, right common carotid artery; SVC, superior vena cava. **(B)** CT image at a level just below the aortic arch, without IV contrast, in a 64-year-old patient with neck and facial swelling indicative of SVC syndrome. Tumor is seen in the region of the SVC (T) and inseparable from it, which revealed small cell lung carcinoma on biopsy. Small bilateral pleural effusions are also present (P). AA, ascending aorta; DA, descending aorta. **(C)** Axial gradient echo MR image in the same patient as in **B**, at approximately the same level in the chest as in Figure 2.6B. No IV contrast was used, and flowing blood appears high in signal (*white*) with this pulse sequence. No normal flow is detected in the expected region of the SVC, which is obliterated by tumor (T). AA, ascending aorta; DA, descending aorta; P, pleural effusion. **(D)** Axial T_1-weighted MR image in a 59-year-old male with chest pain and a large right pleural mass. Biopsy revealed pleural leiomyosarcoma. Heterogeneous tumor (T) is seen in the peripheral right lower chest, along with pleural disease (E), which does not have the expected low signal of simple effusion on this pulse sequence. Note high-signal (*white*) appearance of fat in the subcutaneous regions and mediastinum, as expected on a T_1-weighted sequence. Because fluid is typically low signal on T_1-weighted images, the cerebrospinal fluid (CSF) space appears as a black ring surrounding the higher signal spinal cord (*arrow*). **(E)** Axial T_2-weighted MR image in the same patient as in **D**, at a similar level in the chest. The tumor (T) is again heterogeneous in appearance but of higher signal than on the T_1-weighted image. Signal in the pleural space (E) is similar to that of the tumor, again suggesting pleural spread. Note lower signal (*gray*) appearance of subcutaneous fat in comparison to the T_1-weighted image, as expected on a T_2-weighted sequence. Fluid is typically high in signal on T_2-weighted images, and therefore the CSF space appears as a white ring surrounding the lower signal spinal cord (*arrow*). **(F)** Sagittal T_1-weighted images of the lumbar spine in a 52-year-old female with anemia and low back pain. Normally, the signal in the vertebral bodies is relatively high on T_1-weighted images, due to fat within the marrow. The signal in the vertebral bodies (B) in this patient is similar to that of the intervertebral disks (D), indicating a diffuse infiltrative marrow abnormality. Focal high signal in the L5 vertebral body (*arrow*) is a hemangioma. **(G)** Sagittal T_1-weighted images of the lumbar spine in the same patient as in **F**, after IV administration of gadolinium. The marrow signal in the vertebral bodies does not normally change after IV contrast administration. The signal in the vertebral bodies (B) has increased and is now higher than the signal in the intervertebral disks (D), indicating diffuse enhancement, also suggestive of a diffuse infiltrative process. Bone marrow biopsy revealed evidence of Waldenstrom's macroglobulinemia. Note low signal in CSF (*arrows*), as expected on all T_1-weighted images.

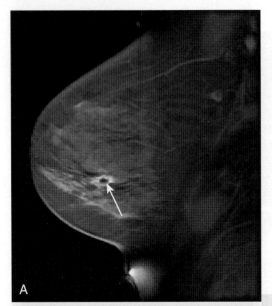

FIGURE 2.12 Use of MRI in management of breast cancer: 43-year-old woman (same patient is in Figure 2.2B–F) with two areas of suspicious microcalcifications in the breast. Stereo core biopsy of one of the groups of calcifications showed ductal carcinoma in situ. Breast MR was performed to assess extent of disease for surgical planning. **(A)** Sagittal breast MR image after administration of IV gadolinium. There is faint enhancement in several areas of the lower breast that is difficult to assess on unprocessed images. A signal void is present (*arrow*) at the site of a metallic marker clip from prior core biopsy. **(B)** Processed image with overlay of quantitative flow information. Blue in the image indicates a suspicious pattern of rapid and significant enhancement. A region of interest (*arrow*) has been selected for graphic analysis. **(C)** Graph of change in signal over time for the voxel indicated by the arrow in **B**. Rapid and significant enhancement pattern indicates probable area of malignancy. **(D)** Selection of control voxel in normal breast tissue (*arrow*), for comparison to abnormal areas. **(E)** Graph of change in signal over time for the voxel indicated by the *arrow* in **D**, in a region of normal breast. Slow and less marked enhancement pattern indicates normal breast tissue. **(F)** Computed volume estimate of tumor in this case, based on regions demonstrating abnormal enhancement pattern. **(G)** Rotating 3D images derived from MR data, showing extensive abnormal enhancement in the left lateral breast. This image sequence shows rotation in the coronal plane and can be helpful in surgical planning. Because of the extent of disease shown on MR, this patient opted for mastectomy rather than lumpectomy.

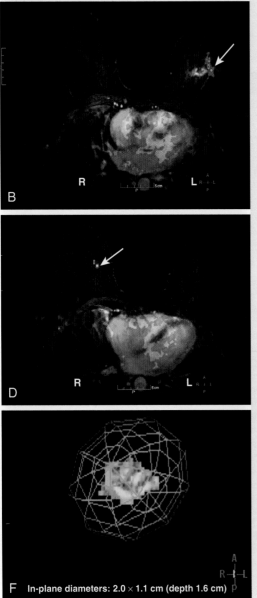

In-plane diameters: 2.0 × 1.1 cm (depth 1.6 cm)

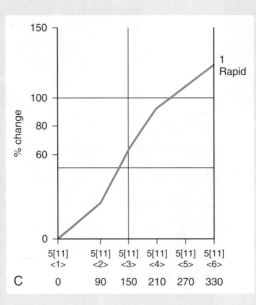

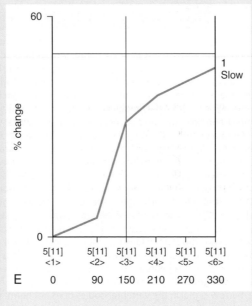

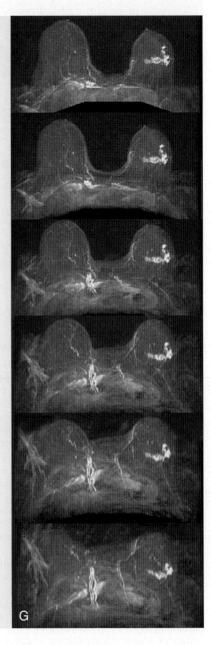

IMAGING COILS

Specialized MR coils have been designed that allow more detailed examination of specific areas of the body. Breast coils allow high-resolution examination of the breast (Harms et al., 1993). Endorectal coils are useful in detection of small lesions of the prostate (Schnall et al., 1991). Phased-array coils or specialized arrangements of multiple detector coils are particularly useful for pelvic imaging (Kier et al., 1993). MR is not currently used for examination of the lung parenchyma, because air does not generate adequate signal; MR also may be less useful than CT in demonstration of some bony abnormalities, because dense bone does not produce a strong signal. Strong signal is obtained from the bone marrow, and MR is the most sensitive study available for surveying marrow involvement by tumor (Negendank and Soulen, 1993). Because MR does not use ionizing radiation, it is an attractive modality for patients requiring frequent repeated imaging. MR is also useful in evaluation of vascular lesions in patients with allergy to CT contrast materials. Most MRI examinations cost from 5 to 6 cost units per study, with extra charges for contrast-enhanced studies.

MRI requires placing the patient in a long, cylindrical gantry, which limits the usefulness of the study in patients with severe claustrophobia. Because the strong magnetic field will have effects on any ferromagnetic metals present within the gantry, the ability to use many patient monitoring devices is somewhat limited, although newer, nonferromagnetic monitoring devices have been developed that avoid this problem (Holshouser et al., 1993). Moderate patient cooperation is required for MR studies, because the images are easily degraded by even minimal patient motion and examinations can take as long as 1–2 hours to complete. MR is more sensitive to patient motion overall than CT, so if a patient has difficulty holding still, CT is generally a better imaging choice than MRI. MRI is contraindicated in patients with certain internal metallic objects (lens implants, intraocular metallic shards, cerebral aneurysm clips, abdominal vascular clips for 3–6 months after surgery, cochlear implants), or particularly in patients with pacemakers. Like CT, MR tables have patient weight limits of 135–160 kg (297–352 lb), and patient diameter may also limit entry of certain patients into the gantry opening. In many areas of the body there is considerable controversy regarding use of CT versus MR for imaging and follow-up. Often either can be used, and other considerations such as cost or ease of scheduling may become the deciding factor. It is important to keep in mind that comparisons between studies will be easier if the same imaging modality is used each time a patient is examined (Table 2.4).

Table 2.4

Uses and Limitations of Various Imaging Procedures in Oncologic Patients

Study	Clinical Utility	Clinical Limitations
Ultrasound	1. Detection of cystic nature of superficial lesions (as in breast) 2. Guidance of biopsy 3. Guidance of thoracocentesis/pericardiocentesis 4. Detection of liver lesions, some characterization (hemangiomas) 5. Real-time imaging 6. Relatively low cost (2–3 cost units for most studies) 7. Can be done portably, intraoperatively 8. No ionizing radiation 9. Does not require IV contrast to demonstrate flowing blood, thrombus 10. Images can be obtained in any plane	1. Limited view of mediastinum 2. Limited view of the pancreas in many patients due to gas 3. Low spatial resolution 4. Images very operator-dependent 5. Limited depth of penetration 6. Not useful in detection of bone lesions 7. Abdominal studies limited in presence of barium in the GI tract from prior fluoroscopy
Computed tomography	1. Better contrast resolution than plain radiographs, sensitive detection of fat and calcification 2. Relatively high spatial resolution 3. Guidance of biopsy/drainages 4. Detection of liver lesions, some characterization (using IV contrast and multiphase imaging) 5. Sensitive in detection of abnormalities of cortical bone 6. Reproducible size measurements (not very operator-dependent) 7. Very rapid imaging possible with MDCT unit, seconds per region 8. Multiplanar reconstructions possible from MDCT data 9. Moderate cost (4–15 cost units, depending on areas included and use of contrast) 10. Relatively insensitive to misregistration and respiratory variation if MDCT	1. Uses ionizing radiation 2. Cannot be performed portably 3. Moderate claustrophobia 4. Limited in the presence of metallic hardware 5. Somewhat limited by patient motion 6. Requires IV contrast to detect flowing blood, thrombus 7. Requires adequate bowel opacification for most abdominal studies (up to 6 hours of preparation time required) 8. Abdominal studies limited in presence of barium in the GI tract from prior procedures
Magnetic resonance imaging	1. No ionizing radiation 2. Less risk of contrast reaction than with CT contrast agents 3. Sensitive in detection of bone marrow infiltration 4. Excellent for survey of spinal cord (cord compression) 5. Most sensitive for detection of CNS metastatic disease 6. Excellent contrast discrimination for soft tissues, joint spaces 7. Does not require IV contrast to detect flowing blood, thrombus 8. Scans can be obtained in any plane 9. Can be used to guide biopsy with specialized coils and equipment 10. Metabolic information can be obtained in some cases with spectroscopy, better tissue characterization	1. Cannot be performed portably 2. Limited ability to monitor patients with older equipment 3. Very limited in patients with severe claustrophobia 4. Very limited by patient motion 5. Limited examination of the bowel 6. High cost (10–20 cost units) 7. Not sensitive in detection of calcification 8. Studies may take 45 minutes to 2 hours to complete 9. Some artifact from metallic hardware

CNS, central nervous system; CT, computed tomography; GI, gastrointestinal; IV, intravenous; MDCT, multidetector CT.

An area of investigation in MR that may have utility in imaging of cancer in the future is MR spectroscopy in vivo to detect signal generated by isotopes other than hydrogen, including phosphorus, nitrogen, sodium, and fluorine. The abundance of these isotopes is less than that of hydrogen in the body, and the signal they generate is also lower, limiting the quality of the images that can be generated with lower-field-strength equipment (Partain and Patton, 1994). Use of magnets with higher field strength increases the signal detectable from these isotopes and improves clinical imaging, but it may also increase artifacts in images. MR spectroscopy using phosphorus may give insight into energy metabolism in tumors (Barker et al., 1993).

Image-Guided Biopsy

Interventional radiology is a rapidly changing field, with many procedures that previously required surgical intervention (such as inferior vena cava filter or gastrostomy tube placement) now performed by radiologists using ultrasound, angiographic, MR, or CT guidance. A description of the many interventional radiologic procedures that may be useful in cancer patients is beyond the scope of this chapter. This section will focus instead on a discussion of biopsy using image guidance.

Percutaneous biopsy can be performed with fine-gauge needles (18–22 gauge) for cytologic aspiration specimens. Using such small needles, safe entry can be made into very deep structures, sometimes passing through bowel, liver, or vessels without complications (Wittenberg et al., 1982). Larger-caliber cutting needles (18–20 gauge) can be used to collect tissue specimens for histologic examination but are only safe for relatively peripheral lesions. Automated core or biopsy guns use 14- to 18-gauge needles to collect even larger specimens and may be particularly useful in breast lesions, lymphoma, or mesothelioma. Such large needles are not suitable for most deeper lesions.

For percutaneous procedures, certain laboratory values are generally checked, similar to those for bronchoscopy: platelets usually must be >50,000, with a normal prothrombin time and partial thromboplastin time. For biopsy of lesions in the lung most nodules must be ≥1 cm in diameter, although smaller lesions may sometimes be biopsied if they are peripheral in location. Biopsy of basilar lesions is more difficult than of lesions in the upper lungs, because the lung bases move more with respiration and relatively small inconsistencies in breath holding may move a lower lobe lesion out of the scan plane and needle track. Consultation with an interventional radiologist with review of all imaging is useful before scheduling percutaneous biopsies, to assess accessibility of lesions and to plan the approach. In most cases it is helpful to obtain a complete cross-sectional imaging series through the lesion (CT or MR) before the biopsy to localize any nearby structures that should be avoided, such as nerves, vessels, or pleural fissures. Either CT or fluoroscopy can be used for guidance of biopsies in the chest. Fluoroscopy is generally easier and faster but may not be appropriate for very central lesions. Most abdominal biopsies use CT or ultrasound guidance. Ultrasound has the advantage of providing real-time visualization of the needle. Ultrasound is limited by requirement for an acoustic "window" to allow imaging and sometimes by depth of penetration of the transducer, particularly in large or obese patients.

Considerable patient cooperation is required for image-guided biopsy procedures. In the chest in particular, the patient must remain still for as long as 30 minutes and must also suspend respiration repeatedly when the needle is in place. If the patient is restless, coughing uncontrollably, or in extreme pain, any image-guided biopsy may be impossible, because each time the patient moves on the scan table, the entire procedure for localizing the lesion must begin again. Most image-guided biopsy procedures can be performed on an outpatient basis. For outpatient chest biopsies, patients are usually monitored for 2–4 hours after the procedure for pneumothorax before being sent home. Ultrasound-guided biopsies may be performed at the bedside. Radiation dose will vary depending on the modality used for guidance. Cost will also vary, with ultrasound generally the least expensive. A cytologic wet reading is often obtained at the time of sample collection, to determine if more samples are needed. This increases the rate of success in obtaining a diagnosis and may also decrease complications through a decrease in the total number of samples collected (Johnsrude et al., 1985).

Image-Guided Therapy

TUMOR ABLATION

In the quest for less invasive options for the treatment of cancer, radiologists have led the wave of new image-guided ablative techniques, most of which are currently used in the palliative setting rather than as curative treatments. Radio waves can be emitted from the tip of a specialized catheter and can produce severe damage to surrounding tissues, which is the basis for radiofrequency ablation techniques. Most are performed under CT guidance. The first such procedures were done for unresectable liver metastases, because surrounding liver parenchyma can contain the fluid and breakdown products from the ablation process. The minimally invasive nature of this procedure allows it to be used repeatedly, and relatively long-term survival is possible in some patients (Thanos et al., 2007). Similar image-guided methods have been used in the lung (Matsuoka and Okuma, 2007), breast (Bland et al., 2007), and kidneys (Hafron and Kaouk, 2007). Ablation of tumor can also be performed with other methods of inducing tissue damage, including heat, cold, or chemical injections (Liapi and Geschwind, 2007).

INTERVENTIONAL MAGNETIC RESONANCE IMAGING

Several recent developments in MR technology have clinical utility in the cancer patient. Open-configuration MR design (Jolesz and Blumenfeld, 1994) allows ready access to patients during MR scans, allowing interventional MR (Fig. 2.13) to be performed. MR has advantages over CT in monitoring the progress of ablation procedures, because imaging can detect chemical changes in tissues related to viability and can also directly monitor tissue temperature changes (Kurumi et al., 2007). In combination with nonferromagnetic needles and innovative coil designs, MR is now routinely used to guide biopsies, drainages, and other interventions. Breast biopsy under MR guidance is a routine procedure and is necessary particularly for lesions that may only be visible on MR images.

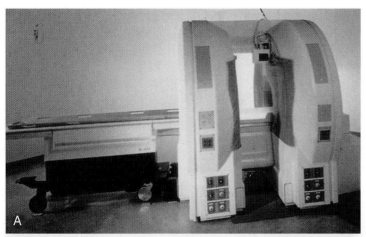

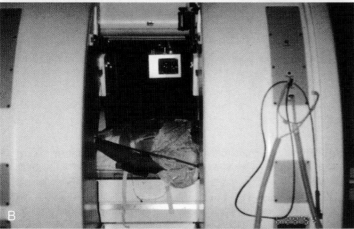

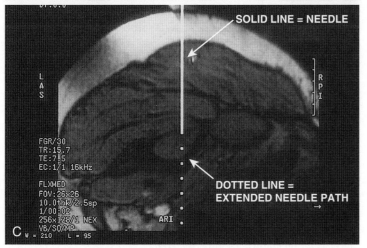

SOLID LINE = NEEDLE

DOTTED LINE =
EXTENDED NEEDLE PATH

FIGURE 2.13 INTERVENTIONAL MR. (A) The open-configuration interventional MR scanner at Brigham and Women's Hospital in Boston, Massachusetts. The magnet gantry is constructed to provide access to the patient during scanning. **(B)** Open-configuration MR scanner with patient in place, demonstrating degree of access available to the radiologist for interventional procedures. **(C)** Specialized rapid MR acquisition (spoiled gradient echo) obtained during an interventional procedure, showing planned needle path for biopsy of a lesion in the left iliac bone. The MR biopsy was nondiagnostic, yielding only bloody material. At final pathology after a surgical biopsy, a primary vascular tumor of bone was diagnosed, an epithelioid hemangio-endothelioma. In such tumors needle aspirates are rarely diagnostic, because they will only yield bloody fluid, as seen here.

Conclusions

Imaging has always played an important role in the initial diagnosis of cancer as well as in the determination of success or failure of treatment regimens. With the development of new targeted treatments for cancer, such as epidermal growth factor receptor–tyrosine kinase inhibitors, we can hope to see more dramatic responses and longer survival in patients, even those who present with extensive disease (Fig. 2.14). Some of these new therapeutic agents may lead to development of more targeted imaging modalities based on the molecular biology of tumors. As more

sensitive and specific imaging modalities are developed, we may be able to screen more effectively for common cancers, detecting them at an earlier stage. Radiologists may also play a larger role in the future in treatment of cancer, through interventional procedures. Whereas these interventions are currently reserved for palliation, they may ultimately become a part of the primary treatment of certain malignancies. Imaging also plays an important role in the detection of complications of treatment, such as radiation fibrosis, drug toxicity, and secondary infection. Radiologists and oncologists should continue to work together closely toward the ultimate goal of early detection and minimally invasive cure of malignancies of all types.

FIGURE 2.14 DRAMATIC RESPONSE OF ADVANCED LUNG CANCER TO ORAL TARGETED TREATMENT (ERLOTINIB). (A) Digital frontal chest radiograph of a 75-year-old woman with advanced lung cancer, with large right hilar mass, large right pleural effusion, and enlarged cardiac silhouette suggesting pericardial fluid. Several other standard treatment regimens had resulted in failure. **(B)** Digital frontal chest radiograph after the same patient received an oral targeted agent, erlotinib. There has been a dramatic decrease in pleural fluid and shrinkage of the hilar mass, and the heart size now appears normal. The degree of response is clear even on plain radiography.

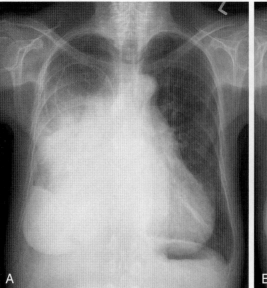 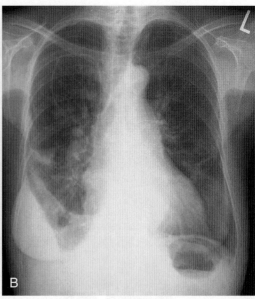

References and Suggested Readings

Atlas SW: MR angiography in neurologic disease, *Radiology* 193:1–16, 1994.

Barker PB, Glickson JD, Bryan RN: In vivo magnetic resonance spectroscopy of human brain tumors, *Topics MRI* 5:32–45, 1993.

Barrett T, Kobayashi H, Brechbiel M, Choyke PL: Macromolecular MRI contrast agents for imaging tumor angiogenesis, *Eur J Radiol* 60:353–366, 2006.

Bielen D, Kiss G: Computer-aided detection for CT colonography: update 2007, *Abdom Imaging* 32(5):571–581, 2007.

Bird RE, Wallace TW, Yankaskas BC: Analysis of cancers missed at screening mammography, *Radiology* 184:613–617, 1992.

Bland KL, Gass J, Klimberg VS: Radiofrequency, cryoablation, and other modalities for breast cancer ablation, *Surg Clin North Am* 87:539–550, 2007.

Botet JF, Lightdale CJ, Zauber AG, et al: Preoperative staging of esophageal cancer: comparison of endoscopic US and dynamic CT, *Radiology* 181:419–425, 1991.

Bressler EL, Alpern MB, Glazer GM, et al: Hypervascular hepatic metastases: CT evaluation, *Radiology* 162:49–51, 1987.

Broadbent MV, Hubbard LB: Science and perception of radiation risk, *Radiographics* 12:381–392, 1992.

Cao Y, Sundgren PC, Tsien CI, et al: Physiologic and metabolic magnetic resonance imaging in gliomas, *J Clin Oncol* 24:1228–1235, 2006.

Caro JJ, Trinidade E, McGregor M: The risks of death and of severe nonfatal reactions with high- vs. low-osmolality contrast media: a meta-analysis, *Am J Roentgenol* 156:825–832, 1991.

Chang RF, Huang SF, Moon WK, et al: Solid breast masses: neural network analysis of vascular features at three-dimensional power Doppler US for benign or malignant classification, *Radiology* 243:56–62, 2007.

Chevalier M, Moran P, Ten JI, et al: Patient dose in digital mammography, *Med Phys* 31:2471–2479, 2004.

Choplin RH, Boehme JM, Maynard CD: PACS mini refresher course: picture archiving and communication systems: an overview, *Radiographics* 12:127–129, 1992.

Clarke MP, Kane RA, Steele G, et al: Prospective comparison of preoperative imaging and intraoperative ultrasonography in the detection of liver tumors, *Surgery* 106:849–855, 1989.

Cowen AR, Workman A, Price JS: Physical aspects of photostimulable phosphor computed radiography, *Br J Radiol* 66:332–345, 1993.

Davis PC, Hudgins PA, Peterman SB, Hoffman Jr JC: Diagnosis of cerebral metastases: double-dose delayed CT vs. contrast-enhanced MR imaging, *Am J Neuroradiol* 12:293–300, 1991.

Diekmann F, Bick U: Tomosynthesis and contrast-enhanced digital mammography: recent advances in digital mammography, *Eur Radiol* 17(12):3086–3092, 2007.

Diller L, Medeiros Nancarrow C, Shaffer K, et al: Breast cancer screening in women previously treated for Hodgkin's disease: a prospective cohort study, *J Clin Oncol* 20:2085–2091, 2002.

Einstein AJ, Henzlova MJ, Rajagopalan S: Estimating risk of cancer associated with radiation exposure from 64-slice computed tomography coronary angiography, *JAMA* 298:317–323, 2007.

Eklund GW, Busby RC, Miller SH, Job JS: Improved imaging of the augmented breast, *Am J Roentgenol* 151:469–473, 1988.

Feig SA: Mammography equipment: principles, features, selection, *Radiol Clin North Am* 25:897–911, 1987.

Gofman JW, O'Connor E: *X-rays: health effects of common exams*, San Francisco, 1985, Sierra Club Books.

Haar GT, Coussios C: High intensity focused ultrasound: physical principles and devices, *Int J Hyperthermia* 23:89–104, 2007.

Hafron J, Kaouk JH: Ablative techniques for the management of kidney cancer, *Nat Clin Pract Urol* 4:261–269, 2007.

Harms SE, Flamig DP, HesleyKL, et al: Fat-suppressed three-dimensional MR imaging of the breast, *Radiographics* 13:247–267, 1993.

Hendrick RE, Haacke EM: Basic physics of MR contrast agents and maximization of image contrast, *J Magn Reson Imaging* 3:137–148, 1993.

Henschke CI, Yankelevitz DF, Altorki NK: The role of CT screening for lung cancer, *Thorac Surg Clin* 17:137–142, 2007.

Hillner BE, Siegel BA, Liu D, et al: Impact of positron emission tomography/computed tomography and positron emission tomography (PET) alone on expected management of patients with cancer: initial results from the national oncologic PET registry, *J Clin Oncol* 26:2155–2161, 2008.

Holland R, Hendricks JH, Mravunac M: Mammographically occult breast cancer: a pathologic and radiologic study, *Cancer* 52:1810–1819, 1983.

Holshouser BA, Hinshaw DB, Shellock FG: Sedation, anesthesia, and physiologic monitoring during MR imaging: evaluation of procedures and equipment, *J Magn Reson Imaging* 10:287–298, 1993.

Jackson VP: The role of US in breast imaging, *Radiology* 177:305–311, 1990.

Johnsrude IS, Silverman JF, Weaver MD, McConnal RW: Rapid cytology to decrease pneumothorax incidence after percutaneous biopsy. *Am J Roentgenol* 144:793–794, 1985.

Jolesz F, Blumenfeld S: Interventional use of magnetic resonance imaging, *Magn Reson Q* 10:85–96, 1994.

Kelly JF, Patterson R, Lieberman P, et al: Radiographic contrast media studies in high-risk patients, *J Allergy Clin Immunol* 62:181–184, 1978.

Khurana A, Runge VM, Narayanan M, et al: Nephrogenic systemic fibrosis: a review of six cases temporally related to gadodiamide injection (omniscan), *Invest Radiol* 42:139–145, 2007.

Kier R, Wain S, Troiano R: Fast spin-echo MR images of the pelvis obtained with a phased-array coil: value in localizing and staging prostatic carcinoma, *Am J Roentgenol* 161:601–606, 1993.

Knutson D, Steiner E: Screening for breast cancer: current recommendations and future directions. *Am Fam Physician* 75:1660–1666, 2007.

Krishna MC, Subramanian S, Kuppusamy P, Mitchell JB: Magnetic resonance imaging for in vivo assessment of tissue oxygen concentration, *Semin Radiat Oncol* 11:58–69, 2001.

Kuehl H, Velt P, Rosenbaum SJ, et al: Can PET/CT replace separate diagnostic CT for cancer imaging? Optimizing CT protocols for imaging cancers of the chest and abdomen, *J Nucl Med* 48(Suppl 1):45S–57S, 2007.

Kurumi Y, Tani T, Naka S, et al: MR-guided microwave ablation for malignancies, *Int J Clin Oncol* 12:85–93, 2007.

Liapi E, Geschwind JF: Transcatheter and ablative therapeutic approaches for solid malignancies, *J Clin Oncol* 25:978–986, 2007.

Marten K, Engelke C: Computer-aided detection and automated CT volumetry of pulmonary nodules, *Eur Radiol* 17:888–901, 2007.

Matsuoka T, Okuma T: CT-guided radiofrequency ablation for lung cancer, *Int J Clin Oncol* 12:71–78, 2007.

Nathanson SD, Burke M, Slater R, Kapke A: Preoperative identification of the sentinel lymph node in breast cancer, *Ann Surg Oncol* 14(11):3102–3110, 2007.

Negendank W, Soulen RL: Magnetic resonance imaging in patients with bone marrow disorders, *Leuk Lymphoma* 10:287–298, 1993.

Nishizawa S, Shinsuke K, Teramukai S, et al: Prospective evaluation of whole-body cancer screening with multiple modalities including [18F] fluorodeoxyglucose positron emission tomography in a healthy population: preliminary report, *J Clin Oncol* 27:1767–1773, 2009.

Partain CL, Patton JA: Magnetic resonance imaging systems. In Taveras JM, Ferrucci JT, editors: *Radiology: diagnosis-imaging-intervention*, vol X, Philadelphia, 1994, Lippincott, pp 33.

Pennes DR, Glazer GM, Wimbish KJ, et al: Chest wall invasion by lung cancer: limitations of CT evaluation, *Am J Roentgenol* 144:507–511, 1985.

Petersen RP, Harpole Jr DH: Computed tomography screening for the early detection of lung cancer, *J Natl Compr Canc Netw* 4:591–594, 2006.

Rothenberg LN, Pentlow KS: Radiation dose in CT, *Radiographics* 12:1225–1243, 1992.

Rouviere O, Souchon R, Salomir R, et al: Transrectal high-intensity focused ultrasound ablation of prostate cancer: effective treatment requiring accurate imaging, *Eur J Radiol* 63(3):317–327, 2007.

Rutten A, Prokop M: Contrast agents in x-ray computed tomography and its applications in oncology, *Anticancer Agents Med Chem* 7:307–316, 2007.

Schnall MD, Imai Y, Tomaszewski J, et al: Prostate cancer: local staging with endorectal surface coil MR imaging, *Radiology* 178:797–802, 1991.

Silverman PM: Liver metastases: imaging considerations for protocol development with multlislice CT (MSCT), *Cancer Imaging* 6:175–181, 2006.

Singletary SE: Multidisciplinary frontiers in breast cancer management: a surgeon's perspective, *Cancer* 109:1019–1029, 2007.

Smart CR: Mammographic screening: efficacy and guidelines, *Curr Opin Radiol* 4:108–117, 1992.

Smith RC, McCarthy S: Physics of magnetic resonance, *J Reprod Med* 37:19–26, 1992.

Sone S, Li F, Yang ZG, et al: Results of three-year mass screening programme for lung cancer using mobile low-dose spiral computed tomography scanner, *Br J Cancer* 84:25–32, 2001.

Stanford W, Galvin JR, Weiss RM, et al: Ultrafast computed tomography in cardiac imaging: a review, *Semin Ultrasound CT MR* 12:45–60, 1991.

Stewart EA, Gostout B, Rabinovici J, et al: Sustained relief of leiomyoma symptoms by using focused ultrasound surgery, *Obstet Gynecol* 110(2 Pt 1):279–287, 2007.

Stomper PC: *Cancer imaging manual*, Philadelphia, 1993, Lippincott.

Stomper PC, Fung CY, Socinski MA, et al: Detection of retroperitoneal metastases in early-stage nonseminomatous testicular cancer: analysis of different CT criteria, *Am J Roentgenol* 149:1187–1190, 1987.

Strijkers GJ, Mulder WJ, van Tilborg GA, Nicolay K: MRI contrast agents: current status and future perspectives, *Anticancer Agents Med Chem* 7:291–305, 2007.

Swensen SJ, Aughenbaugh GL, Douglas WE, Myers JL: High-resolution CT of the lungs: findings in various pulmonary diseases, *Am J Roentgenol* 158:971–979, 1992.

Tanenbaum LN: Clinical 3T MR imaging: mastering the challenges, *Magn Reson Imaging Clin North Am* 14:1–15, 2006.

Thanos L, Mylona S, Nikita A, et al: Long-term outcome of a hepatocellular carcinoma 7 1/2 years after surgery and repeated radiofrequency ablation: case report and review of the literature, *Cardiovasc Intervent Radiol* 30:289–292, 2007.

Torigian DA, Huang SS, Houseni M, Alavi A: Functional imaging of cancer with emphasis on molecular techniques, *CA Cancer J Clin* 57:206–224, 2007.

Ueda T, Mori K, Minami M, et al: Trends in oncological CT imaging: clinical application of multi-detector-row CT and 3D-CT imaging, *Int J Clin Oncol* 11:268–277, 2006.

Vanel D, Stark D, editors: *Imaging strategies in oncology*, New York, 1993, John Wiley.

Vossen JA, Butjs M, Kamel IR: Assessment of tumor response on MR imaging after locoregional therapy, *Tech Vasc Interv Radiol* 9:125–132, 2006.

Wagner LK: Absorbed dose in imaging: why measure it? *Radiology* 178:622–623, 1991.

Wilson R: Analyzing the daily risks of life, *Technol Rev* 81:41–46, 1979.

Wittenberg J, Mueller PR, Ferrucci JT, et al: Percutaneous core biopsy of abdominal tumors using 22 gauge needles: further observations, *Am J Roentgenol* 139:75–80, 1982.

Wong TZ, Paulson EK, Nelson RC, et al: Practical approach to diagnostic CT combined with PET, *Am J Roentgenol* 188:622–629, 2007.

Woolfenden JM, Pitt MJ, Burie BGM, Moon TE: Comparison of bone scintigraphy and radiography in multiple myeloma, *Radiology* 134:723–728, 1980.

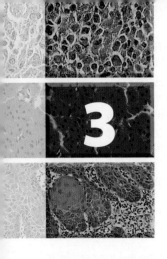

3

Nuclear Medicine in Oncology

STEVEN BURRELL • ANNICK D. VAN DEN ABBEELE

Nuclear medicine has long played a significant role in cancer imaging, and the recent widespread clinical applications of positron emission tomography (PET) have further increased its importance. As the prototype of molecular imaging, nuclear medicine interrogates metabolic and physiologic processes, rather than anatomy, and provides important in vivo information regarding tumor metabolism. Molecular imaging with nuclear medicine can now be performed on hybrid systems that combine a nuclear medicine device such as a PET scanner or a SPECT (single photon emission computed tomography) scanner with a computed tomography (CT) scanner, providing unique functional and anatomic information in one setting and a very complementary assessment of tumor status. As outlined in Table 3.1, nuclear medicine has proven effective in oncology in a number of roles spanning the course of the disease, including the characterization of a mass, staging, restaging, monitoring of therapeutic response, follow-up, various therapeutic applications, and the monitoring of toxicity to nontarget organs.

Nuclear medicine studies are based on imaging the distribution of radioactive tracers, known as radiopharmaceuticals. Radiopharmaceuticals possess two general properties. First, they have some desired physiologic or pathophysiologic property, such as their ability to target tumor cells. Second, they contain a radioactive component (a radioisotope) that emits energy that can be captured by an imaging device such as a gamma camera or a PET camera. These emissions can be transformed into images that visualize the in vivo distribution of the radiopharmaceutical. Usually these two properties are conferred by two different components of the radiopharmaceutical. With the common bone scanning agent technetium-99m–methylene diphosphonate (^{99m}Tc-MDP) for example, the physiologic property is provided by MDP, which is incorporated into areas of osteogenesis, a physiologic response to tumor invasion, whereas the radioactive component is provided by the radioisotope ^{99m}Tc, which has a half-life of 6.03 hours and emits imaging-amenable gamma photons at an energy of 140 keV. Sometimes both properties are provided by the same component, for example iodine-131 (^{131}I), administered as sodium iodide (NaI). Iodine-131 possesses the desired physiologic property of being incorporated into well-differentiated thyroid cancer cells, and it emits gamma photons (365 keV) that allow for in vivo imaging, as well as beta particles (maximum 606 keV) that allow systemic radiation therapy to be performed. Table 3.2 summarizes some common radiopharmaceuticals used in oncologic applications. Nuclear medicine images may be acquired with gamma-emitting radiotracers on stationary cameras, resulting in a 2D planar image, or on cameras slowly rotating around the patient, resulting in 3D tomographic data sets, a form of acquisition known as SPECT. Whereas the planar nuclear medicine image is analogous to the familiar x-ray radiograph, SPECT is analogous to x-ray CT. In PET, the process is different. The radioactive decay of PET radiotracers does not directly yield imaging-amenable photons, but rather the emission of a positively charged subnuclear particle, a positron. The positron collides with a nearby electron, resulting in the annihilation of both particles and the emission of two 511-KeV photons at 180 degrees to one another. It is these photons that are detected by the PET scanner. PET scanners typically consist of stationary rings of small detector elements arranged in a cylindrical geometry around the patient, simultaneously detecting the photons emitted in all directions, yielding a 3D data set of the distribution of the radiopharmaceutical throughout the patient.

Table 3.1	
Roles of Nuclear Medicine in Oncology	
Roles	**Examples**
Diagnosis	FDG-PET in evaluation of solitary pulmonary nodule
	MIBG in suspected neuroblastoma
Staging and restaging	Sentinel node
	Bone scan
	FDG-PET
	Gallium-67
Assessment of therapeutic response	FDG-PET
	Gallium-67
Surveillance	Bone scan
	FDG-PET
Therapy	Iodine-131 for thyroid cancer
	Radiolabeled monoclonal antibodies for lymphoma
	Alleviation of pain in patients with skeletal metastases
Monitoring of non–target organ toxicity	Wall motion study to monitor chemotherapy-induced cardiotoxicity

FDG-PET, 2-deoxy-2-[^{18}F]fluoro-D-glucose–positron emission tomography; MIBG, m-iodobenzylguanidine.

Table 3.2

Some Single-Photon (non-PET) Radiopharmaceuticals Used in Cancer Imaging

Radioisotope	Half-Life	Energy (keV)	Radiopharmaceutical	Clinical Applications
Technetium-99m	6.03 hr	140	^{99m}Tc-MDP ^{99m}Tc-sulfur colloid	Bone scan Sentinel node
Iodine-131	8.06 days	364	^{131}I ^{131}I-MIBG	Thyroid cancer scan and therapy Neuroendocrine tumor imaging and therapy
Iodine-123	13.0 hr	159	^{123}I ^{123}I-MIBG	Thyroid cancer scan Neuroendocrine tumor imaging
Gallium-67	78.1 hr	93, 184, 296	^{67}Ga citrate	Lymphoma
Indium-111	67 hr	172, 247	^{111}In-pentetreotide	Neuroendocrine tumor imaging

MDP, methylene diphosphonate; MIBG, *m*-iodobenzylguanidine.

Bone Scan

The whole-body bone scan is one of the most commonly performed nuclear medicine cancer imaging procedures. It has been established as a sensitive technique for diagnosing and monitoring osseous metastases. Although a variety of radiopharmaceuticals have been used for bone scanning, the vast majority are performed today using a diphosphonate such as methylene diphosphonate labeled with ^{99m}Tc (^{99m}Tc-MDP). These agents are incorporated into bone undergoing osteogenesis, which, in the setting of a focal osseous insult such as neoplasm, fracture, or osteomyelitis, is usually substantially increased.

Typically, osseous metastases begin in the axial skeleton, a reflection of the preferential blood flow and predominance of red marrow, a favorable site of hematogenous metastases. Metastases are generally random in distribution and configuration (Fig. 3.1). As the disease progresses, metastatic involvement expands to the appendicular skeleton and discrete lesions yield to a confluence of metastases. Occasionally an atypical distribution is seen with metastases primarily occurring in the appendicular skeleton (Fig. 3.2A to C). This initial spread to the distal skeleton is more commonly seen in the setting of primary tumors such as lung, breast, and renal cell carcinomas.

Another atypical pattern is the solitary metastasis. Only 50% of solitary lesions are metastases, even in patients with known malignancy. An area of particular interest is the sternum in patients with breast cancer. Mild to moderate uptake in the sternomanubrial joint is a common variant. However, uptake that is intense or asymmetrical should be considered suspicious and correlated with CT (Fig. 3.3A, B). Some of these sternal lesions may derive from a lymph node metastasis within the internal mammary lymph node chain or from soft tissue recurrence and subsequent bone invasion.

As defined radiographically, metastases may be lytic, sclerotic, or mixed. Purely sclerotic lesions are less common and typically occur in metastases from prostate cancer, some breast cancers, and carcinoid tumors. Regardless, most metastases are evident on bone scanning. Even lytic lesions, which result primarily in bone destruction, lead to bone repair and osteogenesis, resulting in some increased uptake on the bone scan (Fig. 3.4A, B). Cases of lytic metastases causing purely "cold" lesions on bone scans are rare and are most frequently seen in multiple myeloma.

With disease progression, osseous metastases become much more numerous and more confluent. This results in increased uptake within innumerable metastases, so that the presence of individual lesions becomes less obvious. This markedly increased uptake of radiopharmaceutical in the skeleton leads to decreased uptake within other organs, including urinary collecting systems and peripheral soft tissues. This pattern has been described as a "superscan." Paradoxically, because there are fewer discrete lesions (Fig. 3.5A to E), this pattern of disease progression may incorrectly be perceived as improvement. A clue to the presence of a superscan is the relatively reduced uptake in the kidneys and soft tissues. Correlation with prior bone scans can be very helpful.

Metastases often involve the ribs. However, rib fractures are common and can be mistaken for metastases. Punctate uptake in several ribs in a linear distribution is highly suggestive of fractures, particularly in the absence of other suspicious lesions, and the clinical history may confirm a recent fall. Appearances suggestive of metastases include random distribution and elongated foci. An exception is in the setting of lung cancer, where direct invasion of contiguous ribs overlying the tumor can result in uptake within adjacent ribs in the absence of distal metastases (Fig. 3.6A, B). Again, correlation with the clinical history and other radiographic studies is important in evaluating any finding on bone scan.

In addition to its value in staging, the bone scan is used to follow response to therapy and for long-term surveillance. A reduction in the number and/or in the intensity of uptake of the tracer in known lesions implies improvement, while an increase in the intensity of uptake and/or in the number of lesions generally indicates progression. However, soon after hormonal therapy or chemotherapy, a successful tumor response may paradoxically appear as a worsening bone scan with more intense uptake seen in known lesions and new lesions, a phenomenon known as "flare." This occurs because the bone scan does not directly image tumor viability but instead the osseous response to the tumor. In the setting of bone healing, an osteoblastic reaction will appear as an area of increased uptake of the tracer. New lesions may be appreciated in the context of flare, because they were previously small and/or lytic but become more prominent in the context of bone healing. It may be challenging to differentiate the flare phenomenon from true progression strictly based on the bone scan, but the clinical history and timing of the new therapy relative to that of the bone scan may help raise this possibility, particularly when the patient is in no pain and other tumor markers are decreasing. A repeat bone scan a couple of months later will confirm the healing with subsequent decrease in the intensity of tracer uptake and in the number of lesions. Additional radiologic features that may favor flare are transition of formerly lytic lesions to a   sclerotic appearance on plain radiographs or CT, and reduction in the size of other nonosseous (soft tissue) metastases.

An interesting bone scan finding in the setting of malignancy is seen in the case of hypertrophic osteoarthropathy. This systemic phenomenon results in increased uptake in the cortices of the long bones, i.e., the "tram track" appearance (Fig. 3.7A, B). This results from the production of humoral factors and does not represent local neoplastic involvement.

Although the main use of the bone scan in oncology is in the evaluation of metastases from nonosseous tumors, it is also useful in the staging of primary bone malignancies (Fig. 3.8A, B). The bone scan is of limited utility in the assessment of the likelihood of malignancy in the primary lesion, because the degree of uptake on the bone scan is not necessarily indicative of aggressiveness. In this setting the extent of local primary tumor involvement is better assessed with magnetic resonance imaging (MRI).

Finally, it should be noted that focal uptake on a bone scan is not necessarily indicative of metastases. Common mimics include focal uptake at the site of osteomyelitis, degenerative/arthritic changes, fractures, and Paget's disease (Fig. 3.9). Recognition of common patterns substantially increases specificity, and correlation with clinical history and anatomic imaging can be diagnostic.

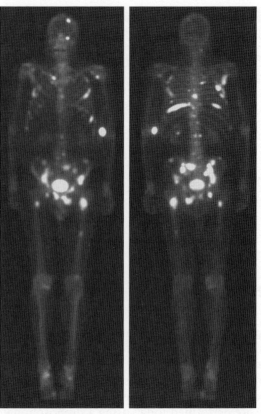

FIGURE 3.1 TYPICAL METASTATIC PATTERN. Anterior and posterior whole-body views of a bone scan in a patient with prostate cancer demonstrating numerous foci of abnormal increased uptake with random distribution and morphology, predominantly confined to the axial skeleton. The focus seen in the left antecubital fossa is related to infiltration at the injection site.

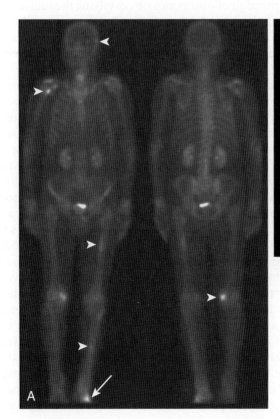

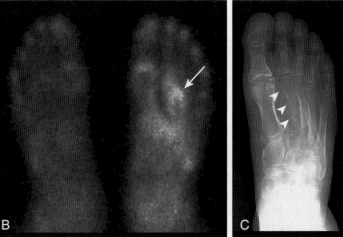

FIGURE 3.2 ATYPICAL PATTERN OF DISTAL OSSEOUS METASTASES. (A) Anterior and posterior whole-body views of a bone scan in a patient with non–small cell lung cancer demonstrating multiple peripheral metastases (*arrowheads*). **(B)** Spot views of the feet demonstrate metastases within the shafts of the left second and third metatarsals. A focal more intense focus (*arrow*) probably represents a superimposed pathologic fracture. **(C)** These lesions correlate with destructive lesions on the correlative radiograph (*arrowheads*), indicative of acral metastases.

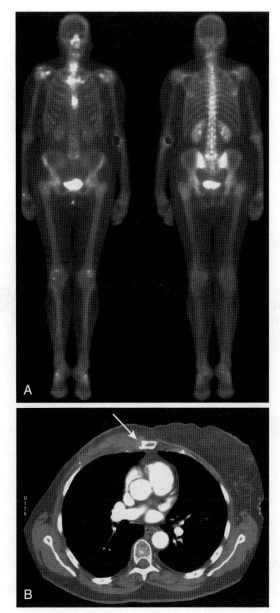

FIGURE 3.3 SOLITARY METASTASIS. (A) Anterior and posterior whole-body views of a bone scan revealing a focus of uptake in the right border of the sternum in a patient with breast cancer. **(B)** CT scan reveals that there has been a previous right mastectomy. There is now a recurrent soft tissue mass, with direct invasion of the sternum (*arrow*), resulting in the uptake on the bone scan.

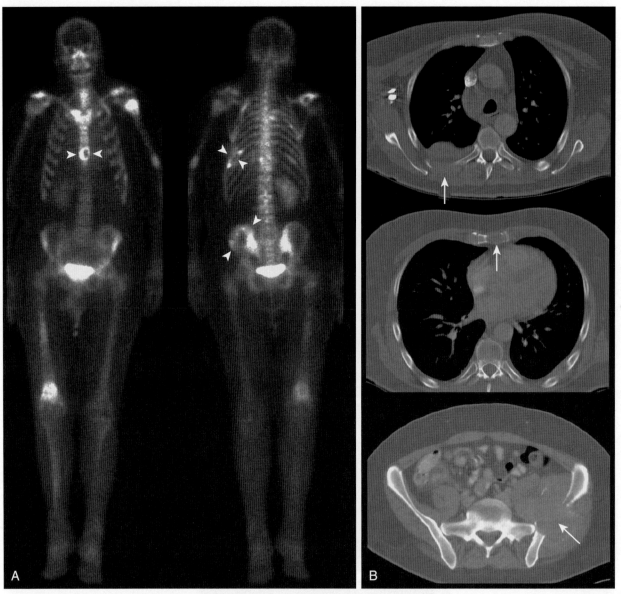

FIGURE 3.4 **LYTIC METASTASES.** **(A)** Anterior and posterior whole-body views of a bone scan in a patient with renal cell carcinoma revealing several metastases with a pattern of expansion and increased uptake surrounding a photopenic center (*arrowheads*) within the left eighth rib, the sternum, and the left iliac bone. There are also several more typical metastases showing focal increased uptake in the long bones and rib cage bilaterally. **(B)** CT confirms expansile destructive lesions in these locations (*arrows*). Note that even purely lytic lesions on radiographs tend to demonstrate some increased uptake on bone scans.

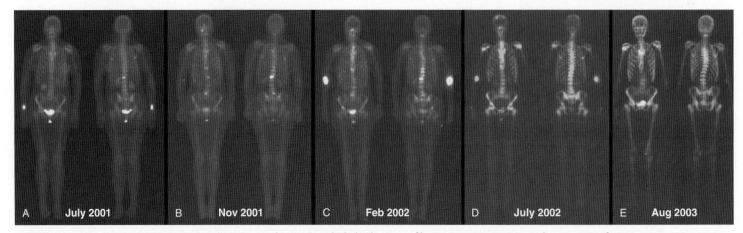

FIGURE 3.5 **EVOLUTION OF A SUPERSCAN.** Serial anterior and posterior whole-body views of bone scans in a patient with metastases from prostate cancer. Initially in July 2001 **(A)** there is limited metastatic disease, with abnormal uptake seen in L1 and L5 (the focus seen in the midline below the pelvis is related to urinary contamination, and the focus in the right wrist is related to the injection site). Over the next two time points in November 2001 and February 2002 **(B, C)** there is an increase in the number of metastatic lesions throughout the axial skeleton. By the fourth time point in July 2002 **(D)** the metastases have become confluent, though still predominantly confined to the axial skeleton. Uptake in the kidneys and other soft tissues has decreased because of the intense osseous uptake. Finally, in August 2003 **(E)** there is quite confluent intense uptake throughout much of the skeleton, with very little renal or soft tissue uptake, consistent with widespread skeletal and marrow involvement throughout the entire skeleton.

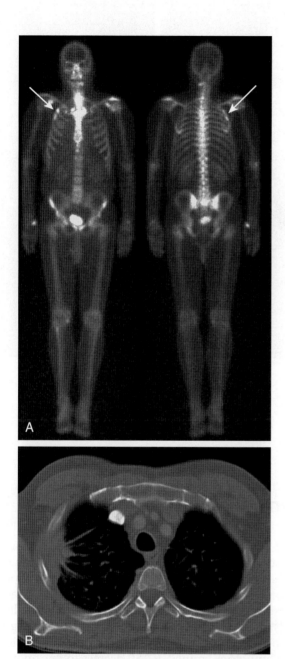

FIGURE 3.6   **CONTIGUOUS RIB ABNORMALITIES NOT DUE TO FRACTURES. (A)** Anterior and posterior whole-body views of a bone scan revealing foci of abnormal increased uptake in the right second and third ribs in a patient with lung cancer. **(B)** CT scan confirms that this is related to direct invasion of these ribs by the primary lung cancer.

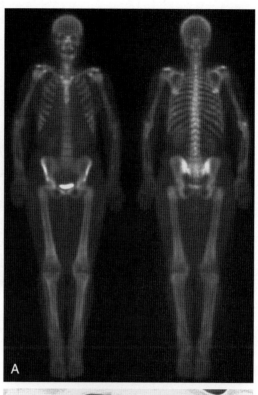

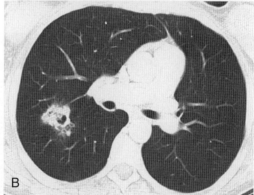

FIGURE 3.7   **HYPERTROPHIC OSTEOARTHROPATHY. (A)** Anterior and posterior whole-body views of a bone scan demonstrating homogeneous uptake along the cortices of the long bones, consistent with hypertrophic osteoarthropathy. **(B)** CT scan reveals that this patient has a cavitated lung cancer.

FIGURE 3.8 OSTEOSARCOMA. (A) Anterior and posterior whole-body views of a bone scan of a patient with a history of osteosarcoma demonstrating intense uptake throughout the primary lesion in the left femur, as well as metastases to the adjacent tibial plateau and pubic bone, and distal metastases to the left iliac bone and right glenoid. **(B)** Correlative radiograph of the distal left femur and proximal tibia demonstrates extensive sclerotic lesions and periosteal reaction.

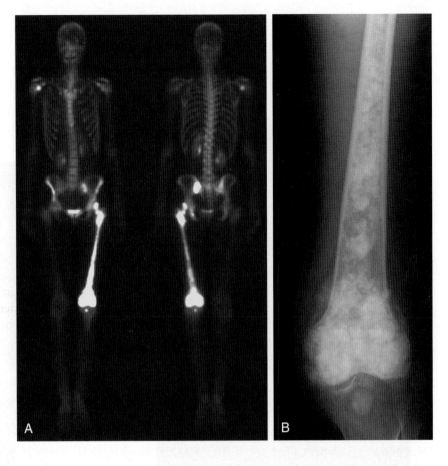

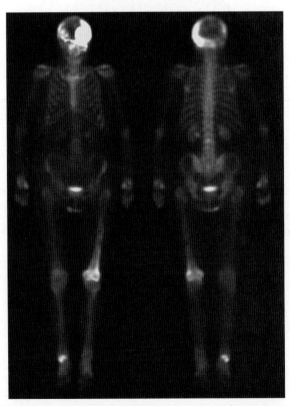

FIGURE 3.9 LESIONS SIMULATING METASTASES. Anterior and posterior whole-body views of a bone scan demonstrating multiple areas of intense uptake throughout the skull and along the left femur mimicking metastatic disease. These areas of uptake are actually due to Paget's disease.

Positron Emission Tomography

Initially used as a research tool, PET has definitely transitioned to widespread clinical use in oncology and indeed has now become the standard of care in many oncologic applications. PET radioisotopes decay by emission of a positron (β$^+$ particle). The positron travels a short distance (0.22 mm for fluorine-18 [^{18}F]) and then interacts with an electron, resulting in the annihilation of both particles and the release of two high-energy gamma photons emitted at 180 degrees to one another that are captured by a PET scanner. The imaging of these annihilation photons results in better sensitivity, spatial resolution, and quality of the images compared with standard gamma camera–based nuclear medicine techniques. In addition, the use of positron-emitting isotopes has yielded an expanded repertoire of imaging radiopharmaceuticals, including the glucose analog 2-deoxy-2-[^{18}F]fluoro-D-glucose (^{18}F-FDG), by far the most widely used PET radiopharmaceutical. Malignant tumors have an increased rate of aerobic glycolysis compared with normal tissues, and ^{18}F-FDG is taken up into tumor cells due to increased glucose transporters such as GLUT-1, increased hexokinase, and decreased glucose-6-phosphatase, resulting in the retention of ^{18}F-FDG in many tumor types. The rate of uptake of ^{18}F-FDG by tumor cells is proportional to their metabolic activity.

Although ^{18}F-FDG is the predominant PET radiopharmaceutical, other ^{18}F-labeled tracers are or could be available soon. These include ^{18}F-fluoride for imaging skeletal metastases, ^{18}F-choline to image prostate cancer, ^{18}F-fluorothymidine to measure cell proliferation, ^{18}F-DOPA for imaging of primary and metastatic neuroendocrine tumors as well as low-grade brain tumors, ^{18}F-fluoroimidazole to assess tumor hypoxia, and others (Table 3.3). Of note, other positron-emitting radionuclides such as oxygen-15, nitrogen-13, and carbon-11 can also be used for PET imaging. However, their short half-lives (20 minutes or less) require an on-site cyclotron facility. With its half-life of approximately 110 minutes, ^{18}F can be produced in off-site cyclotron facilities and easily distributed to imaging centers located within a few hours of traveling distance from the cyclotron facility. The recent production of hybrid scanners combining multislice CT scanners with PET devices, which allow acquisition and display of anatomic and physiologic images in one setting, has further enhanced and expanded the utility of PET imaging.

The application of ^{18}F-FDG and PET (FDG-PET) to the management of oncology patients has resulted in an overall change in patient management in 30% of patients across all cancers. The Centers for Medicaid and Medicare Services (CMS) have recognized the utility of FDG-PET in the management of patients with cancer and have approved reimbursement for the initial and subsequent treatment strategies of patients with many malignancies, including lymphomas; non–small cell lung, esophageal, colorectal, breast, ovary, cervical, head and neck, and thyroid cancers; melanoma; and multiple myeloma; and for the characterization of solitary pulmonary nodules (SPNs). CMS is also supporting other indications under a Coverage with Evidence Development program (CED). Cancer imaging with FDG-PET is now one of the most dynamic and rapidly growing areas of contemporary clinical imaging.

A major application of FDG-PET is in lung cancer, including the evaluation of SPNs (Fig. 3.10A, B). In distinguishing benign from malignant SPNs, PET has shown 96.8% sensitivity, generally obviating the need for biopsy, and is considered a cost-saving as well as cost-effective method for the characterization of indeterminate pulmonary nodules, resulting in a decrease in the number of unnecessary biopsies. The negative predictive value of FDG-PET in the SPN evaluation is much higher (greater than 95%) than its positive predictive value, as ^{18}F-FDG uptake is also seen in a variety of inflammatory and infectious conditions resulting in a lower specificity (77.8%). Therefore, ^{18}F-FDG uptake in a SPN does require further workup. Another application of FDG-PET in lung cancer is staging. With respect to locoregional staging, FDG-PET has proven

more accurate than CT in staging the mediastinum (Fig. 3.11A to C). This modality is also very helpful in assessing distant metastases because of its whole-body imaging capability. This whole-body imaging capability in one setting is a theme that carries across many cancer types.

Another major application of FDG-PET is in lymphoma. FDG-PET is particularly helpful in staging, monitoring of response to therapy, and follow-up of patients with Hodgkin disease and aggressive non-Hodgkin lymphomas (Fig. 3.12). Following therapy, it is not uncommon for lymphomatous masses to persist on anatomic imaging (CT). FDG-PET is a reliable method for distinguishing viable from nonviable residual tumor.

In breast cancer, FDG-PET is generally not indicated for primary tumor diagnosis or locoregional staging; mammography with or without ultrasound and/or MRI, and sentinel node lymphoscintigraphy remain the standards of care, respectively, in most circumstances. However, FDG-PET is very useful in staging distant metastases (Fig. 3.13A to C), restaging at the end of treatment, or in the context of increased tumor markers, and is approved by the CMS for the monitoring of response to therapy.

In head and neck cancers, FDG-PET is used in a number of applications. The majority of these cancers are squamous cell carcinomas, which tend to be very FDG-avid. FDG-PET is used for primary tumor localization in the setting of a metastasis of unknown primary. As with other malignancies, FDG-PET is also very helpful in staging, assessing response to therapy, and monitoring for recurrence (Fig. 3.14A, B).

FDG-PET has proven efficacious in a variety of gastrointestinal malignancies, including gastric, esophageal (Fig. 3.15A to C), colorectal, hepatocellular, and pancreatic carcinomas, as well as gastrointestinal stromal tumors (GISTs). Particularly dramatic therapeutic responses can be seen early within hours or days on FDG-PET following therapy of GIST tumors with tyrosine kinase inhibitors, although no significant changes in the size of these tumors are seen on CT (Fig. 3.16A to D). These observations are leading to several national and international efforts focusing on reassessing the traditional criteria used to define response to therapy in patients treated with molecularly targeted therapy, because metabolic changes within tumor masses do precede significant anatomic changes in patients responding to the treatment.

PET is not routinely used in thyroid cancer. Most thyroid cancers are well differentiated, retaining the ability to concentrate

Table 3.3				
Some PET Radiopharmaceuticals Used in Oncology Imaging				
Radioisotope	Half-Life (min)	Energy (keV)	Radiopharmaceutical	Tumor or Function Assessed
Fluorine-18	109	511	^{18}F-fluoride	Bone
			^{18}F-FDG	Glucose metabolism
			^{18}F-choline	Prostate cancer
			^{18}F-DOPA	Neuroendocrine and brain tumors
			^{18}F-fluorothymidine	Cell proliferation
			^{18}F-fluoromisonidazole	Hypoxia
Carbon-11	20.3	511	^{11}C-methionine	Protein synthesis
			^{11}C-choline	Cell membrane metabolism
Oxygen-15	2	511	$H_2{}^{15}O$	Blood flow
Nitrogen-13	9.97	511	^{13}N-ammonia	Regional blood flow
			^{13}N-L-glutamate	Osteogenic sarcoma

DOPA, 3,4-dihydroxyphenylalanine; FDG, 2-deoxy-2-[^{18}F] fluoro-D-glucose.

Table 3.4

Some Radiopharmaceuticals Used in Oncology Therapy

Radioisotope	Half-Life	Energy*	Radiopharmaceutical	Applications
Iodine-131	8.06 days	0.61	131I	Thyroid cancer
			131I-MIBG	Neuroendocrine tumors
			131I-tositumomab	Lymphoma
Yttrium-90	64 hr	2.3	90Y-ibritumomab	Lymphoma
Strontium-89	50.5 days	1.4	89Sr	Bone metastases
Samarium-153	46.3 hr	0.81	153Sm-EDTMP	Bone metastases

*Energy refers to maximum energy of beta particle in units of MeV.
EDTMP, ethylene diamine tetramethylene phosphonate; MIBG, *m*-iodobenzylguanidine.

iodine, and yet exhibiting low ^{18}F-FDG uptake, and thus most patients are well served with standard radioiodine imaging, as discussed in the following section. However, some thyroid cancers are not iodine-avid; these tend to be less differentiated and more aggressive, and as such exhibit higher ^{18}F-FDG uptake, rendering PET effective in the setting of iodine-negative thyroid cancer (Fig. 3.17A, B).

Despite relatively high ^{18}F-FDG uptake in the normal brain, a reflection of natural high glucose use, FDG-PET is useful in assessing brain tumors because many tumors will exhibit uptake greater than the surrounding normal parenchyma. Initial assess-

ment for the presence of a primary or metastatic brain tumor is still best performed with MRI. However, once a lesion is known, PET has shown utility in determining tumor grade when biopsy is difficult, in determining response to therapy, and in particular in differentiating tumor necrosis from recurrence, because MRI may show nonspecific contrast enhancement, which can reflect either tumor recurrence or simply inflammation (Fig. 3.18). Though less widely available, other PET radiopharmaceuticals such as ^{11}C-methionine might become very useful in the context of brain tumors because of its low uptake in normal brain tissue, yielding higher tumor-to-background ratios.

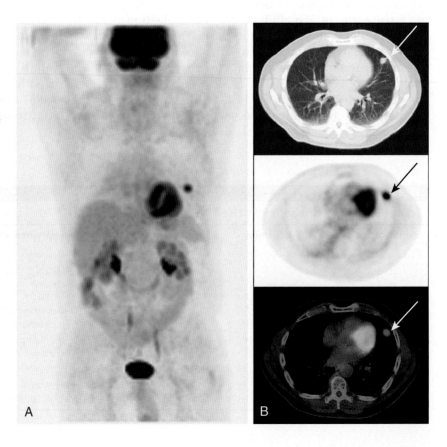

FIGURE 3.10 **SOLITARY PULMONARY NODULE ON FDG-PET.**
(A) Whole-body maximal intensity projection (MIP) image demonstrating a focus of intense FDG uptake within the left lung just lateral to the heart. There is otherwise normal physiologic uptake of FDG in the brain, myocardium, urinary collecting system, liver, spleen, and bowel. Transaxial slices from **(B)** CT (*top*), PET (*middle*), and fused PET/CT (*bottom*) show that the intense uptake is within a pulmonary nodule (*arrows*), highly suggestive of malignancy and confirmed by biopsy.

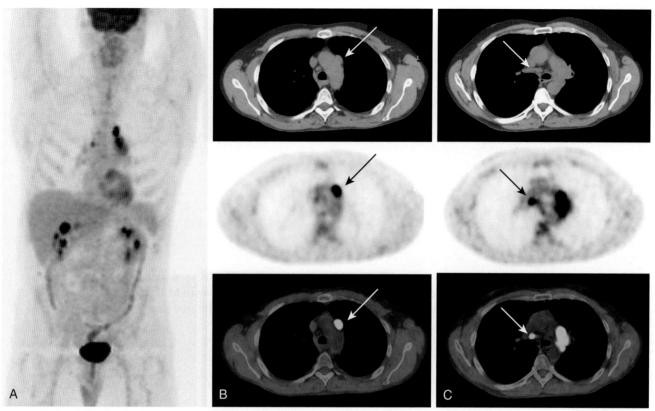

FIGURE 3.11 LUNG CANCER STAGING WITH FDG-PET. (A) Whole-body MIP image demonstrating contiguous foci of intense FDG uptake in the left hilum and mediastinum and a small focus in the right hilum. There is otherwise normal physiologic uptake of FDG in the brain, myocardium, urinary collecting system, genitals, liver, spleen, and bowel. **(B)** Transaxial CT, PET, and fused PET/CT slices depicting the uptake in one of the left-sided lymph nodes (*arrows*) in the prevascular region. **(C)** Transaxial CT, PET, and fused PET/CT slices depicting intense uptake in a small lymph node (*arrows*) in the right hilum. This subcentimeter node would not have been considered positive by standard CT criteria.

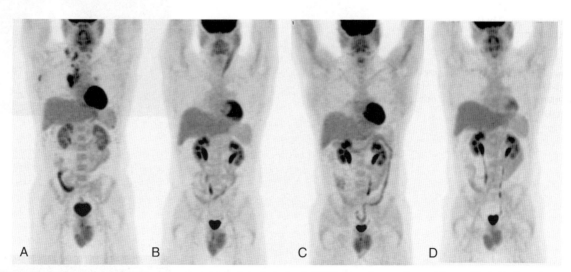

FIGURE 3.12 THERAPY MONITORING IN LYMPHOMA WITH FDG-PET. Serial whole-body MIP images in a patient with non-Hodgkin lymphoma at staging **(A)** revealing pathologic FDG uptake within lymph nodes in the supraclavicular regions, mediastinum, and right axilla. FDG-PET performed after three cycles of chemotherapy **(B)** shows complete resolution of the abnormal uptake. The linear uptake seen in the left neck is consistent with physiologic uptake within muscle. The remainder of FDG biodistribution is physiologic. Restaging at the end of treatment after six cycles of chemotherapy **(C)** shows normal biodistribution of the tracer that persists in the follow-up scan 20 months after diagnosis **(D)**. All scans are performed following a 4- to 6-hour fasting period, but myocardial uptake can vary over time.

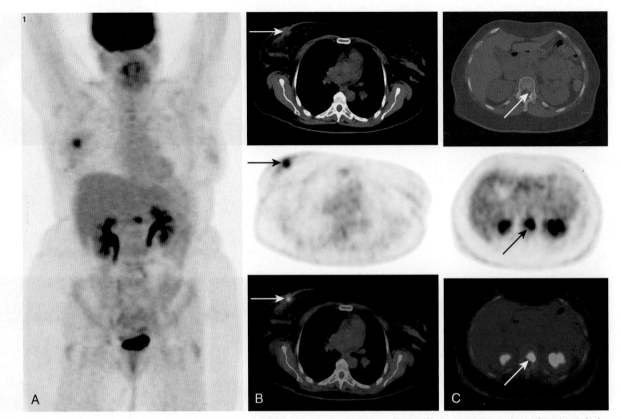

FIGURE 3.13 **BREAST CANCER STAGING WITH FDG-PET. (A)** Whole-body MIP image demonstrating a focus of intense FDG uptake within the right breast, as well as an intense focus projecting between the kidneys. **(B)** Transaxial CT, PET, and fused PET/CT slices confirm the uptake in a right breast mass (*arrows*), the primary malignancy. **(C)** Transaxial CT, PET, and fused PET/CT slices demonstrate that the second focus of uptake is within the T12 vertebral body, extending into the left pedicle (*arrows*), upstaging the patient to stage 4 disease. On the CT scan only a subtle area of lucency is appreciated.

FIGURE 3.14 **RECURRENCE OF HEAD AND NECK CANCER ON FDG-PET. (A)** Whole-body MIP image revealing a small but intense focus of uptake in the lower right neck, lateral to the physiologic uptake seen in the laryngeal muscles, confirming recurrence of this patient's head and neck cancer. **(B)** Transaxial CT, PET, and fused PET/CT slices confirm that the uptake is within a small nodule (*cursors*).

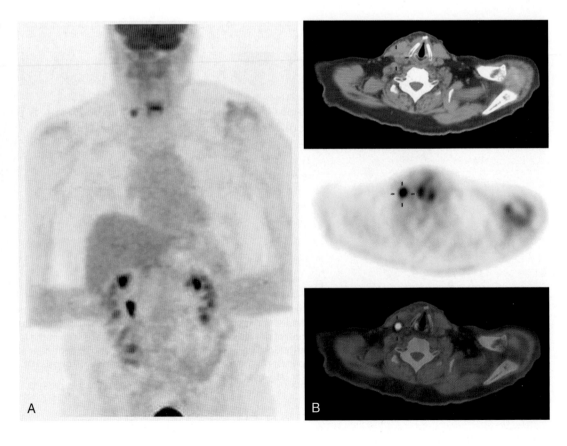

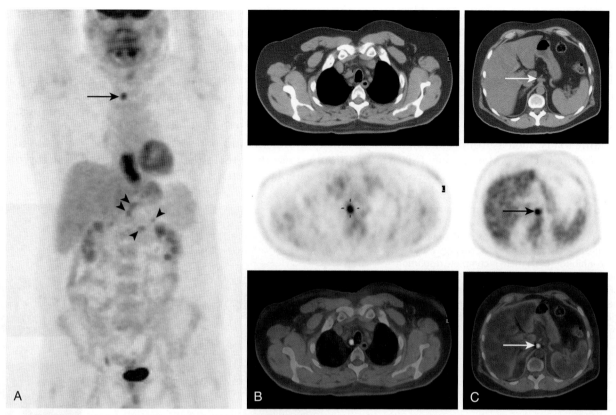

FIGURE 3.15 STAGING IN ESOPHAGEAL CANCER WITH FDG-PET. (A) Whole-body MIP image demonstrating intense uptake throughout the distal esophagus, the primary malignancy. There is also evidence of metastatic FDG-avid lymphadenopathy in a solitary upper paratracheal lymph node (*arrow*) and several celiac axis nodes (*arrowheads*), projecting between the physiologic renal uptake. Transaxial CT, PET, and fused PET/CT slices confirm the abnormal FDG uptake in **(B)** a small upper paratracheal node (*cursors*) and **(C)** one of the celiac axis nodes (*arrows*).

Thyroid Cancer

Evaluation of the thyroid was the first clinical application of nuclear medicine. In 1928 Hertz, Roberts, and Evans measured thyroid uptake in animals using ^{128}I. In 1931, thyroid cancer metastases were assessed with ^{130}I, and the first radioisotope therapy was performed in 1942 using ^{130}I. Today nuclear medicine remains a mainstay of thyroid cancer management, with applications in diagnosis, therapy, and surveillance.

With respect to diagnosis, the nuclear medicine thyroid scan may be used in the assessment of a thyroid nodule discovered clinically or incidentally on ultrasound or CT (Fig. 3.19). In today's practice the thyroid scan is performed using either ^{123}I, which is trapped and organified by the thyroid, or ^{99m}Tc-pertechnetate, which is trapped but not organified. A pinhole collimator is used to enhance spatial resolution. The premise of the scan is that thyroid cancers are less efficient at taking up ^{123}I or ^{99m}Tc-pertechnetate than normal thyroid tissue, so that thyroid cancers show up as a cold nodule on the scan (Fig. 3.19A to C). Overall, 10% to 20% of cold nodules will be malignant, and hence a fine-needle aspiration (FNA) or biopsy is indicated. Conversely, less than 1% of all hot nodules (Fig. 3.20) will be malignant, so further workup is usually not indicated. Nodules isointense to the remainder of the thyroid, so-called warm nodules, pose an intermediate (less than 10%) likelihood of malignancy, and so, as with the cold nodule, further evaluation is indicated. In clinical practice, nuclear medicine scanning is of limited utility in the routine evaluation of thyroid nodules, because the majority (80% to 85%) of nodules will be cold and require further evaluation anyway. Still, the thyroid scan is recommended in the evaluation of a nodule larger than 1–1.5 cm

if the thyroid-stimulating hormone (TSH) concentration is suppressed (because of the greater likelihood of a hot nodule), if a previous FNA or biopsy was indeterminate, or in the setting of a multinodular goiter to assess which nodule(s) should be sampled with FNA or biopsy.

Most thyroid cancers are well differentiated and retain several attributes of the normal thyroid, including the ability to concentrate iodine through the NaI symporter. Although the degree of uptake is less than the normal thyroid, it is usually sufficient to allow visualization of metastases and to provide radioiodine therapy. Radioiodine therapy is further discussed below under "Radioisotope Therapy."

The whole-body scan is performed using either ^{131}I or ^{123}I. Scans may be obtained at several time points. Many centers obtain a scan before radioiodine therapy to assess for unknown metastases (Fig. 3.21), which may result in a change in patient management. This scan is performed 2–3 days after oral administration of a tracer dose of 2 mCi of ^{131}I or ^{123}I. Larger doses are not recommended, because they may result in "thyroid stunning," resulting in decreased uptake of the subsequent therapy dose of ^{131}I. Scanning is generally performed a few days after administration of the therapy dose of 100–200 mCi of ^{131}I to assess for metastases. The higher dose results in greater sensitivity than the pre-therapy scan, and metastases may be discovered on the post-therapy scans that were not identified on the pre-therapy scan. Finally, scans are obtained at various intervals over the following months and years to assess for the adequacy of the thyroid ablation and to monitor for cancer recurrence. The radioiodine therapy should result in ablation of residual normal thyroid tissue. Failure to do so, as demonstrated on the radioiodine scan, may require retreatment with ^{131}I, depending on the amount of uptake seen in the residual tissue and on local practice.

The sensitivity of radioiodine thyroid cancer scans and the effectiveness of radioiodine therapy are optimized by decreasing the circulating levels of endogenous iodine, which can compete with the radioiodine for uptake into tumor cells, and by maximizing TSH, thus increasing the radioiodine uptake. To minimize endogenous iodine levels, patients should undertake a low-iodine diet for 2 weeks before the scan or therapy. Patients should not have received any large iodine loads, such as from IV radiographic contrast, for 6 weeks before therapy. Maximizing TSH has traditionally been achieved through induction of hypothyroidism, by having the patient withhold thyroxine (T_4) replacement for 4 weeks and triiodothyronine (T_3) replacement for 2 weeks. More recently, human recombinant TSH has become available and can be used to increase TSH levels without inducing hypothyroidism. This is particularly useful in patients who have medical conditions that could make it unsafe to induce hypothyroidism, patients who have sustained significant side effects in response to a previous episode of hypothyroidism, and patients who have been unable to adequately raise their TSH in response to withholding thyroid hormone replacement.

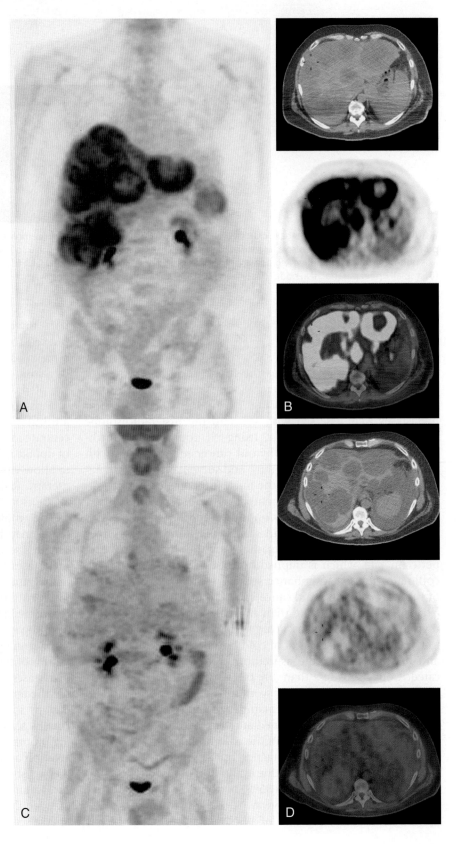

FIGURE 3.16 THERAPY RESPONSE IN GIST WITH FDG-PET. (A) Whole-body MIP image and (B) transaxial CT, PET, and fused PET/CT slices demonstrating intense FDG uptake in multiple large liver metastases. Following therapy with a tyrosine kinase inhibitor (C, D) there is complete resolution of the abnormal uptake previously seen on FDG-PET, indicative of successful therapy. Note that there is no significant reduction in tumor size by standard criteria on the CT images but that there is a change in the density of the tumor masses.

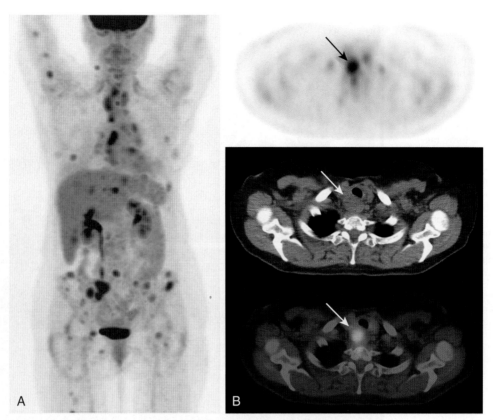

FIGURE 3.17 **METASTATIC MEDULLARY THYROID CANCER ON FDG-PET.** **(A)** Whole-body MIP image demonstrating numerous abnormal foci of FDG uptake consistent with extensive metastatic disease. **(B)** Transaxial CT, PET, and fused PET/CT slices showing focal increased FDG uptake within a thyroid nodule (*arrows*), the primary malignancy.

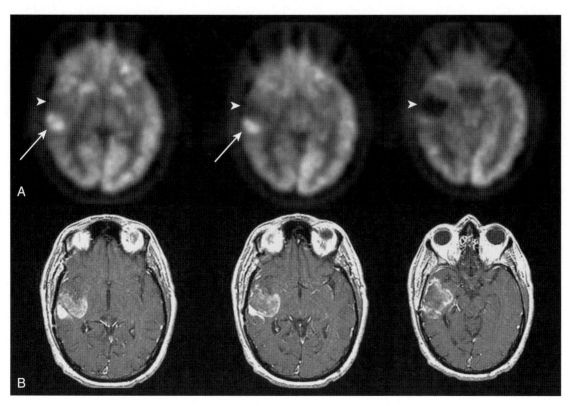

FIGURE 3.18 **BRAIN TUMOR RECURRENCE ON FDG-PET.** Three consecutive transaxial slices from **(A)** FDG-PET scan (*top*) and **(B)** corresponding co-registered MRI transaxial slices (*bottom*, T1, gadolinium-enhanced) in a patient with a history of glioblastoma multiforme. The MRI shows nonspecific enhancement adjacent to the surgical bed. The FDG-PET scan shows physiologic uptake throughout much of the brain and decreased uptake in the surgical bed (*arrowheads*). There is, however, a focal area of intense FDG uptake in the posterior aspect of the surgical bed (*arrows*) matching the nodular area of enhancement seen on MRI, consistent with tumor recurrence at that site.

FIGURE 3.19 THYROID CANCER. (A) Transaxial CT slice demonstrating a thyroid nodule (*arrow*) with a necrotic center arising from the thyroid isthmus (*arrowhead*). **(B)** Anterior planar view from a ^{99m}Tc-pertechnetate scan reveals that this nodule (*arrowheads*) is photopenic, or "cold," and that malignancy cannot therefore be excluded. Subsequent biopsy revealed a papillary thyroid cancer. Following near-total thyroidectomy, the patient underwent ^{131}I scanning from head to mid thighs **(C)** in advance of radioiodine thyroid ablation. Anterior whole-body image demonstrates the typical pattern of uptake in the thyroid remnant but no evidence of distal metastases. There is physiologic uptake within salivary glands, stomach, and bladder. The intense uptake seen to the left of the head is activity within an external standard used for dosimetry calculation purposes.

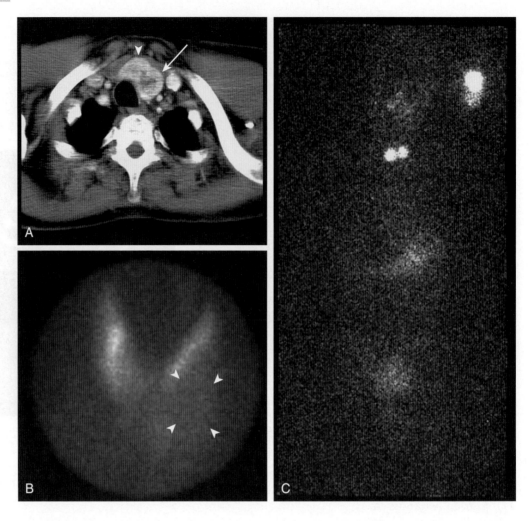

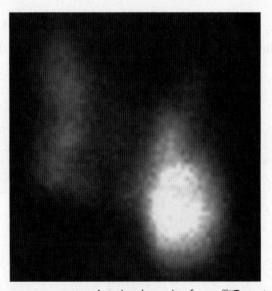

FIGURE 3.20 HOT THYROID NODULE ON A [99M]TC-PERTECHNETATE SCAN. Anterior planar view from a ^{99m}Tc-pertechnetate scan demonstrating a large exophytic hyperactive or "hot" nodule arising from the lower pole of the left thyroid lobe. Malignancy is effectively excluded.

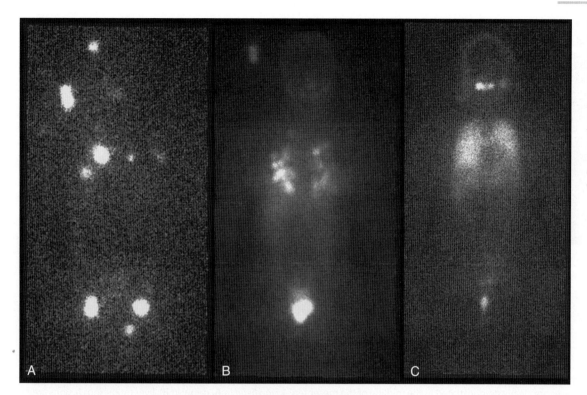

FIGURE 3.21 **THYROID CANCER METASTASES SEEN ON** ^{131}**I SCANS IN THREE DIFFERENT PATIENTS WITH A HISTORY OF THYROID CANCER REVEALING THREE PATTERNS OF METASTASES. A,** numerous bone metastases, **(B)** bilateral discrete lung metastases, and **(C)** diffuse fine lung metastases. Uptake seen to the right of the head in patients **A** and **B** is within an external standard used for dosimetry calculation purposes.

Neuroendocrine Tumors

OVERVIEW

Neoplasms arising from the neuroendocrine system are an interesting group of tumors characterized by uptake of amine precursors and synthesis of bioactive compounds.

Nuclear medicine studies have proven very useful in locating, staging, and following neuroendocrine tumors. The most commonly used agents interrogate unique properties of neuroendocrine tumors, including amine uptake mechanisms (^{123}I- or ^{131}I-metaiodobenzylguanidine (MIBG)), or specific cell receptors, such as somatostatin receptors (^{111}In-pentetreotide). More recently, PET scanning has been applied to assessment of neuroendocrine tumors. However, uptake of the most widely available PET agent, ^{18}F-FDG, is often low in neuroendocrine tumors, a reflection of their low metabolic rate. Consequently, it is usually recommended that FDG-PET imaging be used only when the traditional imaging agents give negative results. More specific, but less widely available, PET radiopharmaceuticals such as ^{18}F-DOPA and ^{11}C-hydroxyephedrine have shown promising results in the evaluation of neuroendocrine tumors, and may play a significant clinical role in the near future.

^{111}In-PENTETREOTIDE

^{111}In-pentetreotide is a conjugate of octreotide, an analog of somatostatin, a 14–amino acid regulatory neuropeptide present in neurons and endocrine cells. The biologic half-life of somatostatin is only 1–3 minutes, but the 8–amino acid analog octreotide has a longer biologic half-life of 90–120 minutes, which makes it more amenable to imaging and therapy. Octreotide is bound to ^{111}In via a diethylenetriaminepentaacetic acid (DTPA) bridge to form the radiopharmaceutical ^{111}In-pentetreotide. Many neuroendocrine cells express somatostatin receptors, and tumors arising from these cells often overexpress them, making this an effective imaging agent.

^{111}In-pentetreotide binds mainly to somatostatin receptor subtypes 2 and 5. Applications of ^{111}In-pentetreotide imaging in neuroendocrine tumors include localizing the primary lesion when other modalities are unable to do so, staging, restaging, assessing response to therapy, assessing for recurrence, aiding intraoperative tumor localization using a gamma probe, and establishing somatostatin receptor status in vivo for potential therapy with somatostatin analogs.

^{111}In-pentetreotide imaging has high sensitivity for most neuroendocrine tumors, including carcinoid tumors (Fig. 3.22A to E) and most pancreatic islet cell tumors (Fig. 3.23A, B). Insulinomas are an exception, however, with a sensitivity of only 61%.

In addition to neuroendocrine tumors, ^{111}In-pentetreotide may also be taken up in other tumors expressing high levels of somatostatin receptors, including lymphoma, breast cancer, and melanoma, and in some inflammatory conditions, including granulomatous and autoimmune diseases.

METAIODOBENZYLGUANIDINE

MIBG, a combination of the benzyl group of bretylium and the guanidine group of guanethidine, is similar in structure and function to norepinephrine. As a result, MIBG is taken up in cells of neural crest origin. Uptake is predominantly via an active uptake-1 mechanism, and once inside the cytoplasm, MIBG is stored in vesicles from which it may be released and become available for reuptake by the same mechanism. MIBG can be labeled with ^{123}I or ^{131}I, yielding an effective imaging and therapeutic agent for tumors derived from neural crest cells, such as pheochromocytomas, ganglioneuromas, and neuroblastomas. Other neuroendocrine tumors, including paragangliomas, medullary thyroid carcinomas, and carcinoid tumors, may also be positive on MIBG scans, though less frequently so.

MIBG is generally recommended for the assessment of pheochromocytomas and neuroblastomas, whereas ^{111}In-pentetreotide demonstrates higher sensitivity for most other neuroendocrine tumors. However, the two imaging agents can be complementary, in that the avidity of any given

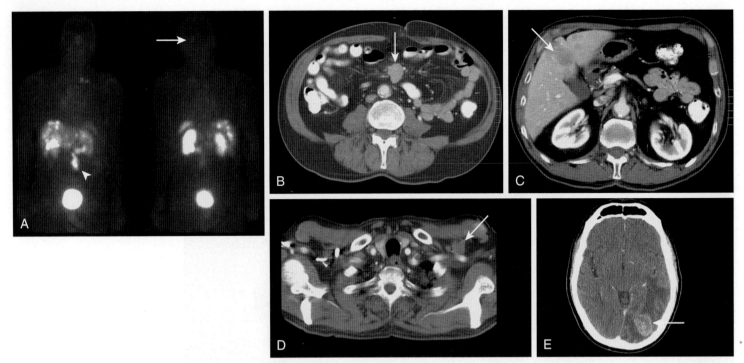

FIGURE 3.22 METASTATIC CARCINOID TUMOR ON ¹¹¹IN-PENTETREOTIDE SCAN. (A) Anterior and posterior whole-body planar ¹¹¹In-pentetreotide images, and **(B–E)** correlative transaxial CT slices. Metastases are clearly demonstrated in the midline of the mesentery (*arrowhead* in **A,** *arrow* in **B**), liver (numerous lesions are seen in **A,** *arrow* in **C**), left supraclavicular lymph nodes (two nodes are seen in **A,** *arrow* in **D**), and brain (*arrows* in both **A** and **E**). Normal physiologic uptake is demonstrated in the kidneys, bladder, spleen, and liver.

tumor can be difficult to predict in advance, and a tumor negative with one imaging agent may be positive with the other.

Image quality with ¹²³I-MIBG (Fig. 3.24A, B) is better than with ¹³¹I-MIBG (Fig. 3.25), because the shorter half-life of ¹²³I and absence of beta-particle emission allow a higher dose to be administered to the patient, and because the lower-energy photons of ¹²³I are more favorable for detection by gamma cameras. These factors also allow SPECT imaging to be performed with ¹²³I-MIBG but not with ¹³¹I-MIBG. ¹²³I-MIBG detects more sites of disease than ¹³¹I-MIBG but is not as widely available.

In pediatrics, MIBG is effective in imaging patients with neuroblastoma (Fig. 3.26A to D). MIBG imaging can be helpful in establishing a tentative diagnosis in a child with a mass, staging the disease, assessing response to therapy, and for subsequent surveillance. Because neuroblastoma may metastasize to bone, a bone scan is part of the standard diagnostic workup. Unlike the case with most tumors, the radiopharmaceutical is taken up by both the primary tumor and the soft tissue metastases, which are frequently depicted on the bone scan.

Gallium-67 and ⁹⁹ᵐTc-SestaMIBI

In addition to the common nuclear medicine studies discussed above, a variety of other radiopharmaceuticals have been useful in cancer evaluation. Although these have largely been replaced by FDG-PET, some remain of interest when FDG-PET is not available or in select circumstances.

Gallium-67, injected as ⁶⁷Ga citrate, has been used in oncology for many years, largely in the setting of lymphoma, where it has played an important role in patient management. In addition to its oncology applications, which include lymphoma and to a lesser extent melanoma and hepatocellular carcinoma, ⁶⁷Ga scanning is also used in the evaluation of a variety of infectious and inflammatory conditions. ⁶⁷Ga is a group IIIA metal that behaves somewhat like iron, and as such binds to a number of proteins including

transferrin receptors, which is its primary uptake mechanism in tumors. Other factors contributing to tumor uptake include binding to lactoferrin (present in large amounts in lymphomas) and to tumor-associated inflammatory cells. Uptake is further enhanced through the nonspecific mechanisms of increased blood flow and capillary permeability associated with tumors.

At the time of staging, ⁶⁷Ga scanning complements CT staging and confirms ⁶⁷Ga avidity for subsequent follow-up (Fig. 3.27). In non-Hodgkin lymphomas, ⁶⁷Ga avidity varies with tumor grade, with aggressive lymphomas showing higher avidity than low-grade tumors. The majority of Hodgkin lymphomas are gallium-avid. ⁶⁷Ga scanning is particularly useful in assessing residual masses during or following therapy (Fig. 3.28A to D). CT is less reliable in this setting, because response to therapy is judged predominantly based on tumor size changes, which may not accurately reflect the presence of residual viable tumor or, conversely, scar tissue. Residual ⁶⁷Ga uptake is indicative of viable tumor and has been shown to correlate with poorer outcomes. ⁶⁷Ga imaging is also efficacious in longer-term surveillance for recurrence. However, it should be emphasized that FDG-PET is superior to ⁶⁷Ga scintigraphy in the initial staging and in predicting prognosis during and after chemotherapy in both Hodgkin disease and non-Hodgkin lymphomas. Hence, if available, FDG-PET should be considered the metabolic imaging technique of choice in the management of patients with lymphomas.

⁹⁹ᵐTc-methoxy-isobutyl-isonitrile (⁹⁹ᵐTc-sestaMIBI) is another radiopharmaceutical occasionally used in oncology imaging. Better known as a myocardial perfusion agent, ⁹⁹ᵐTc-sestaMIBI is a lipophilic cation that passively enters cells and becomes incorporated into mitochondria through electrostatic attraction. It thus concentrates in cells with high mitochondrial concentrations, including many tumors. ⁹⁹ᵐTc-sestaMIBI is still used in select circumstances, particularly where assessment is not hindered by the rather extensive physiologic uptake of ⁹⁹ᵐTc-sestaMIBI. This includes breast imaging when mammography is inconclusive (scintimammography) and in assessing the skeleton in multiple myeloma (Fig. 3.29A, B).

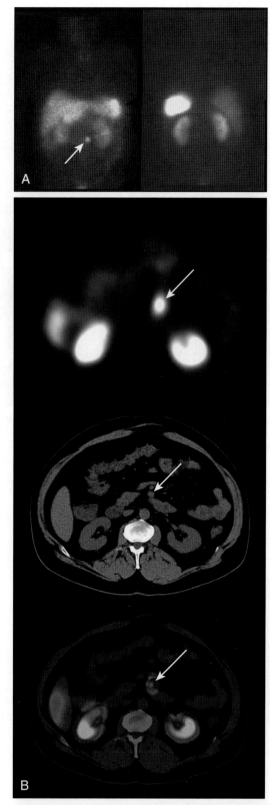

FIGURE 3.23 ¹¹¹IN-PENTETREOTIDE SPECT-CT SCAN IN A PATIENT WITH SUSPECTED GASTRINOMA TUMOR AND NEGATIVE ANATOMIC IMAGING. This study was acquired on an integrated SPECT-CT camera, allowing SPECT and CT images to be acquired in one setting without moving the patient between scans, facilitating co-registration of the anatomic images from the CT scan with the metabolic information provided by the SPECT scan. **(A)** Anterior and posterior whole-body planar views from the ¹¹¹In-pentetreotide scan reveal a small yet intense focus of abnormal uptake in the upper abdomen (*arrow*). **(B)** SPECT, CT, and fused SPECT/CT axial slices demonstrate that the uptake is within a tiny nodule in the upper abdomen (*arrows*). ¹¹¹In-pentetreotide scans can be very helpful in localizing suspected neuroendocrine tumors. (Courtesy of Moncton City Hospital, Moncton, New Brunswick, Canada.)

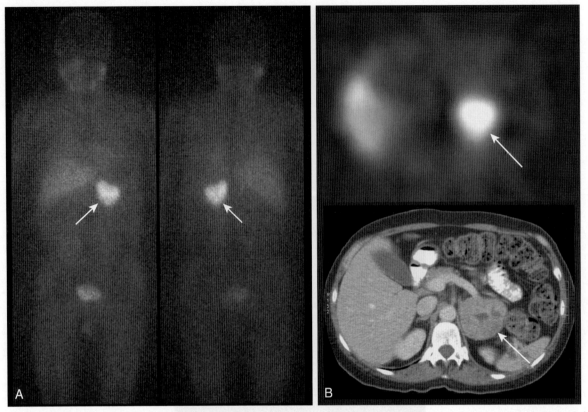

FIGURE 3.24   PHEOCHROMOCYTOMA ON ¹²³I-MIBG SCAN. (A) Anterior and posterior whole-body planar ¹²³I-MIBG images in a patient with a large left-sided pheochromocytoma (*arrows*). There are no distant metastases. **(B)** Transaxial slices from the SPECT acquisition and corresponding CT show that the abnormal uptake correlates with a large suprarenal mass (*arrows*).

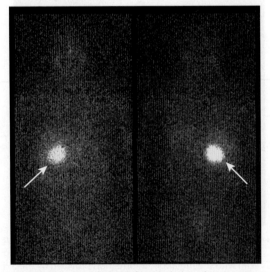

FIGURE 3.25   PHEOCHROMOCYTOMA ON ¹³¹I-MIBG SCAN. This patient has a large right-sided pheochromocytoma. Comparison with Figure 3.24 demonstrates the better image quality seen when using MIBG radiolabeled with ¹²³I rather than ¹³¹I.

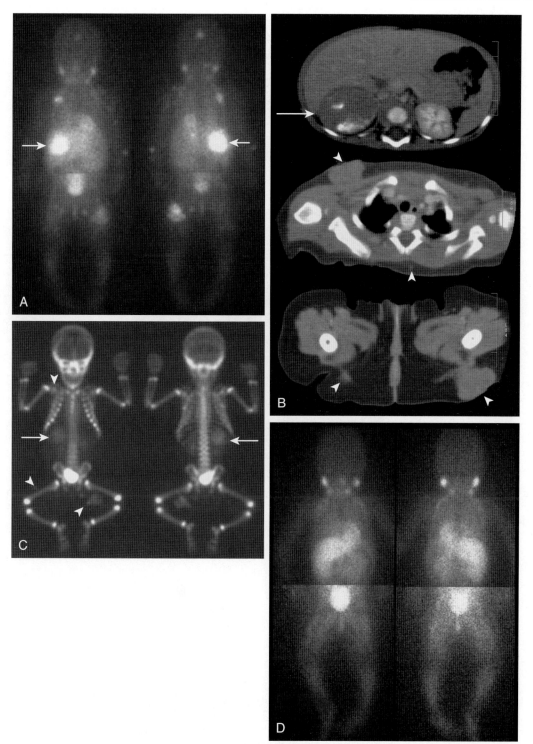

FIGURE 3.26 NEUROBLASTOMA ON ^{123}I-MIBG SCAN AND ^{99M}TC-MDP BONE SCAN. (A) Anterior and posterior whole-body planar images from a ^{123}I-MIBG scan revealing intense uptake within a large right suprarenal mass (*arrows*) and within numerous subcutaneous nodules scattered throughout the body in a young child. **(B)** CT scan demonstrates the large complex suprarenal mass (*top image, arrow*) and several of the subcutaneous nodules (*arrowheads*) at the level of the shoulders (*middle image*) and upper thighs (*lower image*). **(C)** Staging ^{99m}Tc-MDP bone scan in the same child reveals uptake within the suprarenal mass (*arrows*) and some of the larger soft tissue nodules (*arrowheads*). There are no osseous metastases. **(D)** ^{123}I-MIBG scan following therapy reveals complete resolution of pathologic ^{123}I-MIBG uptake. The activity seen within the salivary glands and the remainder of the body is physiologic.

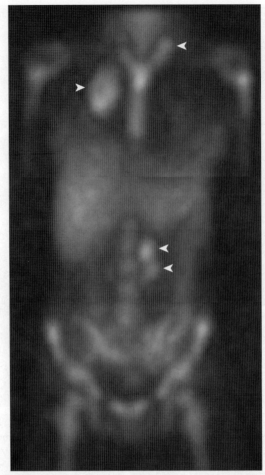

FIGURE 3.27 STAGING ⁶⁷GA SCAN IN A PATIENT WITH HODGKIN DISEASE. Whole-body maximal intensity projection image reveals abnormal increased uptake (*arrowheads*) above and below the diaphragm, including the left neck, a large conglomeration of nodes in the right mediastinum, and left retroperitoneal nodes, indicating Stage 3 disease.

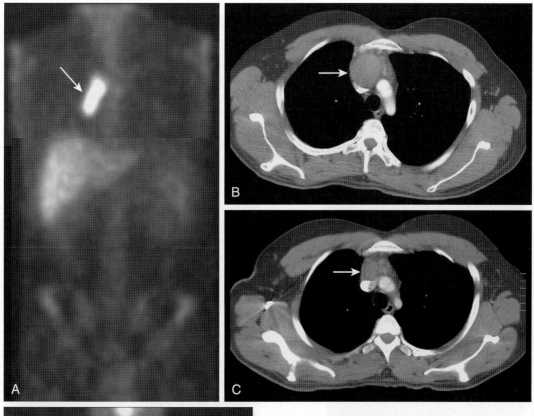

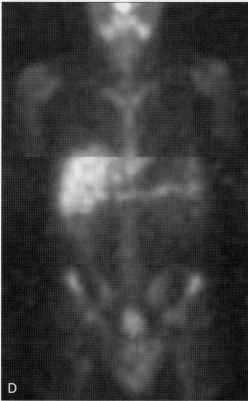

FIGURE 3.28 MONITORING THERAPY RESPONSE WITH ^{67}GA SCANS. (A) Staging ^{67}Ga scan in a patient with Hodgkin disease reveals intense uptake in right mediastinal lymphadenopathy (*arrow*). There are no other abnormalities, confirming stage 1 disease. **(B)** Correlative CT scan reveals the 4.9-cm lymph node (*arrow*) responsible for the ^{67}Ga uptake. **(C)** Follow-up CT scan after two cycles of chemotherapy demonstrates that the enlarged node has shrunk to 2.6 cm (*arrow*), but there is still an anatomic abnormality. **(D)** Follow-up ^{67}Ga scan at the same time reveals no residual ^{67}Ga uptake, indicating a good response to therapy despite the presence of a residual mass.

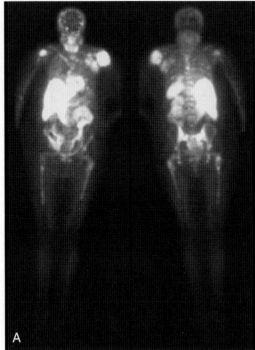

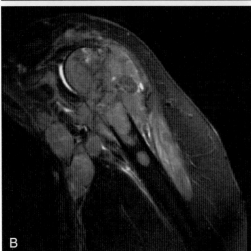

FIGURE 3.29 **99ᴹTC-SESTAMIBI SCAN IN MULTIPLE MYELOMA. (A)** Anterior and posterior planar whole-body images from a 99mTc-sestaMIBI scan demonstrate pathologic uptake of the tracer throughout the axial skeleton, skull, and proximal long bones. Particularly large and intense uptake seen in the left shoulder correlates on MRI **(B)** with abnormal marrow signal (*light areas*) and extension into adjacent soft tissues including axillary lymph nodes. Uptake within salivary glands, myocardium, bowel, liver, and spleen is physiologic.

Sentinel Nodes

In many cancers, knowledge of regional lymph node involvement is critical in determining prognosis and in decisions regarding adjuvant therapy. Determination of lymph node status traditionally required complete dissection of a lymph node basin, which is associated with significant morbidity. Because of earlier detection, nodal involvement in breast cancer has decreased to approximately 30%, and hence 70% of patients undergo complete axillary lymph node dissection needlessly. In some cancers such as melanoma, the primary draining nodal basin cannot always be reliably predicted, particularly when tumors are located in lymphatic watershed areas. The sentinel node study presents an accurate method of identifying the draining basin and assessing its status with minimally invasive techniques.

The premise of the study is that lymphatic drainage from a tumor is orderly and consistent. If a tracer is injected near the tumor, the first node that it would drain to is referred to as the sentinel node. Hence, removal and pathologic evaluation of that node alone will indicate whether there has been nodal spread.

Sentinel node studies were first performed with blue dye and subsequently with radiolabeled colloids. In North America the most widely used radiopharmaceutical is 99mTc-sulfur colloid. The sentinel node study has been most widely used in breast cancer (Fig. 3.30) and in melanoma (Fig. 3.31), though with increasing application in other malignancies such as vulvar cancer and head and neck cancers. In the context of melanoma, injections of the radiolabeled colloid are usually performed intradermally around the primary cancer site. For breast cancer, injections of the tracer can be done in a peritumoral, intradermal, or subareolar location; there is currently no consensus on the best approach. Subsequent imaging will reveal the site of the sentinel node(s). A gamma probe is then used in the operating room to identify and remove the sentinel node(s) using a minimally invasive procedure.

FIGURE 3.30 **SENTINEL NODE IN BREAST CANCER. (A)** Anterior and **(B)** right anterior oblique planar images from a breast sentinel node study clearly demonstrating a solitary sentinel node (*arrowhead*) in the right axilla. Intense uptake seen in the right breast is related to the 99mTc-sulfur colloid injections.

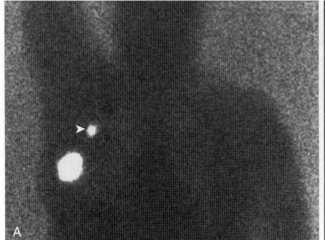

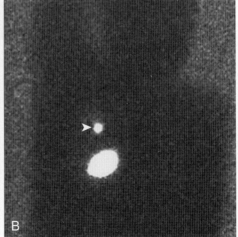

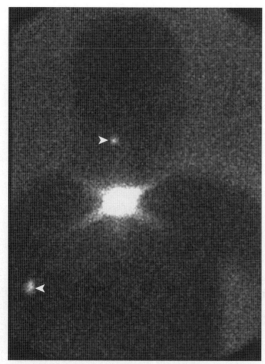

FIGURE 3.31 **SENTINEL NODES IN MELANOMA.** Anterior planar view from a melanoma sentinel node study revealing sentinel nodes in two nodal basins, one in the right axilla and the other in the right cervical region (*arrowheads*). Intense uptake projecting over the thorax is due to the intradermal ^{99m}Tc-sulfur colloid injections at the site of the primary melanoma lesion.

Radioisotope Therapy

The systemic introduction of tumor-seeking radiopharmaceuticals allows not only tumor imaging but also the potential for systemic radiation therapy. As with imaging radiopharmaceuticals, therapeutic radiopharmaceuticals possess two general properties: relevant physiology that governs their biodistribution and tumor uptake, and radioactive decay, resulting in emission of particles or photons that induce tumor cell death, generally through DNA damage. Most therapeutic radioisotopes decay by emission of a beta particle, with ranges of 1–12 mm, depending on the energy of emission. Thus, not all tumor cells have to take up the radiopharmaceutical, as neighboring cells can be killed by the "cross-fire" effect. Less common therapeutic radioisotopes cause cell damage through emission of auger electrons, conversion electrons, or alpha particles. Table 3.4 lists some therapy radiopharmaceuticals.

The most common application of radioisotope therapy is in thyroid cancer. As previously discussed, well-differentiated thyroid cancers retain the ability to concentrate iodine, and hence are amenable to therapy with ^{131}I, a beta emitter. Radioiodine therapy is undertaken with two potential goals: the ablation of normal thyroid tissue in postsurgical remnants and destruction of any residual or recurrent thyroid cancer. Residual normal thyroid tissue is targeted, because it can interfere with attempts to monitor for disease recurrence through production of thyroglobulin, interfering with the ability to use this biomarker to monitor for thyroid cancer, and through uptake of radioiodine on scans (Fig. 3.32), potentially limiting uptake in tumor. Incorporation of radioiodine therapy into the management of patients with well-differentiated thyroid cancer has resulted in improved survival and recurrence rates.

Another long-standing radioisotope therapy has been the palliative treatment of bone pain from osseous metastases. Originally performed with ^{32}P-sodium phosphate, the therapy is currently most commonly performed with Strontium-89 (^{89}Sr) chloride and Samarium-153–ethylene diamine tetramethylene phosphonate (^{153}Sm-EDTMP). Injected intravenously, these agents are incorporated into bone similarly to bone scanning agents like ^{99m}Tc-MDP, and therefore concentrate in areas of osseous metastases. These radioisotopes decay by beta emission, delivering local radiation therapy. ^{153}Sm-EDTMP also emits a gamma photon, allowing imaging to be performed (Fig. 3.33). Approximately 75% of patients attain some symptom relief. The main side effect is bone marrow suppression, which is transient.

Recently, therapies have been developed using monoclonal antibodies (MoAbs) to deliver radioisotopes to targeted receptors on tumor cells, a process known as radioimmunotherapy (RIT). The most successful have been radiolabeled anti-CD20 MoAbs, used primarily in low-grade non-Hodgkin lymphomas. Two agents are available: ^{90}Y-ibritumomab tiuxetan (Zevalin; Fig. 3.34A–C) and ^{131}I-tositumomab (Bexxar). Clinical trials have shown significant response rates in patients receiving RIT after failed chemotherapy and after failed nonradiolabeled MoAb therapy. The specific indications for RIT are still evolving.

In neuroendocrine tumors radioisotope therapy may be performed using larger doses of imaging radiopharmaceuticals. In particular, ^{131}I-MIBG has been used as therapy for a variety of MIBG-avid tumors, most notably pheochromocytomas, neuroblastomas, and carcinoids (Fig. 3.35). Patients whose neuroendocrine tumors are not MIBG-avid but are octreotide-avid are occasionally treated with high doses of ^{111}In-octreotide, although this is done in only a few centers.

FIGURE 3.32 **TYPICAL EVOLUTION OF** ^{131}**I SCANS IN A PATIENT WITH THYROID CANCER.** On the pre-therapy scan **(A)** there is intense uptake in the post-surgical thyroid remnant, as well as physiologic uptake in the colon and bladder. The immediate post-therapy scan **(B)** again reveals intense uptake in the thyroid remnant, as well as physiologic uptake, most notably in the salivary glands. On the 6-month follow-up scan **(C)** there is no longer activity in the thyroid bed, indicating successful ablation of the thyroid remnants. Activity seen within the colon and bladder is physiologic. There was no evidence of iodine-avid metastases at any time point. The focal uptake seen to the right of the head in **A** and **C** is within an external standard used for dosimetry calculation purposes.

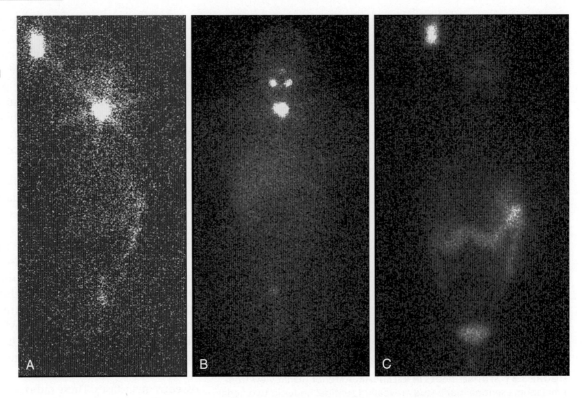

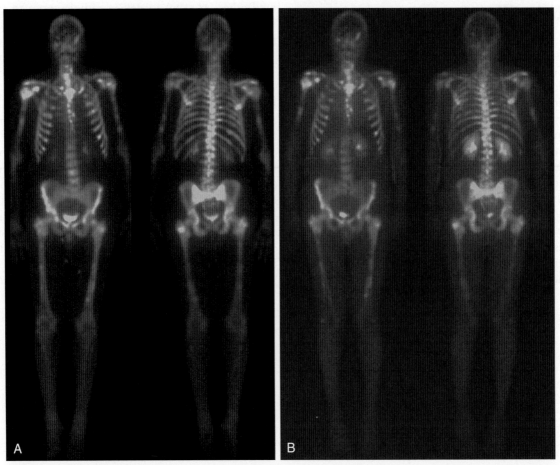

FIGURE 3.33 **PATIENT UNDERGOING RADIOISOTOPE THERAPY FOR PAINFUL BONE METASTASES. (A)** Standard anterior and posterior whole-body views of a ^{99m}Tc-MDP bone scan revealing extensive osseous metastatic disease throughout the axial skeleton extending into the proximal aspects of all four extremities, resulting in pain at multiple sites. **(B)** Images obtained within an hour following injection of a therapeutic dose of ^{153}Sm-EDTMP showing uptake in the osseous metastases paralleling the uptake seen on the bone scan, confirming delivery of the therapeutic agent to the sites of metastatic disease. The patient experienced pain relief in multiple sites within a week after the administration of the therapeutic dose.

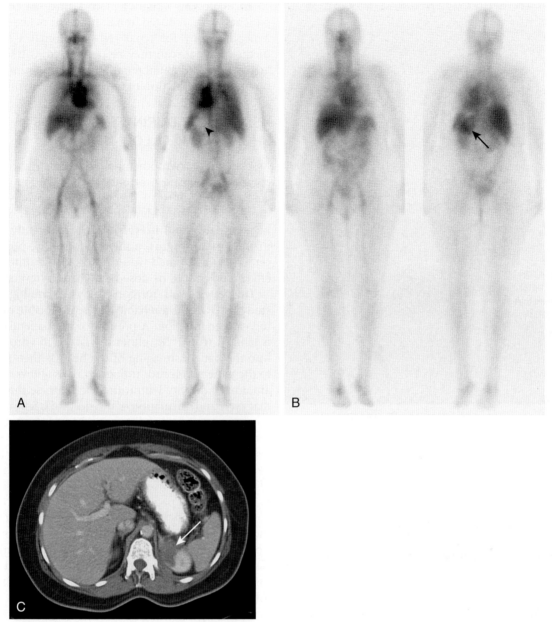

FIGURE 3.34 **PATIENT UNDERGOING RIT FOR NON-HODGKIN LYMPHOMA.** Anterior and posterior whole-body images **(A)** 2 hours and **(B)** 48 hours following
[111]In-ibritumomab tiuxetan infusion in a patient with non-Hodgkin lymphoma being evaluated for eligibility of therapy with ^{90}Y-ibritumomab tiuxetan.
These images are obtained before therapy to confirm normal biodistribution of the tracer, because the therapeutic radioisotope, yttrium-90, does not emit
a gamma photon and hence cannot be imaged. Note that there is a defect in the left suprarenal region on the early images (*arrowhead*) that fills in on the
delayed images (*arrow*). This correlates with the tumor mass (*arrow*) seen on CT **(C)**. The biodistribution was normal and the patient proceeded to receive
the ^{90}Y-ibritumomab tiuxetan therapeutic dose a week later. Of note, both the diagnostic and therapeutic doses are administered following infusion of
nonradiolabeled rituximab (Rituxan) to minimize nonspecific binding of the radiolabeled antibody.

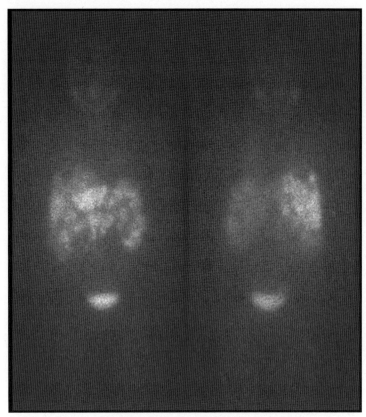

FIGURE 3.35 ^{131}I-MIBG SCAN IN A PATIENT UNDERGOING ^{131}I-MIBG THERAPY. Anterior and posterior whole-body views in a patient with multiple liver metastases from a carcinoid tumor confirming that the tumors are MIBG-avid. The patient went on to two cycles of therapy with high-dose ^{131}I-MIBG, resulting in symptomatic relief.

Assessing Nontarget Organ Response to Therapy

Nuclear medicine studies can also help assess nontarget organ response to therapy and suitability for particular procedures. These studies can be performed before therapy, during therapy, in short-term follow-up, and in the longer term to assess for delayed complications.

ASSESSMENT BEFORE THERAPY

Lung perfusion studies may be performed in patients scheduled to undergo lobectomy or pneumonectomy for lung cancer. These studies are performed using ^{99m}Tc-macroaggregated albumin (MAA) and are used in patients with compromised pulmonary function as indicated by pulmonary function spirometry and lung capacity testing. Such workup is typically not required if preoperative forced expiration volume in the first second (FEV1) is greater than 2 L or more than 80% of predicted FEV1 in patients destined to undergo pneumonectomy, or FEV1 is greater than 1.5 L in patients destined to undergo lobectomy. If these criteria are not met, then the expected postoperative lung function should be predicted using a ^{99m}Tc-MAA scan (Fig. 3.36A, B) or by correcting the preoperative function by the ratio of number of postoperative lobes to preoperative lobes. Predicted postoperative FEV1 less than 40% or diffusing capacity of the lung for carbon monoxide (DLCO) less than 40% indicates a high risk for perioperative death and cardiopulmonary complications.

An analogous situation occurs in renal cell carcinoma. In patients with reduced renal function scheduled to undergo a nephrectomy for renal cell carcinoma, a standard nuclear medicine renal scan may be performed, with semiquantitative analysis of differential renal function, to estimate the influence on total renal function of removal of the involved kidney.

ASSESSMENT DURING THERAPY OR IN SHORT-TERM FOLLOW-UP

Assessment of chemotherapy-induced cardiotoxicity is the most common application of nuclear medicine in assessing nontarget organ response to therapy. Cardiotoxicity has been commonly associated with anthracycline therapy, where it tends to be cumulative and irreversible. More recently introduced trastuzumab (Herceptin), a therapy for HER2-positive breast cancer, is also associated with cardiotoxicity, although this adverse effect tends not to be dose-related and is reversible.

The gated wall motion study, or multigated acquisition study (MUGA), is a reliable and reproducible method of assessing cardiac function. A portion of the patient's red blood cells is labeled with ^{99m}Tc, either in vivo or in vitro with reinjection into the patient. Imaging of the heart is then performed, gated to the patient's electrocardiogram. This allows assessment of the amount of activity within the left ventricle throughout the cardiac cycle and calculation of the ejection fraction (EF) (Fig. 3.37). There are a number of different protocols for monitoring cardiac function with wall motion studies. Commonly used criteria for a significant decline in cardiac function include a decrease of EF by 10 percentage points to below 50% in patients with baseline EF greater than 50%, and a decrease by 10 percentage points or to below 30% in patients with baseline EF less than 50%.

Nephrotoxicity is a potential complication of a variety of chemotherapeutic agents. Decreased renal function can also result from radiation therapy and from nephrectomy. An accurate assessment of renal function may be required before therapy for purposes of dose calculation, or for monitoring purposes following therapy. Reliable monitoring of renal function can be performed using the nuclear medicine glomerular filtration rate (GFR) study. The GFR analysis is performed using either ^{99m}Tc-DTPA or ^{51}Cr-EDTA. Both agents are processed by the kidneys primarily through filtration, such that assessment of the rate of removal from the circulation, assessed through subsequent blood sampling, reflects the GFR.

In patients receiving chemotherapy through an indwelling central line, a potential complication is obstruction of the central line due to thrombosis or a fibrin sheath. There may also be obstruction of the veins of the upper extremities, subclavian and brachiocephalic veins, or superior vena cava. Radionuclide venography is a rapid and minimally invasive means of assessing upper extremity and central line patency. ^{99m}Tc-pertechnetate is injected sequentially through a vein in the arm ipsilateral to the central line, followed by injection into a vein in the contralateral arm, and finally through the central line itself. Dynamic imaging of the chest and upper extremities is performed throughout this process and reviewed for evidence of obstruction.

Lymphedema is a potential complication of therapy, either due to surgery, such as axillary node dissection, or due to radiation. When symptoms such as extremity swelling occur in this setting, a lymphoscintigraphy study may be performed. Subdermal injections of a radiolabeled colloid, typically filtered ^{99m}Tc-sulfur colloid, are placed distally in the affected extremity and in the contralateral extremity as a control. The colloid is picked up by the lymphatics, and serial imaging demonstrates the proximal migration of the tracer along lymphatic vessels into the various nodal groups draining that area in the physiologic setting as well as the dermal backflow or cutaneous flare pathognomonic of lymphedema in the affected limb (Fig. 3.38).

LONG-TERM FOLLOW-UP

Although nuclear medicine techniques are not routinely indicated in long-term follow-up of patients for nontarget organ problems, in certain situations they may play a role. For example, in patients suspected of having developed a secondary malignancy because of prior radiation therapy, or in patients with a hereditary predisposition for developing a malignancy, specific nuclear medicine studies, such as an FDG-PET scan, may be indicated.

Patients having previously undergone chest radiation therapy are at increased risk of coronary artery disease. In the presence of clinical suspicion, a nuclear medicine myocardial perfusion study may be indicated to assess for the presence, extent, and severity of coronary artery disease.

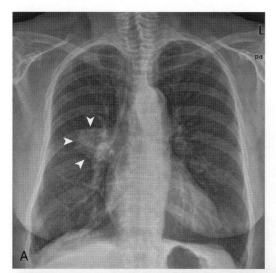

FIGURE 3.36 **QUANTITATIVE LUNG PERFUSION STUDY BEFORE PNEUMONECTOMY FOR LUNG CANCER. (A)** Chest radiograph demonstrating a large bronchogenic carcinoma in the right hilar region (*arrowheads*). **(B)** Quantitative lung perfusion study with ^{99m}Tc-MAA. Each lung has been divided into upper (Lu, Ru), middle (Lm, Rm), and lower (Ll, Rl) thirds on both the posterior (*left*) and anterior (*right*) images. The geometric mean values (*middle columns*) of the counts from the anterior and posterior images best represent the actual activity in the lungs. The left lung contributes 46.5% of the total function versus 53.5% from the right lung: the postoperative FEV1 and DLCO can be expected to decrease by 53.5% following the planned right pneumonectomy. A perfusion defect from the tumor is seen on the anterior images (*arrowheads*), correlating with the chest radiograph.

	Posterior Kct		Geometric mean values				Anterior Kct	
			Left Lung		Right Lung			
	Left	Right	%	Kct	%	Kct	Right	Left
Upper zone:	58.85	54.47	13.4	62.12	11.9	55.18	55.89	65.56
Middle zone:	97.37	121.77	21.6	100.04	24.3	112.64	104.19	102.78
Lower zone:	60.23	79.25	11.5	53.28	17.3	80.32	81.41	47.14
Total lung:	216.45	255.49	46.5	215.44	53.5	248.14	241.50	215.49

B

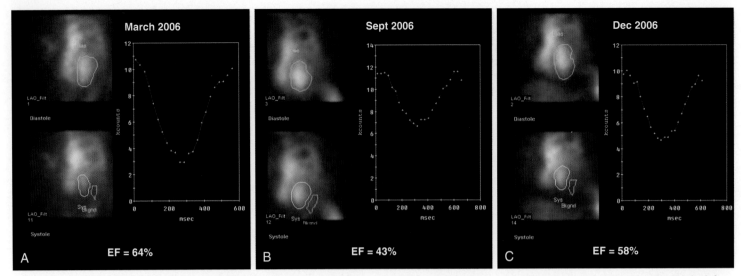

FIGURE 3.37 **SERIAL CARDIAC WALL MOTION STUDIES IN A PATIENT ON TRASTUZUMAB THERAPY FOR BREAST CANCER.** On the baseline study in March 2006 **(A)** the left ventricular ejection fraction (LVEF) was normal at 64%. On a follow-up study 6 months later in September 2006 while the patient was taking trastuzumab **(B)** the LVEF had dropped to 43%, leading to discontinuation of this drug. Further monitoring 3 months later in December 2006 **(C)** showed that the LVEF had recovered to 58%, and trastuzumab therapy was reinstituted.

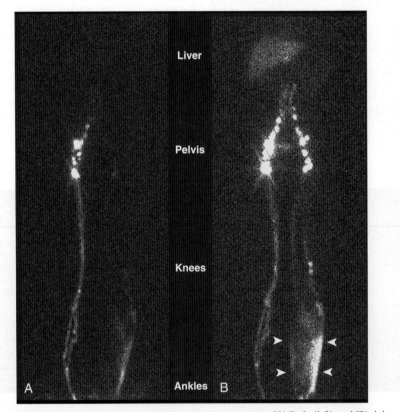

FIGURE 3.38 **LYMPHOSCINTIGRAPHY STUDY OF THE LOWER EXTREMITIES TO EVALUATE LEFT LEG SWELLING. (A)** Early (*left*) and **(B)** delayed (*right*) anterior views of the abdomen and lower extremities following intradermal injection of the tracer in the dorsum of both feet demonstrating normal lymphatic drainage along the right lower extremity in deep lymphatic vessels into the right inguinal and iliac lymph node basins. The drainage in the left lower extremity is delayed relative to the right. Furthermore diffuse uptake is noted within the soft tissues of the left calf, often referred to as "cutaneous flare" or "dermal backflow" (*arrowheads*), that is pathognomonic for lymphedema.

References and Suggested Readings

Cases JA, Surks MI: The changing role of scintigraphy in the evaluation of thyroid nodules, *Semin Nucl Med* 30:81–87, 2000.

Colice GL, Shafazand S, Griffen JP, et al: Physiologic evaluation of the patient with lung cancer being considered for resectional surgery: ACCP evidence-based clinical practice guidelines, 2nd ed. *Chest* 132(Suppl 3):161S–177S, 2007.

Cooper DS, Doherty GM, Haugen BR, et al: Management guidelines for patients with thyroid nodules and differentiated thyroid carcinoma, *Thyroid* 16:109–142, 2006.

Elgazzar AH, Ibrahim EM: Neoplastic bone diseases. In Elgazzar AH, editor: *Orthopedic Nuclear Medicine*, Berlin, 2004, Springer-Verlag, p 143.

Gambhir SS, Czernin J, Schwimmer J, et al: A tabulated summary of the FDG PET literature, *J Nucl Med* 42(Suppl 5):1S–93S, 2001.

Gould MK, MacLean CC, Kuschner WG, et al: Accuracy of positron emission tomography for diagnosis of pulmonary nodules and mass lesions: a meta-analysis, *JAMA* 285:914–924, 2001.

Hillner BE, Siegel BA, Liu D, et al: Impact of positron emission tomography/computed tomography and positron emission tomography (PET) alone on expected management of patients with cancer: initial results from the National Oncologic PET Registry, *J Clin Oncol* 26:2155–2161, 2008.

Hoefnagel CA: Metaiodobenzylguanidine and somatostatin in oncology: role in the management of neural crest tumours, *Eur J Nucl Med* 21:561–581, 1994.

Mazzaferri EL, Jhiang SM: Long-term impact of initial surgical and medical therapy on papillary and follicular thyroid cancer, *Am J Med* 97:418–428, 1994.

Rosenthal DI: Radiologic diagnosis of bone metastases, *Cancer* 80(Suppl): 1595–1607, 1997.

Seregni E, Chiti A, Bombardieri E: Radionuclide imaging of neuroendocrine tumours: biological basis and diagnostic results, *Eur J Nucl Med* 25:639–658, 1998.

Shulkin BL, Shapiro B: Current concepts on the diagnostic use of MIBG in children, *J Nucl Med* 39:679–688, 1998.

Thrall JH: Molecular imaging and molecular biology, *Acad Radiol* 11:S5–S6, 2004.

Van den Abbeele AD, Lechpammer S, Tetrault RJ, et al: Nuclear medicine. In Mauch PM, Armitage JO, Coiffier B, et al, editors: *Non-Hodgkin's Lymphomas*, Philadelphia, 2004, Lippincott Williams & Wilkins, pp 155–169.

Veronesi U, Paganelli G, Viale G, et al: A randomized comparison of sentinel-node biopsy with routine axillary dissection in breast cancer, *N Engl J Med* 349:546–553, 2003.

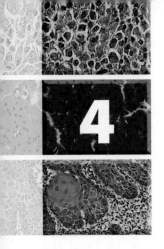

4

Cancer of the Head and Neck region

ROBERT HADDAD • JOHN R. CLARK • JAMES N. SUOJANEN •
A. DIMITRIOS COLEVAS • MARSHALL POSNER

Cancers of the lips, oral cavity, oropharynx, nasopharynx, hypopharynx, larynx, nasal and paranasal sinuses, neck, ear, and salivary glands, as well as those of regional soft tissues and supporting bones, are customarily grouped as cancers of the head and neck. Consequently, a large variety of neoplasms may be encountered, including sarcomas of any type, adenocarcinomas of major or minor salivary gland origin, and squamous cell carcinomas of the mucosal lining of the upper aerodigestive tract. Squamous cell carcinoma (SCCHN) is the most common head and neck cancer, occurring in over 90% of cases. Thus, the term head and neck cancer is most often equated with squamous cell carcinoma.

Estimates provided by the American Cancer Society suggest that more than 48,000 new cases of head and neck cancer were diagnosed in the United States in 2008, and approximately 30% of these patients will die of their disease (Jemal et al., 2008). SCCHN represents approximately 5% of cancers in men and 2% of cancers in women. Even though more than 70% of patients present with disease apparently confined to the head and neck region, 5-year survival rates for whites and blacks are 56% and 34%, respectively, for cancers of the oral cavity and pharynx. Because disease of the larynx tends to become apparent at an earlier stage, 5-year survival rates at this site are slightly better—66% and 53% for whites and blacks, respectively. Squamous cell carcinoma of the aerodigestive tract is directly related to tobacco and alcohol use. Tobacco is the more important of these two substances, but they appear to be synergistic. Individuals who consume substantial quantities of both tobacco and alcohol are 20 times more likely to develop SCCHN than nonusers of these substances (Lewin et al., 1998). The cessation of both alcohol and tobacco consumption is associated with a decreased subsequent risk for all upper aerodigestive neoplasms.

Additional risk factors for cancer of the upper aerodigestive tract include exposure to ionizing radiation and occupational and environmental exposure to carcinogens other than tobacco. For instance, workers involved in plastic fabrication, metal working, and textile processing, as well as individuals occupationally or environmentally exposed to asbestos, show an increased incidence of head and neck cancers. Similarly, nasal and sinus cancers are more common in workers in the furniture industry exposed to the dust of hardwoods. Given that the entire mucosa of the upper aerodigestive tract is exposed in such instances, multicentric lesions are not uncommon and may occur either simultaneously or sequentially. With time, the risk for a second, related cancer can exceed that for direct recurrence of the original tumor. The concept that a focus of cancer is but part of a generally "sick mucosa" is essential to the management of these tumors. The term "field cancerization" is often used to describe this phenomenon.

Viral etiologies are well described in head and neck cancer. Indeed it is accepted now that more than 50% of oropharyngeal cancers are linked to human papillomavirus (HPV) infection, in particular HPV-16. These HPV tumors seem to respond better to treatment than other oropharyngeal cancers and thus have a favorable prognosis (D'Souza et al., 2007; Fakhry et al., 2008). Nasopharyngeal cancer is also linked to Epstein-Barr virus (EBV) and is endemic in various parts of the world.

Histology

EPITHELIAL LESIONS

Two types of premalignant epithelial lesions are recognized based on their clinical appearance: leukoplakia and erythroplasia. Leukoplakia, commonly referred to as smoker's keratosis, is marked by raised, white patches that microscopically represent hyperkeratosis or parakeratosis with varying degrees of atypia and associated mucosal atrophy. The atypia can be graded, in a manner similar to changes seen in the uterine cervix, as mild, moderate, or severe, based on the degree of mucosal involvement by disorderly cells with nuclear abnormalities. There are many causes of leukoplakia. Although the majority of such lesions are innocent and secondary to chronic irritation such as tobacco exposure or dental trauma, 3% to 15% of persistent raised white lesions within the oral cavity and oropharynx represent premalignant dysplastic leukoplakia. Therefore, even leukoplakia on mucous membranes should be considered dysplastic and potentially premalignant until proved otherwise. These lesions always contain some degree of cellular atypia, the severity of which is impossible to determine without biopsy.

Erythroplasia is a mucosal abnormality of greater concern. Visually, the lesions consist of superficial or slightly depressed areas of denuded mucosa where cellular atypia has reached the mucosal surface; they appear red and velvet-like. It should be assumed that they represent at least carcinoma in situ, because over 80% of such lesions at the time of biopsy exhibit pleomorphic squamous cells with full-thickness atypia of the

Table 4.1

Classification of Premalignant and Malignant Epithelial Tumors

Tumor Type	Typical Location
Premalignant Lesions	
Leukoplakia	Floor of mouth
	Ventral and lateral surfaces of tongue
	Buccal space
Erythroplasia	Same as for leukoplakia
Malignant Lesions	
Squamous cell carcinoma	
Well differentiated	All sites, especially oral cavity
Moderately well differentiated	All sites
Poorly differentiated	All sites
Verrucous carcinoma (variant of well differentiated)	Oral cavity
Spindle cell carcinoma*	All sites
Undifferentiated carcinoma (includes lymphoepithelioma)	Nasopharynx and Waldeyer's ring
Nonkeratinizing epithelial carcinoma	Nasopharynx and Waldeyer's ring

*Spindle cell carcinoma is also known as pleomorphic carcinoma, pseudosarcoma, and sarcomatoid squamous cell carcinoma.

Table 4.2

Salivary Gland Tumors and Their Frequency

Type	Location	Type	Frequency (%)
Major	Parotid	Benign	75
		Malignant	25
	Submandibular	Benign	40
		Malignant	60
	Sublingual	Benign	15
		Malignant	85
Minor	Throughout mucous membranes of upper aerodigestive tract	Benign	45
		Malignant	55

Table 4.3

Classification of Malignant Parotid Tumors and Their Frequency

Type	Frequency (%)
Mucoepidermoid carcinoma	29
High grade (26%)	
Low grade (74%)	
Adenocarcinoma	14
Adenoid cystic carcinoma	13
Malignant mixed tumor	13
Undifferentiated carcinoma	11
Squamous cell carcinoma	8
Acinic cell carcinoma	6
Malignant lymphoma	2
Melanoma	<1
Other	3

mucosa. With in situ lesions the basement membrane separating the mucosa from the underlying stroma is intact, but early microinvasion of the basement membrane with extension into the adjacent stroma can also clinically present as erythroplasia. Locations at high risk for erythroplasia include the central floor of the mouth, the ventrolateral surface of the tongue, the buccal mucosa, the anterior tonsillar pillars, and the soft palate.

In the vast majority (90%) of cases, malignant neoplasms of the head and neck arise from the surface epithelium and are therefore squamous cell carcinomas or one of its many variants, including undifferentiated carcinoma, lymphoepithelioma, spindle cell carcinoma, and verrucous carcinoma (Table 4.1). Malignant transformation is accompanied by varying degrees of differentiation of the squamous cells, ranging from well- and moderately well differentiated to poorly differentiated and anaplastic lesions. As a general rule, less differentiated tumors have a higher incidence of infiltration into neighboring glands, muscles, and loose connective tissue, as well as regional spread to lymph nodes of the neck. Bone, cartilage, ligaments, vessels, and nerves, however, offer higher resistance to tumor infiltration. In advanced cancers the morphologic picture may vary considerably in different regions of the lesion. Therefore, surface biopsy specimens may not necessarily represent the entire lesion.

Salivary Gland Tumors

Salivary gland neoplasms may arise from any of the paired major salivary glands—the parotid, submandibular, or sublingual glands—or from one of the many minor salivary glands present throughout the mucosal surfaces of the upper aerodigestive system. These tumors may be benign or malignant, and the probability that a given lesion is malignant varies among sites (Table 4.2). Parotid gland tumors, which are relatively common, are usually benign, pleomorphic adenomas being the most frequently encountered. Other benign salivary tumors

include papillary cystadenoma lymphomatosum (Warthin's tumor or adenolymphoma) and benign lymphoepithelial lesions, such as Godwin's tumor. Malignant parotid tumors are less common, but a spectrum of malignant histologic types may be encountered (Table 4.3). Histologic classification of salivary gland cancers is difficult because of the wide extent of morphologic variation within each tumor type (van der Wal et al., 1998). The same spectrum of benign and malignant histologic types of neoplasms as are found in the parotid gland may be encountered in the other major salivary glands and the minor salivary glands.

Less Frequently Encountered Neoplasms

Esthesioneuroblastomas (olfactory neuroblastomas) arise from the respiratory epithelium about the cribriform plate and nasal septum. They may occur at any age but are most commonly seen in the second and third decades. Histologically, these lesions are composed of rather uniform small blue cells of neuroectodermal origin. They may be confused with undifferentiated carcinoma, undifferentiated lymphoma, or rhabdomyosarcoma. (See also discussions and illustrations of PNET in Chapter 12 and non-CNS PNET in Chapter 16.)

Chemodectomas or non-chromaffin paragangliomas are a group of uncommon, slow-growing neoplasms that may originate wherever glomus bodies are found. Most often they arise from the carotid artery and temporal bone and only rarely from the orbit, nasopharynx, larynx, nasal cavity, paranasal sinuses, tongue, jaw, and trachea. In 10% to 20% of cases, glomus tumors may occur in multiple sites, especially in families with a history of this tumor. The histologic picture of these benign lesions is marked by nests of epithelioid cells within stroma containing thin-walled blood vessels and nonmyelinated nerve fibers; the relative amounts of epithelioid and vascular tissue may vary. The criterion of malignancy is based on the clinical progress of the disease rather than the histologic appearance. Metastases are infrequent (<5% of cases). Endocrine activity has been reported, and serotonin has been identified on histochemical staining, thus confirming the tumor's origin from primitive neuroectodermal cells.

Extramedullary plasmacytomas may occur throughout the body, but 80% of these malignancies are located in the head and neck, most notably in the upper air passages and associated structures: nasopharynx, tonsil, maxillary sinus, nasal vestibule, and trachea. The majority of patients are in their sixth to eighth decades. Up to 25% of patients present with cervical lymph node involvement, and 10% to 40% eventually progress to multiple myeloma. Histologically identical to the osseous form of plasmacytoma, these extramedullary tumors consist of sheets and aggregates of plasma cells.

Inverting papillomas are low-grade neoplasms that are generally considered to be benign. Most frequently affecting the nasal cavity and paranasal sinuses, they are clinically aggressive lesions characterized by extensive bone destruction, intracranial extension, and multiple recurrences. There is an association with squamous cell carcinoma in 10% to 15% of cases. The histologic picture is that of a papilloma that is growing into the stroma rather than outward.

Mucosal melanomas of the head and neck represent 0.5% to 2% of all malignant melanomas. The most common location within the head and neck is the nasal cavity, where melanomas represent up to 18% of all malignant tumors. Though varying in their gross appearance, they are usually solid, polypoid lesions about 3.5 cm in diameter. Approximately one third are amelanotic. The histologic picture is similar to that of cutaneous melanoma, although lymphocytic infiltration is rare.

Midline lethal nonhealing granuloma is a nonspecific term encompassing a variety of histologic and clinical entities that lead to progressive destruction of the nose, paranasal sinuses, hard palate, and contiguous structures. Midline lethal granuloma has been subdivided into three different entities: midline malignant (polymorphic) reticulosis, malignant lymphoma (usually diffuse large cell lymphoma), and Wegener's granulomatosis. (See "Staging of Head and Neck Cancers" and "Clinical Manifestations.")

Molecular Biology

The molecular biology of head and neck cancers has not been defined systematically except for lesions arising from squamous epithelium. Efforts are being made to determine the genetic events associated with, and perhaps responsible for, the conversion of normal squamous epithelium to dysplastic leukoplakia or erythroplasia, to carcinoma in situ, and finally, to invasive cancer. These studies attempt to define environmental and genetic differences between patients with isolated mucosal lesions and those with multiple neoplastic abnormalities, so-called "field carcinogenesis." Related studies are in progress to define the incidence of known oncogenes and tumor suppressor genes in invasive epithelial tumors and to determine their influence on clinical events such as tumor growth rate, potential for metastatic spread, response to therapy, and prognosis after treatment.

The most commonly deleted chromosomal region in SCCHN is 9p21. This region encodes the tumor suppressor p16 (INK4A/MTS-1/CDKN2A), a cyclin-dependent kinase inhibitor (Reed et al., 1996). The loss of p16 is seen early in the evolution of SCCHN, suggesting it may play a part in the early carcinogenic process. Additionally, mutations of the tumor suppressor gene TP53 are also common both in malignant and premalignant mucosal lesions of the head and neck, as well as the histologically normal mucosa of patients with treated squamous cell cancers of the oral cavity and oropharynx (Boyle et al., 1993).

Mutations of TP53 within invasive head and neck squamous carcinomas are frequent. Loss of p53 function due to mutations results in a progression from premalignant lesions to invasive cancer, and approximately half of all SCCHNs contain a mutation of the TP53 gene located at 17p13. Gene amplifications of known oncogenes, though less frequently encountered than TP53 mutations, have also been associated with a poor prognosis.

Cytogenetic evidence for genetic instability and gene amplification of DNA markers on chromosome 11 band q13 has been identified in many invasive head and neck cancers. Moreover, the presence of 11q13 rearrangements has been associated with poor clinical outcome and younger patient age at presentation. This is of interest, in that amplification of several oncogenes located in 11q13, such as int-2, bcl-1, prad-1, and cyclin D1, has been reported in this cancer. Amplification of cyclin D1 in particular has been identified in up to 20% of head and neck cancers and is independently associated with tobacco exposure and poor prognosis (Jares et al., 1994).

Several studies have reported overexpression of epidermal growth factor receptor (EGFR) and transforming growth factor α in many invasive head and neck squamous cancers. These findings suggest growth stimulation in these tumors by autocrine or paracrine mechanisms, and overexpression of EGFR family members is associated with a worse prognosis (Todd and Wong, 1999; Almadori et al., 1999). EGFR inhibitors have been developed and are used in treating head and neck cancer. Whereas tobacco and alcohol environmentally induce the majority of head and neck cancers, viral infection has been suggested as contributory in many patients. HPV-16 has been detected by polymerase chain reaction in more than 50% of oropharyngeal cancers (D'Souza et al., 2007; Fakhry et al., 2008). The molecular profile of HPV-positive tumors is different from the HPV-negative tumors, reflecting what is probably a different disease. EBV DNA has similarly been detected in most nasopharyngeal carcinomas and in some non-nasopharyngeal squamous head and neck cancers (Raab-Traub et al., 1987; Kieff, 1995). In addition, human herpesvirus 6, previously isolated from patients with lymphoproliferative disorders and acquired immunodeficiency syndrome, can be detected in up to 80% of oral SCCHNs (Yadav et al., 1997). Oral carcinogenesis is probably a multistep process with a multifactorial etiology. Some oncogenic viruses, perhaps acting synergistically with chemical carcinogens and a patient's underlying genetic predisposition, could facilitate the transformation process to carcinoma.

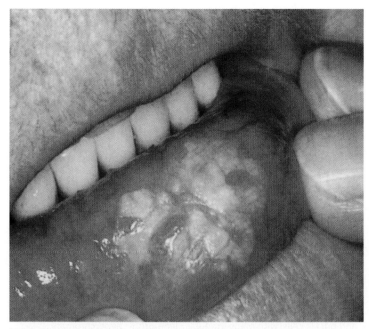

FIGURE 4.1 LEUKOPLAKIA. Also known as smoker's keratosis, this premalignant tumor is marked by extensive, irregular, white thickening or plaques. The woman shown here habitually allowed cigarettes to burn down to the end against her lip. A carcinoma subsequently developed in this area.

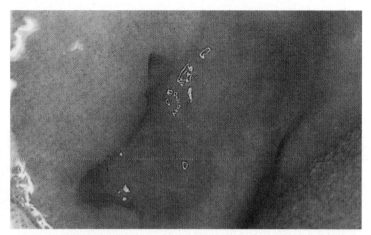

FIGURE 4.2 ERYTHROPLASIA. An extensive red lesion of the buccal mucosa lies either level with or depressed below the surface of the surrounding epithelium due to atrophy of the overlying tissue layers. Biopsy showed severe dysplasia.

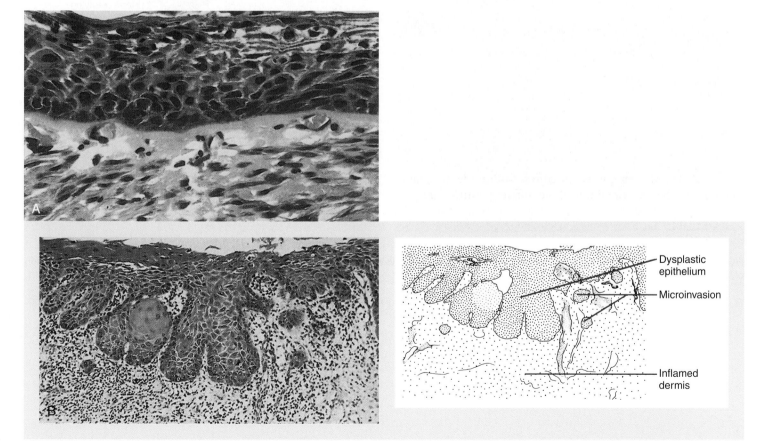

FIGURE 4.3 The microscopic presentation of this lesion is variable, ranging from **(A)** maturation disarray of the mucosal surface with complete disorder of the squamous cells (dysplasia of atrophic epithelium) to **(B)** early finger-like extension into the underlying stroma (microinvasion or early carcinoma in situ).

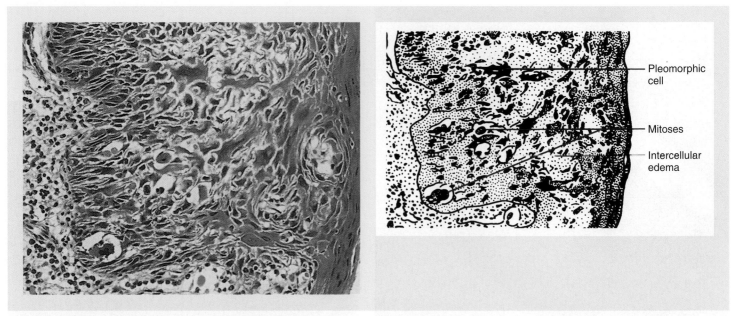

FIGURE 4.4 **SEVERE DYSPLASIA.** There is total loss of differentiation between basal and prickle cells, with many irregular pleomorphic hyperchromatic, including giant, nuclei. The dysplastic changes are confined to the epithelium, which is completely disorganized. Because there is no invasion, this appearance can also be called carcinoma in situ.

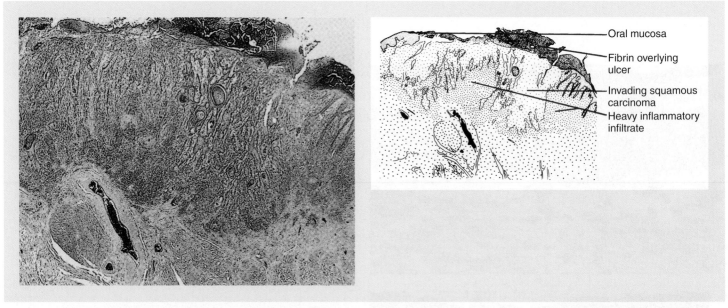

FIGURE 4.5 **SQUAMOUS CELL CARCINOMA.** Low-power microscopic section shows an early invasive lesion of the lip. Note the epithelial proliferation and invasion of the underlying tissue by strands and islands of tumor cells.

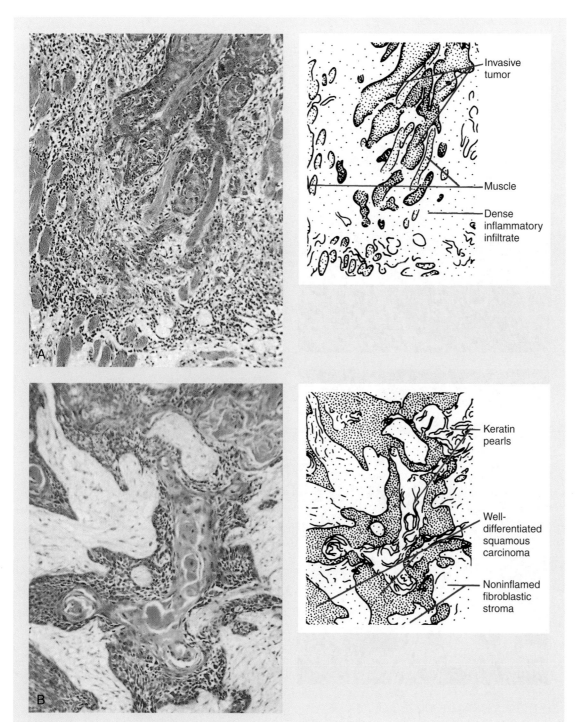

FIGURE 4.6 **SQUAMOUS CELL CARCINOMA.** These well-differentiated tumors demonstrate the variable stromal response that may be encountered, ranging from **(A)** a heavy, chronic inflammatory infiltrate surrounding the invasive tumor to **(B)** an inflammation-free stroma marked by fibroblastic proliferation. Note the presence of numerous keratin pearls.

Invasive tumor

Muscle

Dense inflammatory infiltrate

Keratin pearls

Well-differentiated squamous carcinoma

Noninflamed fibroblastic stroma

FIGURE 4.7 **SQUAMOUS CELL CARCINOMA.** In moderately well differentiated tumors **(A)** individual cell keratinization may be present; in this instance the stroma also shows a heavy inflammatory infiltrate. **(B)** A moderately high mitotic rate is a common feature. In this section there is no evidence of keratinization or an inflammatory response.

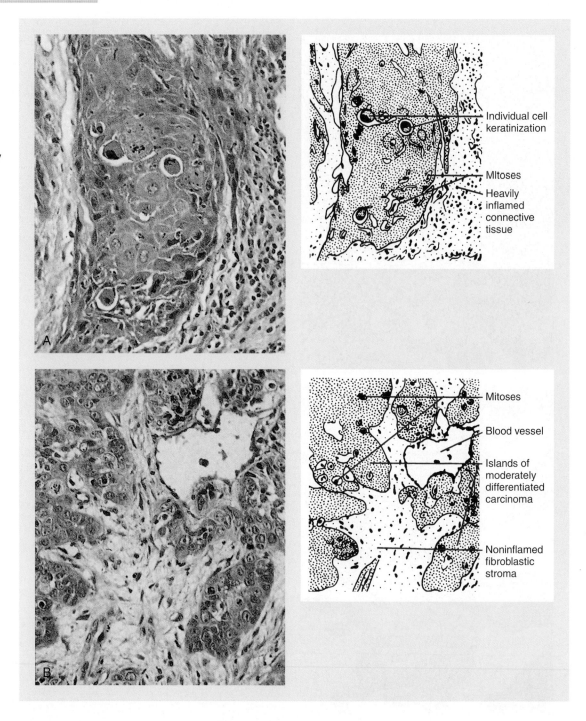

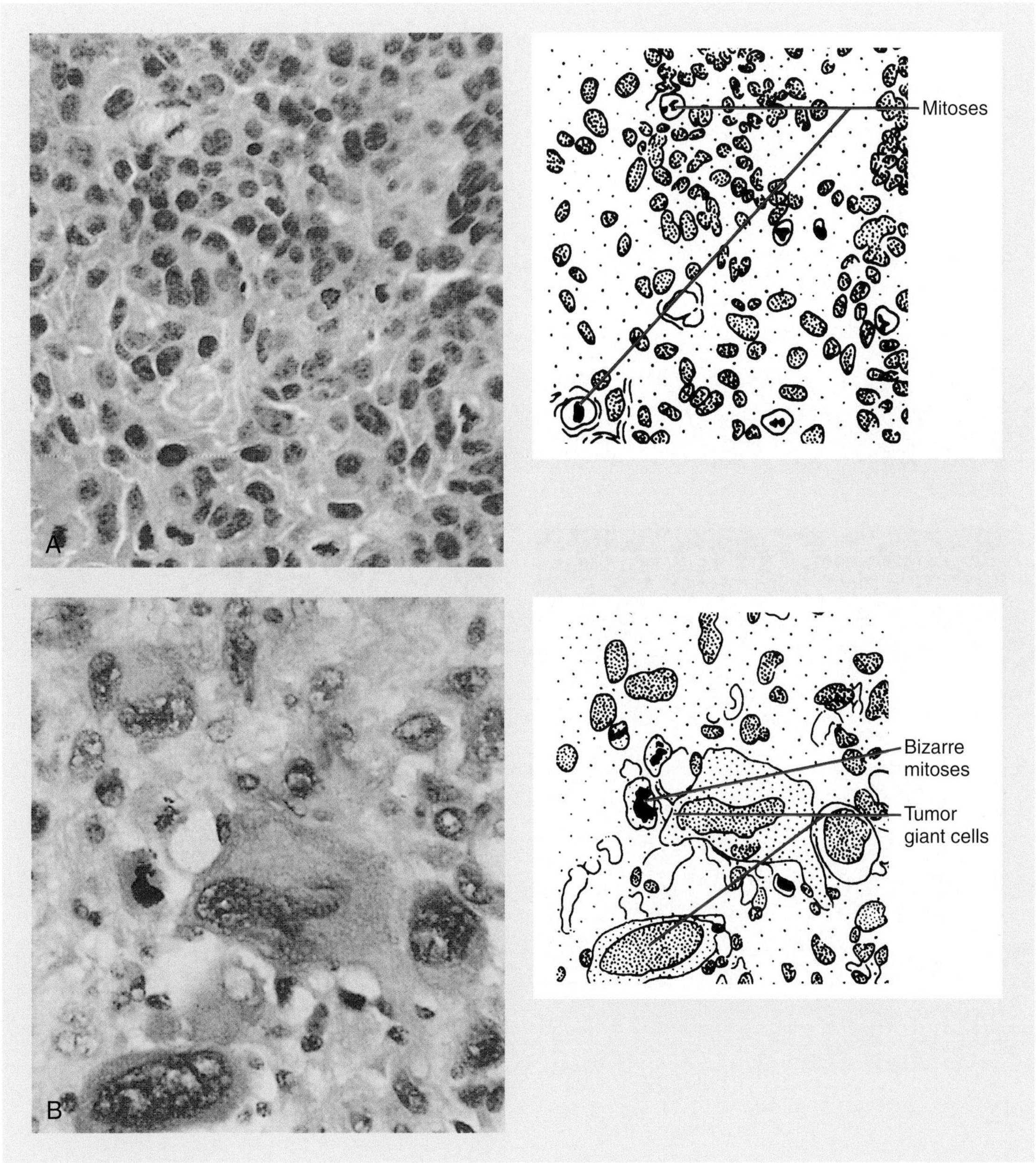

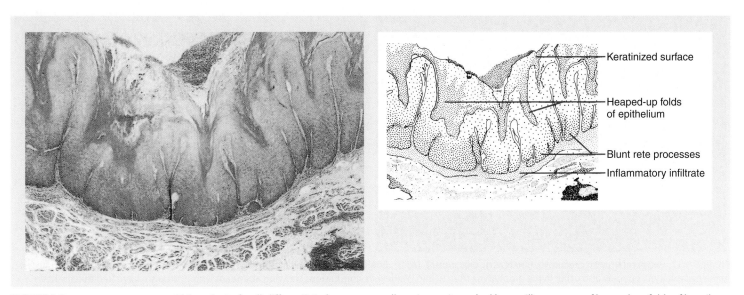

FIGURE 4.8 **SQUAMOUS CELL CARCINOMA.** Poorly differentiated tumors are marked by **(A)** sheets of immature cells and no evidence of keratinization. **(B)** Neoplastic cells show extreme degrees of pleomorphism, often with bizarre mitoses. Tumor giant cells may also be observed.

FIGURE 4.9 **VERRUCOUS CARCINOMA.** This variant of well-differentiated squamous cell carcinoma is marked by papillary masses of heaped-up folds of heavily keratinized epithelium separated by deep cleftlike spaces. The advancing edge of the lesion consists of blunt rete ridges forming a characteristic "pushing margin." An intact basement membrane makes this by definition an in situ lesion. Below the tumor is a dense chronic inflammatory infiltrate.

FIGURE 4.10 SPINDLE CELL CARCINOMA. (A) Low-power photomicrograph shows sheets of neoplastic cells arising from dysplastic epithelium. **(B)** At high power, the lesion is composed of uniform spindle-shaped cells. This variant of a poorly differentiated carcinoma is also referred to as a pleomorphic carcinoma, pseudocarcinoma, or sarcomatoid squamous cell carcinoma. Its reputation as "radiation resistant" is probably unfounded; its natural history is that of a poorly differentiated squamous cell carcinoma.

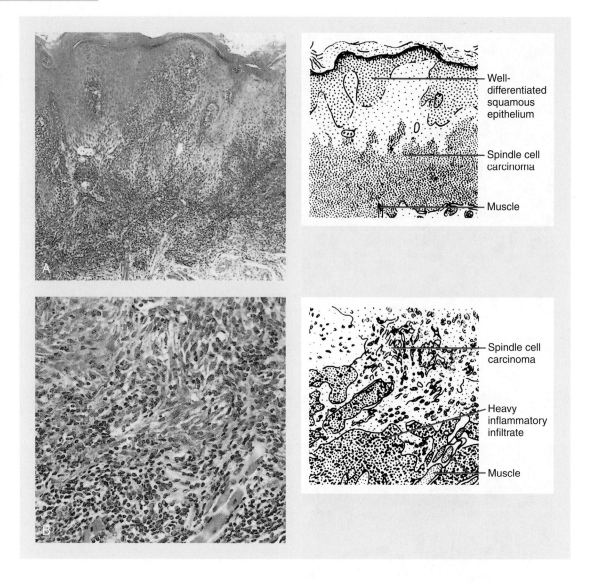

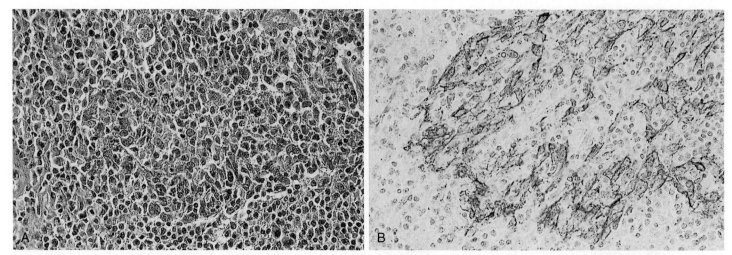

FIGURE 4.11 UNDIFFERENTIATED CARCINOMA (ANAPLASTIC CARCINOMA). (A) Undifferentiated epithelial tumors of the head and neck are frequently encountered in the nasopharynx but may also occur in the oropharynx from within Waldeyer's ring. Lesions showing abundant lymphotropism have traditionally been referred to as lymphoepitheliomas, whereas similar lesions without lymphocytes are designated as anaplastic carcinomas. **(B)** Positive immunoperoxidase staining for keratin confirms the epithelial origin of the tumor.

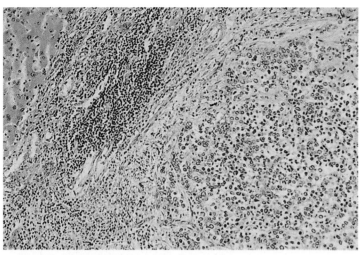

FIGURE 4.12 **UNDIFFERENTIATED CARCINOMA (LYMPHOEPITHELIOMA).** This metastatic lesion in the liver, composed of undifferentiated epithelial cells and numerous small lymphocytes, is identical to that of the primary tumor. Its lymphotropism is remarkable and supports the contention that a lymphoepithelioma of the nasopharynx is more than an undifferentiated carcinoma passively infiltrating neighboring lymphoid tissue.

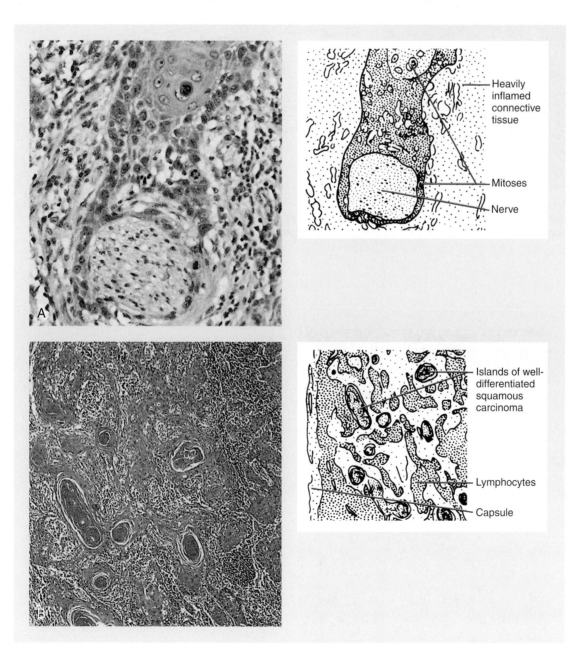

FIGURE 4.13 **SQUAMOUS CELL CARCINOMA.** These tumors are locally aggressive lesions, frequently invading **(A)** regional nerves, blood vessels, or **(B)** lymphatic channels. Perineural invasion by tumor accounts for the rare pattern of relapse along the course of an invaded nerve proximal to the site of the original lesion.

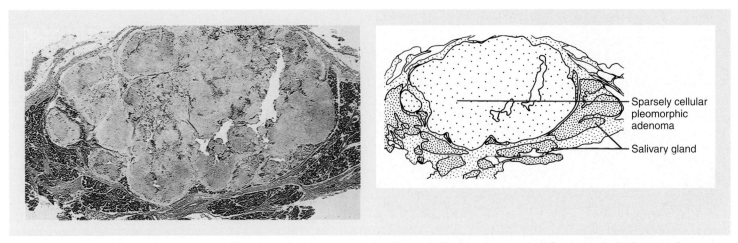

FIGURE 4.14 PLEOMORPHIC ADENOMA. Low-magnification section shows a sparsely cellular, ovoid mass with a poorly defined capsule displacing and compressing adjacent normal gland tissue.

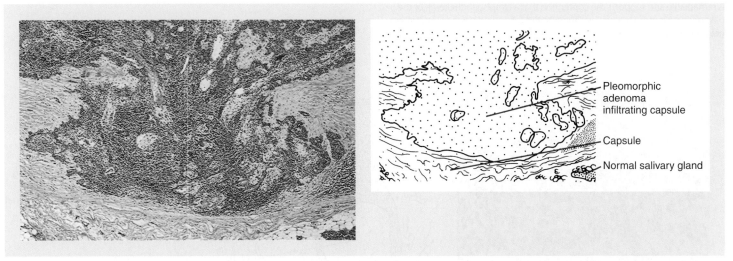

FIGURE 4.15 PLEOMORPHIC ADENOMA. Extracapsular invasion is a common feature of this tumor and is not inconsistent with benign behavior. However, this tendency accounts for the high frequency (at least 20% of cases) of local recurrence of this slow-growing lesion following simple enucleation or excision without wide surgical margins.

FIGURE 4.16 PLEOMORPHIC ADENOMA. Strands of epithelium and individual cells in a myxoid stroma are very common in these tumors. Other morphologic variants include areas of cartilage-like tissue, double-layered ductlike structures, and spindle cells; the latter are probably the result of the proliferation of myoepithelial cells.

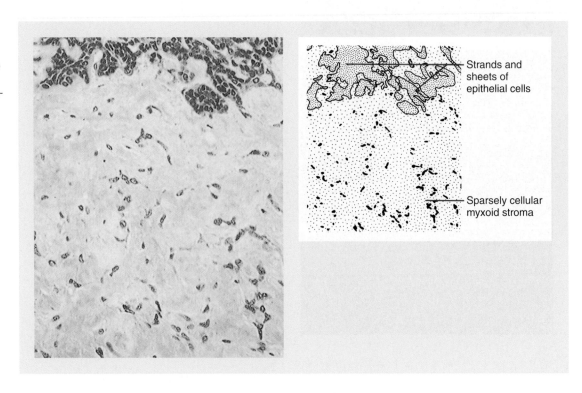

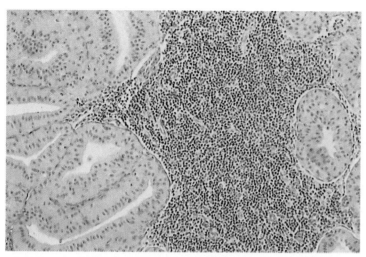

FIGURE 4.17 PAPILLARY CYSTADENOMA LYMPHOMATOSUM (WARTHIN'S TUMOR).
Microscopically, both epithelial and lymphoid elements are present in this
benign lesion, which probably arises from ductal inclusions in intra- or
periparotid lymph nodes. Epithelial cells form tubules, cysts, and solid nests
that are arranged in a characteristic double layer. The lymphoid component
represents lymph node. Accounting for 5% to 10% of all parotid neoplasms,
it occurs predominantly in the tail of the gland in older men. In about 10%
of cases it is bilateral and may be multiple in one or both sides. Recurrence is
rare after excision.

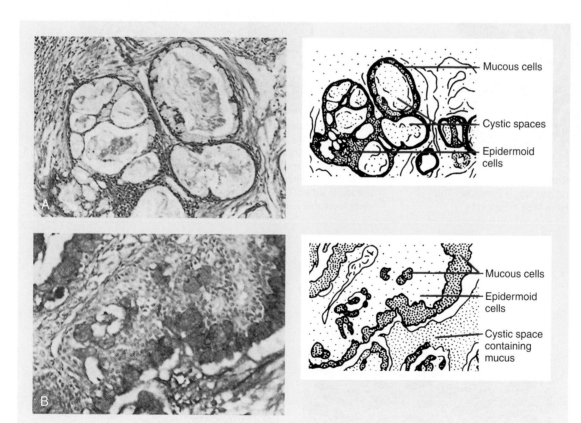

**FIGURE 4.18 MUCOEPIDERMOID
CARCINOMA. (A)** Tumors of
low-grade malignancy consist
predominantly of mucous and
epidermoid cells, as seen here
forming well-defined microcysts
in a fibrous stroma. **(B)** The
mucous cells are obvious with
periodic acid–Schiff staining.
Although these tumors are
generally well circumscribed
(and thus readily cured by
wide excision), in this instance
there is little or no capsule
about the lesion. Occasionally,
mucoepidermoid tumors act
aggressively, widely infiltrating
the normal gland or becoming
fixed to skin. Cervical metastases
are rare.

FIGURE 4.19 MUCOEPIDERMOID CARCINOMA. Squamoid (epidermoid) cells can be seen lining a cyst. Intercellular bridges and keratin pearl formation may also be present, although they are not readily evident here. Mucus-secreting cells also line the cyst where their secretions are discharged.

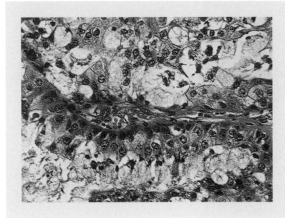
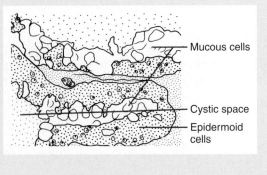

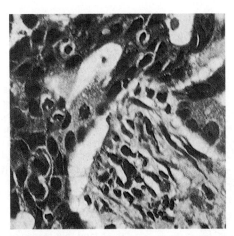

FIGURE 4.20 ADENOCARCINOMA OF PAROTID GLAND. The infiltrative growth pattern of this tumor is marked by gland and tubule formation. This moderately well differentiated tumor has a brisk mitotic rate.

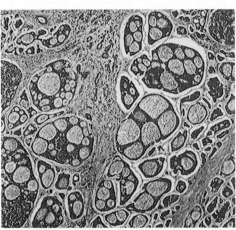

FIGURE 4.21 ADENOID CYSTIC CARCINOMA. This neoplasm is relatively uncommon in the parotid gland, but it is the most common malignant tumor of the submandibular and sublingual glands and the minor salivary glands. It is composed of small, dark-staining myoepithelial cells and cells resembling the lining of normal ducts arranged around cystic spaces. Lesions with a predominance of the cribriform pattern, as shown here, appear to have a more favorable natural history.

FIGURE 4.22 ADENOID CYSTIC CARCINOMA. A variant histologic presentation shows solid masses of cells, often with central necrosis. The absence of a predominant cribriform pattern in this instance suggests a less favorable natural history than that for the tumor shown in Figure 4.21.

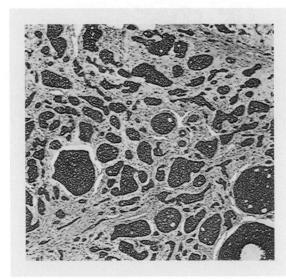
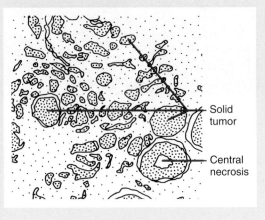

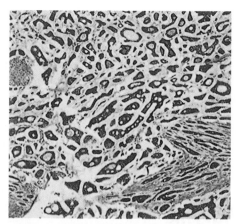

FIGURE 4.23 **ADENOID CYSTIC CARCINOMA.** Perineural and intraneural spread is typical of this tumor.

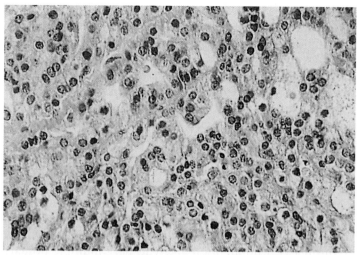

FIGURE 4.25 **ACINIC CELL CARCINOMA.** This slow-growing, low-grade variant of a well-differentiated adenocarcinoma arises from the terminal acinus of a salivary duct. Note the groups of closely packed cells with clear or finely granular cytoplasm and small nuclei.

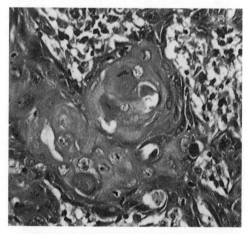

FIGURE 4.24 **SQUAMOUS CELL CARCINOMA OF PAROTID GLAND.** The absence of mucus and the abundance of keratin characterize this well-differentiated tumor. A rare salivary lesion, squamous cell carcinoma probably arises from salivary ducts, a Warthin's tumor, or a lymphoepithelial lesion. It tends to recur locally or in regional lymph nodes (70% of cases); distant metastases are rare.

Staging of Head and Neck Cancers

Tumors of the head and neck are staged according to a site-specific TNM system (see Figs. 4.26, 4.27, 4.28) (Greene et al., 2002). The multiple TNM combinations are ultimately grouped into four stages (Table 4.4), each having a progressively lower survival rate. At best, this anatomically dependent system provides a rapid estimate of a patient's prognosis, facilitates the formation of a treatment plan, and assures the uniform reporting of treatment outcomes. Unfortunately, TNM staging is complex, and the concordance in staging between any two physicians is low. The greatest utility of this imperfect measure of disease potential is restricted to the definition of patients with limited lesions and a good prognosis.

Recommended staging procedures for determining a patient's TNM classification include direct and indirect (mirror or fiberoptic) inspection and palpation of all accessible mucosal surfaces in the head and neck and radiologic investigation. Radiographs or radionuclide scanning of the mandible may be appropriate in selected cases; however, computed tomography (CT) or magnetic resonance imaging (MRI) is standard for exact anatomic localization of primary lesions and facilitates quantification of regional lymph node involvement and parapharyngeal spread of disease. In addition, CT scanning and MRI may be helpful in identifying the site of an occult primary lesion in patients with a solitary neck mass.

Table 4.4

Stage Grouping for Cancer of the Head and Neck Sites Excluding Nasopharynx

Stage	T (Primary Tumor)	N (Regional Nodes)	M (Metastases)
0	Tis	N0	M0
I	T1	N0	M0
II	T2	N0	M0
III	T3	N0	M0
	T1, T2, or T3	N1	M0
IV	T1, T2, or T3	N2 or N3	M0
	T4	Any N	M0
	Any T	Any N	M1

Greene F, Page D, Fleming I, et al, editors, for the American Joint Committee on Cancer: *AJCC cancer staging manual*, ed 6, New York, 2002, Springer.

There is considerable debate about the necessity for "triple endoscopy" in staging patients with head and neck cancers. The addition of bronchoscopy and esophagoscopy to direct laryngoscopy may be appropriate for patients with tumors of the oropharynx, hypopharynx, or larynx that are inadequately evaluated by indirect means. The time, risk, and expense of these additional procedures are negligible given the incidence (as high as 5% in some series) for multiple synchronous primary tumors of the head and neck, lung, and esophagus. On the other hand, the value of triple endoscopy remains controversial in most patients with localized lesions of the oral cavity that can adequately be staged by indirect, noninvasive means (Forastiere et al., 1998). Triple endoscopy is particularly important for patients with intraoral lesions associated with diffuse mucosal abnormalities such as leukoplakia or erythroplasia, who are more likely to have multiple primary tumors.

Clinical Manifestations

The clinical manifestations and natural history of head and neck cancers depend on the site from which they arise. Thus, considerable variability exists and certain characteristic features for the several primary anatomic locations are discussed separately.

Occasionally, patients present with solitary, asymptomatic cervical adenopathy, usually in the upper neck. The primary cancer may be asymptomatic but will usually be discovered on a detailed head and neck examination. Pain may be the first manifestation, usually representing more locally advanced disease. Surprisingly, some patients have large lesions that cause minimal, if any, symptoms.

Lips

Cancer of the lips accounts for 15% of all head and neck cancers. In 95% of cases, the lesion occurs on the lower lip and may involve the vermilion and mucosal surfaces. It typically presents as a recurrent scab or a persistent or slow-growing sore, blister, or ulcer. Because of its location, it is discovered early and lymphatic spread of squamous cell carcinoma to submental and submaxillary lymph nodes occurs in only 5% to 10% of patients. The approximate 5-year survival after standard treatment is greater than 90% for all stages, because most lesions are quite limited. Survival falls to 65% for patients with locally advanced lesions of the upper lip or with regional adenopathy.

Oral Cavity

The oral cavity encompasses the floor of the mouth, oral tongue, buccal mucosa, gingiva, retromolar trigone, and hard palate. Cancers involving these structures account for 20% of all head and neck malignancies. Typically, cancers of the oral cavity present as asymptomatic lesions noted on routine dental examination, as painful ulcers with or without referred otalgia or in association with ill-fitting dentures, difficulty in swallowing or chewing, or altered speech. The principal sites of involvement are the ventrolateral surface of the tongue and the floor of the mouth. In as many as 40% of patients, adenopathy may be present in the upper jugular and submandibular lymph nodes. Carcinomas of the middle and posterior thirds of the mobile tongue have the greatest metastatic potential.

Nasopharynx

Cancers of the nasopharynx are unique in their histology (frequently an undifferentiated or nonkeratinizing epithelial cancer), biology, and epidemiology. They are minimally associated with tobacco use but are 25 times more prevalent in patients of southern Chinese descent. The EBV serum titer is typically elevated, and molecular biologic techniques reveal EBV incorporation into the genome in the majority of tumors. These lesions occur in a younger population than patients with SCCHN at other sites and are best known for their propensity for early spread to regional and distant sites and their relative sensitivity to chemotherapy and radiation therapy.

Nasopharyngeal cancers of epithelial origin typically arise from the lateral pharyngeal wall adjacent to the orifice of the eustachian tube. Cancers similar to those of the nasopharynx may occur in other areas of Waldeyer's ring (a ring of lymphoid tissue encircling the nasopharynx and oropharynx). Although many of these lesions are asymptomatic and found incidentally during evaluation of an upper neck mass of unknown origin, limited lesions may present in association with epistaxis, nasal obstruction, or unilateral hearing loss due to eustachian tube obstruction. More advanced lesions may present with headache, direct osseous involvement of the parasphenoid region, or multiple cranial neuropathies due to tumor extension behind the sphenoid (cranial nerves II through VI) or along the base of the skull about the hypoglossal foramen (cranial nerves XI and XII). The metastatic potential of these lesions is well known. Malignant adenopathy involving the retropharynx and lateral pharyngeal wall is present in 80% of patients at presentation. Bilateral adenopathy is common, and involvement of the posterior cervical chain is characteristic.

Table 4.5			
Stage Grouping for Nasopharyngeal Cancer			
Stage	**T (Primary Tumor)**	**N (Regional Nodes)**	**M (Metastases)**
0	Tis	N0	M0
I	T1	N0	M0
IIA	T2a	N0	M0
IIB	T1, T2a, or T2b	N1	M0
	T2b	N0	M0
III	T1, T2a, or T2b	N2	M0
	T3	N0, N1 or N2	M0
IVA	T4	N0, N1, or N2	M0
IVB	Any T	N3	M0
IVC	Any T	Any N	M1

The nasopharynx may also be involved in nonepithelial malignancies, including sarcomas, minor salivary gland carcinomas, esthesioneuroblastomas, or other neuroectodermal lesions, and unusual tumors such as angiofibromas. Presenting features may mimic those of the more common squamous cell carcinoma, and adequate biopsy specimens must therefore be obtained in all cases.

Oropharynx

Accounting for 10% of all head and neck malignancies, oropharyngeal cancers may involve the tonsillar fossa or pillars, soft palate, base of the tongue, or lateral or posterior pharyngeal wall. They may be clinically silent until they present as advanced tumors with local pain, odynophagia, dysphagia, referred otalgia, or trismus. Tonsillar and base-of-tongue carcinomas have the greatest metastatic potential, with upper jugular (subdigastric or jugulodigastric) lymphadenopathy present in up to 70% of cases. These areas therefore require careful visual inspection and digital palpation during evaluation of a patient with either pharyngeal symptoms consistent with carcinoma or an upper neck mass of unknown origin. CT scanning is standard for tumors presenting at this site.

The oropharynx is rich in lymphatic tissue belonging to Waldeyer's ring. Occasionally, primary Waldeyer's ring lymphomas arise, typically non-Hodgkin's lymphomas of the diffuse large cell type. These tumors are often difficult to distinguish from epithelial tumors on clinical grounds. After histologic and immunologic confirmation, staging procedures for a Waldeyer's ring lymphoma should include bone marrow aspiration and biopsy; CT scan of the chest, abdomen, and pelvis; and, given the high incidence of concurrent gastric involvement, radiographic or endoscopic visualization of the stomach.

Hypopharynx

Hypopharyngeal carcinomas, which occur primarily in the pyriform sinus, account for 5% of head and neck cancers. At presentation patients typically have locally advanced lesions, with odynophagia, dysphagia, referred otalgia, or evidence of laryngeal involvement, including cough, hoarseness, or repeated aspirations. Hypopharyngeal cancers are biologically aggressive; metastases to retropharyngeal or midjugular lymph nodes are common (up to 80% of patients). The 5-year survival of patients with hypopharyngeal carcinomas is reported to be as low as 20% to 30%.

Larynx

Cancers of the larynx, which may arise from the supraglottic, glottic, or subglottic larynx, are the most frequently encountered head and neck cancers in the United States, accounting for 33% of cases. They affect men more commonly than women, most often in the sixth and seventh decades. Chronic inflammation and cigarette smoking are known risk factors. Hoarseness is

the most common presenting symptom, but otalgia, dysphagia, or odynophagia may occur. The natural history of these lesions is variable.

The supraglottic structures include the epiglottis, the arytenoid cartilage, the aryepiglottic folds, and the false vocal cords, all of which are rich in lymphatic channels. Tumors of the supraglottic larynx present late in comparison with other laryngeal tumors and are associated with malignant middle or upper jugular adenopathy in 40% of patients. The glottis, on the other hand, which is rich in elastic tissue, has few lymphatic channels and nodal metastases are rare (<5% of cases) with either limited or advanced primary lesions. Glottic carcinomas arise from the true vocal cords, which anatomically represent a modified tracheal ring. These tumors tend to be well-differentiated lesions presenting early because of hoarseness or a change in voice. Subglottic carcinomas, the least common tumors of the larynx, are essentially tracheal lesions that arise immediately beneath the true vocal cords. They commonly present with hemoptysis, change in voice, or dyspnea. Lymph node metastases to the low neck or retrosternal region are occasionally present in patients with limited lesions, but they may be found in up to 40% of patients with advanced tumors.

Nasal Cavity and Paranasal Sinuses

Squamous cell carcinomas of the nasal cavity and paranasal sinuses are uncommon, constituting less than 5% of head and neck cancers. Sarcomas, plasmacytomas, lymphomas, minor salivary gland carcinomas, and esthesioneuroblastomas may also occur at these sites, as well as histologically benign lesions, such as mucoceles and inverted papillomas that mimic carcinomas. The maxillary antrum is the most frequently involved location within the paranasal sinuses. Tumors at this site typically present with signs and symptoms suggesting inflammatory sinusitis, such as local pain and tenderness, toothache, nasal discharge, or nasal obstruction. Evidence for more invasive disease would include looseness of teeth, ill-fitting dentures, visual disturbances or proptosis, ulcerations of the hard or soft palate, or cheek swelling. Lymph node involvement is present in 15% of patients, a relatively low percentage given the aggressiveness of many primary lesions.

Major and Minor Salivary Glands

Tumors of the parotid, submandibular, and sublingual glands account for 3% to 4% of all head and neck neoplasms. About 80% of major salivary gland lesions occur in the parotid, but the majority of these tumors are benign. In contradistinction are the tumors of the minor salivary glands. Though less common than tumors of the parotid, the majority of these tumors are malignant. Most malignant tumors present as painless masses. With time, local pain, referred pain along the path of an adjacent nerve, or nerve palsy may develop. The latter symptom strongly suggests malignancy.

Malignant salivary gland tumors are heterogeneous in their tendency to infiltrate neighboring tissues and to spread to regional lymph nodes or distant sites. High-grade tumors frequently metastasize to the neck or distantly. For example, up to 25% of patients with salivary adenocarcinomas, which are aggressive tumors, have clinical (20%) or occult (5%) lymph node metastases at presentation. In patients with adenoid cystic carcinomas, metastases to regional nodes are much less common than distant metastases, which may develop in up to 75% of cases. Perineural involvement is a characteristic finding with these tumors, leading to infiltration along nerve trunks; in the case of parotid lesions, facial nerve paralysis may be present at the time of presentation. In patients with slow-growing tumors, adenoid cystic carcinomas may recur months to years after primary treatment. Similarly, acinic cell carcinomas, which microscopically invade contiguous bone, nerve, skin, and blood vessels, are known to recur locally in up to 35% of cases following inadequate excision; relapse may occur as long as 25–30 years after initial treatment.

Minor salivary gland tumors are uncommon, accounting for less than 2% of malignant tumors of the head and neck. They may occur anywhere throughout the upper aerodigestive system, but they are typically located in the oral cavity, nasal cavity, and paranasal sinuses. Benign mixed tumors are the most common benign lesions, and adenoid cystic carcinomas account for two thirds of malignant minor salivary gland tumors. Although presenting symptoms depend on the site of origin and local extension, they are usually those of a mass lesion.

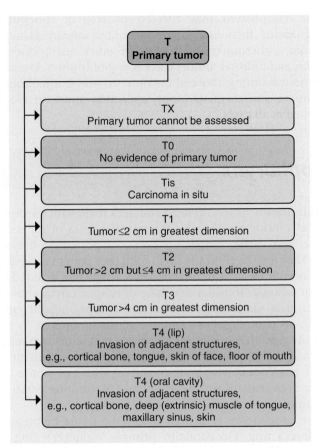

FIGURE 4.26 T categories for cancer of the lip and oral cavity (Greene F, Page D, Fleming I, et al, editors, for the American Joint Committee on Cancer: *AJCC cancer staging manual*, ed 6, New York, 2002, Springer.)

FIGURE 4.27 N and M categories for cancer of the head and neck sites, including the lip and oral cavity, pharynx, larynx, paranasal sinuses, and major and minor salivary glands. For nasopharynx, see Figure 4.28 (Greene F, Page D, Fleming I, et al, editors, for the American Joint Committee on Cancer: *AJCC cancer staging manual*, ed 6, New York, 2002, Springer.)

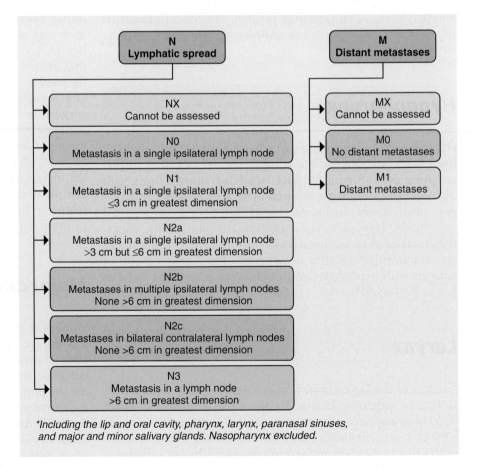

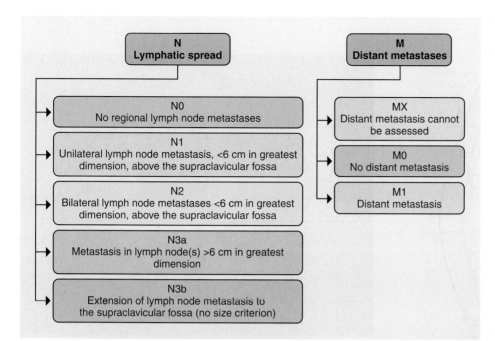

FIGURE 4.28 N and M categories for nasopharyngeal cancer (Greene F, Page D, Fleming I, et al, editors, for the American Joint Committee on Cancer: *AJCC cancer staging manual*, ed 6, New York, 2002, Springer.)

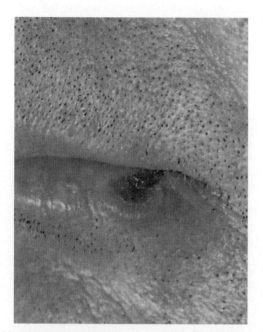

FIGURE 4.29 **SQUAMOUS CELL CARCINOMA.** A central ulcer with an indurated margin is present on the lower lip.

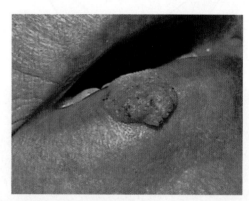

FIGURE 4.31 **SQUAMOUS CELL CARCINOMA.** Although this lesion has a white surface at the rim, it is heaped up and forms an ulcerated nodule.

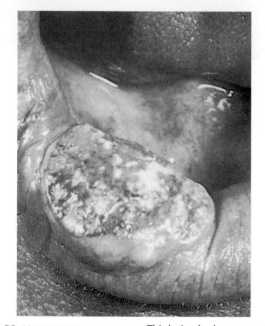

FIGURE 4.30 **SQUAMOUS CELL CARCINOMA.** This lesion had a warty, crusted surface, but the base was firm and suspicious for malignant disease.

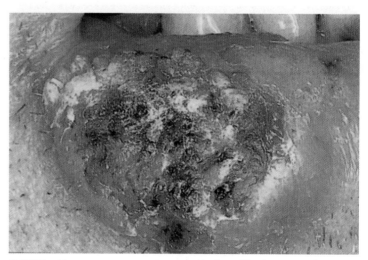

FIGURE 4.32 **SQUAMOUS CELL CARCINOMA.** Neglected by the patient for about a year, this advanced lesion shows the typical thickened, rolled edge and necrotic, scabbing floor.

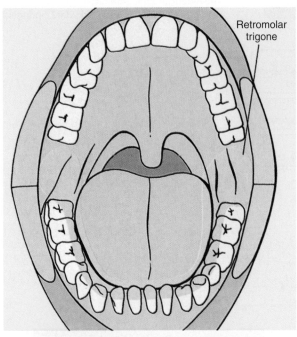

FIGURE 4.33 **INTRAORAL CARCINOMA.** The majority of intraoral tumors are concentrated in the relatively small "drainage" areas (*highlighted in blue*) where saliva pools.

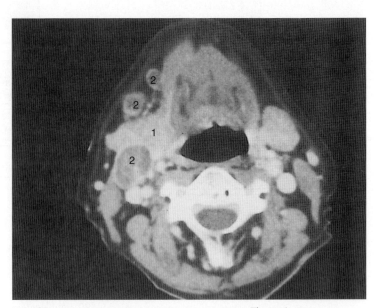

FIGURE 4.36 **SQUAMOUS CELL CARCINOMA OF TONGUE.** The patient was a 57-year-old man who presented with tongue swelling. This contrast-enhanced CT scan reveals extension of the tumor mass into (1) the submandibular region and several lymph nodes (2). The size and peripheral enhancement of the nodes suggest metastatic spread. Surgery confirmed the latter.

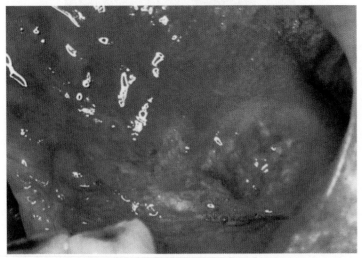

FIGURE 4.34 **SQUAMOUS CELL CARCINOMA OF TONGUE.** Located on the lateral border of the tongue, as is common with these tumors, this nodular lesion was painless despite its being a well-established invasive tumor.

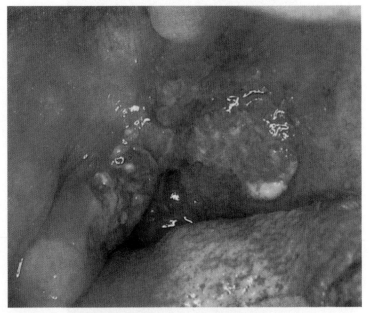

FIGURE 4.37 **SQUAMOUS CELL CARCINOMA OF RETROMOLAR REGION AND SOFT PALATE.** The lesion on the alveolar ridge shows the typical features of a malignant ulcer, but that of the soft palate appears only as a white patch.

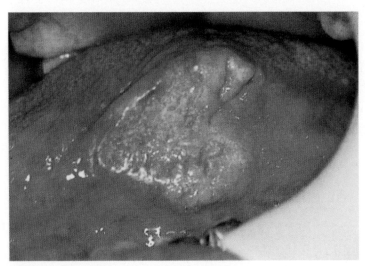

FIGURE 4.35 **SQUAMOUS CELL CARCINOMA OF TONGUE.** This more advanced lesion shows the classic but late features of this malignancy, namely raised, rolled margins and a granulating floor.

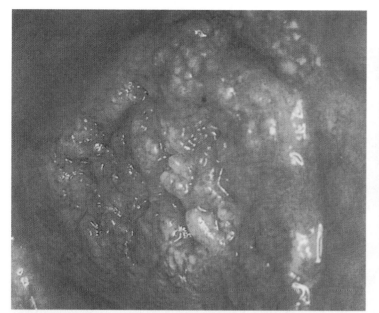

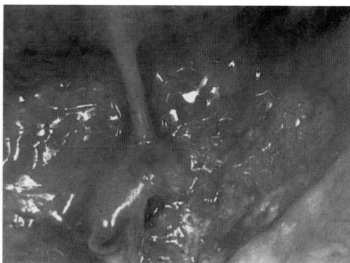

FIGURE 4.40 **SQUAMOUS CELL CARCINOMA OF FLOOR OF MOUTH.** This typical malignant ulcer erodes the base of the lingual frenulum.

FIGURE 4.38 **SQUAMOUS CELL CARCINOMA OF BUCCAL MUCOSA.** The characteristic features of an extensive malignant ulcer, in particular the rough granulating floor, are apparent.

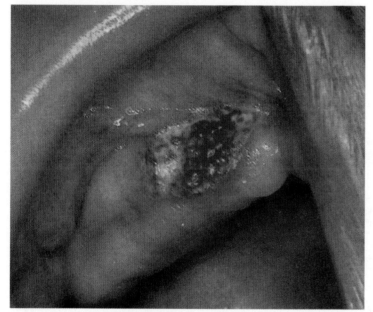

FIGURE 4.39 **SQUAMOUS CELL CARCINOMA OF ALVEOLAR RIDGE.** This relatively early lesion is marked by a predominantly red area without obvious ulceration at this stage.

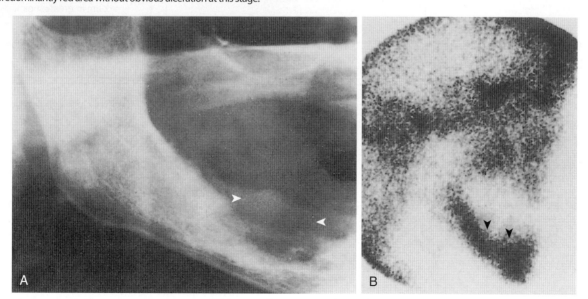

FIGURE 4.41 **SQUAMOUS CELL CARCINOMA OF FLOOR OF MOUTH. (A)** Panoramic tomogram shows a localized area of bone destruction (*arrowheads*) in the body of the mandible. **(B)** Bone scan reveals the true extent of the tumor. The photodeficient area (*arrowheads*) corresponds to the area of bone destruction seen on the tomogram. The area of increased uptake, indicating the actual extent of bone invasion, is much greater, encompassing most of the mandible. (Reproduced with permission from Noyek A, Wortzman G, Kassel E. Diagnostic imaging in rhinology. In Goldman J, editor: *Modern Rhinology*, New York, 1987, John Wiley.)

FIGURE 4.42 **(A)** CT scan of squamous cell carcinoma involving the mandible (*arrows*). **(B)** Spiral CT reconstruction of the lesion localizes the extent of bone involvement and facilitates planning for surgical resection (*arrows*).

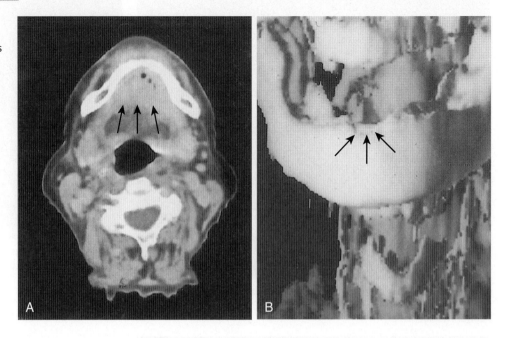

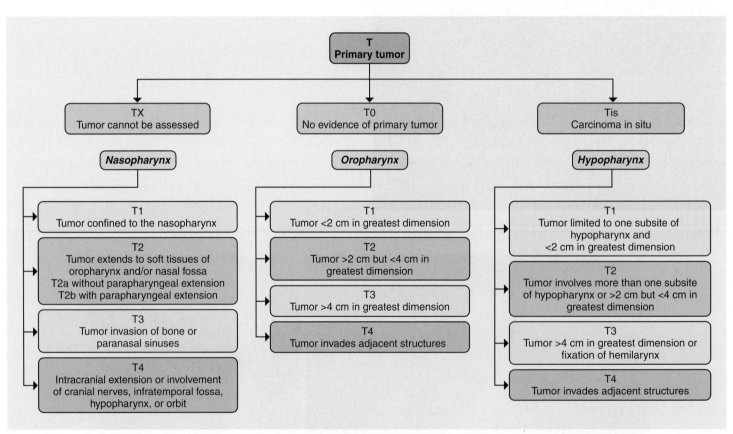

FIGURE 4.43 T categories for cancer of the pharynx (see Fig. 4.27 and Table 4.4 for N and M categories and stage grouping of head and neck cancers) (Greene F, Page D, Fleming I, et al, editors, for the American Joint Committee on Cancer: *AJCC cancer staging manual*, ed 6, New York, 2002, Springer.)

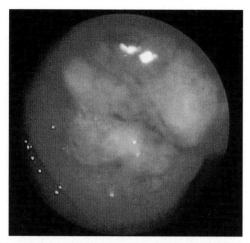

FIGURE 4.44 SQUAMOUS CELL CARCINOMA OF NASOPHARYNX. Persistent or recurrent serous effusion of the middle ear in adults is suspicious for a nasopharyngeal tumor. A Hopkins rod nasopharyngeal telescope reveals a carcinoma arising from the posterior wall of the nasopharynx.

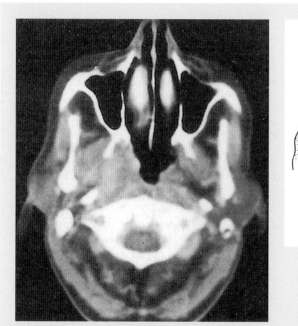

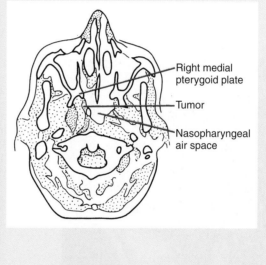

Right medial pterygoid plate

Tumor

Nasopharyngeal air space

FIGURE 4.45 SQUAMOUS CELL CARCINOMA OF NASOPHARYNX. A 64-year-old woman presented with a persistent serous effusion of the right middle ear. An axial CT scan demonstrates a soft tissue mass in the right lateral aspect of the nasopharynx in the region of the fossa of Rosenmüller. The tumor infiltrates deeply and involves the eustachian tube. Note that the fascial planes have been destroyed by the advancing neoplasm (compare with normal left side).

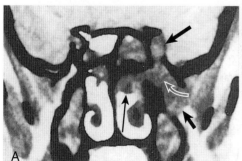

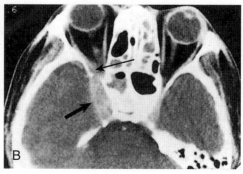

FIGURE 4.46 SQUAMOUS CELL CARCINOMA OF NASOPHARYNX. (A) Coronal CT section shows a tumor extending into the middle cranial fossa (*medium arrow*) and inferiorly through the inferior orbital fissure (*short, thick arrow*), which is markedly widened (*open arrow*). Tumor is also present in the superior aspect of the nasal cavity (*thin arrow*). There is a soft tissue thickening within the sphenoid sinus. **(B)** The axial projection shows tumor at the apex of the right orbit (*thin arrow*) and extending as an enhancing mass into the right cavernous sinus (*thick arrow*). (Courtesy of EE Kassel.)

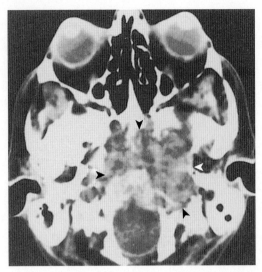

FIGURE 4.47   SQUAMOUS CELL CARCINOMA OF NASOPHARYNX. A 57-year-old woman presented with chronic headaches and dysfunction of cranial nerves IX through XI. This CT scan demonstrates extensive erosion of the base of the skull, with destruction of the petrous bone and the greater wing of the sphenoid by a soft tissue lesion (*arrowheads*).

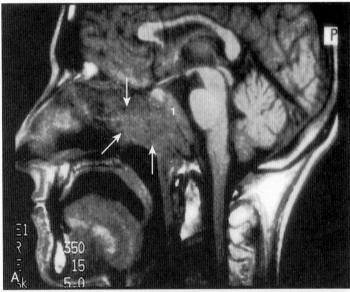

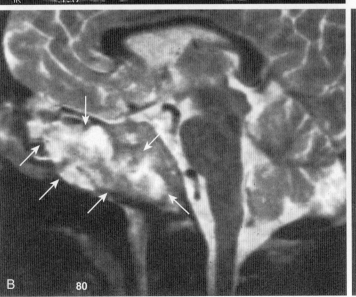

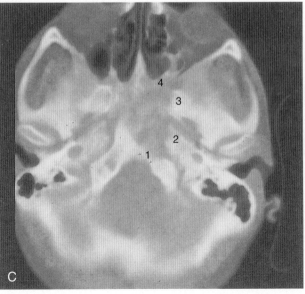

FIGURE 4.48   SQUAMOUS CARCINOMA OF NASOPHARYNX. A 35-year-old woman complained of nasal stuffiness. **(A)** Sagittal T$_1$-weighted MR image shows a large soft tissue mass (*arrows*) involving the sphenoid sinus, ethmoid sinus, and clivus (1). **(B)** Sagittal T$_2$-weighted MR image shows the extent of the primary tumor mass (*arrows*) with destruction of local structures. **(C)** CT scan shows the extent of bony involvement of clivus (1), petrous temporal bone (2), sphenoid bone (3), and ethmoid (4).

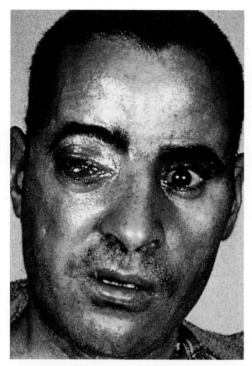

FIGURE 4.49 SQUAMOUS CELL CARCINOMA OF NASOPHARYNX (PARASELLAR SYNDROME). Parasellar structures are frequently affected by invasive nasopharyngeal tumors. In this instance the lesion has invaded the orbit via the superior orbital fissure, leading to severe right proptosis.

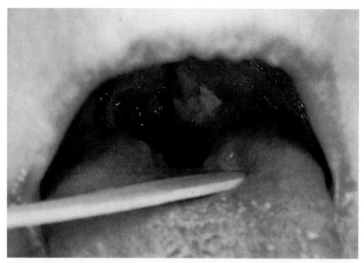

FIGURE 4.50 SQUAMOUS CELL CARCINOMA OF OROPHARYNX. A 56-year-old woman presented with chronic pharyngeal pain and difficulty in swallowing of several months' duration. Clinical examination reveals a bulging necrotic lesion of the left tonsil with involvement of the neighboring soft palate and displacement of the uvula. Biopsy yielded the histologic diagnosis.

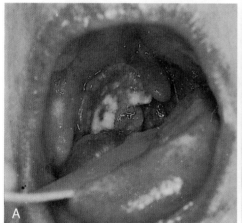
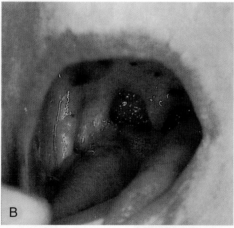

FIGURE 4.51 SQUAMOUS CELL CARCINOMA OF OROPHARYNX. A 63-year-old woman presented with difficulty in swallowing and otalgia. (**A**) Examination reveals an extensive lesion of the right tonsil that involves the lateral pharyngeal wall, as well as the soft palate and uvula. After biopsy, which confirmed the diagnosis, the lesion was outlined (tattooed) with India ink and treated with combination chemotherapy and radiation therapy. (**B**) This photograph, taken after chemotherapy but before radiation therapy, shows complete clinical regression of the tumor.

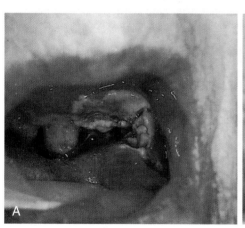
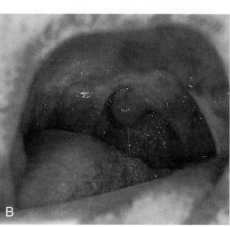

FIGURE 4.52 SQUAMOUS CELL CARCINOMA OF OROPHARYNX. A 53-year-old woman presented with odynophagia and nasal regurgitation of food. (**A**) Examination reveals a large, exophytic, ulcerative lesion of the left tonsil that diffusely involves the soft palate and uvula. Palatal insufficiency resulted from a fistula in the right soft palate extending into the nasopharynx. (**B**) After treatment with combination chemotherapy the lesion completely regressed, replaced by fibrous tissue, and the fistula closed. Treatment continued with definitive radiation therapy. The patient remains free of disease in long-term follow-up.

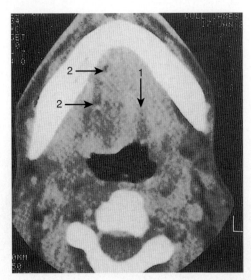

FIGURE 4.53 **SQUAMOUS CELL CARCINOMA OF OROPHARYNX.** A 48-year-old man presented with unilateral otalgia. Clinical examination revealed no obvious tumor. Axial CT scan through the base of the tongue shows an ill-defined T4 mass (1) in the left side of the tongue that obliterates the normal fat planes on the right (2). The tumor crosses the midline. Biopsy of the lesion yielded the histologic diagnosis.

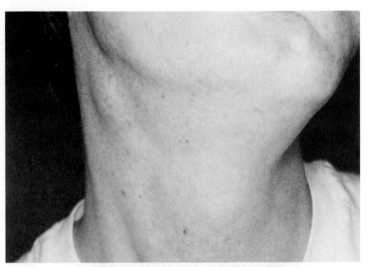

FIGURE 4.55 **DIFFUSE LARGE CELL LYMPHOMA OF OROPHARYNX.** Additional evaluation of this 33-year-old man who presented with right tonsillar enlargement revealed only this jugulodigastric mass; biopsy yielded the histologic diagnosis. For clinical stage II disease, he received six cycles of combination chemotherapy, which resulted in a complete response. He remains disease-free 8 years after treatment.

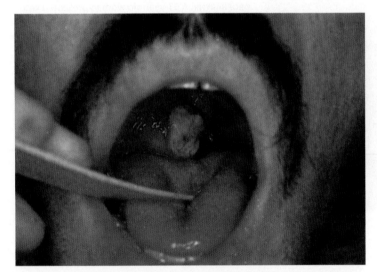

FIGURE 4.54 **DIFFUSE LARGE CELL LYMPHOMA OF OROPHARYNX.** A 24-year-old man, a nonsmoker, presented with a 3-week history of odynophagia and fatigue refractory to a trial of antibiotics. A massive necrotic lesion of the right tonsil is apparent. Intraoral biopsy yielded the histologic diagnosis.

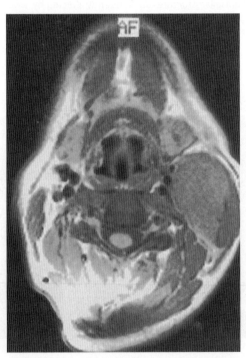

FIGURE 4.56 **DIFFUSE LARGE CELL LYMPHOMA INVOLVING THE NECK (CLINICAL STAGE I DISEASE).** This axial MR scan reveals a soft tissue mass within the neck consistent with malignant regional adenopathy. The homogeneous texture of the lesion favors a diagnosis of lymphoma, which was confirmed after an initial, unremarkable evaluation of the head and neck mucosal surfaces under anesthesia by a head and neck surgeon and subsequent excisional biopsy of the neck lesion.

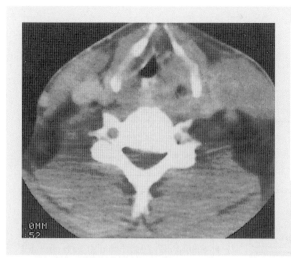

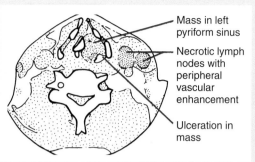

Mass in left
pyriform sinus

Necrotic lymph
nodes with
peripheral
vascular
enhancement

Ulceration in
mass

FIGURE 4.57 **SQUAMOUS CELL CARCINOMA OF HYPOPHARYNX.** Contrast-enhanced axial CT scan in a 45-year-old man shows that the left pyriform sinus is filled with necrotic tumor (note the central ulceration). In addition, two large, centrally necrotic lymph nodes are apparent, with minimal but definite peripheral vascular enhancement.

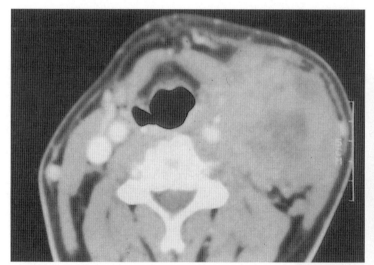

FIGURE 4.58 **SQUAMOUS CELL CARCINOMA OF THE HYPOPHARYNX.** A 56-year-old man presented with a bulky cervical mass. Indirect laryngoscopy revealed bulging of the lateral pharyngeal wall with obliteration of the pyriform sinus. An axial CT revealed a massive neck lesion involving the carotid sheath and the parapharyngeal space. A primary site lesion was suggested on CT. Needle aspiration of the neck mass showed squamous cell carcinoma. Direct laryngoscopy confirmed a small primary site tumor in the pyriform sinus.

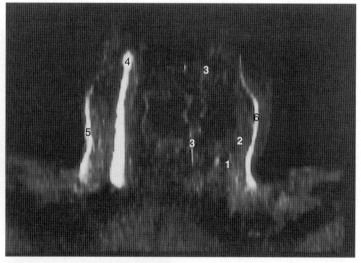

FIGURE 4.59 **SQUAMOUS CELL CARCINOMA OF THE HYPOPHARYNX.** MR venography reveals obstruction of the ipsilateral internal jugular vein (1) by tumor (2). Note collateral veins (3) and normal right internal jugular vein (4), right external jugular vein (5), and left external jugular vein (6).

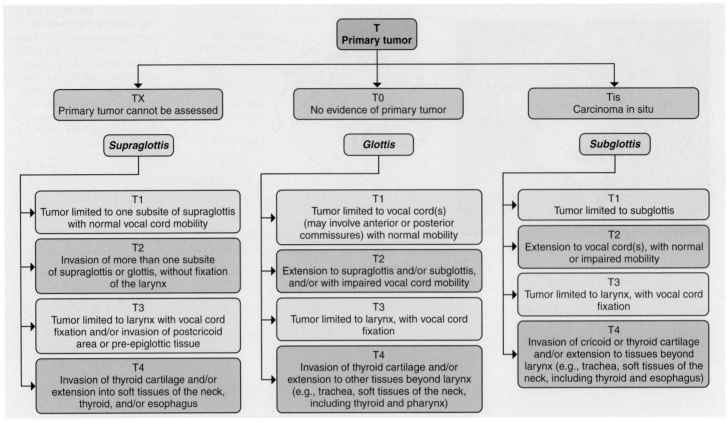

FIGURE 4.60 T categories for cancer of the larynx (see Fig. 4.27 and Table 4.4 for the N and M categories and stage grouping of head and neck cancers) (Greene F, Page D, Fleming I, et al, editors, for the American Joint Committee on Cancer: *AJCC cancer staging manual*, ed 6, New York, 2002, Springer.)

FIGURE 4.61 SQUAMOUS CELL CARCINOMA OF LARYNX. A 68-year-old man presented with a long history of alcohol and tobacco use and progressive dysphagia and hoarseness of several months' duration. **(A)** Laryngoscopy reveals a large exophytic lesion of the supraglottic larynx that involves the aryepiglottic fold, the false vocal cord, and the infrahyoid epiglottis. The true glottis is obscured but immobile. With the discovery of several small ipsilateral cervical lymph nodes, the patient was felt to have stage IV (T3N2b) disease. Radiation therapy was administered when the patient refused surgical resection. **(B)** Twenty-eight months after radiation therapy there is no evidence of tumor. (Courtesy of Dr J. Parsons, University of Florida, Gainesville.)

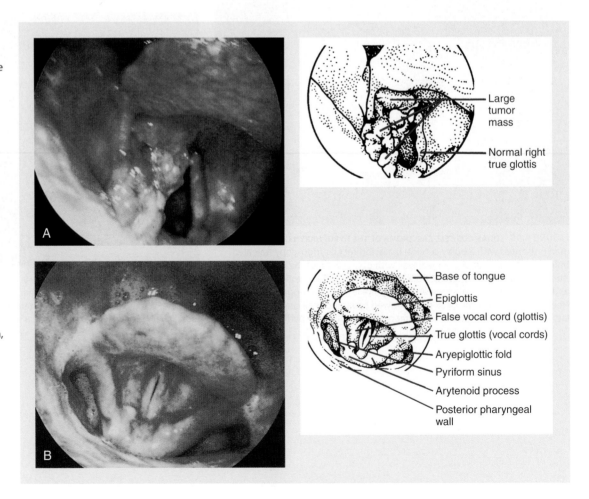

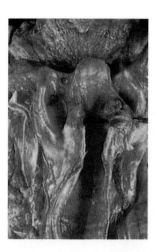

FIGURE 4.62 SQUAMOUS CELL CARCINOMA
OF LARYNX. The trachea and larynx have
been opened posteriorly to reveal a small
fungating supraglottic tumor arising in the
right aryepiglottic fold.

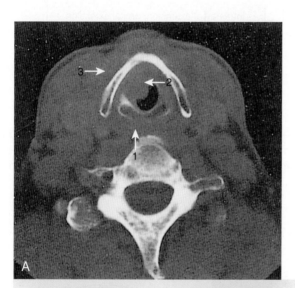

FIGURE 4.63 SQUAMOUS CELL CARCINOMA OF LARYNX. **(A)**
Axial CT scan at the level of the posterior lamina of the
cricoid cartilage (*arrow 1*) in a 58-year-old man shows
subglottic extension of an intralaryngeal tumor mass
(*arrow 2*). The thyroid cartilage is indicated (*arrow 3*).
(B) Section through the glottis (about 1 cm cephalad to
the previous scan) shows that necrotic tumor extends
anteriorly into the soft tissue of the neck. The central
portion of the thyroid cartilage has been destroyed. The
tumor encroaches on the airway and has obliterated the
anterior commissure. This is classified as a T4 lesion.

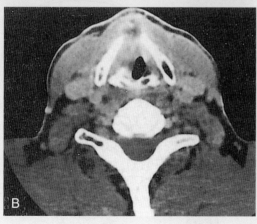

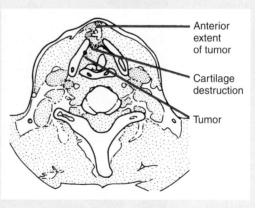

Anterior
extent
of tumor

Cartilage
destruction

Tumor

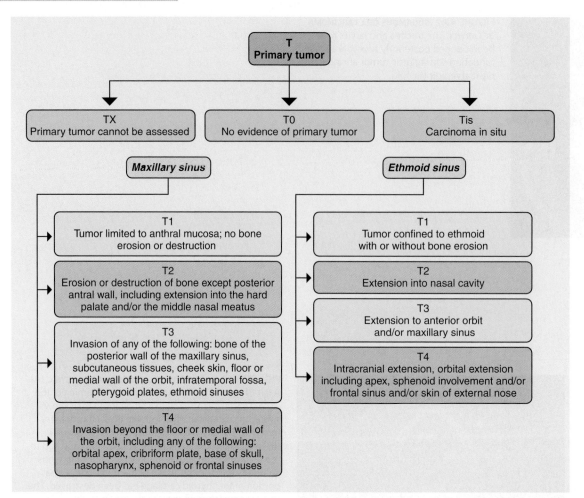

FIGURE 4.64 T categories for cancer of the paranasal sinuses (see Fig. 4.27 and Table 4.4 for the N and M categories and stage grouping of head and neck cancers). (Greene F, Page D, Fleming I, et al, editors, for the American Joint Committee on Cancer: *AJCC cancer staging manual*, ed 6, New York, 2002, Springer.)

FIGURE 4.65 **SQUAMOUS CELL CARCINOMA OF MAXILLARY SINUS.** Coronal CT scan shows intraorbital extension from a large carcinoma arising in the right maxillary sinus. The tumor extends medially into the nasal cavity, superiorly into the ethmoid labyrinth, and anterolaterally into the oral cavity. There is obvious extension of tumor into the orbit with destruction of the normal bony landmarks; the floor of the orbit (roof of the maxillary sinus) is fragmented (compare with left orbit). In this plane the bony floor of the anterior cranial fossa appears intact. A fluid level is present in the left maxillary sinus.

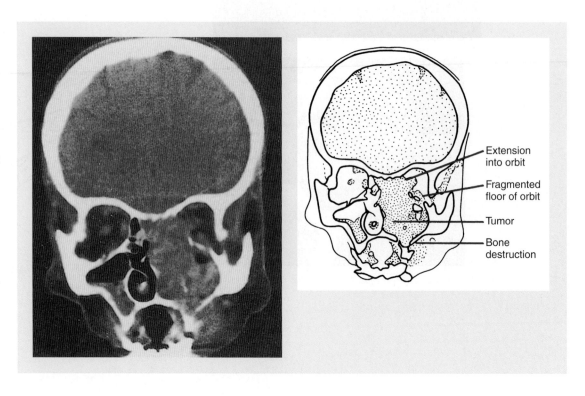

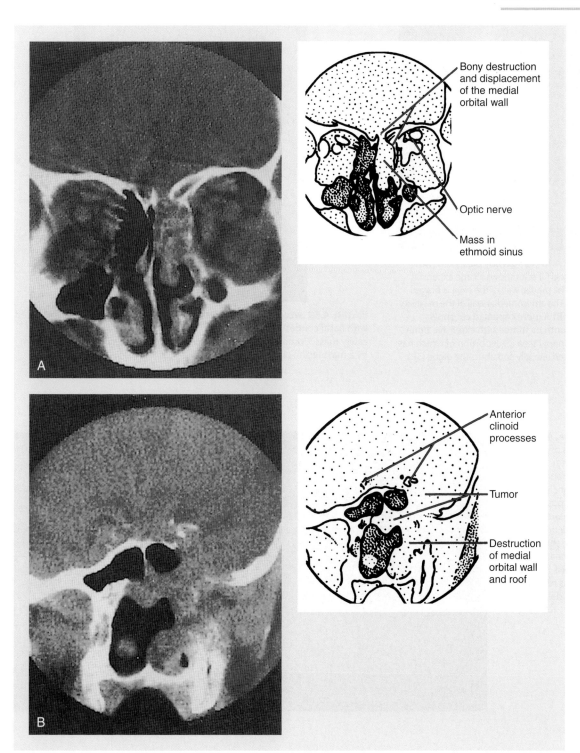

FIGURE 4.66 **CARCINOMA OF ETHMOID SINUS. (A, B)** CT scans show a tumor expanding the ethmoid sinus, destroying the medial orbital wall, and invading posteriorly into the middle cranial fossa.

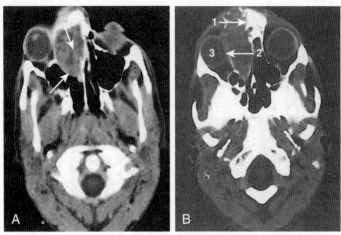

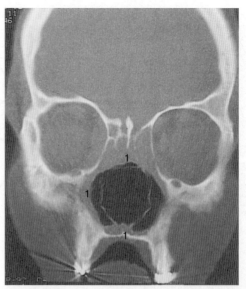

FIGURE 4.67 ESTHESIONEUROBLASTOMA. A 16-year-old boy presented with nasal obstruction of recent onset. **(A)** Axial CT scan shows a large expansile mass (*arrows*) in the right nasal cavity. The medial wall of the orbit is bowed outward, displacing the globe laterally. The anteromedial wall of the maxillary sinus is displaced but appears intact. **(B)** A more cephalad cut shows expansion of the entire ethmoid labyrinth by tumor with extensive bone destruction (1) anteriorly. The lamina papyracea (2), a portion of which has been destroyed by the tumor, is displaced laterally and abuts the globe (3).

FIGURE 4.69 WEGENER'S GRANULOMATOSIS. This 39-year-old female presented with nasal congestion and epistaxis. Examination revealed an erosive nasal cavity mass. Coronal CT scan revealed gross destruction of the nasal septum by a mass lesion (1).

FIGURE 4.68 ESTHESIONEUROBLASTOMA. A 55-year-old male presented with several years of nasal congestion and recent unilateral change in vision. **(A)** Axial T_1-weighted gadolinium-enhanced MR image with fat saturation shows enhancing tissue within the ethmoid air cells (1) with a posterior area of nonenhancement (2). The enhancing tissue could represent either normal mucosa or tumor mass. **(B)** Axial T_2-weighted MR image shows a central low-signal area within the enhancing tissue which represents the tumor mass (1). The bright tissue surrounding it represents retained secretions within surrounding ethmoidal air cells.

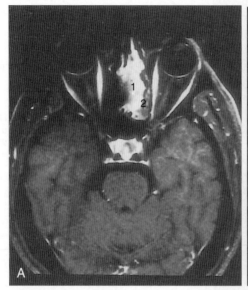

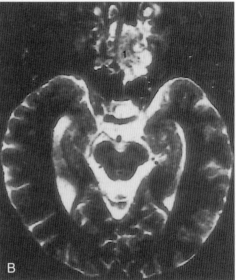

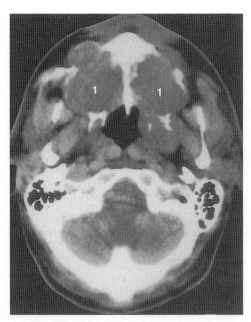

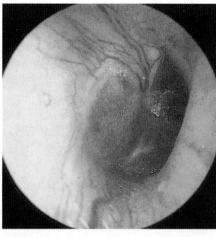

FIGURE 4.72 **GLOMUS JUGULARE TUMOR OF MIDDLE EAR.** Otoscopic view shows a nonulcerated, smooth tumor filling the inferior half of the right middle ear; it is beginning to extend through the tympanic membrane. Note the adjacent dilated blood vessels.

FIGURE 4.70 **SOLITARY PLASMACYTOMA OF PARANASAL SINUSES.** This 69-year-old female presented with head and nasal congestion and clear nasal discharge. Examination revealed a nasal cavity mass. (1) Axial CT scan indicated an extensive lesion involving both maxillary sinuses as well as the nasal cavity. Biopsy of the nasal cavity mass confirmed the diagnosis. Subsequent bone marrow aspiration and biopsy failed to reveal evidence for multiple myeloma.

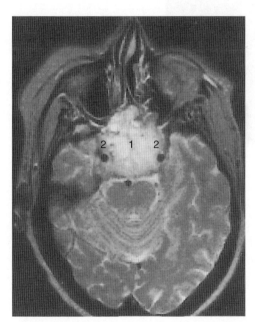

FIGURE 4.71 **BREAST CARCINOMA METASTATIC TO SPHENOID SINUS.** This 62-year-old patient with known breast carcinoma metastatic to the axial skeleton presented with bitemporal headache of several months' duration. Axial T_2-weighted MRI shows an expansile mass within the sphenoid sinus (1) extending into the cavernous sinuses (2).

FIGURE 4.73 GLOMUS VAGALE TUMOR OF PARAPHARYNGEAL SPACE. (A) Contrast-enhanced axial CT scan demonstrates a large mass (1) in the right parapharyngeal space that encroaches on the nasopharynx and extends into the deep fascial spaces of the neck, displacing the internal carotid artery laterally (2). The periphery of the mass enhances, but the central portion is relatively hypodense.
(B) Conventional carotid arteriogram shows a tangle of small vessels (3) supplied by branches of the external carotid artery. The vascular tumor abuts the internal carotid artery, which is bowed anteriorly (4).

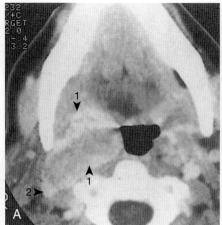
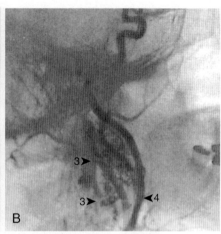

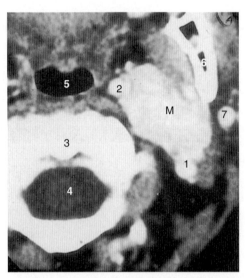

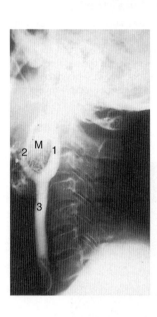

FIGURE 4.75 GLOMUS JUGULARE TUMOR INVOLVING NECK (see Fig. 4.74). Angiogram showing displacement of the internal and external carotid arteries by a hypervascular mass (M). Note the internal (1), external (2), and common (3) carotid arteries.

FIGURE 4.74 GLOMUS JUGULARE TUMOR INVOLVING THE NECK. Axial contrast-enhanced CT image demonstrates an intensely enhancing mass (M) that separates the internal (1) and external (2) carotid arteries. Note the cervical spine (3), spinal cord (4), oropharynx (5), angle of mandible (6), and jugular vein (7).

FIGURE 4.76 GLOMUS JUGULARE TUMOR. (A) This tumor consists of a dense network of thin-walled sinusoidal capillaries that surround glomerular or alveolar-like nests of tumor cells ("Zellballen"). **(B)** The nests or groups of tumor cells contain 5–20 epithelioid cells, which have a moth-eaten, clear, or eosinophilic granular cytoplasm and round vesicular nuclei with prominent nucleoli.

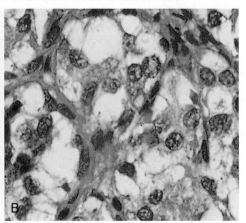

```
                    ┌─────────────────┐
                    │        T        │
                    │  Primary tumor  │
                    └─────────────────┘
```

T
TX Tumor cannot be assessed
T0 No evidence of primary tumor
Tis Carcinoma in situ
T1 Tumor <2 cm in greatest dimension without extraparenchymal extension
T2 Tumor >2 cm but <4 cm in greatest dimension without extraparenchymal extension
T3 Tumor >4 cm but <6 cm in greatest dimension and/or extraparenchymal extension without cranial nerve VII involvement
T4 Tumor >6 cm or invades base of skull and/or cranial nerve VII

Stage	T (primary tumor)	N (regional nodes)	M (metastases)
I	T1 or T2	N0	M0
II	T3	N0	M0
III	T1 or T2	N1	M0
IV	T4	N0 or N1	M0
	T3	N1	M0
	Any T	N1 or N2	M0
	Any T	Any N	M1

FIGURE 4.77 T categories and stage grouping for cancer of the major salivary glands (see Fig. 4.27 for N and M categories). (Greene F, Page D, Fleming I, et al, editors, for the American Joint Committee on Cancer: *AJCC cancer staging manual*, ed 6, New York, 2002, Springer.)

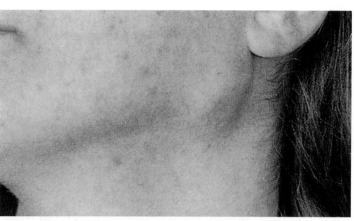

FIGURE 4.78 **PLEOMORPHIC ADENOMA OF PAROTID GLAND.** Clinically, as is common with these tumors, there is a painless swelling; in this instance, the tumor involves the lower pole of the gland.

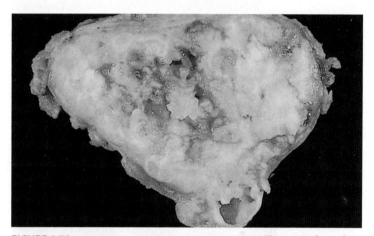

FIGURE 4.79 **PLEOMORPHIC ADENOMA OF PAROTID GLAND.** The cut surface of this fairly well circumscribed, multinodular tumor has a myxoid cartilaginous appearance, and there are small foci of cystic change and hemorrhage. These tumors tend to recur locally, most often as a consequence of spread through the capsule, which results in incomplete surgical excision.

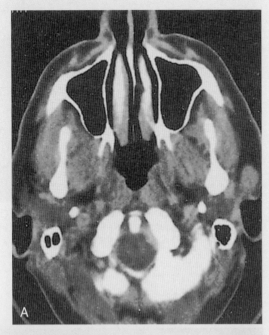

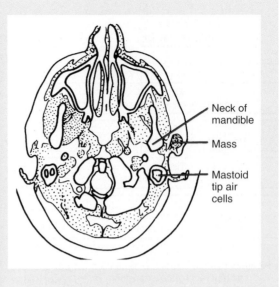

Neck of
mandible

Mass

Mastoid
tip air
cells

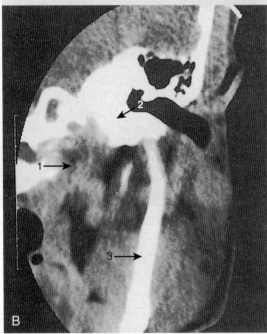

FIGURE 4.80 **PLEOMORPHIC ADENOMA OF PAROTID GLAND.**
(A) Axial CT scan shows a well-circumscribed mass within
the left parotid gland of a 57-year-old man. **(B)** Coronal
CT section shows that the tumor (*arrow 1*) is sharply
demarcated from the rest of the parotid gland and does
not involve deeper structures. The internal auditory
canal (*arrow 2*) and the mandibular ramus (*arrow 3*) are
indicated.

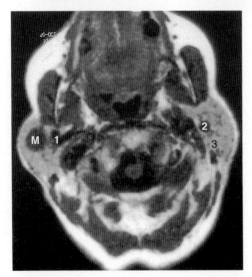

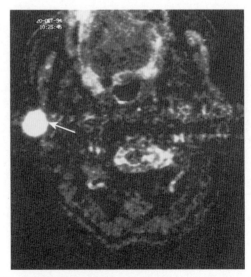

FIGURE 4.81 **PLEOMORPHIC ADENOMA OF PAROTID GLAND.** Pleomorphic
adenoma in the right parotid (M) is a well-defined, low-signal intensity mass
on the axial T_1-weighted MRI. Note displacement of the retromandibular vein
(1) medially by the mass compared with the normal left retromandibular vein
(2). The left facial nerve (3) branching through the normal left parotid is seen.

FIGURE 4.82 **PLEOMORPHIC ADENOMA OF PAROTID GLAND.** Same patient as
Figure 4.81; the lesion has high but slightly mixed signal intensity on the axial
T_2-weighted image with fat saturation (*arrow*).

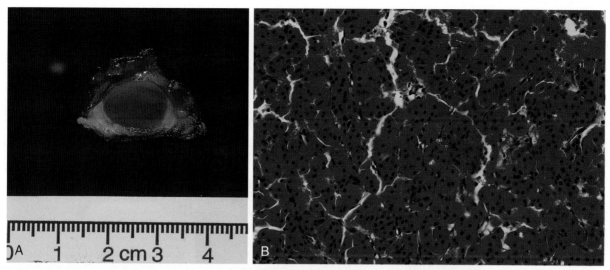

FIGURE 4.83 **ONCOCYTOMA OF SALIVARY GLAND. (A)** Gross photo of a resected parotid gland oncocytoma. It is a benign tumor of elderly patients characterized by a solid or organoid proliferation of polygonal cells with deeply eosinophilic granular cytoplasm. **(B)** This characteristic cytoplasmic staining pattern is due to abundant mitochondria, which may be demonstrated by electron microscopy or staining with phosphotungstic acid–hematoxylin. The tumor may occasionally recur after excision, especially when multifocal at presentation.

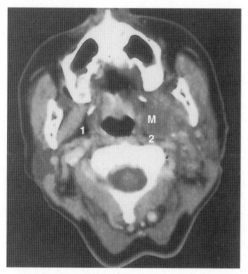

FIGURE 4.84 **ADENOCARCINOMA OF PAROTID GLAND.** This 72-year-old male complained of jaw pain and had some left parotid fullness. Poorly differentiated adenocarcinoma of the parotid gland appears on axial CT scan image as a large heterogeneous mass (M) projecting from the deep lobe of the parotid into the parapharyngeal space. Note the normal right parapharyngeal space (1) compared with the effaced space on the left (2).

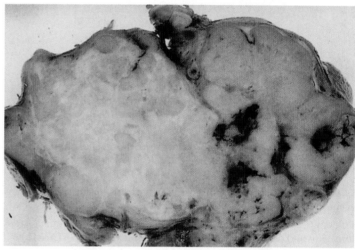

FIGURE 4.86 **CARCINOMA ARISING IN PLEOMORPHIC ADENOMA OF SUBMANDIBULAR GLAND.** This specimen was excised from a 73-year-old man who had noticed a small lump under the jaw for 25 years. A rapid increase in size of the lesion prompted him to see his doctor. The tumor, measuring 10 by 7 by 6 cm in the fresh state, appears encapsulated, is multinodular, and contains gelatinous and hemorrhagic foci. Although it shows features very similar to a benign pleomorphic adenoma, there was unequivocal histologic evidence of malignancy.

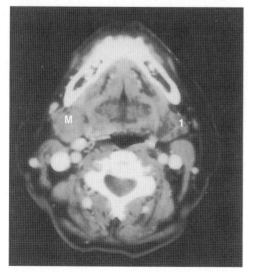

FIGURE 4.85 **MYOEPITHELIAL CARCINOMA OF PAROTID GLAND.** This 55-year-old woman presented with swelling underneath her jaw. The enlarged, slightly heterogeneous right submandibular gland (M) seen on CT scan contained a myoepithelial carcinoma. Note the normal ovoid left submandibular gland (1).

FIGURE 4.87 PAPILLARY CYSTADENOMA LYMPHOMATOSUM (WARTHIN'S TUMOR) OF PAROTID GLAND. Axial CT-sialogram demonstrates a mass in the right parotid gland of a 78-year-old man. Normal glandular tissue (opacified by the contrast agent) surrounds the mass. The deep surface of the parotid tumor is sharply demarcated from the fat-containing parapharyngeal space.

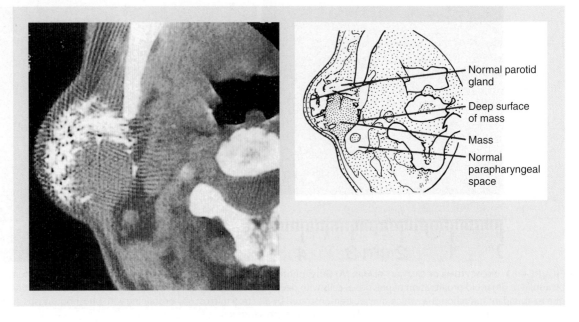

Normal parotid gland

Deep surface of mass

Mass

Normal parapharyngeal space

References and Suggested Readings

Almadori G, Cadoni G, Galli J, et al: Epidermal growth factor receptor expression in primary laryngeal cancer: an independent prognostic factor of neck node relapse, *Int J Cancer* 84:188–191, 1999.

Boyle J, Hakim J, Koch W, et al: The incidence of p53 mutations increases with progression of head and neck cancer, *J Otolaryngol Head Neck Surg* 53:4477–4480, 1993.

Choong N, Vokes E: Expanding role of the medical oncologist in the management of head and neck cancer, *CA Cancer J Clin* 58:32–53, 2008.

D'Souza G, Kreimer AR, Viscidi R, et al: Case-control study of human papillomavirus and oropharyngeal cancer, *N Engl J Med* 356:1944–1956, 2007.

Fakhry C, Westra WH, Li S, et al: Improved survival of patients with human papillomavirus-positive head and neck squamous cell carcinoma in a prospective clinical trial, *J Natl Cancer Inst* 100:261–269, 2008.

Forastiere A, Goepfert H, Goffinet D, et al: NCCN practice guidelines for head and neck cancer. National Comprehensive Cancer Network, *Oncology (Huntingt)* 12:39–147, 1998.

Greene F, Page D, Fleming I, et al, editors, for the American Joint Committee on Cancer: *AJCC cancer staging manual,* ed 6, New York, 2002, Springer.

Grégoire V, DeNeve W, Eisbruch A, et al: Intensity-modulated radiation therapy for head and neck carcinoma, *Oncologist* 12:555–564, 2007.

Jares P, Fernandez P, Campo E, et al: PRAD-1/cyclin D1 gene amplification correlates with messenger RNA overexpression and tumor progression in human laryngeal carcinomas, *Cancer Res* 54:4813–4817, 1994.

Jemal A, Siegel R, Ward E, et al: Cancer statistics, 2008, *CA Cancer J Clin* 58:71–96, 2008.

Kieff E: Epstein-Barr virus—increasing evidence of a link to carcinoma, *N Engl J Med* 333:724–726, 1995.

Layfield L, Cibas E, Gharib H, Mandel S: Thyroid aspiration cytology: current status, *CA Cancer J Clin* 59:99–110, 2009.

Lewin F, Norell SE, Johansson H, et al: Smoking tobacco, oral snuff, and alcohol in the etiology of squamous cell carcinoma of the head and neck, *Cancer* 82:1367–1375, 1998.

Marur S, Forastiere AA: Head and neck cancer: changing epidemiology, diagnosis, and treatment, *Mayo Clin Proc* 83(4):489–501, 2008.

Noyek A, Wortzman G, Kassel E. Diagnostic imaging in rhinology. In Goldman J, editor: *Modern Rhinology,* New York, 1987, John Wiley.

Raab-Traub N, Flynn K, Pearson G, et al: The differentiated form of nasopharyngeal carcinoma contains Epstein-Barr virus DNA, *Int J Cancer* 39:25–29, 1987.

Reed A, Califano J, Cairns P, et al: High frequency of p16 (CDKN2/MTS-1/INK4A) inactivation in head and neck squamous cell carcinoma, *Cancer Res* 56:3630–3633, 1996.

Todd R, Wong D: Epidermal growth factor receptor (EGFR) biology and human oral cancer, *Histol Histopathol* 14:491–500, 1999.

van der Wal JE, Leverstein H, Snow G, et al: Parotid gland tumors: histologic reevaluation and reclassification of 478 cases, *Head Neck* 20:204–207, 1998.

Yadav M, Arivananthan M, Chandrashekran A, et al: Human herpesvirus-6 (HHV-6) DNA and virus-encoded antigen in oral lesions, *J Oral Pathol Med* 26:393–401, 1997.

Figure Credits

The following books published by Gower Medical Publishing are sources of figures in the present chapter. The figure numbers given in the listing are those of the figures in the present chapter. The page numbers (or slide numbers) given in parentheses are those of the original publication.

Cawson RA, Eveson JW: *Oral pathology and diagnosis*, London, 1987, Heinemann Medical Books/Gower Medical Publishing: Figs. 4.1 (p. 12.8), 4.2 (p. 12.11), 4.3 (p. 12.22), 4.4 (p. 12.25), 4.5 (p. 13.8), 4.6 (p. 13.13), 4.7 (p. 13.12), 4.8 (p. 13.12), 4.9 (p. 13.14), 4.10 (p. 13.14), 4.13 (p. 14.13), 4.14 (p. 14.13), 4.15 (p. 14.13), 4.16 (p. 14.15), 4.18 (p. 14.19), 4.19 (p. 14.19), 4.20 (p. 14.22), 4.21 (p. 14.21), 4.22 (p. 14.21), 4.23 (p. 14.22), 4.24 (p. 14.22), 4.32 (p. 13.8), 4.33 (p. 13.6), 4.34 (p. 13.9), 4.35 (p. 13.9), 4.36 (p. 13.9), 4.37 (p. 13.10), 4.38 (p. 13.10), 4.39 (p. 13.10), 4.66 (p. 14.12). du Vivier A: *Atlas of clinical dermatology*, Edinburgh/London, 1986, Churchill Livingstone/Gower Medical Publishing: Figs. 4.29 (p. 7.16), 4.30 (p. 7.16), 4.31 (p. 4.13).

Fletcher CDM, McKee PH: *An atlas of gross pathology*, London, 1987, Edward Arnold/Gower Medical Publishing: Figs. 4.56 (p. 13), 4.67 (p. 23).

Hawke M, Jahn AF: *Diseases of the ear: clinical and pathologic aspects*, Philadelphia/New York, 1987, Lea and Febiger/Gower Medical Publishing: Figs. 4.42 (p. 3.49), 4.62 (p. 3.100), 4.64 (p. 3.102).

Kassner EG, editor: *Atlas of radiology imaging*, Philadelphia/New York, 1989, Lippincott/Gower Medical Publishing: Figs. 4.40 (p. 12.27), 4.43 (p. 12.19), 4.44 (p. 12.23), 4.50 (p. 12.40), 4.53 (p. 12.45), 4.57 (p. 12.38), 4.59 (p. 12.20), 4.61 (p. 12.26), 4.63 (p. 12.43), 4.68 (p. 12.31), 4.70 (p. 12.30).

Perkin GD, Rose FC, Blackwood W, et al: *Atlas of clinical neurology*, Philadelphia/London, 1986, Lippincott/Gower Medical Publishing: Fig. 4.46 (p. 12.12).

Price AB, Morson BC, Scheuer PJ, editors: Alimentary system. In Turk JL, Fletcher CDM, editors: *RSCI slide atlas of pathology*, London, 1986, Gower Medical Publishing: Fig. 4.69 (slide 35).

Spalton DJ, Hitchings RA, Hunter PA: *Atlas of clinical ophthalmology*, Philadelphia/New York, 1984, Lippincott/Gower Medical Publishing: Fig. 4.60 (p. 29.19).

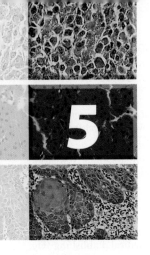

5

Lung Cancer and Tumors of the Heart and Mediastinum

RAVI SALGIA • RAMON BLANCO • ARTHUR T. SKARIN

Lung Cancer

INCIDENCE AND ETIOLOGY

Lung cancer is the most common cancer in the world, with about 1.2 million new cases per year (WHO, 2003). The estimate for new cases of lung cancer in the United States in men for 2009 is 129,710 and among women, 107,280 (Jemal et al., 2009). Lung cancer will still be the leading cause of death from malignancy in both sexes in the United States, resulting in 71,550 estimated deaths in women in 2009 and 92,240 deaths in men. Lung cancer is responsible for 25% of all cancer deaths and for 5% of all deaths in the United States. The vast majority of cases (85% or more) are due to chronic cigarette smoking. Other etiologic factors include asbestos (shipyard workers, insulators, etc.), radon gas (underground mining, etc.), ionizing radiation, and certain industrial agents and compounds (chloromethyl ether, arsenic, nickel-cadmium, and chromium). Tobacco smoking is thought to be synergistic with the latter elements. Tobacco smoke contains oxidants that are believed to be important in biologic damage of DNA, proteins, and lipids, leading to lung cancer. Genetic abnormalities as well as underlying lung disease (chronic obstructive pulmonary disease) also predispose patients to lung cancer.

Whereas lung cancer is one of the easiest cancers to prevent, it is one of the most difficult to cure, as a result of the early dissemination in many cases and therapeutically refractory disease when metastases occur. The overall rate of cure for all patients is about 16%, although there is a wide range of cure rates related mainly to stage of disease. If a patient survives the initial cancer the risk of subsequent lung cancer increases to 3% to 7% per year. By discontinuing cigarette smoking, the patient lowers the risk for primary lung cancer as well as subsequent cancer, but 15–20 years must pass before the risk approaches that of nonsmokers. Still, at 15 years after quitting smoking the risk is 1.5 times that of a person who never smoked. Passive smoking accounts for 3% to 5% of all cases of lung cancer. According to the U.S. Surgeon General, 5000–10,000 of the 160,000 deaths due to lung cancer each year occur in patients exposed to sidestream smoke.

LUNG CANCER, GENDER, AND AGE

Lung cancer rates in women have risen dramatically, both worldwide and in the United States. Population-based data by the National Cancer Institute (NCI) Surveillance, Epidemiology and End Results (SEER) Program have shown that the age-adjusted rate for lung cancer for all race/sex groups has risen sharply since 1950. The incidence started rising in the mid-1930s and overtook breast cancer as the leading cause of cancer deaths among women in the late 1980s. This observation correlates with the increase in the number of women who smoke. The male-to-female ratio is 3.47 in patients over 45 years of age and 1.7 in patients younger than 45. Adenocarcinoma is the most common type in young patients and squamous cell carcinoma in the older age group. Notably, adenocarcinoma is increasing in women, especially nonsmokers. Reasons for this are multiple, including genetic factors, increased susceptibility to lung cancer carcinogens as compared with men, and secondary or passive smoking exposure (Colson et al., 2007).

HISTOPATHOLOGY

Over 95% of lung neoplasms are of epithelial origin (carcinomas), comprising four main types (see below) (Table 5.4). Based on clinical features and biologic properties from studies of cultured malignant cells, these carcinomas can be separated into two major categories: non–small cell lung cancer (squamous cell, adenocarcinoma, and undifferentiated large cell types) and small cell lung cancer (Minna et al., 1989). About 5% of lung cancers are composed of rare mixed epithelial types or neoplasms arising from bronchial glands and other tissues (Table 5.4).

Preinvasive Lesions

In the new World Health Organization (WHO)/International Association for the Study of Lung Cancer (IASLC) 1999 classification, preinvasive lesions include squamous dysplasia/carcinoma in situ (leading to squamous cell carcinoma), atypical adenomatous hyperplasia (characterized by discrete ill-defined bronchioloalveolar proliferation, leading to adenocarcinomas), and diffuse idiopathic pulmonary neuroendocrine cell hyperplasia (characterized by proliferation of neuroendocrine cells throughout the peripheral airways, leading to carcinoids) (Travis et al., 1999).

Non–Small Cell Lung Cancer

Non–small cell lung cancer (NSCLC) comprises about 85% of all lung cancers. They are subdivided into three groups. Squamous cell carcinoma (SCC) is characterized by keratin formation (cytokeratin proteins are intermediate filaments).

Table 5.1

Lesions Causing a Mass on Chest Radiography

Neoplastic	Infective	Miscellaneous
Malignant	Bacterial	Sarcoidosis
Primary lung carcinoma	Pneumonia	Rheumatoid nodules
Carcinoid tumor	Lung abscess	Pseudolymphoma
Lymphoma	Empyema	Wegener's
Plasmacytoma	Tuberculosis	granulomatosis
Thymoma	Tuberculoma	Bronchocentric
Germ cell tumor	Fungal	granulomatosis
Sarcoma	Aspergilloma	Echinococcal cyst
Metastatic carcinoma	Allergic	Pseudotumor (fluid)
Benign	aspergillosis	Bronchial lymph node
Neurofibroma	Histoplasmoma	
Hamartoma	Mycetoma	
Thymoma		
Cyst		
Arteriovenous		
malformation		

Keratin may appear under the light microscope as "keratin pearls" (see Fig. 5.6) or as desmosomes (a type of tight junction seen as "intercellular bridges"; Fig. 5.6). The incidence of this type of lung cancer is decreasing in the United States. Most SCCs arise from the central or proximal tracheal-bronchial tree in areas of squamous cell metaplasia, dysplasia, and carcinoma in situ. SCCs grow slowly and tend to cavitate in about 20% of cases. About one third of SCCs are poorly differentiated and, as such, show a greater potential for distant spread, especially to the liver and small intestine. Poorly differentiated SCCs may acquire a spindle cell morphology that may mimic a sarcoma; identification of such tumors is based on finding a transition zone between the epithelial-appearing tumor cells and the spindle cells and/or on the demonstration of keratin in the spindle cells by immunohistochemistry.

Adenocarcinoma is characterized by definite gland formation (well and moderately differentiated) or by the presence of mucus production in a solid tumor (poorly differentiated) as determined by mucin stains (mucicarmine and D-PAS) (see Fig. 5.10). Adenocarcinomas are increasing in frequency in the United States: at most medical centers they are now more common than squamous cell carcinomas. In about two thirds of cases adenocarcinomas originate in peripheral airways and alveoli. Classically, they were thought to arise from scars ("scar carcinoma"). This view is no longer accepted: the "scar tissue" (desmoplasia) is now thought to be induced by the neoplastic

Table 5.2

Diagnostic Methods for Assessment of Mass Lesions*

Fiberoptic Bronchoscopy	Radiology	Transthoracic Biopsy
Bronchial tree secretions: bacteriology and cytology	Plain posteroanterior and lateral views	Fine-needle aspiration Cutting-needle biopsy
Bronchial biopsy	Computed tomography Magnetic resonance imaging	Video-assisted thoracoscopic biopsy/resection
Transbronchial biopsy	Gallium citrate (Ga-67) scanning	
Transbronchial needle aspiration	Angiography (not often used)	
Selective bronchial brushing		
Bronchioalveolar lavage		

*When the biopsy studies given here are negative, mediastinoscopy or mediastinotomy may be indicated in selected patients.

Table 5.3

WHO Classification of Bronchioloalveolar Carcinoma (BAC)

A. Noninvasive with lepidic spread (5%)
  1. Nonmucinous (Clara/pneumocyte type II)
  2. Mucinous
  3. Mixed mucinous and nonmucinous (intermediate cell type)
B. Invasive with stromal vascular or pleural involvement (95%)
  Adenocarcinoma with BAC features

Modified from Brambilla E, Travis WD, Colby TV, et al: The new World Health Organization classification of lung tumors, *Eur Respir J* 18:1059–1068, 2001.

cells (see Fig. 5.9). Around one third of cases arise centrally, in larger bronchi, from either the surface epithelium or the submucosal glands. Adenocarcinomas frequently present as subpleural nodules, often with a malignant effusion. These cases must be differentiated by means of special stains from malignant mesothelioma, which lacks mucin (see Table 6.1). Metastases from adenocarcinoma to distant sites occur early (e.g., before symptoms or diagnosis) in most patients. Adenocarcinoma arising from sites other than lung can also look very similar to adenocarcinoma arising in the lung. Cytokeratins (7 vs 20) can aid in distinguishing adenocarcinoma from lung as opposed to other sites (in the case of lung, cytokeratin 7 is usually positive and cytokeratin 20 usually negative). TTF-1 (thyroid transcription factor-1) marker is found in adenocarcinoma of the lung and thyroid cancer and is useful in the differential diagnosis of metastatic adenocarcinoma from an unknown primary site (see Table 5.13) (Ordonez, 2000).

Bronchioloalveolar carcinoma (BAC) is a subtype of well-differentiated adenocarcinoma, constituting about 3% of cases (pure type) as compared with 20% for mixed types. It is increasing in frequency and is the one subtype of lung carcinoma (in addition to carcinoid tumors) that is not strongly associated with cigarette smoking. BAC arises from the peripheral bronchioles or alveoli. About 50% of BACs are mucin-secreting tumors consisting of tall columnar cells, whereas the remaining 40% have little or no mucin and consist of peg-shaped ("hobnail") cells with variable degrees of pleomorphism. They are thought to arise from Clara cells or type II pneumocytes, respectively.

Table 5.4

Histopathologic Classification of Epithelial Lung Carcinoma, with Relative Frequencies

Type	Subtype*
Non–small cell carcinoma (85%)	• Squamous cell (epidermoid) carcinoma (40%) WD, MD, PD, and PD spindle-cell variant • Adenocarcinoma[†] (47%) WD, MD, PD, and BAC • Large cell undifferentiated carcinoma (13%) Neuroendocrine, clear cell, basaloid
Small cell carcinoma (10% to 15%)	• Pure small cell (90%) • Mixed small/large cell type (about 5%) • Combined small cell/squamous cell or small cell/adenocarcinoma (about 5%)
Others (5%)	• Adenosquamous carcinoma • Adenocystic carcinoma • Mucoepidermoid carcinoma • Carcinoid tumor • Miscellaneous

*WD, well differentiated; MD, moderately differentiated; PD, poorly differentiated. BAC, bronchioloalveolar cell carcinoma.
[†]World Health Organization subtypes: acinar, papillary, bronchioloalveolar, solid with mucin production, mixed and variants.
Modified from Mountain et al, (1987); Hirsch et al, (1988); Brambilla et al, (2001).

Some adenocarcinomas may contain a small proportion of tumor cells with BAC morphology, typically in the periphery of the tumor. It is, however, generally designated as adenocarcinoma with BAC features. In the World Health Organization (WHO) classification, true BAC has growth in a lepidic fashion with lack of invasive growth (Travis et al., 1999). BAC tends to spread throughout air passages while preserving (or recapitulating) the septal and lobular architecture. The tumor is slow-growing and usually metastasizes late in the course of the disease. It may induce a characteristic voluminous clear sputum production (bronchorrhea). Prognosis is related to stage of disease, but because BAC may be mistaken for chronic infection or diffuse interstitial disease, there may be a long delay in diagnosis.

Undifferentiated large cell carcinoma is characterized by large cells with vesicular nuclei, prominent eosinophilic nucleoli, moderate to abundant cytoplasm, distinct cytoplasmic membrane, and no evidence of squamous or glandular differentiation by light microscopy. Some of these tumors may contain features of either squamous and/or glandular differentiation as evidenced by immunohistochemistry or electron microscopy, implying some heterogeneity in this group. Giant cell and clear cell variants are uncommon. A giant cell variant may mimic an anaplastic large cell lymphoma (Ki-1 lymphoma), in that the latter tends to proliferate in lymph node sinuses (similar to metastatic cancer), unlike the usual lymphoma proliferation within the lymph node itself. Clinically, most patients with large cell lung cancer present with bulky, peripheral tumors. Metastases occur early, preferentially to the central nervous system (CNS), and the 5-year survival is under 5%.

Small Cell Lung Cancer

Small cell lung cancer (SCLC) represents about 15% of all lung tumors, is extremely aggressive, is frequently associated with distant metastases, and has the poorest prognosis of all lung neoplasms. The incidence is decreasing for unknown specific reasons; however, it may be related to the greater use of cigarette smokers. SCLC is highly related to cigarette smoking (98% or more of cases). SCLC has a central origin in most cases, although 10% of these tumors are found in the peripheral lung field. The tumors have a white-tan appearance, are friable, and show extensive necrosis. Histologically they are characterized by scant cytoplasm or high nuclear-to-cytoplasmic ratio, fine chromatin, and "nuclear molding." Small cells are characterized as "small blue cell tumor" and must be distinguished from lymphoma, carcinoid tumors, Ewing's sarcoma, and primitive neuroepithelial tumors (PNET). The rapid growth and scanty cytoplasm of small cell carcinomas make them unusually susceptible to ischemic necrosis, as well as crush artefact, during handling and fixation. Although not pathognomonic, the so-called Azzopardi effect (crushed DNA material encrusted around blood vessels) is very characteristic (Fig. 5.21B). The subclassification of small cell carcinoma into oat cell, intermediate cell, and combined oat cell carcinoma has been dropped from the new WHO classification, and the only subtype of SCLC is combined SCLC. Less than 10% of SCLCs are admixed with non–small cell lung carcinoma (NSCLC) components (with large cells 4% to 6%, 1% to 3% with adenocarcinoma or squamous cell carcinoma).

Most SCLCs contain dense-core granules (which contain among other molecules, amines, peptide products, and L-dopa decarboxylase), indicating neuroendocrine differentiation. Immunohistochemical studies demonstrate the presence of neuron-specific enolase (NSE), chromogranin A, Leu-7 (a natural killer cell antigen also present in some neuroendocrine cells), and synaptophysin. Other antigens that may also be expressed are carcinoembryonic antigen (CEA), adrenocorticotrophic hormone (ACTH), and "big" ACTH. "Big" ACTH is a physiologically inactive form of ACTH produced by certain tumors as a paraneoplastic product that is larger and more acidic than "little" (normal) ACTH but immunochemically indistinguishable. SCLC cells, as with most carcinomas, express keratin proteins.

SCLCs produce and release into the circulation a variety of functioning polypeptide hormones that can cause paraneoplastic syndromes (Table 5.8). They also grow in a submucosal pattern with a high frequency of lymphatic and vascular invasion; for this reason they do not often cause hemoptysis. Thus, they may not be readily identified on bronchoscopy. Prominent mediastinal adenopathy is often present. Almost 70% of patients have metastatic disease at the time of diagnosis. Almost any organ can be involved, but preferential sites include the liver, bone, bone marrow, CNS, adrenal glands, abdominal lymph nodes, pancreas, skin, and endocrine organs.

Carcinoid Tumor and the Spectrum of Neuroendocrine Tumors of the Lung

The classification of neuroendocrine neoplasms of the lung has evolved substantially over the past two decades. Initially there were only two categories: carcinoid and SCLC. The latter is discussed above.

Typical carcinoid or carcinoid tumors (bronchial carcinoid tumors) are similar to tumors arising in the gastrointestinal tract and elsewhere. They are characterized by small (0.7–3.5 cm), well-circumscribed solid tan/yellow nodules with no necrosis or hemorrhage. Usually they are centrally seen, less commonly peripheral in location. By light microscopy tumor cells are round and uniform in size, with finely granular eosinophilic cytoplasm. The nucleus is centrally placed with finely granular or stippled chromatin and small nucleoli. The cells arrange themselves in an organoid pattern (cords, nests, and acini may be formed). Mitoses are rare and necrosis is not seen. By electron microscopy numerous cytoplasmic membrane-bound, dense-core granules (90–450 nm) are usually seen. By immunohistology they are usually positive for NSE, chromogranin A, Leu-7, synaptophysin, bombesin, CEA, ACTH, calcitonin, and keratin. Carcinoid tumors may be responsible for ectopic hormone secretion, particularly 5-hydroxytryptamine, ACTH, vasopressin, and insulin. Typical carcinoid tumors have low malignant potential. They are not usually associated with cigarette smoking.

Atypical carcinoid is a third category described in 1972. Atypical carcinoid is similar to typical carcinoid but usually larger (1.5–2.3 cm) and contains foci of necrosis and mitoses (usually 3–4/10 high-power fields [HPF]). Atypical carcinoids can follow a more aggressive clinical course than typical carcinoid and have metastatic potential. Atypical carcinoids represent approximately 10% of all carcinoid tumors.

The fourth category is large cell neuroendocrine carcinoma (LCNEC). LCNEC is a malignant neuroendocrine neoplasm composed of large polygonal cells with a relatively low nuclear-to-cytoplasmic ratio, coarse nuclear chromatin, frequent nucleoli, high mitotic rate (>10/10 HPF), and frequent necrosis. The cells in LCNEC are larger than cells in SCLC and have more abundant eosinophilic cytoplasm. However, the biology and prognosis of both of these neuroendocrine malignancies is poor as a result of the metastatic disease that occurs early in the natural history and may be refractory to curative treatment.

CHROMOSOMES, GENES, AND LUNG CANCER

The evolution to cancer in general is currently understood as a multistep process. Insight into this evolution has been gained through recent advances in cytogenetics, cell biology, and mainly molecular biology. It has become apparent that mutations in a limited number of genes, which control cell proliferation and differentiation, are key events in this process. Proto-oncogenes ("activated" by a particular mutation) and tumor suppressor genes ("deactivation" unleashes unregulated proliferation of cells) have major roles in malignant transformation of cells and may be prognostic forms (see Tables 5.5 and 5.6). Diagrams for molecular and biochemical abnormalities in lung cancer and mechanisms for metastatic spread are given in Figures 5.1 and 5.2.

Chromosomal Abnormalities and Telomerase Activation

Using both actual tumor specimens and cell lines, various chromosomal and oncogene abnormalities have been identified. In NSCLC chromosomal aberrations have been described on 3p, 8p, 9p, 11p, 15p, and 17p with deletions of chromosomes 7, 11, 13, or 19. Also, in SCLC, chromosomal abnormalities have been described on 1p, 3p, 5q, 6q, 8q, 13q, or 17p. One of the most consistent chromosomal abnormalities in lung cancer has been the loss of the short arm of chromosome 3 (3p14–p25). The loss of alleles at 3p is observed in more than 90% of SCLC tumors and approximately 50% of NSCLC tumors. As many as three tumor suppressor genes may contribute to SCLC pathogenesis.

Other genetic losses have, though not consistently, been identified in lung cancer. In NSCLC these include genetic loss at chromosome 8p (21.3–p22) and may be abnormal in 50% of tumor samples. Genetic loss at 9p (21–p22) could potentially involve the p16 (MTS1/p16INK4A) and p15 (MTS2/p15INK4B) tumor suppressor genes, which are involved in cell cycle regulation at the G_1 checkpoint by inhibiting cyclin-dependent kinase CDK4 and may be affected in 67% of tumor samples. Genetic loss at 11p (p13 and p15) may involve the Wilms' tumor suppressor gene at region p13 and can be affected in 20% to 46% of tumor samples.

Telomeres, which are genetic elements at the ends of linear eukaryotic chromosomes consisting of tandem repeats of simple DNA sequences, are important in stabilizing chromosomes from degradation, illegitimate recombination, or cellular senescence. Longer telomeres are present in germ cells and in most cancer cells, via the telomerase enzyme, and these maintain the ability of the cells to divide indefinitely. Telomerase activity has been directly correlated with malignant and metastatic phenotype of a wide array of solid tumors. In one study 80% of tumor tissue from lung cancer had telomerase activity (Hiyama et al., 1995).

Proto-Oncogenes in NSCLC

Amplification of the RAS genes (*KRAS*, *HRAS*, and *NRAS*), especially *KRAS*, is frequent in NSCLC. The level and frequency vary with the tumor type, ranging from about 30% in adenocarcinoma as compared with 10% in other cell types. There is evidence of linking mutations in the RAS family with a poor prognosis in patients undergoing surgery. There is a correlation between *KRAS* mutations in adenocarcinomas and smoking history. In particular, mutations of the *KRAS* oncogene involving codon 12 may be a specific target of tobacco smoke and may occur early and irreversibly during carcinogenesis in adenocarcinomas of the lung (Westra et al., 1993). Amplification of c-*MYC* is found in about 10% of NSCLC of all types.

The *erb*B-1 (epidermal growth factor receptor, EGFR) protein is overexpressed in approximately 60% to 80% of NSCLC, with high expression in squamous cell carcinomas. The EGFR can be mutated somatically in certain subsets of NSCLC (especially adenocarcinomas). The frequency of mutations is highest in the tyrosine kinase domain, nonsmokers, females, and certain ethnic populations (such as Asians). There is also a truncation mutation, EGFR-vIII, that can occur in squamous cell carcinomas. EGFR overexpression can be a prognostication for lung cancer, and the mutations can be a predictive marker for therapeutic response to small molecule tyrosine kinase inhibitors. In certain subsets of NSCLC, EGFR can also be amplified.

The c-*erb*B-2 (HER2/neu) gene encodes a transmembrane tyrosine-specific protein kinase, p185neu. Frequency of abnormal expression of c-*erb*B-2 is approximately 25%. This gene is frequently amplified in adenocarcinomas and squamous cell carcinomas; in adenocarcinomas p185neu expression tends to be found in older patients and is usually associated with shorter survival.

The c-MET gene can also be overexpressed in lung cancer. In particular subsets of patients there are also activating mutations and/or amplification that will have prognostic and predictive biomarker implications.

Tumor Suppressor Genes in NSCLC

The *TP53* gene encodes a 53-kDa nuclear phosphoprotein identified as a transcriptional activator. High levels of the wild-type gene product inhibit growth, possibly by acting as a checkpoint for DNA damage at the G_0–G_1 transition in cell division. Mutations in *TP53* are very common features in different types of cancer and are present in NSCLC and have been detected in preinvasive lesions of the bronchus (Sundaresan et al., 1992). The frequency of mutations varies with the type of NSCLC: about 67% of squamous cell carcinomas and 37% of adenocarcinomas contain *TP53* mutations. Mutations are also present in undifferentiated large cell carcinomas. No significant correlation has been found between *TP53* mutations and age, sex, histopathology, clinical stage, or lymph node involvement. G:C-to-T:A transversions, found in about 50% of NSCLC, are remarkably uncommon in other types of human cancer. Because one of the components of cigarette smoking is benzo[*a*]pyrene, a potent mutagen that causes G:C-to-T:A transversions, the implication is that smoking may be responsible for these mutations. Interestingly, mutations in both *TP53* and *KRAS* are most commonly G-to-T transversions in lung cancer versus G-to-A transitions in other cancers (Johnson and Kelley, 1993).

The retinoblastoma gene (*RB1*) encodes a DNA-binding protein of 110 kDa that is involved in important events of cell division. Inactivation of this gene by deletion and loss of heterozygosity has been found in several cancers, with abnormalities in NSCLC approximately 15%. In NSCLC, an inverse correlation exists between p16INK4A expression and *RB1* expression, thereby implicating a key role of these proteins in growth suppression.

Table 5.5

Prognostic Factors in Stage I Non–Small Cell Lung Cancer*

Variable	Favorable	Unfavorable
Histopathologic Markers		
1. Tumor status	T1	T2
2. Histologic subtype	Squamous	Large cell[†]
3. Degree of tumor differentiation	WD	PD[‡]
4. Lymphatic and/or blood vessel invasion	Absent	Present
5. Mitotic index	Low	High
6. Plasma cell infiltration	Present	Absent or minimal
7. Tumor giant cells	Absent	Present
8. WHO subtype of adenocarcinoma	Bronchoalveolar or acinar or papillary	Solid tumor with mucus formation
Molecular Genetic Markers		
1. *KRAS* oncogene activation	No point mutation	Point mutation at codon 12
2. *RAS* gene protein product expression	Absent p21 staining	Strong p21 staining[§]
3. C-*erb*-2 protein expression	Normal	Increased
4. *TP53* tumor suppressor gene	No mutation	Gene mutation present
5. p53 protein product expression	Normal p53	Overexpression of p53
6. Retinoblastoma (RB) protein expression	RB-positive	RB-negative
7. BCL2 protein expression	BCL2-positive	BCL2-negative
Differentiation Markers		
1. Expression of blood group antigen on tumor cells	Conserved expression of blood group antigens	Altered expression of blood group antigens
2. Expression of H/Ley/Leb antigens	Negative staining with MIA-15-5	Positive staining with MIA-15-5
Proliferation Markers		
1. DNA content (flow cytometry)	Diploid	Aneuploid
2. S-phase fraction (flow cytometry)	Low	High
3. Mitotic index	<13 mitoses per 10 HPF	≥13 mitoses per 10 HPF
4. Proliferation index (PI) using Ki-67 nuclear antigen	<3.5	>3.5
5. Thymidine labeling index (TLI)	<2.9	>2.9
6. Number of nucleolar organizing regions	Mean <3.80/cell	Mean >3.80/cell
7. Proliferating cell nuclear antigen staining	<5% of tumor cells stained	>5% of tumor cells stained
Markers of Metastatic Propensity in Stage I NSCLC		
1. Intensity of angiogenesis	Low microvessel count and density grade	High microvessel
2. Basement membrane deposition (squamous cell carcinoma)	Extensive deposition	Limited deposition[¶]
3. Ability to establish in vitro cell lines	In vitro cell lines not established	Independent cell lines
4. Soluble interleukin-2 receptor	Postoperative value less than preoperative	Postoperative value greater than preoperative

HPF, high-power fields; PD, poorly differentiated; WD, well-differentiated.

[†]Adenocarcinoma is intermediate prognosis.
[‡]Moderately differentiated is intermediate prognosis.
[§]Moderate staining is intermediate prognosis.
[¶]Moderate deposition is intermediate prognosis.

*Additional poor prognostic factors have been recently identified, including location of lung cancer in the non–upper lobes (Ou et al., 2007), visceral pleural invasion (Shimizue et al., 2005), circulating c-MET messenger RNA (Cheng et al., 2005), loss of expressin of p16 gene (Tanaka et al., 2005), postoperative CEA level >5 (Sawabata et al., 2004; Inoue et al., 2006). In addition, improved methodology in lung cancer genomic profiling has led to prognostic information that may be useful for adjuvant chemotherapy in patients at high risk of relapse (Potti et al., 2006; Chen et al., 2007a).

From Strauss GM, Kwiat Kowski DJ, Harpole DH, et al: Molecular and pathologic analysis of stage I non-small cell carcinoma of the lung: implications for the future, *J Clin Oncol* 13:1265–1279, 1995.

Proto-Oncogenes In SCLC

Mutations in *RAS* genes are absent in SCLC. Gene amplification of all three types of *MYC* genes has been observed in SCLC. Amplification of *MYC* genes has been observed more frequently in patients who have undergone chemotherapy, but cell lines established from SCLCs before and after chemotherapy did not alter their status of *MYC* gene copy number. It is unclear whether chemotherapy can actually cause *MYC* gene amplification. Increased expression of N-*MYC* gene has been reported to correlate with poor subsequent response to chemotherapy, rapid tumor growth, and short survival times. c-KIT and c-MET receptor tyrosine kinases are also overexpressed in SCLC.

Tumor Suppressor Genes in SCLC

The *RB1* gene (chromosome 3q) is absent or aberrant in over 90% of patients. This was the first identification of a recessive oncogene participating in the pathogenesis of lung cancer (Otterson et al., 1992). RB1 gene protein has important functions in the regulation of growth stages of cell cycle events, by maintaining cells in a quiescent or growth-arrested state.

Mutations of the *TP53* gene are present in over 75% of SCLCs and are considered an early event in carcinogenesis. Structural abnormalities have been detected in some cell lines, but in the absence of RB1 messenger RNA and p105 RB protein.

Table 5.6

Chromosomes, Genes, and Lung Cancer

Type	Subtype	Cytogenic Abnormalities	Proto-Oncogenes	Onco-suppressor Genes
NSCLC	Not specified	1p13, 3p13	c-MYC (10%)	TP53 (50%)
		8p11–q11	BCL-2	
		8p11–q11		
		15p11–q11		
		17p11		
		Chrs. 7, 13, 19		
	Squamous cell carcinoma	Chr. 11	erbB-1	TP53 (67%)
		3p17q	c-erbB-2	
			c-FOS	
			c-JUN (AP-1)	
	Adenocarcinoma	3p21.3 (<50%)	KRAS (30%)	TP53 (37%)
		3p14.1–12.1	c-erbB-2 (25%)	
			c-FOS	
			c-JUN (AP-1)	
Small cell carcinoma		3p21.3–3p25 (90%)	c-RAF1	
		3p14		
		5q21 (APC)	c-FMS	TP53 (80%)
		6q24	c-MYB	
		8q24	c-MYC	
		1p32	L-MYC	
		13q14		RB (90%)
		17q13		

Chr., chromosome; NSCLC, non–small cell lung carcinoma.
*Frequency (%) of abnormalities among the types of lung cancer is indicated.
Data adapted from Anderson M, Spandidos D: Oncogenes and onco-suppressor genes in lung cancer, *Respir Med* 87: 413–420, 1993.

Chromosomal abnormalities in SCLC mainly consist of chromosome 3 short-arm deletions, in three different regions between 3p21 and 3p25, occurring in over 90% of cases.

Growth Factor Abnormalities in SCLC

In SCLC many of the tumor cells produce neuroendocrine peptides, such as gastrin-releasing peptide (GRP), and respond to them in an autocrine or paracrine fashion. GRP binds to the receptor (G-protein family member) and transduces intracellular signal with proliferation of SCLC cells. Another growth factor, insulin-like growth factor I, is elevated in more than 95% of SCLCs and modulates mitogenic signaling. Also, Steel factor, the ligand for the proto-oncogene tyrosine kinase receptor c-KIT, supports growth and survival of immature hematopoietic cells of multiple lineages. In SCLC, c-KIT and Steel factor are simultaneously expressed, thus forming an autocrine loop.

Metastatic Mechanisms in Lung Cancer

Paget initially observed that metastasis of tumor cells occurred when certain tumor cells ("seed") had special affinity for the growth environment provided by certain specific organs ("soil"). Tumor cells are heterogeneous and have different angiogenic, invasive, and metastatic properties. Inducing angiogenesis may be an important mechanism for a tumor cell to proliferate and eventually metastasize. Angiogenesis has been shown to be a prognostic factor in stage I NSCLC (Harpole et al., 1996). Tumor cells can also penetrate pre-existing vessels, thereby leading to metastasis. In one study 15% of patients with tumor invasion of peripheral, node-negative NSCLC had a poor survival rate and a higher recurrence rate (Macchiarini et al., 1992).

Angiogenesis is an important part for tumor growth and metastasis. Neoangiogenesis appears to be a significant prognostic factor in patients with resected NSCLC in most, but not all, clinical studies. As an example, one study of tumors from 275 patients with stage I NSCLC analyzed overall survival via multivariate analysis of angiogenesis, proto-oncogene *HER2/neu*, tumor suppressor gene *TP53*, and the proliferation marker Ki-67 (see "HER-2/neu (c-erbB-2) oncogene and protein expression" above and see "TP53 tumor suppressor gene" above). Of these factors, excessive angiogenesis was the most significant adverse prognostic factor. Others have reported a correlation between MVD, PD-ECGF, and VEGF expression, neovascularity, and prognosis in resected NSCLC.

Staging of Lung Cancer

The most widely used system is the International Staging System (ISS) using TNM, categories to place patients into stages I–IV, each having a progressively lower survival rate (Fig. 5.34). It was revised in 1997 with additional stage subgroupings (Mountain, 1997; see also Figs. 5.36 and 5.37). Only 30% of patients present with stage I or II disease; 15% to 20% have potentially resectable stage IIIA disease and the remainder have advanced unresectable stage IIIB or metastatic stage IV disease. Although the ISS can be applied to all cell types, SCLC is often categorized as limited disease (stage I, II, or III) or extensive disease (stage IV) for therapeutic purposes. New changes in the TNM classification were first proposed by the International Association for the Study of Lung Cancer (IASCL) at the international meeting in Seoul, Korea, in August 2007 and also in San Francisco, U.S.A., at the thirteenth annual World Conference on Lung Cancer in August 2009. The changes have been accepted by the American Joint Committee on Cancer (AJCC) and the International Union Against Cancer (UICC) and are summarized in Figures 5.31 and 5.32, along with the survival in a large number of patients according to the pathologic stage (Fig. 5.33). The latter should be compared to survival based on clinical stage (Fig. 5.34) based upon preoperative studies (Goldstraw, 2009).

Survival for patients with SCLC seems to have improved over the last 15 years. However, 2- to 3-year survival still occurs in only 10% to 25% of patients with limited disease and 1% to 2% of patients with extensive disease. Moreover, relapse of SCLC and development of other neoplasms are common in patients surviving beyond 2 years. Prognostic indicators (disease stage) should help target individual SCLC patients for specific intensive treatments designed to prolong survival and achieve cure (Skarin, 1993).

Staging procedures consist of computed tomography (CT) scan of the chest and upper abdomen to include liver and adrenals. Assays for tumor markers (e.g., CEA, CA 125, and NSE; Salgia et al., 2001), if elevated, may be of prognostic value and also allow for monitoring of disease status. Several studies are ongoing to determine the role of molecular markers. A bone scan and head CT scan with contrast magnetic resonance imaging (MRI) should be performed in all patients except for those with stage I NSCLC who are asymptomatic with normal chemistries. In these patients the likelihood of early (occult) metastases is under 5%. Positron-emission tomography (PET) scans are also of value in initial assessment and follow-up restaging or search for metastases (see Chapter 2). Whole-body PET using [18F]fluorodeoxyglucose as a tracer is a new imaging technique based upon the increased metabolism of glucose in malignant cells. PET has a 95% sensitivity for detecting primary lung cancers and mediastinal lymph node involvement (Pieterman et al., 2000). The threshold of detection is around 3–5 mm. It may more accurately predict the likelihood of long-term survival than chest CT does (Dunagan et al., 2001). It is also useful to differentiate benign from malignant pulmonary nodules, assess response to treatment and recurrence, and assist in radiotherapeutic planning (Marom et al., 2000). Bone marrow involvement as the only stage IV manifestation is unusual, however, and occurs in approximately 5% of cases with limited thoracic disease in SCLC.

Invasive staging procedures include thoracoscopy, cervical (suprasternal) mediastinoscopy, and anterior mediastinoscopy (Chamberlain procedure). One or more may be carried out to evaluate mediastinal nodal stations (see Fig. 5.30) or suspicious sites of disease in resectable patients, particularly when multimodality treatment protocols are utilized. Video-assisted thoracoscopic surgery (VATS) is being used for staging as well as management in selected cases (see Fig. 5.56). VATS has minimal mortality and greatly reduces hospitalization time compared with traditional thoracotomy (Mentzer and Sugarbaker, 1994).

CLINICAL MANIFESTATIONS

The signs and symptoms of lung cancer are related directly to the primary malignancy or to distant metastases. Indirect signs and symptoms may be encountered as a result of the secretion of biologically active polypeptides and hormones.

Manifestations of early thoracic disease depend on the location of the primary cancer. Central (proximal) lesions such as squamous cell carcinoma often erode the bronchus, causing hemoptysis and cough. Chest pain is a common symptom in early-stage lung cancer. As the tumor spreads, bronchial obstruction with atelectasis and pneumonia often occurs. Hilar adenopathy and cavitation of the primary cancer may also develop. Although small cell cancers are central in origin, they grow submucosally and thus rarely cause hemoptysis. Due to lymphatic invasion, mediastinal adenopathy occurs in most cases. Extension into the recurrent laryngeal nerve results in hoarseness, and involvement of the phrenic nerve causes a paralyzed (elevated) diaphragm. Stridor, caused by invasion of the trachea or bilateral vocal cord

paralysis, results from compromise of the lumen of the trachea. Invasion and compression of the superior vena cava leads to the superior vena cava (SVC) syndrome (see Fig. 5.62); this can occur either with isolated stage IIIB disease or as part of stage IV (metastatic) disease. Extension of malignancy into the pericardium results in pericardial effusion and acute cardiac tamponade.

Cancers that arise in the peripheral lung fields, such as adenocarcinoma and large cell carcinoma, cause chest pain and cough due to involvement of the pleura, often with malignant pleural effusion and resultant dyspnea. Undifferentiated large cell tumors may reach enormous size before symptoms occur. Widespread metastases develop in most cases.

Cancers arising in the apex of the lung grow into the adjacent soft tissues, resulting in a Pancoast tumor or superior sulcus tumor syndrome, the features of which may vary. Histologically, Pancoast tumors are usually squamous cell carcinomas, although other non–small cell types of cancer can occur; the rarest cause is small cell (oat cell) lung cancer. Persistent symptoms can result from early lesions that may be missed on routine radiographs, unless apical views or tomograms are obtained. CT scans can detect early lesions and define the extent of regional disease. The advanced syndrome is marked by shoulder pain radiating to the ulnar nerve distribution, rib and vertebral body destruction, and Horner's syndrome (enophthalmos, ptosis, miosis, and ipsilateral loss of sweating) due to invasion of the sympathetic nerves. With early involvement, mydriasis (pupillary dilatation) may be the first clue. Unilateral supraclavicular adenopathy is a sign of advanced local disease.

Metastatic disease can occur to any organ, and thus a variety of clinical and laboratory manifestations may be encountered. At autopsy the frequency of extrathoracic metastases related to histologic type of lung cancer is as follows: squamous cell carcinoma, 25% to 54%; adenocarcinoma, 50% to 82%; large cell carcinoma, 48% to 86%; and small cell carcinoma, 74% to 96%. With advanced disease there are no particular selective sites for metastases related to histologic type. Lymphangitic spread of the tumor through the parenchyma of the lung is characterized by progressive dyspnea, cough, and hypoxia.

Indirect manifestations of lung cancer vary from severe weight loss and cachexia, seen in up to one third of patients, to one or more of several paraneoplastic syndromes. The latter are due to the secretion of biologically active polypeptide hormones or to unknown factors often related to certain histologic cell types (see Table 5.8). Patients may initially present with these problems, which can be misinterpreted—for example, joint pains due to clubbing being mistaken for arthritis. Hypertrophic osteoarthropathy can occur with symptoms of swelling and pain in the joints and extremities. These manifestations, however, should also be viewed as clues to an underlying lung cancer. In some patients the initial chest film may fail to show an obvious lesion, a scenario occasionally seen in SCLC. In this situation CT scanning may reveal a small tumor mass or bronchoscopy may yield the correct diagnosis.

Tumors of the Heart

Primary tumors of the heart are rare. The incidence varies from 0.0017% to 0.28% in autopsy studies. Cardiac myxomas are by far the most common, up to 30%, arising most often in adulthood, equally in either sex. Patients with myxomas typically present either with the features of mitral valve disease or with systemic emboli; they often remain asymptomatic. Unusual clinical features include polyarthralgia, Reynaud's phenomenon, malaise, and weight loss. The great majority of cardiac myxomas develop as pedunculated tumors in the left atrium (75% to 80%); the right atrium is the second most common site; the ventricles are only rarely affected. The precise nature of these benign lesions has been a source of controversy. Once viewed as representing simply organized, rather myxoid thrombi, myxomas are currently regarded as true neoplasms derived from subendocardial tissue. Histologically, they show only primitive mesenchymal differentiation.

The most common primary malignancy of the heart is angiosarcoma, which occurs mainly in the right atrium. Most patients present with congestive heart failure, and the diagnosis may not even be established until autopsy. There is no effective therapy in the vast majority of cases.

In contrast, metastatic tumors to the heart are relatively common. Lung cancer often spreads to the pericardium, resulting in malignant pericardial effusion and acute tamponade, but metastases can also develop in the endocardium and myocardium, producing arrhythmias and cardiac failure. Rarely, coronary artery metastases occur, with resultant angina or acute myocardial infarction. Other malignancies that often spread to the heart include malignant melanoma, breast cancer, lymphoma, leukemia, soft tissue sarcomas, renal cell carcinoma, choriocarcinoma, and hepatocellular carcinoma. Kaposi's sarcoma may also involve the heart, particularly in patients with acquired immunodeficiency syndrome.

Tumors of the Mediastinum

The mediastinum is formed laterally by the parietal pleura, anteriorly by the sternum and attached muscles, and posteriorly by the thoracic spine. Its upper limit is the first thoracic vertebra and the manubrium; its lower limit is the diaphragm. For descriptive purposes the mediastinum is usually divided into four major compartments: superior, anterior, middle, and posterior (see Fig. 5.101). Clinical manifestations of the various disorders of the mediastinum are related mainly to pressure or invasion of the structures within each division.

The mediastinum is the site of a variety of primary and metastatic tumors. The latter are quite common, most frequently originating from lymphomas or from carcinomas of the lung, breast, intestinal tract, and testes. In some cases the original cancer may be occult. Primary tumors of the mediastinum, on the other hand, are quite rare. The majority of tumors, about 75%, are benign; of these, most are neurogenic tumors or primary cysts (bronchogenic, pericardial, enteric, and others).

HISTOLOGY

Germ Cell Tumors

All types of germinal tumors found in the testes are known to occur in the mediastinum. Primary seminomas, less than 5% of which occur in women, constitute half of all cases. Nonseminomatous tumors may be pure or mixed germ cell tumors. About 60% to 70% of patients have elevated levels of β-human chorionic gonadotrophin (choriocarcinomatous elements) and/or α-fetoprotein (embryonal and endodermal sinus elements). Benign teratomas, which account for about 20% of anterior mediastinal tumors, occur with equal frequency in men and women. The teratoma, which is cystic in nature, is often referred to as a dermoid cyst, and it is entirely comparable with ovarian dermoid tumors. Histologic sections usually reveal tissues arising from all three germ cell layers. The tumors contain hair, sebaceous material, bone, cartilage, and other tissues. Calcifications are present in 75% of lesions and may be seen on radiographs. Malignant transition to teratocarcinoma occurs in 10% to 20% of cases.

Thymic Tumors

Thymic tumors most frequently occur in the superior mediastinum but may develop in the anterior mediastinum as well. Thymomas are often large and encapsulated, and show fibrous septae on cut section. These tumors are composed of neoplastic epithelial cells with a variable admixture of T lymphocytes. The WHO classification for thymic epithelial tumors, commonly used, includes six histologic categories (see Table 5.11). The classification scheme correlates with invasiveness: types A and AB are usually clinically benign and encapsulated, type B is more likely invasive, and type C is usually invasive. The Masaoka staging system is generally used with six prognostic groups (see Table 5.12). Prognosis for thymomas is generally good, with 5- and 10-year survival rates over 60% and 50%, respectively. Poor prognostic features include predominantly epithelial histology, large tumor size and local invasion at surgery (about one third of cases), and metastases. About 30% to 40% of all patients develop myasthenia gravis (most common in the mixed cell type), whereas 10% have other paraneoplastic syndromes including pure red cell aplasia, hypogammaglobulinemia, polymyositis, and positive lupus erythematosus tests. Of patients with myasthenia gravis, 65% show thymic follicular hyperplasia whereas 10% have a thymoma.

Other primary tumors of the thymus are rare. These include thymic squamous carcinomas, carcinoids, and neuroendocrine tumors, as well as germ cell tumors and lipomas. Malignant lymphoma and other hematopoietic tumors may rarely arise within the thymus.

Table 5.7

Causes of Interstitial Lung Disease*

Neoplastic	Immunologic	Occupational	Infectious	Drug-related	Rare
Multiple metastatic deposits	Collagen-vascular diseases	Asbestosis	Miliary tuberculosis	Amiodarone	Hemosiderosis
Bronchioalveolar carcinoma	Cryptogenic fibrosing alveolitis	Silicosis	Fungal infection (e.g., candidiasis)	Cytotoxic drugs	Eosinophilic granuloma
Lymphangitis carcinomatosa	Extrinsic allergic alveolitis	Siderosis	Protozoan infection (e.g., *Pneumocystis*)	Paraquat	Alveolar proteinosis
Leukemia	Pulmonary eosinophilia	Talcosis	Viral infection (e.g., cytomegalovirus)		
Lymphoma	Granulomatous disorders				

*The finding of an interstitial pattern on chest radiography may be the result of numerous causes, among them lung neoplasia.

Table 5.8

Manifestations of Selected Paraneoplastic Syndromes in Lung Cancer Patients by Type of Manifestation and Frequency

Type of Manifestation	Frequency (%)
Systemic	
Anorexia–cachexia	31
Fever	21
Suppressed immunity	–
Skeletal	
Digital clubbing	29
Periostitis (hypertrophic pulmonary osteoarthropathy)—commonly associated with adenocarcinoma	1–10
Endocrine	
Hypercalcemia (ectopic parathyroid hormone)— commonly associated with squamous cell carcinoma	
Hyponatremia (inappropriate secretion of antidiuretic hormone)—commonly associated with small cell carcinoma	
Cushing syndrome (ectopic corticotrophin secretion) — commonly associated with small cell carcinoma	
Hematologic	8
Anemia	
Granulocytosis	
Eosinophilia	
Leukoerythroblastosis	
Coagulation—thrombotic	1–4
Venous thrombosis (migratory thrombophlebitis, Trousseau's syndrome)	
Arterial embolism (nonbacterial thrombotic endocarditis)	
Hemorrhage (disseminated intravascular coagulation)	
Neurologic—myopathic	1
Eaton-Lambert syndrome (myasthenia)—commonly associated with small cell carcinoma	
Peripheral neuropathy	
Subacute cerebellar degeneration	
Cortical degeneration	
Polymyositis	
Neurologic—cutaneous	1
Dermatomyositis	
Acanthosis nigricans	
Renal	<1
Nephrotic syndrome	
Glomerulonephritis	

Modified from Minna JD, Pass H, Glatstein EJ: Cancer of the lung. In DeVita Jr VT, Hellman S, Rosenberg SA, editors: *Cancer: principles and practices of oncology*, ed 3, Philadelphia, 1989, Lippincott, pp 591–724.

Table 5.9

Tumors and Cysts of the Heart and Pericardium

Type	Frequency (%)	Type	Frequency (%)
Benign tumors		Malignant tumors	
Myxoma	24.4	Angiosarcoma	7.3
Lipoma	8.4	Rhabdomyosarcoma	4.9
Papillary fibroelastoma	7.9	Mesothelioma	3.6
Rhabdomyoma	6.8	Fibrosarcoma	2.6
Fibroma	3.2	Malignant lymphoma	1.3
Hemangioma	2.8	Extraskeletal osteosarcoma	<1
Teratoma (dermoid cyst)	2.6	Neurogenic sarcoma	<1
Mesothelioma of atrioventricular node	2.3	Malignant teratoma	<1
		Thymoma	<1
		Leiomyosarcoma	<1
Granular cell tumor	<1%	Liposarcoma	<1
		Synovial sarcoma	<1
Neurofibroma	<1		
Lymphangioma	<1		
Cyst			
Pericardial cyst	15.4		
Bronchogenic cyst	1.3		

Modified from McAllister HA Jr, Fenoglio JJ Jr: *Tumors of the cardiovascular system*, Washington, DC, 1978, Armed Forces Institute of Pathology.

Table 5.10

General Manifestations of Neoplastic Heart Disease

Pericardial Involvement	Myocardial Involvement	Intracavity Tumor
Pericarditis pain	Arrhythmias, ventricular and atrial	Cavity obliteration
Pericardial effusion	Electrocardiographic changes	Valve obstruction and valve damage
Radiographic evidence of enlargement	Radiographic evidence of enlargement (generalized, localized)	Embolic phenomena (systemic, neurologic, coronary)
Arrhythmia, predominantly atrial	Conduction disturbances and heart block	Constitutional manifestations
Tamponade	Congestive heart failure	
Constriction	Coronary involvement (angina, infarction)	

Reproduced with permission from Hall R, Cooley D: Neoplastic heart disease. In Hurst J, editor: *The heart: arteries and veins*, ed 6, New York, 1986, McGraw-Hill.

Neurogenic Tumors

Neurogenic tumors characteristically arise in the posterior mediastinum near the paravertebral gutter. They occur at all ages, but the malignant variants are often present in childhood. The lesions arise from nerve cells of the sympathetic nervous system, peripheral nerve sheaths, or embryonal neurogenic rests. Types of tumors include neurofibromas (singly or in association with von Recklinghausen's disease), neurilemmomas (from the nerve sheath or Schwann's membrane), ganglioneuromas (from the sympathetic chain), and neuroblastomas.

CLINICAL MANIFESTATIONS

Mediastinal tumors, even when massive, may be asymptomatic and are often detected incidentally on routine chest radiography. However, symptoms occur in about two thirds of patients,

Table 5.11

World Health Organization (WHO) Classification System for Thymic Tumors (1999)

WHO Classification	Description
A	Medullary; spindle-cell thymoma
AB	Mixed thymoma
B1	Predominantly cortical; lymphocyte-rich; lymphocytic, organoid thymoma
B2	Cortical
B3	Epithelial; squamous; atypical thymoma; well-differentiated thymic carcinoma
C	Thymic carcinoma

With permission from Riedel RF, Burfeind WR: Thymoma: benign appearance, malignant potential, *Oncologist* 11: 887–894, 2006.

Table 5.12

Masaoka Staging System for Thymoma (1981)

Masaoka Stage	Criteria
I	Encapsulated tumor
IIA	Microscopic capsular invasion
IIB	Macroscopic invasion into fatty tissue
III	Invasion into great vessels, pericardium, or lung
IVA	Pleural and/or pericardial dissemination
IVB	Lymphatic or hematogenous metastases

From Riedel RF, Burfeind WR: Thymoma: benign appearance, malignant potential, *Oncologist* 11: 887–894, 2006.

consisting of retrosternal pain, dyspnea, and other respiratory complications in anterior mediastinal tumors. In the posterior medi-astinum symptoms vary greatly. Compression of the trachea and bronchi results in cough and dyspnea, whereas esophageal compression causes dysphagia. Other presenting problems include paralysis of the diaphragm, hoarseness, Horner's syndrome, and SVC syndrome in tumors involving the superior mediastinum.

Diagnostic evaluation includes standard radiologic studies, as well as esophagograms in some cases. CT and MRI scanning are approximately equivalent in assessing the primary lesion and any regional metastases. Combined CT-PET scanning is under evaluation for assessing activity and regional spread as well as possible distant metastases of the mediastinal tumors. A specific diagnosis can be established by several procedures, including needle biopsy, mediastinoscopy, mediastinotomy, or in some cases thoracotomy with resection of the lesion.

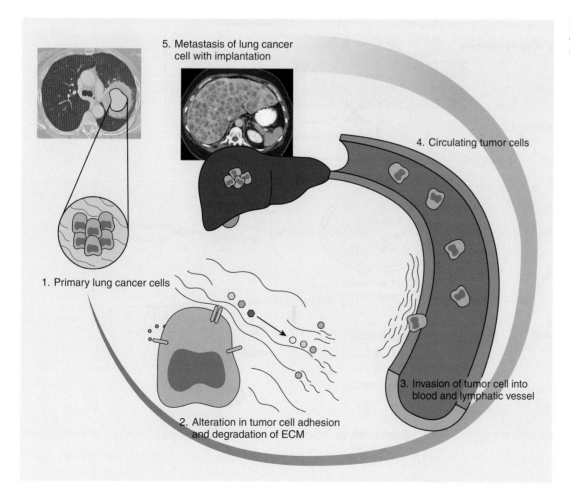

FIGURE 5.1 Mechanisms of lung cancer metastasis. ECM, extracellular matrix.

5. Metastasis of lung cancer cell with implantation

4. Circulating tumor cells

1. Primary lung cancer cells

3. Invasion of tumor cell into blood and lymphatic vessel

2. Alteration in tumor cell adhesion and degradation of ECM

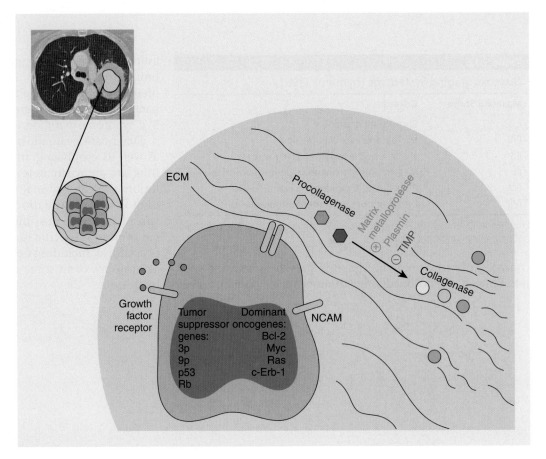

FIGURE 5.2 Mechanisms and biochemical abnormalities in a lung cancer cell and its interaction with the ECM. TIMP, tissue inhibitor of metalloproteinase.

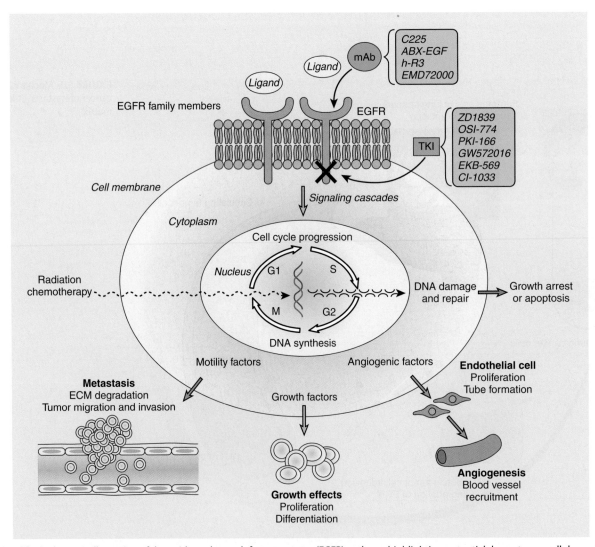

FIGURE 5.3 Simplified schematic illustration of the epidermal growth factor receptor (EGFR) pathway highlighting potential downstream cellular and tissue effects of EGFR signaling inhibition. The receptor action site for molecular EGFR inhibitors is depicted for monoclonal antibodies (mAbs) and tyrosine kinase inhibitors (TKIs). (Adapted with permission from Harari P, Huang S: Radiation response modification following molecular inhibition of epidermal growth factor receptor signaling, *Semin Radiat Oncol* 11: 281, 2001. Redrawn from Harari P, Huang S: Searching for reliable epidermal growth factor receptor response predictors, *Clin Cancer Res* 10: 428–432, 2004.)

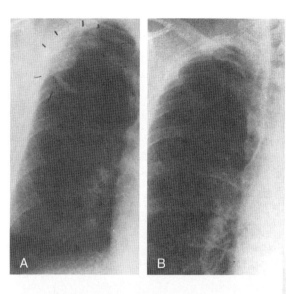 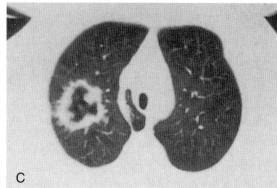

FIGURE 5.4 **SQUAMOUS CELL CARCINOMA.** A 58-year-old man who presented with increasing cough was found to have a large cavitating lesion in the right upper lung (**A**). (**B**) Chest film obtained 4 years earlier shows a small nodule that most likely represents the primary cancer. (**C**) CT scan shows a localized cavitating lesion. Squamous cell carcinoma often presents with cavitation due to tumor necrosis.

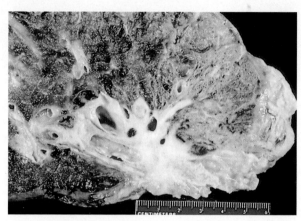

FIGURE 5.5 **SQUAMOUS CELL CARCINOMA.** A 66-year-old woman had a long-standing history of cigarette smoking and presented with metastatic disease. Bronchoscopy was positive for squamous cell carcinoma. Death resulted from widespread metastases. Midcoronal section of the left lung shows local invasion of the large bronchi and hilum. Most squamous cell lung tumors are of central origin. (Courtesy of Pathology Department, Brigham and Women's Hospital, Boston, MA.)

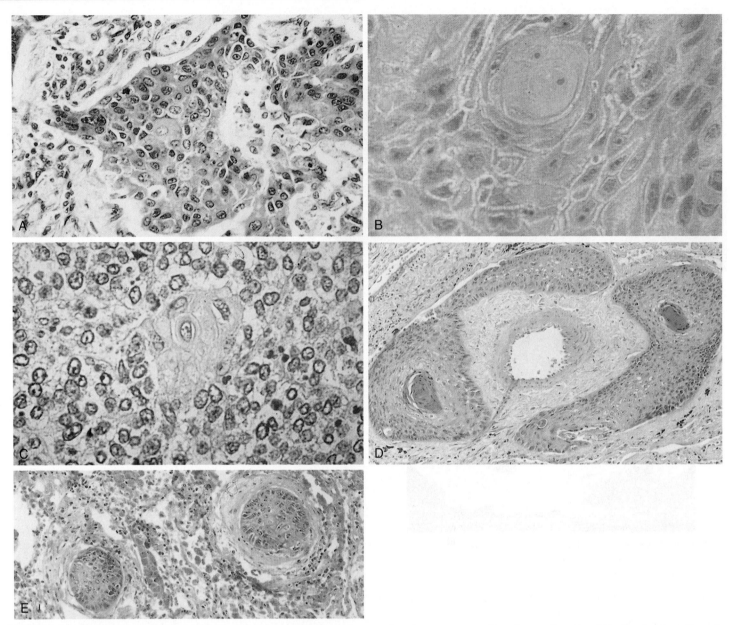

FIGURE 5.6 **SQUAMOUS CELL CARCINOMA.** (**A**) Low-power photomicrograph shows an invasive squamous cell carcinoma. Note the distinction between the cells at the periphery and the keratinized cells in the center of the island of tumor. (**B**) This high-power view shows the classic appearance of a keratin pearl and intercellular bridges diagnostic for squamous cell carcinoma. (**C**) This poorly differentiated tumor shows a focal central keratinized area. Immunoperoxidase staining for keratin protein was positive (not shown). (**D**) Squamous cell carcinoma invading and extending through lymphatic vessels surrounding a small blood vessel. (**E**) Squamous cell carcinoma in blood vessels. A section through the upper lobe shows a variety of features: brick-red parenchymal pigmentation with focal fibrosis, a pale mass arising in the upper lobe bronchus that has infiltrated the upper lobe, small foci of caseous necrosis at the base of the upper lobe, and an organized thrombus in the upper lobe branch of the pulmonary artery. Tuberculosis, as well as bronchial carcinoma, is a not uncommon complication of hematite lung. The carcinoma may frequently develop away from the bronchial wall in an area of scarring. It is thought that the increased radioactivity in hematite mines may be responsible for this neoplastic change.

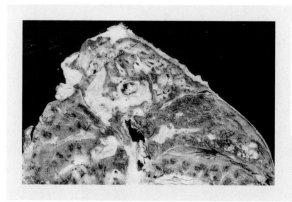

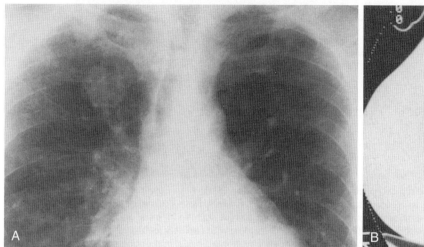

Tumor
Tumor mass in bronchus
Parenchymal pigmentation due to iron deposition
Thrombus

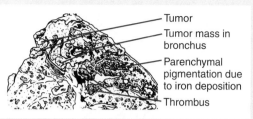

FIGURE 5.7 **HEMATITE PNEUMOCONIOSIS WITH SQUAMOUS CELL CARCINOMA AND TUBERCULOSIS.** This postmortem lung specimen was taken from a 61-year-old man who had been an iron ore miner for 20 years and had required numerous hospital admissions for deteriorating respiratory function.

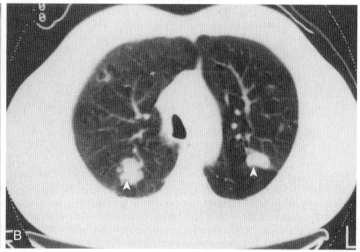

FIGURE 5.8 **ADENOCARCINOMA.** (**A**) On routine medical examination the chest film of a 64-year-old man shows bilateral primary lung tumors in the upper lobes; the lesion on the left side is partly obscured by the clavicle. (**B**) CT scan clearly defines the irregularly shaped primary lesions (*arrows*). Synchronous primary lung cancers occur in about 3% to 5% of patients and can be of different histologic subgroups.

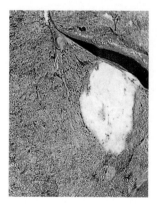

FIGURE 5.9 **ADENOCARCINOMA.** Just beneath the pleura of the oblique interlobar fissure of this lung specimen is an irregular, well-demarcated, pale tumor situated well away from the main bronchial tree. Most peripheral primary pulmonary malignancies are adenocarcinomas, which constitute about 30% to 35% of all lung cancers. Some peripheral lesions may be associated with scarring, mainly considered to be induced by the tumor itself.

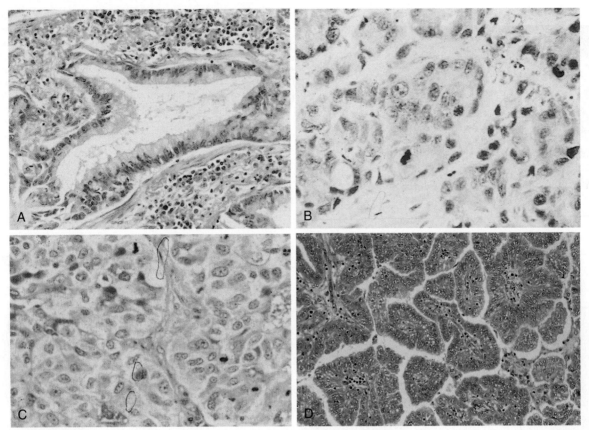

FIGURE 5.10 **ADENOCARCINOMA.** (**A**) Microscopic section shows the typical appearance of a gland formation. (**B**) On high-power view, this poorly to moderately differentiated adenocarcinoma shows clusters of cells with eccentric nuclei and abundant cytoplasm. Note a cluster of tumor cells with a central lumen in the lower left of the field. (**C**) This poorly differentiated adenocarcinoma shows positive mucicarmine staining for intra- and extracytoplasmic mucin. (**D**) Papillary adenocarcinoma of lung. Low-power view of a moderately well differentiated adenocarcinoma with papillary features. Metastases from ovary, thyroid, breast, or kidney cancer should be considered in the differential diagnosis of papillary adenocarcinoma. Special immunoperoxidase stains may aid in the differential diagnosis of these different tumors (see Table 5.13).

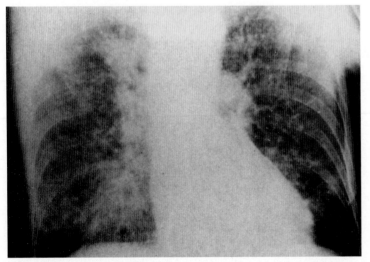

FIGURE 5.11 **BRONCHIOLOALVEOLAR CARCINOMA.** A 60-year-old female presented with the classic features of advanced disease: increasing dyspnea on exertion with a frequent cough that produced large amounts of frothy sputum. Chest radiograph shows extensive metastases throughout the lung fields with hilar and mediastinal adenopathy. In some cases infiltrative lesions termed GGOs (ground-glass opacities) are often seen with bronchioloalveolar carcinoma. The GGOs are often misdiagnosed as benign, particularly when the growth rate is quite slow.

Table 5.13

Use of Modern Immunoperoxidase Markers in the Differential Diagnosis of Metastatic Malignancies*†‡§

	CK7	CK20	TTF-1	CDX-2	SMAD4	P63
Lung adenocarcinoma	+	–	+ (nuclear)	–	+	–
Lung squamous carcinoma	+	–/+	–/+	–	+	+
Ovarian cancer	+	–	–	–	+	–
Gastric cancer	+/–	+/–	–	+/–	+	–
Pancreatic cancer	+	+	–	+/–	–	–/+
Appendiceal cancer	–/+	+	–	+	+	–
Colonic cancer	–	+	–	+	+	–
Uterine cancer	+	–	–	–	+	–

*Results may differ due to variable expression of the markers. Courtesy of Waichin Foo, M.D., Ph.D., Department of Pathology, Brigham and Women's Hospital.
†CK7, cytokeratin 7; CK20, cytokeratin 20; TTF-1, thyroid transcription factor 1; CDX-2, nuclear transcription factor involved in intestinal development; SMAD, 4 transcriptional regulator expressed in normal tissues; P63, nuclear transcription factor.
‡Interpretation: +, mostly positive stain; –, mostly negative stain; –/+, either positive or negative stain; SMADA: +, means retained; –, means lost.
§See also Tables 1.1 – 1.3 in Chapter 1.

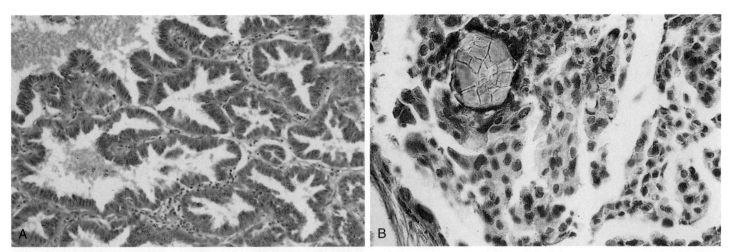

FIGURE 5.12 **BRONCHIOLOALVEOLAR CARCINOMA.** (**A**) Lower-power photomicrograph shows tall columnar peg-shaped cells growing in a "picket-fence" pattern on the alveolar walls. (**B**) On high-power view, a typical psammoma body, characterized by concentric laminations, is evident.

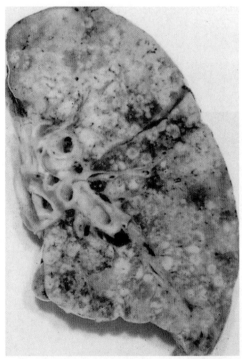

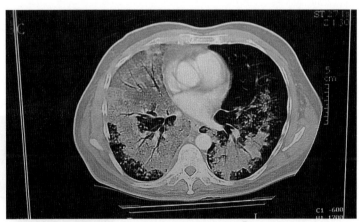

FIGURE 5.14 **BRONCHIOLOALVEOLAR CARCINOMA.** CT scan shows bilateral lung lesions in this 48-year-old woman with cough and excessive sputum production. Note the classic air bronchograms.

FIGURE 5.13 **BRONCHIOLOALVEOLAR CARCINOMA.** This is a postmortem specimen from a 45-year-old man who presented with a 2-year history of cough and malaise. Chest radiography suggested tuberculosis. Despite empirical treatment his condition deteriorated with increasing dyspnea and hemoptysis, and he died. At autopsy, except for a single involved lymph node at the carina, there was no evidence of metastasis elsewhere. A coronal section through the right lung shows widespread, diffuse infiltration by pale tumor, which has a nodular appearance in places. Very little normal parenchyma remains.

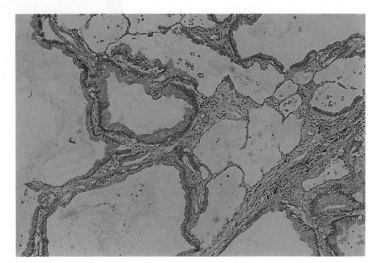

FIGURE 5.15 **BRONCHIOLOALVEOLAR CELL CARCINOMA.** Microscopic view shows lepidic (scalelike) growth along alveolar septa.

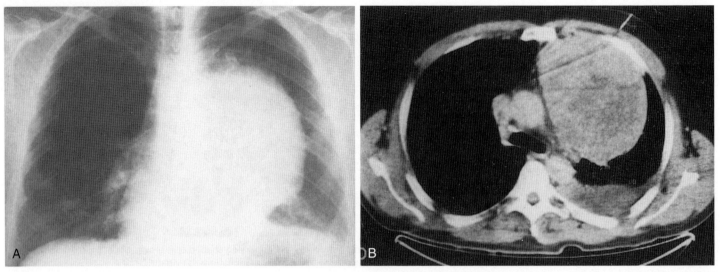

FIGURE 5.16 **LARGE CELL CARCINOMA.** A 45-year-old man with a long history of cigarette smoking developed increasing chest pain and cough. (**A**) Radiograph shows a huge primary mass. (**B**) CT scan shows the mass extending into the left anterior chest wall; a small pleural effusion is also apparent. Note the biopsy needle.

FIGURE 5.17 **LARGE CELL CARCINOMA.** (**A**) Surgical specimen from a 60-year-old man shows a primary malignancy arising in the periphery of the lung. In this case the tumor, which is well circumscribed with focal central areas of necrosis, is associated with subpleural cyst formation. (**B**) Microscopic section reveals mainly undifferentiated large cells with ovoid to spindly shapes. Note the discrete cell borders and prominent nucleoli. In some patients with the giant cell variant of large cell undifferentiated carcinoma, a diagnosis of Ki-1 anaplastic large cell lymphoma must be considered. Appropriate immunoperoxidase stains will establish the correct diagnosis (see Fig. 16.56).

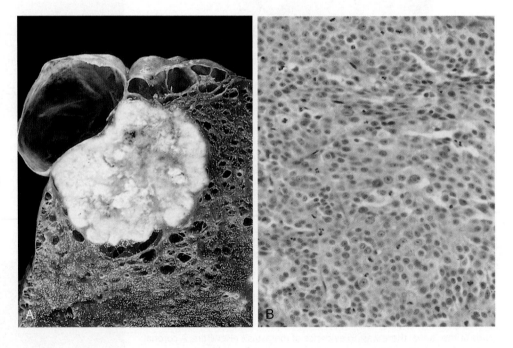

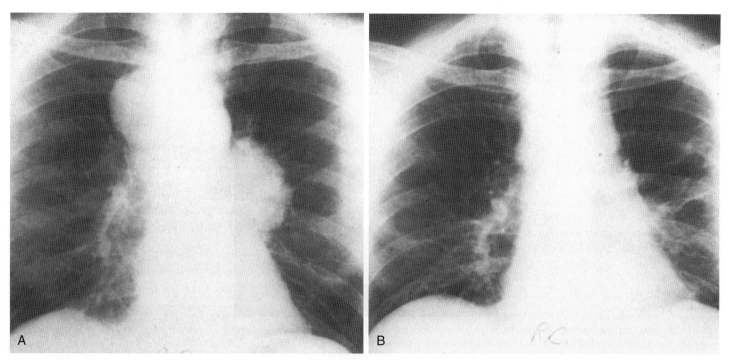

FIGURE 5.18 **SMALL CELL CARCINOMA.** (**A**) Chest radiograph of a 46-year-old man who presented with a cough and chest pain shows bilateral mediastinal nodal metastases. Bronchoscopy was positive for small cell lung cancer. Combination chemotherapy followed by mediastinal irradiation resulted in complete remission. (**B**) On follow-up examination 18 months later a chest film shows continuing remission.

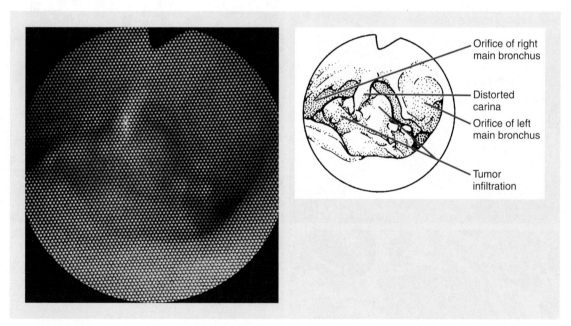

FIGURE 5.19 **SMALL CELL CARCINOMA.** A 66-year-old woman presented with a 5-month history of wheeze, sputum-producing cough, and episodic right-sided chest pain. In addition she had lost 6 kg in weight in that period and had recently experienced upper abdominal pain; her liver was enlarged. She had smoked 30 cigarettes a day for over 40 years. Her chest radiograph showed signs of right lower lobe collapse. Laboratory findings revealed elevated liver enzymes, as well as severe airway obstruction. On fiberoptic bronchoscopy the upper airway appeared normal but, as seen in this view, the carina is involved posteriorly by tumor. The tumor has broadened the carina and infiltrated it bilaterally, making it immobile. Tumor occluded the right upper lobe bronchus and partially obstructed the main bronchus, which could not be entered. The histology of the biopsy specimen showed a small cell (oat cell) carcinoma.

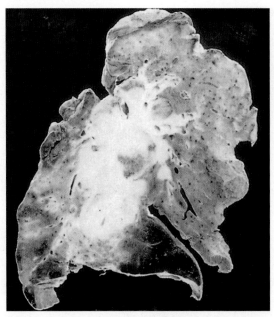

FIGURE 5.20 SMALL CELL CARCINOMA. This specimen was excised from a 40-year-old man who presented with a 6-week history of a dry cough and pleuritic chest pain. Radiographs showed collapse and consolidation of the left lower lobe, and bronchoscopy showed rigid infiltration of the left lower lobe bronchus. Mediastinal lymph node involvement was noted during a left pneumonectomy. This coronal section through the left lung shows a large, irregularly infiltrative, pale neoplasm arising at the lung hilum. The lower lobe bronchus is virtually obliterated, and the hilar lymph nodes are invaded in continuity with the main tumor mass. Extensive infarction of the remainder of the lower lobe suggests vascular occlusion or disruption by tumor. Microscopic examination of the tumor revealed a small cell anaplastic (oat cell) carcinoma. With modern management, radical surgery would not be carried out with locally advanced disease, but reserved for selected cases with stage I or II and rarely stage IIIA disease as part of multi-modality therapy.

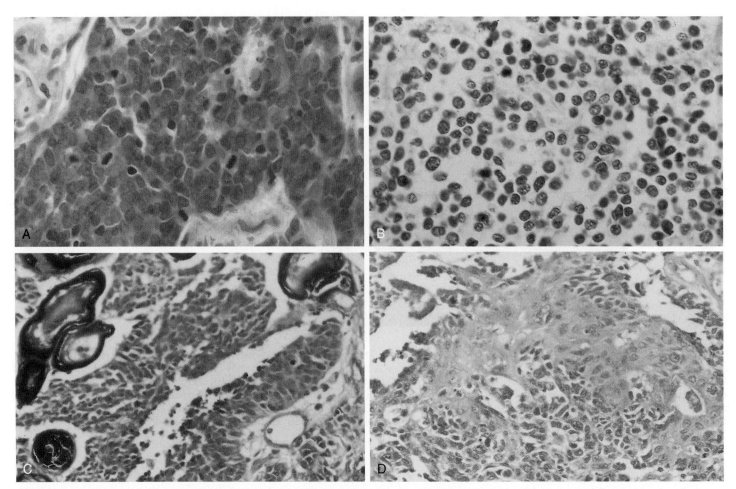

FIGURE 5.21 SMALL CELL CARCINOMA. (A) Photomicrograph shows the classic appearance of "oatlike" cells. Each cell is approximately twice the size of a lymphocyte and has scant cytoplasm, finely dispersed chromatin, and an inconspicuous nucleolus. Note characteristic "molding" of cells and a high mitotic rate. **(B)** In another case the cells have a "lymphocyte-like" appearance. Such tumors are included in the category of small cell lung cancer. Other malignancies that have a "small cell" appearance include lymphomas, Merkel cell tumor, carcinoid tumors, rhabdomyosarcoma, Ewing's sarcoma, and neuroblastoma. **(C)** Small cell carcinoma. This low-power view shows the Azzopardi effect, due to crushed DNA material encrusted around blood vessels, which is characteristic though not pathognomonic of small cell carcinoma. **(D)** Small cell carcinoma, mixed subtype. This tumor shows small cell and squamous cell components.

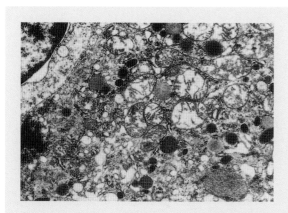
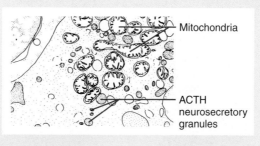

FIGURE 5.22 **SMALL CELL CARCINOMA.** Electron micrograph shows the ultrastructure of a small cell tumor of the lung associated with Cushing syndrome. Secretory granules containing ACTH are less frequent than they are in the islet cell tumor; nevertheless, they are also characteristic of neuroendocrine cells.

FIGURE 5.23 **CARCINOID TUMOR.**
(**A**) Routine chest radiograph of an 18-year-old woman reveals a prominence in the right hilar region. Three years later she was treated for tuberculosis, although test results were negative. Four years afterward she developed increased breathlessness and backache, and on examination was found to have abnormal facial hair, dyspnea at rest, and signs of mitral incompetence. Echocardiography showed a thickened interventricular septum, reduced left ventricular cavity size, and systolic posterior cusp prolapse. Pulmonary function tests indicated a marked restrictive defect. (**B**) Chest radiograph at this time shows a prominent right hilum and diffuse bilateral pulmonary metastases. (**C**) Fiberoptic bronchoscopy, using a rigid bronchoscope for clarity, reveals a lesion in the apical segment of the right lower lobe bronchus showing the typical appearance of a carcinoid tumor (bronchial "adenoma"). Bronchial and transbronchial biopsies were performed, revealing a carcinoid tumor infiltrating the lung. (**D**) Transbronchial specimen shows lymphatic infiltration by tumor (*arrowhead*). The diagnosis was supported by finding a whole-blood 5-hydroxytryptamine level of 705 ng/mL (normal range: 100–250 ng/mL) and an elevated 24-hour urinary 5-hydroxyindoleacetic acid level of 56 mg (normal range: <20 mg). (**C,** Courtesy of Dr. P. Stradling.)

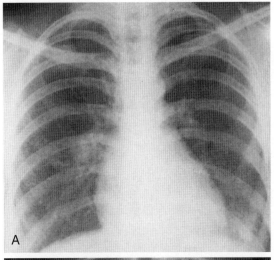

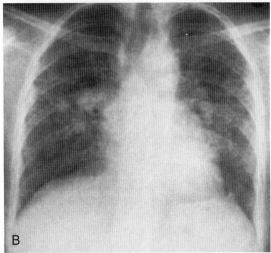

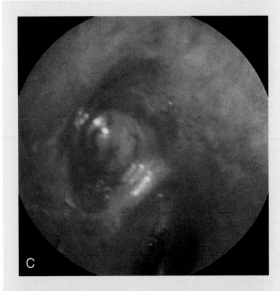

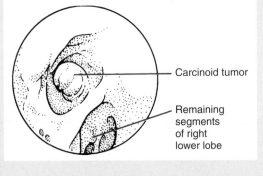

Carcinoid tumor

Remaining segments of right lower lobe

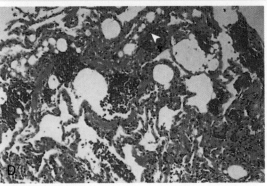

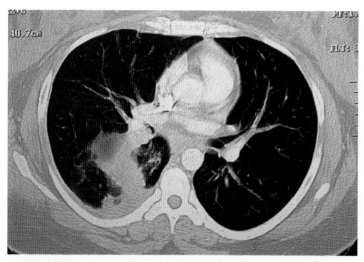

FIGURE 5.24 CARCINOID TUMOR. CT scan shows an endobronchial mass filling the bronchus intermedius of this 24-year-old woman with a history of recurrent asthma and episodes of pneumonia. Note large area of consolidation due to the obstructing lesion.

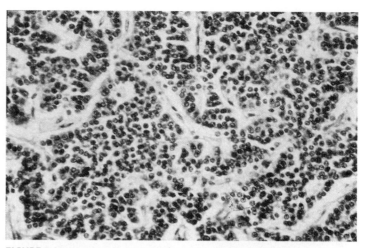

FIGURE 5.25 CARCINOID TUMOR. High-power photomicrograph shows a uniform population of small, bland "blue" cells with delicate nuclear chromatin and small amounts of cytoplasm. Note the organized arrangement of the tumor cells.

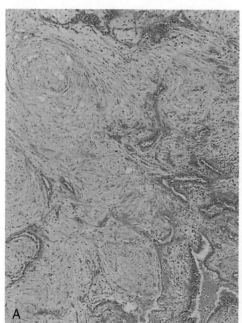
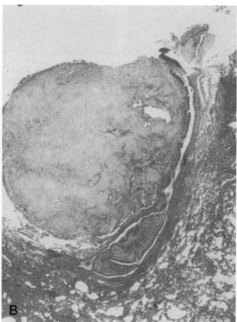

FIGURE 5.26 BRONCHIAL HAMARTOMA. A 70-year-old man with a history of cigarette smoking and a cough presented with a nodule in the left lower lung. A VAT resection revealed a bronchial hamartoma. (**A**) Low power at *right* reveals nodular growth. (**B**) High power at *left* displays benign cartilaginous growth with embedded epithelial elements. The term *hamartoma* means "tumor-like malformation," indicating a benign proliferation composed of tissue normally found in a location but present in excess or disarray. Recently, cytogenetic abnormalities have been observed in bronchial hamartomas involving chromosomes 18 and 6p21, suggesting a clonal origin (Fletcher et al., 1992.)

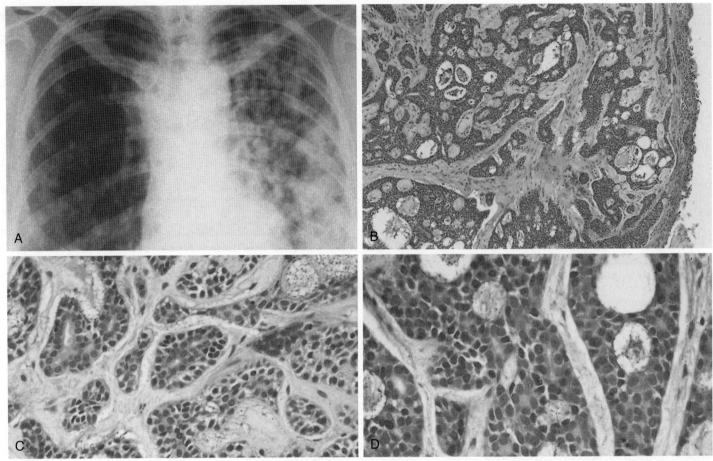

FIGURE 5.27   ADENOID CYSTIC CARCINOMA. (**A**) Chest film of a 40-year-old woman, who had resection of a primary adenoid cystic carcinoma of the right upper lobe 4 years earlier and developed multiple bilateral metastases with slowly progressive increase in size of the lesions. The upper mediastinum is slightly widened, suggesting adenopathy. Her symptoms were only mild dyspnea on exertion. (**B**) Adenoid cystic carcinoma may arise in bronchial mucous glands of the lung. The tumor cells form branching ductal structures with round, "punched-out" spaces, giving the tumor a lacelike pattern. (**C**) In this case the stroma separating cell clusters contains dense homogeneous eosinophilic basement membrane–like material, (**D**) but may also contain bubbly, bluish, mucoid material. The round spaces are filled by either material and surrounded by tumor cells with round to ovoid nuclei, coarse chromatin, and scant cytoplasm. Adenoid cystic carcinoma (also called cylindroma) occurs mainly in the upper aerodigestive tract (see Chapter 4). Involvement of the lung is unusual. The tumor shows histologic features that resemble salivary glands but are more aggressive than salivary gland cylindromas. Metastases to regional nodes and distant sites are common, and perineural involvement is characteristic. Occurrence in the respiratory tract may result in obstructive symptoms including recurrent wheezing, often leading to a misdiagnosis of asthma (which also occurs in the bronchial carcinoid tumors).

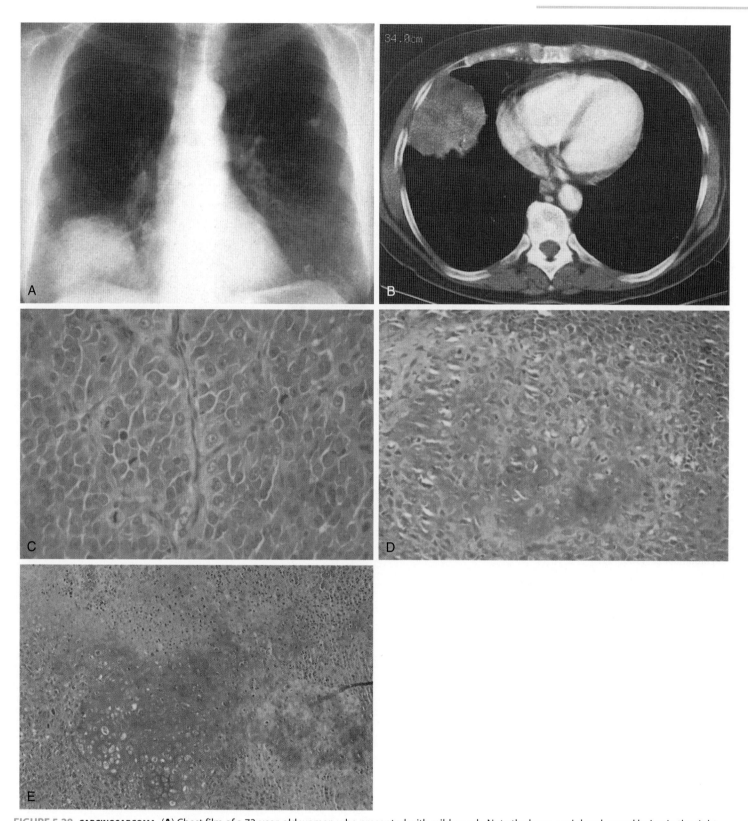

FIGURE 5.28 CARCINOSARCOMA. (A) Chest film of a 73-year-old woman who presented with mild cough. Note the large, peripheral, round lesion in the right lung. **(B)** CT scan shows a heterogeneous mass with a tiny peripheral focus of calcification. Evaluation revealed no metastases, and complete resection was carried out. **(C)** High-power view of the tumor mass reveals large epithelial cells with abundant cytoplasm, large vesicular nuclei, and occasionally prominent nucleoli. **(D)** High-power view of a different area reveals a malignant mesenchymal component (chondrosarcoma). **(E)** High-power view of malignant mesenchymal component stained with mucicarmine highlights in red the cartilaginous ground substance (rich in mucopolysaccharides). Carcinosarcoma is an uncommon lung malignancy, generally with a poor prognosis unless it is completely resected. The mesenchymal component may be fibrosarcoma, osteosarcoma, and, less frequently, chondrosarcoma or rhabdosarcoma. Metastases may consist of either carcinomatous and/or sarcomatoid elements. Historically, carcinosarcomas were thought to arise from primitive cells that can differentiate into carcinomatous and sarcomatous elements. However, current ultrastructural, cell culture, and immunohistochemical data support a monoclonal origin and suggest that "sarcomatoid carcinoma" is a more accurate designation for this neoplasm (Wick and Swanson, 1993).

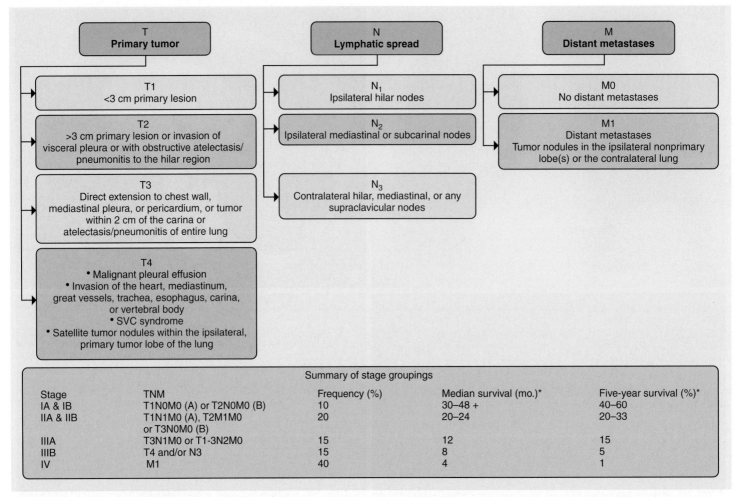

Summary of stage groupings				
Stage	TNM	Frequency (%)	Median survival (mo.)*	Five-year survival (%)*
IA & IB	T1N0M0 (A) or T2N0M0 (B)	10	30–48 +	40–60
IIA & IIB	T1N1M0 (A), T2M1M0 or T3N0M0 (B)	20	20–24	20–33
IIIA	T3N1M0 or T1-3N2M0	15	12	15
IIIB	T4 and/or N3	15	8	5
IV	M1	40	4	1

FIGURE 5.29 **INTERNATIONAL STAGING SYSTEM FOR LUNG CANCER.** The frequency of each clinical stage varies, depending upon patient referral patterns. Survival is based upon clinical staging. Survival for surgically staged patients is higher in resected cases. Not indicated above: TX, malignant cells in bronchopulmonary secretions but primary cancer not otherwise visualized; T0, no evidence of primary tumor; Tis, carcinoma in situ. (Adapted and simplified from Mountain CF, 1986, 1993.)

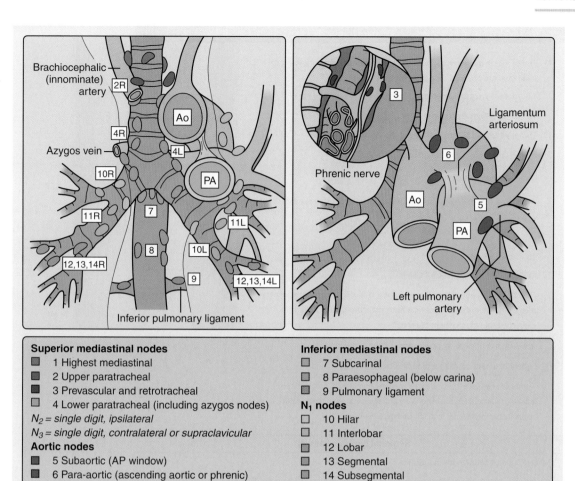

FIGURE 5.30 Regional nodal stations for lung cancer staging. (From Mountain CF: Revisions in the international system for staging lung cancer, *Chest* 111: 1710–1717, 1997.)

Superior mediastinal nodes
- ◼ 1 Highest mediastinal
- ◼ 2 Upper paratracheal
- ◼ 3 Prevascular and retrotracheal
- ☐ 4 Lower paratracheal (including azygos nodes)

N₂ = single digit, ipsilateral

N₃ = single digit, contralateral or supraclavicular

Aortic nodes
- ◼ 5 Subaortic (AP window)
- ◼ 6 Para-aortic (ascending aortic or phrenic)

Inferior mediastinal nodes
- ☐ 7 Subcarinal
- ☐ 8 Paraesophageal (below carina)
- ☐ 9 Pulmonary ligament

N₁ nodes
- ☐ 10 Hilar
- ☐ 11 Interlobar
- ▨ 12 Lobar
- ▨ 13 Segmental
- ☐ 14 Subsegmental

Primary tumor (T)
T1 - Tumor ≤3 cm diameter, surrounded by lung or visceral pleura, without invasion more proximal than lobar bronchus
T1a - Tumor ≤2 cm in diameter
T1b - Tumor >2 cm in diameter
T2 - Tumor >3 cm but ≤7 cm, with any of the following features:
Involves main bronchus, ≥2 cm distal to carina
Invades visceral pleura
Associated with atelectasis or obstructive pneumonitis that extends to the hilar region but does not involve the entire lung
T2a - Tumor ≤5 cm
T2b - Tumor >5 cm
T3 - Tumor >7 cm or any of the following:
Directly invades any of the following: chest wall, diaphragm, phrenic nerve, mediastinal pleura, parietal pericardium, main bronchus <2 cm from carina (without involvement of carina)
Atelectasis or obstructive pneumonitis of the entire lung
Separate tumor nodules in the same lobe
T4 - Tumor of any size that invades the mediastinum, heart, great vessels, trachea, recurrent laryngeal nerve, esophagus, vertebral body, carina, or with separate tumor nodules in a different ipsilateral lobe

Regional lymph nodes (N)
N0 - No regional lymph node metastases
N1 - Metastasis in ipsilateral peribronchial and/or ipsilateral hilar lymph nodes and intrapulmonary nodes, including involvement by direct extension
N2 - Metastasis in ipsilateral mediastinal and/or subcarinal lymph node(s)
N3 - Metastasis in contralateral mediastinal, contralateral hilar, ipsilateral or contralateral scalene, or supraclavicular lymph node(s)

Distant metastasis (M)
M0 - No distant metastasis
M1 - Distant metastasis
M1a - Separate tumor nodule(s) in a contralateral lobe; tumor with pleural nodules or malignant pleural or pericardial effusion
M1b - Distant metastasis

Stage groupings			
Stage IA:	T1a to T1b	N0	M0
Stage IB:	T2a	N0	M0
Stage IIA:	T1a to T2a	N1	M0
	T2b	N0	M0
Stage IIB:	T2b	N1	M0
	T3	N0	M0
Stage IIIA:	T1a to T3	N2	M0
	T3	N1	M0
	T4	N0 to N1	M0
Stage IIIB:	T4	N2	M0
	T1a to T4	N3	M0
Stage IV:	Any T	Any N	M1a or M1bN

FIGURE 5.31 Proposed seventh edition TNM staging system for lung cancer. (Adapted from Goldstraw P, Crowley J, Chansky K, et al: The IASLC Lung Cancer Staging Project: proposals for the revision of the TNM stage groups in the forthcoming (seventh) edition of the TNM classification of malignant tumours. *J Thorac Oncol* 2: 706–714, 2007.)

Primary tumor (T):
T1 lesions are divided based upon size into T1a ($\leq$ 2 cm) and T1b (>2 cm but <3 cm)
T2 lesions are divided into T2a ($\leq$5 cm) and T2b (>5 cm but $\leq$7 cm)
T2 tumors >7 cm are reclassified as T3
T4 tumors with satellite nodules in the same lobe as the primary tumor are reclassified as T3
Additional nodules in a different lobe of same lung are reclassified as T4 rather than M1
Malignant pleural or pericardial effusions or pleural nodules are now classified as metastasis (M1a) rather than T4

Regional nodes (N)
No changes

Metastasis (M)
Subdivided into M1a (malignant pleural or pericardial effusion, pleural nodules, nodules in contralateral lung) and M1b (distant metastasis)

Stage grouping
T2aN1M0 lesions are classified as IIA rather than IIB.
T2bN0M0 lesions are classified as IIA rather than IB.
T3 (>7 cm), N0M0 lesions are classified as IIB rather than IB.
T3 (>7 cm), N1M0 lesions are classified as IIIA rather than IIB.
T3N0M0 (nodules in same lobe) lesions are classified as IIB rather than IIIB.
T3N1M0 or T3N2M0 (nodules in same lobe) lesions are classified as IIIA rather than IIIB.
T4M0 (ipsilateral lung nodules) lesions are classified as IIIA (if N0 or N1) and IIIB (if N2 or N3) rather than stage IV.
T4M0 (direct extension) lesions are classified as IIIA (if N0 or N1) rather than IIIB.
Malignant pleural effusions (M1a) are classified as IV rather than IIIB.

FIGURE 5.32 Changes in the proposed seventh edition of TNM classification of lung tumors. (Adapted from Groome PA, Bolejack V, Crowley JJ, et al: The IASLC Lung Cancer Staging Project: validation of the proposals for revision of the T, N, and M descriptors and consequent stage groupings in the forthcoming (seventh) edition of the TNM classification of malignant tumours, *J Thorac Oncol* 2: 694, 2007; and Goldstraw P, Crowley J, Chansky K, et al: The IASLC Lung Cancer Staging Project: proposals for the revision of the TNM stage groups in the forthcoming (seventh) edition of the TNM classification of malignant tumours. *J Thorac Oncol* 2: 706–714, 2007.)

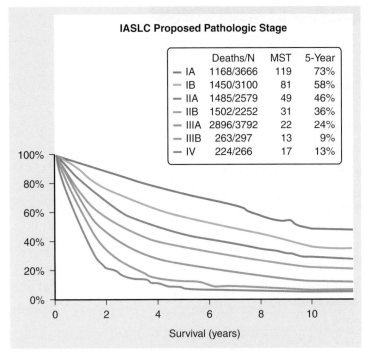

IASLC Proposed Pathologic Stage

	Deaths/N	MST	5-Year
— IA	1168/3666	119	73%
— IB	1450/3100	81	58%
— IIA	1485/2579	49	46%
— IIB	1502/2252	31	36%
— IIIA	2896/3792	22	24%
— IIIB	263/297	13	9%
— IV	224/266	17	13%

FIGURE 5.33 Overall survival, expressed as median survival time (MST) and 5-year survival, by pathologic stage using the proposed International Association of the Study of Lung Cancer recommendations. (Modified and used with permission from Goldstraw P, Crowley J, Chansky K, et al: The IASLC Lung Cancer Staging Project: proposals for the revision of the TNM stage groups in the forthcoming (seventh) edition of the TNM classification of malignant tumours. *J Thorac Oncol* 2: 706–714, 2007.)

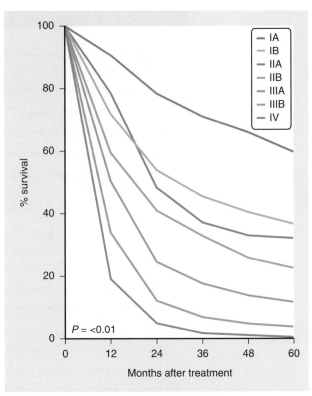

FIGURE 5.34 Cumulative proportion of patients expected to survive following treatment according to clinical estimates of the stage of disease. (From Mountain CF: Revisions in the international system for staging lung cancer, *Chest* 111: 1710–1717, 1997.)

FIGURE 5.35 T1N0 (STAGE I) SQUAMOUS CELL CARCINOMA. Fiberoptic bronchoscopy reveals a 2-mm–diameter lesion in the posterior segment of the right upper lobe bronchus.

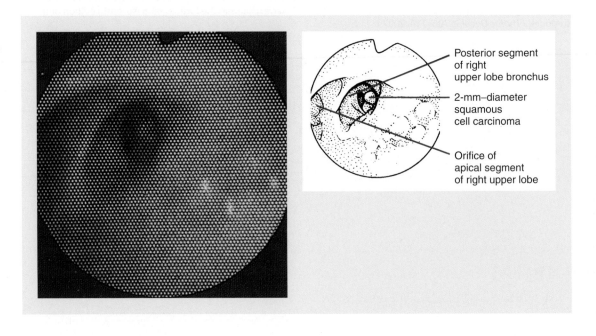

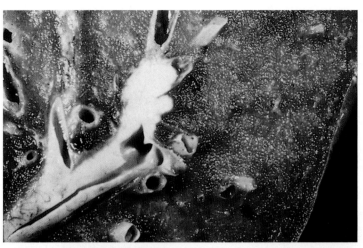

FIGURE 5.36 T1N0 (STAGE I) SQUAMOUS CELL CARCINOMA. Surgical specimen from a 60-year-old woman who presented with hemoptysis shows the bronchial origin of the tumor. No regional or distant metastases were present.

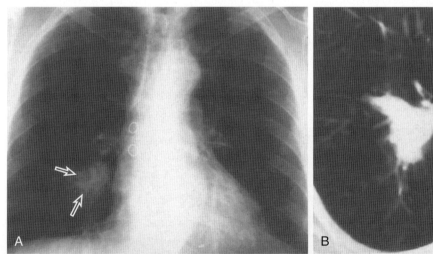

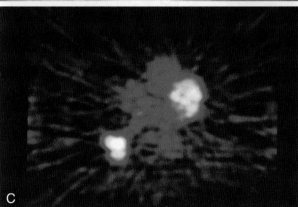

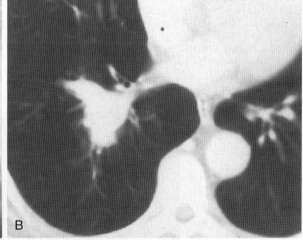

FIGURE 5.37 T1N0 (STAGE I) ADENOCARCINOMA. (A) Posteroanterior chest film in a 60-year-old man with hemoptysis demonstrates a poorly defined, spiculated 2.5-cm mass in the right lower lobe (RLL) (*arrows*). The patient had a prior sternotomy and coronary artery bypass graft.
(**B**) CT confirms the radiographically indeterminate RLL mass.
(**C**) Axial PET image at the level of the mass demonstrates significantly increased uptake within the tumor, which was proven to be an adenocarcinoma by bronchoscopy. Note the normal increased activity in the left ventricle myocardium. Staging studies showed no metastases, and a successful lobectomy was carried out. (Courtesy of Dr. E.F. Patz Jr.)

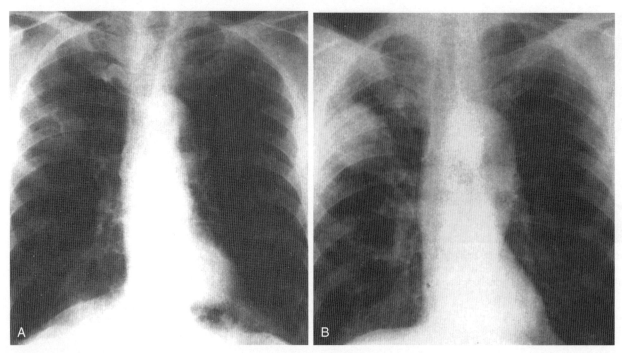

FIGURE 5.38 **T2N0 (STAGE IB) SQUAMOUS CELL CARCINOMA.** A 77-year-old man had a history of heavy alcohol intake and presented with right-sided pleuritic pains. (**A**) Chest radiograph shows right upper lobe shadowing, which in view of the patient's heavy smoking was provisionally diagnosed as peripheral bronchial carcinoma. Because there was no obvious evidence of metastatic disease, a transbronchial biopsy was attempted under radiographic screening. At fiberoptic bronchoscopy, a hard, irregular mass was found in the orifice of the right intermediate bronchus; it was not possible to inspect the distal lobar bronchi. Superficially the mass resembled a tumor, but as attempts were made to take a biopsy, it became clear that it was a foreign body embedded in granulation tissue. The mass was removed using a rigid bronchoscope with general anesthesia. The foreign body was subsequently identified as a vertebra from a rabbit. The patient had no explanation for its presence in his bronchial tree, but he had presumably inhaled it during one of his drinking bouts. The diagnosis was therefore revised to a pneumonic process in the right upper lobe resulting from proximal obstruction by a foreign body. Paradoxically, the initial diagnosis proved to be correct. (**B**) Chest film obtained 1 year later shows enlargement of the peripheral shadow despite removal of the foreign body. Subsequent investigations indicated the presence of a 4-cm squamous cell carcinoma.

FIGURE 5.39 **T2N0 (STAGE I) LUNG CANCER.** At the apex of the left lower lobe of this pneumonectomy specimen is a partly necrotic, pale, 3.5-cm neoplasm that has obliterated the lower lobe bronchus. Distally the smaller bronchi are grossly dilated (bronchiectasis), and the remaining parenchyma shows consolidation; the adjacent middle lobe shows confluent bronchopneumonia. These common complications of obstructive bronchial carcinoma may also be accompanied by collapse or abscess formation.

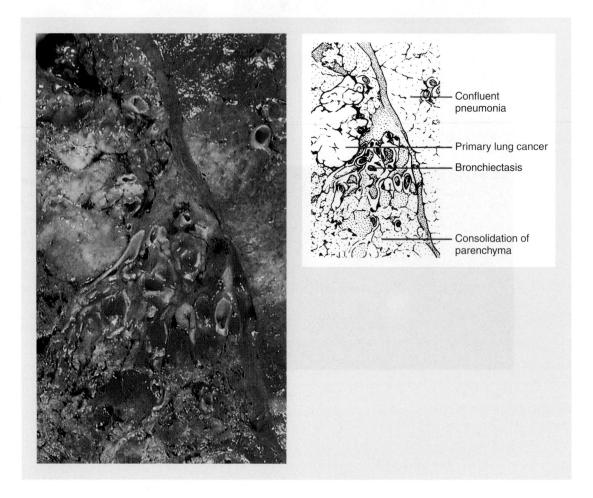

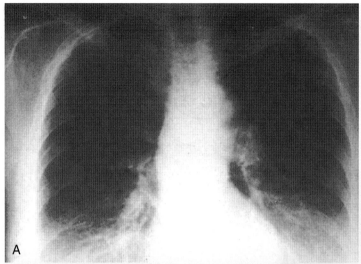

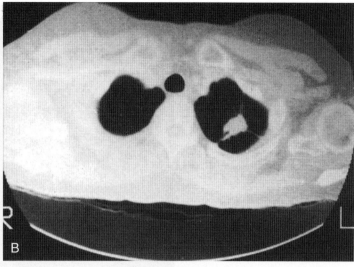

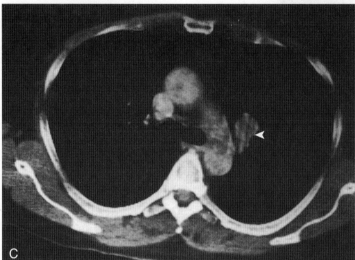

FIGURE 5.40 T1N1 (STAGE II) POORLY DIFFERENTIATED ADENOCARCINOMA. This 56-year-old woman presented with recent onset of cough. (**A**) Chest radiograph shows left hilar adenopathy and a small lesion in the left upper lobe. CT scans confirm (**B**) a 1.5- to 2.0-cm primary lesion in the left upper lobe, and (**C**) an enlarged left hilar node (*arrowhead*). No mediastinal adenopathy was present, and the tumor was successfully resected.

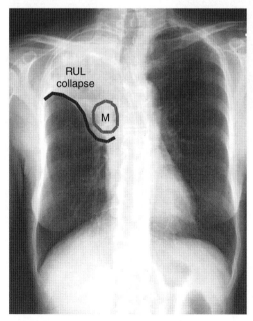

FIGURE 5.41 T1N1 (STAGE IIA) ADENOCARCINOMA. This posteroanterior chest radiograph shows classic features of right upper lobe (RUL) collapse due to a central obstructing hilar mass (M). The combination of lobar volume loss sharply outlined by the elevated minor fissure and the rounded density of the hilar mass results in the reverse S-sign of Golden, as seen in this case.

FIGURE 5.42 **T3 (STAGE IIIA)**
LUNG CANCER. Bronchoscopy
demonstrates extrinsic
compression of the left lower
trachea and distortion of the
carina and right bronchus by
tumor. The cancer was within
2 cm of the carina but without
invasion of the carina or trachea.
This image was made via a rigid
bronchoscope for clarity; it is
oriented for a bronchoscopist
standing in front of the subject.
(Courtesy of Dr. P. Stradling.)

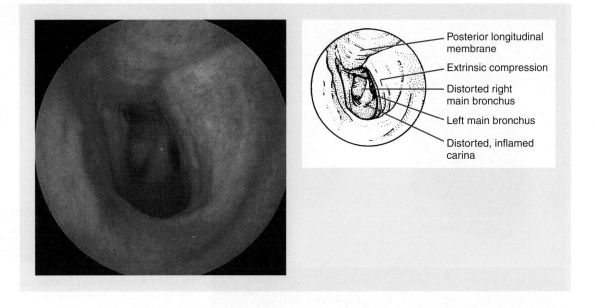

FIGURE 5.43 **T3 (STAGE IIB) LUNG CANCER.** A 27-year-old woman presented with increasing cough and sudden shortness of breath. (**A**) Chest radiograph shows complete collapse of the left lung. At bronchoscopy a tumor was identified at the orifice of the left main bronchus. (**B**) Chest film following treatment shows re-expansion of the upper lobe. Involvement of the proximal bronchus within 2 cm of the carina, but not involvement of the carina itself, constitutes T3 (stage IIB) disease that is marginally resectable.

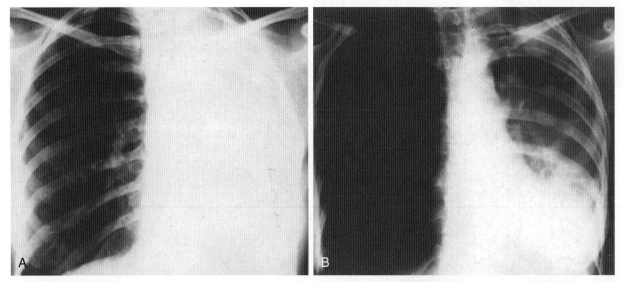

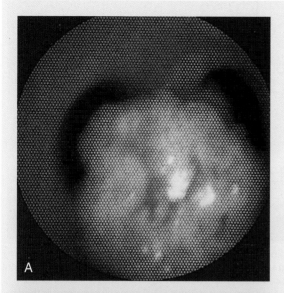

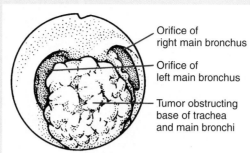

Orifice of
right main bronchus

Orifice of
left main bronchus

Tumor obstructing
base of trachea
and main bronchi

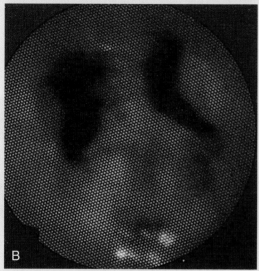

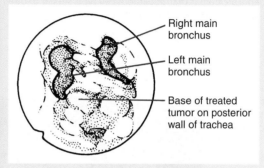

Right main
bronchus

Left main
bronchus

Base of treated
tumor on posterior
wall of trachea

FIGURE 5.44 T4 (STAGE IIIB) TRACHEAL CARCINOMA. A 66-year-old man presented with a 6-week history of rapidly increasing breathlessness that had originally been attributed to asthma. As his stridor became more obvious, bronchoscopy was performed and tumor was found at the main carina, causing severe obstruction of the orifices of both main bronchi (**A**). The tumor was cut back by laser photoresection to its base on the carina and posterior tracheal wall, resulting in substantial improvement in the airway (**B**). Both main bronchi are now clearly seen. Pulmonary function tests showed great improvement. Subsequent investigations showed that the tumor was confined to the base of the trachea and main carina. Eventually, the patient underwent surgery for resection of the carina and lower trachea with anastomosis to the main bronchi. Unfortunately, overall prognosis for squamous cell carcinoma of the trachea is poor due to recurrent regional disease as well as distant metastases. Adenoid cystic carcinomas are less common and less aggressive with improved survival after surgery and/or irradiation (Allen MS: Malignant tracheal tumors, *Mayo Clin Proc* 68: 680–684, 1993).

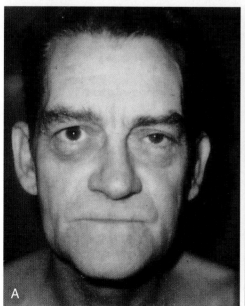

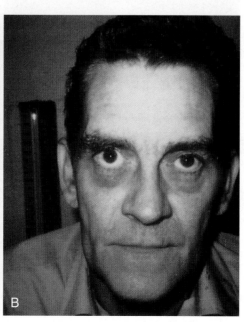

FIGURE 5.45 T3N0 (STAGE IIB) PANCOAST TUMOR. (**A**) This 58-year-old man presented with chronic left arm and shoulder pain along with progressive weakness of his lower arm and hand. Physical examination showed clinical findings of a superior sulcus (Pancoast) tumor: ptosis of the left eyelid, miosis of the pupil, decreased sweating of the left face, arm, and upper chest (Horner's syndrome), and a tumor mass in the lung apex that involved the brachial plexus and adjacent rib. (**B**) After radiation therapy the manifestations of Horner's syndrome have resolved. There was also improvement in his pain and neurologic symptoms. Survival is poor with Pancoast tumors (under 30% at 5 years) as a result of progressive regional disease but also distant metastases.

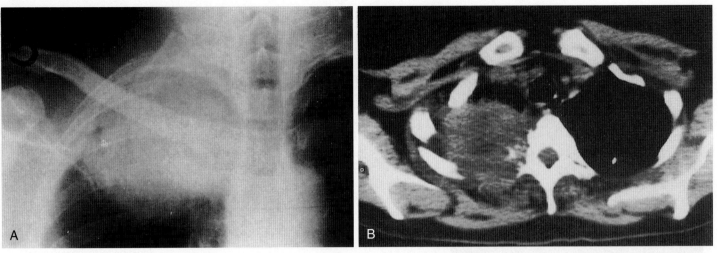

FIGURE 5.46 **T4N0 (STAGE IIIA) PANCOAST TUMOR.** A 52-year-old woman presented with long-standing right shoulder and back pain. (**A**) Her chest film shows a large tumor of the right upper lobe that has destroyed the adjacent rib. (**B**) CT scan reveals rib and soft tissue involvement as well as destruction of an adjacent vertebral body. Biopsy showed a squamous cell carcinoma. Whereas in the past Pancoast (superior sulcus) tumors were mostly squamous cell carcinomas, many centers are now reporting more adenocarcinomas than squamous cell type, similar to other lung cancers (see Table 5.4). Large cell carcinoma is third in frequency, whereas small cell carcinoma rarely presents as a Pancoast tumor.

FIGURE 5.47 **T4N2 (STAGE IIIB) PANCOAST TUMOR.**
(**A**) A 60-year-old man developed increasing right shoulder, back, and arm pain. Chest radiograph (not shown) revealed a mass in the right lung apex. Fine-needle aspiration was positive for poorly differentiated adenocarcinoma. T_1-weighted MR image in the coronal plane through the region of the thoracic inlet shows a Pancoast tumor on the right (T). The tumor directly invades one of the upper thoracic vertebral bodies (*arrow*). (**B**) A 48-year-old woman presented with severe pain in the shoulder and arm with marked arm weakness. T_1-weighted MR image in the sagittal plane to the right of midline shows tumor (T) growing into the region of several adjacent neural foramina.

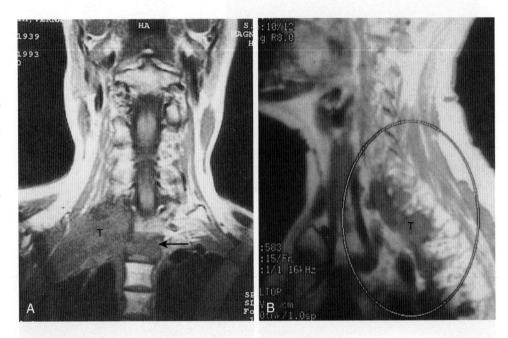

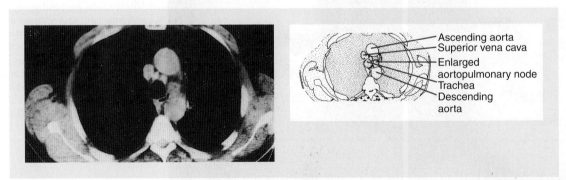

FIGURE 5.48 **N2 (STAGE IIIA) ADENOCARCINOMA.** A 47-year-old man with a primary tumor of the left upper lobe presented with hoarseness. Indirect laryngoscopy showed paralysis of the left vocal cord. This CT scan reveals an enlarged lymph node in the aortopulmonary window that was not seen on chest radiography. Anterior mediastinotomy (Chamberlain procedure) confirmed a metastatic tumor in the mediastinal node that compressed the recurrent laryngeal nerve, resulting in hoarseness.

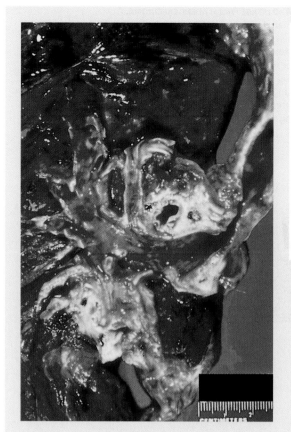

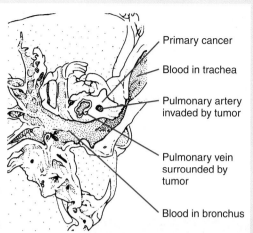

FIGURE 5.49 **T4N0 (STAGE IIIA) SQUAMOUS CELL CARCINOMA (PULMONARY ARTERY INVASION).** This autopsy specimen was taken from a 64-year-old man who died 1 day after a diagnosis was established by bronchoscopy. Exsanguination occurred when the malignancy eroded into the pulmonary artery. It is interesting to note that this patient had been cured of a diffuse large cell lymphoma after combination chemotherapy 4 years earlier. He was a heavy cigarette smoker.

(Labels on diagram: Primary cancer; Blood in trachea; Pulmonary artery invaded by tumor; Pulmonary vein surrounded by tumor; Blood in bronchus)

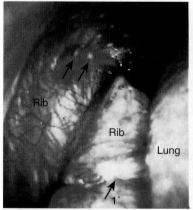

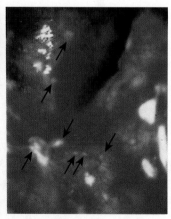

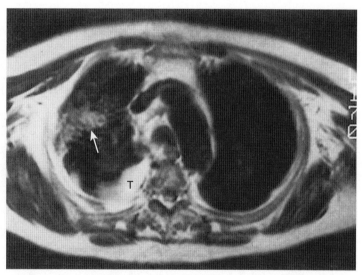

FIGURE 5.50 **T4 (STAGE IVM1a) ADENOCARCINOMA.** A 44-year-old woman presented with increasing cough, and chest radiograph (not shown) revealed a 2-cm infiltrative lesion in the left lower lobe (*left panel*, primary tumor). CT scan showed no mediastinal adenopathy, but some small pleural densities were present (not shown). VATS was carried out and revealed multiple small visceral and parietal pleural nodules (*arrows; right panel*). Biopsies were positive for metastatic adenocarcinoma unresectable stage IIIB disease. The patient was spared a formal thoracotomy by the staging VATS procedure.

FIGURE 5.51 **T4 (STAGE IVM1a) ADENOCARCINOMA.** A 76-year-old man with chronic obstructive pulmonary disease and previous asbestos exposure presented with increasing pulmonary complaints. Chest radiographs showed chronic scarring and infiltrates in the right lung along with multiple pleural lesions (not shown). In this patient a T_1-weighted MR image in the axial plane at the level of the aortic arch shows tumor in the pleural space posteriorly (T) with extension into the major fissure on the right (*arrow*). Fine-needle aspiration biopsy with special immunoperoxidase stains (see Fig. 5.53) was diagnostic for poorly differentiated adenocarcinoma of the lung. The lesion originated in the peripheral lung and extended throughout the pleura.

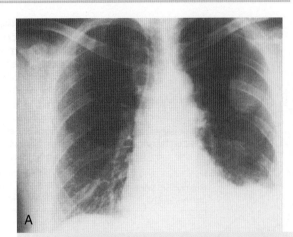

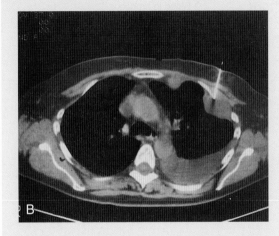

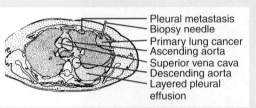

FIGURE 5.52 **T4N0 (STAGE IVM1a) ADENOCARCINOMA.** A 61-year-old woman developed increasing left chest wall pain with dyspnea on exertion. (**A**) Chest radiograph shows a pleural-based tumor mass with a pleural effusion. (**B**) CT scan confirms these findings and reveals a second small pleural metastasis. CT-guided needle biopsy showed a non–small cell lung cancer; thoracocentesis was positive for a poorly differentiated adenocarcinoma. Mammograms and other staging studies were normal.

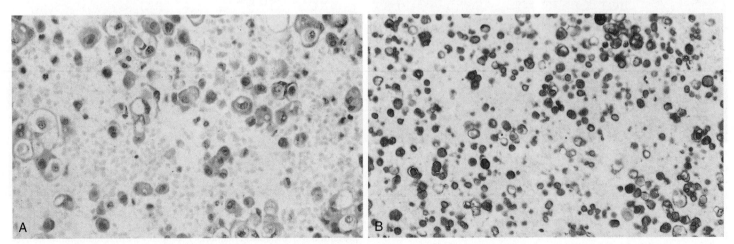

FIGURE 5.53 **T4 (STAGE IVM1a) ADENOCARCINOMA.** Histopathologic studies of the same patient as shown in Figure 5.53 reveal (**A**) positive mucicarmine stain (red) for intracytoplasmic mucin and (**B**) positive immunoreactive immunoperoxidase stain (brown) for callus cytokeratin. The peripheral pattern of staining is characteristic of adenocarcinoma, as opposed to mesothelioma, which has perinuclear and cytoplasmic staining. Immunoperoxidase stains were also positive for (cytokeratin-7, thyroid transcription factor-1, epithelial membrane antigen, and CEA, confirming the epithelial origin of the tumor.

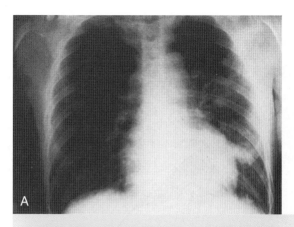

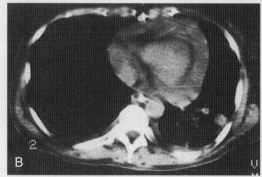

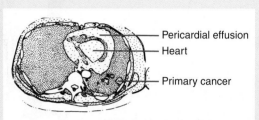

Pericardial effusion
Heart
Primary cancer

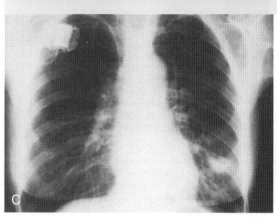

FIGURE 5.54 T4N0 (STAGE IVM1a) ADENOCARCINOMA. A 62-year-old woman presented with severe dyspnea at rest. (**A**) Chest film shows a tumor mass in the left lower lobe associated with cardiomegaly due to pericardial effusion with acute tamponade, findings that are confirmed on CT scan (**B**). Histopathologic specimens obtained by pericardiocentesis showed poorly differentiated adenocarcinoma cells. Radiation therapy was administered. (**C**) Follow-up chest film reveals improvement in heart size but persistence of the primary tumor mass.

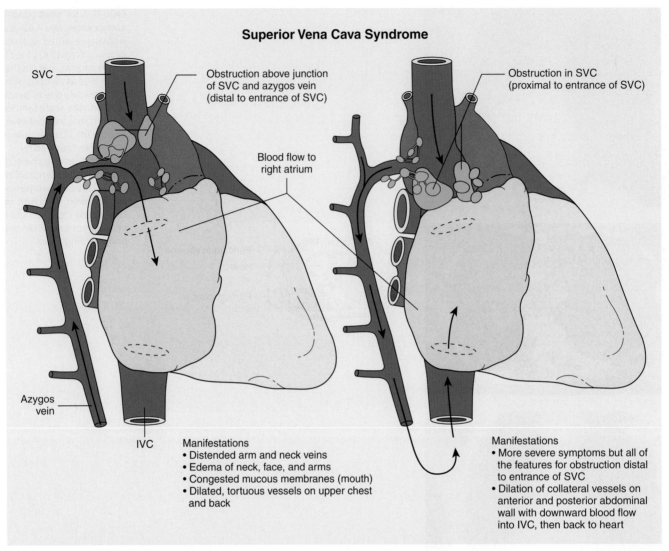

Superior Vena Cava Syndrome

SVC

Obstruction above junction of SVC and azygos vein (distal to entrance of SVC)

Obstruction in SVC (proximal to entrance of SVC)

Blood flow to right atrium

Azygos vein

IVC

Manifestations
• Distended arm and neck veins
• Edema of neck, face, and arms
• Congested mucous membranes (mouth)
• Dilated, tortuous vessels on upper chest and back

Manifestations
• More severe symptoms but all of the features for obstruction distal to entrance of SVC
• Dilation of collateral vessels on anterior and posterior abdominal wall with downward blood flow into IVC, then back to heart

FIGURE 5.55 T4 (STAGE IIIA OR B OR IV) LUNG CANCER (SVC SYNDROME). Compression and/or invasion of the superior vena cava by a tumor mass or mediastinal lymph node metastases leads to increased venous pressure and a variety of manifestations depending on the level of obstruction. SVC syndrome can occur as an isolated finding in stage IIIA lung cancer or as a part of metastatic disease (stage IV). The syndrome occurs in 3% to 5% of patients with lung cancer. It is seen most commonly in those with small cell lung cancer (15% to 45%), followed by squamous cell cancer (20% to 25%), adenocarcinoma (5% to 25%), and large cell carcinoma (4% to 30%). IVC, inferior vena cava.

FIGURE 5.56 T4N2 (STAGE IIIB) SQUAMOUS CELL CARCINOMA (SVC SYNDROME). (A) A 56-year-old woman with diagnosed lung cancer presented with marked facial edema characteristic of SVC syndrome. **(B)** After radiation therapy the swelling regressed markedly.

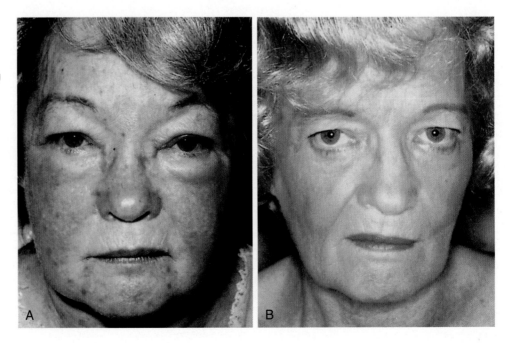

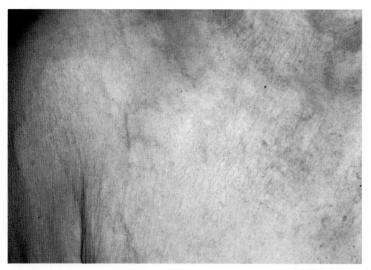

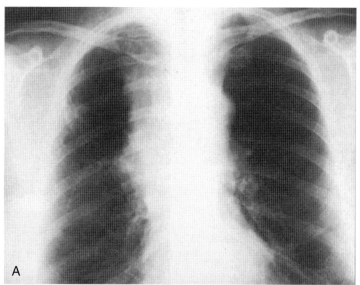

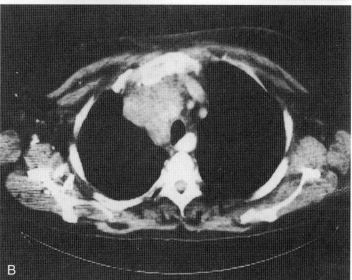

FIGURE 5.57 T4N0 (STAGE IIIA) LARGE CELL CARCINOMA (SVC SYNDROME). Dilatation of superficial collateral veins, as noted on the chest wall of this 70-year-old patient, is a common clinical finding in SVC syndrome. Collateral veins may also develop in the lower chest wall and upper abdomen.

FIGURE 5.58 T4N2 (STAGE IIIB) SQUAMOUS CELL CARCINOMA (SVC SYNDROME). A 45-year-old woman developed increasing facial edema, distended neck veins, enlarged breasts, and shortness of breath. (**A**) Chest radiograph reveals a large mass in the right upper lung and mediastinum. (**B**) CT scan shows encasement of the superior vena cava by the primary tumor mass.

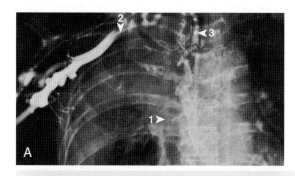

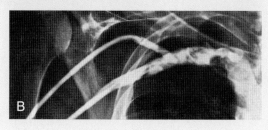

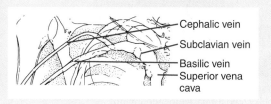

FIGURE 5.59 T4N2 (STAGE IIIB) BRONCHOGENIC CARCINOMA (SVC SYNDROME). (**A**) Upper extremity venogram performed on a patient with SVC syndrome due to large bronchogenic tumor (*arrowhead 1*) in the right lung shows complete obstruction of the subclavian vein (*arrowhead 2*) and filling of venous collaterals (*arrowhead 3*) bypassing the obstructed SVC. (**B**) By contrast, this normal right subclavian venogram demonstrates filling of the basilic and cephalic veins, which then fill the subclavian vein and finally the normal SVC. The lucent defects within the contrast-filled subclavian vein represent inflow of unopacified blood from venous tributaries.

FIGURE 5.60 **T4 (STAGE IIIB) SMALL CELL CARCINOMA (SVC SYNDROME).** A 48-year-old woman presented with slowly progressive facial edema. Chest radiography suggested mediastinal widening, which was confirmed by CT scan. Bronchoscopy was positive for small cell lung cancer. Radionuclide imaging was performed as a safe and rapid means of establishing a diagnosis of SVC syndrome. (**A**) This scan, obtained following injection of 0.3 mL of technetium with a saline flush into the basilic arm vein, shows total obstruction of the SVC, with filling of collateral vessels. (**B**) For comparison a normal SVC flow study is shown. (Courtesy of William Kaplan, MD, Department of Nuclear Medicine, Dana-Farber Cancer Institute, Boston, MA.)

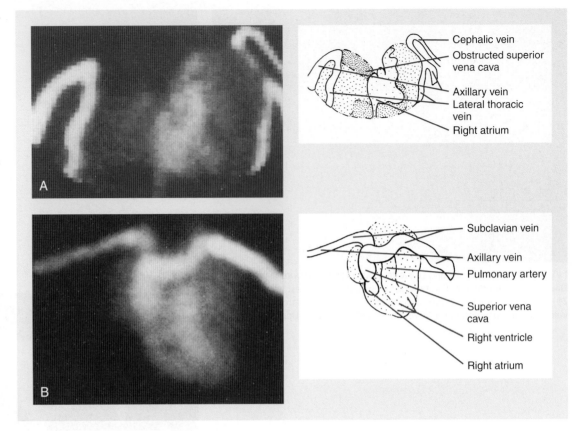

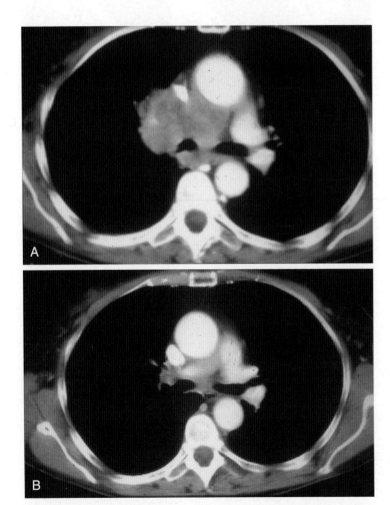

FIGURE 5.61 **N3 (STAGE IIIB) POORLY DIFFERENTIATED ADENOCARCINOMA.** In this 59-year-old woman, CT scan showed bulky mediastinal lymphadenopathy (**A**), which regressed markedly after systemic chemotherapy with a taxane- and platinum-based regimen (**B**).

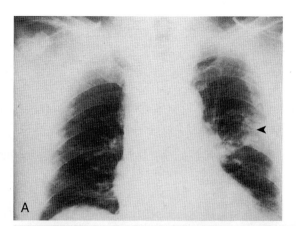

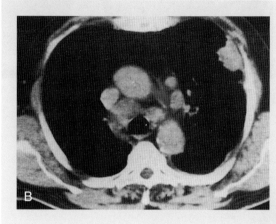

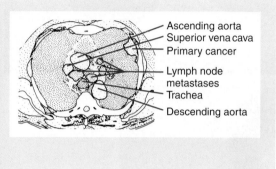

FIGURE 5.62 **N3 (STAGE IIIB) POORLY DIFFERENTIATED ADENOCARCINOMA.** A 67-year-old man complained of increasing cough, chest discomfort, and weight loss. (**A**) Chest radiograph shows a lesion (*arrowhead*) in the left upper lobe. (**B**) CT scan confirms a 2- to 3-cm primary lung tumor (T2) based in the pleura and reveals in addition bilateral mediastinal lymph node metastases. Bronchoscopy was negative, but needle biopsy of the primary lesion yielded the histologic diagnosis.

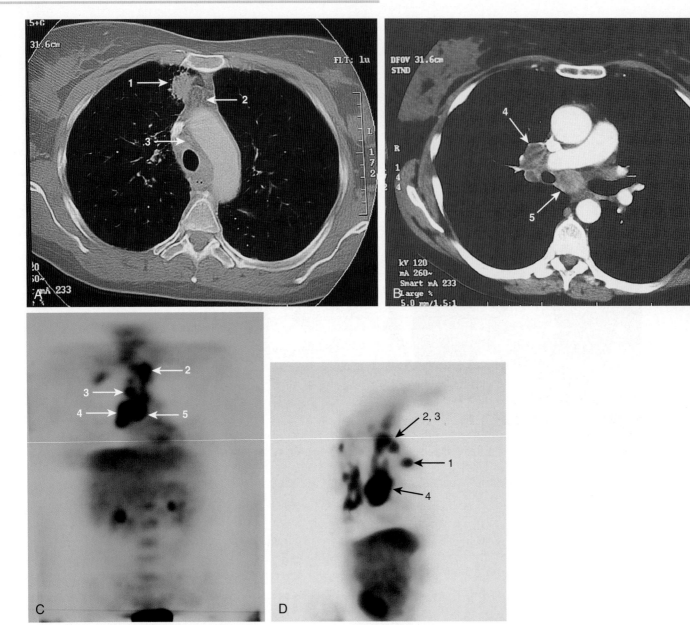

FIGURE 5.63 **T1N3 (STAGE IIIB) ADENOCARCINOMA OF THE LUNG.** A 44-year-old woman presented with an enlarged supraclavicular lymph node mass. Biopsy showed metastatic adenocarcinoma that was positive for thyroid transcription factor-1 (TTF-1) and cytokeratin 7 but negative for cytokeratin 20, consistent with lung cancer. At age 18 she had been treated for stage IIIB Hodgkin disease with MOPP chemotherapy followed by mantle field irradiation (Chapter 16). CT scan shows (**A**) the primary cancer in the medial right upper lobe (1), and left (2) and right (3) mediastinal nodes; (**B**) right hilar (4) and subcarinal (5) nodes. A staging PET scan reveals (**C**) coronal image: right hilar (4), subcarinal (5), and upper mediastinal (2, 3) nodes; (**D**) sagittal image: primary cancer (1), and upper mediastinal (2, 3) and right hilar (4) nodes. Normal liver uptake and renal excretion are noted. No other metastases were evident. The diagnostic role of TTF-1 is discussed by Ordonez (2000), whereas the value of PET staging is reviewed by Pieterman et al. (2000). MOPP, mustargen oncovin procarbazine prednisone. (Courtesy of Milos Janicek, MD, PhD, Department of Radiology, Brigham and Women's Hospital and Dana-Farber Cancer Institute, Boston, MA.)

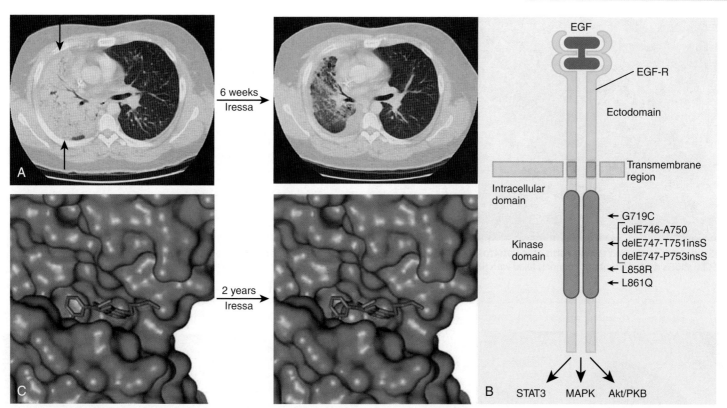

FIGURE 5.64 **NON–SMALL CELL LUNG CANCERS RESPONSIVE TO IRESSA TREATMENT.** (**A**) A minority of patients with refractory non–small cell lung cancers (NSCLCs)— tumors that have failed to respond or no longer respond to standard chemotherapy—show marked responses to treatment by Iressa (gefitinib, a tyrosine kinase inhibitor). These CT radiographic images reveal a large mass in the right lung (*left*) of a patient that underwent marked regression following 6 weeks of Iressa treatment (*right*). (**B**) A substantial proportion of NSCLCs that respond to Iressa treatment have been found to carry mutations in the gene encoding the EGFR that affect the cytoplasmic domain of the receptor and include both deletions ("del") and point mutations. These alterations in EGFR structure deregulate and activate the tyrosine kinase function of the receptor, thereby stimulating the downstream Akt/PKB and STAT signaling pathways, which protect these tumor cells from apoptosis. (**C**) Eventually, patients with some of the indicated mutations relapse from Iressa (gefitinib) or Tarceva (erlotinib) therapy. As is the case with acquired resistance to Gleevec (imatinib), the EGFRs in these NSCLC patients often acquire structural changes that block drug binding. Here a patient, whose tumor-associated EGFR showed a delE747-P753insS mutation (**B**), enjoyed a remission achieved by Iressa therapy; after 2 years, however, his tumor regrew. Sequencing of the EGFR gene in the relapsed tumor showed that the binding site present in the wild-type receptor (*left*) was now partially occluded by a threonine-to-methionine substitution (*right*), causing the bulkier methionine side chain (*orange sphere*) to block binding of Iressa. (Modified from Weinberg R: Textbook of molecular biology, 2008. **A, B,** from Lynch TJ, Bell DW, Sordella R, et al: Activating mutations in the epidermal growth factor receptor underlying responsiveness of non–small-cell lung cancer to Gefitinib, *N Engl J Med* 350: 2129–2139, 2004; **C** from Kobayashi S, Boggon TJ, Dayaram T, et al: EGFR mutation and resistance of non–small-cell lung cancer to Gefitinib, *N Engl 15 Med* 352: 786–792, 2005.)

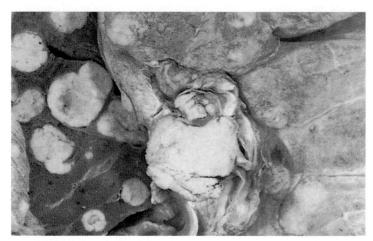

FIGURE 5.65 **METASTATIC DISEASE (STAGE IVM1b) MULTIPLE PULMONARY METASTASES.** Beneath the pleura and in the lung parenchyma are numerous pale, umbilicated nodules of tumor. Up to a third of patients dying of malignant disease have pulmonary metastases, the most common sources of which are primary tumors of the breast, colon, stomach, and lung itself. The extensive vascular and lymphatic system of the lungs is responsible for the predilection that metastases show for this site.

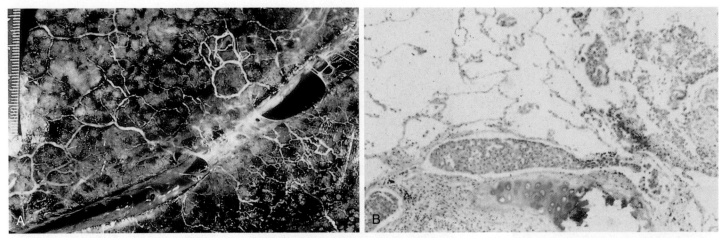

FIGURE 5.66 **PULMONARY LYMPHANGITIS CARCINOMATOSA.** (**A**) The pleural surface of this autopsy specimen from a patient who died of a poorly differentiated NSCLC shows dilated lymphatic channels filled with tumor. (**B**) Microscopic section of the lung demonstrates malignant cells infiltrating lymphatic channels.

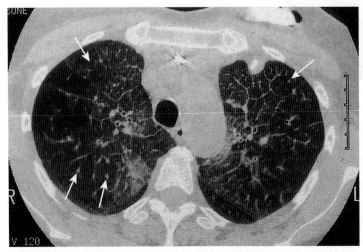

FIGURE 5.67 **PULMONARY LYMPHANGITIS CARCINOMATOSA.** A 49-year-old woman with previous resection of a poorly differentiated adenocarcinoma of the lung presented with increasing dyspnea on exertion. Chest radiograph showed nondiagnostic features. CT image at the level of the aortic arch displayed with lung windows shows bilateral thickening of interlobular septae consistent with lymphangitic tumor spread. The thickened septae (*arrows*) form polygons containing a central dot, representing a pulmonary vein.

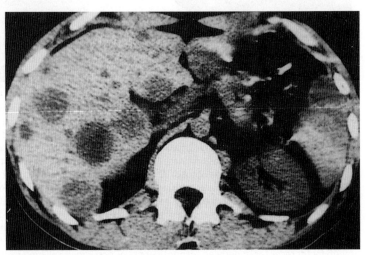

FIGURE 5.69 **LIVER METASTASES.** CT scan of a 28-year-old man with metastatic atypical carcinoid tumor shows numerous metastatic liver deposits that developed after control of his primary pulmonary malignancy by surgery. CT is quite accurate in detecting early metastases, and use of contrast with CT helps rule out benign cysts, which do not enhance with contrast. Ultrasound can also differentiate cystic from solid lesions. These lesions would also be evident by technetium sulfur colloid scanning.

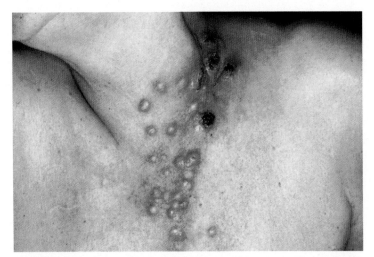

FIGURE 5.68 **CUTANEOUS METASTASES.** A 48-year-old woman with a small cell (oat cell) lung cancer developed numerous skin lesions. Generalized skin or subcutaneous metastases, which may be quite painful, often occur, and they may be seen in all histologic subtypes. In some patients a solitary early skin metastasis may be the presenting sign of an underlying lung tumor.

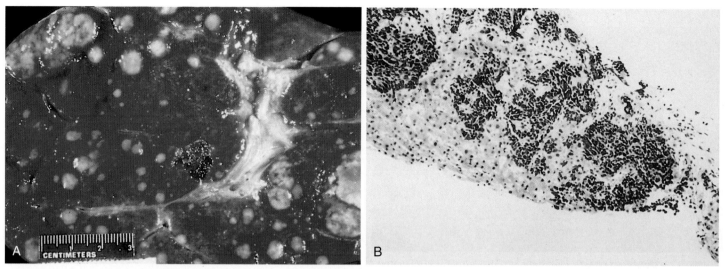

FIGURE 5.70 **LIVER METASTASES.** (**A**) Autopsy specimen from a patient who died of widespread small cell (oat cell) lung cancer shows numerous lesions ranging in size from a few millimeters to 1–2 cm. A similar pattern can be seen with non–small cell carcinomas. (**B**) Photomicrograph of a liver biopsy specimen from a patient with small cell lung tumor shows marked involvement by clumps of undifferentiated dark-staining cells.

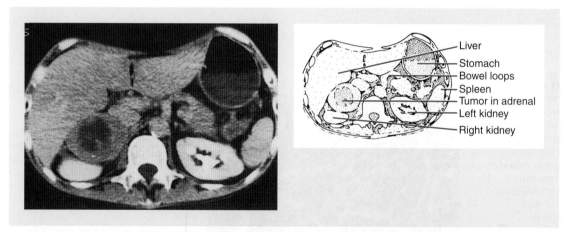

FIGURE 5.71 **ADRENAL METASTASES.** Abdominal CT scan of a patient with a NSCLC, a large metastatic lesion in the right adrenal gland; central tumor necrosis is also evident. This patient was considered for surgery before the adrenal lesion was detected. About 5% to 10% of patients with localized lung cancer on chest radiography have asymptomatic adrenal metastases. Carcinoma of the lung is by far the most common source of adrenal metastases, followed by carcinoma of the breast and malignant melanoma. In general, adrenal metastases are bilateral and most often appear first in the medulla. Cortical involvement is also common, and in rare cases such metastatic spread may give rise to Addison's disease.

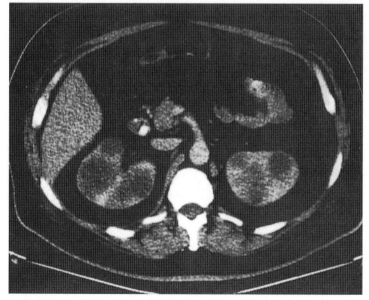

FIGURE 5.72 **KIDNEY METASTASES.** CT scan shows bilateral renal metastases in a 63-year-old man who also had liver and bone involvement by a primary adenocarcinoma of the lung. Renal cysts can usually be ruled out by ultrasound.

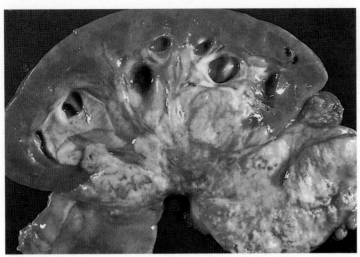

FIGURE 5.73 **KIDNEY METASTASES.** Metastatic SCLC has extensively infiltrated the renal hilum, producing moderate hydronephrosis. Ureteral and periureteral metastases may also occur, resulting in urinary tract obstruction and infection. Because primary renal cell carcinoma is not uncommon in older patients, it should also be considered in the differential diagnosis, especially when there are no other sites of metastatic lung cancer.

FIGURE 5.74 **KIDNEY METASTASES.** Hematogenous spread of a lung carcinoma is evident in this glomerulus, which contains a nodule of metastatic adenocarcinoma in the capillary tuft, as well as malignant cells in Bowman's space. (Reproduced with permission from Schumann GB, Weiss MA: *Atlas of renal and urinary tract cytology and its histopathologic bases*, Philadelphia, 1981, Lippincott.)

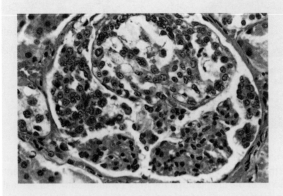

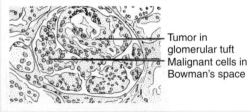

Tumor in glomerular tuft
Malignant cells in Bowman's space

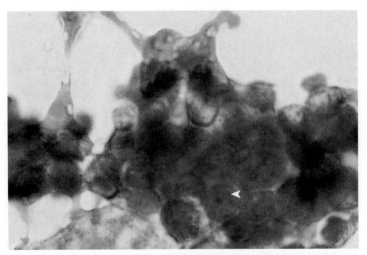

FIGURE 5.75 **KIDNEY METASTASES.** Fine-needle aspiration biopsy specimen from the kidney shown in Figure 5.72 contains loose aggregates of small malignant cells with the cytologic characteristics typical of small cell (oat cell) carcinoma—nuclei with moderately granular chromatin, small, inconspicuous nucleoli, scant cytoplasm, and prominent nuclear molding (*arrowhead*). Fine-needle aspiration is a useful diagnostic procedure for differentiating metastatic tumors from primary urinary tract malignancies (Papanicolaou stain).

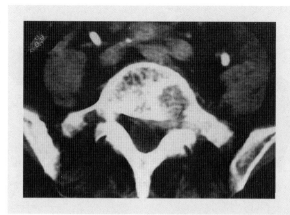
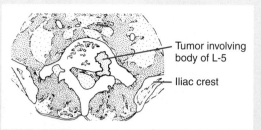

Tumor involving
body of L-5

Iliac crest

FIGURE 5.76 BONE METASTASES.
A 74-year-old woman presented with pain and weakness of the left leg. A right lower lobe mass was noted on her chest radiograph, and a diagnosis of adenocarcinoma was subsequently made by bronchoscopy. CT scan shows compression of the cauda equina by tumor involving the body of L5. Her leg pain and weakness markedly improved after radiation therapy.

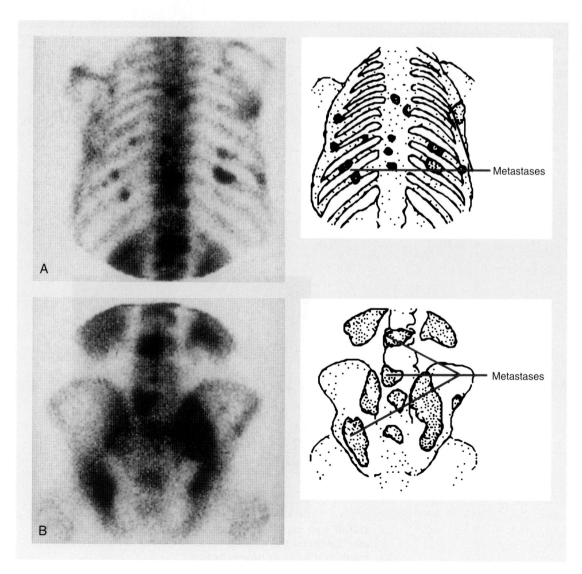

Metastases

Metastases

A

B

FIGURE 5.77 BONE METASTASES.
Radiograph of the lumbar spine in a patient who had a bronchial carcinoma and complained of back pain indicates no abnormality. However, radionuclide bone scans (**A, B**) reveal multiple metastases in the lumbar spine and pelvis, as well as deposits in the thoracic vertebrae and ribs.

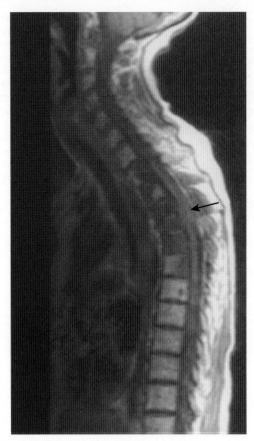

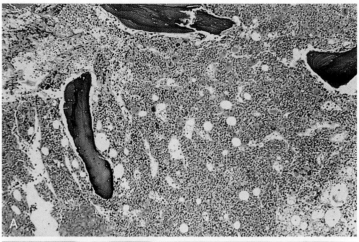

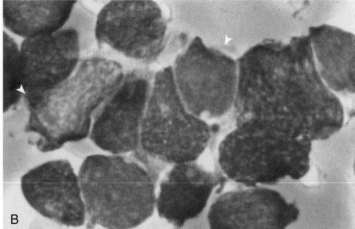

FIGURE 5.78 **BONE MARROW METASTASES.** A 62-year-old woman presented with upper back pain and neurologic findings diagnostic of early spinal cord compression. Normal bone marrow appears white on this T_2-weighted MRI scan because of fat content, except in the upper spine where metastatic lung cancer has replaced the bone marrow and appears black. The spinal cord appears white and shows an area of displacement due to compression by tumor invading through the intervertebral space (*arrow*).

FIGURE 5.79 **BONE MARROW METASTASES.** (**A**) Low-power photomicrograph of a bone marrow biopsy specimen shows focal involvement by metastatic small cell (oat cell) lung cancer. (**B**) High-power view of a bone marrow aspirate shows a cluster of malignant small cells with prominent nuclear molding (*arrowheads*). The differential diagnosis of this cytology includes other small blue cell malignancies (e.g., Ewing's sarcoma, neuroblastoma, rhabdomyosarcoma, and lymphoma). Bone marrow involvement as the only site of metastatic disease occurs in 5% to 10% of cases; the incidence rises to 40% or greater when metastases are found at other sites.

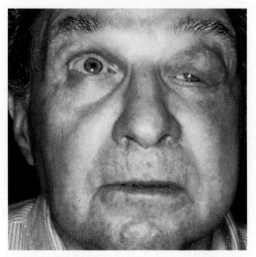

FIGURE 5.80 **ORBITAL METASTASES.** This 62-year-old man had a lung adenocarcinoma that metastasized to the retro-orbital space, resulting in proptosis and limitation in eye motion.

FIGURE 5.81 ORBITAL METASTASES. A 75-year-old woman presented with retro-orbital pain and a cranial nerve VI palsy. Later, proptosis developed, with downward and outward deviation of the globe. (**A**) CT scan shows a high-density lesion in the left retro-orbital space. (**B**) Chest film demonstrates a mass below the left hilum (*arrowhead*), which on aspiration biopsy proved to be an adenocarcinoma.

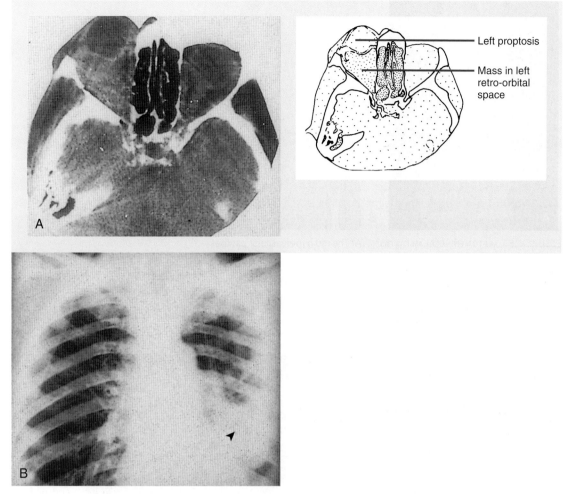

Left proptosis

Mass in left retro-orbital space

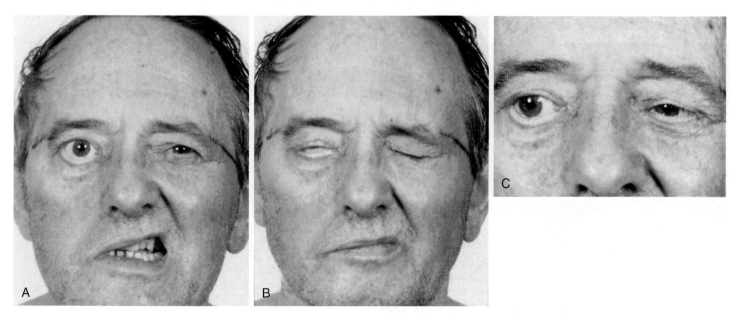

FIGURE 5.82 CRANIAL NERVE METASTASES. This 61-year-old man presented with loss of feeling in the left leg, left facial numbness, and ataxias. CT scan demonstrated multiple cerebral metastases of a bronchial carcinoma. Involvement of the right cranial nerves VI and VII is reflected in the weakness of the orbicular muscle of the right eye (**A**) and that of the right side of the mouth (**B, C**). Incomplete abduction of the right eye is also apparent.

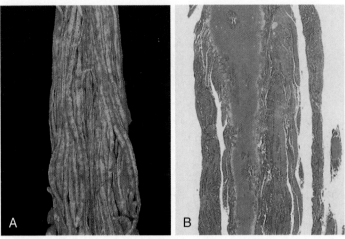

FIGURE 5.83 **LEPTOMENINGEAL METASTASES. (A)** The red hypervascular patches on the nerve roots of the cauda equina in this fresh specimen represent leptomeningeal deposits of a metastatic lung carcinoma. The cauda equina is a favorite location for this process. **(B)** Whole-mount section of the specimen, which better demonstrates the extent of infiltration, shows ropy thickening of individual nerve roots by dense, blue-staining tumor cell nuclei. Minor extension of tumor into the spinal cord is also evident.

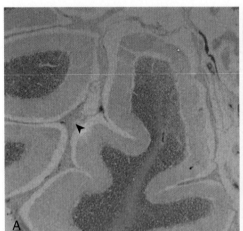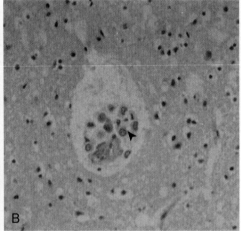

FIGURE 5.84 **LEPTOMENINGEAL METASTASES.** A 55-year-old man was diagnosed with an undifferentiated large cell lung cancer. Two months later, he presented with headache followed by numbness of the hands. Examination showed diplopia, dysarthria, nystagmus, palsies of the left VI and right VII cranial nerves, bilateral limb ataxia, areflexia, and gait ataxia. **(A)** Section of cerebellum shows infiltration of the leptomeninges by malignant cells (*arrowhead*) and, on high-power view **(B)**, invasion of the Virchow-Robin space (*arrowhead*).

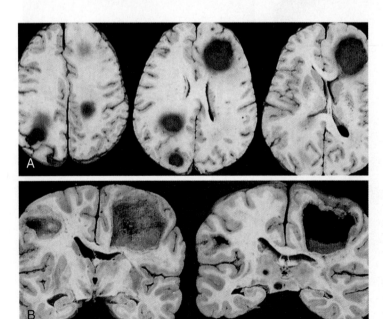

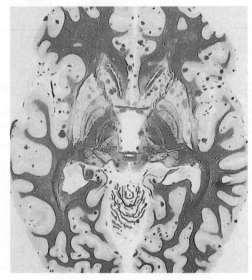

FIGURE 5.86 **BRAIN METASTASES.** Horizontal whole-mount section of a brain shows metastatic SCLC as miliary cerebral metastases. Many are situated in gray matter or at the gray-white matter junction. The ventricular surface is also involved. Note the relative sparing of white matter and the absence of edema.

FIGURE 5.85 **BRAIN METASTASES. (A)** Gross specimens show metastatic deposits of an undifferentiated large cell lung carcinoma. The metastases form essentially necrotic masses with peripheral enhancement and peritumoral edema. **(B)** Occasionally, extensive necrosis transforms metastases into cysts lined by only a thin rim of viable tumor.

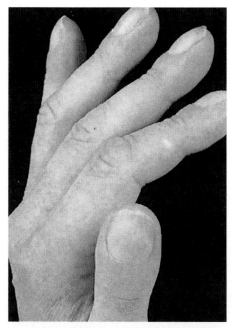

FIGURE 5.87 **HYPERTROPHIC PULMONARY OSTEOARTHROPATHY (HPO; DIGIT CLUBBING).** A characteristic manifestation of HPO, digit clubbing occurs in about 10% of lung cancer patients of all histologic subgroups, but particularly in adenocarcinoma. The disease may be early or advanced. Benign tumors, inflammatory disease, and liver disease are also associated with clubbing. Although the pathophysiology is poorly understood, digital clubbing, painful joints, and tender extremities—features commonly seen in HPO—often reverse markedly after successful thoracotomy, radiation therapy, or chemotherapy.

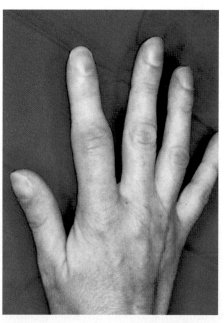

FIGURE 5.88 **HYPERTROPHIC PULMONARY OSTEOARTHROPATHY AND DIGITAL METASTASES.** This 45-year-old woman presented with HPO and also pain and swelling of her right index finger. Radiographs showed lytic lesions in the phalanx and bone scan was positive in this area (not shown). Biopsy was positive for metastatic, poorly differentiated adenocarcinoma from the lung. Metastases to bone beyond the humerus and/or femur are unusual in any type of primary cancer.

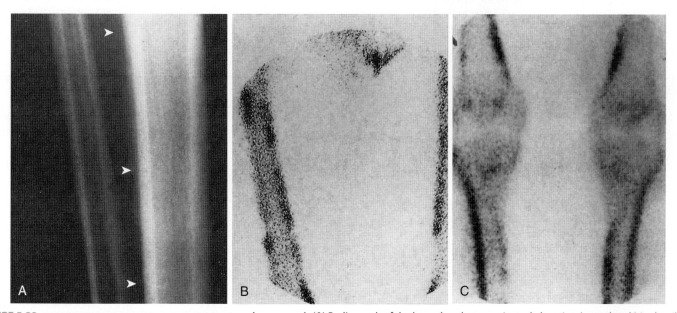

FIGURE 5.89 **HYPERTROPHIC PULMONARY OSTEOARTHROPATHY (PERIOSTITIS).** (**A**) Radiograph of the lower leg shows periosteal elevation (*arrowheads*) in the tibia of a patient who presented with joint pain of the lower legs and feet. Evaluation subsequently showed a primary lung adenocarcinoma of the right upper lobe. (**B, C**) Bone scans show focal increased uptake of radiopharmaceutical in both legs in areas of new bone formation; no bone metastases are evident.

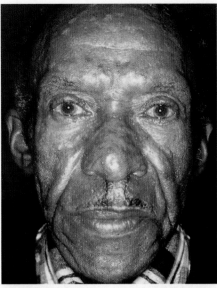

FIGURE 5.90 HYPERTROPHIC PULMONARY OSTEOARTHROPATHY (PACHYDERMOPERIOSTITIS). This 60-year-old man with squamous cell lung cancer developed HPO and changing facial features resembling acromegaly. His appearance became progressively coarser, with deepening facial and scalp furrows. Thickening of the legs and forearms, with the development of spadelike hands and feet, may also occur in this paraneoplastic syndrome.

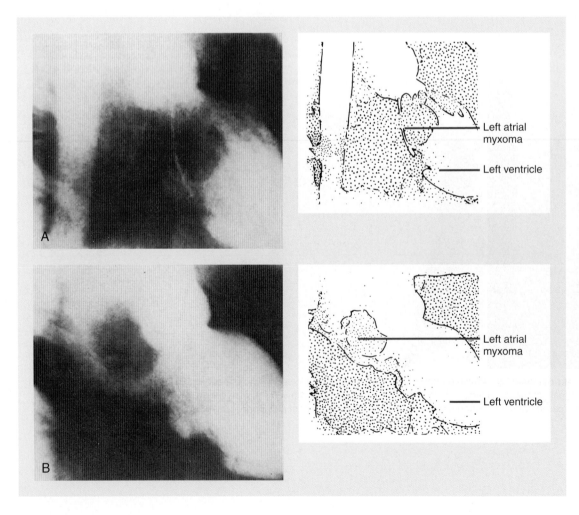

FIGURE 5.91 LEFT ATRIAL MYXOMA. (**A**) Left ventriculogram in the right anterior oblique projection shows a mobile left atrial myxoma as a space-filling defect within the mitral valve in diastole. (**B**) Sufficient mitral regurgitation is present to delineate the myxoma in the left atrium in systole. (Reproduced with permission from Hall R, Cooley D: Neoplastic heart disease. In Hurst J, editor: *The heart: arteries and veins*, ed 6, New York, 1986, McGraw-Hill.)

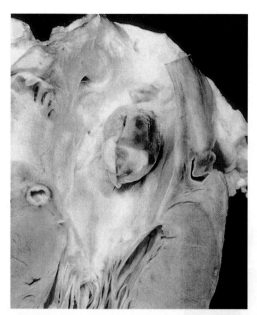

FIGURE 5.92 **LEFT ATRIAL MYXOMA.** The left side of the heart has been opened to show a rounded, polypoid, gelatinous tumor (1.5 cm in diameter) arising from the interatrial septum below the oval fossa. This was an incidental finding at autopsy of a 66-year-old hypertensive woman who died of a cerebral hemorrhage. Note the marked left ventricular hypertrophy, a probable consequence of hypertension.

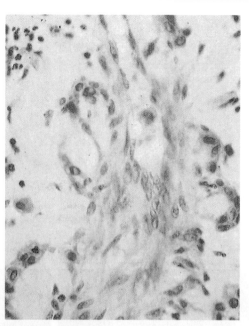

FIGURE 5.94 **CARDIAC MYXOMA.** Histologic section of a tumor shows polygonal cell strands within a mucoid stroma.

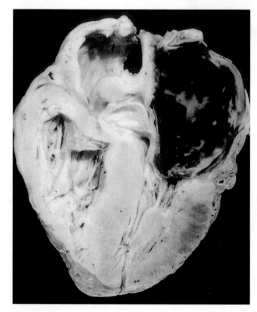

FIGURE 5.93 **LEFT ATRIAL MYXOMA.** This autopsy specimen from a 46-year-old woman who died after being admitted with severe congestive heart failure and atrial fibrillation has been sectioned to reveal a 7-cm hemorrhagic mass filling the left atrium. Originating near the oval fossa, the tumor occludes the mitral valve orifice and projects through it. The myocardium of both ventricles is hypertrophied.

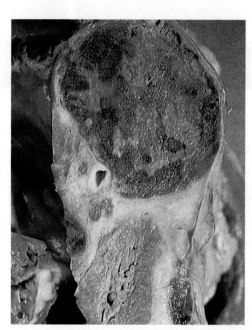

FIGURE 5.95 **ANGIOSARCOMA.** This specimen shows an angiosarcoma of the heart localized in the atrioventricular groove. Note the characteristic hemorrhagic appearance.

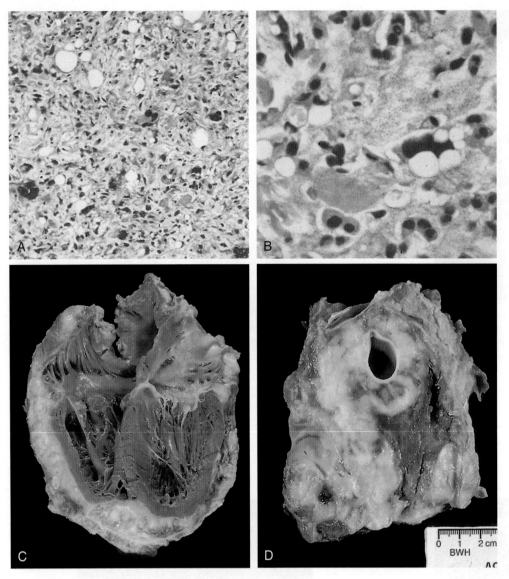

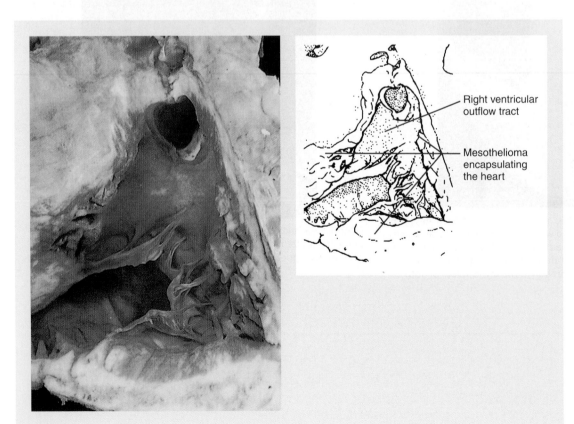

FIGURE 5.96 CARDIAC LIPOSARCOMA.
A 23-year-old man presented with an anterior mediastinal mass. Biopsy demonstrated a high-grade sarcoma with many pleomorphic cells (**A**, low-power). At high power (**B**) a lipoblast with fat-containing intracytoplastic vacuoles, indenting on a hyperchromatic nucleus, can be seen. These features are diagnostic of liposarcoma. He had a rapid downhill course despite attempts at therapy. At autopsy the heart and large vessels were encased in tumor (24 cm in maximal dimension). (**C, D**) The tumor appeared to arise from the epicardial/pericardial tissue. (Gross pictures courtesy of Dr. Klaus Busam, Brigham and Women's Hospital, Boston, MA.)

FIGURE 5.97 MESOTHELIOMA.
The right side of the heart has been opened to reveal a primary mesothelioma of the pericardium. The tumor presents as a thick pericardial layer covering the heart, with local invasion into the myocardium. Some malignant mesotheliomas may originate in the central pleural areas and then spread throughout the rest of the pleura. Usually, however, they spread from the outer lung pleura to other sites in one or both pleural spaces (see Chapter 6).

Right ventricular outflow tract

Mesothelioma encapsulating the heart

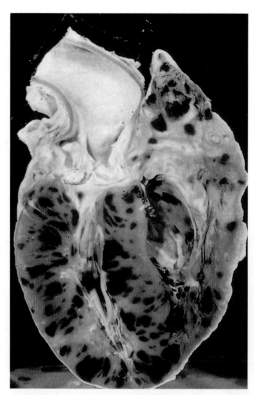

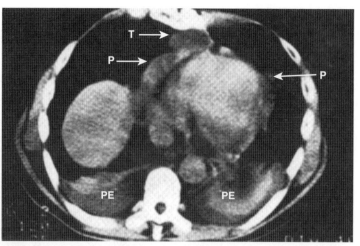

FIGURE 5.99 **METASTATIC RENAL CELL CARCINOMA.** CT scan of the chest at the level of the heart in a patient with renal cell carcinoma reveals metastases to the anterior mediastinum (T) and the pericardium (P). Bilateral pleural effusions (PE) also are evident. (Courtesy of F. Parker Gregg, MD, Houston, TX. Reproduced with permission from Hall R, Cooley D: Neoplastic heart disease. In Hurst J, editor: *The heart: arteries and veins*, ed 6, New York, 1986, McGraw-Hill.)

FIGURE 5.98 **METASTATIC MALIGNANT MELANOMA.** An adult male who had undergone excision of a primary cutaneous malignant melanoma over the right iliac crest 18 months previously developed lymph node and hepatic metastases, followed by bony and cutaneous deposits with terminal melanuria. This section through the heart shows numerous pigmented deposits of metastatic melanoma throughout the myocardium.

FIGURE 5.100 **METASTATIC RENAL CELL CARCINOMA.** A 54-year-old man had a renal cell carcinoma with positive nodes resected 6 years previously but subsequently developed jaundice and other evidence of widespread metastases. (**A**) Autopsy showed a single, large metastasis to the right ventricle protruding into the lumen. (**B**) High-power photomicrograph reveals the renal cell carcinoma, papillary type, invading cardiac muscle. The patient had not developed any cardiac symptoms.

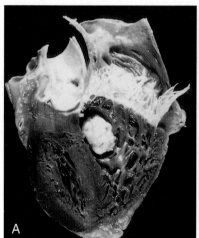

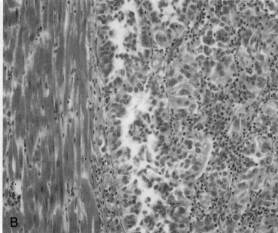

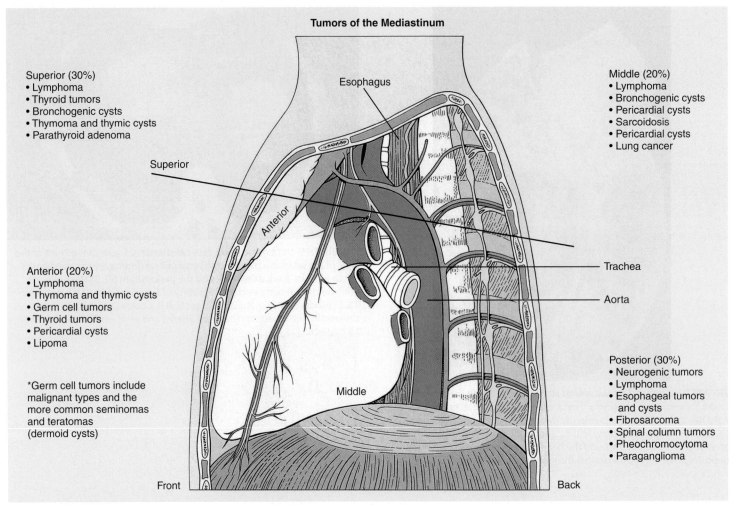

Tumors of the Mediastinum

Esophagus

Superior

Anterior

Trachea

Aorta

Middle

Front

Back

Superior (30%)
• Lymphoma
• Thyroid tumors
• Bronchogenic cysts
• Thymoma and thymic cysts
• Parathyroid adenoma

Anterior (20%)
• Lymphoma
• Thymoma and thymic cysts
• Germ cell tumors
• Thyroid tumors
• Pericardial cysts
• Lipoma

*Germ cell tumors include
malignant types and the
more common seminomas
and teratomas
(dermoid cysts)

Middle (20%)
• Lymphoma
• Bronchogenic cysts
• Pericardial cysts
• Sarcoidosis
• Pericardial cysts
• Lung cancer

Posterior (30%)
• Neurogenic tumors
• Lymphoma
• Esophageal tumors
  and cysts
• Fibrosarcoma
• Spinal column tumors
• Pheochromocytoma
• Paraganglioma

FIGURE 5.101 TUMORS OF THE MEDIASTINUM. The customary subdivisions of the mediastinum are illustrated, together with a partial listing of mediastinal tumors and the relative frequency of occurrence of tumors in the various mediastinal divisions. About 25% of mediastinal tumors are malignant. There is some overlap in cell types.

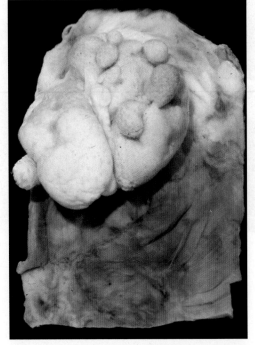

FIGURE 5.102 MEDIASTINUM: DERMOID CYST (BENIGN TERATOMA). This specimen was excised from a 28-year-old woman who presented with dull chest pain and dyspnea. At operation, a large mass arising in the mediastinum was found to occupy much of the right side of the thoracic cavity. This is part of the wall of this very large cystic teratoma. Projecting from the inner surface there is a nodular mass, measuring 4 cm in maximum dimension, which is covered in clearly recognizable skin bearing short pale hairs. The resemblance to normal epidermal structures is admirably demonstrated in this example.

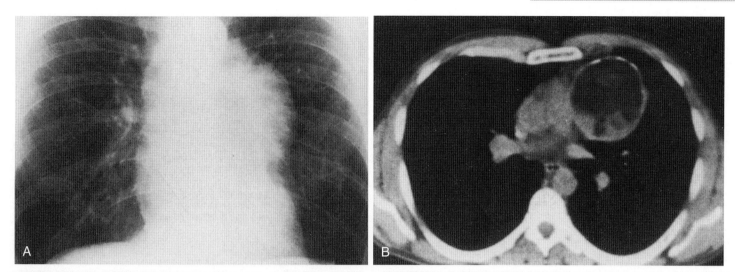

FIGURE 5.103 **BENIGN TERATOMA.** A 30-year-old man developed mild chest discomfort. (**A**) Chest radiograph reveals a large mass in the anterior mediastinum. (**B**) CT scan shows a thin-walled cystic lesion. The tumor was completely resected at thoracotomy.

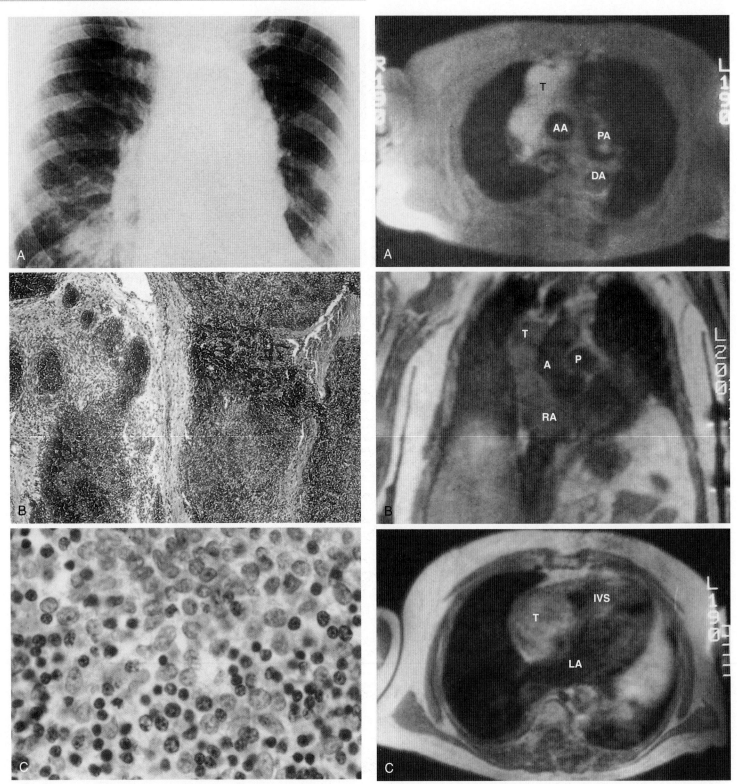

FIGURE 5.104 **THYMOMA.** A 50-year-old woman presented with severe anemia due to pure red cell aplasia. (**A**) Chest radiograph demonstrates an anterior mediastinal mass. A locally invasive thymoma was resected, but small pleural metastases were found. (**B**) Low-power photomicrograph of the lesion shows fibrous septae separating tumor nodules. (**C**) On high-power view, neoplastic epithelial cells are evident with an admixture of T lymphocytes, which are probably non-neoplastic. The epithelial cells are positive for keratin. Metastases are uncommon within the chest and even moreso outside the chest. Thymic carcinomas, however, are more invasive and often metastasize to rare distant sites.

FIGURE 5.105 **THYMOMA INVADING THE HEART.** A 67-year-old man presented with early features of SVC syndrome (see Fig. 5.55). He also had increasing cough and several syncopal episodes. He suffered cardiac arrest in the emergency room but was resuscitated and received radiation therapy with improvement. Chest radiograph showed an anterior mediastinal mass. (**A**) T_1-weighted MR image in the axial plane at the level of the main pulmonary artery (PA) with a lobular mediastinal mass (T) on the right wrapping around the ascending aorta (AA). DA, descending aorta. (**B**) T_1-weighted image in the coronal plane through the ascending aorta (A) with tumor extending from the upper right mediastinum (T) down into and filling the right atrium (RA). P, main pulmonary artery. (**C**) T_1-weighted MR image in the axial plane at the level of the left atrium (LA) with tumor filling the right atrium (T). IVS, interventricular septum.

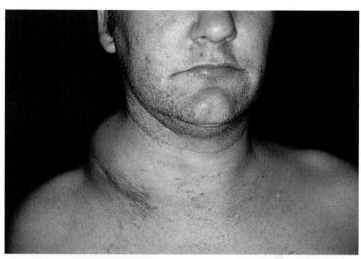

FIGURE 5.106 THYMOMA. This 38-year-old man with recurrent malignant thymoma had disease progression directly into the supraclavicular and cervical lymph node sites, that was refractory to both chemotherapy and radiation therapy.

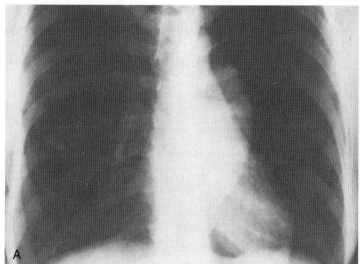 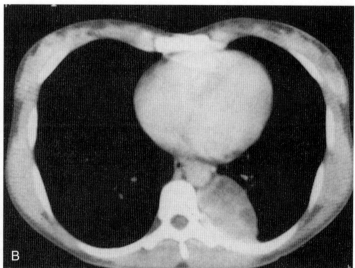

FIGURE 5.107 GANGLIONEUROMA. (A) During evaluation for an unrelated problem, chest radiography in a 24-year-old woman revealed an asymptomatic posterior mediastinal mass. **(B)** CT scan shows the classic location of a neurogenic tumor in the posterior mediastinum. The lesion is multicystic. Curative resection revealed a ganglioneuroma.

References and Suggested Readings

Allen MS: Malignant tracheal tumors, *Mayo Clin Proc* 68:680–684, 1993.

Anderson M, Spandidos D: Oncogenes and onco-suppressor genes in lung cancer, *Respir Med* 87:413–420, 1993.

Brambilla E, Travis WD, Colby TV, et al: The new World Health Organization classification of lung tumors, *Eur Respir J* 18:1059–1068, 2001.

Bryant A, Cerfolio RJ: Differences in epidemiology, histology, and survival between cigarette smokers and never-smokers who develop non–small cell lung cancer, *Chest* 132:185–192, 2007.

Chen AM, Jahan TM, Jablons DM, et al: Risk of cerebral metastases and neurological death after pathological complete response to neoadjuvant therapy for locally advanced nonsmall-cell lung cancer. *Cancer* 109:1668–1675, 2007a.

Chen HY, Yu SL, Chen CH, et al: A five-gene signature and clinical outcome in non-small-cell lung cancer, *N Engl J Med* 356:11–20, 2007b.

Cheng TL, Chang MY, Huang SY, et al: Overexpression of circulating c-Met messenger RNA is significantly correlated with nodal stage and early recurrence in non-small cell lung cancer, *Chest* 128:1453–1460, 2005.

Cicin I, Karagol H, Uzunoglu S, et al: Extrapulmonary small-cell carcinoma compared with small-cell lung carcinoma, *Cancer* 110:1068–1076, 2007.

ColsonY, Sanders J, Skarin A: Gender-specific differences in lung cancer: commentary on the International Early Lung Cancer Action Project, *Am J Hematol Oncol* 6:2–5, 2007.

Demmy TL: Tumor of the heart and pericardium. In Aisner J, Arriagada R, Green MR, et al, editors. *Comprehensive textbook of thoracic oncology*, Chap. 32, Philadelphia, Williams & Wilkins, 1996, pp 681–710.

Dunagan DP, Chin Jr R, McCain TW, et al: Staging by positron emission tomography predicts survival in patients with non-small cell lung cancer, *Chest* 119:333–339, 2001.

Fischer B, Lassen U, Mortensen J, et al: Preoperative staging of lung cancer with combined PET-CT, *N Engl J Med* 361:32–39, 2009.

Fletcher JA, Pinkus GS, Donovan K, et al: Clonal rearrangement of chromosome band:6p21 in mesenchymal component of pulmonary chondroid hamartoma, *Cancer Res* 52:6224–6228, 1992.

Gauger J, Patz EF, Coleman RE, et al: Clinical stage I non–small cell lung cancer including FDG-PET imaging: sites and time to recurrence, *J Thorac Oncol* 2:499–505, 2007.

Goldstraw P, for the International Association for the Study of Lung Cancer: Staging manual in Thoracic Oncology, Orange Park, Florida, Editoral Rx Press, 2009.

Groome PA, Bolejack V, Crowley JJ, et al: The IASLC Lung Cancer Staging Project: validation of the proposals for revision of the T, N, and M descriptors and consequent stage groupings in the forthcoming (seventh), edition of the TNM classification of malignant tumours, *J Torac Oncol* 2:694–705, 2007.

Hall R, Cooley D: Neoplastic heart disease. In Hurst J, editor: *The heart: arteries and veins*, ed 6, New York, McGraw-Hill, 165–275, 1986.

Harpole D, Richards W, Herndon J, et al: Angiogenesis and molecular biologic substaging in patients with stage I non-small cell lung cancer, *Ann Thorac Surg* 61:1470–1476, 1996.

Hartman TE: Lung cancer screening results: easily misunderstood, *Mayo Clin Proc* 82:14–15, 2007.

Heffner JE, Klein JS: Recent advances in the diagnosis and management of malignant pleural effusions, *Mayo Clin Proc* 88(2):235–250, 2008.

Hirsch RF, Matthews MJ, Aisner S, et al: Histopathologic classification of small cell lung cancer, *Cancer* 62:973–977, 1988.

Hiyama K, Ishioka S, Shirotani Y, et al: Alterations in telomeric repeat length in lung cancer are associated with loss of heterozygosity in p53 and RB, *Oncogene* 10:937–944, 1995.

Huang Y-T, Heist RS, Chirieac LR, et al: Genome-wide analysis of survival in early-stage non–small-cell lung cancer, *J Clin Oncol* 27:2660–2667, 2009.

Inoue M, Minami M, Shiono H, et al: Clinicopathologic study of resected, peripheral, small-sized, non-small cell lung cancer tumors of 2 cm or less in diameter: pleural invasion and increase of serum carcinoembryonic antigen level as predictors of nodal involvement, *J Thorac Cardiovasc Surg* 131:988–993, 2006.

Jackman DM, Chirieac LR, Janne PA, et al: Bronchioloalveolar carcinoma: a review of the epidemiology, pathology and treatment, *Semin Respir Crit Care Med* 26:342–352, 2005.

Jemal A, Siegel R, Ward E, et al: Cancer statistics 2009, *CA Cancer J Clin* 59:225–249, 2009.

Johnson BE, Kelley MJ: Overview of genetic and molecular events in the pathogenesis of lung cancer, *Chest* 103:1S–3S, 1993.

Kimura T, Sato T, Onodera K: Clinical significance of DNA measurements in small cell lung cancer, *Cancer* 72:3216–3222, 1993.

Kobayashi S, Boggon TJ, Dayaram T, et al: EGFR mutation and resistance of non–small-cell lung cancer to gefitinib, *Engl J Med* 352:786–792, 2005.

Lee J, Yoon A, Kalapurakal S, et al: Expression of p53 oncoprotein in non-small cell lung cancer: a favorable prognostic factor, *J Clin Oncol* 13:1893–1903, 1995.

Lim E, Goldstraw P, Nicholson AG, et al: Proceedings of the IASLC international workshop on advances in pulmonary neuroendocrine tumors 2007, *J Thoracic Oncol* 3:1194–1201, 2008.

Lynch TJ, Bell DW, Sordella R, et al: Activating mutations in the epidermal growth factor receptor underlying responsiveness of non–small-cell lung cancer to Gefitinib, *N Engl J Med* 350:2129–2139, 2004.

Macchiarini P, Fontanini G, Hardin J, et al: Most peripheral, node-negative, non-small-cell lung cancers have low proliferative rates and no intratumoral and peritumoral blood and lymphatic vessel invasion, *J Thorac Cardiovasc Surg* 104:892–899, 1992.

Marks JL, Broderick S, Zhou Q, et al: Prognostic and therapeutic implications of EGFR and KRAS mutations in resected lung adenocarcinoma, *J Thoracic Oncol* 3:111–116, 2008.

Marom EM, Erasmus JJ, Patz Jr EF: Lung cancer and positron emission tomography with fluorodeoxyglucose, *Lung Cancer* 28:187–202, 2000.

Masaoka A, Monden Y, Nakahara K, et al: Follow-up study of thymomas with special reference to their clinical stages, *Cancer* 48:2485–2492, 1981.

Matsumoto H, Muramatsu H, Shimotakahara T, et al: Correlation of expression of ABH blood group carbohydrate antigens with metastatic potential in human lung carcinomas, *Cancer* 72:75–81, 1993.

McAllister HA Jr, Fenoglio Jr JJ: *Tumors of the cardiovascular system*, Washington, DC, 1978, Armed Forces Institute of Pathology.

Mentzer SJ, Sugarbaker DJ: Thoracoscopy and video-assisted thoracic surgery. In Brooks DC, editor: *Current techniques in laparoscopy*, Philadelphia, 1994, Current Medicine, pp 20.1–20.12.

Minna JD, Pass H, Glatstein EJ: Cancer of the lung. In DeVita Jr VT, Hellman S, Rosenberg SA, editors: *Cancer: principles and practice of oncology*, ed 3, Philadelphia, 1989, Lippincott, pp 591–724.

Mitsudomi T, Oyama T, Kusano T, et al: Mutations of the p53 gene as a predictor of poor prognosis in patients with non-small cell lung cancer, *J Natl Cancer Inst* 85:2018, 1993.

Mountain CF: Lung cancer staging classification, *Clin Chest Med* 14:48–53, 1993.

Mountain CF: A new international staging system for lung cancer, *Chest* 89(Suppl):225–233, 1986.

Mountain CF: Revisions in the international system for staging lung cancer, *Chest* 111:1710–1717, 1997.

Nishino M, Ashiku SK, Kocher ON, et al: The thymus: a comprehensive review, *Radiographics* 26:335–348, 2006.

Ordonez NG: Value of thyroid transcription factor-1, E-cadherin, BG8, WT1, and CD44S immunostaining in distinguishing epithelial pleural mesothelioma from pulmonary and nonpulmonary adenocarcinoma, *Am J Surg Pathol* 24:598–606, 2000.

Otterson G, Lin A, Kaye F, et al: Genetic etiology of lung cancer, *Oncology* 6:97–107, 1992.

Ou SH, Zell JA, Ziogas A, et al: Prognostic factors for survival of stage I non-small cell lung cancer patients, *Cancer* 110:1532–1541, 2007.

Pezzella F, Turley H, Kuzu I, et al: bcl-2 protein in non-small cell lung carcinoma, *N Engl J Med* 329:690–694, 1993.

Pieterman RM, van Putten JWG, Meuzelaar JJ, et al: Preoperative staging of non-small cell lung cancer with positron-emission tomography, *N Engl J Med* 343:254–261, 2000.

Potti A, Mukherjee S, Petersen R, et al: A genomic strategy to refine prognosis in early-stage non-small-cell lung cancer, *N Engl J Med* 355:570–580, 2006.

Riedel RF, Burfeind WR: Thymoma: benign appearance, malignant potential, *Oncologist* 11:887–894, 2006.

Rosai J: *Histological typing of tumours of the thymus*, End edition, Berlin and Heidelberg, 1999, Springer-Verlag.

Rusch VW, Asamura H, Watanabe H, et al, for the International Association for the Study of Lung Cancer Staging Committee: The IASLC lung cancer staging project: a proposal for a new international lymph node map in the forthcoming seventh edition of the TNM classification for lung cancer, *J Thoracic Oncol* 4:568–577, 2009.

Salgia R, Harpole D, Herndon D, et al: Role of serum markers CA125 and CEA in non-small cell lung cancer, *Anticancer Res* 21:1241–1246, 2001.

Salgia R, Skarin AT: Molecular abnormalities in lung cancer, *J Clin Oncol* 16:1207–1217, 1998.

Sato M, Shames DS, Gazdar AF, et al: A translational view of the molecular pathogenesis of lung cancer, *J Thorac Oncol* 2:327–343, 2007.

Sawabata N, Maeda H, Yokota S, et al: Postoperative serum carcinoembryonic antigen levels in patients with pathologic stage IA nonsmall cell lung carcinoma, *Cancer* 101:803–809, 2004.

Skarin A: Multimodality treatment of lung cancer. In Skarin A, editor: Multimodality treatment of lung cancer, New York, 2000, Marcel Dekker.

Skarin AT: Analysis of long-term survivors with small-cell lung cancer, *Chest* 103:440S–444S, 1993.

Skarin AT, Jochelson M, Sheldon T, et al: Neoadjuvant chemotherapy in marginally resectable stage III MO non-small cell lung cancer: long term follow-up in 41 patients, *J Surg Oncol* 40:266–274, 1989.

Sozzi G, Veronese M, Negrini M, et al: The FHIT gene at 3p14.2 is abnormal in lung cancer, *Cell* 85:17–26, 1996.

Strauss GM, Kwiatkowski DJ, Harpole DH, et al: Molecular and pathologic analysis of stage I non-small cell carcinoma of the lung: implications for the future, *J Clin Oncol* 13:1265–1279, 1995.

Sun Z, Aubry MC, Deschamps C, et al: Histologic grade is an independent prognostic factor for survival in non-small cell lung cancer: an analysis of 5018 hospital- and 712 population-based cases. *J Thorac Cardiovasc Surg* 131:1014–1020, 2006.

Sundaresan V, Ganly P, Hasleton P, et al: p53 and chromosome 3 abnormalities, characteristic of malignant lung tumors, are detectable in preinvasive lesions of the bronchus, *Oncogene* 7:1989–1997, 1992.

Tanaka R, Wang D, Morishita Y, et al: Loss of function of p16 gene and prognosis of pulmonary adenocarcinoma, *Cancer* 103:608–615, 2005.

Travis WD, Colby TV, Corrin B, et al: *Histological typing of lung and pleural tumors*, ed 3, Berlin, 1999, Springer Verlag.

Vansteenkiste JF, Stroobants SS: PET scan in lung cancer: current recommendations and innovation, *J Thorac Oncol* 1:71–73, 2006.

Westra WH, Slebos RJC, Offerhaus GJA, et al: K-ras oncogene activation in lung adenocarcinomas from former smokers, *Cancer* 72:432–438, 1993.

Wick MR, Swanson PE: Carcinosarcomas: current perspectives and an historical review of nosological concepts, *Semin Diag Pathol* 10:118–127, 1993.

Wilson LD, Detterbeck FC, Yahalom J, et al: Superior vena cava syndrome with malignant causes, *N Engl J Med* 356:1862–1869, 2007.

World Health Organization (WHO): *Global cancer rates could increase by 50% to 15 billion by 2020.* Available at: <http://www.who.int/mediacentre/news/releases/2003/pr27/en> 2003. Accessed on 18 July 2006.

Figure Credits

The following books published by Gower Medical Publishing are sources of figures in the present chapter. The figure numbers given in the listing are those of the figures in the present chapter. The page numbers (or slide numbers) given in parentheses are those of the original publication.

Anderson RH, editor: Cardiovascular system. In Turk JL, Fletcher CDM, editors: *RCSE slide atlas of pathology*. London, 1986, Gower Medical Publishing: Figs. 5.92 (slide 72); 5.93 (slide 73); 5.97 (slide 76).

Becker AF, Anderson RH: *Cardiac pathology.* Edinburgh/London, 1983, Churchill Livingstone/Gower Medical Publishing: Fig. 5.96 (p 8.4).

Besser GM, Cudworth AG: *Clinical endocrinology.* Philadelphia/London, 1987, Lippincott/Gower Medical Publishing: Fig. 5.22 (p 19.7).

Dieppe PA, Bacon PA, Bamji AN, et al: *Atlas of clinical rheumatology.* Philadelphia/London, 1986, Lea & Febiger/Gower Medical Publishing: Fig. 5.77 (p 21.6); Table 5.8 (p 21.2).

du Bois RM, Clarke SW: *Fibreoptic bronchoscopy in diagnosis and management.* Philadelphia/London, 1987, Lippincott/Gower Medical Publishing: Table 5.1 (p 3.2); Table 5.2 (p 3.2); Figs. 5.19 (p 3.12); 5.23A, B (p 3.15); 5.23C, D (p 3.16); 5.35 (p 3.8); 5.38 (p 6.4); 5.42 (p 3.11); 5.43 (p 6.18); 5.44 (p 6.15); Table 5.7 (p 4.2).

Fletcher CDM, McKee PH: *An atlas of gross pathology.* London, 1987, Edward Arnold/ Gower Medical Publishing: Figs. 5.9 (p 21); 5.39 (p 21), 5.65 (p 21).

Hurst JW, editor: *Atlas of the heart.* New York, 1988, McGraw-Hill/Gower Medical Publishing: Table 5.9 (p 13.2); Table 5.10 (p 13.2); Figs 5.11 (p 13.9); 5.96 (p 4.31); 5.97 (p 13.9); 5.99 (p 3.11).

Kassner EG, editor: *Atlas of radiologic imaging.* Philadelphia/New York, 1989, Lippincott/Gower Medical Publishing: Fig. 5.59 (p 8.8).

Okazaki H, Scheithauer BW: *Atlas of neuropathology.* Philadelphia/New York, 1988, Lippincott/Gower Medical Publishing: Figs. 5.83 (p 168); 5.85 (p 171); 5.86 (p 170).

Perkin GD, Rose FC, Blackwood W, et al: *Atlas of clinical urology.* Philadelphia/London, 1986, Lippincott/Gower Medical Publishing: Figs. 5.81 (p 7.13); 5.82 (p 7.13); 5.84 (p 9.8).

Spencer H, editor: Respiratory system. In Turk JL, Fletcher CDM, editors: *RCSE slide atlas of pathology.* London, 1986, Gower Medical Publishing: Figs. 5.5 (slide 68); 5.8 (slide 91); 5.20 (slide 87).

Weiss MA, Mills SE: *Atlas of genitourinary tract disorders.* Philadelphia/New York, 1988, Gower Medical Publishing: Figs. 5.73 (p 8.21), 5.74 (p 11.55), 5.75 (p 8.21).

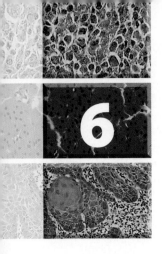

6

Malignant Mesothelioma

PASI A. JÄNNE • DAVID WU • LUCIAN R. CHIRIEAC

Malignant mesothelioma is a rare malignancy arising from the mesothelial cells of the pleural or peritoneal surfaces. Mesothelioma can arise from the pleura (pleural mesothelioma), peritoneum (peritoneal mesothelioma), pericardium (pericardial mesothelioma), or tunica vaginalis (testicular mesothelioma). In the United States there are approximately 3000 new cases of mesothelioma reported annually. Approximately 80% of these occur as pleural mesothelioma.

The development of mesothelioma is most clearly associated with prior asbestos exposure (Hodgson and Darnton, 2000). Asbestos was (and continues to be in some parts of the world) an important and affordable industrial resource as a result of its resistance to heat and combustion. Asbestos was used in shipbuilding, in car brakes, in the production of cement, and as insulation. There are two main forms of asbestos known as amphiboles and chrysotile. Amphiboles are long, thin asbestos fibers and are believed to be the most carcinogenic of the asbestos fibers. Chrysotile asbestos has also been associated with mesothelioma, although the frequency may be less than with amphibole asbestos (Hodgson and Darnton, 2000). The latency period between the time of asbestos exposure to development of mesothelioma can be 20–40 years. These unique features reflect the population of patients who develop mesothelioma including asbestos miners, plumbers, pipefitters, or those who worked in shipbuilding industries. In the United States mesothelioma is a disease of Caucasian men, reflecting the population of asbestos workers in the 1960s and early 1970s. The median age of patients diagnosed with mesothelioma is the mid-60s, although in the Surveillance Epidemiology and End Results database from the United States the median age is over 70. Approximately 80% of patients who develop mesothelioma are men. Women who develop mesothelioma also may have worked in industries that used asbestos, although there are reports of secondary exposure, for example, from clothing of spouses who worked directly with asbestos (Miller, 2005). The estimated incidence of mesothelioma worldwide also reflects the use of asbestos in different regions of the world. A second, but very controversial factor thought to have a role in the development of mesothelioma is simian virus 40 (SV40). SV40 is an oncogenic polyomavirus in human cells, and infection with it leads to inactivation of tumor suppressor genes *TP53* and the retinoblastoma gene (*RB1*) (De Luca et al., 1997). SV40 may have been transmitted to humans inadvertently as a contaminant in the polio vaccine 30–40 years ago. However, epidemiologic studies have not found a greater incidence of mesothelioma in those who received the polio vaccine during that time period (Strickler et al., 2003). Although SV40 viral sequences have been detected in mesotheliomas (and not in normal adjacent lung tissues), this has not been a consistent finding and, as suggested by some investigators, may even be a false-positive finding (Lopez-Rios et al., 2004). Other etiologic factors leading to mesothelioma include prior ionizing radiation and rare familial forms reported to occur in Cappadocia, Turkey (Weissmann et al., 1996; Roushdy-Hammady et al., 2001).

Clinical Presentation

The most common clinical presentation of malignant pleural mesothelioma includes dyspnea on exertion and shortness of breath. These clinical symptoms often lead physicians to obtain a chest radiograph wherein a unilateral pleural effusion is noted (Fig. 6.1). Mesothelioma is rarely an incidental finding on a routine chest radiograph. Patients can also present with nonpleuritic chest pain. This symptom is important to elicit from patients, because those who present with chest pains often have disease extending into the chest wall and thus are not surgical candidates. Other presenting signs and symptoms include discordant chest wall expansion, weight loss, night sweats, and the presence of a palpable subcutaneous mass (Fig. 6.2).

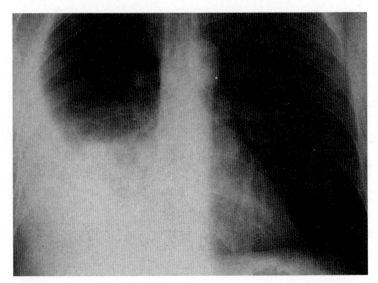

FIGURE 6.1 **MESOTHELIOMA.** A 60-year-old shipyard worker developed increasing dyspnea. On chest radiography he was found to have a large right pleural effusion. Pleural biopsy confirmed the diagnosis of malignant mesothelioma.

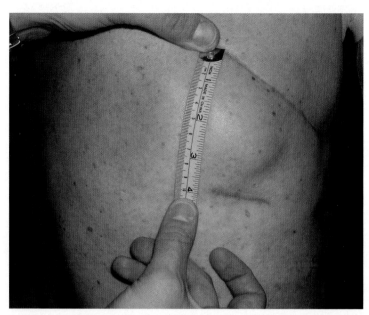

FIGURE 6.2 SUBCUTANEOUS CHEST WALL MASS. This painful subcutaneous mass appeared in a patient with mesothelioma a few months following surgical exploration.

Diagnostic Evaluation

Three main imaging modalities, computed tomography (CT), positron emission tomography (PET), and magnetic resonance imaging (MRI), are used to evaluate patients with newly diagnosed mesothelioma. Contrast-enhanced CT scanning often reveals a thickened lobulated circumferential pleural rind (Figs. 6.3, 6.4) with or without the presence of a concurrent pleural effusion. CT scanning can also help identify the presence of pleural plaques (Fig. 6.5), a sign of previous asbestos exposure, and whether the disease extends into the interlobar fissures. In addition, a contrast-enhanced CT scan can help determine the presence of mediastinal lymph nodes (Fig. 6.3). 2-[^{18}F]-fluoro-2-deoxy-D-glucose (FDG)-PET scanning has also recently been evaluated for its clinical utility, in that most mesotheliomas are PET-avid (Fig. 6.6). Analogous to lung cancer, FDG-PET scanning can identify occult metastatic disease in patients who are otherwise potential surgical candidates (Flores et al., 2003). However, its utility in defining locoregional disease and the role of FDG-PET scanning in advanced mesothelioma remain to be determined. MRI can also be useful in the evaluation of mesothelioma, because it can identify chest wall or transdiaphragmatic invasion and involvement of the intralobular fissures (Fig. 6.7). Peritoneal mesothelioma is more difficult to image accurately. CT scanning often reveals a thickened omentum and/or the presence of ascites (Fig. 6.8A to C). FDG-PET scanning has also been used in the evaluation of peritoneal mesothelioma. The peritoneal cavity is also a common site of mesothelioma recurrence in patients who have undergone prior surgical resection of their thoracic disease (Fig. 6.8D).

The presentation of a patient with a new pleural effusion often leads to a thoracentesis to evaluate the nature of the effusion. The pleural effusions in mesothelioma are often cytologically negative, and patients frequently undergo repeated thoracenteses to establish the diagnosis of mesothelioma or before performing a more invasive evaluation. Because of the frequent nature of cytologically negative effusions, cytology is

not a reliable method of diagnosing mesothelioma. In addition, cytologic specimens are often insufficient to determine the histologic subtype of mesothelioma, which itself provides prognostic information. The diagnostic procedure of choice for mesothelioma is a thoracoscopic biopsy. There are several advantages to this approach. First, it provides the surgeon the ability to visualize the extent of involvement of the mesothelioma to determine whether it is located on the parietal and/or visceral pleural surfaces. Second, a biopsy specimen of the involved area can be obtained under direct visualization. This is critical for making an accurate histologic diagnosis. Finally, thoracoscopy provides the ability to also perform a pleurodesis, which can help control recurrent pleural effusions.

On gross pathologic evaluation mesothelioma can be seen as a pale infiltrative tumor that encases the lung (Fig. 6.9). It can also infiltrate the underlying lung parenchyma and/or involve local and regional lymph nodes (Fig. 6.10). The most common histologic subtype is epithelioid mesothelioma and accounts for approximately 60% of all mesotheliomas (Fig. 6.11A to C). Other subtypes of mesothelioma include sarcomatoid mesothelioma (Fig. 6.12) and mixed-type (containing components of both epithelioid and sarcomatoid) mesothelioma (Figs. 6.13, 6.14). The main reason to determine the histologic subtype of mesothelioma is that patients with sarcomatoid mesothelioma often have a much worse prognosis than those with epithelial mesothelioma. The microscopic pathologic diagnosis of malignant mesothelioma can sometimes be more challenging, because the disease can be confused pathologically with adenocarcinoma of the lung. However, several tumor markers can help distinguish adenocarcinoma from malignant mesothelioma (Table 6.1). Mesotheliomas express the Wilms' tumor protein (WT1) and calretinin, which are not expressed by lung adenocarcinomas (Amin et al., 1995; Ordonez, 1998). Unlike adenocarcinomas, mesotheliomas do not express thyroid transcription factor 1 (TTF1) or carcinoembryonic antigen (CEA). These immunohistochemical features help distinguish mesothelioma from adenocarcinoma (Fig. 6.15). In addition, electron microscopy has been used in the diagnosis of mesothelioma (Fig. 6.16). Furthermore, two serum markers, osteopontin and soluble mesothelin-related (SMR) proteins, have also recently emerged as potential diagnostic markers in mesothelioma and are being evaluated in several prospective series (Robinson et al., 2003; Pass et al., 2005). These serum markers may help in screening individuals who were exposed to asbestos and thus at risk for developing mesothelioma before clinical and/or radiographic evidence of mesothelioma.

Table 6.1

Immunohistochemical Markers Used to Distinguish Malignant Mesothelioma from Lung Adenocarcinoma

Marker	Mesothelioma	Adenocarcinoma
Cytokeratin	Positive	Positive
CEA	Negative	Positive
TTF-1	Negative	Positive*
Calretinin	Positive	Negative
WT-1	Positive	Negative

CEA, carcinoembryonic antigen; TTF-1, thyroid transcription factor 1; WT-1, Wilms' tumor antigen.

*TTF-1 is positive in lung adenocarcinomas and negative in adenocarcinomas arising in other organs and metastasizing to pleura.

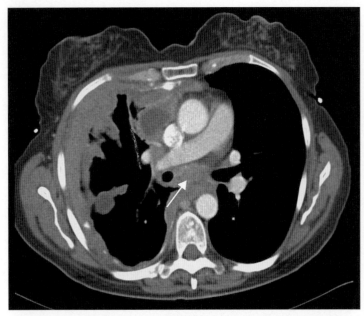

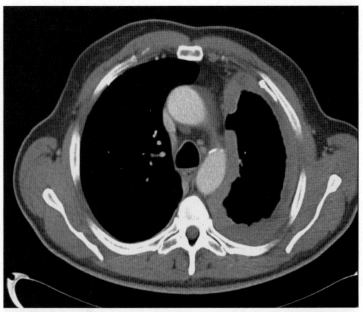

FIGURE 6.3 **CT APPEARANCE OF MESOTHELIOMA.** A thickened circumferential right-sided pleural rind is seen on chest CT in this patient with epithelial mesothelioma. This tumor also involves the mediastinal lymph nodes (*arrow*).

FIGURE 6.4 **CT APPEARANCE OF SARCOMATOID MESOTHELIOMA.** A thickened circumferential left-sided pleural rind is seen on chest CT in this patient with sarcomatoid mesothelioma.

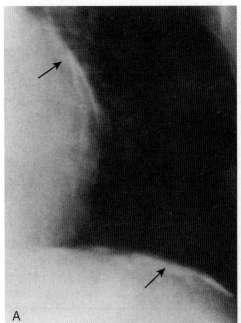

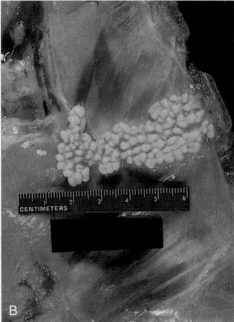

FIGURE 6.5 **(A)** Chest radiograph showing the left lower lung of a 57-year old man demonstrates pericardial and pleural plaques (*arrows*), representing fibrous thickening. These features are common findings indicating pulmonary asbestosis. **(B)** Autopsy features of calcified pleural plaques are quite striking. This specimen from a patient with mesothelioma shows focal calcifications on the lateral pleural surface. (Courtesy of Pathology Department, Brigham and Women's Hospital, Boston, MA.)

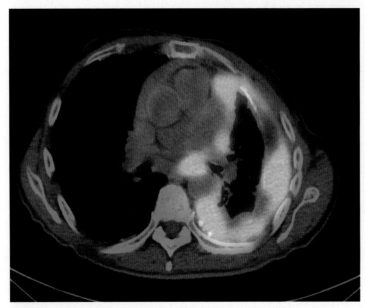

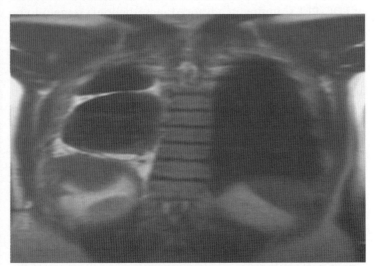

FIGURE 6.6 Fused CT and FDG-PET images from a patient with newly diagnosed mesothelioma. The mesothelioma is very FDG-avid.

FIGURE 6.7 Coronal image of the hemithorax of a patient with newly diagnosed malignant mesothelioma. The pleural rind is easily visualized (*arrows*) and demonstrates extension into the intralobular fissure in the right lung.

FIGURE 6.8 PERITONEAL MESOTHELIOMA.
(A) Peritoneal thickening (*arrows*) in a patient with peritoneal mesothelioma. **(B)** Right lower quadrant intraperitoneal mass (*arrow*) in a 52-year-old female with long-standing peritoneal mesothelioma. **(C)** Large-volume ascites (*arrow*) in a 63-year-old male with peritoneal mesothelioma. **(D)** Intra-abdominal recurrence in a patient with pleural mesothelioma 3.5 years after an extrapleural pneumonectomy. The recurrence involves the celiac lymph nodes (*arrow*) and the chest wall (*circle*).

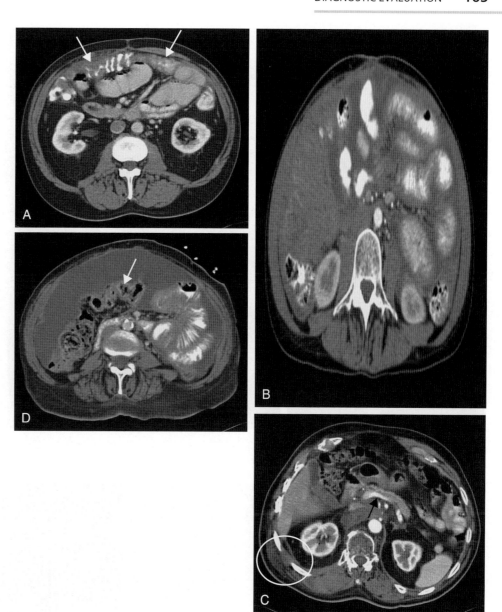

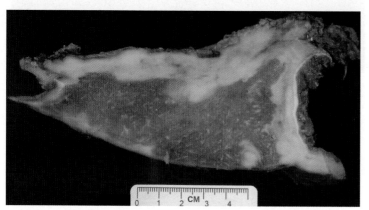

FIGURE 6.9 MESOTHELIOMA GROSS PATHOLOGY SPECIMEN. The lung is encased in a pale infiltrating tumor that arises from the pleura.

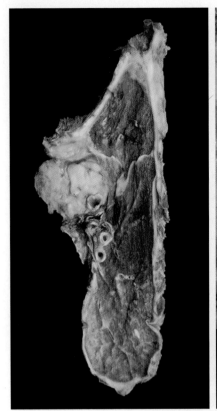
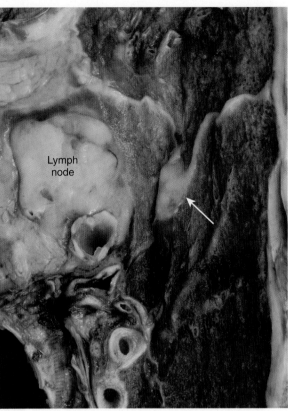

FIGURE 6.10 **MESOTHELIOMA GROSS PATHOLOGY SPECIMEN.** Low- (*left*) and high- (*right*) power views of a surgical specimen from a patient who has undergone an extrapleural pneumonectomy for mesothelioma. The tumor involves the hilar lymph nodes and the intralobular fissure (*arrow*).

Lymph
node

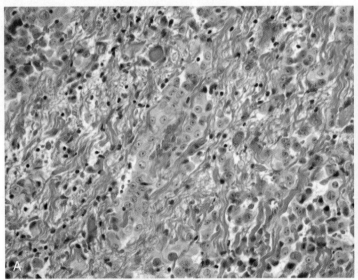
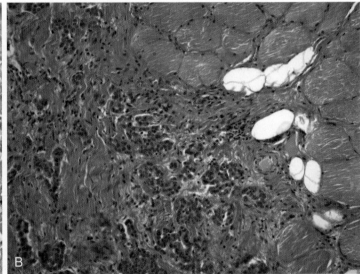

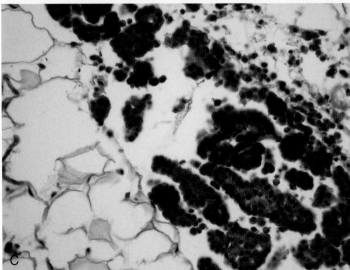

FIGURE 6.11 **(A)** Epithelioid mesothelioma (hematoxylin and eosin [H&E], 400×). **(B)** Epithelioid malignant mesothelioma with a tubular, infiltrative growth pattern. Tumor cells with a tubular pattern and invasion into the skeletal muscle (H&E, 400×). **(C)** Epithelioid mesothelioma with a tubulopapillary pattern invading the adipose tissue (H&E, 400×).

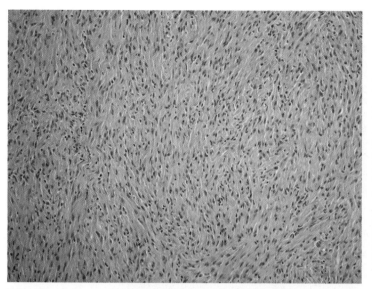

FIGURE 6.12 Sarcomatoid mesothelioma composed of spindle-shaped cells arranged in sheets or fascicles that form nonspecific architectural patterns that resemble those seen in various sarcomas (H&E, 400×).

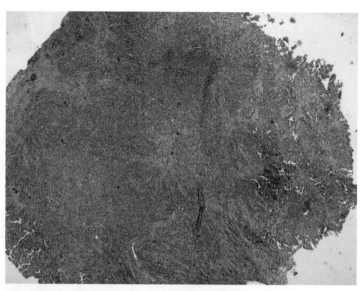

FIGURE 6.13 **BIPHASIC MESOTHELIOMA.** Low-power view of a biphasic mesothelioma containing components of both epithelioid and sarcomatoid mesothelioma.

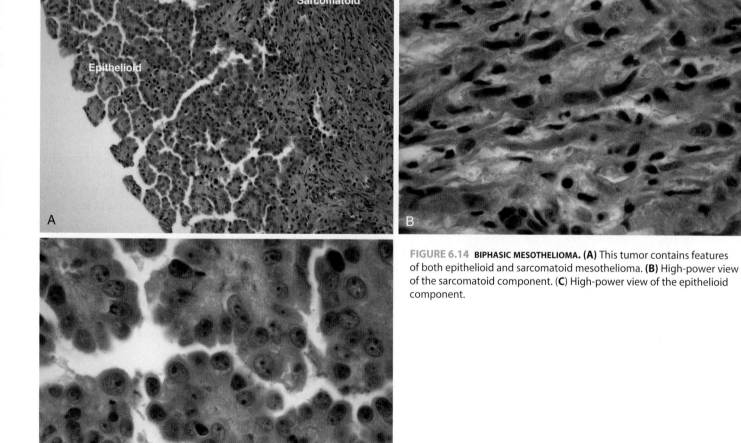

FIGURE 6.14 **BIPHASIC MESOTHELIOMA. (A)** This tumor contains features of both epithelioid and sarcomatoid mesothelioma. **(B)** High-power view of the sarcomatoid component. **(C)** High-power view of the epithelioid component.

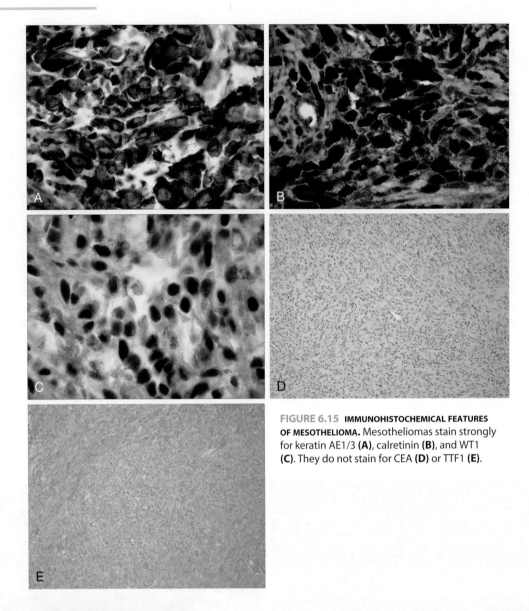

FIGURE 6.15 **IMMUNOHISTOCHEMICAL FEATURES OF MESOTHELIOMA.** Mesotheliomas stain strongly for keratin AE1/3 **(A)**, calretinin **(B)**, and WT1 **(C)**. They do not stain for CEA **(D)** or TTF1 **(E)**.

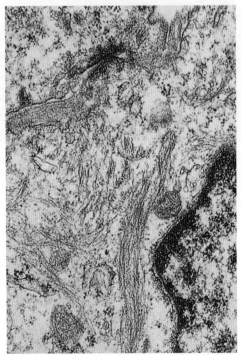

FIGURE 6.16 Electron microscopy reveals the cells of epithelial variant to be polygonal with numerous long, slender, branching surface microvilli, abundant tonofilaments, desmosomes, and intracellular lumen formation. In contrast, adenocarcinomas have short, stubby surface microvilli, fewer tonofilaments, and microvillous rootlets or lamellar bodies.

Staging

Whereas multiple staging systems have been described for pleural mesothelioma, there is no staging system for peritoneal mesothelioma. The goal of staging is to stratify prognosis and to identify patients who are potential candidates for surgery. The most commonly and widely accepted staging system is the International Mesothelioma Interest Group system, which is a modified tumor-node-metastases (TNM) staging system (Rusch et al., 1995). Mesothelioma is a difficult disease to stage accurately on the basis of radiographic imaging, and often staging is only possible at the time of surgery. Some staging systems, such as the Brigham and Women's Hospital staging system, are based solely on findings at the time of surgery (Sugarbaker et al., 1993).

Prognostic Factors

There is no known curative modality for mesothelioma. The median survival of newly diagnosed patients ranges from 6 to 18 months. The disease course (even untreated) can be highly variable, and thus several prognostic systems have been developed to identify patient subsets with different prognoses.

The two main prognostic systems are the Cancer and Leukemia Group B prognostic groups and the European Organization for Research and Treatment of Cancer prognostic factors and prognostic scores (Curran et al., 1998; Herndon et al., 1998). Patients with sarcomatoid mesothelioma, those with a poor performance status, and those who present with chest pain (indicative of disease invasion into the chest wall) are ones with a poor prognosis. In addition, patients with evidence of a systemic inflammatory response to their mesothelioma, manifested by either an increased white blood cell count or platelet count also tend to have a poorer prognosis.

Treatment

There is no standard therapeutic approach for malignant mesothelioma. One of the limitations in this disease is the lack of randomized clinical trials comparing different treatment modalities. Treatment approaches to mesothelioma vary significantly and range from palliative care to chemotherapy to aggressive surgical approaches based on the patient's age, co-morbid medical conditions, and performance status.

Surgery

Surgery is a therapeutic option for some patients with malignant mesothelioma. One of the rationales for performing surgery is that mesothelioma is a disease that tends to spread locally into adjacent structures such as the chest wall and the mediastinum before spreading to systemic sites. Thus, local treatments such as surgery may offer therapeutic and palliative benefits to patients. Two main surgical approaches, an extrapleural pneumonectomy (EPP) and a pleurectomy/decortication (P/D), have been used to treat mesothelioma (Sugarbaker et al., 1999). An EPP is an en bloc resection of the parietal pleura, lung, pericardium, and diaphragm (Sugarbaker et al., 2004). The diaphragm and pericardium are then reconstructed with the use of a Gor-Tex patch. In contrast, a P/D is a resection of the parietal and mediastinal pleura and involved visceral and diaphragmatic pleura and pericardium. The lung, however, remains in place. There have been no randomized studies comparing the two different surgical approaches. The patients most likely to benefit from an EPP are those with epithelial histology mesothelioma with negative resection margins in whom there is no N2 lymph node involvement (Sugarbaker et al., 1999). In general, patients who are eligible for this operation are younger with appropriate cardiopulmonary reserve. Patients who undergo a P/D are often older with other co-morbid medical illnesses. In addition, patients with minimal pleural disease and those whose tumors do not extend into the interlobular pleural surfaces may be more appropriate candidates for a P/D operation.

Chemotherapy

Until recently mesothelioma was considered a disease refractory to systemic chemotherapy. In fact, most if not all chemotherapy agents have been tested in clinical trials for patients with mesothelioma (Jänne, 2003). The agents with the most consistent single-agent antitumor activity include antifolates, platinum agents (cisplatin and carboplatin), vinorelbine, and gemcitabine. The largest (and only adequately powered) phase III clinical trial in mesothelioma compared the combination of cisplatin and pemetrexed to cisplatin alone as initial treatment for patients with malignant mesothelioma. This study demonstrated a response rate of 41% and a median survival rate of 12.1 months for the combination arm, which were significantly better than rates in the cisplatin-alone arm (16.7% and 9.3 months, respectively) (Vogelzang et al., 2003). This trial was the basis for the U.S. Food and Drug Administration's approval of cisplatin/pemetrexed in malignant mesothelioma and helped establish this combination as one standard treatment approach for mesothelioma patients. There are virtually no data on second-line treatments of mesothelioma, and this remains an active area of clinical investigation.

Irradiation

Irradiation has a limited therapeutic role for most patients with mesothelioma. Irradiation is often used either in the palliative setting or to decrease the likelihood of tumor invasion into surgical or biopsy sites. In addition, for patients who undergo an EPP, irradiation is used in the postoperative treatment of the hemithorax (Yajnik et al., 2003). Because the surgical margins following EPP are often involved with mesothelioma (or in very close proximity), radiation therapy provides an opportunity to decrease local recurrence. Patients treated with early-stage mesothelioma and hemithorax irradiation have a low chance of recurrence within the operated thoracic cavity but a much greater chance of systemic recurrence. Many such patients are often treated with the combination of surgery, chemotherapy, and radiation therapy.

References and Suggested Readings

Amin KM, Litzky LA, Smythe WR, et al: Wilms' tumor 1 susceptibility (WT1) gene products are selectively expressed in malignant mesothelioma, *Am J Pathol* 146:344–356, 1995.

Curran D, Sahmoud T, Therasse P, et al: Prognostic factors in patients with pleural mesothelioma: the European Organization for Research and Treatment of Cancer experience, *J Clin Oncol* 16:145–152, 1998.

De Luca A, Baldi A, Esposito V, et al: The retinoblastoma gene family pRb/p105, p107, pRb2/p130 and simian virus-40 large T-antigen in human mesotheliomas, *Nat Med* 3:913–916, 1997.

Fasola G, Belvedere O, Aita M, et al: Low-dose computer tomography screening for lung cancer and pleural mesothelioma in an asbestos-exposed population: baseline results of a prospective, nonrandomized feasibility trial—an Alpe-Adria Thoracic Oncology Multidisciplinary Group Study (ATOM 002), *Oncologist* 12:1215–1224, 2007.

Flores RM, Akhurst T, Gonen M, et al: Positron emission tomography defines metastatic disease but not locoregional disease in patients with malignant pleural mesothelioma, *J Thorac Cardiovasc Surg* 126:11–16, 2003.

Gaissert HA, Piyavisetpat N, Mark EJ: Case 14-2009: A 36-year-old man with chest pain, dysphagia, and pleural and mediastinal calcifications, *N Engl J Med* 360:1886–1895, 2009.

Herndon JE, Green MR, Chahinian AP, et al: Factors predictive of survival among 337 patients with mesothelioma treated between 1984 and 1994 by the Cancer and Leukemia Group B, *Chest* 113:723–731, 1998.

Hodgson JT, Darnton A: The quantitative risks of mesothelioma and lung cancer in relation to asbestos exposure, *Ann Occup Hyg* 44:565–601, 2000.

Jänne PA: Chemotherapy for malignant pleural mesothelioma, *Clin Lung Cancer* 5:98–106, 2003.

Lopez-Rios F, Illei PB, Rusch V, et al: Evidence against a role for SV40 infection in human mesotheliomas and high risk of false-positive PCR results owing to presence of SV40 sequences in common laboratory plasmids, *Lancet* 364:1157–1166, 2004.

Miller A: Mesothelioma in household members of asbestos-exposed workers: 32 United States cases since 1990, *Am J Ind Med* 47:458–462, 2005.

Ordonez NG: Value of calretinin immunostaining in differentiating epithelial mesothelioma from lung adenocarcinoma, *Mod Pathol* 11:929–933, 1998.

Pass HI, Lott D, Lonardo F, et al: Asbestos exposure, pleural mesothelioma, and serum osteopontin levels, *N Engl J Med* 353:1564–1573, 2005.

Roberts HC, Patsios DA, Paul NS, et al: Screening for malignant pleural mesothelioma and lung cancer in individuals with a history of asbestos exposure, *J Thorac Oncol* 4:620–628, 2009.

Robinson BW, Creaney J, Lake R, et al: Mesothelin-family proteins and diagnosis of mesothelioma, *Lancet* 362:1612–1616, 2003.

Roushdy-Hammady I, Siegel J, Emri S, et al: Genetic-susceptibility factor and malignant mesothelioma in the Cappadocian region of Turkey, *Lancet* 357:444–445, 2001.

Rusch VW: A proposed new international TNM staging system for malignant pleural mesothelioma. From the International Mesothelioma Interest Group, *Chest* 108:1122–1128, 1995.

Strickler HD, Goedert JJ, Devesa SS, et al: Trends in U.S. pleural mesothelioma incidence rates following simian virus 40 contamination of early poliovirus vaccines, *J Natl Cancer Inst* 95:38–45, 2003.

Sugarbaker DJ, Flores RM, Jaklitsch MT, et al: Resection margins, extrapleural nodal status, and cell type determine postoperative long-term survival in trimodality therapy of malignant pleural mesothelioma: results in 183 patients, *J Thorac Cardiovasc Surg* 117:54–65, 1999.

Sugarbaker DJ, Jaklitsch MT, Bueno R, et al: Prevention, early detection, and management of complications after 328 consecutive extrapleural pneumonectomies, *J Thorac Cardiovasc Surg* 128:138–146, 2004.

Sugarbaker DJ, Strauss GM, Lynch TJ, et al: Node status has prognostic significance in the multimodality therapy of diffuse, malignant mesothelioma, *J Clin Oncol* 11:1172–1178, 1993.

Vogelzang NJ, Rusthoven JJ, Symanowski J, et al: Phase III study of pemetrexed in combination with cisplatin versus cisplatin alone in patients with malignant pleural mesothelioma, *J Clin Oncol* 21:2636–2644, 2003.

Weissmann LB, Corson JM, Neugut AI, et al: Malignant mesothelioma following treatment for Hodgkin's disease, *J Clin Oncol* 14:2098–2100, 1996.

Yajnik S, Rosenzweig KE, Mychalczak B, et al: Hemithoracic radiation after extrapleural pneumonectomy for malignant pleural mesothelioma, *Int J Radiat Oncol Biol Phys* 56:1319–1326, 2003.

Cancer of the Gastrointestinal Tract and Neuroendocrine Tumors

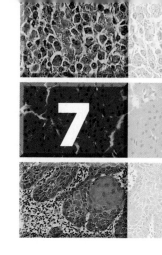

7

JEFFREY A. MEYERHARDT • MATTHEW H. KULKE • JERROLD R. TURNER

Esophageal Cancers

The prevalence of esophageal cancer varies over 20-fold throughout the world. Esophageal cancer is most common in central Asia and remains relatively rare in the United States. Approximately 14,000 new cases of esophageal cancer occur annually in the United States, where 75% of esophageal cancers develop in men and only 25% in women.

HISTOLOGY OF ESOPHAGEAL CANCER

Worldwide, 90% of esophageal cancers are squamous cell carcinomas. The risk of esophageal squamous cell carcinoma is related closely to excessive alcohol consumption and chronic cigarette smoking. The squamous cell carcinomas, including spindle cell and verrucous variants, are most prevalent in the upper esophagus. Interestingly, in the past two decades the relative incidence of squamous cell carcinoma and adenocarcinoma of the esophagus has shifted markedly in both the United States and Europe. In these regions squamous cell carcinoma has become somewhat less common, whereas the incidence of esophageal adenocarcinoma has increased to a considerable degree. In Caucasian males in the United States, for example, the incidence of adenocarcinoma now exceeds the incidence of squamous cell carcinoma. Adenocarcinomas of the esophagus generally occur in the distal third of the esophagus and are particularly common at the gastroesophageal junction. The risk of esophageal adenocarcinoma has been closely linked to the presence of chronic gastroesophageal reflux and Barrett's esophagus.

In addition to tobacco and alcohol, other risk factors for squamous cell esophageal cancer include achalasia, history of cancer treated with radiation therapy in the mid- to upper chest region (e.g., breast cancer), tylosis, caustic injury to the esophagus, and Plummer-Vinson syndrome. In contrast, risk factors for the development of adenocarcinoma of the esophagus include gastroesophageal reflux disease, Barrett's esophagus, obesity, prior radiation exposure to the mid- to upper chest, and smoking. Rare undifferentiated small cell carcinomas occur in the lower and middle esophagus. Risk factors for these unusual lesions have not been established. These highly malignant tumors behave like small cell lung cancers, occasionally producing paraneoplastic syndromes.

STAGING OF ESOPHAGEAL CANCERS

The unique structure of the esophagus is significant to the biologic understanding and clinical management of malignant disease. There is a rich lymphatic drainage throughout the length of the esophagus and a discontinuous serosa. Therefore, "skip areas" of micrometastases occur that necessitate wide surgical resection of operable tumors. Lymph node drainage varies within the esophagus (cervical vs thoracic). Nodal metastases frequently develop in mediastinal, para-aortic, and celiac lymph nodes.

In the TNM staging system (tumor, node, metastasis) commonly used for esophageal carcinoma, stages I and II represent operable disease, stage III denotes marginally resectable disease, and stage IV signifies inoperable cancer. The last stage is characterized by metastases (M1). About 15% of cancers originate in the upper third of the esophagus (cervical and upper thoracic esophagus), 50% in the middle third, and 35% in the lower third. The site of the primary tumor is critically important, because it relates to clinical behavior (adjacent organ involvement, nodal metastases) and technical resectability. Primary surgical resection is possible in about 40% to 50% of cases. About one third of patients are candidates for palliative surgery, and 20% to 30% present with unresectable stage III or IV disease. The 5-year survival rate is less than 5% for stage IV disease but is about 70% for stage I cancers.

Staging procedures involve triple endoscopy, including detailed ear-nose-throat examination as well as bronchoscopy and esophagoscopy, because there is a high potential for development of other aerodigestive cancers because of similar risk factors. Mediastinoscopy, laparoscopy, and computed tomography (CT) scans of the chest, liver, and upper abdomen are important to determine the presence of nodal or visceral metastases. Endoscopic ultrasound is helpful to determine the extent of invasion through the esophageal wall and involvement of regional lymph nodes. Positron emission tomography (PET) scanning has been shown to be highly sensitive in detecting occult metastases from esophageal cancer and is being increasingly used as a staging procedure.

CLINICAL MANIFESTATIONS

About 90% of patients present with dysphagia and weight loss, often accompanied by pain on swallowing (odynophagia). These symptoms characteristically appear with advanced disease, because difficulty in swallowing arises when at least

60% of the esophageal circumference is infiltrated by cancer. Other symptoms include regurgitation or emesis and discomfort in the throat, substernal area, or epigastrium. In advanced disease, local invasion of the trachea, bronchi, lung, or even aorta may result in aspiration pneumonia, massive hemorrhage, pleural effusion, or superior vena cava syndrome. Moreover, the development of one or more tracheo- or bronchoesophageal fistulae may also occur, as well as esophageal perforation and mediastinitis. Occasionally patients present with supraclavicular lymph node, bone, or liver metastases.

TREATMENT CONSIDERATIONS

Treatment of esophageal cancers is dependent on the stage of disease as well as whether the health of the patient allows him or her to undergo surgery. For patients with resectable cancers, options would include surgery alone, combined-modality chemotherapy and radiation therapy followed by surgery, or chemoradiation alone. Despite lack of definitive data supporting this approach, for tumors with at least moderate invasion into the esophageal wall and/or regional lymph node involvement, most patients in the United States are treated with chemoradiation followed by surgery. For patients not deemed operative candidates, who refuse surgery, or who have nonresectable disease but lack distant metastases, combined-modality chemotherapy and radiation therapy is the treatment of choice and can lead to a cure in select patients. Finally, patients with metastatic disease should be considered for palliative therapies, including chemotherapy, radiation therapy, and/or esophageal stenting.

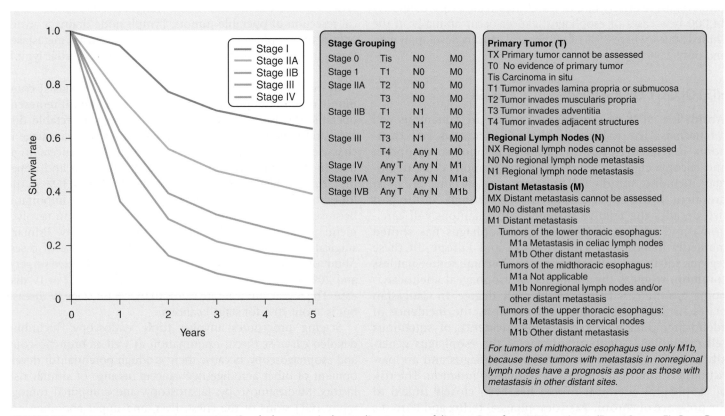

FIGURE 7.1 STAGING OF ESOPHAGEAL CARCINOMA. Graph shows survival according to stage of disease. Data from 5071 patients. (From Greene FL, Page D, Fleming I, et al, editors, for the American Joint Committee on Cancer: *AJCC cancer staging handbook*, ed 6, New York, 2002, Springer.)

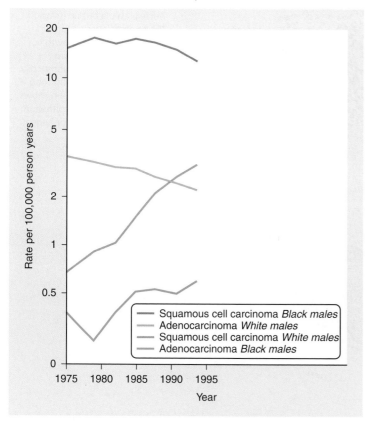

FIGURE 7.2 Trends in age-adjusted incidence rates for esophageal carcinoma among U.S. males by race and cell type, 1974–1976 to 1992–1994. (From Devesa SS, Blot WJ, Fraumeni J: Changing patterns in the incidence of esophageal and gastric carcinoma in the United States, *Cancer* 83(10): 2049–2063, 1998.)

FIGURE 7.3 **SQUAMOUS CELL CARCINOMA**. Endoscopic view of the esophagus shows a tiny, early ulcer that proved on biopsy to be malignant.

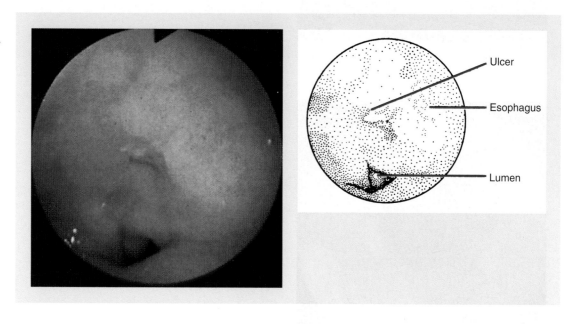

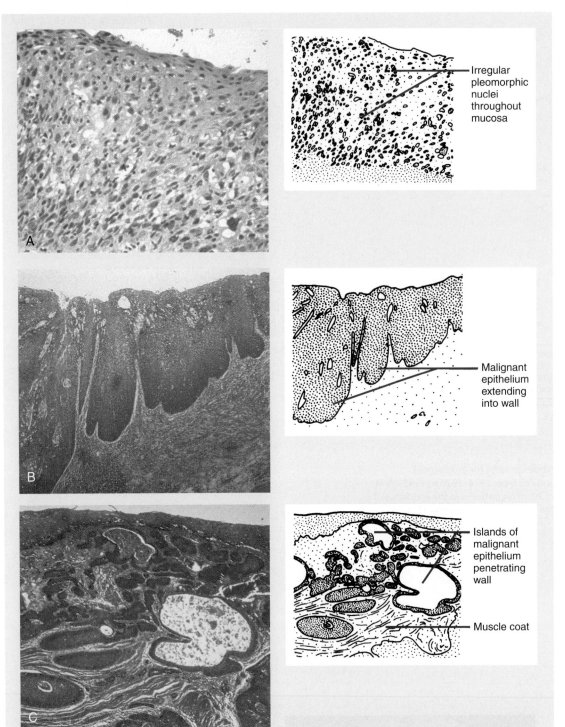

FIGURE 7.4 **SQUAMOUS CELL CARCINOMA.** **(A)** An esophageal lesion in situ shows full-thickness nuclear atypia but no invasion. **(B)** An early invasive tumor is marked by downgrowth of malignant epithelium encroaching on the submucosa. **(C)** An established, infiltrating, well-differentiated lesion shows islands of malignant epithelium invading deep into esophageal muscle.

Irregular pleomorphic nuclei throughout mucosa

Malignant epithelium extending into wall

Islands of malignant epithelium penetrating wall

Muscle coat

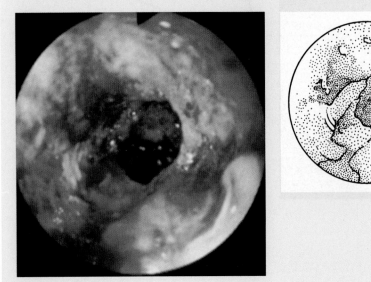
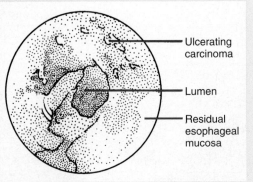

FIGURE 7.5 **SQUAMOUS CELL CARCINOMA.** Endoscopic view shows circumferential involvement of the esophagus with friable tumor. Note the narrowed lumen.

Ulcerating carcinoma

Lumen

Residual esophageal mucosa

FIGURE 7.6 SQUAMOUS CELL CARCINOMA. Endoscopy shows a tracheoesophageal fistula caused by an ulcerating esophageal squamous cancer. The orifice of the fistula tract is clearly visible.

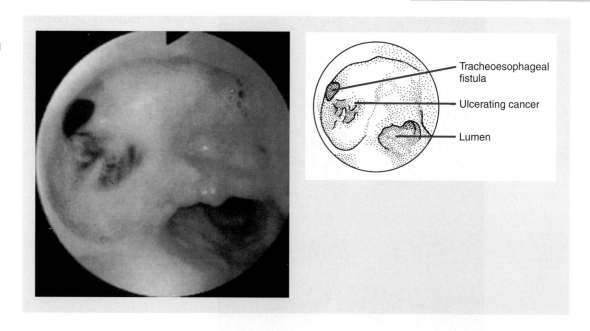

Tracheoesophageal fistula

Ulcerating cancer

Lumen

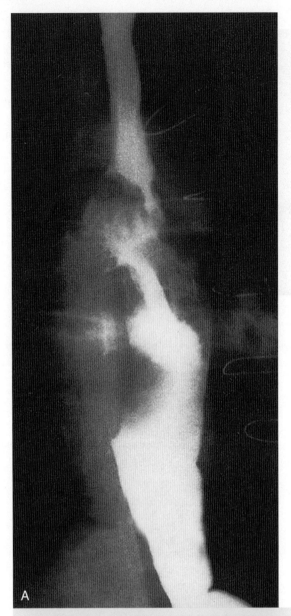

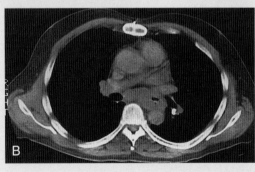

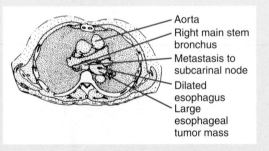

FIGURE 7.7 SQUAMOUS CELL CARCINOMA. A 62-year-old man with progressive dysphagia and marked weight loss was found on endoscopy to have a poorly differentiated tumor of the middle third of the esophagus. **(A)** Barium swallow film shows narrowing of the esophagus with mucosal destruction, consistent with esophageal cancer. **(B)** CT scan reveals regional metastases and a large primary mass obstructing the esophagus. Complete clinical remission was achieved in 3 months after combination chemotherapy plus radiation therapy. Unfortunately, liver metastases subsequently occurred.

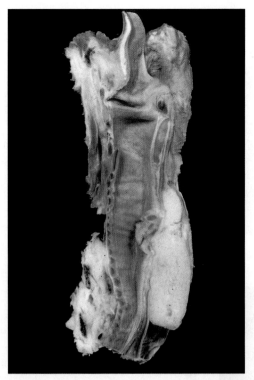

FIGURE 7.8 **SQUAMOUS CELL CARCINOMA.** This sagittal section through the larynx, trachea, and anterior wall of the esophagus (on the right) was obtained at autopsy of a 57-year-old man who presented with a short history of dysphagia. A barium swallow revealed neoplastic obstruction of the esophagus; the patient died soon afterward from bronchopneumonia. A solid, raised, pale tumor (6 × 2 × 2 cm), arising in the esophagus, has infiltrated the posterior wall of the trachea, forming a nodular projection into the tracheal lumen. Anthracotic paratracheal lymph nodes are extensively infiltrated by pale tumor. This case clearly demonstrates the spread of esophageal carcinoma.

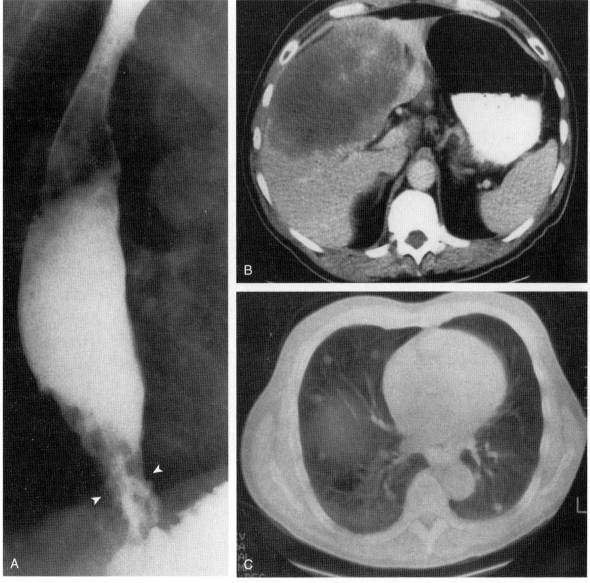

FIGURE 7.9 **ADENOCARCINOMA.** Weight loss and right upper abdominal pain, with minimal dysphagia, developed in a 58-year-old man. Esophagoscopy showed a constricting, poorly differentiated lesion of the lower third of the esophagus. **(A)** Barium swallow film defines the extent of the lesion (*arrowheads*). On CT scan, **(B)** a large liver metastasis and **(C)** early pulmonary metastases are noted.

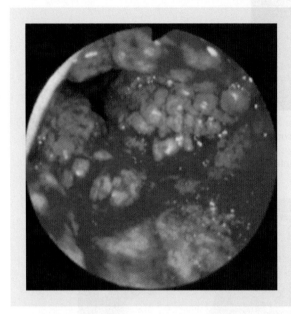

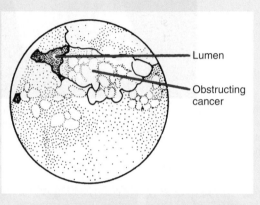

FIGURE 7.10 ADENOCARCINOMA. This ulcerating tumor arose at the gastroesophageal junction where, as in this case, it is often impossible to distinguish an esophageal carcinoma from one arising in the gastric fundus and growing upward to involve the distal esophagus.

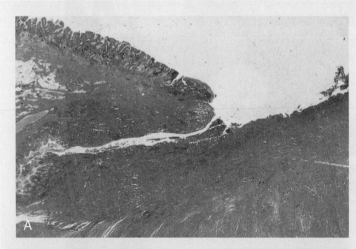

FIGURE 7.11 ADENOCARCINOMA IN BARRETT'S METAPLASIA. Endoscopic view demonstrates an extensive lesion arising in an area of Barrett's metaplasia; the lumen is obstructed by a bleeding and polypoid exophytic mass.

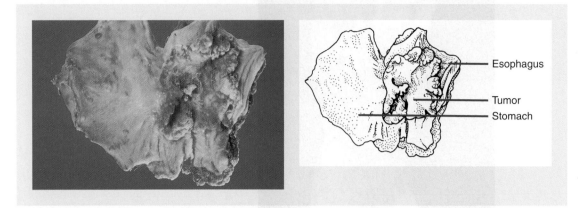

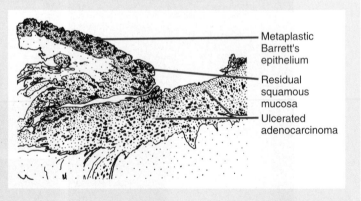

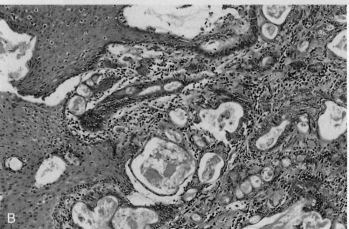

FIGURE 7.12 ADENOCARCINOMA IN BARRETT'S METAPLASIA. (A) Low-power photomicrograph shows esophageal tissue with metaplastic Barrett's epithelium, with columnar cells and villous changes. There is some residual esophageal squamous mucosa adjacent to an area of ulcerated adenocarcinoma. **(B)** High-power view shows glands of tumor encroaching on the squamous epithelium.

Gastric Cancers

There is a marked variation in the incidence of gastric cancer worldwide. Death rates are highest in Costa Rica and Japan, about 10-fold greater than those in the United States. Nonetheless, both the incidence and the mortality rate of gastric cancer have decreased worldwide over the past 50 years. In 1930 gastric cancer was the leading cause of cancer-related deaths in men, with a rate of 37 per 100,000 in the United States, as compared with the current U.S. rate of less than 6 per 100,000. The incidence of gastric cancer increases after age 50 and is highest in lower socioeconomic groups. The male-to-female ratio of 3:2 is less than observed in esophageal cancer.

Many etiologic influences have been proposed to explain the decreasing incidence of gastric cancer, mostly concerning dietary and environmental factors and the increased availability of refrigeration, which reduces the growth of nitrate-producing bacteria in food. Another factor, loss of gastric acidity, may predispose to stomach cancer. This condition can be caused by partial gastrectomy, atrophic gastritis, or achlorhydria with subsequent pernicious anemia. Chronic gastritis is frequently associated with gastric cancer, and the presence of intestinal metaplasia further elevates the risk of gastric cancer. Recent studies suggest that infection with *Helicobacter pylori* is associated with gastric cancer, leading some to postulate a pathogenic role. Other premalignant lesions include adenomas, 40% of which may progress to carcinoma. Hereditary diffuse gastric cancer is associated with mutations in the E-cadherin gene.

HISTOLOGY

About 90% of gastric malignancies are adenocarcinomas, with the remainder comprising malignant gastrointestinal (GI) stromal tumors (GISTs; leiomyosarcomas) and lymphomas. Histologically, adenocarcinomas are classified as intestinal or diffuse. Intestinal-type cancers are characterized by cohesive neoplastic cells that form glandlike tubular structures resembling colonic adenocarcinomas. They are often preceded by premalignant changes (chronic atrophic gastritis and intestinal metaplasia) and may result in ulcerative lesions, particularly in the antrum or the lesser curvature. Diffuse-type cancers are composed of infiltrating gastric mucous or "signet-ring" cells that infrequently form masses or ulcers. They tend to occur throughout the stomach, often resulting in a linitis plastica ("leather bottle") appearance. Much of the decline in gastric cancer rates has been due to decreases in the intestinal type. Consequently, the diffuse-type adenocarcinomas have become relatively more common, accounting for up to one third of cases. Diffuse-type malignancies are associated with a very poor prognosis, with a survival rate of less than 2%. Much of the pale "tumor" tissue in this variant actually represents fibrosis of the submucosa and muscle.

Macroscopically, gastric cancers are classified into five categories. The ulcerative variant (25% of cases) may resemble a benign gastric ulcer. About 7% and 36% are polypoid and fungating tumors, respectively, and are nodular tumors that can reach a large size. The remaining 26% of gastric cancers show a scirrhous pattern caused by thickening and rigidity of the gastric wall due to diffuse infiltration by signet-ring cells. The marked fibrous reaction results in the appearance of linitis plastica. The least common gross appearance is the superficial type, representing less than 6% of cases. The normal mucosa is replaced by sheet-like collections of malignant cells that do not invade beyond the submucosa. This type is categorized as early gastric cancer and represents potentially resectable (for cure) cancers.

STAGING OF GASTRIC CANCERS

A TNM staging system is used for gastric cancers. Prognosis is dependent both on stage of disease and location within the stomach. Proximal tumors (within the cardia and fundus) have a worse prognosis than distal tumors (antrum and pylorus). The 5-year survival rate is 45% to 80% for the uncommon cases that are detected in stage I of the disease, 25% to 40% for stage II, less than 20% for stage III, and 5% for stage IV.

Extensive local invasion by gastric cancer is common and most often involves the pancreas, omentum, transverse colon, liver, or spleen; direct contiguous spread into the esophagus or duodenum is also common. Moreover, because gastric cancer so often penetrates the serosa, it is particularly prone to transperitoneal dissemination. Spread also occurs via lymphatics and blood vessels. Gastric cancer can lead to drop metastases to the large and small bowel, pelvic floor, and ovary. Staging studies include endoscopy with or without endoscopic ultrasound, chest imaging; CT scans of liver, abdomen, and pelvis should be obtained.

CLINICAL MANIFESTATIONS

Because early gastric cancer is asymptomatic, many patients present with advanced disease. Symptoms include ulcer-related pain, anorexia, weight loss, and vague epigastric distress. Development of left supraclavicular adenopathy (Virchow's node), an ovarian mass (Krukenberg tumor), hepatomegaly, ascites, or anemia may be the initial manifestation. Gastric carcinoma is also a well-recognized cause of secondary pyloric stenosis in adulthood.

TREATMENT CONSIDERATIONS

Up to 50% of patients diagnosed with gastric cancer are considered inoperable, and treatment should be directed toward palliation. Options for palliation include best supportive care only, systemic chemotherapy, radiation therapy (usually limited to control bleeding and obstructive systems), and endoscopic stenting. For patients with resectable disease, growing evidence supports the role of either postoperative adjuvant therapy (with combination of chemotherapy and chemoradiotherapy) or neoadjuvant chemotherapy followed by surgery followed by further adjuvant chemotherapy.

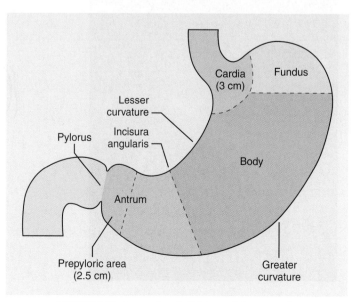

FIGURE 7.13 Anatomic subdivisions of the stomach.

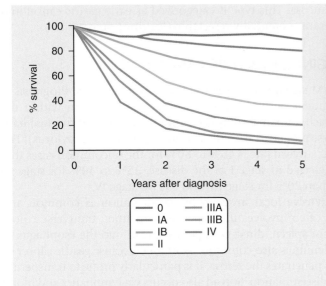

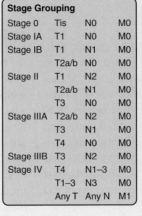

Stage Grouping			
Stage 0	Tis	N0	M0
Stage IA	T1	N0	M0
Stage IB	T1	N1	M0
	T2a/b	N0	M0
Stage II	T1	N2	M0
	T2a/b	N1	M0
	T3	N0	M0
Stage IIIA	T2a/b	N2	M0
	T3	N1	M0
	T4	N0	M0
Stage IIIB	T3	N2	M0
Stage IV	T4	N1–3	M0
	T1–3	N3	M0
	Any T	Any N	M1

Definition of TNM

Primary Tumor (T)
TX Primary tumor cannot be assessed
T0 No evidence of primary tumor
Tis Carcinoma in situ: intra-epithelial tumor
      without invasion of the lamina propria
T1 Tumor invades lamina propria or submucosa
T2 Tumor invades muscularis propria or subserosa*
T2a Tumor invades muscularis propria
T2b Tumor invades subserosa
T3 Tumor penetrates serosa (visceral peritoneum)
      without invasion of adjacent structures[+,‡]
T4 Tumor invades adjacent structures[+,‡]

*Note: A tumor may penetrate the muscularis propria
with extension into the gastrocolic or gastrohepatic
ligaments, or into the greater or lesser omentum
without perforation of the visceral peritoneum
covering these structures. In this case the tumor is
classified T2. If there is perforation of the visceral
peritoneum covering the gastric ligaments or the
omentum, the tumor should be classified T3.
[+]Note: The adjacent structures of the stomach
include the spleen, transverse colon, liver, diaphragm,
pancreas, abdominal wall, adrenal gland, kidney,
small intestine, and retroperitoneum.
[‡]Note: Intramural extension to the duodenum or
esophagus is classified by the depth of greatest
invasion in any of these sites, including the stomach.

Regional Lymph Nodes (N)
NX Regional lymph node(s) cannot be assessed
N0 No regional lymph node metastasis
N1 Metastasis in 1 to 6 regional lymph nodes
N2 Metastasis in 7 to 15 regional lymph nodes
N3 Metastasis in more than 15 regional
      lymph nodes

Distant Metastasis (M)
MX Distant metastasis cannot be assessed
M0 No distant metastasis
M1 Distant metastasis

FIGURE 7.14 STAGING OF GASTRIC CARCINOMA. Graph of disease-specific survival data taken from the Commission on Cancer Patient Care Evaluation Study (Wanebo HJ, Kennedy BJ, Chmiel J, et al: Cancer of the stomach: a patient care study by the American College of Surgeons, *Ann Surg* 218:583–592, 1993). (From Greene FL, Page D, Fleming I, et al, editors, for the American Joint Committee on Cancer: *AJCC cancer staging handbook*, ed 6, New York, 2002, Springer.)

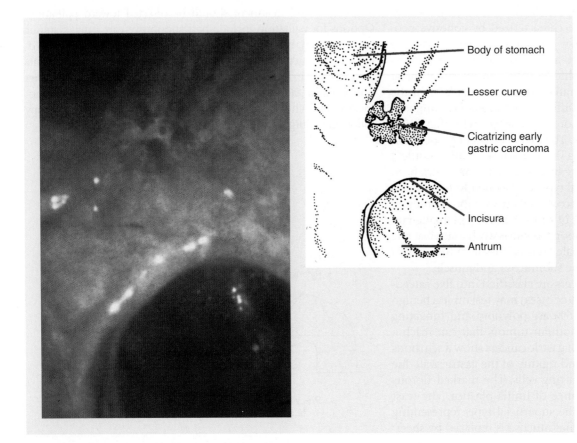

FIGURE 7.15 EARLY ADENOCARCINOMA. Endoscopic view shows an early gastric lesion arising between the lesser curvature and antrum. Note the irregular area of elevation and scarring.

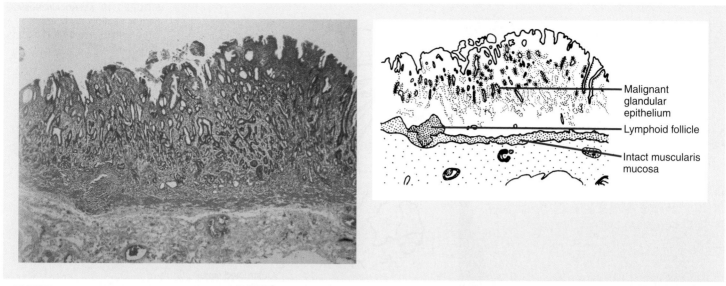

FIGURE 7.16 **EARLY ADENOCARCINOMA.** An intestinal-type lesion extends throughout the mucosa and submucosa but not through the muscularis mucosa.

FIGURE 7.17 **ADENOCARCINOMA.** Endoscopic view shows a lesion extending from the cardia into the distal esophagus.

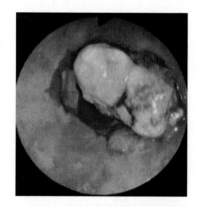

Table 7.1	
Distribution of Malignancies among Subdivisions of the Stomach	
Subdivision	**Frequency (%)**
Antrum and prepylorus	≥50
Cardia and fundus	−25
Lesser curvature	20
Greater curvature	3–5
Entire stomach	5–10

*Approximately 2% of patients may have cancers in multiple sites.

FIGURE 7.18 **ADENOCARCINOMA.** Infiltrating glands of tumor extend upward from the stomach underneath the esophageal squamous lining.

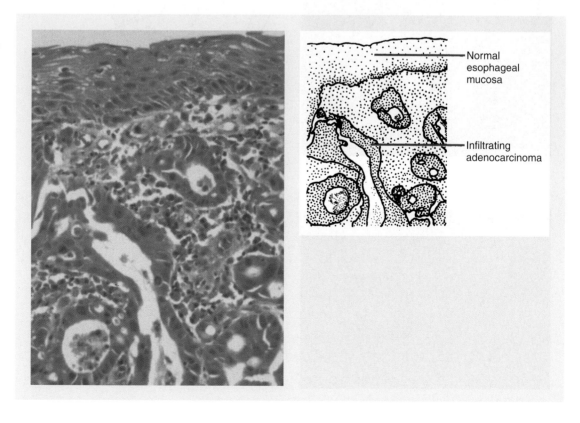

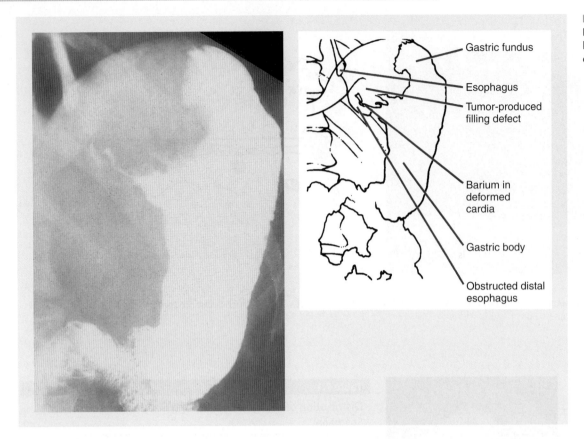

FIGURE 7.19 ADENOCARCINOMA. Barium swallow study shows a large fundal carcinoma. (Courtesy of H. Shawdon.)

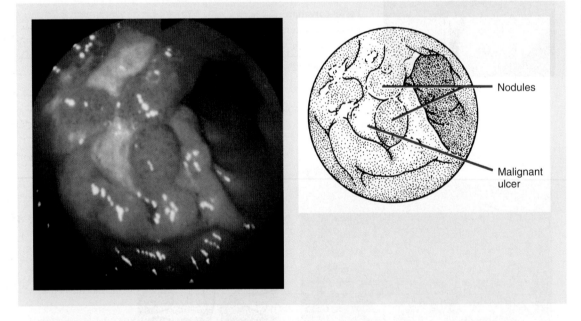

FIGURE 7.20 MALIGNANT GASTRIC ULCER. This antral lesion shows heaped-up nodular margins, particularly suggestive of malignancy.

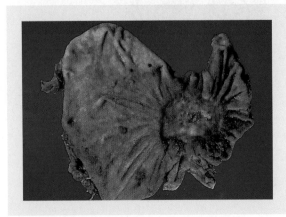

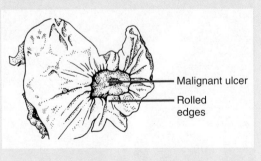

FIGURE 7.21 MALIGNANT GASTRIC ULCER. Partial gastrectomy specimen shows a large malignant ulcer of the lesser curvature, with raised, rolled margins.

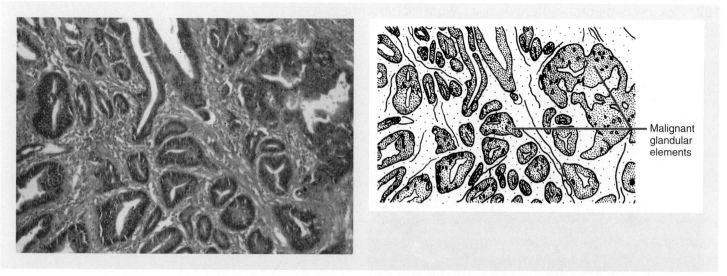

FIGURE 7.22 ADENOCARCINOMA. This intestinal-type tumor shows well-formed malignant glandular elements.

Malignant glandular elements

FIGURE 7.23 ADENOCARCINOMA (POLYPOID TYPE). Barium swallow study reveals a large polypoid lesion in the body of the stomach, causing a filling defect.

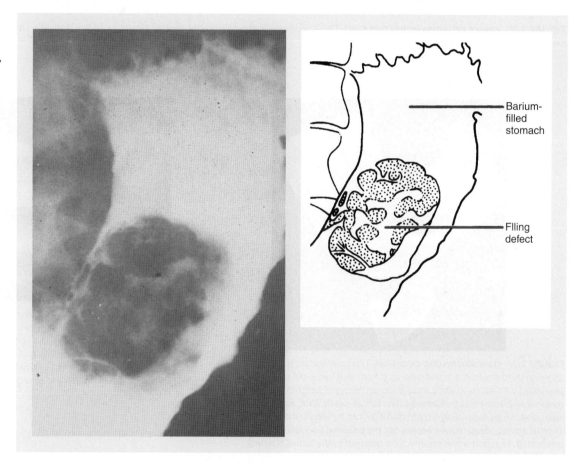

Barium-filled stomach

Flling defect

FIGURE 7.24 ADENOCARCINOMA (FUNGATING TYPE). Endoscopic view reveals a hemorrhagic tumor near the lesser curvature, with ulceration and necrosis.

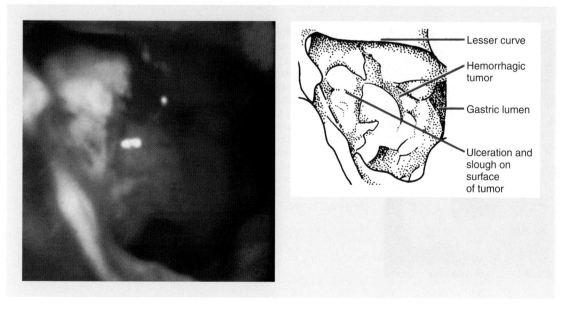

Lesser curve

Hemorrhagic tumor

Gastric lumen

Ulceration and slough on surface of tumor

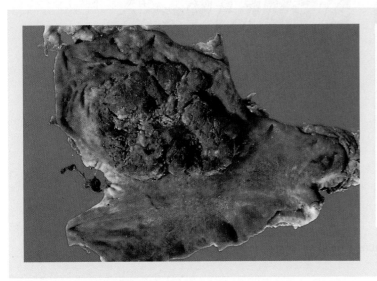
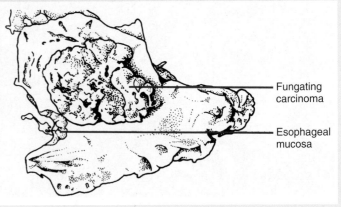

FIGURE 7.25 ADENOCARCINOMA (FUNGATING TYPE). This specimen, opened along the greater curvature of the stomach, shows a large, fungating tumor occupying the lesser curvature.

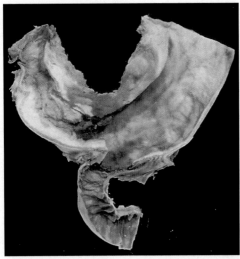

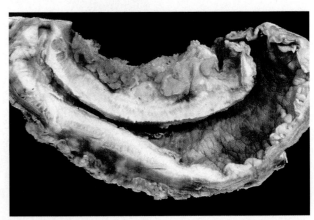

FIGURE 7.28 DIFFUSE ADENOCARCINOMA (LINITIS PLASTICA). This gastrectomy specimen, opened anteriorly, is from a 64-year-old man who had a 3-year history of dyspepsia. Barium swallow and endoscopy revealed a gastric carcinoma. There is diffuse infiltration of the pylorus and body of the stomach by pale tumor, as well as marked luminal narrowing, although the tumor has no exophytic component. Note the irregular infiltration of the muscle coat.

FIGURE 7.26 STENOSING PYLORIC CARCINOMA. This postmortem specimen, showing the distal stomach and pylorus, is from an 84-year-old woman who presented with severe anemia and a 3-month history of weight loss. Palliative gastroenterostomy was performed 4 days before death. A localized, nodular, stenosing tumor, measuring 6 cm in diameter, can be seen in the pyloric canal. There is obvious deep mural invasion, but the proximal duodenum is completely unaffected. The gastroenterostomy, 2 cm proximal to the tumor, is patent.

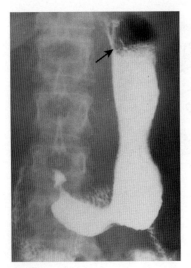

FIGURE 7.27 DIFFUSE ADENOCARCINOMA (LINITIS PLASTICA). Barium study (erect view) shows the typical appearance of an extensive linitis plastica involving the entire stomach, which appears fixed and narrowed. No peristalsis was observed, and barium flowed out of the stomach quickly. The mucosal edge is only slightly irregular; ulceration of the mucosa may be minimal or absent in this type of carcinoma. (*Arrow* indicates the gastric fundus.)

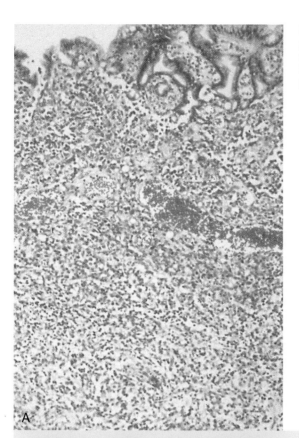

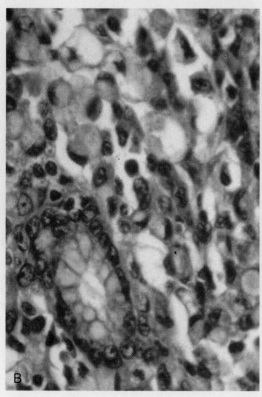

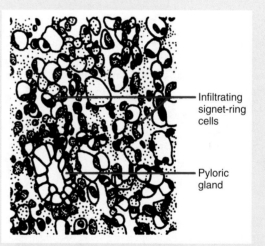

Infiltrating signet-ring cells

Pyloric gland

FIGURE 7.29 **DIFFUSE ADENOCARCINOMA. (A)** No tubular pattern can be seen in the low-power view. **(B)** Higher magnification reveals the discrete nature of the mucin-laden tumor cells (signet-ring cells) in contrast to the residual benign pyloric gland.

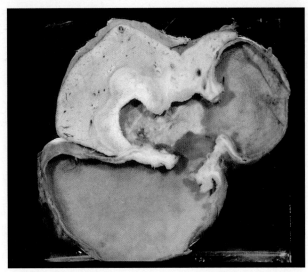

FIGURE 7.30 **LIVER INVASION.** This specimen, showing the stomach opened anteriorly, is from a 62-year-old man who presented with a 6-month history of epigastric pain, vomiting, and weight loss, as well as a palpable epigastric mass. Total gastrectomy with partial hepatic lobectomy was performed. An ulcerating neoplasm of the lesser curvature has spread extensively into the adherent hepatic parenchyma. Extensive local invasion by gastric cancer is common.

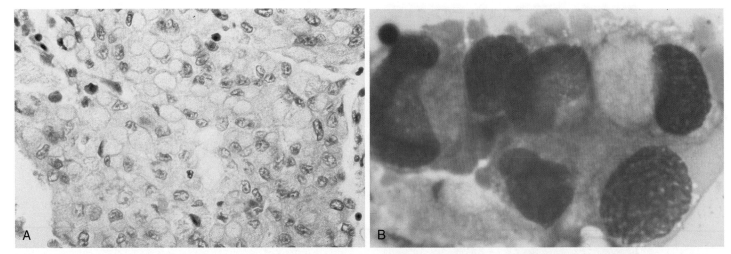

FIGURE 7.31 **BONE MARROW METASTASES.** A 60-year-old man presented with microangiopathic hemolytic anemia (MAHA). **(A)** Bone marrow biopsy specimen shows metastatic mucin-producing adenocarcinoma. **(B)** High-power view of a bone marrow aspirate demonstrates a clump of malignant cells. Further evaluation revealed a primary gastric cancer. Chemotherapy led to a complete clinical remission lasting 9 months. Cancer-related MAHA is most commonly seen with gastric carcinoma. Fragmentation of red blood cells is due to many factors, including the shearing effect of fibrin strands secondary to disseminated intravascular coagulation (associated with mucin-producing adenocarcinomas) or shearing by direct contact with intravascular tumor cells or with secondary proliferation of pulmonary arterioles.

Pancreatic Cancers

The increasing incidence of exocrine pancreatic cancers in the United States reflects the aging of the population. About 32,000 new cases are diagnosed each year, with nearly as many deaths. It is the fourth most common cause of cancer-related mortality in adults in the United States. The median age of patients with these tumors is approximately 70 years, with one third of cases occurring in persons aged 75 years or older. About one quarter of patients are younger than 60 years. The etiology remains obscure, except for a known association with cigarette smoking; pancreatic cancer is two to four times more common in heavy smokers than in nonsmokers. Other risk factors include diabetes mellitus and rare hereditary syndromes (e.g., ataxia-telangiectasia, Peutz-Jeghers syndrome, and hereditary chronic pancreatitis). Data are mixed regarding the risk of alcohol abuse and chronic pancreatitis in the development of pancreatic cancer.

HISTOLOGY

About 75% of pancreatic malignancies are ductal adenocarcinomas, of which approximately 70% occur in the head of the pancreas. A variety of uncommon types of pancreatic carcinoma have been described, including acinar, adenosquamous, anaplastic, papillary, mucous, and microadenocarcinomas, each of which composes less than 5% of the total. All of these have similarly poor prognoses and are treated in a similar fashion. Also uncommon are mucinous cystic neoplasms (cystadenoma/cystadenocarcinoma) of the pancreas, which occur most frequently in middle-aged women. These are typically located in the tail of the pancreas. Clinical behavior can be difficult to predict pathologically, leading some to conclude that all mucinous cystic neoplasms of the pancreas have malignant potential. Complete surgical resection results in cure rates of 30% to 60%. The remaining 5% to 10% of pancreatic neoplasms are predominantly islet cell–derived (see Chapter 10). Other rare neoplasms include pancreatoblastomas, most of which occur in children, and the solid and cystic neoplasms. The latter occurs most frequently in young women and carries an excellent prognosis following resection.

STAGING OF PANCREATIC CANCERS

Pancreatic cancer most commonly presents at an advanced stage. Early or local disease (stage I), with cancer confined to the pancreas, is unusual. Regional disease (stage II or III) is more common and includes tumor invasion into the bile duct, duodenum, adjacent peripancreatic tissue, or adjacent lymph nodes. Extensive disease (stage IV) signifies either invasion of tumor into the stomach, colon, spleen, or blood vessels, or the presence of distant metastases. More practically, pancreatic cancer can be divided into three stages: local/resectable, locally advanced (considered unresectable but without distant metastases), and metastatic. The overall prognosis of pancreatic carcinoma (excluding mucinous cystic neoplasms) is dismal, with a median survival time of 4–6 months and a 5-year survival rate of 2% to 3%.

Staging procedures include ultrasonography, CT scanning, and magnetic resonance imaging (MRI). A diagnostic laparoscopy may also be performed to detect peritoneal disease that is not visible radiologically. Regardless of these studies, an accurate histologic diagnosis is necessary to distinguish benign disease from carcinoma, islet cell tumors, and retroperitoneal lymphomas, because of the major therapeutic and prognostic differences among these disease entities. When liver metastases are present, fine-needle aspiration biopsy is often successful in establishing a diagnosis of metastatic disease. In the case of locally advanced disease, endoscopic retrograde cholangiopancreatography or fine-needle aspiration may be used. In the setting of a resectable pancreatic mass, biopsy may be deferred in favor of proceeding directly with surgical resection. Criteria for surgical resection include absence of metastatic disease and absence of invasion of prominent local blood vessels.

CLINICAL MANIFESTATIONS

Carcinoma of the head of the pancreas leads to jaundice caused by biliary obstruction. The gallbladder is usually distended (Courvoisier sign). Carcinomas of the body and tail are accompanied by severe pain resulting from retroperitoneal invasion and infiltration of the celiac ganglia and splanchnic nerves. However, body and tail lesions are often detected at later stages because symptoms do not occur until the disease has advanced more than pancreatic head tumors. About 75% of patients present with pain and progressive weight loss. Splenomegaly, due to encasement and obstruction of the splenic vein, may also occur. Other features include depression, diabetes mellitus (5% to 10% of cases), alterations in bowel function (particularly obstipation), and venous thrombosis with migratory thrombophlebitis (Trousseau sign; see "Hepatobiliary Cancers").

TREATMENT CONSIDERATIONS

Treatment of pancreatic cancer is dependent on the clinical stages described earlier—local/resectable, locally advanced, and metastatic. For resectable disease surgery remains the treatment of choice (although recurrence rates are >80%). The use and choice of adjuvant therapy remain controversial but may include chemotherapy alone or combined-modality chemotherapy and radiation therapy. For patients with locally advanced disease either chemoradiotherapy or chemotherapy alone should be considered. Patients with metastatic disease should be considered for chemotherapy; however, the benefits for most patients remain limited.

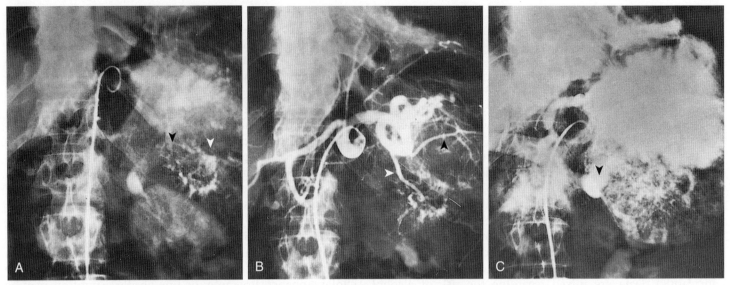

FIGURE 7.32 CYSTADENOMA-CYSTADENOCARCINOMA. Cystadenomas and cystadenocarcinomas are often quite large at the time of clinical detection. **(A)** As their names imply, both tumors contain cystic elements and both frequently show internal calcification, often in a stellate pattern (*arrowheads*). **(B, C)** The tumor is typically hypervascular; angiography demonstrates hypertrophied pancreatic branches (*arrowheads*) of the splenic artery feeding the lesion in the tail of the pancreas.

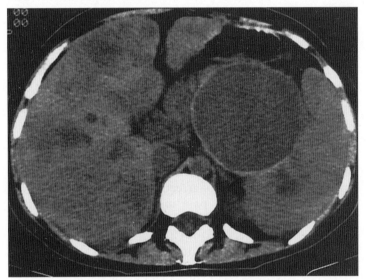

FIGURE 7.33 CYSTADENOCARCINOMA. CT scan of a 33-year-old woman who presented with metastatic disease shows one of several large pancreatic cysts and many liver metastases.

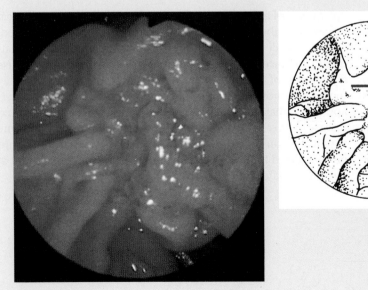

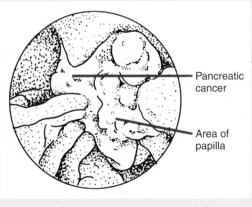

FIGURE 7.34 PANCREATIC CARCINOMA. Endoscopic view shows a tumor invading the duodenal wall just above the papilla of the pancreatic duct. The folds are irregular and nodular.

Pancreatic cancer

Area of papilla

FIGURE 7.35 **PANCREATIC CARCINOMA.** Barium study shows a tumor mass in the head of the pancreas invading the duodenal loop and producing changes in the fold pattern.

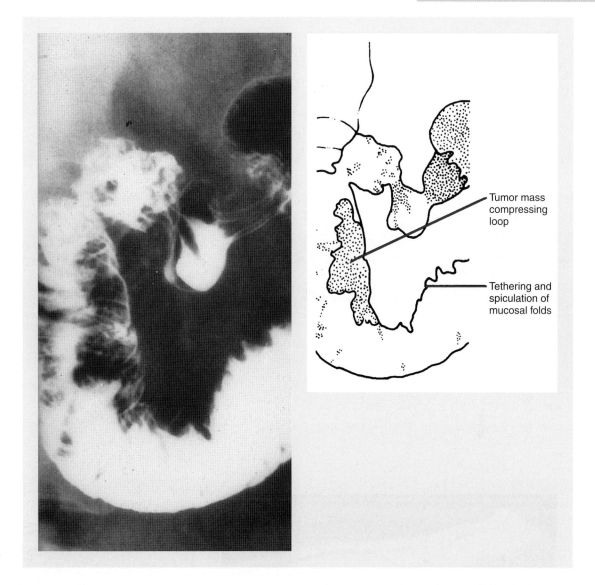

Tumor mass compressing loop

Tethering and spiculation of mucosal folds

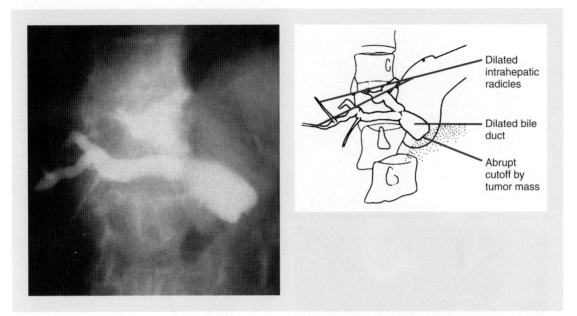

FIGURE 7.36 PANCREATIC CARCINOMA. Percutaneous transhepatic cholangiogram demonstrates obstruction of the common bile duct by tumor, which produced jaundice in this patient.

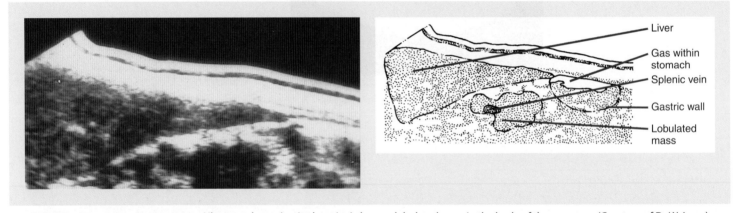

FIGURE 7.37 PANCREATIC CARCINOMA. Ultrasound scan (sagittal section) shows a lobulated mass in the body of the pancreas. (Courtesy of Dr W. Lees.)

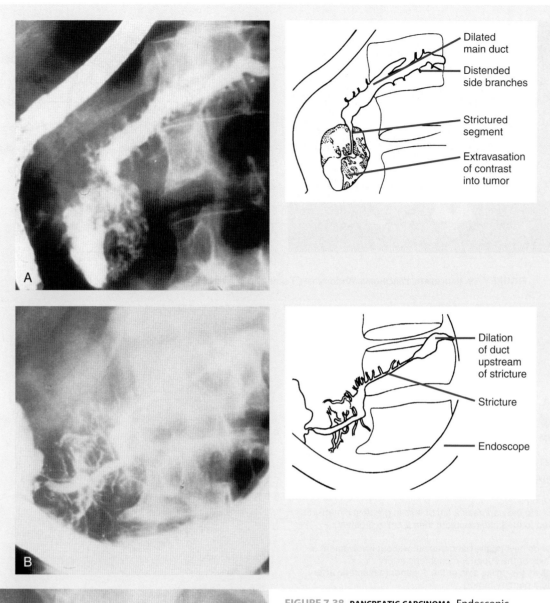

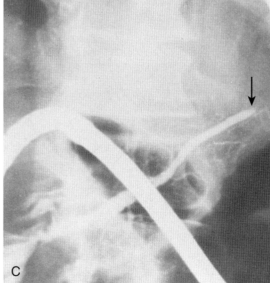

FIGURE 7.38 PANCREATIC CARCINOMA. Endoscopic retrograde cholangiopancreatography shows stricture of the pancreatic duct with dilatation upstream due to carcinoma. Shown are examples of carcinoma of the head (**A**), body (**B**), and tail (**C**) of the pancreas producing obstruction of the pancreatic duct (*arrow*).

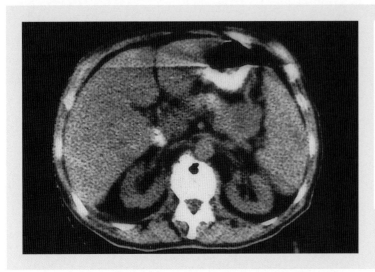
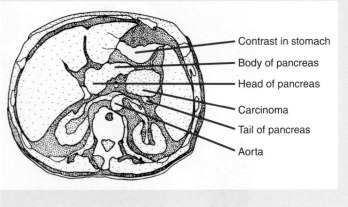

Contrast in stomach
Body of pancreas
Head of pancreas
Carcinoma
Tail of pancreas
Aorta

FIGURE 7.39 **PANCREATIC CARCINOMA.** Abdominal CT scan shows a large focal mass in the tail of the pancreas.

Definition of TNM

Primary Tumor (T)

TX   Primary tumor cannot be assessed
T0   No evidence of primary tumor
Tis   In situ carcinoma
T1   Tumor limited to the pancreas 2 cm or less in greatest dimension
T2   Tumor limited to the pancreas more than 2 cm in greatest dimension
T3   Tumor extends beyond the pancreas but without involvement of the celiac axis or the superior mesenteric artery
T4   Tumor involves the celiac axis or the superior mesenteric artery (unresectable primary tumor)

Regional Lymph Nodes (N)

NX   Regional lymph nodes cannot be assessed
N0   No regional lymph node metastasis
N1   Regional lymph node metastasis

Distant Metastasis (M)

MX   Distant metastasis cannot be assessed
M0   No distant metastasis
M1   Distant metastasis

Stage grouping

Stage 0	Tis	N0	M0
Stage IA	T1	N0	M0
Stage IB	T2	N0	M0
Stage IIA	T3	N0	M0
Stage IIB	T1–3	N1	M0
Stage III	T4	Any N	M0
Stage IV	Any T	Any N	M1

FIGURE 7.40 Staging of pancreatic carcinoma. (From Greene FL, Page D, Fleming I, et al, editors, for the American Joint Committee on Cancer: *AJCC cancer staging handbook*, ed 6, New York, 2002, Springer.)

FIGURE 7.41 BENIGN VERSUS MALIGNANT PANCREATIC CYTOLOGY. In contrast to **(A)** a sheet of benign ductal cells, **(B)** malignant cells show the usual characteristics of malignancy: an increased nucleus-to-cytoplasm ratio, hyperchromatic nuclei, and irregular nuclear contours. Note the uniform distribution of the benign, as compared with the malignant cells.

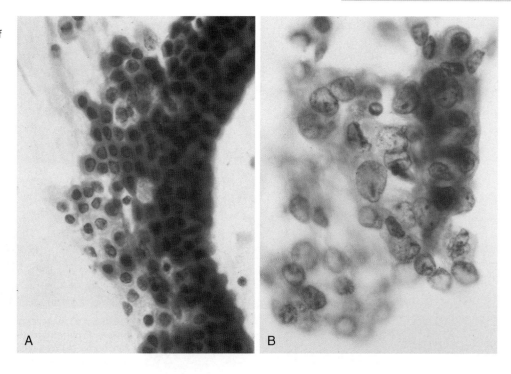

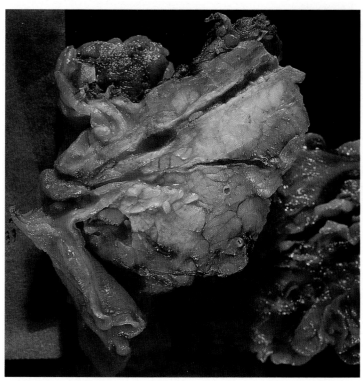

FIGURE 7.42 Adenocarcinoma of the pancreas often appears as a diffuse infiltrative, tan/white fibrotic lesion effacing the normal lobular architecture of the pancreatic parenchyma, as shown here in the head of the pancreas (between the pancreatic and common bile ducts) in a Whipple resection specimen. (1) ampulla, (2) common bile duct, (3) cancer, (4) pancreatic duct, (5) duodenal wall.

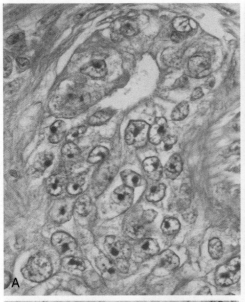

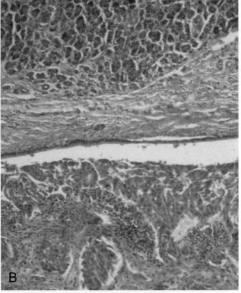

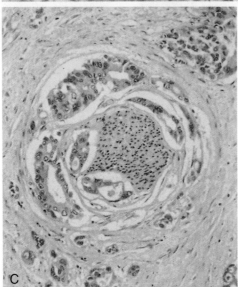

FIGURE 7.43 **PANCREATIC CARCINOMA.** Three histologic patterns may be found in pancreatic carcinoma. **(A)** Well-differentiated tumors are marked by well-formed glands of tumor cells. **(B)** In this moderately differentiated lesion, nests of tumor cells produce a squamoid configuration. **(C)** Pancreatic carcinomas typically induce an intense desmoplastic response. Perineural tumor invasion is also a frequent finding. In some cases diagnosis of malignancy from a needle biopsy that samples only the desmoplastic stroma may be difficult to distinguish from dense fibrosis in chronic pancreatitis.

FIGURE 7.44 PANCREATIC CARCINOMA. These autopsy specimens demonstrate **(A)** a carcinoma invading the head of the pancreas, infiltrating the duodenum, and destroying the pancreatic duct, and tumors **(B)** of the body (*arrows*) and **(C)** tail. Note the well-demarcated masses and areas of necrosis. (**A**, Courtesy of M. Knight; **B**, courtesy of Dr J. Newman.)

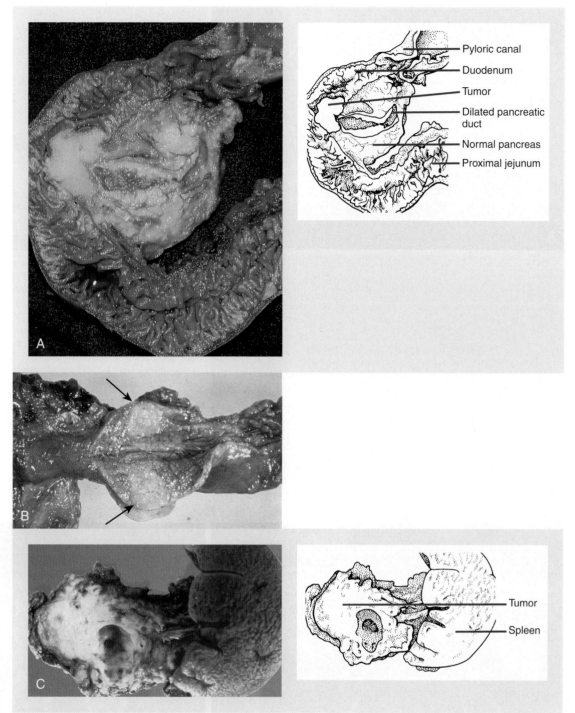

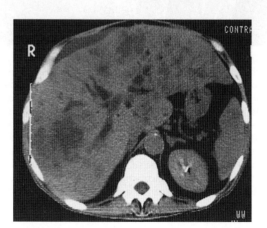

FIGURE 7.45 LIVER METASTASES. Abdominal CT scan in a patient with pancreatic carcinoma shows an enlarged, abnormal-looking liver, with dilated bile ducts centrally (to which the patient's jaundice can be ascribed) and widespread metastases more peripherally. Other CT sections showed a mass in the head of the pancreas.

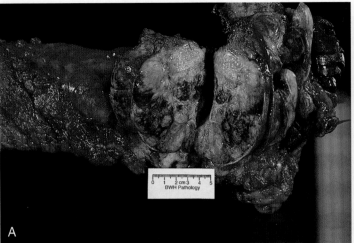

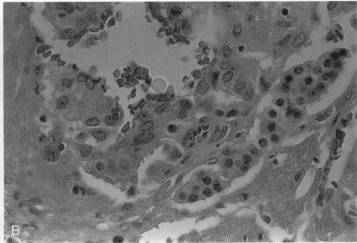

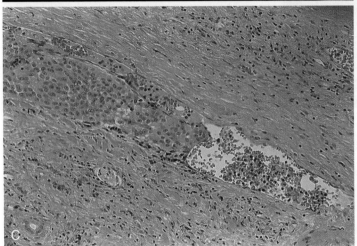

FIGURE 7.46 **(A)** Solid pseudopapillary tumor of the pancreas, as shown here in the tail of the pancreas abutting the spleen, typically has hemorrhagic/necrotic foci on gross examination; occasionally such foci impart a pseudocystic appearance (not shown). The tumor is classically encountered as an incidental finding or as a cause of abdominal pain in young adult females. The cytologic appearance on direct smears prepared from fine-needle aspirates is characteristic: loosely cohesive tumor cells appear to show off a "pseudopapilla," that is, a core of myxoid stroma containing a central capillary. Although more than 95% of patients are cured by excision alone, this case showed cytologic atypia **(B)**, vascular invasion **(C)**, and frequent mitoses (not shown), warranting designation as the malignant variant of solid pseudopapillary tumor. An isolated metastasis in the lesser sac was identified at the time of resection (not shown).

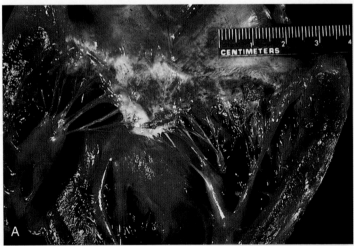

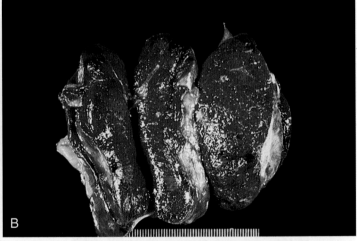

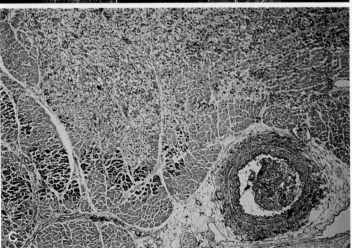

FIGURE 7.47 **(A)** Nonbacterial thrombotic endocarditis (NBTE). A 70-year-old man with pancreatic cancer developed fatal pulmonary and cerebral emboli. Autopsy findings included classic features of NBTE, characterized by sterile thrombi without inflammation at the lines of closure of cardiac valve leaflets. This complication is associated with the hypercoaguable state classically referred to as the Trousseau syndrome in patients with mucinous adenocarcinoma. The thrombi may embolize or disseminated intravascular coagulation may supervene, leading to vascular occlusion in end organs such as the spleen, which displays wedge-shaped hemorrhagic infarcts **(B)**, or the heart, where microscopy reveals a thrombus in a small muscular artery supplying an organizing, infarcted zone of myocardium **(C)**.

Hepatobiliary Cancers

LIVER CANCERS

Hepatocellular carcinoma is less common in the United States, although in parts of Africa and Asia it is one of the most common forms of malignant disease—a difference probably attributable to environmental influences (including diet and the increased incidence of viral hepatitis). In the United States, about 60% to 80% of cases are preceded by and associated with hepatic cirrhosis. In contrast, in areas of high incidence, hepatocellular carcinoma often occurs without cirrhosis in middle-aged patients. Risk factors include hereditary hemochromatosis, hepatitis B or C viral infection, and other causes of cirrhosis, including alcohol abuse, schistosome infestation, and homozygous α_1-antitrypsin deficiency. Noncirrhotic causes include chronic ingestion of food containing aflatoxins (metabolites of the mold *Aspergillus flavus*), plant derivatives found in "bush tea" (cycasin and pyrrolizidine), and possibly long-term use of androgens or oral contraceptives.

Hepatocellular carcinomas (hepatomas) have a wide range of histologic appearances, from well-differentiated tumors (which may be difficult to distinguish from regenerative nodules) to anaplastic malignancies. Diagnostic studies include CT-guided needle core biopsy and fine-needle aspiration biopsy, radionuclide scanning, ultrasonography, liver CT scanning, and determination of α-fetoprotein (AFP) level. The AFP is elevated in about 70% of cases, usually above 400 ng/mL (normal 20–40 ng/mL). Unfortunately, AFP is also increased in certain benign diseases (e.g., hepatitis) and in other malignancies (germ cell tumors and gastric, pancreatic, and pulmonary cancers). Hepatic angiography can be informative, showing a hypervascular tumor, and can also delineate the anatomic distribution for evaluating the possibility of successful resection.

The American Joint Committee on Cancer staging system for hepatocellular carcinoma is based on tumor size, number of tumor nodules, involvement of one or more liver lobes, vascular invasion, nodal metastases, and presence or absence of distant metastases. In Africa one proposed clinical staging system is based on risk factors, the presence or absence of ascites, weight loss, portal hypertension, and jaundice. In general, surgical resectability is the most important factor, because hepatocellular carcinomas are highly resistant to chemotherapy. The ability to resect the tumor completely while leaving adequate liver to support life is critical. The highest success rates have been in patients with incidental hepatocellular carcinomas discovered at transplantation for chronic liver disease. Survival rates with unresectable tumors vary from less than 2 months for advanced disease to 3 or more months for early hepatoma. Selected patients with resectable tumors may do significantly better, with some series reporting 10-year survival rates of nearly 20%.

Clinical manifestations depend on the presence or absence of underlying cirrhosis. In the latter case the presence of hepatoma may be heralded by sudden deterioration of hepatic function, leading rapidly to death. The most frequent presenting symptom, however, is weight loss associated with a painful mass in the epigastrium or right upper quadrant. The sudden development of ascites may be due to a Budd-Chiari syndrome (hepatic vein obstruction or thrombosis). Clinically evident metastases are not common and occur mainly to the lung and bones. Hepatic cancer may be accompanied by any of several paraneoplastic syndromes, including erythrocytosis, hypercalcemia, hypoglycemia, dysfibrinogenemia, and thrombocytosis.

For patients not deemed to have surgically resectable disease, options for treatment include transarterial chemoembolization, radiofrequency ablation, cryoablation, or systemic therapy. The most studied localized procedure, transarterial chemoembolization, has mixed data on the impact of such a modality on overall survival. Systemic therapy has been disappointing overall; no standard cytotoxic chemotherapies were even able to stabilize disease for the majority of patients. Recent data suggest certain targeted agents affecting angiogenesis may benefit some good-performance-status patients with unresectable disease.

BILIARY TRACT CANCERS

Carcinoma of the gallbladder and bile ducts is relatively uncommon, causing about 5000 deaths per year in the United States. Gallbladder cancer is most often an incidental pathologic finding at the time of cholecystectomy for cholelithiasis and is present in 0.2% to 5% of patients who undergo cholecystectomy; there is a female predominance. The presence of gallstones is strongly associated with gallbladder cancer, particularly gallstones of large size. However, the incidence of gallbladder carcinoma in patients with gallstones is only 1%.

Over half the gallbladder cancers that are discovered at an early stage originate in the fundus of the gallbladder. These early cases have an increased chance of long-term survival. Unfortunately, the majority of patients present with involvement of the entire gallbladder, and the 5-year survival rate is only 5%. Histologically, 85% to 95% of cases are adenocarcinomas, with the remainder comprising squamous cell carcinomas and other rare malignancies. Most patients die as the result of liver involvement either by direct invasion or hematogenous spread, although metastases to other sites, particularly regional lymph nodes, may occur.

Cholangiocarcinomas, which are more commonly extrahepatic than intrahepatic in origin, are primary carcinomas of the bile ducts. They may be located in the common duct (40% of cases), the confluence of the cystic, common, and hepatic ducts (24%), hepatic ducts and bifurcation (19%), common hepatic duct (10%), and cystic duct (7%). This tumor typically arises in late adult life, in either sex, and, unlike carcinoma of the gallbladder, shows no association with cholelithiasis. In some Asians, biliary infestation with the fluke *Clonorchis sinensis* is a predisposing factor. In other cases an association with choledochal cysts or ulcerative colitis and associated primary sclerosing cholangitis may be present. Virtually all cases are adenocarcinomas, with variable degrees of mucus production, fibroblastic reaction, and in some cases anaplasia. Jaundice is present in most patients, associated with severe pruritus and pain. Cure is rare but is occasionally achieved by radical surgery.

Carcinomas of the ampulla of Vater are uncommon but unique. They have a high potential for cure, in that cases can sometimes be diagnosed at an early stage, because they tend to cause obstructive jaundice early in the course of the disease. Most tumors are papillary and histologically are moderately well to well-differentiated adenocarcinomas. The presenting symptoms include jaundice, pain, pruritus, fever, and weakness due to blood loss. A characteristic sign is caused by incorporation of blood into the acholic and fat-laden stool, which produces the "silver stool" sign of Thomas.

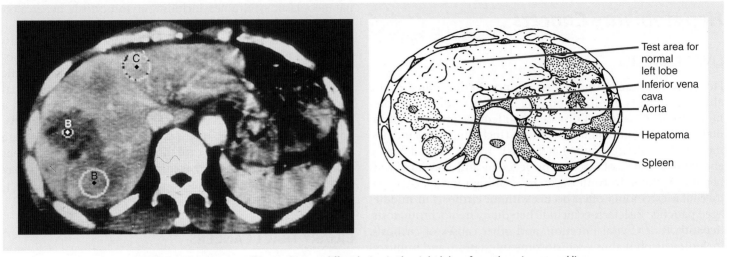

FIGURE 7.48 **HEPATOMA.** CT scan shows a diffuse lesion in the right lobe of an otherwise normal liver.

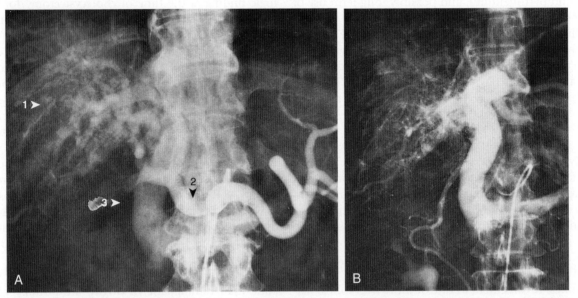

FIGURE 7.49 **HEPATOCELLULAR CARCINOMA WITH ESOPHAGEAL VARICES.** A 72-year-old man presented with massive upper GI bleeding. **(A)** Celiac arteriogram shows a hypervascular mass in the liver (*arrowhead 1*). There is massive shunting from the hepatic artery (*arrowhead 2*) to the main portal vein (*arrowhead 3*). **(B)** Later-phase film shows further filling of the portal vein and hepatofungal flow, causing the variceal bleeding.

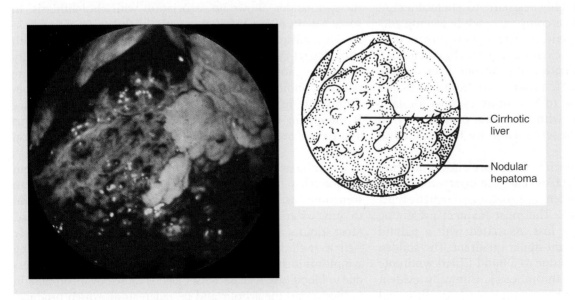

FIGURE 7.50 **HEPATOCELLULAR CARCINOMA.** Laparoscopic view shows a cirrhotic liver with a nodular hepatoma.

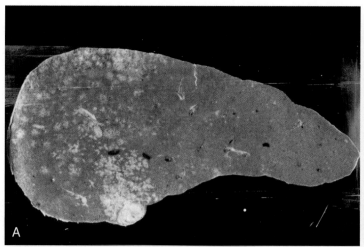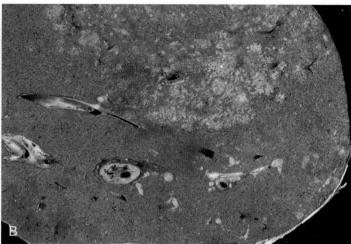

FIGURE 7.51 MULTIFOCAL HEPATOCELLULAR CARCINOMA IN HEMOCHROMATOSIS. A 61-year-old man with hemochromatosis and a 12-year history of hepatomegaly and diabetes mellitus died after developing liver failure with ascites. **(A)** Section through the right lobe of the liver shows an ill-defined micronodular cirrhosis, associated with deep brick-red parenchymal pigmentation. Scattered throughout the posterior region are many pale nodules of carcinoma. **(B)** The right main portal vein and its branches are occluded by similar pale neoplastic tissue. Multifocal hepatocellular carcinoma is the most common type of malignancy (about two thirds of cases) arising in cases of long-standing hemochromatosis.

FIGURE 7.52 Staging of hepatocellular carcinoma (including intrahepatic bile ducts). (From Greene FL, Page D, Fleming I, et al, editors, for the American Joint Committee on Cancer: *AJCC cancer staging handbook*, ed 6, New York, 2002, Springer.)

Definition of TNM

Primary Tumor (T)

TX	Primary tumor cannot be assessed
T0	No evidence of primary tumor
T1	Solitary tumor without vascular invasion
T2	Solitary tumor with vascular invasion, or multiple tumors, none more than 5 cm
T3	Multiple tumors more than 5 cm or tumor involving a major branch of the portal or hepatic vein(s)
T4	Tumor(s) with direct invasion of adjacent organs other than the gallbladder or with perforation of visceral peritoneum

Regional Lymph Nodes (N)

NX	Regional lymph nodes cannot be assessed
N0	No regional lymph node metastasis
N1	Regional lymph node metastasis

Distant Metastasis (M)

MX	Distant metastasis cannot be assessed
M0	No distant metastasis
M1	Distant metastasis

Stage grouping

Stage I	T1	N0	M0
Stage II	T2	N0	M0
Stage IIIA	T3	N0	M0
Stage IIIB	T4	N0	M0
Stage IIIC	Any T	N1	M0
Stage IV	Any T	Any N	M1

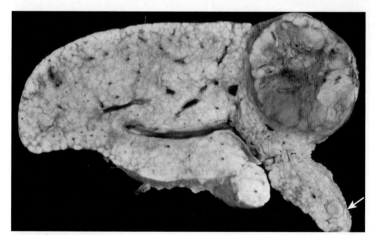

FIGURE 7.53 UNINODULAR HEPATOCELLULAR CARCINOMA. Autopsy of a 77-year-old man who collapsed and died while undergoing treatment in a psychiatric hospital revealed rupture of a hepatic tumor through the visceral peritoneum; death resulted from exsanguination with hemoperitoneum. The cut surface of the liver shows fine, uniform, micronodular cirrhosis. A rounded, apparently well circumscribed, partly bile-stained tumor (6.5 cm in diameter) arises near the diaphragmatic surface. A smaller nodule of similar tumor is apparent at the bottom right (*arrow*). The uninodular type of hepatocellular carcinoma represents about 30% of cases. An encapsulated type, which is rare in the United States but common in Japan, has a slightly better prognosis.

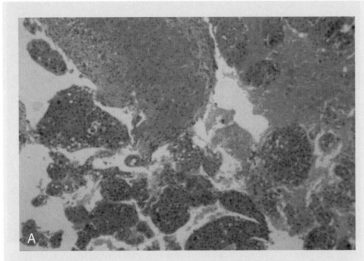

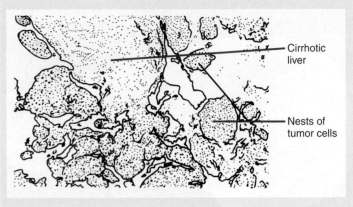

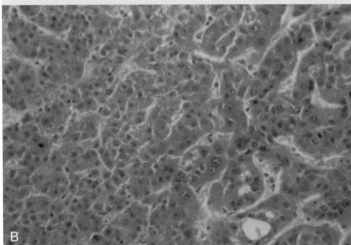

FIGURE 7.54 **HEPATOCELLULAR CARCINOMA.** Primary hepatic angiosarcoma. **(A)** Low-power photomicrograph shows a typical fragmented biopsy specimen, with nests of tumor cells and a fragment of cirrhotic liver. The malignant cells resemble normal liver cells and may be well differentiated. **(B)** At higher magnification, however, the cells are often pleomorphic, with prominent nucleoli. Immunoperoxidase stains for AFP, a_1-antitrypsin, carcinoembryonic antigen, and cytokeratins are useful in distinguishing hepatocellular carcinoma from metastatic tumors.

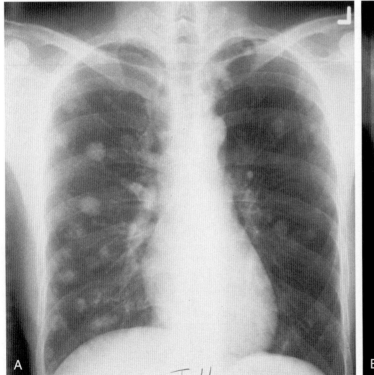

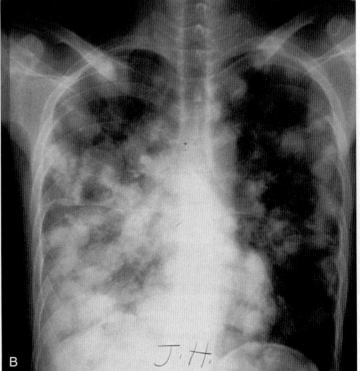

FIGURE 7.55 **LUNG METASTASES. (A)** Chest film of a 19-year-old Asian man who presented with hepatocellular carcinoma shows the well-defined pulmonary nodules characteristic of metastatic deposits. **(B)** Rapid disease progression occurred within 2 months. Metastases are unusual with hepatoma but do occur to the bones, lung, and brain.

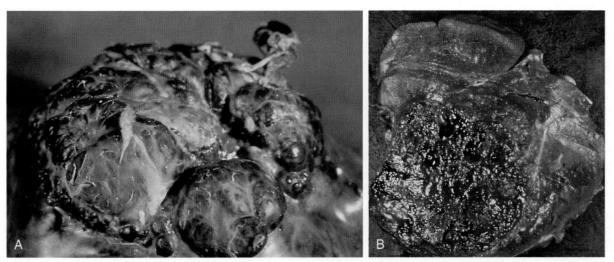

FIGURE 7.56 Typically, these tumors may appear as **(A)** a surface vascular tumor or **(B)** a hemorrhagic tumor mass. They are associated with industrial exposure to vinyl chloride and the radiographic contrast agent Thorotrast and usually comprise multicentric hemorrhagic nodules. (Courtesy of Prof. K. Weinbren.)

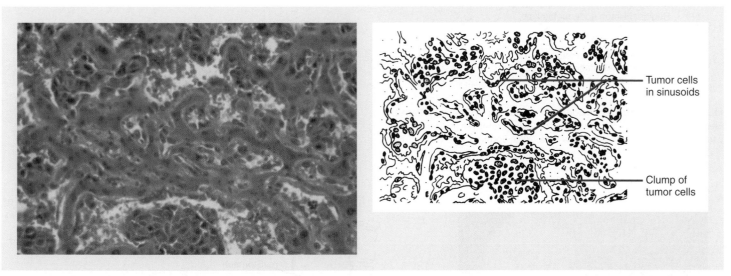

FIGURE 7.57 **PRIMARY HEPATIC ANGIOSARCOMA.** Its characteristic pattern is marked by growth of tumor cells along the sinusoids.

Stage grouping

Stage 0	Tis	N0	M0
Stage IA	T1	N0	M0
Stage IB	T2	N0	M0
Stage IIA	T3	N0	M0
Stage IIB	T1–3	N1	M0
Stage III	T4	Any N	M0
Stage IV	Any T	Any N	M1

Definition of TNM

Primary Tumor (T)

TX   Primary tumor cannot be assessed
T0   No evidence of primary tumor
Tis   Carcinoma in situ
T1   Tumor invades mucosa or muscle layer
        T1a Tumor invades the mucosa
        T1b Tumor invades the muscle layer
T2   Tumor invades the perimuscular connective tissue; no
        extension beyond the serosa or into the liver
T3   Tumor perforates the serosa (visceral peritoneum) and/or
        directly invades the liver and/or one other adjacent organ
        or structure, such as the stomach, duodenum, colon or
        pancreas, omentum, or extrahepatic bile ducts
T4   Tumor invades main portal vein or hepatic artery or invades
        multiple extrahepatic organs or structures

Regional Lymph Nodes (N)

NX   Regional lymph nodes cannot be assessed
N0   No regional lymph node metastasis
N1   Regional lymph node metastasis

Distant Metastasis (M)

MX   Presence of distant metastasis cannot be assessed
M0   No distant metastasis
M1   Distant metastasis

FIGURE 7.58 Staging of gallbladder carcinoma. (From Greene FL, Page D, Fleming I, et al, editors, for the American Joint Committee on Cancer: *AJCC cancer staging handbook*, ed 6, New York, 2002, Springer.)

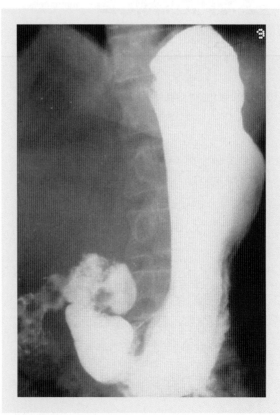
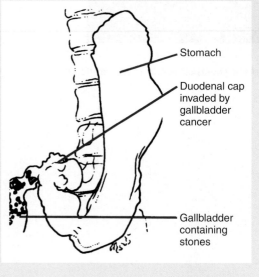

Stomach

Duodenal cap invaded by gallbladder cancer

Gallbladder containing stones

FIGURE 7.59 **ADENOCARCINOMA OF GALLBLADDER.** Barium study shows invasion of the duodenum by a gallbladder tumor, accompanied by a fistula.

FIGURE 7.60 ADENOCARCINOMA OF GALLBLADDER. Nests of tumor cells can be seen invading the gallbladder wall.

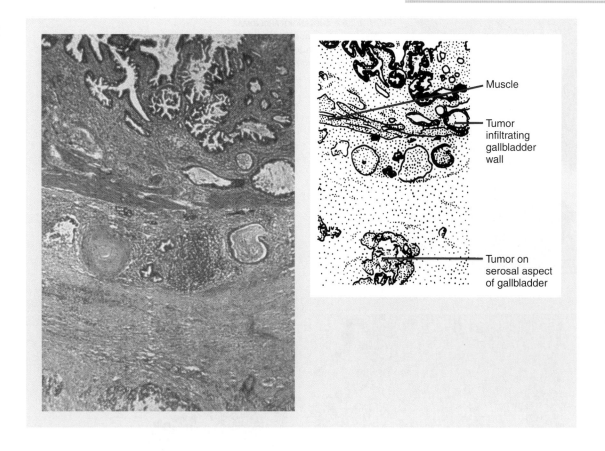

Muscle

Tumor infiltrating gallbladder wall

Tumor on serosal aspect of gallbladder

FIGURE 7.61 ADENOCARCINOMA OF NECK OF GALLBLADDER. These tumors are frequently associated with gallstones, as shown here. Most cases of gallbladder malignancy are associated with a long-standing history of cholelithiasis and cholecystitis.

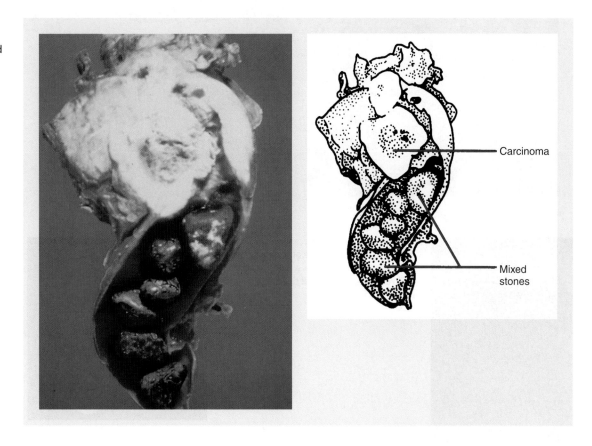

Carcinoma

Mixed stones

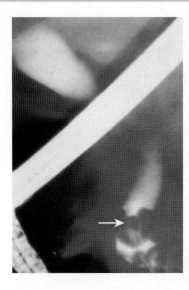

FIGURE 7.62 CHOLANGIOCARCINOMA.
Endoscopic retrograde cholangiogram shows a lesion obstructing the common bile duct (*arrow*).

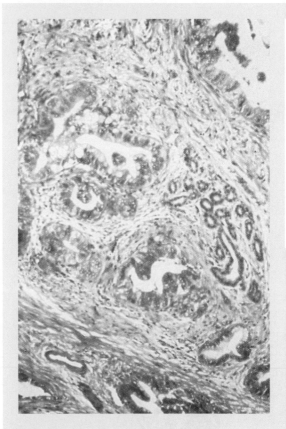

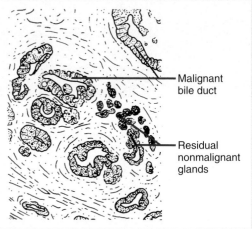

Malignant bile duct

Residual nonmalignant glands

FIGURE 7.63 CHOLANGIOCARCINOMA.
In this moderately differentiated adenocarcinoma, glands of malignant bile duct epithelium can be seen adjacent to benign structures. When intrahepatic, such tumors may be indistinguishable from metastatic adenocarcinoma arising at other sites. (Courtesy of Prof. K. Weinbren.)

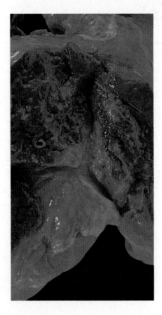

FIGURE 7.64 Cholangiocarcinoma arising at the confluence of the right and left main hepatic ducts is a pale, locally infiltrative tumor. Each of the ducts is markedly dilated.

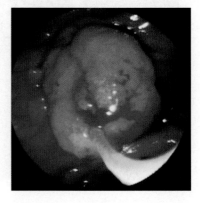

FIGURE 7.65 ADENOCARCINOMA OF AMPULLA OF VATER. Endoscopic view shows a periampullary lesion with an area of minimal bleeding in the center. The tumor is cannulated for endoscopic retrograde cholangiopancreatography to determine the extent of obstruction.

FIGURE 7.66 ADENOCARCINOMA OF AMPULLA OF VATER. Pancreatic duct is dilated secondary to obstruction by tumor. The partially filled and dilated bile duct can also be seen. The gallbladder is palpable in 30% of such cases, with painless jaundice.

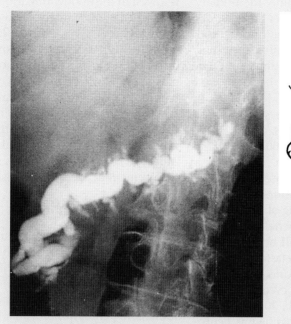

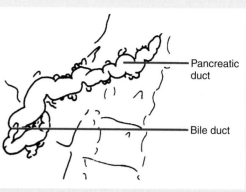

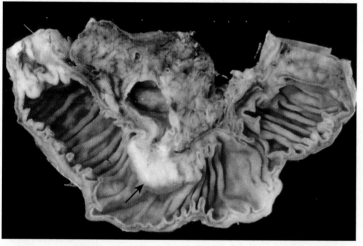

FIGURE 7.67 ADENOCARCINOMA OF AMPULLA OF VATER. This specimen is from a 56-year-old man who presented with a 3-week history of jaundice, itching, and slight fever. Radiologic studies were normal, but at laparotomy the gallbladder and common bile duct were found to be distended by distal obstruction. Pancreaticoduodenectomy and cholecystojejunostomy were performed. The head of the pancreas, the duodenum, and the distal common bile duct are dissected to reveal a small, nodular, pale neoplasm arising in the ampulla of Vater beneath the duodenal mucosa (*arrow*). The tumor (1.5 cm in diameter) has obstructed the orifice of the ampulla, leading to marked dilatation of the common bile duct (*middle right*).

Cancers of the Small Intestine

Each year approximately 5640 cases of small bowel cancer are diagnosed in the United States and approximately 1090 patients die of the disease. Among 14,253 patients with small bowel cancer who were identified in the National Cancer Data Base, adenocarcinoma (35.1%) was the most common histology, followed by carcinoid (27.6%), lymphoma (20.8%), and sarcoma (10.1%). Whereas adenocarcinomas occur most commonly in the duodenum, carcinoid tumors and lymphomas occur more commonly in the distal small intestine. In the National Cancer Data Base, 63% of small bowel adenocarcinomas originated in the duodenum, 20% in the jejunum, and 15% in the ileum. Tumors of all four histologies have the potential to metastasize.

The treatment of small bowel tumors differs significantly depending on the tumor type and stage of disease.

SMALL BOWEL ADENOCARCINOMA

The optimal management of locally advanced small bowel adenocarcinomas has not been clearly defined. Among 4995 patients with small bowel adenocarcinoma, 5-year disease-specific survival was 30.5%. Based on similarities in both natural history and treatment response between small bowel and large bowel adenocarcinomas, many investigators have suggested that small bowel adenocarcinoma should be treated in the same stage-specific manner as large bowel adenocarcinoma. Nonetheless, when compared to large bowel adenocarcinoma, patients with small bowel adenocarcinoma were more likely to present with stage IV disease (32% vs 19%) and less likely to present with stage I disease (12% vs 23%). Moreover, in these studies, 5-year disease-specific survival was lower for small bowel adenocarcinoma as compared with colorectal cancer for all stages. These differences may relate to the lack of a successful screening program for small bowel adenocarcinoma and the tendency for patients with small bowel adenocarcinoma to present with symptoms of obstruction, bleeding, and abdominal pain. Alternatively, small bowel adenocarcinoma may simply represent a biologically more aggressive malignancy (Kulke and Fuchs, 2006).

SMALL BOWEL CARCINOID TUMORS

Small bowel carcinoid tumors compose approximately one third of small bowel tumors in surgical series (Barclay and Schapira, 1983). Patients with small bowel carcinoids generally present in the sixth or seventh decade of life, most commonly with abdominal pain or small bowel obstruction; these symptoms are commonly misdiagnosed as "irritable bowel syndrome" (Barclay and Schapira, 1983; Makridis et al., 1990; Hellman et al., 2002). Approximately 5% to 7% will present with the carcinoid syndrome, at which time hepatic metastases are usually also present (Moertel et al., 1961; Burke et al., 1997). The difficulty in diagnosing small bowel carcinoids is compounded by the fact that standard imaging techniques such as CT scan and small bowel barium contrast studies only rarely identify the primary tumor. When detected and surgically removed they are most frequently located in the distal ileum and are often multicentric, occasionally appearing as dozens of lesions lining the small bowel (Moertel et al., 1961). Tumor size is an unreliable predictor of metastatic disease, and metastases have been reported even from tumors measuring less than 0.5 cm (Makridis et al., 1990). The 5-year survival rate is 60% for patients with localized disease, 73% for those with regional metastases, and 21% for patients with distant metastases (Modlin et al., 2003).

Mesenteric fibrosis and associated ischemia, caused by a characteristic desmoplastic reaction, are often present in association with small bowel carcinoids. These tumors are also frequently associated with "buckling" or tethering of the intestine due to extensive mesenteric involvement (Moertel et al., 1961; Eckhauser et al., 1981). Resection of the small bowel primary tumor, together with associated mesenteric metastases, leads to significant reduction in tumor-related symptoms of pain and obstruction, and is therefore recommended even in patients with known metastatic disease (Hellman et al., 2002). Because small intestinal carcinoid tumors are now classified as neuroendocrine tumors, considerable interest and research in this area have occurred, especially in the development of new therapeutic agents, as is detailed in a recent review (Kulke et al., 2006).

SMALL BOWEL LYMPHOMA

Lymphomas may be localized or diffuse and may occur throughout the GI tract. They are most common in the stomach (up to 60%), and nearly 35% occur in the small intestine. The frequency is lowest in the duodenum, moderate in the jejunum, and highest in the ileum. Primary small intestinal lymphomas are most often solitary lesions, with multiple separate lesions present in up to 20% of cases. The lymphomas are typically large at time of discovery, averaging 8 cm. Histologically, primary small intestinal lymphomas are similar to lymphomas of mucosal-associated lymphoid tissue (MALTomas) in the remainder of the GI tract and the respiratory system. In children most GI lymphomas are histiocytic (large cell) or Burkitt's (undifferentiated) types, with a predilection for the terminal ileum and the ileocecal valve. Although systemic lymphomas may involve the small intestine, involvement by Hodgkin disease is quite rare.

SMALL BOWEL SARCOMA

Malignant GISTs constitute about 15% of small bowel malignancies; they appear to have a slight predilection for the duodenum and jejunum (see further detailed discussion of GISTs, pp. ?). They often reach large sizes (≥20 cm) before diagnosis, and the tumor mass may be predominantly extraluminal. Perforation with abscess formation, peritonitis, or fistula formation is an unusual but dramatic event. Most patients present with abdominal pain, with or without GI bleeding. Regional lymph node involvement is rare, but hematogenous metastases, directly related to the histologic aggressiveness of the tumor, develop in many patients. Among other small bowel sarcomas leiomyosarcomas are most common, but fibrosarcomas, liposarcomas, and malignant neural tumors may also occur. These may arise anywhere along the small bowel; they metastasize most commonly to the liver and lungs. Involvement of the regional lymph nodes occurs in less than 15% of cases.

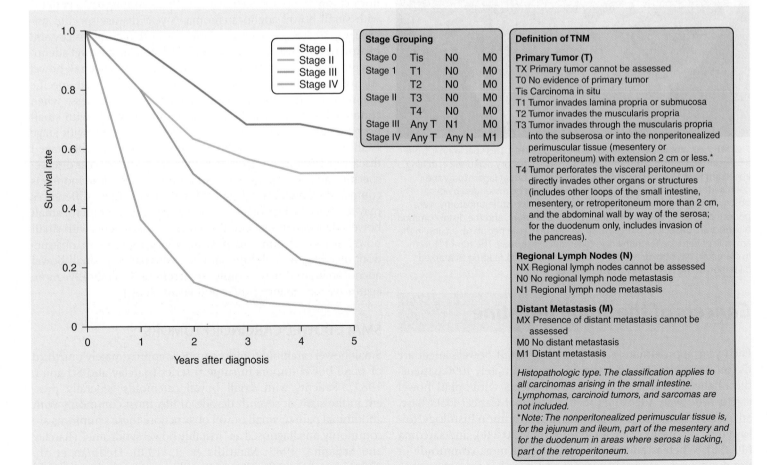

FIGURE 7.68 **STAGING OF CANCERS OF THE SMALL INTESTINE.** Histopathologic type: the classification applies to all carcinomas arising in the small intestine. Lymphomas, carcinoid tumors, and sarcomas are not included. Graph shows relative survival rates according to stage of disease. Data based on 250 cases recorded in the Surveillance Epidemiology and End Results Program of the National Cancer Institute. Stage I includes 13 cases; stage II, 77; stage III, 56; and stage IV, 104. (From Greene FL, Page D, Fleming I, et al, editors, for the American Joint Committee on Cancer: *AJCC cancer staging manual,* ed 6, New York, 2002, Springer.)

FIGURE 7.69 HAMARTOMATOUS POLYP IN PEUTZ-JEGHERS SYNDROME. Endoscopic view shows a broad-based polyp in the duodenum in a patient with Peutz-Jeghers syndrome. These small intestinal polyps only rarely become malignant. This syndrome is an autosomal-dominant condition that is also marked by deposits of melanin on the buccal mucosa, lips, and digits. Ovarian neoplasms arise in almost 5% of women with this syndrome.

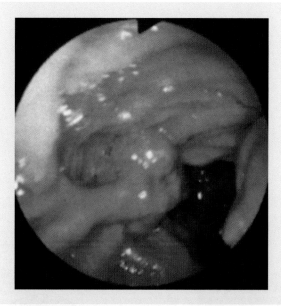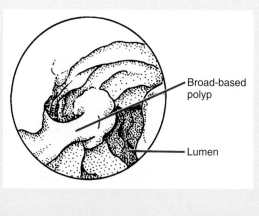

FIGURE 7.70 DIFFUSE ADENOMATOSIS IN FAMILIAL ADENOMATOUS POLYPOSIS. The proximal small intestine has been almost entirely affected by adenomatous (dysplastic) changes. Note the difference in color between adenomatous tissue and uninvolved Kerckring's folds.

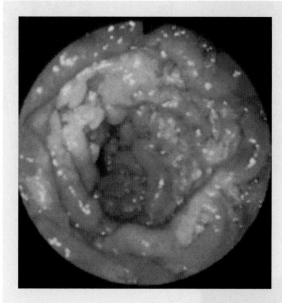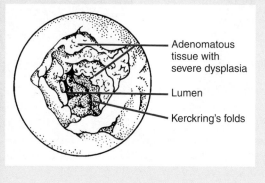

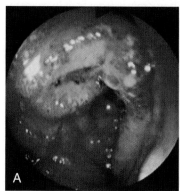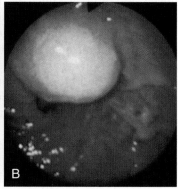

FIGURE 7.71 MALIGNANT GIST OF DUODENUM. Endoscopy demonstrates **(A)** destruction of the duodenal wall by tumor and **(B)** a tumor mass compressing the antrum.

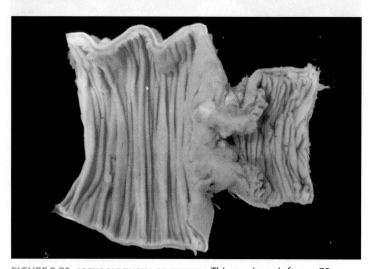

FIGURE 7.72 ADENOCARCINOMA OF JEJUNUM. This specimen is from a 75-year-old woman who presented with a 6-week history of profuse vomiting. A barium study was not diagnostic, and laparatomy was performed. A segment of jejunum has been opened to show an annular, stenosing tumor, extending over a length of 1.5 cm; it has infiltrated the full thickness of the bowel wall. The intestine is markedly dilated proximal to the obstruction and shows muscle hypertrophy.

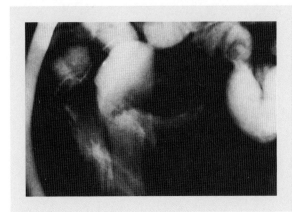

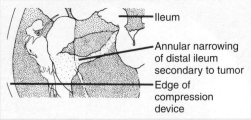

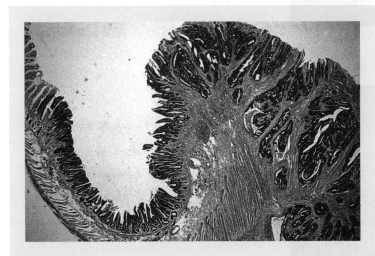

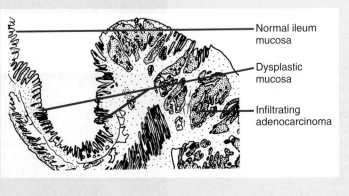

FIGURE 7.74 **ADENOCARCINOMA OF ILEUM.** Low-power photomicrograph demonstrates a gradual transition from normal mucosa through dysplasia to invasive adenocarcinoma.

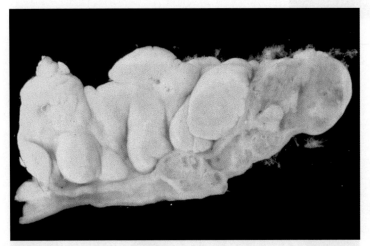

FIGURE 7.75 **MUCINOUS CYSTADENOCARCINOMA OF APPENDIX.** This specimen is from an 83-year-old man who died of peritoneal carcinomatosis; the primary tumor site was not identified before death. The appendix is diffusely expanded by a multilocular cystic tumor largely composed of pale, mucinous material. Adenocarcinoma of the appendix is extremely rare and is usually of the mucinous type. The elderly are typically affected and may present with symptoms of acute appendicitis. The clinical behavior and prognostic features are the same as those of cecal adenocarcinoma. These tumors occasionally give rise to pseudomyxoma peritonei, a condition marked by progressive accumulation of intra-abdominal pearly, gelatinous, mucoid material grossly indistinguishable from ruptured benign mucocele. (Courtesy of the Gordon Museum, Guy's Hospital Medical School, London, UK.)

NEUROENDOCRINE TUMORS OF THE GASTROINTESTINAL TRACT

Gastrointestinal neuroendocrine tumors are divided into carcinoid tumors (see above) or pancreatic tumors. Histologically, these tumors are generally well differentiated with few mitoses and are comprised of similar "small blue cells" with round nuclei, and indistinct nucleoli. They are positive for silver stains and neuroendocrine markers, including neuron specific enolase, synaptophysin and chromogranin. In the basophilie cytoplasm, numerous membrane-bound neurosecretory granules are seen (best on electron microscopy) which contain a variety of hormones and biogenic amines. The release of proteins like serotonin, insulin, gastrin, glucagon, and insulin into the blood results in various syndromes associated with neuroendocrine tumors.

Table 7.2 lists the clinical presentations of pancreatic neuroendocrine tumors (Kulke, 2006). Other features of interest include secretory cell type, incidence of metastases and extra pancreatic locations. Table 7.3 focuses specifically on location of carcinoid neuroendocrine tumors and also lists the major symptoms when present.

FIGURE 7.76 **ADENOCARCINOMA OF APPENDIX.** (**A**, **B**) A mucin-secreting adenocarcinoma has penetrated the full thickness of the appendiceal wall (**A**, Alcian blue; **B**, hematoxylin & eosin).

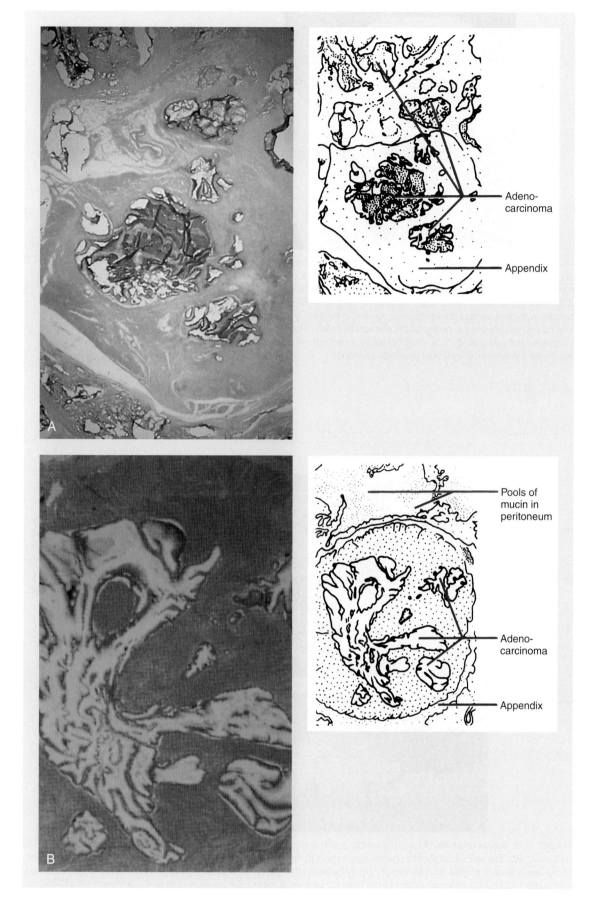

Adeno-carcinoma

Appendix

Pools of mucin in peritoneum

Adeno-carcinoma

Appendix

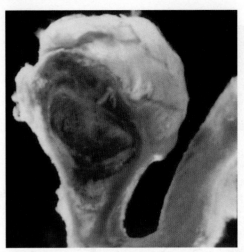

FIGURE 7.77 **CARCINOID TUMOR OF APPENDIX.** This tumor was found incidentally during cholecystectomy in a 59-year-old woman. The appendix has been mounted to show a pear-shaped, yellow-brown tumor (2.5 cm in length) at the distal end. The appendix is the single most common primary site of GI carcinoid tumors, with carcinoids of the ileum being second in frequency. Appendiceal lesions are typically seen in young adults and usually follow a benign course, in contrast to those arising in the small bowel. As a consequence, the carcinoid syndrome is a rare complication of appendiceal lesions.

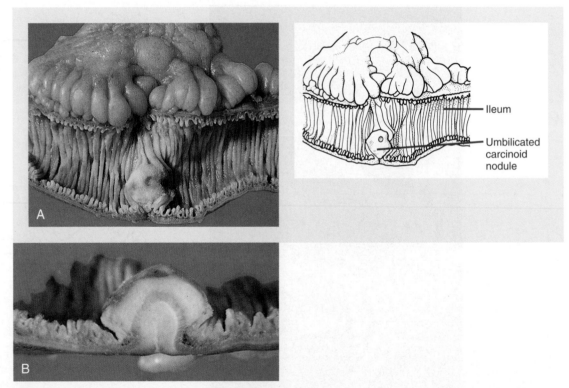

FIGURE 7.78 **TUMOR OF ILEUM. (A)** A small, umbilicated carcinoid nodule from a patient with carcinoid syndrome arises from the submucosa, as seen on sectioning **(B)**. The yellow color of the tumor is the result of formalin fixation. Such tumors may not be detectable on barium examination. Carcinoid tumors of the ileum show a predilection for men, typically between the ages of 50 and 70. An indolent clinical course is common, but the majority of these tumors eventually metastasize to lymph nodes or the liver. These lesions secrete 5-hydroxytryptamine, which is normally metabolized in the liver and therefore has no systemic effects. However, the development of liver metastases circumvents this metabolic process, and the carcinoid syndrome may then ensue. Thus, the clinical development of the carcinoid syndrome in a patient with a history of small intestinal carcinoid tumor should suggest the likelihood of extraintestinal metastases.

FIGURE 7.79 LYMPHOMA.
Barium film in a patient with celiac disease shows a small bowel lymphoma giving rise to a large mesenteric mass in the right lower quadrant. The tumor displaces and compresses several ileal loops, which show effacement of the fold pattern, as well as nodular irregularity indicating mucosal invasion. (Courtesy of Dr R. Dick.)

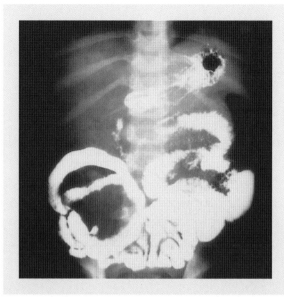

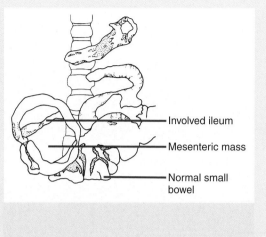

Involved ileum

Mesenteric mass

Normal small bowel

Table 7.2

Clinical Presentation of Pancreatic Neuroendocrine Tumors

Tumor	Symptoms or Signs	Cell Type	Incidence of Metastases	Extrapancreatic Location
Insulinoma	Hypoglycemia resulting in intermittent confusion, sweating, weakness, nausea. Loss of consciousness may occur in severe cases	β-cell	<15%	Rare
Glucagonoma	Rash (necrotizing migratory erythema), cachexia, diabetes, deep venous thrombosis	α-cell	majority	Rare
VIPoma, Verner-Morrison Syndrome, WDHA Syndrome	Profound secretory diarrhea, electrolyte disturbances	Non-β-cell	majority	10%
Gastrinoma, Zollinger-Ellison Syndrome	Acid hypersecretion resulting in refractory peptic ulcer disease, abdominal pain, and diarrhea	Non-β-cell	<50%	Frequently in duodenum
Somatostatinoma	Diabetes, diarrhea, cholelithiasis	δ-cell	majority	Rare
PPoma "Nonfunctioning"	May be first diagnosed due to mass effect			

From Kelson D, Daly JM, Kern SE, et al, editors: *Gastrointestinal oncology: principles and practice*, ed 2, New York, 2002, Lippincott, Williams & Wilkins, pp 873–898.

Table 7.3

Clinical Presentation of Carcinoid Tumors

Tumor	Symptom
Foregut	
Bronchial Carcinoids	Cough, hemoptysis, post-obstructive pneumonia, Cushing's syndrome. Carcinoid syndrome rare.
Gastric Carcinoids	Usually asymptomatic and found incidentally.
Midgut	
Small Intestine Carcinoids	Intermittent bowel obstruction or mesenteric ischemia. Carcinoid syndrome common when metastatic.
Appendiceal Carcinoids	Usually found incidentally. May cause carcinoid syndrome when metastatic.
Hindgut	
Rectal Carcinoids	Either found incidentally or discovered due to bleeding, pain, and constipation. Rarely cause hormonal symptoms, even when metastatic.

From Kelson D, Daly JM, Kern SE, et al, editors: *Gastrointestinal oncology: principles and practice*, ed 2, New York, 2002, Lippincott, Williams & Wilkins, pp 873–898.

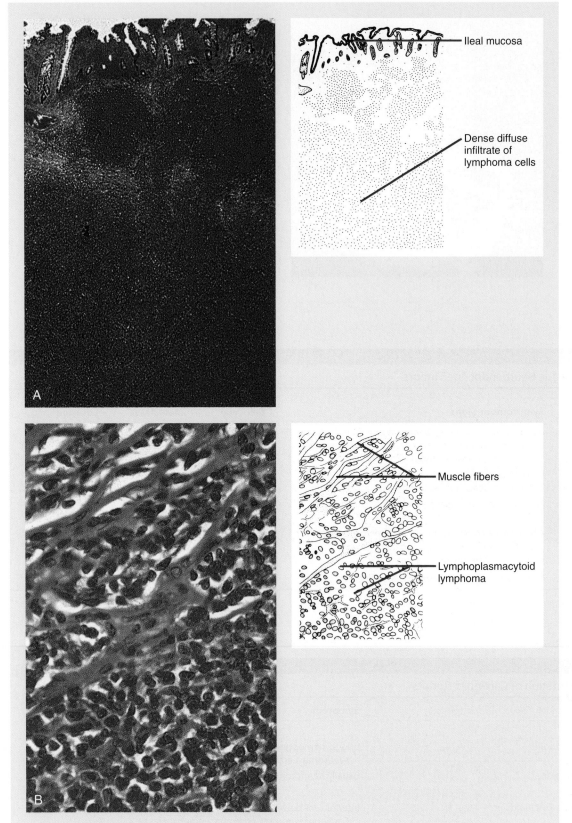

FIGURE 7.80 LYMPHOMA.
(A) Low-power photomicrograph of a small bowel tumor shows sheets of small, blue-staining tumor cells infiltrating the submucosa and muscle; the mucosa is relatively spared.
(B) High magnification reveals infiltration of well-differentiated lymphoplasmacytoid lymphoma cells between the muscle fibers of the ileal wall.

FIGURE 7.81 LYMPHOMA.
Plaquelike growths of a large cell lymphoma have infiltrated the ileal wall; note the smaller intervening nodule. In such instances intestinal obstruction is the most common presentation.

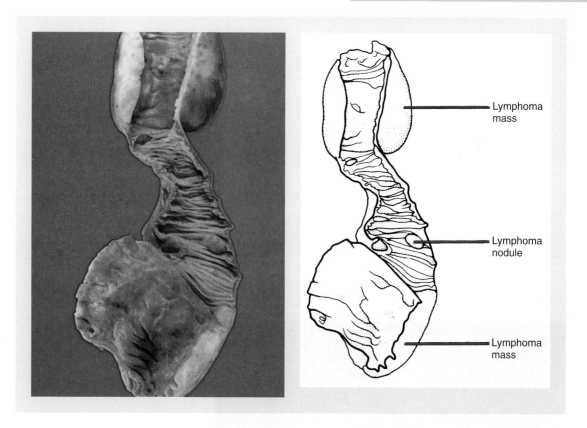

Lymphoma mass

Lymphoma nodule

Lymphoma mass

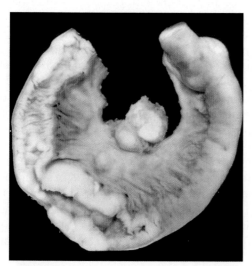

FIGURE 7.82 METASTATIC MALIGNANT MELANOMA OF ILEUM. This specimen is from a 60-year-old man who presented with a change in bowel habits, weight loss, and frequent vomiting. The case was initially believed to represent a multicentric lymphoma. However, the source of his primary tumor was not detected before signs of intestinal obstruction developed and laparotomy was performed. This partly opened loop of small bowel shows three separate pale amelanotic infiltrative deposits of tumor, along with several enlarged mesenteric nodes, which are replaced by further metastases. The propensity of malignant melanoma to metastasize to almost any site is well known. Such lesions, when amelanotic, may be misdiagnosed both clinically and pathologically. In general, metastasis of any tumor to the small bowel is uncommon.

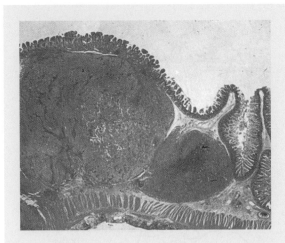

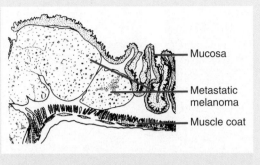

FIGURE 7.83 METASTATIC MALIGNANT MELANOMA OF JEJUNUM. Metastatic deposits of tumor can be seen in the submucosa of the jejunum. The lesion is predominantly amelanotic. Radiographic studies in such instances may reveal "target" or "bull's-eye" lesions.

Mucosa

Metastatic melanoma

Muscle coat

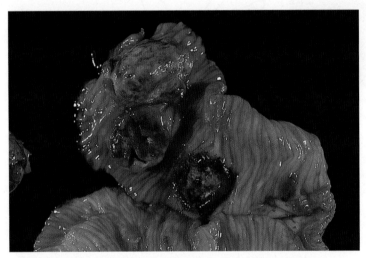

FIGURE 7.84 The small bowel is a favored site for metastases from melanoma. This jejunal resection specimen shows the typical appearance of multiple pigmented nodules; some show surface ulceration and associated central necrosis. These appear as "target" lesions on radiographic contrast studies.

Colorectal Cancers

Colorectal cancer is the fourth most common malignancy and the second most frequent cause of cancer-related death in the United States. Annually, an estimated 148,000 cases of colorectal cancer will be diagnosed and 55,000 people will die from this disease. Worldwide, colorectal cancer is the fourth most commonly diagnosed malignancy, with an estimated 1,023,152 new cases and 529,978 deaths in 2002. Approximately 70% of these cancers will arise in the colon, whereas 30% will occur in the rectum. Overall mortality from colorectal cancer has declined progressively in the past two decades, partially as a result of detection of disease at an earlier stage and of more effective treatments, particularly adjuvant therapy.

RISK FACTORS

The incidence of colon cancer is highest in industrialized regions such as the United States and Europe. As a result, epidemiology studies have focused on identifying factors prevalent in these populations that relatively increase and decrease one's risk of developing colorectal cancer. In addition to family history and certain medical conditions, a host of dietary and lifestyle factors have been consistently shown to modify this risk.

FAMILY HISTORY

Up to 25% of all patients with colorectal cancer have a family history of the disease. Several hereditary syndromes are associated with an increased risk for colon cancer. Familial adenomatous polyposis (FAP) is a rare autosomal-dominant condition that is characterized by the development of numerous polyps throughout the colon. Virtually all patients with FAP will develop colon cancer by age 40 unless prophylactic colectomy is performed. FAP is caused by germline mutations in the tumor suppressor gene *APC*. Variants of FAP include Gardner's syndrome (in which prominent extraintestinal lesions like desmoid tumors and sebaceous or epidermoid cysts are seen in addition to extensive polyposis) and Turcot's syndrome (brain tumors, particularly medulloblastomas, in addition to colonic tumors). The importance of *APC* is emphasized by the observation that it is mutated in colon tumors (but not the germline) of some patients with sporadic (i.e., nonhereditary) colon cancer.

Hereditary nonpolyposis colon cancer (HNPCC), another inherited syndrome, is characterized by the early onset of colon cancer, often involving the right side of the colon, and typically occurring in the absence of numerous colonic polyps. Several germline defects responsible for HNPCC have been identified; the most common of these are mutations in *MLH1* and *MSH2*. These genes are essential components of a nucleotide mismatch repair system. HNPCC is also associated with the development of extracolonic tumors, including malignancies of the endometrium, ovary, stomach, and small bowel. Genetic screening for individuals at risk for HNPCC is available.

In addition to familial syndromes, a family or personal history of colorectal cancer or adenomatous polyps increases one's risk of developing colorectal cancer. This risk is modified by number of family members affected and age of diagnosis of family members, particularly first-degree relatives.

ASSOCIATED DISEASES

Patients with inflammatory bowel disease have an increased risk of colorectal cancer that can be up to 10-fold higher than the general population. Although initial observations suggested that such a risk was limited to patients with ulcerative colitis, recent evidence also implicates Crohn's disease as a risk factor. Extent of disease involvement of the colon and rectum and duration of disease are the main determinants of the increased risk. In general, patients with ulcerative colitis do not have an appreciable increase in risk until about 8–10 years from time of diagnosis of inflammatory bowel disease.

Diabetes mellitus has also been associated with a risk of colorectal cancer. The potential mechanism is related to insulin and insulin-like growth factor (IGF), stimulants of colonic cell growth. Case-control and cohort studies have suggested that diabetic patients have a 1.3- to 1.5-fold increased risk of colorectal cancer, compared to nondiabetics. However, given the prevalence of diabetes, such a relative risk is clinically significant.

Individuals with acromegaly have a 2.5-fold increased risk of colorectal cancer. Although the mechanism of this increased risk is not entirely clear, the elevated levels of growth factor and IGF-1 characteristic of acromegaly probably stimulate colonic mucosa proliferation.

DIETARY AND LIFESTYLE FACTORS

Epidemiology studies have demonstrated dietary factors that contribute to the risk of developing colorectal cancer. Prospective cohort studies link high intake of red meat, low intake of folic acid, and decreased calcium and vitamin D to increased risk of developing colorectal cancer. Fiber intake and fruit and vegetables have been studied extensively as risk factors, although the majority of studies show little or no association except in the case of very low intake of these dietary factors.

Obesity and physical activity have consistently been shown to influence the risk of colorectal cancer. Increasing body mass index and lower levels of physical activity increase the risk of developing colorectal cancer up to twofold. Recent hypotheses have linked physical activity, obesity, and adipose distribution to circulating insulin and free IGF-1.

An association between alcohol consumption and an increased risk of colorectal cancer has been observed in several studies. A pooled analysis of eight cohort studies estimated a 40% increased risk of colorectal cancer in those whose alcohol consumption exceeded 45 g/day. The amount of alcohol in 12 ounces of beer, 4 ounces of wine, and 1.5 ounces of 80-proof liquor was estimated to be 13 g, 11 g, and 14 g, respectively. Cigarette smoking has been associated both with an increased incidence of colorectal cancer and an increased mortality rate from colorectal cancer.

PREVENTATIVE AGENTS

Preclinical, epidemiologic, and intervention studies support a protective effect of aspirin, nonsteroidal anti-inflammatory drugs, and selective COX-2 inhibitors on the risk of colorectal cancer and adenomas. Recently, the use of 3-hydroxy-3-methylglutaryl coenzyme A reductase inhibitors, commonly known as statins, has been tested as also providing a protective effect against colorectal cancer development. Thus far, study results have been mixed and the potential benefit remains unclear.

HISTOLOGY

More than 98% of cancers of the large bowel are adenocarcinomas. Characteristic subgroups include mucinous or colloid tumors and signet-ring cell tumors. Adenocarcinomas are classified as well, moderately, or poorly differentiated, each category having a distinct prognostic implication. Most colorectal carcinomas originate from adenomatous polyps. Pathologically, progression from early adenomatous proliferations through adenomatous polyp, high-grade dysplasia, and, ultimately, invasive carcinoma occurs as a continuum. This progression coincides with the accumulation of genetic alterations within the neoplasm as originally described by Fearon and Vogelstein (1990). These alterations include mutations of tumor suppressor genes (e.g., *TP53*, *DCC*, and *APC*), as well as activation and/or overexpression of oncogenes (e.g., c-*MYC* and k-*RAS*. Although the order of occurrence of these genetic changes may vary, the quantitative accumulation of defects correlates with biologic and histologic parameters of neoplastic progression, suggesting a multistep model of tumorigenesis. The majority of bowel cancers arise in the rectum and sigmoid colon; however, recent studies show that, for unknown reasons, the proportion of cancers arising in the rectum is decreasing, whereas the percentage of those originating in the cecum and ascending colon is increasing. The remaining 2% of colorectal cancers consist of lymphomas, leiomyosarcomas, and miscellaneous tumors.

STAGING

Colorectal cancers are generally staged at the time of surgery. CT scans of the abdomen and pelvis and chest radiographs are usually also performed to evaluate for metastatic disease. Bone scans are not routinely carried out in the absence of bone pain, because of a low incidence of bone metastases. Extension of primary rectal cancers into adjacent soft tissues can often be assessed by pelvic MRI or endorectal ultrasound.

Several systems have been used in staging colorectal cancer. The initial staging system was introduced by Dukes and subsequently modified by Kirklin and colleagues, Astler and Coller, and others. These classifications were based on three prognostic variables: depth of tumor invasion through the bowel wall, regional lymph node involvement, and distant metastases. Unlike other cancers, the size of the primary colon carcinoma does not in itself affect prognosis. These systems have largely been replaced by the more universal cancer TNM staging system. The sixth edition of the American Joint Commission on Cancer staging manual (Greene et al., 2002) revised the TNM staging classification, where new subcategories of stage II and III colorectal cancer are included to differentiate tumors based on the extent of invasion through the bowel wall and the number of involved lymph nodes (one to three vs four or more). As recent studies have shown, the 5-year survival rate for each stage of disease, except for stage IV, has improved. The reasons for this trend may not necessarily be related to improvements in early detection and in surgical technique but instead to more thorough and accurate staging.

Colorectal cancers spread by direct invasion, through lymphatic channels, along hematogenous routes, and by implantation. Spread of colon cancers through the portal venous circulation leads to liver metastases, which are present in about two thirds of patients at autopsy. Cancers that originate below the peritoneal reflection (12–15 cm from the anal verge) are considered rectal cancers. The location of these lesions and the lymphatic drainage of this area necessitate special management decisions. Rectal cancers situated below the peritoneal reflection have a high rate of local recurrence. Cancers of the lower rectum may metastasize via the paravertebral plexus to supraclavicular nodes, lungs, bone, and brain, without liver involvement.

Initial staging remains the most predictive prognostic factor for overall survival. Patients with stage I disease have greater than 90% 5-year survival with surgery. Patients with stage II disease have 70% to 85% 5-year survival (dependent on extent of disease through the bowel wall and existence of other prognostic features such as clinical bowel obstruction, bowel perforation, or poor differentiation, which increase the risk for recurrence). Patients with stage III disease have a variable 5-year survival of 35% to 70% (depending on number of positive lymph nodes and presence of other high-risk features). Finally, patients with stage IV (metastatic) disease have a long-term survival rate of less than 5%.

CLINICAL MANIFESTATIONS

Patients with cancer of the cecum and ascending colon usually present with anemia caused by intermittent GI bleeding. Obstruction is rare, because the bowel wall is more distensible and has a greater circumference than the descending colon. These cancers are often large and may be fungating or friable. Carcinomas of the transverse colon and either the hepatic or the splenic flexure, which account for about 10% of total cases, are somewhat less common than cecal neoplasms and much less common than rectosigmoid tumors. They frequently cause cramping pain, bleeding, and sometimes obstruction or perforation. Large bowel obstruction is the most common complication of colon carcinoma and may lead to proximal ulceration or perforation. Obstruction is the principal reason why up to 30% of cases present as surgical emergencies. Other complications include iron deficiency anemia, hypokalemia (particularly associated with large villous rectal lesions), and intussusception in adults. Tumors of the sigmoid colon and rectum cancers usually cause changes in normal bowel habits, with tenesmus, decrease in stool caliber, secretion of mucus, and hematochezia.

Colorectal cancer is usually initially diagnosed with colonoscopy. A full colonoscopy should be performed in all patients with colorectal cancer to rule out the possibility of second occult primary colon cancers, which occur in about 5% of patients.

TREATMENT CONSIDERATIONS

Treatment for colorectal cancer is dependent on the stage of disease. Surgical resection of the primary colorectal cancer is generally performed either with curative intent or, in patients with metastatic disease, as a palliative procedure to reduce the risk of obstruction and bleeding. For patients with stage I colon or rectal cancer, surgery alone is the usual treatment. For patients with rectal cancer, preoperative staging with either endorectal coil MRI or endoscopic ultrasound should be performed, and patients with stage II or III disease should be considered for neoadjuvant therapy. Options for neoadjuvant therapy include either radiation therapy alone or chemoradiotherapy. The latter is performed by most oncologists in the United States and much

of Europe. Following surgery for stage II or III disease, further adjuvant chemotherapy should be given to patients regardless of the final pathology. Alternatively, chemoradiation therapy and chemotherapy can all be given as adjuvant therapy for those with stage II or III rectal cancer who undergo initial surgery. For patients with colon cancer, surgery should usually be performed first; if the patient has lymph node–positive disease without metastatic spread (stage II), chemotherapy should be offered. If patients have stage II colon cancer, chemotherapy is more controversial but should be considered for those at least with high-risk features. Patients with metastatic disease are generally considered for chemotherapy only, although a select group of such patients may be eligible for localized therapy for their metastatic disease (surgery, ablation, or other such modalities).

Anal Cancers

There are over 4600 new cases of anal carcinoma in the United States annually. As a result of the transitional (columnar to squamous) nature of the epithelium of the anorectal junction and the presence of glandular epithelium, endocrine cells, and melanocytes, several different histologies may develop. These include squamous cell carcinoma (>50%), basaloid carcinoma, colonic-type adenocarcinoma, and, rarely, mucinous carcinoma, melanoma, and small cell carcinoma. The incidence of anal cancer and its precursor lesions (such as anal intraepithelial neoplasia) is increasing, particularly in HIV-positive men and women. The development of anal carcinoma is also strongly associated with human papillomavirus infection. Patients with Crohn's disease and chronic perianal fistulae are also at increased risk. Screening in high-risk persons includes a physical exam, an anal Pap smear, and anoscopy if the Pap smear is abnormal.

Squamous cell carcinomas can be divided into tumors arising in the anal canal, most often above the dentate line, and those arising in the skin at the anal margin. Tumors of the anal canal, which are three times as common as those at the anal margin, tend to spread proximally and to disseminate predominantly to intrapelvic lymph nodes; the 5-year survival rate is about 50%. In contrast, squamous cell cancers arising at the anal margin tend to be more indolent, metastasize to inguinal lymph nodes, and have a favorable prognosis.

Anal malignant melanoma, like squamous carcinoma, can be divided into two types: tumors arising in the anal canal and those arising from anal skin. The latter group is entirely comparable to conventional cutaneous malignant melanomas. Malignant melanoma of the anal canal is fairly rare and tends to present in late adulthood in either sex. It shows a predilection for extensive local invasion and early lymph node metastases and is associated with a poor prognosis.

TREATMENT CONSIDERATIONS

Treatment of cancers arising perianally depends on histology. Adenocarcinomas should be treated like a rectal cancer and anal melanomas like other skin melanomas. For squamous cell variants, the majority of anal cancers without distant spread can be cured with combined-modality chemotherapy and radiation therapy. Following completion of such therapy re-evaluation of the lesion is required, and persistent lesions may still be cured with surgery.

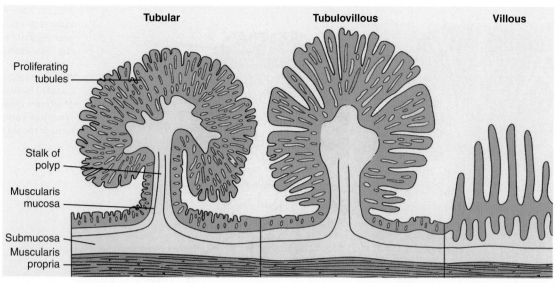

Tubular   **Tubulovillous**   **Villous**

Proliferating tubules

Stalk of polyp

Muscularis mucosa

Submucosa

Muscularis propria

FIGURE 7.85 **PATTERNS OF ADENOMATOUS COLONIC POLYPS.** Polyps may be pedunculated (*left, middle*) or sessile (*right*). The surface epithelium of the stalk may be non-neoplastic (*left*) or adenomatous (*middle*). Polyps may be solitary or multiple; the presence of more than approximately 100 polyps suggests the diagnosis of familial adenomatous polyposis. Although they can arise at any site in the large bowel, the largest and more often symptomatic lesions tend to be situated in the left side of the colon. The diagnosis of adenoma requires the presence of epithelial dysplasia. These polyps are therefore premalignant neoplastic tissue. Factors believed to increase the risk of malignant change include large polyp size (particularly >2 cm in diameter), severe epithelial dysplasia, and villous architecture. Penetration of the muscularis mucosa by dysplastic epithelium with invasion of submucosa is the distinguishing sign of invasive carcinoma.

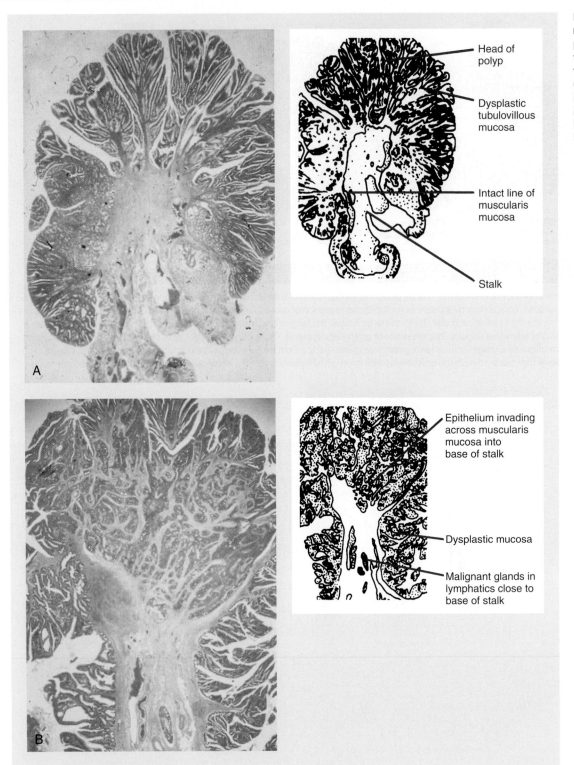

FIGURE 7.86 **ADENOMATOUS LESIONS OF COLON. (A)** In the premalignant neoplastic lesion the muscularis mucosa is intact, whereas in the malignant lesion **(B)** the muscularis is obviously invaded by malignant epithelium. Malignant glands in the lymphatics are seen close to the base of the stalk.

Head of polyp

Dysplastic tubulovillous mucosa

Intact line of muscularis mucosa

Stalk

Epithelium invading across muscularis mucosa into base of stalk

Dysplastic mucosa

Malignant glands in lymphatics close to base of stalk

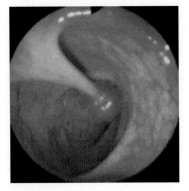

FIGURE 7.87 **TUBULAR ADENOMA.** Endoscopy shows a pedunculated adenomatous polyp of the colon.

FIGURE 7.88 TUBULAR ADENOMA.
(A) Barium enema study shows a pedunculated polyp en face. The two rings formed by the polyp and the stalk are called the "target sign." **(B)** Lateral decubitus view confirms that the polyp is pedunculated.

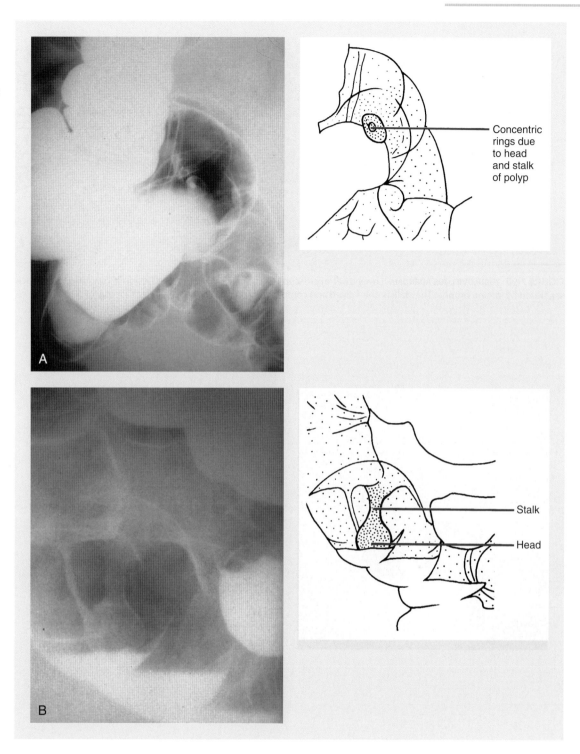

Concentric rings due to head and stalk of polyp

Stalk

Head

FIGURE 7.89 TUBULOVILLOUS ADENOMA. Endoscopic view shows a moderate-sized sessile polyp. Several lobules are evident.

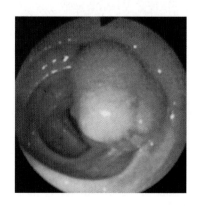

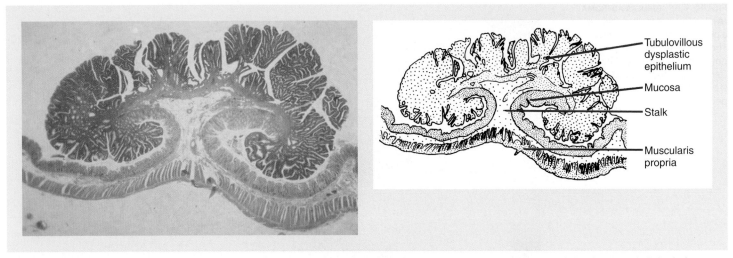

FIGURE 7.90 TUBULOVILLOUS ADENOMA. Low-power microscopic section of a typical stalked lesion shows the closely packed dysplastic epithelial tubules, separated by lamina propria. The stalk is uninvolved and composed of submucosa and normal mucosa.

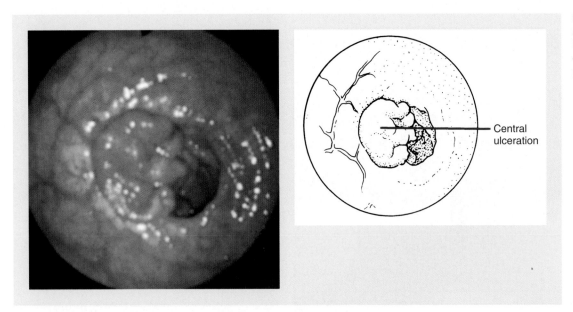

FIGURE 7.91 VILLOUS ADENOMA. Malignant rectal villous polyp. Endoscopy shows superficial central ulceration in this rectal polyp, suggestive of malignancy.

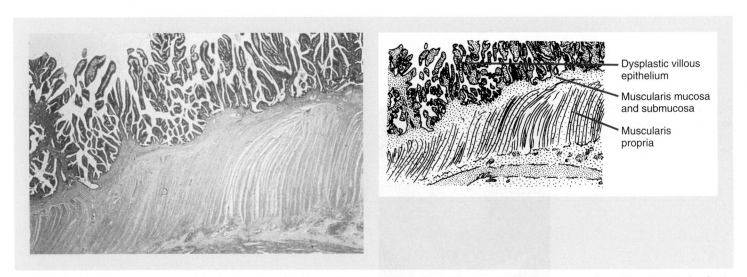

FIGURE 7.92 SESSILE VILLOUS ADENOMA. Histologic section of a villous polyp demonstrates its sessile nature. Note the numerous finger-like villi, with dysplastic epithelium over a core of lamina propria, resting directly on the muscularis mucosa. No invasion is present.

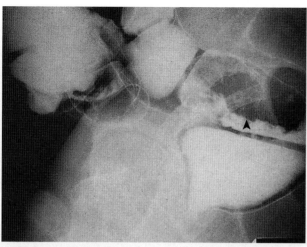

FIGURE 7.93 VILLOUS ADENOMA. A broad rectal lesion can be seen rising posteriorly (*arrowhead*). Histologic examination revealed a villous adenoma. Tumors of this size have a high probability of malignancy and are too large and broad-based for endoscopic removal. Typical symptoms include copious, watery, mucus-containing diarrhea, rectal bleeding, and tenesmus.

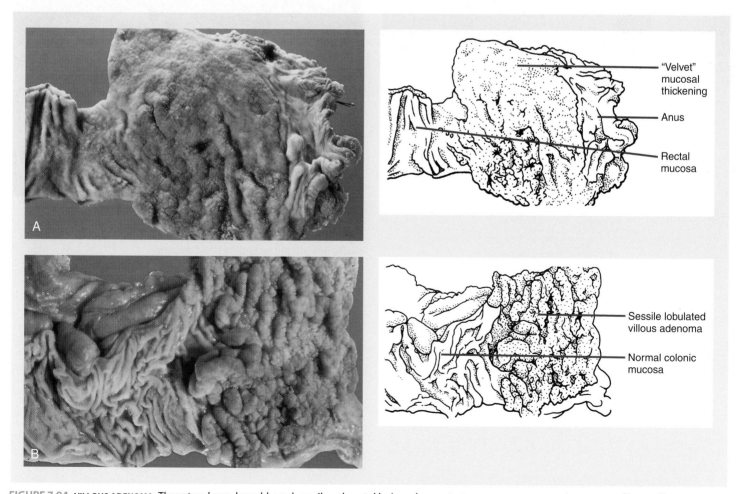

FIGURE 7.94 VILLOUS ADENOMA. These two large, broad-based, sessile colorectal lesions demonstrate common macroscopic patterns of large villous adenomas. **(A)** A fine villous pattern gives the mucosa of this rectal lesion a velvety appearance; this is in contrast to **(B)** the coarser, lobulated pattern seen in this colonic adenoma. The margins of both lesions are ill-defined. Villous adenomas are most common in the rectum, where they tend to be larger and to show more severe dysplasia than tubular adenomas; they therefore more commonly progress to adenocarcinoma. Villous adenomas of the rectum sometimes secrete large amounts of potassium or albumin, giving rise to hypokalemia or hypoalbuminemia.

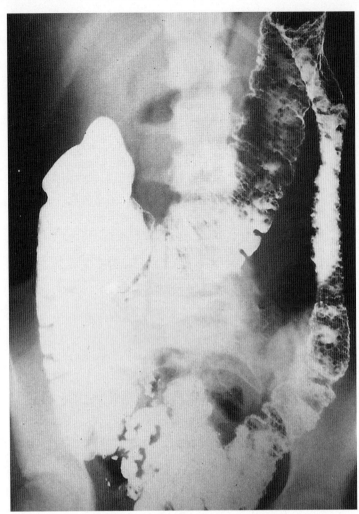

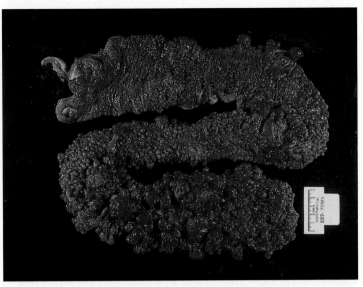

FIGURE 7.96 Familial adenomatous polyposis, with innumerable adenomatous polyps, increasing in size and density from proximal (*upper left*) to distal (*lower right*).

FIGURE 7.95 **FAMILIAL ADENOMATOUS POLYPOSIS.** Barium enema study demonstrates multiple small polyps throughout the colon.

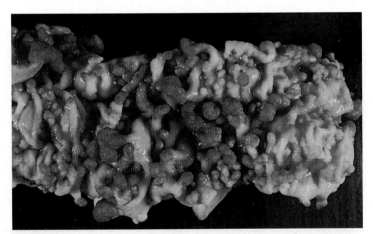

FIGURE 7.97 **FAMILIAL ADENOMATOUS POLYPOSIS.** This disorder is marked by the development of hundreds of large bowel adenomas, as seen in this segment of large bowel, which is covered with adenomas of various sizes. It usually arises in the second and third decades.

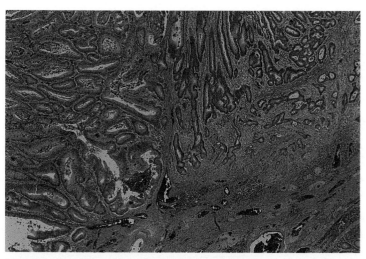

FIGURE 7.98 **FAMILIAL ADENOMATOUS POLYPOSIS.** Section of colon shows innumerable polyps characteristic of FAP. If left untreated the risk of colon cancer in such patients approaches 100% by the age of 40.

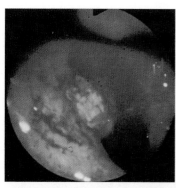

FIGURE 7.99 **POLYPOID EPITHELIAL DYSPLASIA IN ULCERATIVE COLITIS.** Endoscopy reveals epithelial dysplasia with surrounding chronic active colitis in a patient who had ulcerative colitis for nearly 20 years. Histologic examination showed high-grade mucosal dysplasia. The dysplasia is histologically identical to that seen in adenomatous polyps. However, in the setting of ulcerative colitis of more than 10 years' duration, high-grade dysplasia is strongly associated with the development of invasive cancer and should prompt serious consideration of colectomy.

FIGURE 7.100 **INTRAMUCOSAL CARCINOMA IN ULCERATIVE COLITIS.** Frank intramucosal carcinoma is evident in this colon biopsy specimen from a patient with ulcerative colitis. The lesion infiltrates the lamina propria but does not extend beyond the muscularis mucosa. The tumor evolves through ascending grades of dysplasia in nonpolypoid mucosa, as evidenced by the uninvolved mucosa at the left margin.

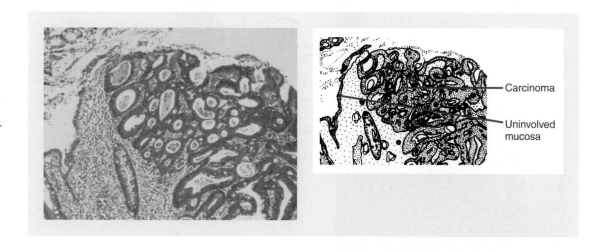

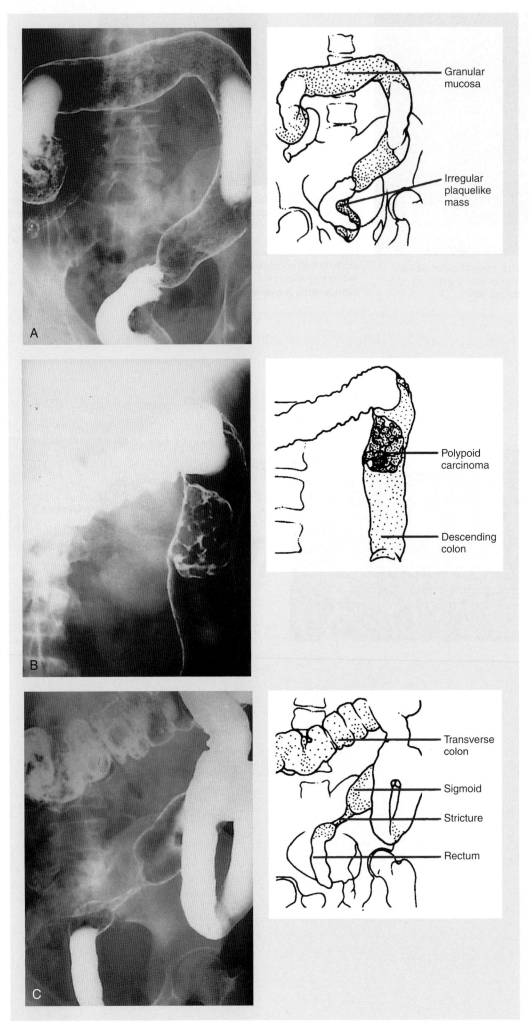

FIGURE 7.101 CARCINOMA IN ULCERATIVE COLITIS. Malignancies developing in ulcerative colitis may present as **(A)** an infiltrative plaque, **(B)** a polypoid mass, or **(C)** a stricture. The cumulative risk of cancer increases dramatically with the duration of ulcerative colitis. After 20 years there is a 15% incidence of colon cancer, which increases to 50% after 40 years.

FIGURE 7.102 **MODIFIED DUKES' STAGING CLASSIFICATION OF COLORECTAL CANCER.** Stages B3 and C3 (not shown) signify perforation or invasion of contiguous organs or structures (T4). The TNM classification provides a more accurate staging system: Dukes' B is a composite of better (T2N0) and worse (T3N0, T4N0) prognostic groups, as is Dukes' C (T × N1 or T × N2).

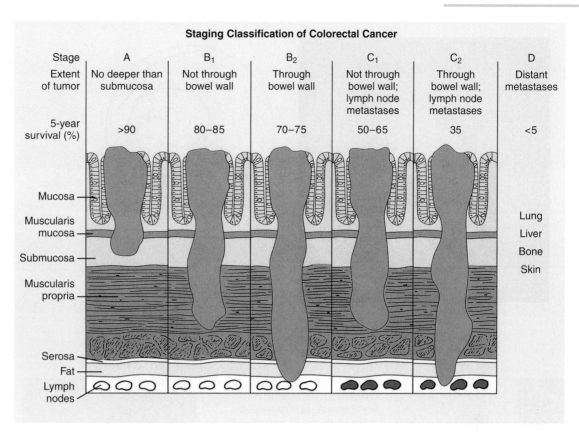

Staging Classification of Colorectal Cancer

Stage	A	B₁	B₂	C₁	C₂	D
Extent of tumor	No deeper than submucosa	Not through bowel wall	Through bowel wall	Not through bowel wall; lymph node metastases	Through bowel wall; lymph node metastases	Distant metastases
5-year survival (%)	>90	80–85	70–75	50–65	35	<5

Mucosa
Muscularis mucosa
Submucosa
Muscularis propria
Serosa
Fat
Lymph nodes

Lung
Liver
Bone
Skin

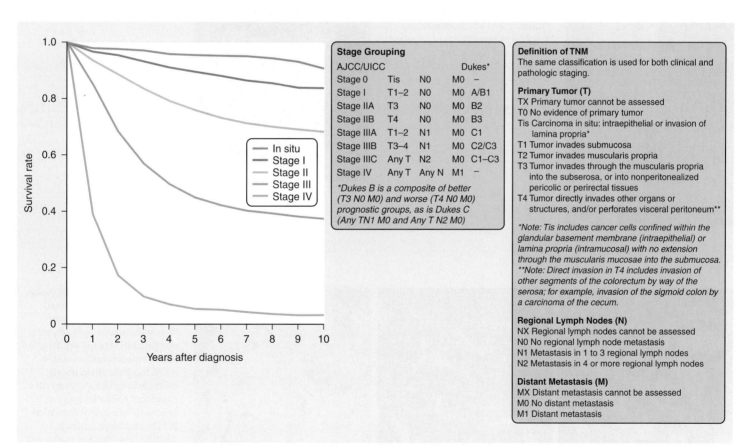

Stage Grouping				
AJCC/UICC				Dukes*
Stage 0	Tis	N0	M0	–
Stage I	T1–2	N0	M0	A/B1
Stage IIA	T3	N0	M0	B2
Stage IIB	T4	N0	M0	B3
Stage IIIA	T1–2	N1	M0	C1
Stage IIIB	T3–4	N1	M0	C2/C3
Stage IIIC	Any T	N2	M0	C1–C3
Stage IV	Any T	Any N	M1	–

*Dukes B is a composite of better (T3 N0 M0) and worse (T4 N0 M0) prognostic groups, as is Dukes C (Any TN1 M0 and Any T N2 M0)

Definition of TNM
The same classification is used for both clinical and pathologic staging.

Primary Tumor (T)
TX Primary tumor cannot be assessed
T0 No evidence of primary tumor
Tis Carcinoma in situ: intraepithelial or invasion of lamina propria*
T1 Tumor invades submucosa
T2 Tumor invades muscularis propria
T3 Tumor invades through the muscularis propria into the subserosa, or into nonperitonealized pericolic or perirectal tissues
T4 Tumor directly invades other organs or structures, and/or perforates visceral peritoneum**

*Note: Tis includes cancer cells confined within the glandular basement membrane (intraepithelial) or lamina propria (intramucosal) with no extension through the muscularis mucosae into the submucosa.
**Note: Direct invasion in T4 includes invasion of other segments of the colorectum by way of the serosa; for example, invasion of the sigmoid colon by a carcinoma of the cecum.

Regional Lymph Nodes (N)
NX Regional lymph nodes cannot be assessed
N0 No regional lymph node metastasis
N1 Metastasis in 1 to 3 regional lymph nodes
N2 Metastasis in 4 or more regional lymph nodes

Distant Metastasis (M)
MX Distant metastasis cannot be assessed
M0 No distant metastasis
M1 Distant metastasis

FIGURE 7.103 **TNM STAGING OF COLORECTAL CANCER.** Graph shows relative survival rates of patients with colon cancer according to the stage of disease. Rates based on 111,110 patients. Data taken from the Surveillance, Epidemiology and End Results Program of the National Cancer Institute for the years 1973 to 1987. Patients were staged according to the current TNM. Stage 0 (in situ) includes 4,841 patients; Stage I, 19,623; Stage II, 33,798; Stage III, 29,615; and Stage IV, 23,233. (From Greene FL, Page D, Fleming I, et al, editors, for the American Joint Committee on Cancer: *AJCC cancer staging handbook*, ed 6, New York, 2002, Springer.)

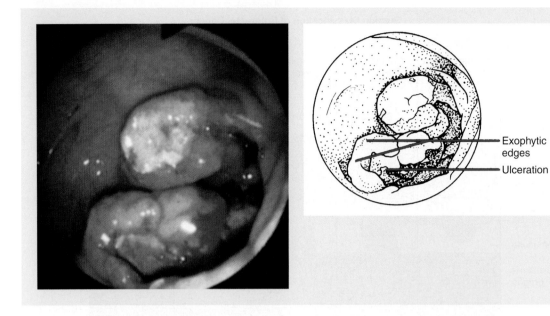

FIGURE 7.104 ADENOCARCINOMA OF CECUM. Endoscopic view shows tumor presenting as a centrally excavated mass with exophytic overhanging edges. The ulceration is typically irregular, deep, and gray or pink, with a necrotic appearance.

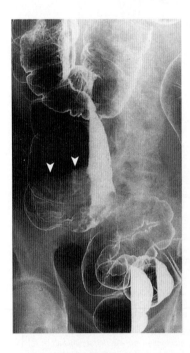

FIGURE 7.105 ADENOCARCINOMA OF CECUM. Intestinal obstruction occurs late in the course of the disease. Although this lesion (*arrowheads*) is relatively large, there was no obstruction to retrograde filling of the ileum and no dilatation of the small intestine. Symptoms may include anemia or dyspepsia and weight loss reminiscent of a benign or malignant gastric ulcer.

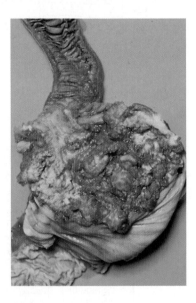

FIGURE 7.106 ADENOCARCINOMA OF CECUM. Large, fungating tumors, as seen here, are a less common presentation of colorectal tumors; they predominate in the cecum.

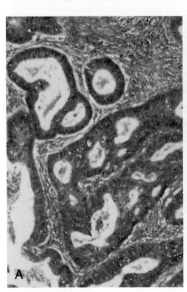
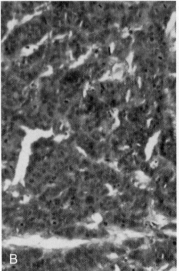
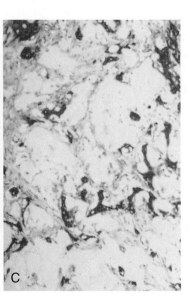

FIGURE 7.107 ADENOCARCINOMA. **(A)** Moderately differentiated tumors are marked by gland (acinar) formation by malignant epithelium; there is considerable nuclear pleomorphism within individual cells. **(B)** In poorly differentiated lesions, sheets of malignant epithelial cells can be seen with little acinar formation. **(C)** The mucinous (colloid) variant shows nests of malignant epithelium in pools of mucin.

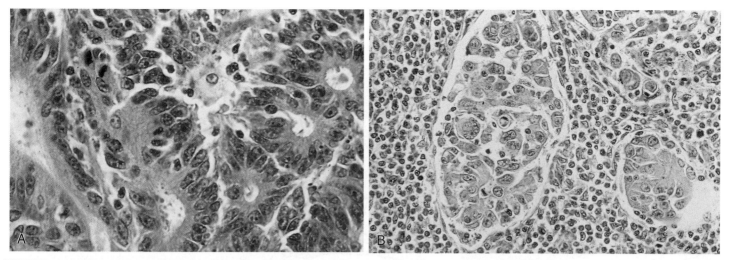

FIGURE 7.108 **ADENOCARCINOMA. (A)** High-power view of a moderately differentiated tumor shows irregular and hyperchromatic nuclei, prominent nucleoli, and several mitoses. **(B)** Metastases are evident in this lymph node biopsy specimen.

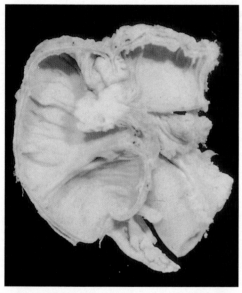

FIGURE 7.109 **ADENOCARCINOMA OF ASCENDING COLON.** This specimen is from a 57-year-old man who presented with a 1-year history of right upper quadrant abdominal pain. Examination revealed a tender mass beneath the right costal margin, and barium enema film showed a tumor just proximal to the hepatic flexure. A right hemicolectomy was performed. The distal ileum, cecum, and ascending colon have been opened to show an annular, stenosing neoplasm at the hepatic flexure; the bowel lumen has been reduced to a narrow cleft. Proximally there is obvious dilatation of the intestine, with some associated muscle hypertrophy.

FIGURE 7.110 **ADENOCARCINOMA OF SIGMOID COLON.** Barium enema film shows an annular stenosing lesion of the distal sigmoid, producing a characteristic "apple core" appearance.

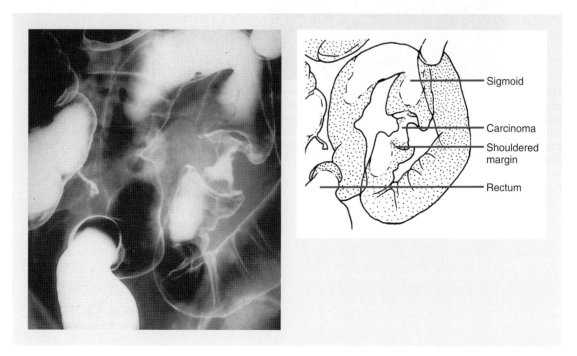

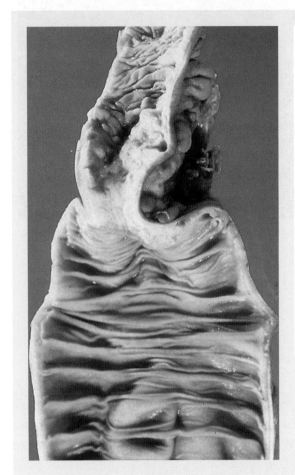

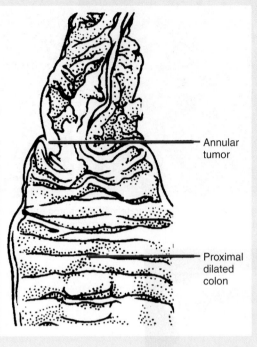

Annular
tumor

Proximal
dilated
colon

FIGURE 7.111 **ADENOCARCINOMA OF COLON.** This specimen shows an annular, stenosing lesion with dilatation of the colon proximal to it. This appearance may be seen at any site and is facilitated by circumferential spread of the tumor through submucosal (or serosal) lymphatic channels.

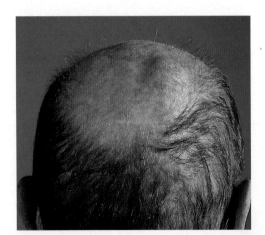

FIGURE 7.112 **METASTATIC COLON CANCER.** A 60-year-old man with previous colectomy for stage III colon cancer 4 years earlier developed a nodule on his posterior scalp. Biopsy was positive for poorly differentiated adenocarcinoma, similar to the original cancer. Carcinoembryonic antigen concentration was elevated at 50 ng/mL. Subsequent studies showed multiple liver metastases. Metastases to skin are not common but have been reported in colon, pancreatic, breast, and lung cancers as well as miscellaneous other malignancies.

FIGURE 7.113 ADENOCARCINOMA OF RECTUM. This lower rectal lesion demonstrates the most common macroscopic appearance of colorectal cancers as well-circumscribed lesions with raised edges and an ulcerated center.

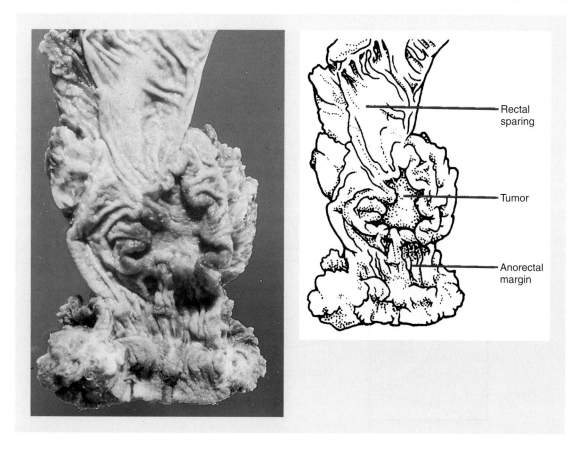

Rectal sparing

Tumor

Anorectal margin

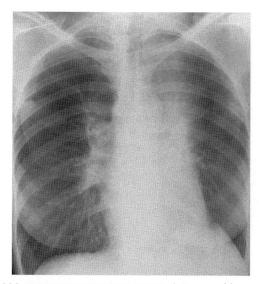

FIGURE 7.114 METASTATIC COLORECTAL CANCER. A 34-year-old woman with prior anteroposterior resection for a stage II rectal cancer 3 years earlier presented with clinical features of superior vena cava syndrome. Chest radiograph showed mediastinal adenopathy and atelactatic changes in the left upper lobe. Chest CT scan and nuclide flow studies (not shown) revealed tumor obstruction of the superior vena cava. Mediastinoscopy was positive for adenocarcinoma with features similar to the original rectal carcinoma. Bronchoscopy showed no intrinsic lesions. Radiation therapy resulted in a partial remission. Liver metastases eventually occurred. Metastatic colorectal carcinoma may spread to the lungs and mediastinum and bypass the liver as a result of lymphatic spread via the paravertebral vascular channels of Batson as well as lower pelvic collaterals.

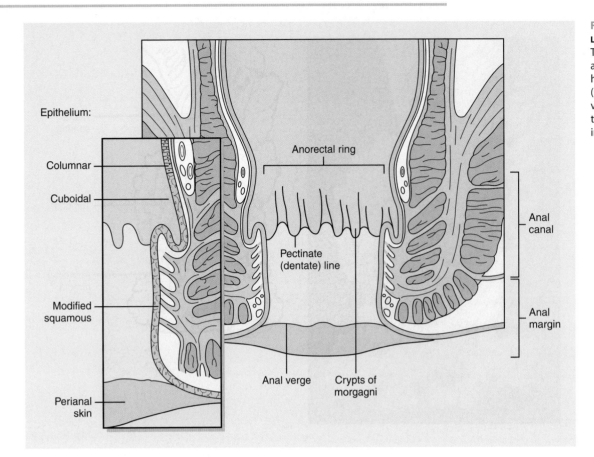

Epithelium:

Columnar

Cuboidal

Modified squamous

Perianal skin

Anorectal ring

Pectinate (dentate) line

Anal verge

Crypts of morgagni

Anal canal

Anal margin

FIGURE 7.115 ANATOMY OF THE LOWER RECTUM AND ANAL CANAL. The anal canal extends from the anorectal ring to an area about halfway between the dentate (pectinate) line and the anal verge. The anal margin consists of the area distal to the anal canal, including the perianal skin.

Definition of TNM

Primary Tumor (T)

TX	Primary tumor cannot be assessed
T0	No evidence of primary tumor
Tis	Carcinoma in situ
T1	Tumor 2 cm or less in greatest dimension
T2	Tumor more than 2 cm, but not more than 5 cm in greatest dimension
T3	Tumor more than 5 cm in greatest dimension
T4	Tumor of any size invades adjacent organ(s), e.g., vagina, urethra, bladder (involvement of sphincter muscles(s) alone is not classified as T4)

Regional Lymph Nodes (N)

NX	Regional lymph nodes cannot be assessed
N0	No regional lymph node metastasis
N1	Metastasis in perirectal lymph node(s)
N2	Metastasis in unilateral iliac and/or inguinal lymph node(s)
N3	Metastasis in perirectal and inguinal lymph nodes and/or bilateral internal iliac and/or inguinal lymph nodes

Distant Metastasis (M)

MX	Presence of distant metastasis cannot be assessed
M0	No distant metastasis
M1	Distant metastasis

Stage grouping

Stage	T	N	M
Stage 0	Tis	N0	M0
Stage I	T1	N0	M0
Stage II	T2	N0	M0
	T3	N0	M0
Stage IIIA	T1	N1	M0
	T2	N1	M0
	T3	N1	M0
	T4	N0	M0
Stage IIIB	T4	N1	M0
	Any T	N2	M0
	Any T	N3	M0
Stage IV	Any T	Any N	M1

FIGURE 7.116 STAGING OF CANCER OF THE ANAL CANAL. The staging system applies to all carcinomas arising in the anal canal, including carcinomas that arise within anorectal fistulae. The classification also includes cloacogenic carcinomas. Melanomas are excluded. (From Greene FL, Page D, Fleming I, et al, editors, for the American Joint Committee on Cancer: *AJCC cancer staging handbook*, ed 6, New York, 2002, Springer.)

FIGURE 7.117 PAGET'S DISEASE OF PERIANAL SKIN. Extramammary Paget's disease is an intraepithelial adenocarcinoma, whereas Bowen's disease is an intraepithelial squamous cell carcinoma. Any abnormal skin in the perianal area should be biopsied to establish the diagnosis and should not be assumed to represent eczema or psoriasis.

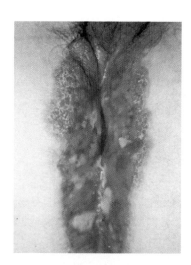

FIGURE 7.118 EXTRAMAMMARY PAGET'S DISEASE. Histologic section of anal tissue shows nests of malignant cells within the epidermis.

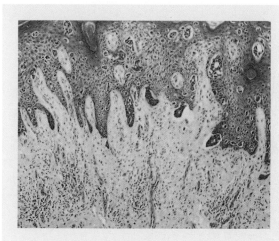
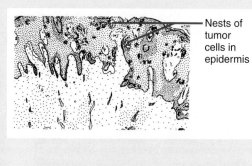

Nests of tumor cells in epidermis

FIGURE 7.119 SQUAMOUS CELL CARCINOMA OF ANAL MARGIN. Squamous cancers of the anus are divided into tumors arising in the anal canal (most often above the dentate line) and those arising in the skin at the anal margin, as shown here. This lesion measures 1 cm across. Neoplasms at this site tend to be slow-growing and metastasize to inguinal lymph nodes. They have a 5-year survival rate of approximately 70%.

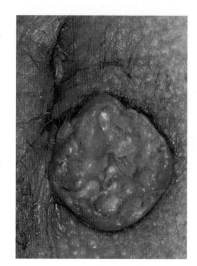

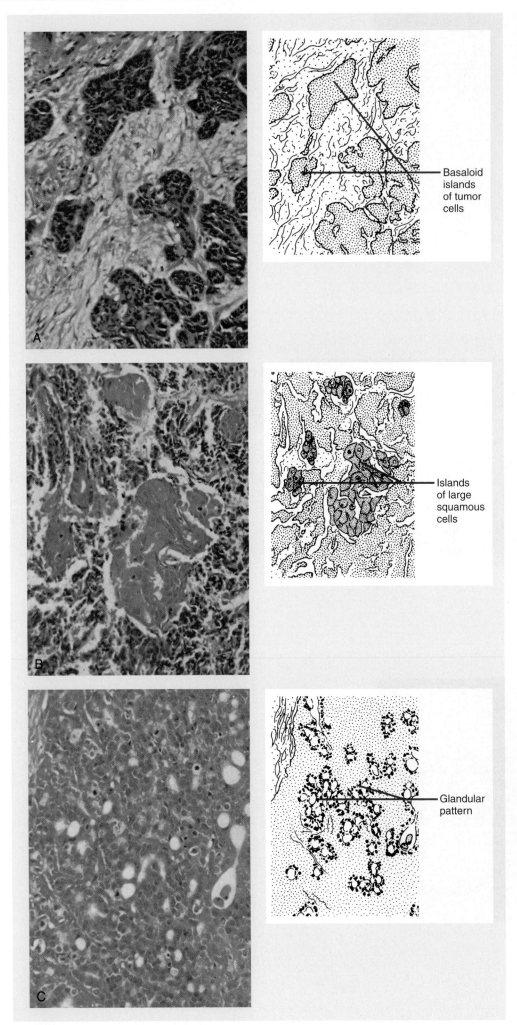

FIGURE 7.120 CARCINOMA OF ANAL CANAL. Besides pure squamous tumors, a range of histologic patterns may be observed from **(A)** basaloid through **(B)** squamous to **(C)** glandular.

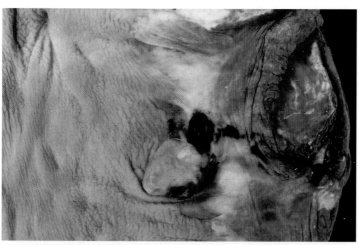

FIGURE 7.121 MALIGNANT MELANOMA OF ANAL CANAL. This specimen is from a 74-year-old woman who presented with a brief history of episodic rectal bleeding. A hard mass was palpable in the lateral wall of the anal canal, and an abdominoperineal resection was performed. The anal canal has been opened to show a flattened, ovoid nodule (2 cm in diameter) arising at about the level of the dentate line. The edge of the tumor shows obvious melanotic pigmentation, and an irregular streak of pigment extends from the nodule to the anal margin. Anorectal melanoma is rare, accounting for about 1% of anal cancers.

Table 7.4		
Classification of Colonic Polyps		
Type	**Histopathology**	**Associated Diseases**
Neoplastic	Adenoma	None (sporadic)
	Tubular adenoma	Familial adenomatous polyposis
	Tubulovillous adenoma	Gardner's syndrome
	Villous adenoma	Turcot syndrome
Non-neoplastic	Hyperplastic polyp	None (sporadic)
		Hyperplastic polyposis
	Hamartomatous polyp	None (sporadic)
		Peutz-Jeghers syndrome
	Inflammatory fibroid polyp	None (sporadic)
	Inflammatory pseudopolyp	Ulcerative colitis, Crohn's disease
		Ischemic colitis
		Infection (amebiasis, schistosomiasis)
		Ulceration
	Juvenile polyp	None (sporadic)
		Juvenile polyposis syndrome
		Cronkhite-Canada syndrome
		None (incidental, reactive)
		Lymphoid polyposis
	Lymphoid polyp	

References and Suggested Readings

Astler VB, Coller FA: The prognostic significance of direct extension of carcinoma of the colon and rectum, *Ann Surg* 139:846–851, 1954.

Barclay T, Schapira D: Malignant tumors of the small intestine, *Cancer* 51:878–881, 1983.

Burke A, Thomas R, Elsayed A, et al: Carcinoids of the jejunum and ileum: an immunohistochemical and clinicopathologic study of 167 cases, *Cancer* 79:1086–1093, 1997.

Chow WH, Blot WJ, Vaughan TL, et al: Body mass index and risk of adenocarcinomas of the esophagus and gastric cardia, *J Natl Cancer Inst* 90:150–155, 1998.

Colli A, Fraquelli M, Casazza G, et al: Accuracy of ultrasonography, spiral CT, magnetic resonance, and alpha-fetoprotein in diagnosing hepatocellular carcinoma: a systematic review, *Am J Gastroenterol* 101:513–523, 2006.

Cunningham D, Allum WH, Stenning SP, et al: MAGIC Trial Participants: perioperative chemotherapy versus surgery alone for resectable gastroesophageal cancer, *N Engl J Med* 355:11–20, 2006.

Dukes CE: Cancer of the rectum — An analysis of 1,000 cases, *J Pathol Bacteriol* 50:527–539, 1940.

Eckhauser F, Argenta L, Strodl W, et al: Mesenteric angiopathy, intestinal gangrene, and midgut carcinoids, *Surgery* 90:720–728, 1981.

Engel LS, Chow WH, Vaughan TL, et al: Population attributable risks of esophageal and gastric cancers, *J Natl Cancer Inst* 95:1404–1413, 2003.

Enzinger PC, Mayer RJ: Esophageal cancer, *N Engl J Med* 349:2241–2252, 2003.

Fearon ER, Vogelstein B: A genetic model for colorectal tumorigenesis, *Cell* 61:759–767, 1990.

Giovannucci E: Diet, body weight, and colorectal cancer: a summary of the epidemiologic evidence, *J Womens Health (Larchmt)* 12:173–182, 2003.

Giovannucci E, Michaud D: The role of obesity and related metabolic disturbances in cancers of the colon, prostate, and pancreas, *Gastroenterology* 132:2208–2225, 2007.

Gore RM, Mehta UK, Berlin JW, et al: Diagnosis and staging of small bowel tumours, *Cancer Imaging* 6:209–212, 2006.

Greene FL, Page D, Fleming I, et al, editors, for the American Joint Committee on Cancer: *AJCC cancer staging handbook*, ed 6, New York, 2002, Springer.

Greene FL, Stewart AK, Norton HJ: A new TNM staging strategy for node-positive (stage III) colon cancer: an analysis of 50,042 patients, *Ann Surg* 236:416–421, 2002.

Hellman P, Lundstrom T, Ohrvall U, et al: Effect of surgery on the outcome of midgut carcinoid disease with lymph node and liver metastases, *World J Surg* 26:991–997, 2002.

Hendriks YM, de Jong AE, Morreau H, et al: Diagnostic approach and management of Lynch syndrome (hereditary nonpolyposis colorectal carcinoma): a guide for clinicians, *CA Cancer J Clin* 56:213–225, 2006.

Jänne PA, Mayer RJ: Chemoprevention of colorectal cancer, *N Engl J Med* 342:1960–1968, 2000.

Kamangar F, Dawsey SM, Blaser MJ, et al: Opposing risks of gastric cardia and noncardia gastric adenocarcinomas associated with *Helicobacter pylori* seropositivity, *J Natl Cancer Inst* 98:1445–1452, 2006.

Kaurah P, MacMillan A, Boyd N, et al: Founder and recurrent CDH1 mutations in families with hereditary diffuse gastric cancer, *JAMA* 297:2360–2372, 2007.

Krok KL, Lichtenstein GR: Colorectal cancer in inflammatory bowel disease, *Curr Opin Gastroenterol*, 20:43–48, 2004.

Kulke MH: Clinical presentation and management of carcinoid tumors, *Hematol Oncol Clin North Am* 21:433–455, 2007.

Kulke MH: Neuroendocrine tumours: clinical presentation and management of localized disease, *Cancer Treat Rev* 29:363–370, 2003.

Kulke MH, Fuchs CS: Cancer of the small bowel and appendix. In Ragharan D, editor:*Textbook of uncommon cancer*, ed 3, Sussex, England, 2006, John Wiley & Sons, pp 410–417.

Kulke MH, Mayer RJ: Carcinoid tumors, *N Engl J Med* 340:858–868, 1999.

Kulke MH, Rait CP: Neuroendocrine tumors of the gastrointestinal tract. In Kelsen D, Daly JM, Kern SE, editors: *Gastrointestinal oncology: principles and practice*, ed 2, New York, Lippincott, Williams & Wilkins, 2006, pp 873–898.

Lowenfels AB, Maisonneuve P: Epidemiology and risk factors for pancreatic cancer, *Best Pract Res Clin Gastroenterol* 20:197–209, 2006.

Lynch HT, de la Chapelle A: Hereditary colorectal cancer, *N Engl J Med* 348:919–932, 2003.

Macdonald JS, Smalley SR, Benedetti J, et al: Chemoradiotherapy after surgery compared with surgery alone for adenocarcinoma of the stomach or gastroesophageal junction, *N Engl J Med* 345:725–730, 2001.

Makridis C, Oberg K, Juhlin C, et al: Surgical treatment of mid-gut carcinoid tumors, *World J Surg* 14:377–385, 1990.

Meyerhardt JA, Mayer RJ: Systemic therapy for colorectal cancer, *N Engl J Med* 352:476–487, 2005.

Modlin I, Lye K, Kidd M: A 5-decade analysis of 13,715 carcinoid tumors, *Cancer* 97:934–959, 2003.

Moertel C, Sauer W, Dockerty M, et al: Life history of the carcinoid tumor of the small intestine, *Cancer* 14:901–912, 1961.

Nelson H, Petrelli N, Carlin A, et al: Guidelines 2000 for colon and rectal cancer surgery, *J Natl Cancer Inst* 93:583–596, 2001.

O'Connell, JB, Maggard MA, Ko CY: Colon cancer survival rates with the new American Joint Committee on Cancer sixth edition staging, *J Natl Cancer Inst* 96:1420–1425, 2004.

Raza SA, Clifford GM, Franceschi S: Worldwide variation in the relative importance of hepatitis B and hepatitis C viruses in hepatocellular carcinoma: a systematic review, *Br J Cancer* 96:1127–1134, 2007.

Ryan DP, Compton CC, Mayer RJ: Carcinoma of the anal canal, *N Engl J Med* 342:792–800, 2000.

Shaheen N, Ransohoff DF: Gastroesophageal reflux, Barrett esophagus, and esophageal cancer: clinical applications, *JAMA* 287:1982–1986, 2002.

Singh P, Patel T: Advances in the diagnosis, evaluation and management of cholangiocarcinoma, *Curr Opin Gastroenterol* 22:294–299, 2006.

Sultana A, Tudur Smith C, Cunningham D, et al: Systematic review, including meta-analyses, on the management of locally advanced pancreatic cancer using radiation/combined modality therapy, *Br J Cancer* 96:1183–1190, 2007.

Uemura N, Okamoto S, Yamamoto S, et al: *Helicobacter pylori* infection and the development of gastric cancer, *N Engl J Med* 345:784–789, 2001.

Urschel JD, Vasan H: A meta-analysis of randomized controlled trials that compared neoadjuvant chemoradiation and surgery to surgery alone for resectable esophageal cancer, *Am J Surg* 185:538–543, 2003.

Wanebo HJ, Kennedy BJ, Chmiel J, et al: Cancer of the stomach: a patient care study by the American College of Surgeons, *Ann Surg* 218:583–592, 1993.

Wang WH, Huang JQ, Zheng GF, et al: Non-steroidal anti-inflammatory drug use and the risk of gastric cancer: a systematic review and meta-analysis, *J Natl Cancer Inst* 95:1784–1791, 2003.

Wei EK, Giovannucci E, Wu K, et al: Comparison of risk factors for colon and rectal cancer, *Int J Cancer* 108:433–442, 2004.

Ye W, Held M, Lagergren J, et al: *Helicobacter pylori* infection and gastric atrophy: risk of adenocarcinoma and squamous-cell carcinoma of the esophagus and adenocarcinoma of the gastric cardia, *J Natl Cancer Inst* 96:388–396, 2004.

Zhu AX: Systemic therapy of advanced hepatocellular carcinoma: how hopeful should we be? *Oncologist* 11:790–800, 2006.

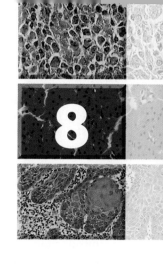

Cancer of the Genitourinary Tract

WILLIAM K. OH • ROBERT ROSS • TONI K. CHOUEIRI • PHILIP W. KANTOFF • CHRISTOPHER CORLESS

Prostate Cancer

Prostate cancer is the most commonly diagnosed noncutaneous malignancy in men in the United States. In 2007, over 218,000 cases will be diagnosed and over 27,000 men will die of the disease. The incidence of prostate cancer increased rapidly in the early 1990s because of the widespread use of the prostate-specific antigen (PSA) test, but subsequently leveled off in the late 1990s. Mortality from prostate cancer has also begun to decline recently, although the cause for this drop is not known.

The incidence of prostate cancer increases rapidly with age, particularly after the age of 50, although the presence of pathologic prostate cancer in men younger than 50 years of age has been demonstrated in autopsy series. Age, race, and family history are the most well established risk factors for prostate cancer. Scandinavians and Americans, and particularly African Americans, have a very high incidence of prostate cancer as compared with Asian men. The results of studies including men who migrate from areas of low incidence to areas of high incidence and acquire intermediate probabilities of developing prostate cancer suggest that environmental factors contribute to these differences. One such factor may be the high-fat diet of the Western developed world. Another potential risk factor may be serum hormone levels, particularly testosterone, although such data are controversial. Recent data from a clinical trial of 5α-reductase (the enzyme that converts testosterone to dihydrotestosterone) support the idea that alterations of the androgen milieu can alter the short-term risk of the development of prostate cancer.

A subset of patients who develop prostate cancer probably do so on the basis of genetic predisposition. Familial prostate cancer may be an important factor among patients who develop prostate cancer at a young age. First-degree relatives of men with prostate cancer have a two- to threefold increased risk of developing prostate cancer compared with the general population. Such data have led to a search for genetic loci that confer an increased risk of prostate cancer, including one on the long arm of chromosome 1 called *HPC1*. Many studies are now evaluating potential candidate genes within this locus, including *RNASEL*, which encodes an enzyme that regulates cell proliferation.

HISTOLOGY

The vast majority of prostate cancers are adenocarcinomas. Most exhibit acinar-type differentiation, but some also have features of ductal differentiation. Pure large duct prostatic adenocarcinomas are uncommon. Typical prostatic adenocarcinomas may contain foci of mucinous differentiation or neuroendocrine differentiation, but the prognostic significance of these features remains uncertain. Small cell undifferentiated carcinoma of the prostate is rare but when present is often associated with areas of adenocarcinoma. Whether presenting in pure form or intermixed with adenocarcinoma, small cell undifferentiated carcinoma in the prostate carries a grave prognosis. Other tumors occurring in the prostate include transitional cell carcinoma (most often by invasion from the urethra), sarcomas of stromal origin, and metastases from other organs.

The putative precursor of invasive adenocarcinoma is prostatic intraepithelial neoplasia (PIN), in which cytologically dysplastic cells are found lining normal ducts and acini. PIN is divided into low and high grades; however, only the latter is geographically associated with invasive adenocarcinoma. Although the natural history of PIN is unknown, many foci of high-grade PIN demonstrate partial loss of the basal cell layer, and a transition to small invasive glands is occasionally observed. A diagnosis of high-grade PIN on needle biopsy should prompt additional studies to rule out invasive tumor.

Small foci of adenocarcinoma are found incidentally at autopsy in more than 30% of men over the age of 50 who die of unrelated causes. Thus, there is a large pool of these so-called latent or "autopsy" prostate cancers present in the older male population. Whether clinical cancers arise from latent tumors or develop by an independent pathway is unknown.

Although a variety of grading schemes for prostate cancer have been developed, the most widely used in the United States is the Gleason grading system, which is based strictly upon architectural rather than cytologic features of the cancer. According to this scheme, the pattern of infiltrating tumor glands is assigned a grade from 1 (well differentiated) to 5 (poorly differentiated). Because many adenocarcinomas show more than one pattern, the grades for the two most common patterns present in a tumor are added together to give a Gleason sum or Gleason score. The prognostic utility of the Gleason grading system has been validated in numerous studies wherein patients diagnosed with low Gleason score cancers have an excellent prognosis, whereas those with high Gleason score cancers have a poor prognosis. The main shortcoming of the Gleason grading system is that the majority of cancers are intermediate in grade. Less than 30% of cancers in most studies are within the Gleason score 2–4 or 8–10 groups. As a result, the Gleason score provides little prognostic information in most cases.

Tissue staining for PSA has become an important adjunct to confirming the diagnosis of prostate cancer. This is particularly useful in poorly differentiated cancers or those cancers that manifest themselves initially at metastatic sites as poorly differentiated carcinoma.

DIAGNOSIS AND STAGING OF PROSTATE CANCER

The detection of prostate cancer has been greatly enhanced by the introduction of the PSA test. Optimal detection of prostate cancer is now achieved through the combination of the digital rectal examination (DRE) and PSA. Biopsies are facilitated by transrectal ultrasound, which allows the physician to locate the areas of abnormality. The morbidity from biopsy is now minimal with the use of spring-loaded biopsy guns. Optimal information is acquired when multiple specially coordinated biopsies are performed. With such biopsies, the grade of the cancer, the number of cores positive for cancer, and the percentage of cancer per core should be determined.

A bone scan should be performed after the diagnosis of prostate cancer is made, particularly in men with a PSA in excess of 20 ng/mL or high Gleason grade disease (Gleason scores of 8–10). Although the incidence of radiographically detected regional lymph nodes is quite low, scanning by computed tomography (CT) or magnetic resonance imaging (MRI) should be considered, particularly in patients with high-grade, high-stage cancers or in those with high PSA serum levels. Recent techniques with newer MRI contrast agents (lymphotrophic nanoparticle-enhanced MRI) may help identify regional lymph node involvement. Endorectal coil MRI should be performed at experienced centers in patients being considered for radical prostatectomy in whom it is necessary to assess the extent of local disease. With the widespread use of PSA, the proportion of localized prostate cancers has increased.

Approximately 80% of cancers arising in the prostate gland arise in the peripheral zones, whereas 20% arise in the periurethral, or transition, zone. Cancers arising in the transition zone traditionally had been diagnosed by transurethral resection of the prostate. However, with increasing use of PSA and of medical therapies for benign prostatic hyperplasia, the frequency of cancers diagnosed in this manner has diminished.

Two systems are commonly used for staging of prostate cancer: the Whitmore-Jewett system (stages A through D) and the American Joint Committee on Cancer (AJCC) tumor/node/metastases (TNM) system last modified in 2002 (see Fig. 8.11). The AJCC TNM system is used more commonly now.

The majority of cancers that are currently diagnosed are detected as a result of an abnormal PSA or DRE, or both. Organ-confined, palpable cancers are classified as T2 (see Fig. 8.11). Cancers diagnosed strictly on the basis of an abnormal PSA with no associated palpable abnormality are currently classified as T1c. Cancers that on physical examination extend into the seminal vesicles or palpably extend beyond the prostate are categorized as T3 cancers. Stage IV cancers are those that have metastasized either to regional lymph nodes (N1) or distant lymph nodes, bone, or viscera (M1) (see Fig. 8.11).

Careful examination of the prostate following its removal at the time of radical prostatectomy provides critical prognostic information. There is good correlation between the grade of cancer found at the time of biopsy and that found at the time of radical prostatectomy; when discrepancy occurs the biopsy results most frequently undergrade the cancer. With careful examination of the prostate, the volume of cancer can be ascertained, as can the degree of local extension. Cancers that are confined within the capsule are less likely to recur than those that invade through the capsule or into the seminal vesicle or demonstrate positive margins. Clinically localized tumors are frequently upstaged into T3 cancers pathologically. The frequency of lymph node involvement at the time of radical prostatectomy has apparently decreased in recent years, perhaps in part because of the more careful selection of surgical patients afforded by the use of the PSA.

CLINICAL MANIFESTATIONS

Most patients diagnosed with prostate cancer are asymptomatic, and the diagnosis is made as a result of an abnormal PSA or DRE. Because the prevalence of benign prostatic hyperplasia in the population of men susceptible to prostate cancer is high, many men will manifest mild degrees of prostatism. With locally advanced prostate cancer, urinary obstruction may occur, as may hematospermia. Carcinoma should be considered when obstructive urinary symptomatology develops over a short period of time. Some patients initially present with symptoms of metastatic disease either from painful bony metastasis or from lymphadenopathy. In such patients, immunostaining for PSA may be of particular value in distinguishing a carcinoma of prostatic origin.

Bladder Cancer

Over 60,000 new cases of bladder cancer are diagnosed in the United States each year, with over 13,000 deaths attributable to this disease (Jemal et al., 2007). Bladder cancer generally arises as a result of exposure to environmental carcinogens. In the United States the most important carcinogen is cigarette smoke, contributing to at least 50% of cases. On a worldwide basis, environmental toxins and *Schistosoma haematobium* have a more significant role. Specific genetic abnormalities have been delineated in association with bladder cancer. Monosomy 9 is frequently associated with superficial papillary transitional cell carcinomas. Tumors associated with a higher malignant potential frequently contain abnormalities on chromosome 17p, including *TP53* abnormalities. On the other hand, tumors with fibroblast growth factor receptor 3 (*FGFR3*) mutations have a much better prognosis and are unlikely to progress to muscle invasive disease (Hernandez et al., 2006).

HISTOLOGY

Ninety percent of bladder cancers are transitional cell carcinomas, also known as urothelial carcinomas. These are designated grade 1 (well differentiated) to grade 3 (poorly differentiated), although in recent staging, tumors are designated simply as low grade or high grade. They often show a papillary architecture when presenting as superficial lesions. High-grade tumors may be localized within the bladder but are sometimes associated with widespread transitional cell carcinoma in situ. Alternatively, patients may present with carcinoma in situ in the absence of grossly recognizable tumor. Both high-grade papillary lesions and carcinoma in situ are associated with a substantial risk for developing muscularis invasion. Some transitional cell carcinomas show areas of squamous or adenocarcinomatous differentiation, the significance of which is uncertain. Pure squamous cell carcinomas and adenocarcinomas of the bladder are much less common than transitional cell carcinomas but are less responsive to therapy.

STAGING OF BLADDER CANCER

Because bladder cancer can metastasize rapidly, sometimes even before symptoms become apparent, staging studies in a patient with this diagnosis are imperative. Chest films, radionuclide bone scanning, tests of liver and renal function, and CT scans are all valuable.

Standard staging systems have been based on intravenous urography, bimanual examination, and transurethral resection. At present, two systems are used: the Jewett-Strong-Marshall (JSM) system and the AJCC system (see Fig. 8.30). Both classify bladder cancers as superficial, invasive, or metastatic. Superficial disease is limited to the mucosa or submucosa (JSM stages O and A or AJCC Ta and T1); this is the most common form of bladder cancer. Lesions that extend through the submucosa and into the muscularis are classified as invasive bladder cancer. These include lesions that involve superficial or deep muscles (JSM stages B1 and B2 or AJCC T2a and T2b). Although it was formerly believed that the depth of muscle invasion (superficial vs deep) was most important, it now seems that the presence of any muscle involvement is prognostically significant. Almost 50% of patients with muscle invasion eventually die of disease, usually associated with distant metastases. Stages III (T3, T4) and IV (N+) denote lesions invading the perivesicular fat and extending beyond it, respectively.

CLINICAL MANIFESTATIONS

The most common symptom of bladder cancer is painless hematuria. Carcinoma in situ can cause symptoms of urinary tract irritation. Endoscopically the bladder mucosa may appear normal; a definitive diagnosis can be established only after a urinary cytologic specimen or a mucosal biopsy specimen is obtained and examined. Urinary obstruction caused by urethral blockage and pain secondary to metastatic disease occur occasionally but are relatively uncommon initial manifestations. Sites of metastases include the liver, lung, lymphatic system, and bones.

Kidney Cancer

In 2007, over 50,000 new cases of kidney cancer will be diagnosed in the United States, resulting in 12,900 deaths (Jemal et al., 2007). Renal cell carcinomas (RCCs), which originate within the renal cortex, constitute 85% to 90% of primary renal neoplasms. Transitional cell carcinomas of the renal pelvis are the next most common kidney cancer subtype (~8%). In the past, RCC was frequently diagnosed when symptoms arose from local extension of disease, metastases, or a variety of paraneoplastic phenomena. However, an increasing proportion of patients are currently diagnosed as a result of an incidental finding on noninvasive radiologic examination performed for other reasons. This change in the pattern of presentation may have contributed to better outcomes in RCC (Gudbjartsson et al., 2005). In the last 5 years, significant progress has been made in understanding the biology of clear cell kidney cancer (the most common histologic subtype), which has led to many treatment advances, particularly the use of anti-angiogenic drugs (Motzer et al., 2007; Escudier et al., 2007).

HISTOLOGY

RCCs constitute a group of heterogeneous tumors (adenocarcinomas) arising from the epithelium of the renal tubules. These tumors have unique pathologic, cytogenetic, and molecular characteristics. They also have distinct biologic behavior, clinical manifestations, and therapeutic response. The current classification, published by the World Health Organization in 2004 (Table 8.1), is based on histomorphology, presumptive histogenic origin, and cytogenetic and molecular characteristics of the renal tumors.

Clear cell carcinoma is by far the most common type of RCC and arises from the proximal tubules. It typically has a deletion in the short arm of chromosome 3, often in the area of the von Hippel-Lindau (VHL) gene. The product of this gene, the VHL protein, plays a crucial role in the "hypoxia-inducible pathway." It forms with several proteins a complex that has ubiquitin ligase activity and targets cellular proteins for ubiquitin-mediated degradation by proteasomes. One of the substrates is hypoxia-inducible factor (HIF), a heterodimeric transcription factor critical for the expression of hypoxia-inducible genes. Under normal conditions, the two isoforms of HIF, HIF1α and HIF2α, are hydroxylated on one of the proline residues. VHL proteins can then bind to and target the hydroxylated HIF for polyubiquitination and eventual degradation. Under hypoxic conditions, or when VHL is mutated or absent, HIF cannot bind to VHL and therefore is not directed for degradation. As the result, HIF accumulates within the cell and activates many hypoxia-inducible genes, such as vascular endothelial growth factor (VEGF), platelet-derived growth factor, and others (Kim, 2003), leading to tumor growth and invasion. Microscopically, tumor cells have "clear" cytoplasm due to the loss of cytoplasmic lipid and glycogen during the processing of the tissue and preparation of slides, although high-grade clear cell RCC often has more eosinophilic and granular cytoplasm. Indicative of a worse prognosis, sarcomatoid differentiation is found in about 5% of the cases.

Papillary RCC (PRCC) is the second most common subtype of RCC. Two types of PRCC are recognized based on the histomorphology. Accounting for about two thirds of PRCCs, type I contains papillae that are lined with a single layer of tumor cells with scant pale cytoplasm and low-grade nuclei. In contrast,

Table 8.1

2004 WHO Classification of Renal Cell Neoplasms

Malignant
Renal cell carcinoma
  Clear cell renal cell carcinoma (75%)
  Multilocular clear cell renal cell carcinoma
  Papillary renal cell carcinoma (105%)
  Chromophobe renal cell carcinoma (5%)
  Carcinoma of the collecting ducts of Bellini
  Renal medullary carcinoma
  Xp11 translocation carcinomas
  Carcinoma associated with neuroblastoma
  Mucinous tubular and spindle cell carcinoma
  Renal cell carcinoma, unclassified

Benign
  Papillary adenoma/renal cortical adenoma
  Oncocytoma (5%)

type II tumor cells have abundant eosinophilic cytoplasm and large pseudostratified nuclei with prominent nucleoli. Type I PRCC has a better prognosis than type II PRCC. Chromosomal gain, including tri- or tetrasomy 7 and 17, and loss of Y chromosome are the most common cytogenetic changes observed in PRCC (Reuter, 2006). On the other hand, papillary adenomas are benign epithelial neoplasms of papillary or tubular architecture, with increased incidence with age, and in patients on long-term dialysis or acquired renal cystic disease.

Chromophobe RCC accounts for approximately 5% of RCCs. It is a malignant tumor characterized by large pale cells with prominent cell membranes and irregular nuclei. The prognosis is significantly better than in clear cell RCC with mortality less than 10%. This subtype shows extensive chromosomal loss, most commonly involving chromosomes 1, 2, 6, 10, 13, 17, and 21 (Reuter, 2006).

Other rare type of RCC include collecting duct and medullary carcinoma (both with very aggressive behavior), oncocytomas (benign tumors), and others (Table 8.1).

Although the majority of RCCs are sporadic in nature, less than 5% of the cases present as part of the inherited cancer syndromes, including VHL syndrome (clear cell RCC), hereditary papillary renal cell carcinoma syndrome, hereditary leiomyomatosis, renal cell cancer (papillary RCC), and Birt-Hogg-Dube syndrome (chromophobe RCC). In general, hereditary cases present at a younger age and are much more likely to be multifocal and bilateral. A comparison of genetic defects between sporadic and hereditary RCC based on histologic appearance is provided in Table 8.2.

STAGING OF KIDNEY CANCER

The most widely used system to assess the extent of invasion and dissemination of RCC is the AJCC staging method that is based upon the TNM classification (Table 8.3). These criteria clearly define the anatomic extent of disease and stage and have been shown to correlate with survival.

The 2002 version of the AJCC staging system separates T1 lesions into T1a (tumors limited to the kidney and <4 cm) and T1b (intrarenal tumors >4 cm and <7 cm) (Greene et al., 2002). This division of T1 reflects the higher rate of survival in patients with T1 tumors smaller than 4 cm and the increasing tendency to use nephron-sparing surgery (such as partial nephrectomy, radiofrequency ablation, cryoablation, and others) in these patients.

Table 8.3

AJCC Kidney Cancer Staging (2002)

Primary Tumor (T)

TX	Primary tumor cannot be assessed.
T0	No evidence of primary tumor
T1	Tumor less than 7 cm in diameter and limited to the kidney
T1a	Tumor 4 cm or less in greatest dimension and limited to kidney
T1b	Tumor more than 4 cm but less than 7 cm, and limited to kidney
T2	Tumor more than 7 cm in greatest dimension limited to the kidney
T3	Tumor extends into major veins or invades the adrenal gland or perinephric tissues, but not beyond Gerota's fascia.
T3a	Tumor directly invades the adrenal gland or perinephric tissues but not beyond Gerota's fascia.
T3b	Tumor grossly extends into the renal vein or its segmental (muscle-containing) branches, or vena cava below the diaphragm.
T3c	Tumor grossly extends into the vena cava above the diaphragm or invades the wall of the vena cava.
T4	Tumor invades beyond Gerota's fascia.

Regional Lymph Nodes (N)

NX	Regional lymph nodes cannot be assessed.
N0	No regional lymph node metastases
N1	Metastasis in a single regional lymph node
N2	Metastases in more than one regional lymph node

Distant Metastasis (M)

MX	Distant metastasis cannot be assessed.
M0	No distant metastasis
M1	Distant metastasis

From Cohen HT, McGovern FJ: Renal-cell Carcinoma, *N Engl J Med* 353:2477–2490, 2005.

CLINICAL MANIFESTATIONS

The classic triad of symptoms—hematuria, flank pain, and abdominal mass—is observed in only about 10% of patients. However, individual symptoms occur in almost half of patients with kidney cancer. A variety of paraneoplastic phenomena can be associated with renal adenocarcinoma, including hypertension and hepatosplenomegaly not caused by metastases.

NOVEL TARGETED AGENTS IN THE TREATMENT OF ADVANCED RENAL CELL CARCINOMA

Although surgery is the mainstay of therapy for RCC in its localized form, advanced disease has been classically treated with

Table 8.2

Sporadic and Hereditary Renal Cell Carcinomas and Genetic Defects According to Histologic Appearance*

	Sporadic Renal Cell Carcinomas			Renal Cell Carcinomas in an Inherited Syndrome	
Histologic Appearance	Incidence (%)	Gene and Frequency (%)		Rare Syndrome*	Gene
Conventional	75	VHL (60)		VHL disease	VHL
				FCRC	Chromosome 3p translocation
				Hereditary paraganglioma	SDHB
Papillary	12	MET (13)		HPRC	MET
		TFE3 (<1)		HLRCC	FH
Chromophobe	4			Birt-Hogg-Dubé syndrome	BHD
Oncocytoma	4			Birt-Hogg-Dubé syndrome	BHD
Collecting duct	<1				
Unclassified	3–5				

FCRC, familial clear cell renal cancer; FH, fumarate hydratase; HLRCC, hereditary leiomyomatosis and renal cell cancer; HPRC, hereditary papillary renal carcinoma; SDHB, succinate dehydrogenase B; VHL, von Hippel–Lindau.
From Cohen HT, McGovern FJ: Renal-cell carcinoma, *N Engl J Med* 353:2477–2490, 2005.
*Additional rare syndromes or infrequent associations are not included.

immunotherapy such as interferon-α and interleukin-2. Responses were modest at best, and long-term disease control was rare. However, over the last few years RCC has become a model disease for targeted therapeutics based on the growing understanding of the underlying molecular pathways in this disease. Clear cell RCC is characterized by the inactivation of the *VHL* tumor suppressor gene, which results in the dysregulation of hypoxia response genes and subsequent promotion of tumor angiogenesis, growth, and metastasis. In advanced RCC substantial clinical activity has been reported with VEGF blockade using a variety of approaches including antibodies (bevacizumab) and small-molecule VEGF receptor inhibitors (sunitinib and sorafenib). These novel agents are replacing immunotherapy as a new standard of care. Several clinical trials are still in progress with the goal of defining the optimal efficacy of these agents as monotherapy or in combination (Choueiri, 2006).

Testicular Cancer

Testicular cancer, which in the United States is diagnosed in over 7000 patients each year, serves as a model of a curable neoplasm. Most patients are young, in their third or fourth decade of life. In patients over the age of 50, testicular neoplasms are usually due to a malignant lymphoma.

HISTOLOGY

Germ cell cancers of the testis can be divided into seminomas and nonseminomas. This distinction is based on the extreme radioresponsiveness of seminomas and their tendency toward localized tissue invasion, as opposed to the tendency of nonseminomas to be more radioresistant and to metastasize via hematogenous routes to the lung or liver. Histologic variants of nonseminoma include embryonal carcinoma, teratoma, choriocarcinoma, and yolk sac tumor (also known as endodermal sinus tumor). Germ cell tumors can also arise from extragonadal sites, including the retroperitoneum and the mediastinum. Mediastinal nonseminomas have a particularly poor prognosis, whereas mediastinal seminomas have a similar prognosis to testicular seminomas.

Fewer than 5% of testicular malignancies originate from the gonadal stroma; these are mainly Leydig cell tumors, which can occur at any age and secrete both testosterone and estradiol, causing sexual precocity in prepubertal boys and gynecomastia in adults. About 10% of Leydig cell tumors metastasize; these demonstrate histologic features of aggressive behavior, such as blood vessel invasion and poor cell differentiation. Sertoli cell tumors are rare (only about 100 cases have been reported) and are also found in all age groups. They may secrete estrogens and thus cause gynecomastia. Metastases occur in 10% to 20% of cases.

Lymphomas, usually of the diffuse large cell type, represent 5% or less of testicular malignancies. They tend to be bilateral and often disseminate, particularly to the central nervous system. Involvement of the testes may occur in systemic lymphomas (about 10% of cases) and in some patients may herald an underlying malignant lymphoma.

STAGING OF TESTICULAR CANCER

The staging evaluation of testicular cancers usually includes an abdominopelvic CT scan and chest radiography; sometimes suspicious abnormalities on a chest film prompt CT scanning of the chest as well. In certain high-risk patients, a bone scan and brain MRI are performed. Stage I nonseminomas are often surgically staged by retroperitoneal lymph node dissection. Circulating biologic markers, such as human chorionic gonadotrophin (β-hCG), lactate dehydrogenase, and α-fetoprotein (AFP), are prognostically important and are useful in following the clinical course.

Cancer confined to the testis, with no clinical, laboratory, or radiologic evidence of distant metastases, constitutes stage I disease (see Fig. 8.69). If there is no disease above the diaphragm but evidence of retroperitoneal adenopathy is demonstrated on CT scan or lymphangiogram, the cancer is classified as stage II disease. Stage III disease is marked by persistence of positive biologic markers after orchidectomy or by subdiaphragmatic visceral involvement (e.g., of the liver, spleen, or inferior vena cava) or supradiaphragmatic metastases to the lung parenchyma or central nervous system. Prognosis can be determined by criteria established by the International Germ Cell Consensus Criteria (Table 8.4).

Table 8.4	
International Germ Cell Consensus Criteria for Testicular Cancer	
Nonseminoma	**Seminoma**
Good Prognosis	
Testis/retroperitoneal primary *and* No nonpulmonary visceral metastases *and* Good markers—all of • AFP < 1000 ng/mL and • hCG < 5000 IU/L (1000 ng/mL) and • LDH < 1.5 × upper limit of normal 58% of nonseminomas 5-year PFS 89% 5-year survival 92%	Any primary site *and* No nonpulmonary visceral metastases *and* Normal AFP, any hCG, any LDH 90% of seminomas 5-year PFS 82% 5-year survival 86%
Intermediate Prognosis	
Testis/retroperitoneal primary *and* No nonpulmonary visceral metastases *and* Intermediate markers—any of • AFP ≥ 1000 and ≤ 10,000 ng/mL or • hCG ≥ 5000 IU/L and ≤ 50,000 IU/L or • LDH ≥ 1.5 × normal and ≤ 10 × normal 28% of nonseminomas 5-year PFS 75% 5-year survival 80%	Any primary site *and* Nonpulmonary visceral metastases *and* Normal AFP, any hCG, any LDH 10% of seminomas 5-year PFS 67% 5-year survival 72%
Poor Prognosis	
Mediastinal primary *or* Nonpulmonary visceral metastases *or* Poor markers—any of • AFP > 10,000 ng/mL or • hCG > 50,000 IU/L (10,000 ng/mL) or • LDH > 10 × upper limit of normal 16% of nonseminomas 5-year PFS 41% 5-year survival 48%	No patients classified as poor prognosis

AFP, α-fetoprotein; hCG, human chorionic gonadotrophin; LDH, lactate dehydrogenase; PFS, progression-free survival.

CLINICAL MANIFESTATIONS

The manifestations of testicular cancer are protean, ranging from detection of an asymptomatic nodule or swelling on self-examination of the testes to the development of symptoms secondary to metastatic disease. Patients who present with a painful lesion in the scrotum are often initially diagnosed and treated for epididymitis before the true diagnosis of cancer is established. Epididymitis often occurs concomitantly in patients with testicular cancer and may explain the associated pain. The sudden, acute appearance of a rapidly enlarging testis, particularly characteristic of choriocarcinoma, is usually associated with hemorrhage into neoplastic tissue. Back or abdominal pain secondary to retroperitoneal adenopathy, dyspnea caused by pulmonary metastases, weight loss, gynecomastia, supraclavicular lymphadenopathy, and urinary obstruction may also be evident at the time of presentation.

Penile Cancer

Cancer of the penis, which occurs almost exclusively in uncircumcised men, is exceedingly uncommon in the United States, representing less than 2% of malignancies of the male genitourinary tract. The highest rate of incidence is seen in men over 45 years of age, with a predominance of African Americans over whites in a ratio of 3:1. A higher incidence of penile cancer is observed in those Eastern nations where circumcision is not routinely practiced.

Although the precise etiology of penile cancer is unknown, a clear link to poor hygiene in the uncircumcised male has been established, implicating the growth of possibly carcinogenic micro-organisms in smegma retained beneath the prepuce. Approximately 20% of patients have a history of past or present venereal disease. An etiologic role for herpes simplex infection has been postulated but not proven.

HISTOLOGY

The vast majority of penile cancers are squamous cell carcinomas. Rare cases of adenocarcinoma, melanocarcinoma, and sarcoma have been reported, the latter being in some instances associated with Kaposi's sarcoma. Metastatic disease of the penis originating from primary tumors of the rectum, prostate, or bladder also occurs but is quite uncommon.

Approximately 50% of penile cancers metastasize via lymphatic vessels to the deep and superficial inguinal nodes. Most of these malignancies are relatively unresponsive to radiation therapy, and a consistently effective chemotherapeutic protocol has yet to be developed. Treatment of penile cancer is therefore heavily reliant on surgery. Depending on the extent of disease, this may involve partial, complete, or radical penectomy, with inguinal lymphadenectomy when necessary to remove affected nodes. In cases of penile cancer detected at an early stage, cure is sometimes achieved by a partial penectomy that preserves a penile stump adequate for sexual activity and urination. The overall 5-year survival for cancer of the penis is 80% for men without nodal involvement, but less than 50% in men with nodal metastases.

CLINICAL MANIFESTATIONS

At the time of presentation, the penile lesion, invariably located in the preputial area, may appear either as a flat ulcer with raised edges, usually extending into the underlying tissues, or as a clustered papillomatous growth resembling the much more common, sexually transmitted condyloma acuminatum. All such penile lesions are suspect and should be biopsied to confirm the histologic diagnosis. Because of overlying psychological factors associated with any abnormality of the penis, patients may delay seeking medical attention until the malignancy is well established. However, most of these lesions are slow to grow and metastasize, and therefore the prognosis even for fairly well advanced cases remains relatively good unless extensive involvement of the inguinal lymph nodes is already present.

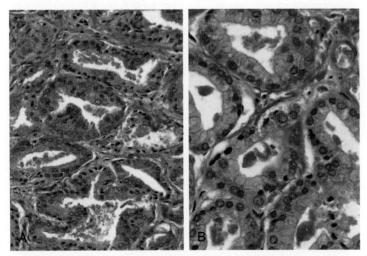

FIGURE 8.1 **ADENOMATOUS HYPERPLASIA.** (**A**) In this atypical example, small, irregular, closely packed glands form a circumscribed nodule. (**B**) At higher power the epithelial cells lack the prominent nucleoli of adenocarcinoma. A two-cell layer is present focally. Distinction of atypical adenomatous hyperplasia from well-differentiated adenocarcinoma may be difficult.

FIGURE 8.2 **PROSTATE CANCER.** Sagittal ultrasonogram demonstrates hypoechoic areas, which are the most common abnormalities seen with prostate cancer. Needle biopsy of hypoechoic lesions can be performed directly under ultrasonographic guidance.

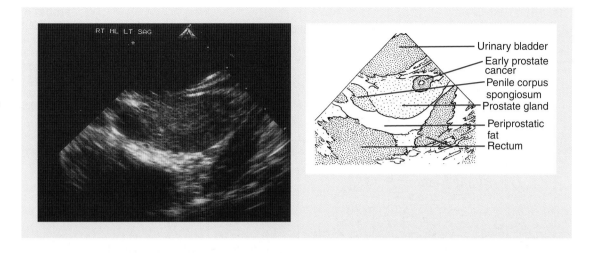

Urinary bladder
Early prostate cancer
Penile corpus spongiosum
Prostate gland
Periprostatic fat
Rectum

FIGURE 8.3 **ADENOCARCINOMA.** (**A**) Many prostatic carcinomas arise in the posterior portion of the gland. Cystic areas in this specimen represent zones of nodular hyperplasia unrelated to the carcinoma. This site of origin is not invariably the case, however. (**B**) A yellow zone of coloration in the periurethral region in this specimen corresponds to a lesion involving both lateral lobes.

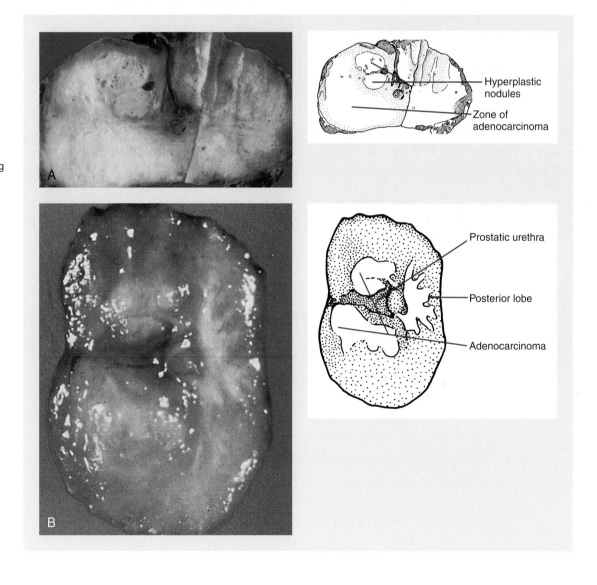

Hyperplastic nodules
Zone of adenocarcinoma

Prostatic urethra
Posterior lobe
Adenocarcinoma

Histologic grading of prostatic adenocarcinoma

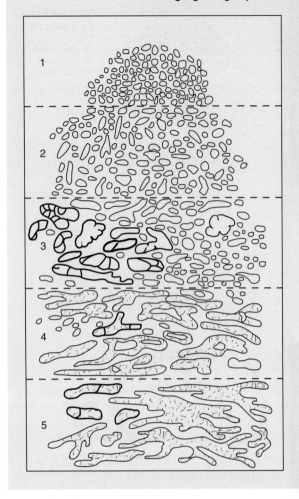

- Sharply circumscribed aggregate of small, closely packed, uniform glands

- Greater variation in glandular size
- More stroma between glands
- More infiltrative margins

- Further variation in glandular size
- Glands more widely dispersed in stroma
- Distinctly infiltrative margins, with loss of circumscription

- "Fused gland" pattern – irregular masses of neoplastic glands coalescing and branching
- Infiltration of prostatic stroma

- Diffusely infiltrating tumor cells with only occasional gland formation

Adapted from Gleason, 1977

FIGURE 8.4 **GLEASON PATTERN SCORES.** This is one of the standard grading systems for prostate adenocarcinomas. Five histologic patterns are identified. Patterns 1 and 2 correspond to well-differentiated cancers. Pattern 3 marks a moderately differentiated cancer, and patterns 4 and 5 correspond to poorly differentiated or anaplastic lesions.

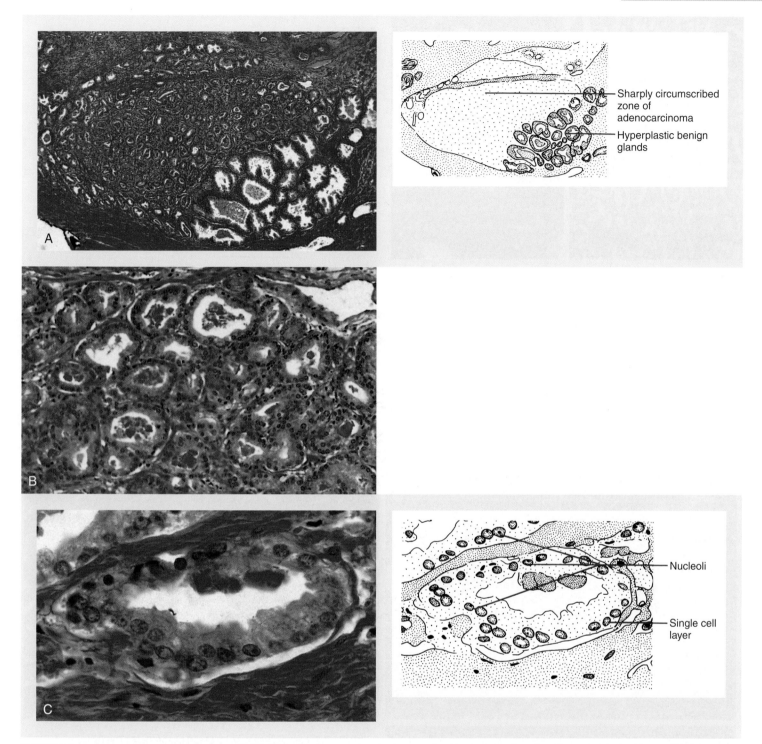

Sharply circumscribed
zone of
adenocarcinoma

Hyperplastic benign
glands

Nucleoli

Single cell
layer

FIGURE 8.5 **ADENOCARCINOMA (GLEASON GRADE 1).** (**A**) This lesion forms a sharply circumscribed aggregate of small, uniform glands. At this magnification, distinction from atypical adenomatous hyperplasia is not possible. The larger surrounding glands are hyperplastic. (**B**) Small, uniform, closely spaced glands are the hallmark of this low-grade malignancy. Note the sharply circumscribed border, with the surrounding stroma at the top left of the field. Intraluminal crystalloids are also present. (**C**) The presence of large nucleoli in the glandular cells has been used to distinguish low-grade carcinoma from atypical adenomatous hyperplasia. This admittedly arbitrary distinction has little if any biologic importance.

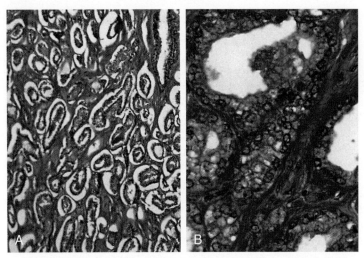

FIGURE 8.6 **ADENOCARCINOMA (GLEASON GRADE 2).** (**A**) This grade shows greater variation in glandular size, more stroma between glands, and a more infiltrative margin than the much less common grade 1 pattern. Distinction of grade 2 lesions from grade 3 is somewhat subjective. (**B**) Carcinomatous glands are composed of a single layer of cells. The nuclei are enlarged and have prominent nucleoli.

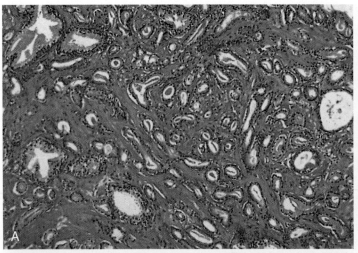

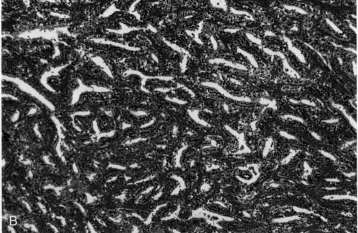

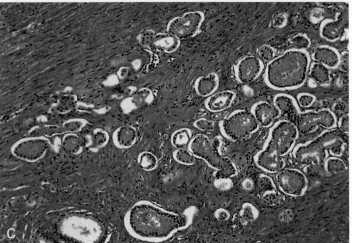

FIGURE 8.7 **ADENOCARCINOMA (GLEASON GRADE 3).** (**A**) The features of this lesion represent an extension of the changes seen in the grade 2 pattern. The glands are even more irregular in size and shape. The tumor is distinctly infiltrative, without any of the circumscription characterizing grade 1 and 2 lesions. (**B**) Glandular size and shape in this example are markedly irregular. (**C**) Diffuse infiltration of single, irregular glands is evident. Small foci such as these are commonly encountered in needle biopsy specimens.

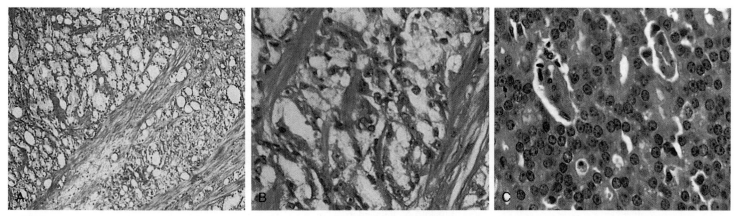

FIGURE 8.8 **ADENOCARCINOMA (GLEASON GRADE 4).** (**A**) The most common grade 4 variant of prostatic adenocarcinoma is the fused-gland pattern seen here. Back-to-back glands without intervening stroma infiltrate the prostate. (**B**) Higher-power view shows back-to-back glands infiltrating the stroma. (**C**) In another example of the fused-gland pattern, the carcinoma grows as an infiltrating sheet of cells containing scattered lumina.

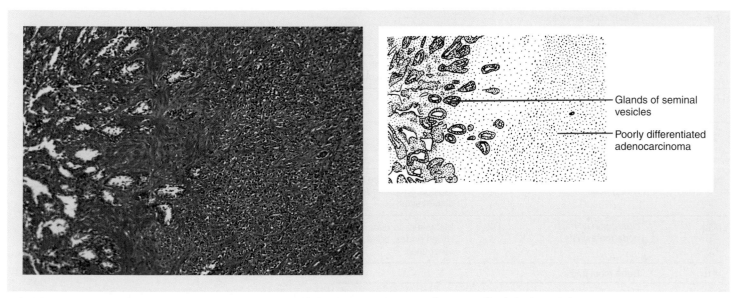

FIGURE 8.9 **ADENOCARCINOMA (GLEASON GRADE 5).** A seminal vesicle has been invaded by single tumor cells of a high-grade lesion.

FIGURE 8.10 **ADENOCARCINOMA (GLEASON GRADE 5).** This lesion shows a comedocarcinomatous pattern. Circumscribed nests of tumor cells are similar to those seen at low power in the cribriform variant of Gleason grade 3. The presence of a central area of necrosis distinguishes this pattern from grade 3. The cells of this variant have pleomorphic, vesicular nuclei.

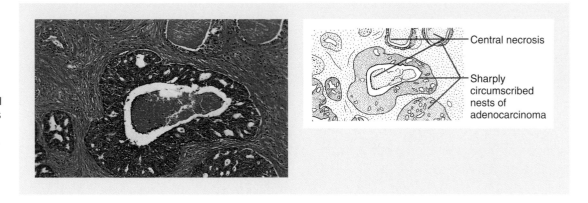

Clinical staging of prostate cancer, using the 2002 AJCC TNM classification and the Whitmore-Jewett system

Note that for patients who are postprostatectomy, a pathologic T stage is often employed (pT) in which there is no pT1 designation

2002 AJCC	Stage		Whitmore-Jewett	
T1a	I	Microscopic tumor in ≤5% of prostatic chips	A	Nonpalpable tumor, detected incidentally
T1b	II	Microscopic tumor in > 5% of prostatic chips		
T1c		Nonpalpable tumor identified by needle biopsy	B	Palpable tumor, confined within the prostate, or detected by prostate-specific antigen
T2a		Tumor confined within the prostate, involves one half of one lobe or less		
T2b		Tumor confined within the prostate, involves more than one half of one lobe, but not both lobes		
T2c		Tumor confined within the prostate, involves both lobes		
T3a	III	Tumor extends through the prostate capsule	C	Tumor extends through the prostate capsule
T3b		Tumor invades the seminal vesicle		
T4	IV	Tumor is fixed or invades adjacent structures other than the seminal vesicle		
N1		Metastasis in regional lymph node	D1	Metastatic disease to regional lymph nodes or distant sites
M1a		Nonregional lymph node metastasis	D2	Metastasis to distant lymph nodes, bone, or other sites
M1b		Bone metastasis		
M1c		Other sites		

FIGURE 8.11 Clinical staging of prostate cancer, using the 2002 AJCC TNM classification and the Whitmore-Jewett system.

FIGURE 8.12 ADENOCARCINOMA.
(**A**) Glands of tumor cells have extended into the capsule but have not penetrated to the pericapsular fat. (**B**) In this instance the lesion has extended through the prostatic capsule and into the surrounding fat, evoking a desmoplastic reaction, which is easily palpable on rectal examination.

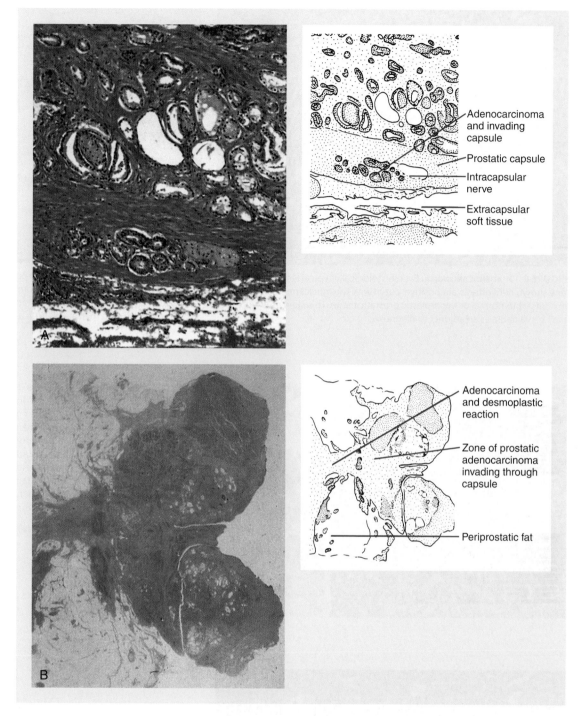

Adenocarcinoma and invading capsule

Prostatic capsule

Intracapsular nerve

Extracapsular soft tissue

Adenocarcinoma and desmoplastic reaction

Zone of prostatic adenocarcinoma invading through capsule

Periprostatic fat

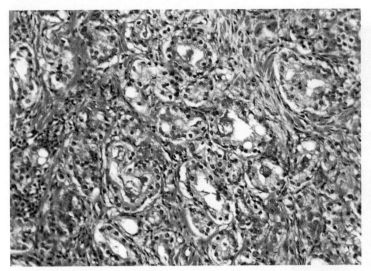

FIGURE 8.13 ADENOCARCINOMA. Even histologically typical lesions like the one shown here often stain positively (*red*) with the mucicarmine technique, in contrast to normal or hyperplastic prostatic tissue. This stain, therefore, may be valuable as an adjunct to diagnosis.

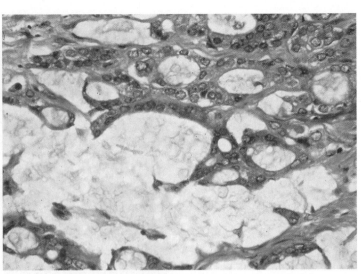

FIGURE 8.14 ADENOCARCINOMA. Some prostatic adenocarcinomas produce abundant extracellular mucin, which forms large pools in the stroma, separating tumor cells. Such carcinomas are not readily amenable to Gleason grading and may be confused with metastases from a primary gastrointestinal tumor.

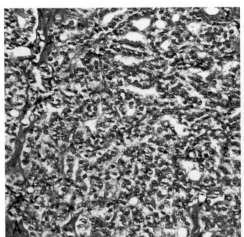
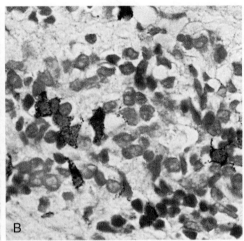

FIGURE 8-15 CARCINOID-LIKE TUMOR. (A) Nests of cells with uniform nuclei show a glandular-trabecular growth pattern resembling gastrointestinal carcinoid tumors. (**B**) Argyrophil stain demonstrates many positive (*brown*) cells in a prostatic carcinoid-like tumor, confirming its neuroendocrine differentiation (Churukian-Schenk stain). The tumor has a more indolent course than undifferentiated small cell carcinoma (see Fig. 8.16).

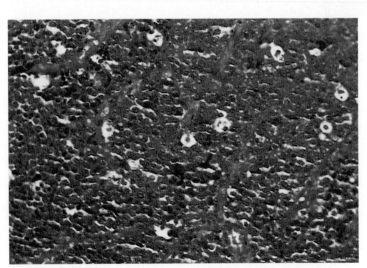

FIGURE 8.16 SMALL CELL CARCINOMA. Carcinomas indistinguishable by light microscopy from pulmonary small cell carcinoma occasionally arise in the prostate. They are usually seen in association with areas of more conventional adenocarcinoma. The small cell carcinoma may respond to chemotherapy, but the biology is similar to other small cell aggressive neuroendocrine tumors, which develop widespread fatal metastases usually within 1 year. Pure small cell carcinomas of the prostate are rare.

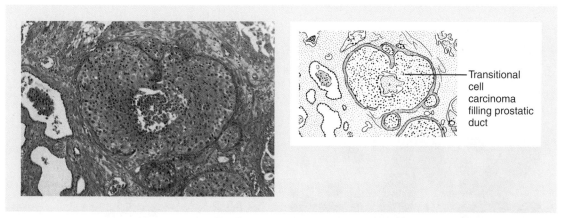

Transitional
cell
carcinoma
filling prostatic
duct

FIGURE 8.17 **TRANSITIONAL CELL CARCINOMA.** This tumor may arise in the prostatic ducts or may extend into the ducts from an initial focus in the prostatic urethra. Cytologically identical to analogous lesions of the bladder and urethra, it is characteristically composed of highly pleomorphic cells without any evidence of squamous or glandular differentiation. The closely packed, irregular contour of the tumor nests and the surrounding fibroplastic stromal reaction suggest that this is an invasive lesion rather than an in situ change in normal ducts.

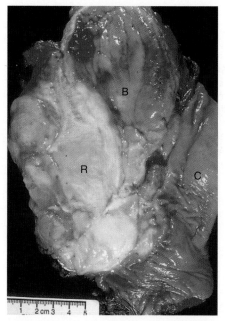

FIGURE 8.18 **RHABDOMYOSARCOMA.** The tumor forms a large, fleshy mass that replaces the prostate gland and invades the bladder and sigmoid colon. B, urinary bladder; C, distal sigmoid colon; R, rhabdomyosarcoma replacing prostate gland.

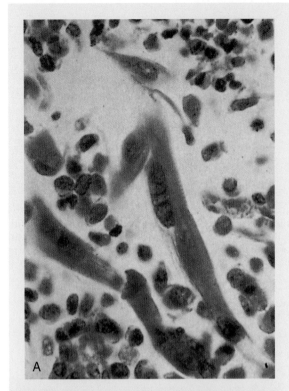

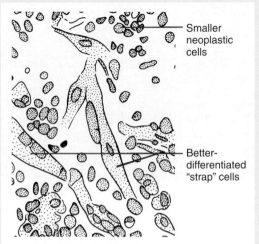

Smaller neoplastic cells

Better-differentiated "strap" cells

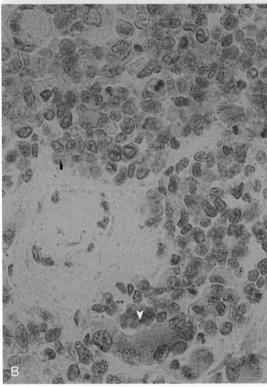

FIGURE 8.19 **RHABDOMYOSARCOMA. (A)** Prostatic rhabdomyosarcomas are usually of the embryonal type and are predominantly composed of small cells with little evidence of differentiation. Rare "strap" cells may be found in some tumors with more obvious skeletal muscle features. **(B)** In questionable cases, staining for skeletal muscle markers such as myoglobin may be helpful. The large, brown-staining cell (*arrowhead*) is positive in this tumor.

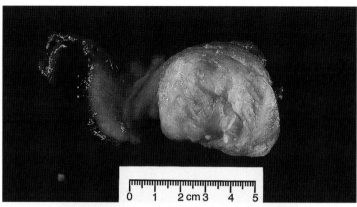

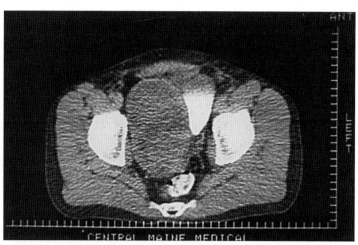

FIGURE 8.20 LEIOMYOSARCOMA OF PROSTATE. Leiomyosarcoma of prostate, though rare (composing less than 0.1% of primary prostatic neoplasms), is the single most common prostatic sarcoma typically occurring in older adults (26% of cases). The tumor is characterized by fascicular arrangements of spindle-shaped cells with brightly eosinophilic cytoplasm and strong immunohistochemical positivity for smooth muscle actin and weaker positivity for desmin. Precise criteria for distinction from (benign) leiomyoma have not been proven reliable. Reactive myofibroblastic/fibroblastic proliferations such as postoperative spindle cell nodule should also be considered in the differential diagnosis.

FIGURE 8.22 PROSTATE SARCOMA. Same patient as in Figure 8.21. CT scan shows large sarcoma of the prostate (S) displacing the urinary bladder, and rectum.

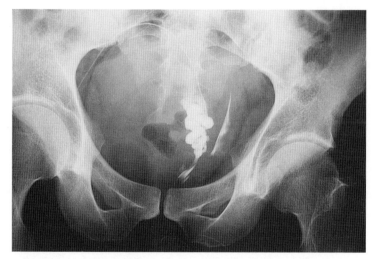

FIGURE 8.21 PROSTATE SARCOMA. A 35-year-old man with an unusual sarcoma of the prostate. Vasogram shows dilated seminal vesicle due to obstruction from the tumor.

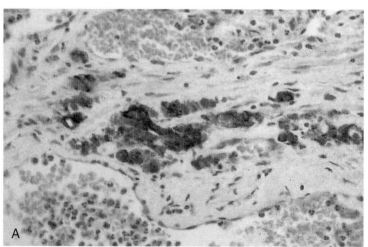

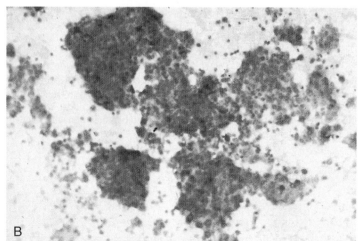

FIGURE 8.23 METASTATIC ADENOCARCINOMA OF PROSTATE. (A) This biopsy specimen containing a high-grade adenocarcinoma stains positively for anti-PSA, strongly supporting a prostatic origin. **(B)** Antibodies directed against PSA and prostatic acid phosphatase in this needle aspiration cytology specimen of lung tissue react positively for the latter, indicating a prostatic origin.

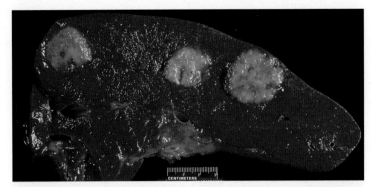

FIGURE 8.24 LIVER METASTASES. In unusual instances, prostate cancer can metastasize to the liver. Discrete nodularity is the most common pattern. (Courtesy of Pathology Department, Brigham and Women's Hospital, Boston, MA.)

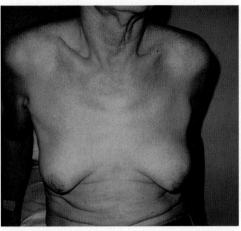

FIGURE 8.26 Gynecomastia in a man treated with diethylstilbestrol (DES) for advanced prostate cancer. Because estrogenic therapies (including the herbal therapy PC-SPES) are now being increasingly used for androgen-independent prostate cancer, recognition of this complication is important. In addition, antiandrogen monotherapy can also lead to significant gynecomastia. A short course of prophylactic breast irradiation may inhibit growth of breast tissue.

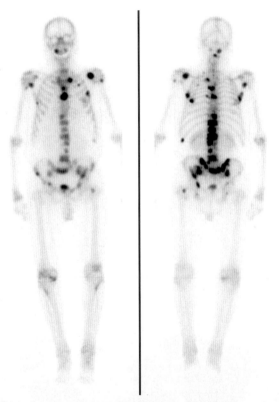

FIGURE 8.25 BONE SCAN TO IDENTIFY METASTATIC PROSTATE CANCER. Anterior and posterior view of a bone scan of a patient with multiple bony metastases from his prostate cancer. This pattern is typical for prostate cancer, with involvement of the thoracic and lumbar spine and bilateral hips, with relative sparing of the long bones of the extremities.

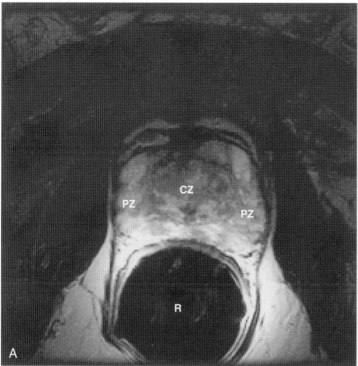 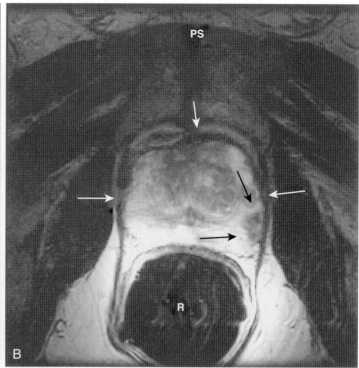

FIGURE 8.27 TWO AXIAL T$_2$-WEIGHTED IMAGES FROM A PROSTATE MR USING AN ENDORECTAL COIL. (**A**) At a relatively superior level in the prostate, the normal differentiation between the lower-signal central zone (CZ) and the higher-signal peripheral zone (PZ) is evident. The rectum (R) is distended by the coil. (**B**) At a lower position in the prostate, a focal area of low signal in the left peripheral zone is seen (*black arrows*), indicating an area of infiltration with tumor. The margins of the prostate capsule (*white arrows*) appear intact. The rectum (R) and pubic symphysis (PS) are marked for orientation.

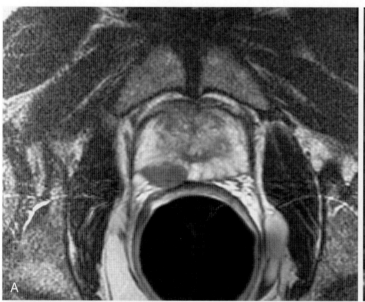 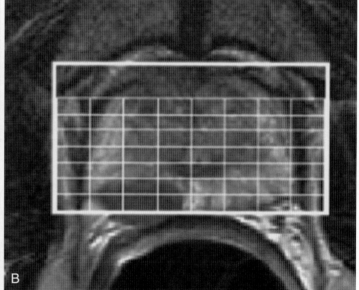

FIGURE 8.28 MR SPECTROSCOPY TO IDENTIFY PROSTATE CANCER. (**A**) T$_2$-weighted endorectal MRI revealing an abnormal region of hypointensity within the right aspect of the peripheral zone of the prostate gland. (**B**) Superimposed upon the T$_2$-weighted image is the localized spectroscopic volume of investigation. Within each voxel the choline and citrate spectra are investigated. (**C**) Localized spectra from each voxel. Voxels that are suspicious for cancer demonstrate increased choline (the first peak on the left) and decreased citrate peaks (highlighted). (Courtesy of Dr. Fergus Coakley, University of California, San Francisco.)

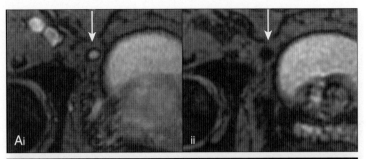

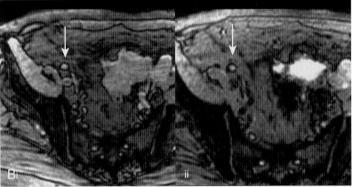

FIGURE 8.29 LYMPHOTROPIC NANOPARTICLE-ENHANCED MRI TO IDENTIFY INVOLVED LYMPH NODES. (A) (i) T_2*-weighted endorectal MR image at the level of the acetabulum before iron oxide nanoparticle contrast displaying a normally enhancing external iliac node. (ii) After iron oxide nanoparticle contrast T_2*-weighted image at the same level demonstrating homogeneous uptake of contrast into the external iliac node (dark), which is normal for an uninvolved lymph node. (B) (i) T_2*-weighted endorectal MR image superior to the acetabulum before iron oxide nanoparticle contrast displaying a normally enhancing external iliac node. (ii) After iron oxide nanoparticle contrast T_2*-weighted image at the same level demonstrating a lack of homogeneous uptake of contrast into the external iliac node (bright), which is consistent with malignant nodal involvement. (Courtesy of Dr. Mukesh Harisinghani, Massachusetts General Hospital, Boston, MA.)

FIGURE 8.30 The Jewett-Strong-Marshall (JSM) and AJCC staging systems for bladder cancer.

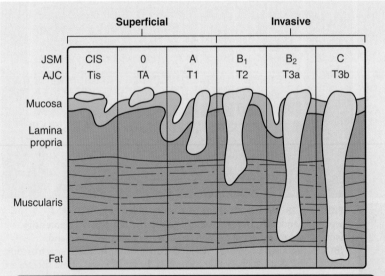

Stage			Features
JSM	AJCC TNM	AJCC Stage	
CIS	Tis	Ois	Carcinoma in situ: tumor limited to mucosa (flat tumor)
0	Ta	Oa	Noninvasive papillary carcinoma
A	T1	I	Tumor invades lamina propria
B1	T2a	II	Tumor invades superficial muscle (inner half)
B2	T2b		Tumor invades deep muscle (outer half)
C	T3a	III	Tumor invades perivesical tissue, microscopically
	T3b		Tumor invades perivesical tissue, macroscopically
	T4a		Tumor invades prostate, uterus, or vagina
	T4b	IV	Tumor invades pelvic or abdominal wall
D1	N1		Metastases in a single lymph node ≤2 cm
	N2		Metastases in a single lymph node 2–5 cm; or multiple lymph nodes, none >5 cm
	N3		Metastases in a lymph node >5 cm
D2	M1		Distant metastases

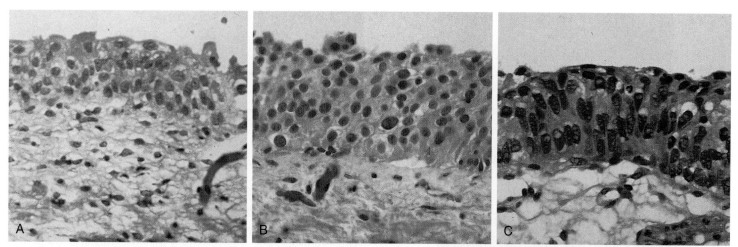

FIGURE 8.31 UROTHELIAL DYSPLASIA. (A) In mild urothelial dysplasia, cell polarity is altered and there is irregular crowding of nuclei, which are enlarged and focally notched. **(B)** Moderate urothelial dysplasia is marked by more evident loss of cytoplasmic clearing, and there are greater numbers of enlarged, slightly irregular, hyperchromatic nuclei. **(C)** Although polarity is not totally lost and there is maturation to superficial cells, the degree of pleomorphism present in this severely dysplastic urothelium approaches carcinoma in situ. It should be considered neoplastic and carries a high risk for invasion.

FIGURE 8.32 CARCINOMA IN SITU. (A) Diffuse mucosal erythema with redness not confined within blood vessels is seen in the foreground of this cystoscopic view. This is one appearance of a diffuse in situ lesion. **(B)** This raised, sessile in situ lesion at the bladder neck shows many round, whitish, submucosal aggregates of cystitis follicularis. The background bladder wall has patches of reddened mucosa and other areas consistent with multifocal carcinoma in situ. (Courtesy of B. Bracken, MD, Cincinnati, OH.)

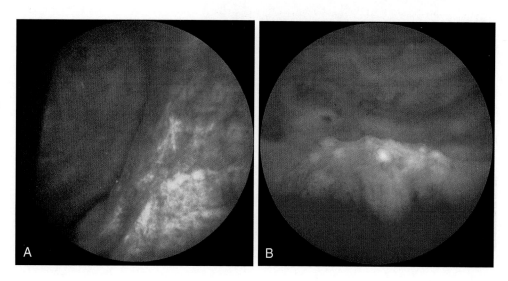

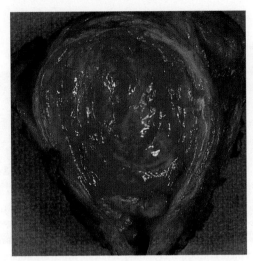

FIGURE 8.33 **CARCINOMA IN SITU.** This cystectomy specimen has a granular and erythematous mucosa, with hemorrhagic areas marking sites of extensive denudation. Numerous poorly defined areas have a cobblestone appearance.

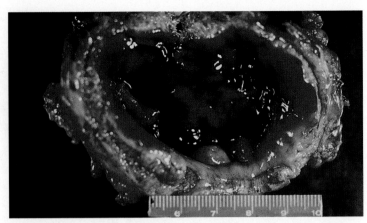

FIGURE 8.35 **HEMORRHAGIC CYSTITIS.** This 70-year-old woman had recurrent episodes of hemorrhagic cystitis over many years related to chronic use of cyclophosphamide. Cystectomy was required for control of symptoms. Note markedly thickened bladder wall. In some cases the presence of the metabolites (especially acrolein) of cyclophosphamide can lead to bladder carcinoma.

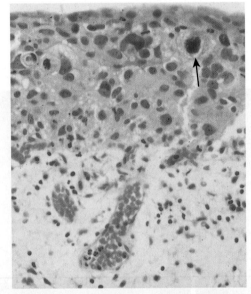

FIGURE 8.34 **TRANSITIONAL CELL CARCINOMA IN SITU.** The cells show loss of polarity with respect to the surface and contain large, irregular nuclei. An atypical mitosis is evident on the right (*arrow*), suggesting possible aneuploidy.

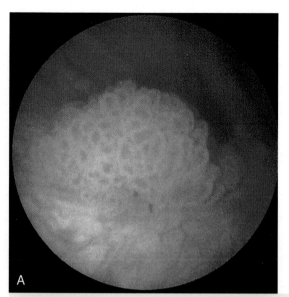

FIGURE 8.36 **TRANSITIONAL CELL CARCINOMA.** Cystoscopic findings are frequently predictive of the histologic grade of tumor and are useful in assessing adjacent urothelium. (**A**) This discrete grade II papillary lesion (TA or T1) is surrounded by normal mucosa. (**B**) Multiple grade II papillary lesions (TA or T1) are poorly defined because of the surrounding mucosal abnormalities. This lack of definition between malignant and benign mucosa makes definitive transurethral resection uncertain. (**C**) A grade II papillary transitional cell carcinoma (TA or T1) is associated with a sessile invasive tumor (T2 or greater), thus forming a "collision tumor." (Courtesy of B. Bracken, MD, Cincinnati, OH.)

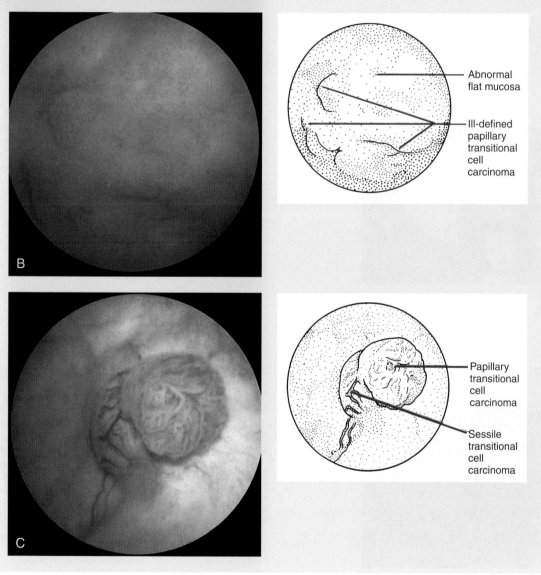

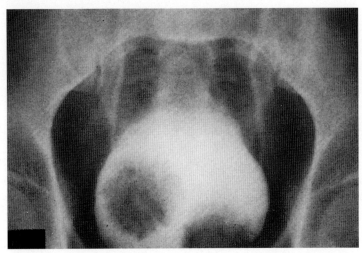

FIGURE 8.37 **TRANSITIONAL CELL CARCINOMA.** The two large, round masses evident in this cystogram represent papillary tumors. The contrast material enters the crypts, causing a fuzzy, ill-defined appearance at the edges of the masses.

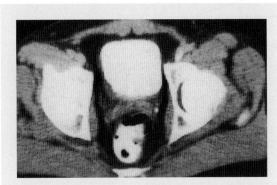

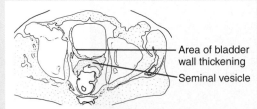

FIGURE 8.38 **TRANSITIONAL CELL CARCINOMA.** Abdominopelvic CT scanning is helpful in staging bladder cancers. In this example the neoplasm has thickened the bladder wall without definite extension into the surrounding fat.

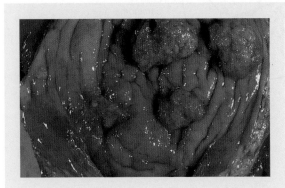

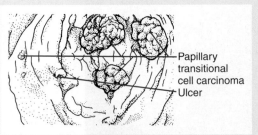

FIGURE 8.39 **TRANSITIONAL CELL CARCINOMA.** This cystectomy specimen shows three large and two small papillary tumors. Transurethral resection of an additional papillary tumor, which documented muscle invasion, has left an ulcerated area in the right posterolateral wall.

FIGURE 8.40 TRANSITIONAL CELL CARCINOMA.
(**A**) This grade I papillary tumor shows well-formed papillae that are covered by hyperplastic urothelium. (**B**) Urothelium shows orderly maturation to superficial cells. The slightly hyperchromatic nuclei are crowded together secondary to mild to moderate enlargement.

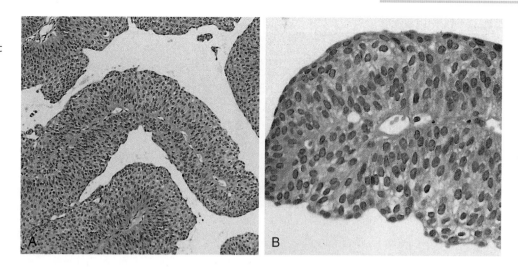

FIGURE 8.41 TRANSITIONAL CELL CARCINOMA. Nests and cords of an infiltrating grade II lesion are present between and within smooth muscle bundles of the bladder wall.

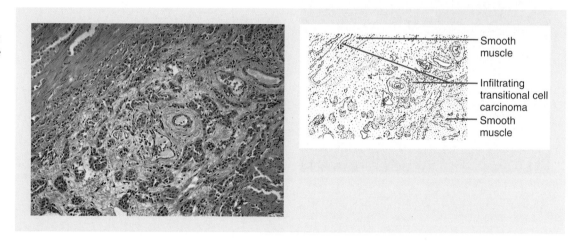

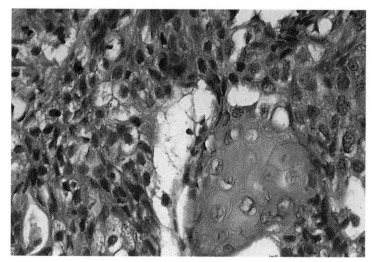

FIGURE 8.42 TRANSITIONAL CELL CARCINOMA. This high-grade tumor shows focal squamous differentiation (*center*). It should not be misdiagnosed as a squamous cell carcinoma, which usually shows intercellular bridging and keratin pearls.

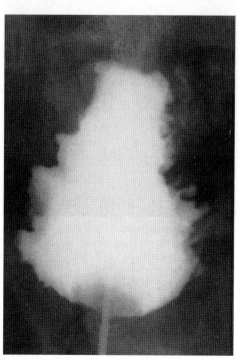

FIGURE 8.43 SQUAMOUS CELL CARCINOMA. An earlier cystogram in this patient demonstrated a typical "Christmas tree" bladder with round diverticula. Six years later the flattening and irregularity of the side walls of the bladder strongly suggest tumor infiltration.

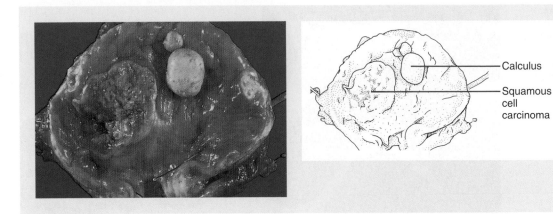

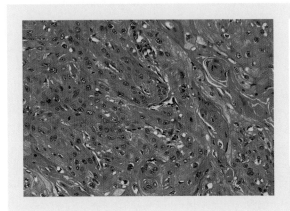

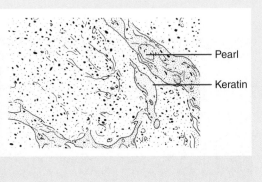

FIGURE 8.44 **SQUAMOUS CELL CARCINOMA.** The ulcerated, necrotic tumor in this cystectomy specimen has raised edges that appear sharply demarcated from the surrounding mucosa. Several bladder calculi are present.

FIGURE 8.45 **SQUAMOUS CELL CARCINOMA.** In this well-differentiated tumor, sheets of polygonal keratinizing cells with intercellular bridges produce extracellular keratin and form pearls.

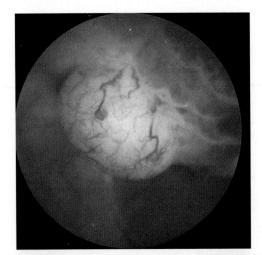

FIGURE 8.46 **ADENOCARCINOMA OF URACHUS.** A tumor in the bladder dome stretches the intact normal mucosa and appears to be invading the bladder from an intramural or extravesical source. These cystoscopic findings are characteristic of a urachal adenocarcinoma.

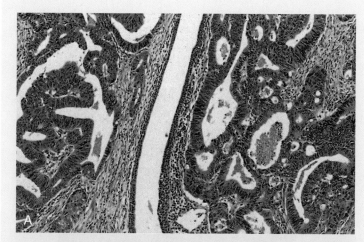

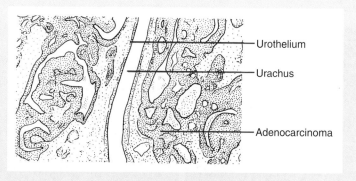

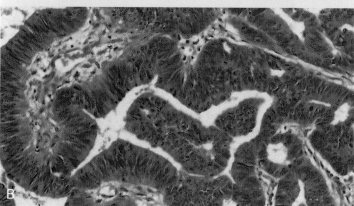

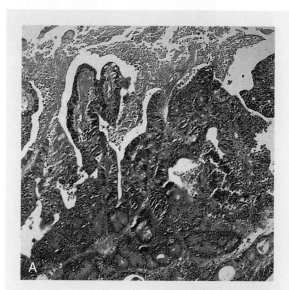

FIGURE 8.47 **ADENOCARCINOMA OF URACHUS.** (**A**) Low-power photomicrograph of a tumor that arose in the wall of the bladder dome shows that the urachus, lined by a thin layer of urothelium, is microscopically patent. (**B**) Papillae and glands are lined by stratified columnar epithelium. (**A,** Courtesy of B. Bracken, MD, Cincinnati, OH.)

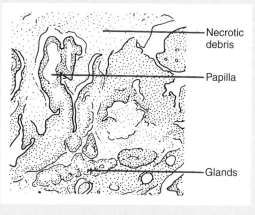

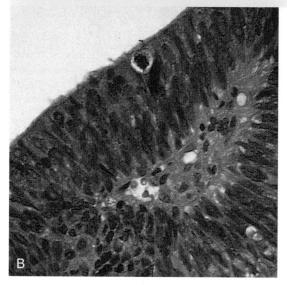

FIGURE 8.48 **ADENOCARCINOMA.** (**A**) These tumors are commonly papillary and glandular, resembling intestinal neoplasms. The luminal surface in this example is covered with necrotic cellular debris and mucin. (**B**) Like urachal adenocarcinoma, papillae and glands contain stratified columnar epithelium. Intracytoplasmic mucin may be absent.

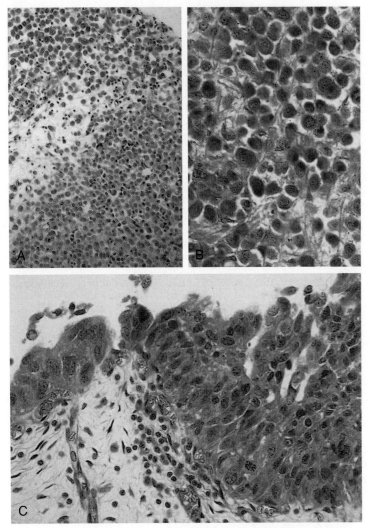

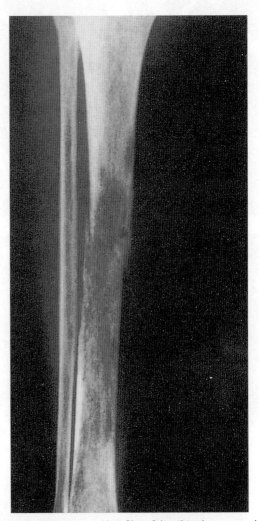

FIGURE 8.49 **SIGNET-RING CELL CARCINOMA.** (**A**) The lamina propria contains a dense infiltrate of neoplastic cells. Overlying urothelium is denuded. (**B**) Many cells contain mucin vacuoles. Cells with displaced nuclei have a signet-ring cell appearance. (**C**) The presence of carcinoma in situ (*on the left*) supports a bladder origin for this cancer.

FIGURE 8.50 **BONE METASTASES.** Plain film of the tibia shows osteolytic metastases in the midshaft in a patient with advanced transitional cell carcinoma of the bladder. Surprisingly, these lesions can undergo healing with intensive combination chemotherapy. If the lesion is isolated and small, it can be surgically resected.

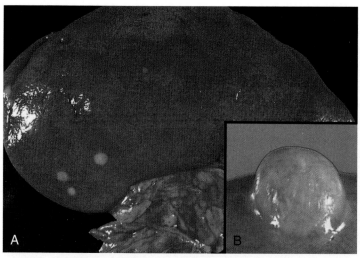

FIGURE 8.51 CORTICAL ADENOMA. This benign lesion is a common incidental finding at autopsy; it may be multiple. (**A**) The three adenomas in this kidney are each less than 5 mm in diameter, slightly raised, sharply demarcated, gray-white, subcapsular nodules. (**B**) An adenoma protrudes from the cortical surface. Although predominantly gray-white, it has multiple yellow areas, indicating that it is composed of both granular and clear cells.

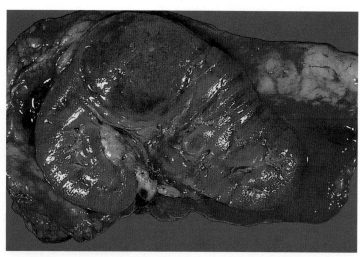

FIGURE 8.53 ONCOCYTOMA. Apparently arising from epithelial cells of the proximal renal tubule, these tumors have a low malignant potential when they are less than 5 cm in diameter and are well circumscribed. They have a characteristic mahogany-brown color. Uncommon focal hemorrhage is also present.

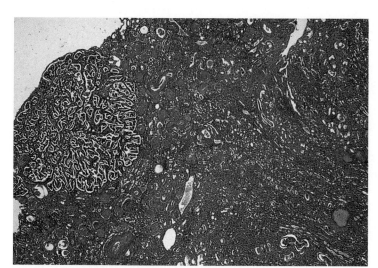

FIGURE 8.52 CORTICAL ADENOMA. An unencapsulated tubular epithelial neoplasm in the subcapsular cortex merges imperceptibly with the surrounding parenchyma. It has a uniform papillary growth pattern and lacks hemorrhage and necrosis.

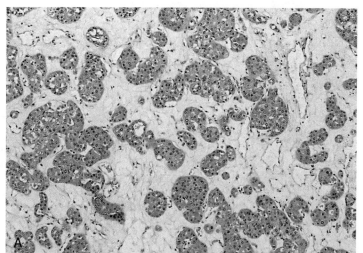

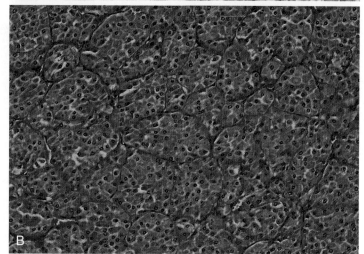

FIGURE 8.54 ONCOCYTOMA. (**A**) The central scar is composed of loose, relatively acellular, fibrous tissue. Organoid packeting of oncocytes is prominent. (**B**) Compact peripheral nests are separated by a delicate fibrovascular stroma. Oncocytomas compose a uniform population of tubular cells with abundant eosinophilic, granular cytoplasm and minimal nuclear atypia.

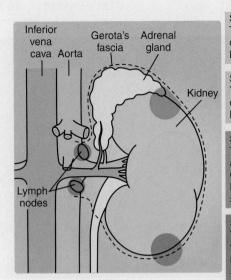

Stage I
Tumor <7 cm in greatest dimension and limited to kidney; 5-year survival, ~95%

Stage II
Tumor >7 cm in greatest dimension and limited to kidney; 5-year survival, ~88%

Stage III
Tumor in major veins or adrenal gland, tumor within Gerota's fascia, or 1 regional lymph node involved; 5-year survival, ~59%

Stage IV
Tumor beyond Gerota's fascia or >1 regional lymph node involved; 5-year survival, ~20%

FIGURE 8.55 CLINICAL STAGING AND PROGNOSIS IN RENAL CELL CARCINOMA. American Joint Committee on Cancer Criteria. (Modified from Cohen HT, McGovern FJ: Renal-cell carcinoma, *N Engl J Med* 353:2477–2490, 2005.)

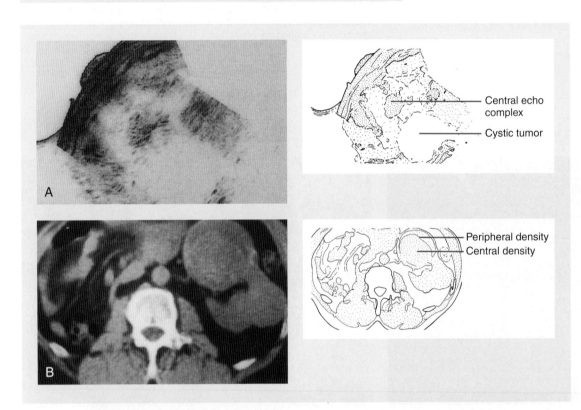

Central echo complex

Cystic tumor

Peripheral density
Central density

FIGURE 8.56 RENAL CELL CARCINOMA. (A) Sonogram of a cystic, hemorrhagic tumor shows an ovoid anechoic area located anterior to the central echo complex. The ill-defined borders and lack of enhanced through-transmission suggest that the lesion is not a simple cyst. **(B)** CT reveals two radiodensities in the mass, an ovoid central density and a more lucent peripheral density, suggesting two components.

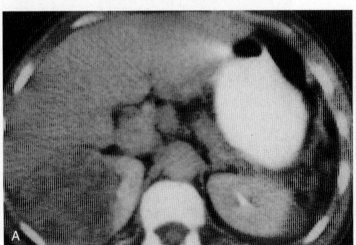

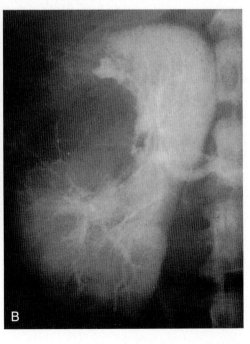

FIGURE 8.57 RENAL CELL CARCINOMA. (A) A solid tumor with areas of hemorrhage or necrosis, which appeared echogenic on sonography, shows mixed density on CT scan. **(B)** Arteriography reveals a hypovascular mass.

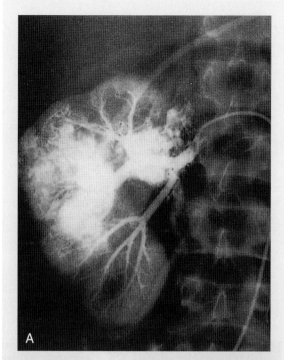

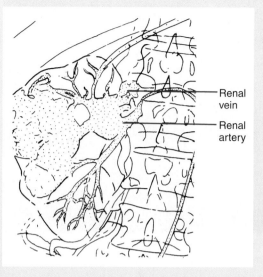

Renal
vein

Renal
artery

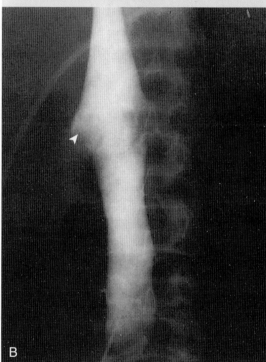

FIGURE 8.58 RENAL CELL CARCINOMA. (A) In addition to renal vein invasion, this arteriogram shows neovascularity in the tumor, as well as in the course of the renal vein. **(B)** On the inferior vena cavagram, the contrast column defines the tumor thrombus on the right (*arrowhead*). There is wash-in from the normal left renal vein flow.

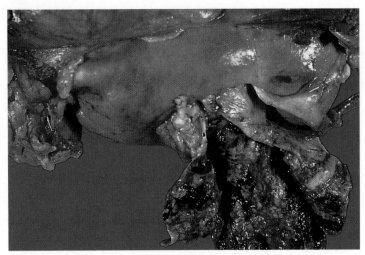

FIGURE 8.59 **RENAL CELL CARCINOMA.** With massive invasion by tumor, the renal vein may become occluded by adherent tumor thrombus.

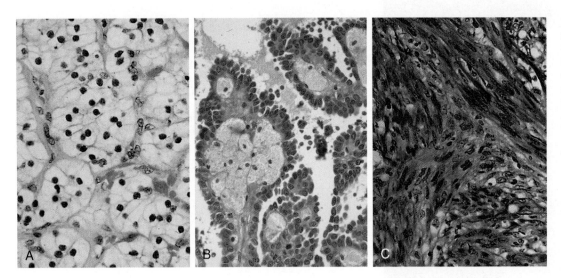

FIGURE 8.60 **RENAL CELL CARCINOMA HISTOLOGY.** (**A**) The classic clear cell variant of renal cell carcinoma is composed of cells with abundant cytoplasm containing lipid and glycogen. (**B**) Tumor cells in the papillary variant are arranged around fibrovascular cores that frequently contain clusters of foamy macrophages. (**C**) Intersecting fascicles of anaplastic spindle cells are present in this sarcomatoid variant.

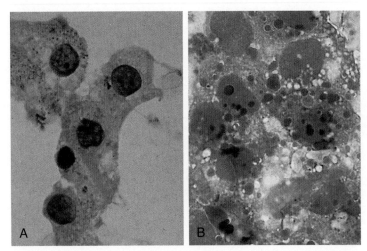

FIGURE 8.61 **RENAL CELL CARCINOMA.** (**A, B**) Fine-needle aspiration biopsy of a well-differentiated tumor shows small sheets and groups of cells with slight nuclear enlargement and hyperchromatism, small nucleoli, and abundant cytoplasm containing hemosiderin granules and lipid vacuoles.

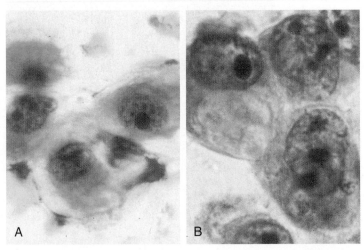

FIGURE 8.62 **RENAL CELL CARCINOMA.** (**A, B**) Fine-needle aspiration biopsy of a poorly differentiated tumor shows cells that have prominent nuclear pleomorphism with chromatin clearing and single or multiple macronucleoli. Nucleus-to-cytoplasm ratios are high. In **A**, perinuclear cytoplasm is distinctly granular. Urine cytology may reveal similar cells.

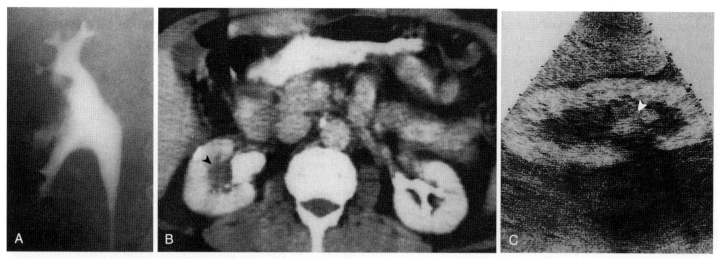

FIGURE 8.63 **TRANSITIONAL CELL CARCINOMA.** (**A**) The urogram reveals a mass with ill-defined margins either arising in or impinging on the lateral portion of the renal pelvis. (**B**) CT shows a minimally enhancing mass in the renal sinus/pelvis displacing the contrast in the pelvis medially (*arrowhead*). (**C**) Because the mass (*arrowhead*) is echogenic on the sonogram, it is solid rather than cystic.

FIGURE 8.64 **SKULL METASTASES.** (**A, B**) This 74-year-old man developed metastatic renal cell cancer to the skull with marked protuberance of the temporal bone. Cranial radiation therapy, administered because of the brain metastases (not seen on this CT scan), was followed by radiation dermatitis.

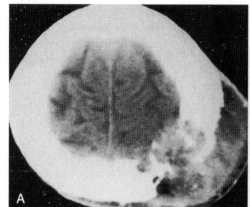

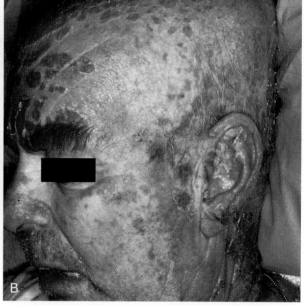

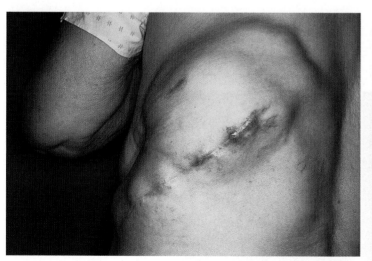

FIGURE 8.65 **RENAL CELL CARCINOMA.** Soft tissue metastases in the lower chest and flank developed in this 57-year-old woman, 1 year after nephrectomy.

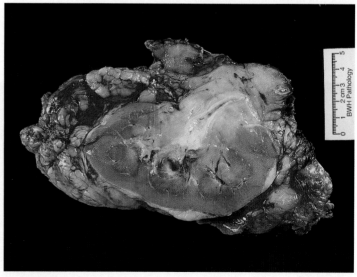

FIGURE 8.66 **RENAL LYMPHOMA.** The kidney and perirenal lymph nodes were secondarily involved by non-Hodgkin lymphoma, predominantly diffuse (focally nodular), large B-cell type, with focal CD10 positivity in nodular areas, consistent with transformation from lower-grade follicular lymphoma (as demonstrated in the separately submitted right retroperitoneal nodes).

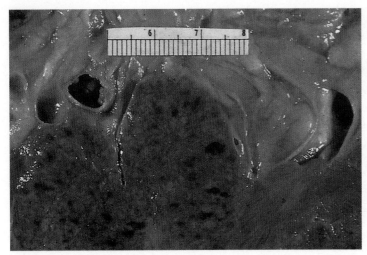

FIGURE 8.67 METASTATIC MALIGNANT MELANOMA. The urinary tract is a common site of metastases. If not amelanotic, the metastatic nodules are brown-black. Urine may also be black.

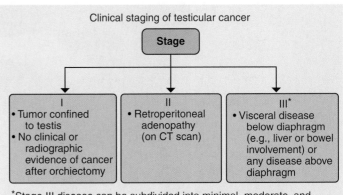

Clinical staging of testicular cancer

Stage

I	II	III*
• Tumor confined to testis • No clinical or radiographic evidence of cancer after orchiectomy	• Retroperitoneal adenopathy (on CT scan)	• Visceral disease below diaphragm (e.g., liver or bowel involvement) or any disease above diaphragm

*Stage III disease can be subdivided into minimal, moderate, and high-risk, depending on the location of tumor and the extent of tumor spread.

FIGURE 8.69 CLINICAL STAGING OF TESTICULAR CANCER. The AJCC TNM staging system is less commonly used, because it is based upon histologic evaluation of the orchidectomy specimen and retroperitoneal peri-aortic lymph node dissection. Because the latter may not be performed in every patient, the clinical staging system is generally more practical.

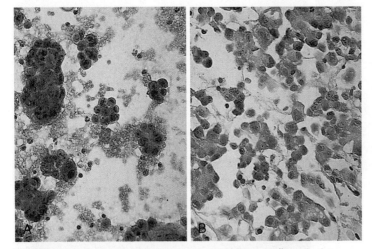

FIGURE 8.68 METASTATIC ADENOCARCINOMA. (A, B) Fine-needle aspiration kidney biopsy specimen from a patient with pulmonary and renal masses contains papillary and glandular epithelial fragments. The presence of intracytoplasmic mucin (**B**, *center*) excludes renal cell carcinoma and is consistent with metastatic adenocarcinoma, in this case originating in the lung.

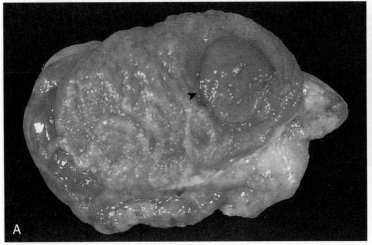

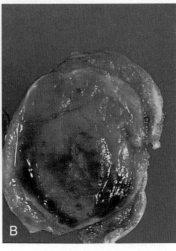

FIGURE 8.70 LEYDIG CELL TUMOR. (A) This tumor forms a small, circumscribed, yellow nodule (*arrowhead*) within the testis. (**B**) An encapsulated, focally hemorrhagic tumor has replaced most of the testicular parenchyma.

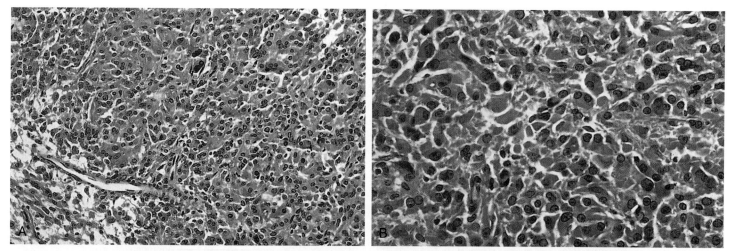

FIGURE 8.71 LEYDIG CELL TUMOR. (A) Sheets of tumor cells with prominent, eosinophilic cytoplasm infiltrate the testicular stroma. **(B)** High-power view reveals that the tumor is composed of polygonal, ovoid, and spindled cells with dense eosinophilic cytoplasm and round to ovoid nuclei. There is moderate nuclear pleomorphism.

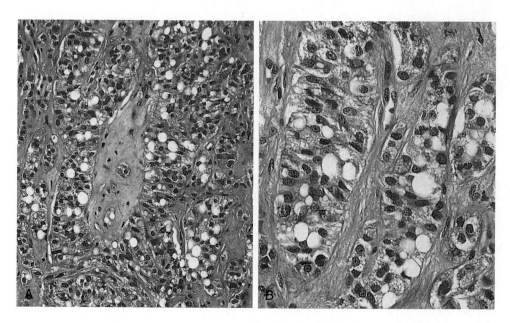

FIGURE 8.72 SERTOLI CELL TUMOR. (A) Low- and **(B)** high-power photomicrographs reveal irregular cords of tumor cells with vacuolated cytoplasm infiltrating the testicular stroma.

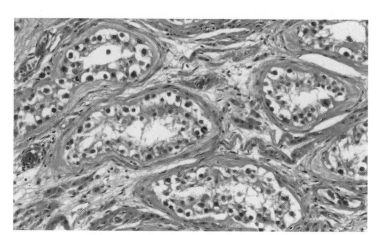

FIGURE 8.73 GERM CELL NEOPLASIA IN SITU. Neoplastic germ cells with abundant, clear cytoplasm line the seminiferous tubules. The nuclei are larger and more hyperchromatic than normal germ cells. Spermatogenesis is decreased or absent.

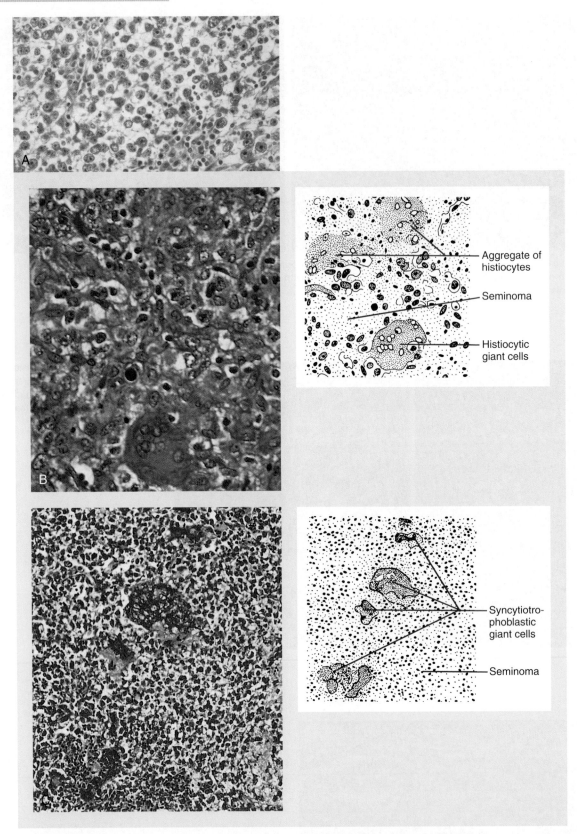

FIGURE 8.74 **SEMINOMA.** (**A**) A lymphatic infiltrate is typical in seminomas. (**B**) Multinucleate histiocytes (giant cells) may be seen in seminomas and should not be confused with syncytiotrophoblastic cells. The nuclei of the giant cells have a uniform vesicular appearance identical to that of mononuclear histiocytes. (**C**) The large, irregular giant cells in this seminoma are syncytiotrophoblastic cells resembling placental syncytial cells and producing the β-subunit of human chorionic gonadotrophin. In the absence of a mixture of cytotrophoblastic and syncytiotrophoblastic elements, choriocarcinoma should not be diagnosed.

FIGURE 8.75 **EMBRYONAL CARCINOMA. (A)** Nests and cords of neoplastic cells are surrounded by zones of necrosis. **(B)** Medium-power view demonstrates highly pleomorphic tumor cells clustering around small blood vessels. **(C)** The degree of nuclear pleomorphism, a high mitotic rate, and eosinophilic cytoplasm distinguish this tumor from seminoma. However, it may be difficult to distinguish it from anaplastic seminoma. **(D)** Perivascular rosettes and irregular lumen-like structures are common. Many of the luminal structures probably form when central cells become necrotic and disappear.

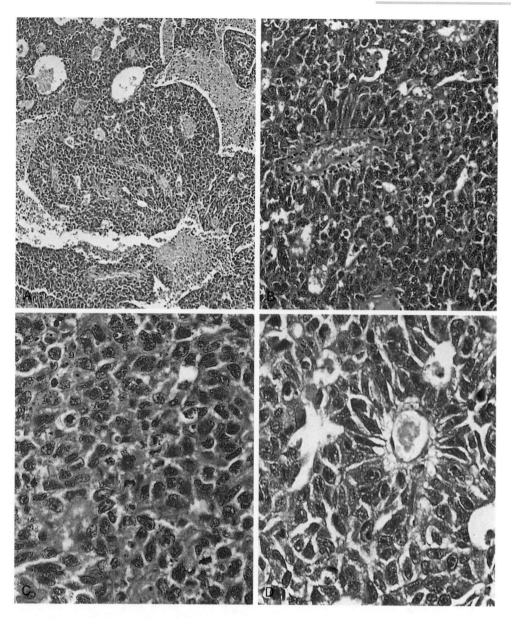

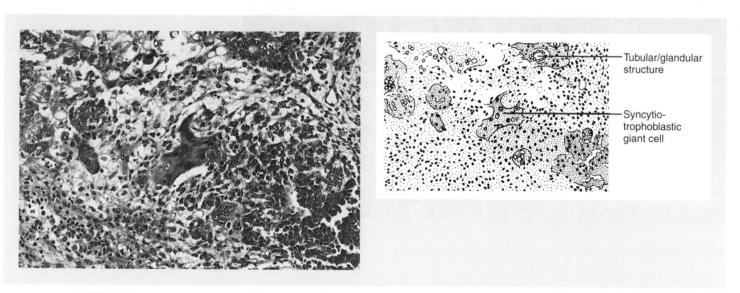

FIGURE 8.76 **EMBRYONAL CARCINOMA.** Like seminoma, this tumor may contain scattered syncytial cells in which β-hCG is found.

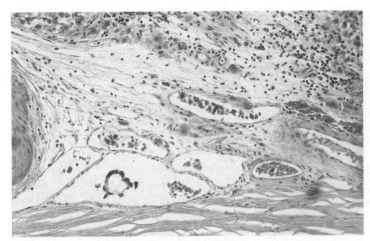

FIGURE 8.77 EMBRYONAL CARCINOMA. Lymphatic invasion, as demonstrated here, is a very important prognostic feature for the subsequent development of retroperitoneal metastases. The possibility should be considered in all patients with primary testicular tumors, especially if retroperitoneal lymph node dissection is contemplated.

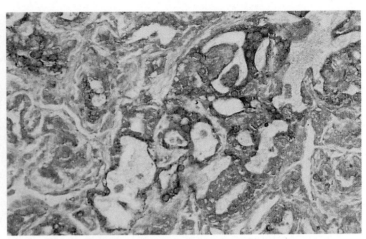

FIGURE 8.79 YOLK SAC (ENDODERMAL SINUS) TUMOR. The brown staining corresponds to deposits of AFP localized by immunocytochemistry.

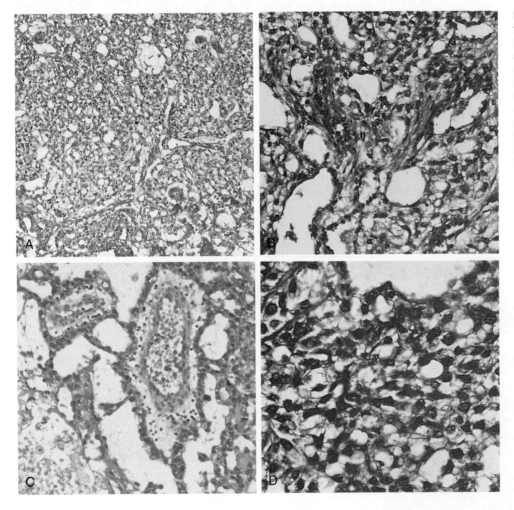

FIGURE 8.78 YOLK SAC (ENDODERMAL SINUS) TUMOR. (A) Low- and **(B)** medium-power photomicrographs show irregular cystic spaces alternating with more solid areas. The cells appear cytologically uniform. **(C)** Diagnostic Schiller-Duval bodies are papillary structures containing a vascular core invested by loose connective tissue and surrounded by a layer of tumor cells. **(D)** Eosinophilic globules are frequently seen in yolk sac tumors. The globules have been shown to contain AFP and α_1-antitrypsin.

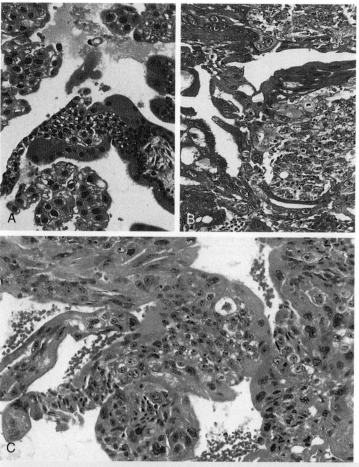

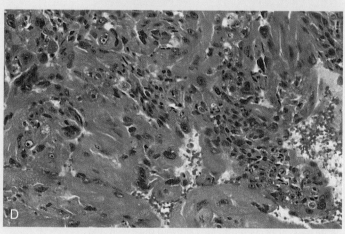

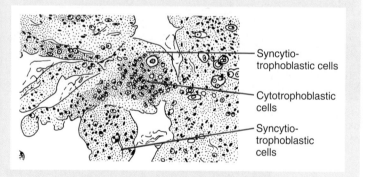

FIGURE 8.80 CHORIOCARCINOMA. Microscopically, developing placental tissue (**A**) closely resembles choriocarcinoma (**B**). The intimate mixture of neoplastic cytotrophoblastic and syncytiotrophoblastic cells is diagnostic. (**C**) Syncytiotrophoblastic cells with abundant eosinophilic cytoplasm surround central aggregates of cytotrophoblastic cells. (**D**) Aggregates of syncytial and cytotrophoblastic cells are associated with stromal hemorrhage.

Syncytio-trophoblastic cells

Cytotrophoblastic cells

Syncytio-trophoblastic cells

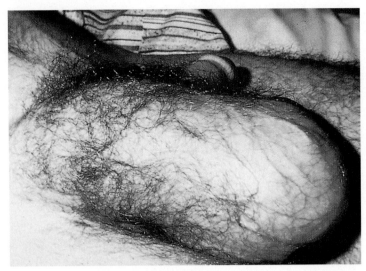

FIGURE 8.81 **TERATOMA.** Testicular teratomas may reach enormous size. (Courtesy of J.E. Fowler Jr, MD, Chicago, IL.)

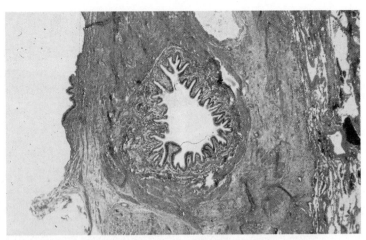

FIGURE 8.84 **METASTATIC TERATOMA.** Microscopic section of a resected pulmonary nodule shows a mature teratoma. The large, fibrous nodule contains blunt papillary projections lined by columnar epithelial cells surrounding a central lumen. A stromal lymphocytic infiltrate (*blue cells*) underlies the papillary mucosa (enteric derived). Mature teratomas recapitulate endodermal, mesodermal, and ectodermal structures, typically showing adult tissue from more than one germ cell line.

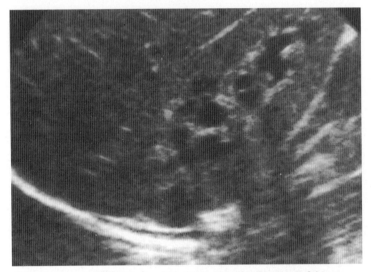

FIGURE 8.82 **TERATOMA.** The multicystic structure in the center of this ultrasonogram is a small teratoma containing several cystic spaces. (Courtesy of T.L. Pope Jr, MD, Charlottesville, VA.)

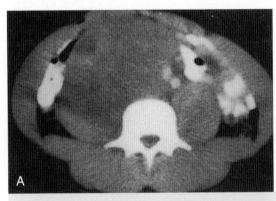

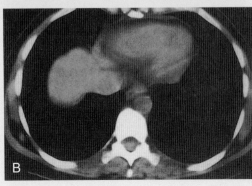

FIGURE 8.83 **MATURE TERATOMA.** A 24-year-old patient with metastatic mixed embryonal cell carcinoma and teratoma (often called teratocarcinoma) and a persistent mass in the abdomen (**A**) and lung (**B**). Biopsy of the large mass after chemotherapy showed pure teratoma without evidence of embryonal cell carcinoma. Though histologically benign, teratomas may increase in size. Surgical resection is indicated, because these tumors are unresponsive to chemotherapy. (Courtesy of T.L. Pope Jr, MD, Charlottesville, VA.)

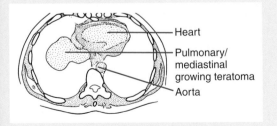

Heart

Pulmonary/ mediastinal growing teratoma

Aorta

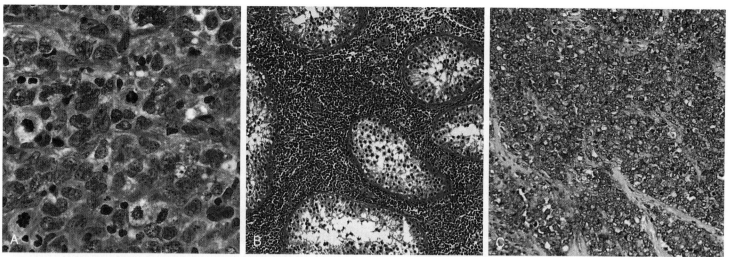

FIGURE 8.85 **PRIMARY LYMPHOMA OF TESTIS. (A)** Most testicular lymphomas are of the diffuse large cell type, characterized by large cells with pleomorphic nuclei and a high mitotic rate. **(B)** The growth of testicular lymphoma around normal seminiferous tubules may be helpful in distinguishing it from seminoma. **(C)** Immunocytochemical localization of leukocyte common antigen (*brown pigment*) is extremely helpful in identifying lymphoma when the distinction from seminoma is difficult.

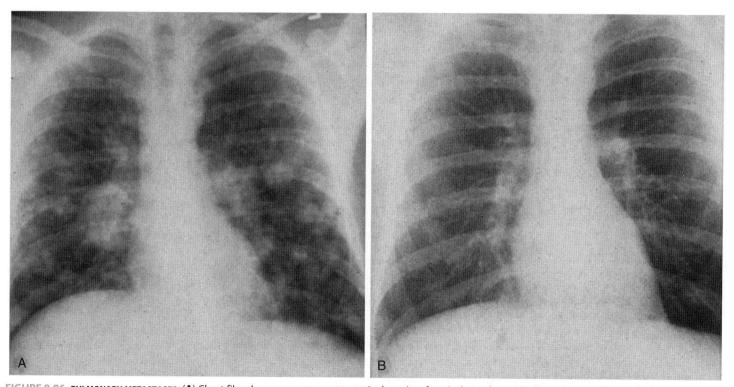

FIGURE 8.86 **PULMONARY METASTASES. (A)** Chest film shows numerous metastatic deposits of testicular embryonal cell carcinoma. **(B)** A marked response can be seen following combination chemotherapy containing cisplatin. This chemotherapeutic protocol achieves over a 90% cure rate for metastatic disease.

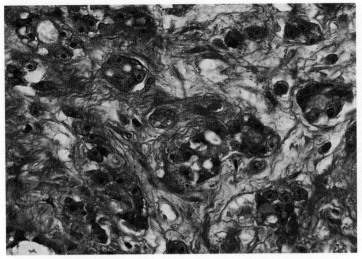

FIGURE 8.87 **METASTATIC ADENOCARCINOMA OF PROSTATE.** Small, glandular clusters of tumor cells can be seen in the testicular interstitium. This is a rare site for metastases.

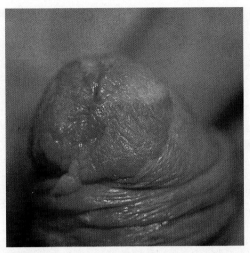

FIGURE 8.89 **CARCINOMA IN SITU.** This lesion presents clinically as a well-demarcated, slightly elevated erythematous plaque. (Courtesy of K.R. Greer, MD, Charlottesville, VA.)

Definition of TNM

Primary tumor (T)

TX	Primary tumor cannot be assessed
T0	No evidence of primary tumor
Tis	Carcinoma in situ
Ta	Noninvasive verrucous carcinoma
T1	Tumor invades subepithelial connective tissue
T2	Tumor invades the corpus spongiosum or cavernosum
T3	Tumor invades the urethra or prostate
T4	Tumor invades the adjacent structures

Regional lymph nodes (N)

NX	Regional lymph nodes cannot be assessed
N0	No regional lymph node metastasis
N1	Metastasis in a single superficial inguinal lymph node
N2	Metastasis in multiple or bilateral superficial inguinal lymph nodes
N3	Metastasis in deep inguinal or pelvic lymph node(s), unilateral or bilateral

Distant metastasis (M)

MX	Presence of distant metastasis cannot be assessed
M0	No distant metastasis
M1	Distant metastasis

Stage grouping

Stage 0	Tis	N0	M0
	Ta	N0	M0
Stage I	T1	N0	M0
Stage II	T1	N1	M0
	T2	N0	M0
	T2	N1	M0
Stage III	T1	N2	M0
	T2	N2	M0
	T3	N0	M0
	T3	N1	M0
	T3	N2	M0
Stage VI	T4	Any N	M0
	Any T	N3	M0
	Any T	Any N	M1

FIGURE 8.88 AJCC staging of penile cancer.

FIGURE 8.90 **SQUAMOUS CELL CARCINOMA.** (**A**) This resection specimen shows a small lesion arising in the coronal sulcus. (**B**) Cut section from the specimen demonstrates two small nodules of invasive tumor.

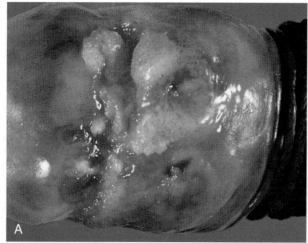
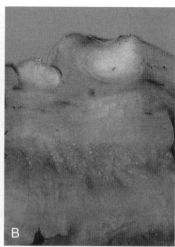

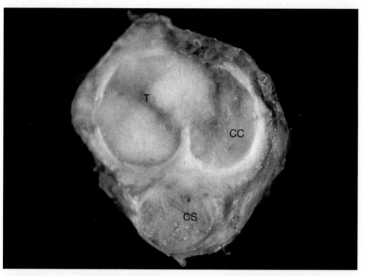

FIGURE 8.91 **SQUAMOUS CELL CARCINOMA.** A cross-section of the penile shaft illustrating replacement of the corpus cavernosum (CC) by tumor (T). CS, corpus spongiosum.

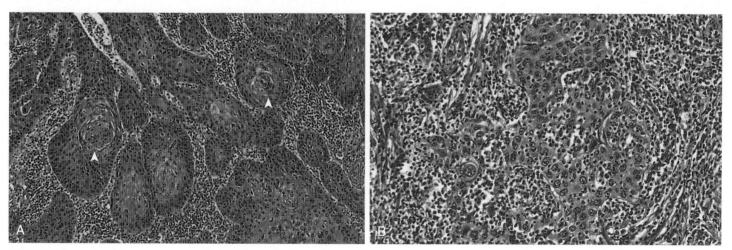

FIGURE 8.92 **SQUAMOUS CELL CARCINOMA.** (**A**) Irregular nests of neoplastic cells invade the underlying tissue. Note the foci of keratinization (*arrowheads*). (**B**) At the point of deepest invasion the squamous carcinoma cells are nonkeratinizing and show considerable pleomorphism, with large vesicular nuclei. Note the associated intense inflammation often seen in invasive carcinoma.

References and Suggested Readings

Abrahamsson PA: Neuroendocrine differentiation in prostatic carcinoma, *Prostate* 39:135–148, 1999.

Albertsen PC, Hanley JA, Gleason DF, et al: Competing risk analysis of men aged 55 to 74 years at diagnosis managed conservatively for clinically localized prostate cancer, *JAMA* 280:975–980, 1998.

Bosl GJ, Motzer RJ: Testicular germ-cell cancer, *N Engl J Med* 337:242–253, 1997.

Bostwick DG, Grignon DJ, Hammond ME, et al: Prognostic factors in prostate cancer. College of American Pathologists Consensus Statement 1999, *Arch Pathol Lab Med* 124:995–1000, 2000.

Carlin BI, Andriole GL: The natural history, skeletal complications, and management of bone metastases in patients with prostate carcinoma, *Cancer* 88(Suppl 12):2989–2994, 2000.

Catalona WJ, Southwick PC, Slawin KM, et al: Comparison of percent free PSA, PSA density, and age-specific PSA cutoffs for prostate cancer detection and staging, *Urology* 56:255–260, 2000.

Choueiri TK, Bukowski RM, Rini BI: The current role of angiogenesis inhibitors in the treatment of renal cell carcinoma, *Semin Oncol* 33:596–606, 2006.

Cohen HT, McGovern FJ: Renal-cell carcinoma, *N Engl J Med* 353:2477–2490, 2005.

Comiter CV, Kibel AS, Richie JP, et al: Prognostic features of teratomas with malignant transformation: a clinicopathological study of 21 cases, *J Urol* 159:859–863, 1998.

Costa LJ, Drabkin HA: Renal cell carcinoma: new developments in molecular biology and potential for targeted therapies, *Oncologist* 12:1404–1415, 2007.

D'Amico AV: Prostate-specific antigen (PSA) and PSA velocity: competitors or collaborators in the prediction of curable and clinically significant prostate cancer, *J Clin Oncol* 26:823–824, 2008.

D'Amico AV, Schnall M, Whittington R, et al: Endorectal coil magnetic resonance imaging identifies locally advanced prostate cancer in select patients with clinically localized disease, *Urology* 51:449–454, 1998.

D'Amico AV, Whittington R, Malkowicz SB, et al: Clinical utility of the percentage of positive prostate biopsies in defining biochemical outcome after radical prostatectomy for patients with clinically localized prostate cancer, *J Clin Oncol* 18:1164–1172, 2000.

Efstahiou E, Logothetis CJ: Review of late complications of treatment and late relapse in testicular cancer, *JNCCN* 4:1059–1070, 2006.

Elgamal AA, Troychak MJ, Murphy GP: ProstaScint scan may enhance identification of prostate cancer recurrences after prostatectomy, radiation, or hormone therapy: analysis of 136 scans of 100 patients, *Prostate* 37:261–269, 1998.

Epstein JI: Gleason score 2–4 adenocarcinoma of the prostate on needle biopsy: a diagnosis that should not be made, *Am J Surg Pathol* 24:477–478, 2000.

Escudier B, Eisen T, Stadler WM, et al: Sorafenib in advanced clear-cell renal-cell carcinoma, *N Engl J Med* 356:125–134, 2007.

Fleming S, O'Donnell M: Surgical pathology of renal epithelial neoplasms: recent advances and current status, *Histopathology* 36:195–202, 2000.

Fuchjäger M, Akin O, Shukla-Dave A, et al: The role of MRI and MRSI in diagnosis, treatment selection, and post-treatment follow-up for prostate cancer, *Clin Adv Hematol Oncol* 7:193, 2009.

George DJ, Kantoff PW: Prognostic indicators in hormone refractory prostate cancer, *Urol Clin North Am* 26:303–310, viii, 1999.

Gleason DF: Histologic grading of prostate cancer: a perspective, *Hum Pathol* 23:273–279, 1992.

Greene FL, Page D, Fleming I, et al, editors, for the American Joint Committee on Cancer: *AJCC cancer staging handbook*, ed 6, New York, 2002, Springer.

Greenlee RT, Hill-Harmon MB, Murray T, et al: Cancer statistics, 2001, *CA Cancer J Clin* 51:15–36, 2001.

Gudbjartsson T, Thoroddsen A, Petursdottir V, et al: Effect of incidental detection for survival of patients with renal cell carcinoma: results of population-based study of 701 patients, *Urology* 66:1186, 2005.

Han M, Walsh PC, Partin AW, et al: Ability of the 1992 and 1997 American Joint Committee on Cancer staging systems for prostate cancer to predict progression-free survival after radical prostatectomy for stage T2 disease, *J Urol* 164:89–92, 2000.

Hernández S, López-Knowles E, Lloreta J, et al: Prospective study of FGFR3 mutations as a prognostic factor in nonmuscle invasive urothelial bladder carcinomas, *J Clin Oncol* 24:3664–3671, 2006.

International Germ Cell Cancer Collaborative Group: International Germ Cell Consensus Classification: a prognostic factor-based staging system for metastatic germ cell cancers, *J Clin Oncol* 15:594–603, 1997.

Jemal A, Siegal R, Ward E, et al: Cancer statistics, 2007, *CA Cancer J Clin* 57:43–66, 2007.

Jones J, Libermann TA: Genomics of renal cell cancer: the biology behind and the therapy ahead, *Clin Cancer Res* 13:685, 2007.

Kim W, Kaelin WG: The von Hippel-Lindau tumor suppressor protein: new insights into oxygen sensing and cancer, *Curr Opin Genet Dev* 13:55–60, 2003.

Motzer RJ, Hutson TE, Tomczak P, et al: Sunitinib versus interferon alpha in metastatic renal-cell carcinoma, *N Engl J Med* 356:125–134, 2007.

Oh WK, Hurwitz M, D'Amico AV, et al: Prostate cancer. In Bast R, Kufe D, Pollock R, et al, editors: *Cancer medicine*, ed 5, Hamilton, Ontario, Canada, 2000, BC Decker.

Oh WK, Kantoff PW: Management of hormone refractory prostate cancer: current standards and future prospects, *J Urol* 160:1220–1229, 1998.

Olumi AF: A critical analysis of the use of p53 as a marker for management of bladder cancer, *Urol Clin North Am* 27:75–82, ix, 2000.

Reuter VE: The pathology of renal epithelial neoplasms, *Semin Oncol* 33:534–543, 2006.

Shuin T, Kondo K, Ashida S, et al: Germline and somatic mutations in von Hippel-Lindau disease gene and its significance in the development of kidney cancer, *Contrib Nephrol* 128:1–10, 1999.

Smith JA, Labasky RF, Cockett AT, et al: Bladder cancer clinical guidelines panel summary report on the management of nonmuscle invasive bladder cancer (stages Ta, T1 and TIS). The American Urological Association, *J Urol* 162:1697–1701, 1999.

Steele GS, Richie JP: Management of low-stage nonseminomatous germ cell tumors of the testis, *Compr Ther* 26:210–219, 2000.

Stein JP, Lieskovsky G, Cote R, et al: Radical cystectomy in the treatment of invasive bladder cancer: long-term results in 1,054 patients, *J Clin Oncol* 19:666–675, 2001.

Truong LD, Caraway N, Ngo T, et al: The diagnostic and therapeutic roles of fine-needle aspiration, *Am J Clin Pathol* 115:18–31, 2001.

Varghese SL, Grossfeld GD: The prostatic gland: malignancies other than adenocarcinomas, *Radiol Clin North Am* 38:179–202, 2000.

Figure Credits

The following books published by Gower Medical Publishing are sources of figures in the present chapter. The figure numbers given in the listing are those of the figures in the present chapter. The page numbers given in parentheses are those of the original publication.

Weiss MA, Mills SE: *Atlas of genitourinary tract disorders.* Philadelphia/New York, 1988, JB Lippincott/Gower Medical Publishing: Figs. 8.1 (p. 13.15), 8.4 (p. 14.8), 8.5 (p. 14.12), 8.6 (p. 14.13), 8.7 (p. 14.13), 8.8 (p. 14.14), 8.9 (p. 14.11), 8.10 (p. 14.16), 8.12 (p. 14.10), 8.13 (p. 14.18), 8.15 (p. 14.20), 8.16 (p. 14.20), 8.17 (p. 14.21), 8.19 (p. 4.24), 8.23 (p. 14.17), 8.31A, B (p. 12.14), 8.31C (p. 12.14), 8.32 (p. 12.9), 8.33 (p. 12.9), 8.36 (p. 12.16), 8.37 (p. 12.6), 8.38 (p. 12.8), 8.39 (p. 12.16), 8.40 (p. 12.17), 8.41 (p. 12.19), 8.42 (p. 12.21), 8.43 (p. 12.7), 8.44 (p. 12.27), 8.45 (p. 12.28),8.46 (p. 12.31), 8.47 (p. 12.31), 8.48 (p. 12.32), 8.49 (p. 12.33), 8.51 (p. 11.2), 8.52 (p. 11.3), 8.53 (p. 11.5), 8.54 (p. 11.7), 8.56 (p. 11.12), 8.57 (p. 11.13), 8.58 (p. 11.10), 8.59 (p. 11.21), 8.60 (p. 11.17), 8.61 (p. 11.8), 8.62 (p. 11.9), 8.63 (p. 11.49), 8.67 (p. 11.55), 8.68 (p. 11.57), 8.70 (p. 16.24), 8.71 (p. 16.24), 8.72 (p. 16.25), 8.74 (p. 16.9), 8.75 (p. 16.13), 8.76 (p. 16.14), 8.78 (p. 16.15), 8.79A, B (p. 16.16), 8.79C, D (p. 16.17), 8.81 (p. 16.18), 8.82 (p. 16.19), 8.83 (p. 16.22), 8.85 (p. 16.31), 8.87 (p. 16.31), 8.89 (p. 19.2), 8.90 (p. 19.8), 8.92 (p. 19.7).

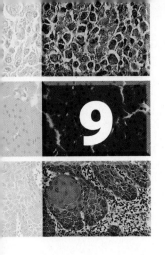

9

Gynecologic Tumors and Malignancies

MICHELLE S. HIRSCH • KAREN J. KRAG • URSULA A. MATULONIS

Ovarian Carcinoma

Though not the most common gynecologic malignancy, epithelial ovarian cancer is the most lethal, affecting approximately 26,000 women per year and causing at least 15,000 deaths in the United States, representing the fifth most frequent cause of cancer death in women (Jemal et al., 2008). The median age of diagnosis is 63, and close to 50% of patients are 65 years of age or older. The risk factors for epithelial ovarian cancer include nulliparity, whereas protective factors include multiple births and use of oral contraceptives. Family history of ovarian cancer is an important risk factor, and compared with the general population, whose lifetime risk is 1.6%, a woman with a single relative affected by ovarian cancer has a 4% to 5% increased risk for developing ovarian cancer. Genes implicated in increased susceptibility if germ-line inheritance occurs in an autosomal-dominant pattern include the *BRCA1* and *BRCA2* genes (hereditary breast-ovarian cancer), and mismatch repair genes such as *MSH2*, *MLH1*, *MSH6*, and *PMS2* (hereditary nonpolyposis colorectal syndrome). For women carrying a mutated high-risk gene, parity lowers risk but protective use of oral contraception remains controversial.

HISTOLOGY

The majority of malignant ovarian tumors are of epithelial origin (Table 9.1). Papillary serous adenocarcinomas, which constitute the majority of these tumors, are classically characterized by papillary fronds and psammoma bodies with cells reminiscent of fallopian tube mucosa. However, because most papillary serous carcinomas are poorly differentiated, architectural changes often include a more solid growth pattern with slitlike spaces and high-grade cytology. The contralateral ovary is involved either grossly or microscopically in at least half of cases. Endometrioid tumors are second in frequency and are less commonly bilateral but may coexist with a synchronous uterine carcinoma in up to 20% of cases. The remaining ovarian epithelial malignancies—mucinous carcinoma, clear cell carcinoma, undifferentiated carcinoma, and malignant Brenner tumors—are all less common. Mixed histologies may occur in the same patient, and squamous differentiation may be present in endometrioid tumors.

With the exception of the poor prognosis associated with advanced clear cell tumors, multivariate analyses have generally not shown histologic subtype to influence survival when com-

Table 9.1	
Classification of Malignant Ovarian Tumors	
Tumor	**Frequency(%)**
Epithelial	
Papillary serous cystadenocarcinoma	38
Mucinous cystadenocarcinoma	11
Endometrioid carcinoma	13
Clear cell carcinoma	5
Malignant Brenner tumor	<0.5
Undifferentiated carcinoma	15
Sex Cord–Stromal	
Granulosa cell tumor	2
Sertoli-Leydig tumor	<1
Mixed tumors	<0.5
Germ Cell	
Immature teratoma	<0.5
Embryonal carcinoma	<0.5
Endodermal sinus tumor	<1
Choriocarcinoma	<0.5
Mixed	<1
Dysgerminoma	2
Stromal	
Sarcomas	<0.5
Miscellaneous	
Metastatic carcinoma	10
Lymphoma	<0.5

paring stage for stage. Instead the grade of tumor contributes more significantly to prognosis, with shorter survival times associated with high-grade tumors. Poorly differentiated carcinomas are usually more chemotherapy-sensitive than lower grade tumors. Borderline epithelial tumors consist of neoplasms with a complex architecture that traditionally show no evidence of stromal invasion; however, occasionally borderline tumors can be associated with microinvasion of the underlying stroma, a finding that does not significantly affect outcome (McKenny et al, 2006a; Hart, 2005). Approximately 90% of borderline tumors are serous and 10% are mucinous; rarely, endometrioid and clear cell varieties are encountered. Patients who carry a mutated *BRCA1* or *BRCA2* gene typically have an improved overall prognosis as compared with patients who do not carry a such a mutation. Borderline tumors have a very long natural history, although they can metastasize and cause death (Longacre et al, 2005; Ayhan et al, 2005). Poorer prognosis is most frequently associated with the presence of micropapillary features and/or invasive implants (noninvasive implants do not affect survival rates) (McKenny et al, 2006b; Prat, 2003; Prat et al, 2002; Rollins et al, 2006).

Germ cell tumors constitute approximately 20% of benign ovarian neoplasms but represent <5% of ovarian malignancies (Ulbright, 2005). They are most common in young women and children, where cure and preservation of fertility are frequently achieved. Mature teratoma, a benign neoplasm, is the most common germ cell tumor of the ovary. Dysgerminoma accounts for nearly half of all malignant germ cell tumors, with a median age at diagnosis of 22 years. Other malignant germ cell tumors include immature teratoma, yolk sac tumor, embryonal carcinoma, and nongestational choriocarcinoma. The malignant ovarian germ cell tumors are all rare but interesting because of their similarity to male testicular cancers in both natural history and responsiveness to chemotherapy.

Other nonepithelial ovarian tumors may be divided into sex cord–stromal tumors (Young, 2005), metastatic malignancies (Hirsch and Lee, 2006; Prat, 2005), and sarcomas (Lerwill et al, 2004; Chang 1993; Irving et al, 2006). Of the sex cord–stromal tumors, granulosa cell tumors are the most common and constitute 2% of all ovarian malignancies. Composed of granulosa cells with or without theca cells, they may be hormonally active, causing resumption of menses in older women or precocious pseudopuberty in the rare young person developing this malignancy. Sertoli-Leydig cell tumors are sex cord–stromal tumors marked by some testicular differentiation and often by androgen production; they are rarely malignant. Metastatic tumors, which represent 10% of ovarian malignancies, most commonly originate from primary sites in the endometrium/cervix, gastrointestinal (GI) tract, and breast. They include Krukenberg tumors of gastric origin, which exhibit a classic mucus-secreting, "signet-ring" cell, metastatic colon carcinomas which often demonstrate characteristic dirty necrosis, and pancreatic carcinomas, which not infrequently mimic a primary ovarian mucinous tumor. Metastases from the appendix can pose a diagnostic challenge, in that the primary tumor may be occult and morphologic features of appendiceal and ovarian neoplasms can be identical. Epithelial neoplasms in the ovary associated with pseudomyxoma peritonei should be considered of appendiceal origin until proven otherwise (Bradley et al, 2007; Young 2005; O'Connell et al, 2002). Immunohistochemical stains can be useful in separating primary and secondary tumors of the ovary (Hart 2005). Primary ovarian sarcomas are very rare and may be classified in a manner similar to that used for uterine sarcomas. The most common sarcomas primary to the ovary include leiomyosarcoma (LMS) (Lerwill et al 2004), endometrial stromal sarcoma (ESS) (Change et al 1993) and fibrosarcoma (Irving et al 2006); metastases from the uterus should always be considered for LMS and ESS. Mixed tumors marked by the presence of both sarcomatous and epithelial elements also occur, and are termed carcinosarcomas (previously called malignant mixed müllerian tumors).

Three types of small cell carcinoma, all with morphologic overlap, can occur in the ovary: (1) small cell carcinoma, pulmonary type; (2) small cell carcinoma, hypercalcemic type; and (3) metastatic small cell (neuroendocrine) carcinomas to the ovary, typically from the cervix, lung, or GI tract. Distinction of primary versus secondary small cell carcinoma can be determined with the aid of ancillary studies, such as immunohistochemistry and human papillomavirus (HPV) testing, in the majority of cases (Carlson et al, 2007; McCluggage 2004).Small cell carcinomas of the ovary are typically very aggressive and have a poor prognosis.

STAGING OF OVARIAN CARCINOMA

Ovarian cancer is staged according to FIGO staging.* Early-stage ovarian carcinoma is confined to the ovary (stage I) or the pelvic organs (stage II) (see Fig. 9.1). However, because of the vague nature of symptoms and the lack of effective screening programs, most women present with spread throughout the peritoneal cavity (stage III). Ovarian carcinomas usually disseminate intraperitoneally. Extraperitoneal dissemination (stage IV) is less common and usually occurs late in the course of the disease, whereas pleural effusions are the most common manifestation of extra-abdominal disease. Although the mechanism for this tendency is unclear, the right hemidiaphragm is commonly involved in stage IV disease, and there are connections between the lymphatic systems above and below the diaphragm. Parenchymal lung involvement is unusual. Nodal spread may also occur to Virchow's node (supraclavicular), the inguinal nodes or Sister Mary-Joseph's node in the para-umbilical region. The FIGO staging system requires assessment of the ovarian capsule, lymph node dissection, and multiple peritoneal/omental biopsies for accurate staging. Without careful surgical evaluation, up to 30% of women may have their disease under-staged.

CLINICAL MANIFESTATIONS

Early-stage epithelial ovarian carcinoma rarely causes symptoms, although large masses may cause pelvic pain, constipation, tenesmus, and urinary frequency or dysuria. Abdominal cramping, flatulence, bloating, and gas pains are more common presenting symptoms, usually due to tumor dissemination throughout the peritoneal cavity. These symptoms unfortunately are often poorly defined and occasionally mild; they may be attributed to benign GI pathology, until the woman has obvious abdominal distention, most often related to increasing ascites or intestinal obstruction. The importance of a pelvic examination in the initial evaluation of any woman with GI complaints cannot be overemphasized. Late in the course of the disease, shortness of breath from pleural effusions may occur. Hematogenous dissemination to the liver, lungs, and left supraclavicular or axillary nodes is a less common occurrence, and bone, brain, or meningeal metastases are rare. However, unusual metastases may occur, especially in patients with a prolonged natural history.

In women with an abnormal pelvic mass, useful diagnostic tests include a transvaginal ultrasound and computed tomography (CT) scan. The CA125 blood test (which measures the concentration of a blood protein known as cancer antigen 125) is not a useful screening tool but is important in monitoring the results of therapy once a diagnosis has been established and thereafter following for recurrence once the patient has completed chemotherapy.

Nonepithelial tumors often present in a fashion similar to epithelial malignancies. Granulosa cell tumors and other stromal neoplasms are usually detected when a woman presents with pelvic discomfort or vague abdominal symptoms; these tumors also may secrete estrogen and cause resumption of menses in the postmenopausal woman; these tumors can also produce inhibin, which can serve as a biomarker. This hyperestrogenic effect may lead to the simultaneous development of endometrial carcinoma. Germ cell tumors are seen almost exclusively in premenopausal women. They are occasionally detected as an asymptomatic pelvic mass, but more commonly they present acutely with symptoms of rapid tumor growth or as abdominal emergencies secondary to hemorrhage, rupture, or torsion.

*The revised FIGO staging is just being released (Mutch, 2009).

FIGURE 9.1 FIGO staging system for carcinoma of the ovary (2000).

FIGO staging system of the ovary

Stage I	Growth limited to ovaries	Stage III	Tumor involving one or both ovaries with peritoneal implants outside the pelvis and/or retroperitoneal or inguinal nodes. Superficial liver metastases equals stage III. Tumor is limited to the true pelvis, but with histologically verified malignant extension to small bowel or omentum.
	Stage IA Growth is limited to one ovary. No ascites; no tumor on external surface; capsule intact		
	Stage IB Growth is limited to both ovaries. No ascites; no tumor on external surface; capsule intact		**Stage IIIA** Tumor grossly limited to true pelvis with negative nodes but with histologically confirmed microscopic seeding of abdominal peritoneal surface
	Stage IC Tumor either stage IA or IB, but with tumor on the surface of one or both ovaries; or with capsule rupture; or with ascites containing malignant cells; or with positive peritoneal washings		**Stage IIIB** Tumor of one or both ovaries with histologically confirmed implants on abdominal peritoneal surfaces, none >2 cm in diameter. Nodes negative.
Stage II	Growth involving one or both ovaries with pelvic extension		
	Stage IIA Extension and/or metastases to uterus and/or tubes		**Stage IIIC** Abdominal implants >2 cm in diameter and/or positive retroperitoneal or inguinal nodes
	Stage IIB Extension to other pelvic tissues	Stage IV	Growth involving one or both ovaries with distant metastases. If pleural effusion is present, there must be positive cytologic test results to assign a case to stage IV. Parenchymal liver metastases equals stage IV.
	Stage IIC Tumor either stage IIA or IIB, but with tumor on the surface of one or both ovaries; or with capsule rupture; or with ascites containing malignant cells; or with positive peritoneal washings		

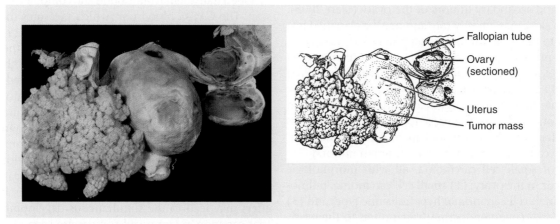

Fallopian tube
Ovary (sectioned)
Uterus
Tumor mass

FIGURE 9.2 **PAPILLARY SEROUS TUMOR OF BORDERLINE MALIGNANCY INVOLVING THE SURFACE OF THE OVARY.** This specimen, from a 29-year-old woman who presented with menorrhagia, consists of the uterus with both tubes and ovaries. The left ovary is largely replaced by a tumor covered by sessile papillae. The uterus is distorted by leiomyomas, and the right ovary contains a follicular cyst and corpus luteum. Both serous and mucinous tumors of borderline malignancy are now well defined histologically and clearly recognized clinically. The median age at presentation is 5–10 years younger than patients with invasive cancer, and borderline malignancies are not unusual in premenopausal women.

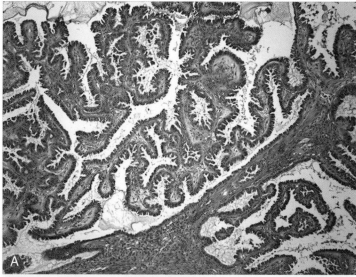

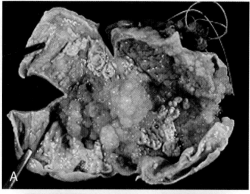

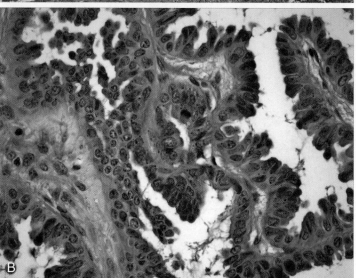

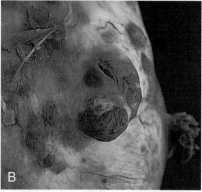

FIGURE 9.4 PAPILLARY SEROUS CYSTADENOMA OF BORDER LINE MALIGNANCY. (**A**) The ovary is replaced by a large, unilocular cystic structure that contains tan, soft papillary excrescences that project into the center of the cyst. (**B**) In a carcinoma, tumor can be seen extending through the surface of the ovary. Capsule excrescences, dense adherence of tumor to peritoneum, the presence of cytologically positive peritoneal fluid, and a high histologic grade are all poor prognostic signs in stage I patients and suggest the necessity for further therapy.

FIGURE 9.3 PAPILLARY SEROUS TUMOR OF BORDERLINE MALIGNANCY. (A) Complex papillary structure. (**B**) Histologic examination at higher magnification reveals mitotic activity and nuclear atypia, together with multilayering and cell proliferation, but the absence of stromal invasion is consistent with borderline/uncertain malignant potential. These tumors may spread throughout the peritoneum and serosal surfaces as either noninvasive or invasive implants; the latter are more common with micropapillary features. The 5-year survival rate is ~95%, but 10-year survival falls to ~75%. A small percentage of tumors are aggressive, and chemotherapy seems to be ineffective.

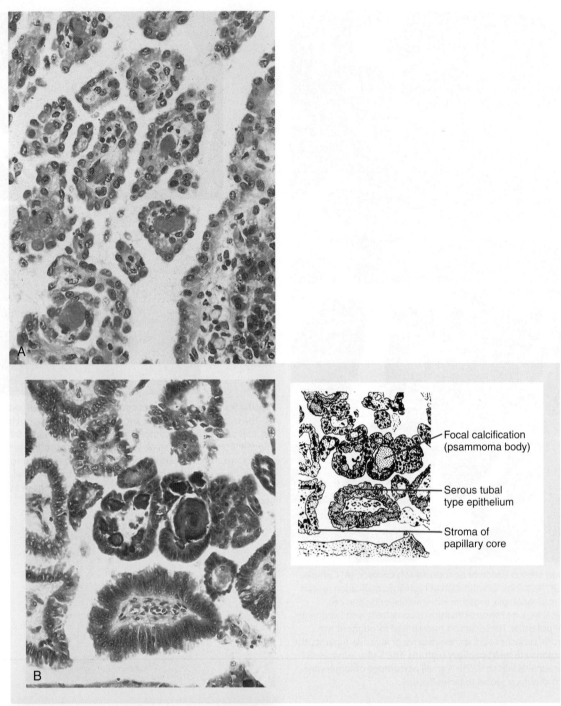

Focal calcification
(psammoma body)

Serous tubal
type epithelium

Stroma of
papillary core

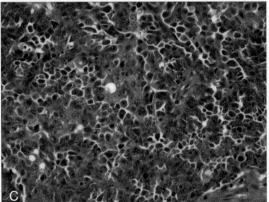

FIGURE 9.5 PAPILLARY SEROUS CYSTADENOCARCINOMA.
Histologically, these tumors range from (**A**) well-
differentiated neoplasms with obvious papillae and
minimal cytologic atypia, to (**B**) moderate differentiation
with more proliferative epithelium, and to (**C**) poorly
differentiated solid nests of cells. Psammoma bodies (as
seen in **B**) can occur in all grades but are more frequent in
well-differentiated tumors.

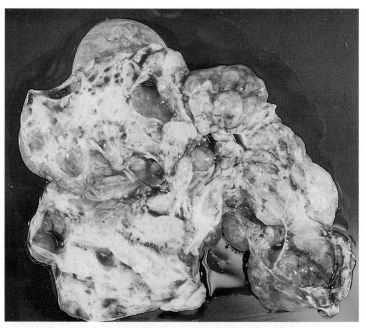

FIGURE 9.6 **MUCINOUS CYSTADENOCARCINOMA.** The ovary is replaced by a multiloculated, partly cystic, partly solid mass. Cystic spaces contain viscid fluid. This tumor arises largely in middle-aged or elderly women. Like its benign counterpart, mucinous cystadenoma, it may attain great size. Although a secondary carcinoma, especially from the GI tract, should be considered when a mucinous tumor involves the ovary, the presence of unilateral disease and size >10 cm favors a primary ovarian tumor.

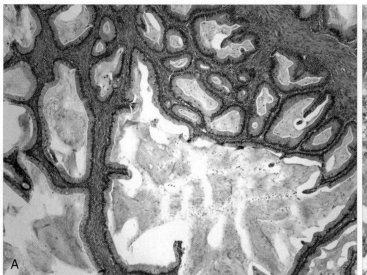

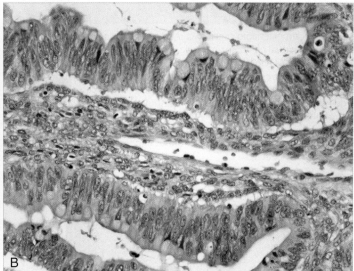

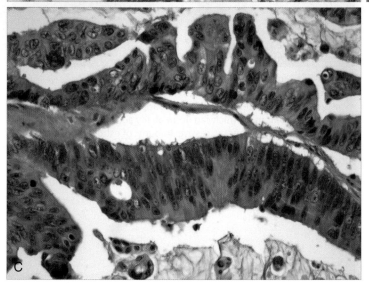

FIGURE 9.7 **MUCINOUS CYSTADENOCARCINOMA.** Mucinous carcinomas may demonstrate expansile or infiltrative patterns of invasion. The neoplastic epithelium can be (**A**) frankly mucinous, lined by columnar cells with basally located nuclei and apical mucinous cytoplasm, or it may resemble a GI carcinoma either (**B**) with or (**C**) without scattered goblet cells.

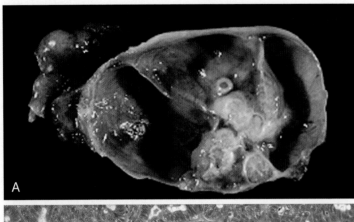

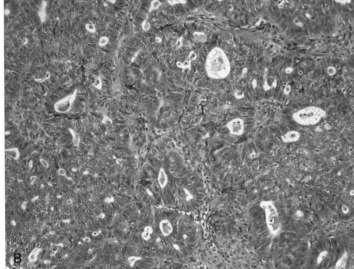

FIGURE 9.8 **ENDOMETRIOID CARCINOMA.** A 44-year-old woman presented with intermenstrual bleeding and underwent surgery for presumed endometriosis. (**A**) A focus of endometrioid carcinoma was discovered inside one endometriotic cyst. There was no disease elsewhere in the abdomen. Endometrioid carcinoma occurs in approximately 0.5% of cases of ovarian endometriosis and is the most common pathologic subtype associated with this condition. The tumor is usually partially cystic and may be filled with a chocolate-brown fluid. (**B**) Microscopically, the glands resemble uterine endometrioid carcinoma, and a synchronous endometrial carcinoma may be seen in ~20% of patients.

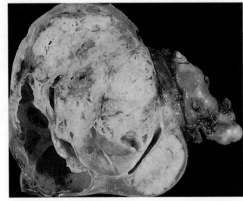

FIGURE 9.9 **CLEAR CELL ADENOCARCINOMA.** Arising in the ovary is a large, predominantly solid, yellowish neoplasm that shows focal cystic change and necrosis. Cystic changes, often representative of endometriosis/endometrioma, are common in these tumors.

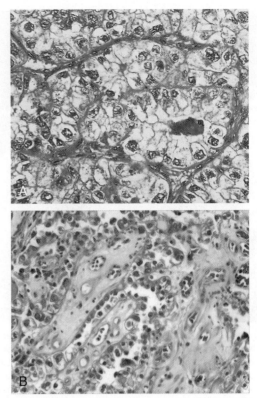

FIGURE 9.10 **CLEAR CELL ADENOCARCINOMA.** The architecture is typically variable, usually including solid sheets or tubular arrangement of cells, but (**A**) cytologically they are all characterized by severely atypical (high-grade) cells with abundant clear cytoplasm, and (**B**) cystic spaces lined by hobnail cells, with nuclei projecting apically. In more than 60% of patients, these tumors are confined to the ovary at presentation, but stage for stage, the prognosis is worse than for other types of ovarian adenocarcinomas, including serous carcinoma. Hematogenous metastases are more frequent, and some patients have a fulminant course.

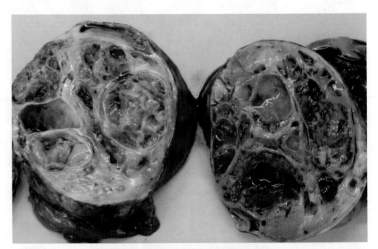

FIGURE 9.11 **GRANULOSA CELL TUMOR.** This specimen is from a 60-year-old woman. This solid and cystic yellowish tumor is well circumscribed and measures 1 cm in greatest dimension. This appearance is typical of this sex cord–stromal tumor, which can occur at any age, including childhood, but most frequently secretes excessive amounts of estrogen, leading to menstrual irregularity or postmenopausal bleeding. All granulosa cell tumors should be regarded as malignant, but the clinical course is often indolent.

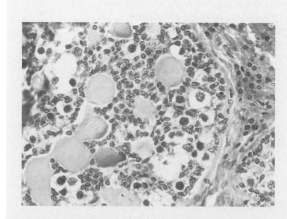

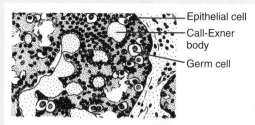

FIGURE 9.12 **GRANULOSA CELL TUMOR.** This tumor is composed of nests of cells with inconspicuous cytoplasm; bland, oval nuclei with little cytologic atypia; and occasional longitudinal nuclear grooves ("coffee bean appearance"). Germ cells and epithelial cells may coexist epithelial cells may form Call-Exner bodies, consisting of pink, inspissated material.

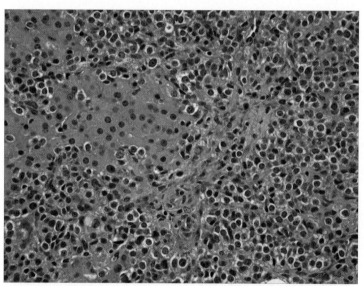

FIGURE 9.13 Sertoli–Leydig cell tumors consist of a biphasic proliferation of Sertoli (*right of image*) and Leydig cells (*left of image*). The latter have very round nuclei with prominent nucleoli and a moderate amount of eosinophilic cytoplasm. Occasionally these cells may be vacuolated and contain lipofuscin. The Sertoli cells infiltrate as nests, cords, and tubules, and the degree of tubular differentiation, as well as cytologic atypia and mitotic activity, are used to grade the tumor. This tumor is consistent with an intermediate grade Sertoli–Leydig cell tumor.

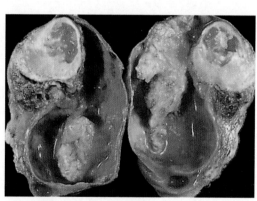

FIGURE 9.14 **MATURE CYSTIC TERATOMA.** The bisected ovary reveals replacement by a multicystic tumor within which sebaceous material and matted hair can be seen.

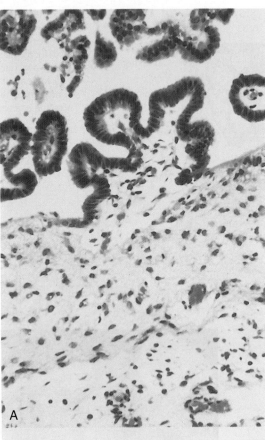

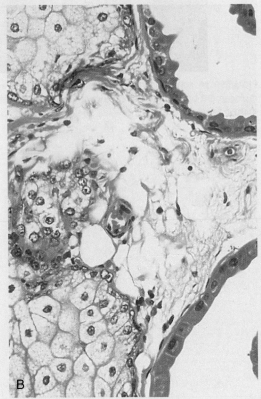

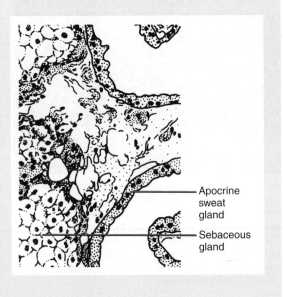

FIGURE 9.15 **MATURE CYSTIC TERATOMA. (A)** A small focus of mature choroid plexus lies above equally mature-appearing brain tissue. **(B)** Normal sebaceous glands below are adjacent to well-developed apocrine sweat glands above. Struma ovarii is an uncommon variant of this germ cell tumor, composed predominantly of thyroid tissue (not shown).

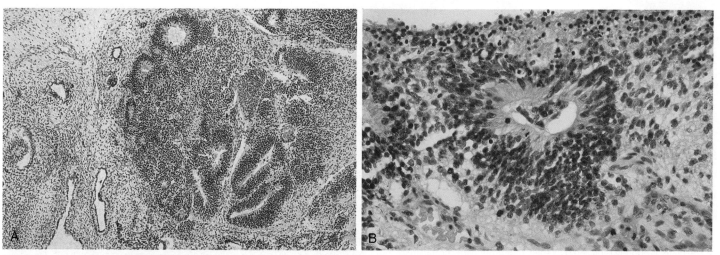

FIGURE 9.16 **IMMATURE TERATOMA.** (**A**) A large region of immature neuroepithelium is present. (**B**) Neuroepithelial rosettes, indicative of embryonic differentiation, are characteristic of immature teratomas.

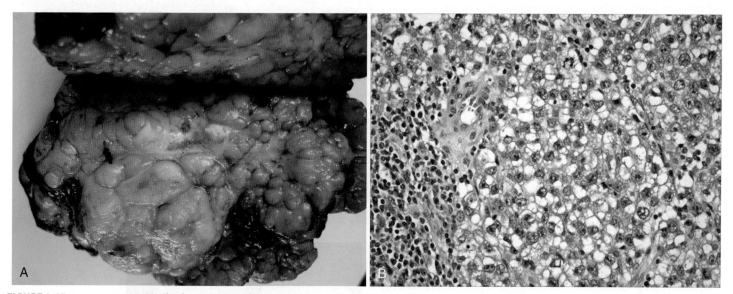

FIGURE 9.17 **DYSGERMINOMA.** (**A**) This large, multinodular whitish/tan tumor arising in the ovary is morphologically similar to testicular seminoma. It typically does not secrete human chorionic gonadotrophin (HCG) nor α-fetoprotein; however, scattered syncytiotrophoblasts present in some of these tumors may account for low levels of serum HCG. Dysgerminomas are extremely sensitive to irradiation and chemotherapy and carry an excellent prognosis, with many patients retaining their fertility. (**B**) Histologically, nests of large, uniform cells with pale to clear cytoplasm and prominent nucleoli are separated by stroma infiltrated by lymphocytes and plasma cells (*lower left*).

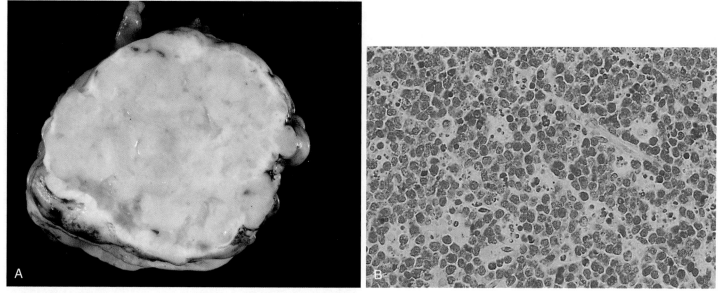

FIGURE 9.18 **BURKITT LYMPHOMA.** (**A**) Occasionally the ovary is the primary site for an extranodal lymphoma. This tumor, which may occur in children, is grossly characterized by diffuse replacement of the ovary by a homogeneous fleshy mass. (**B**) Cytologically, the tumor demonstrates the classic starry-sky pattern marked by large, light-staining benign histiocytes admixed with small, basophilic, undifferentiated malignant cells. The differential diagnosis includes a poorly differentiated carcinoma and small cell carcinoma.

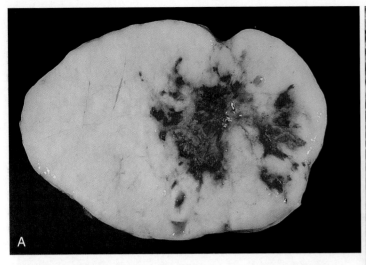

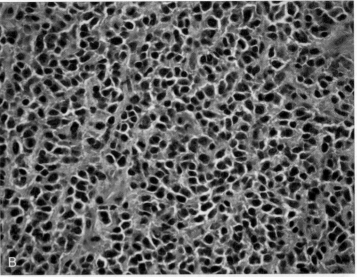

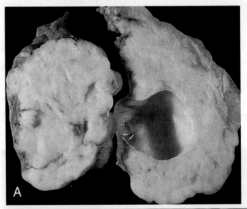

FIGURE 9.19 **SMALL CELL CARCINOMA OF THE OVARY, HYPERCALCEMIC TYPE.**
(**A**) The ovary is entirely replaced by a solid, tan tumor with central areas of hemorrhage, and frequently necrosis. This rare, yet very aggressive neoplasm affects young women and has a poor prognosis.
(**B**) Histologically, there are solid sheets of closely packed, undifferentiated, small cells with scant cytoplasm, round to irregular vesicular nuclei, and numerous mitoses. Because of morphologic overlap, the differential diagnosis includes small cell carcinoma of the ovary, pulmonary type, and a metastatic small cell (neuroendocrine) carcinoma from nonovarian sites such as the lung or GI tract; keratin, neuroendocrine and WT-1 and TTF-1 immunostains can aid in the distinction. (**C**) Microfollicles (fluid-filled spaces lined by tumor cells) are frequently seen in small cell carcinoma, hypercalcemic type; however, similar structures can also be seen in juvenile granula cell tumor, a much less aggressive tumor.

FIGURE 9.20 **METASTATIC BREAST CANCER.** (**A**) Both ovaries are diffusely replaced by pale, rather nodular tumor; a follicular cyst is also present on the right. Bilateral involvement by metastases is common. (**B**) In this case the metastatic breast cancer cells are arranged in long lines perpendicular to the surface of the ovarian cortex; glandular elements can also be seen in metastatic ductal carcinomas.

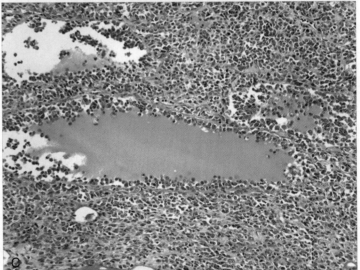

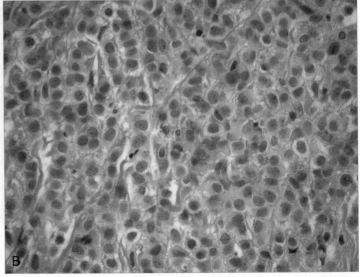

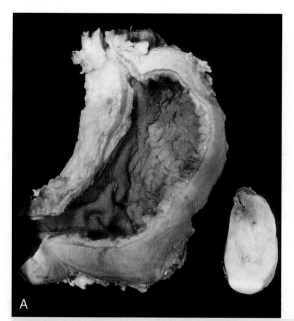

FIGURE 9.21 GASTRIC ADENOCARCINOMA WITH OVARIAN
METASTASIS (KRUKENBERG TUMOR). (**A**) This specimen is from a 65-year-old woman who had a 4-month history of dysphagia. A barium meal revealed a tumor of the gastric fundus, and esophagogastrectomy with resection of a right ovarian tumor was performed. The sectioned ovary at the right shows total replacement by pale tumor. (**B**) When the gastric tumor is a mucus-secreting signet-ring cell adenocarcinoma, the ovarian moiety is known as a Krukenberg tumor. Ovarian involvement may be bilateral. Other primary sources of signet-ring histology are most frequently carcinomas of the breast, colon, and appendix.

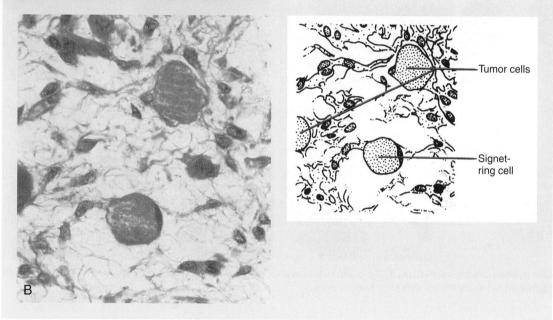

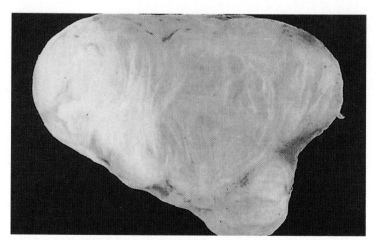

FIGURE 9.22 **FIBROMA.** The ovary is replaced by a pale, lobulated tumor, the cut surface of which is fibrous and whorled. Ovarian fibromas, derived from stromal mesenchyme, usually arise in the fifth or sixth decade, and are almost invariably benign. They are sometimes accompanied by ascites or pleural effusions (Meigs syndrome).

FIGURE 9.23 STAGE III OVARIAN CANCER (ASCITES). CT scan in a 57-year-old woman with recurrent ovarian cancer who presented with ascites shows peritoneal fluid surrounding loops of small bowel.

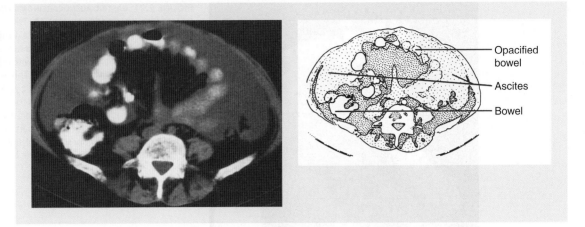

Opacified bowel

Ascites

Bowel

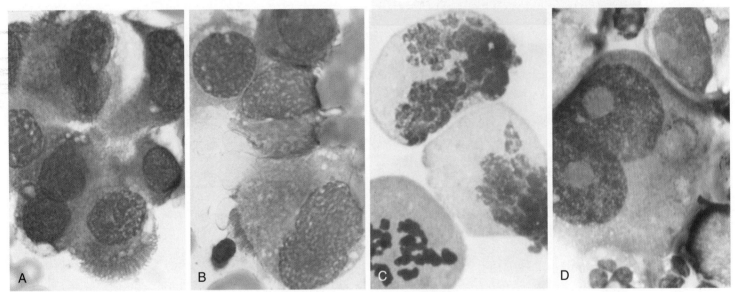

FIGURE 9.24 STAGE III OVARIAN CANCER (ASCITES). (A, B) Malignant cells in ascitic fluid show characteristic brush borders. **(C)** Mitotic figures can also be seen, as well as **(D)** a large, immature binucleate cell with prominent nucleoli.

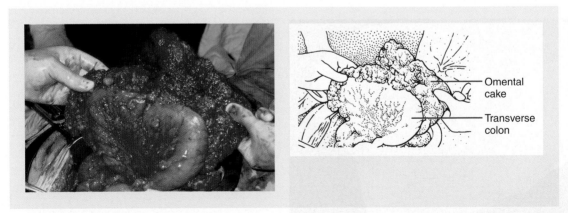

Omental cake

Transverse colon

FIGURE 9.25 STAGE III OVARIAN CANCER (PERITONEAL IMPLANTS). Despite extensive tumor with mesenteric studding, together with a large omental "cake" of tumor, this 55-year-old woman had few symptoms: vague abdominal bloating, increased gas, and a feeling of fullness. Histologic examination showed a papillary serous cystadenocarcinoma. (Courtesy of Howard Goodman, MD, Department of Gynecologic Oncology, Brigham and Women's Hospital, Boston, MA.)

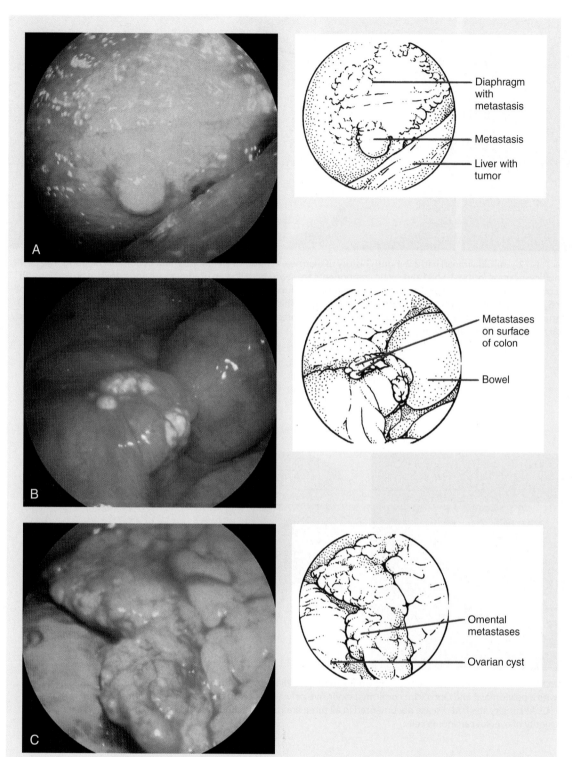

Diaphragm with metastasis

Metastasis

Liver with tumor

Metastases on surface of colon

Bowel

Omental metastases

Ovarian cyst

A

B

C

FIGURE 9.26 **STAGE III OVARIAN CANCER (PERITONEAL IMPLANTS).** Metastases in patients in this stage may be tiny seedlings, as (**A**) in this laparoscopic photograph of the right hemidiaphragm. They may also be (**B**) larger nodules on bowel serosa or (**C**) extensive omental "cakes".

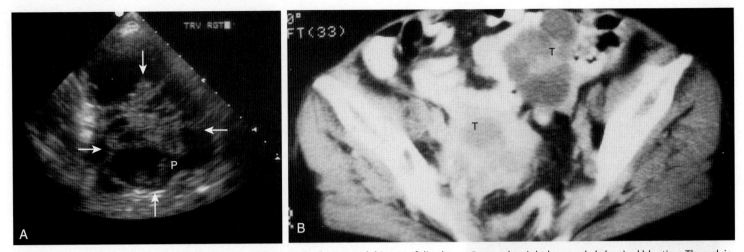

FIGURE 9.27 STAGE III OVARIAN CANCER. This 72-year-old woman had a 2-month history of diarrhea, a 5-pound weight loss, and abdominal bloating. The pelvic ultrasonogram (**A**) shows a complex multicystic mass (*arrows*). Solid and cystic components are seen, as well as an irregular wall and papillary projections (P) within the cystic structures. The most common adnexal mass in the premenopausal woman is a functional cyst, which should resolve over a few weeks; in the postmenopausal patient any cyst over 5 cm or with internal septations must be fully evaluated. This pelvic CT scan (**B**) confirms the large multicystic mass (T). At surgery she had diffuse peritoneal studding, extensive retroperitoneal adenopathy, and an unresectable pelvic mass. She responded well to chemotherapy, with normalization of markers and total regression of her symptoms.

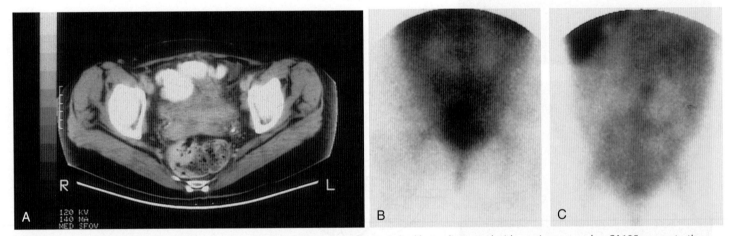

FIGURE 9.28 RECURRENT OVARIAN CANCER. Nine months after this 54-year-old woman had been diagnosed with ovarian cancer, her CA125 concentration began to increase. A CT scan (**A**) showed a pelvic mass, and OncoScint confirmed extensive pelvic disease (**B**) but also showed diffuse peritoneal involvement and para-aortic disease (**C**). At surgery she had disease documented in all three areas. OncoScint is an ^{111}In-labeled monoclonal antibody to TAG-72, an antigen present on the majority of ovarian carcinoma cells.

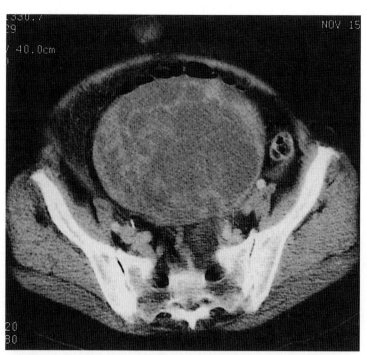

FIGURE 9.29 **OVARIAN GRANULOSA CELL TUMOR.** This axial CT scan was taken of a 72-year-old woman who presented with a several-month history of abdominal pressure. It shows a large pelvic mass, which was resectable at surgery. Pathology demonstrated a granulosa cell tumor, and she had some bloody though cytologically negative ascites. These tumors are usually cystic and filled with serous fluid and blood, and 15% of women present with hemoperitoneum due to partial or complete cyst rupture.

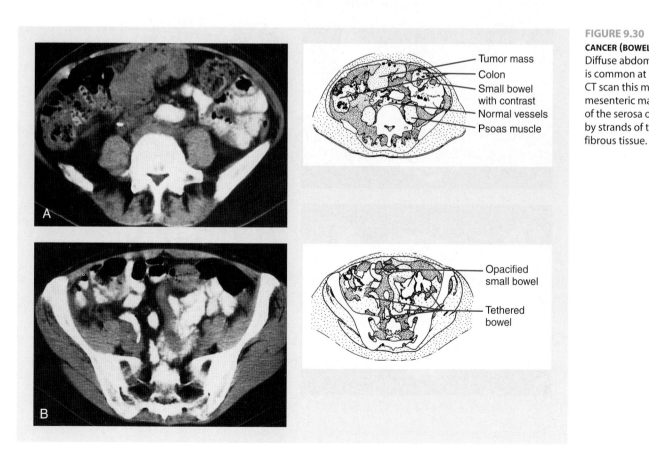

FIGURE 9.30 **STAGE III OVARIAN CANCER (BOWEL TETHERING).** Diffuse abdominal involvement is common at presentation. On CT scan this may be seen as (**A**) a mesenteric mass or (**B**) tethering of the serosa of the small bowel by strands of tumor and reactive fibrous tissue.

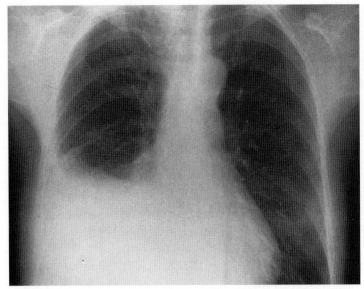

FIGURE 9.31 STAGE IV OVARIAN CANCER (PLEURAL EFFUSION). A 54-year-old nonsmoker presented with shortness of breath; she had no abdominal symptoms. Plain film of the chest demonstrates a large pleural effusion that was cytologically positive for carcinoma. Pelvic examination revealed a large left ovarian mass. Her CA125 concentration was 2000 U/mL (normal is usually <35 U/mL). After six cycles of chemotherapy there was complete resolution of the effusion, the pelvic mass, and the elevated CA125. She remained without evidence of disease 24 months later.

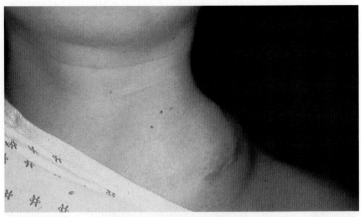

FIGURE 9.32 STAGE IV OVARIAN CANCER. This 35-year-old woman presented with a large supraclavicular mass 10 years after surgery and adjuvant chemotherapy for stage III ovarian carcinoma. Pathologic examination showed papillary serous adenocarcinoma identical to her initial tumor. Although such nodal involvement is occasionally seen at presentation, spread to the left supraclavicular (Virchow's) node or left axillary (Irish's) node, as well as to the liver, lung, or brain, is usually a late occurrence. Even at autopsy, liver or lung metastases are present in only 15% of cases.

FIGURE 9.33 RESPONSE TO CHEMOTHERAPY. A 51-year-old woman presented with a rapid increase in abdominal girth. (**A**) On CT scan she was found to have a 12 × 8 cm ovarian mass with a cystic component; peritoneal involvement was extensive, and 6 L of ascites were removed. Pathologic examination showed a poorly differentiated tumor. The tumor was not resectable, and she was treated with combination chemotherapy. After one cycle of therapy her abdomen returned to normal size. (**B**) A CT scan reveals only a small residual ovarian mass. Surgery after four cycles of chemotherapy showed no gross or microscopic tumor. She received four more cycles of chemotherapy but relapsed 1 year later with abdominal metastases.

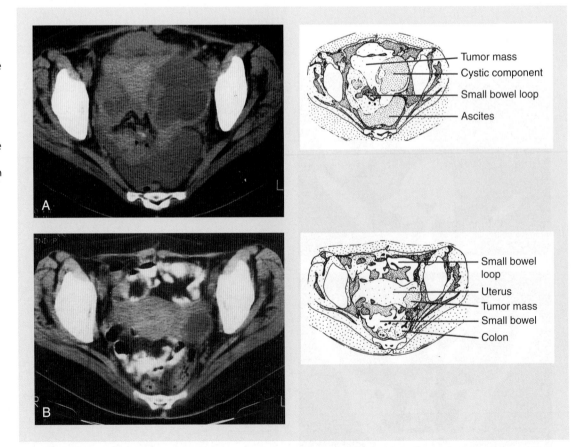

Tumor mass
Cystic component
Small bowel loop
Ascites

Small bowel loop
Uterus
Tumor mass
Small bowel
Colon

Endometrial Carcinoma

Endometrial carcinoma is the most common malignancy of the female genital tract, with up to 40,000 new cases diagnosed each year (Jemal et al., 2008). Despite its prevalence, less than one sixth of these cases (~7000) result in death from disease. Increased survival rates are most likely secondary to patient and physician education, the presence of symptoms at earlier stages of the disease, and ease of obtaining a biopsy specimen. Therefore, cases are diagnosed at an earlier stage than in the past, and death rates are continuing to decrease. The incidence of endometrial cancer peaks late in the sixth decade, and proven associations include obesity (50 pounds overweight increases the risk 10-fold), diabetes mellitus, late menopause, and probably hypertension, as well as other factors such as nulliparity and infertility, which increase estrogenic stimulation to the endometrium. Exogenous estrogens increase the risk for carcinoma, but this can be reversed by cycling estrogens with progestins. Polycystic ovarian disease and other illnesses that cause chronic anovulation increase the risk for this malignancy, and women with these problems may develop endometrial carcinoma before menopause. Sporadic cases of endometrial carcinomas have been shown to be associated with multiple gene mutations, including *TP53* mutations in serous (type II) carcinomas, and *PTEN*, *KRAS*, and β-catenin mutations in endometrioid (type II) carcinomas (Hecht and Mutter, 2006). Endometrial carcinomas associated with mutations in the mismatch repair genes *MSH2* and *MLSH1* can be a sporadic findings but is more commonly associated with hereditary nonpolyposis colorectal cancer (HNPCC) syndrome. Patients known to be affected by HNPCC have an increased risk for developing endometrial carcinoma (as well as colorectal carcinoma) at a younger age; however, there is controversy as to whether the gene mutations affect prognosis (Zighelboim et al, 2007; Prat et al, 2007; An et al, 2007).

There is no effective screening method for detecting endometrial carcinoma. However, on occasion an endometrial cancer may be revealed when malignant or normal endometrial cells are seen in a Papanicolaou (Pap) smear. The presence of the former requires distinction between endocervical and endometrial origins, and the presence of the latter may indicate a carcinoma in approximately 10% of postmenopausal women. Nevertheless, evaluation in these women, as well as in women with postmenopausal bleeding, requires endometrial sampling or dilatation and curettage. The majority of women with well-differentiated stage I endometrial cancers are cured by surgery alone. Radiation therapy and/or more commonly vaginal brachytherapy are being used for higher risk patients (i.e., significant myometrial involvement, high-grade tumors, cervical involvement with cancer) so as to decrease pelvic and vaginal recurrences.

HISTOLOGY

Adenocarcinoma constitutes more than 90% of endometrial cancers, with the endometrioid subtype being the most common. Other subtypes of endometrial carcinoma include serous, mucinous, clear cell, and mixed subtypes. Grossly, these tumors are often polypoid or exophytic; however, a more endophytic invasive growth pattern can also be recognized. The microscopic appearance is marked by architectural irregularity with multiple fused and/or cribriform glands that crowd out supporting stroma, and it is not infrequently associated with endometrial intraepithelial neoplasia (EIN), the endometrioid carcinoma precursor lesion. The cells in an endometrioid carcinoma are more frequently of lower grade, but increased cytologic atypia and pleomorphism can be encountered. Tumor grade, which takes into account cell type, nuclear atypia, and glandular to more solid growth patterns, seems to be an important prognostic feature; lymphatic and vascular space involvement may also be significant for prognosis. In contrast to endometrioid and mucinous carcinomas, which are graded on the basis of architectural features, grade of serous and clear cell carcinomas is based on cytologic findings. Squamous, and less frequently mucinous, differentiation can be seen, especially in endometrioid subtypes. Papillary serous and clear cell adenocarcinomas of the uterus (type II endometrial cancers) are seen less frequently when compared with endometrioid carcinomas, and are highly aggressive types of endometrial cancer. Treatment of early papillary serous and clear cell tumors is controversial. Unlike endometrioid and mucinous carcinomas, noninvasive serous and clear cell carcinomas of the uterus still have a poor prognosis.

Sarcomas, of which leiomyosarcoma (LMS) is the most common, represent approximately 5% of uterine malignancies. Believed to arise de novo and not from leiomyomas, LMSs usually occur in the fifth and sixth decades. They are homologous tumors, containing elements derived from uterine smooth muscle, and are usually intramural in location. Microscopically they are composed of atypical spindle cells associated with necrosis and increased mitotic activity, often with 10 or more mitoses per 10 high-power fields (HPFs). A variant showing 5–10 mitoses per 10 HPFs is of uncertain malignant potential (called a smooth muscle tumor of uncertain malignant potential, or "STUMP") and may possess a long natural history. A diagnosis of STUMP should be made with caution in a myomectomy specimen, because evaluations may be limited. Extrauterine involvement has been seen with both benign and malignant smooth muscle neoplasms: the former is associated with disseminated peritoneal leiomyomatosis, intravascular leiomyomatosis, or benign metastasizing leiomyoma; metastatic spread of LMS connotes a poor prognosis.

Endometrial stromal tumors are homologous tumors, derived from uterine mesenchyme, which resemble proliferative endometrial stroma, demonstrate little cytologic atypia, contain prominent spiral-like arterioles, and have variable numbers of mitotic figures (most frequently fewer than 10 per 10 HPFs). Well-circumscribed stromal neoplasms are termed endometrial stromal nodules, whereas those that infiltrate the myometrium and often demonstrate vascular invasion are termed endometrial stromal sarcomas (ESSs) (previously called endolymphatic stromal myosis or low-grade ESS). Endometrial stromal nodules are benign lesions, whereas ESSs are considered low-grade tumors that have an indolent clinical course and may take up to 10 or so years to recur. ESSs usually have a low mitotic count (<10 per 10 HPFs) and an absence of necrosis.

High-grade malignancies that are thought to be of endometrial stromal origin but no longer resemble endometrial stroma are termed undifferentiated uterine sarcoma (UUSs) (previously called high-grade ESSs). UUSs are associated with a greater degree of nuclear atypia and pleomorphism, extensive necrosis, and numerous mitotic figures (often >10, and frequently as many as 20 mitoses per 10 HPFs including atypical forms). Heterologous tumors, which are extremely rare, are most frequently associated with an epithelial component (carcinosarcomas, see below).

Carcinosarcomas (previously called malignant mixed müllerian tumors) contain both epithelial (carcinoma) and mesenchymal (sarcoma) elements. The epithelial component is most commonly high grade, whereas the sarcomatous portion may be homologous or heterologous (most frequently rhabdomyosarcoma). Carcinosarcomas have a poorer prognosis compared with endometrioid cancers, stage for stage.

STAGING OF ENDOMETRIAL CARCINOMA

Most endometrial malignancies are confined to the uterus at the time of diagnosis (stage I) (see Fig. 9.34). Spread to the cervix marks stage II tumors and should be described as spread to cervical mucosa (stage IIa) and/or cervical stromal (stage IIb). More advanced stages—which include spread to pelvic organs or retroperitoneal lymph nodes (stage III) or hematogenous spread to distant sites (stage IV), usually to the lungs—are occasionally seen; such cases have a worse prognosis.

Preoperative workup in patients with suspected higher risk endometrial cancer would include a chest CT scan to rule out lung metastases and an abdominal/pelvic CT scan to rule out liver, nodal, and other sites of metastases. Depth of invasion of the myometrium as assessed at surgery also is essential for staging. Removal of pelvic and para-aortic lymph nodes is typically recommended for patients with high-risk cancers and can help decide treatment after surgery. These factors provide useful information for determining prognosis and aid in the choice of possible adjuvant therapy.

CLINICAL MANIFESTATIONS

More than 90% of women with endometrial carcinoma present with abnormal vaginal bleeding. Although atrophic vaginitis is the most common cause of vaginal bleeding in low-risk postmenopausal women, patients presenting with this complaint require an endometrial biopsy for proper evaluation. With increasing age, abnormal postmenopausal bleeding is more often associated with carcinoma; overall, about 20% of such women will be found to have a malignancy. Carcinoma in perimenopausal women or anovulatory women may present with heavy or prolonged bleeding; these women may ignore changes in their bleeding pattern, considering them to be signs of approaching menopause. If the tumor spreads outside the uterus, adjacent organs are most commonly involved. Vaginal or suburethral metastases may cause pain, bleeding, or discharge; abdominal distention, and bowel or urinary dysfunction may develop from involvement of the bladder or rectum. Back pain may result from para-aortic nodal involvement. Pulmonary metastases may occur late in the course of disease as a result of hematogenous spread, and brain metastases may occur, but less commonly.

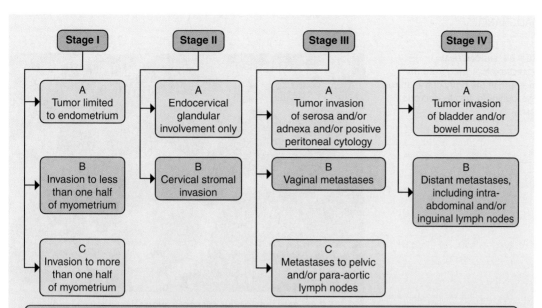

FIGURE 9.34 FIGO staging system for endometrial carcinoma (1990).

Histopathology–degree of differentiation
Cases should be grouped by the degree of differentiation of the adenocarcinoma:
GI 5% or less of a nonsquamous or nonmorular solid growth pattern
GII 6% to 50% of a nonsquamous or nonmorular solid growth pattern
GII More than 50% of a nonsquamous or nonmorular solid growth pattern

Notes on pathologic grading
Notable nuclear atypia, inappropriate for the architectural grade, raise the grade of a grade I or grade II tumor by one. In serous adenocarcinomas, clear cell adenocarcinomas and squamous cell carcinomas, take precedence. Adenocarcinomas with squamous differentiation are graded according to the nuclear grade of the glandular component.

Rules related to staging
Because corpus cancer is now surgically staged, procedures previously used for determination of staging are no longer applicable, such as the finding of fractional D&C to differentiate between stages I and II. It is appreciated that there may be a small number of patients with corpus cancer who will be treated primarily with radiation therapy. If that is the case, the clinical staging adopted by FIGO in 1971 would still apply, but designation of that staging system would be noted. Ideally, width of the myometrium should be measured, along with the width of tumor invasion.

TNM staging compared to the FIGO system

Definition of TNM
Primary tumor (T)*

TNM	FIGO	Definition
TX	–	Primary tumor cannot be assessed
T0	–	No evidence of primary tumor.
T1s	–	Carcinoma in situ
T1	1	Tumor confined to the corpus uten
T1a	IA	Tumor limited to the endometrium
T1b	IB	Tumor invades up to of less than one half of the myometrium
T1c	IC	Tumor invades more than one-half of the myometrium
T2	II	Tumor invades the cervix but not extending beyond the uterus
T2a	IIA	Endocervical glandular involvement only
T2b	IIB	Cervical stromal invasion
T3 and/or N1	III	Local and/or regional spread as specified in T3a, b, NI and FIGO IIIA, B, and C below
T3a	IIIA	Tumor involves the serosa and/or adnexa (direct extension or metastasis) and/or cancer cells in ascites or peritoneal washings
T3b	IIIB	Vaginal involvement (direct extension or metastasis)
N1	IIIC	Metastasis to the pelvic and/or para-aortic lymph nodes
T4	IVA	Tumor invades the bladder mucosa or the rectum and/or the bowel mucosa
M1	IVB	Distant metastasis (excluding metastasis to the vagina, pelvic serosa, or adnexa; including metastasis to intra-abdominal lymph nodes other than para-aortic, and/or inguinal lymph nodes.)

Regional lymph nodes (N)
NX Regional lymph nodes cannot be assessed
NO No regional lymph node metastasis
N1 Regional lymph node metastasis

Distant metastasis (M)

TNM	FIGO	Definition
MX	–	Presence of distant metastasis cannot be assessed
MO	–	No distant metastasis
M1	IVB	Distant metastasis

Stage grouping

AJCC/UICC				FIGO
Stage 0	T1s	N0	M0	
Stage IA	T1a	N0	M0	Stage IA
Stage IB	T1b	N0	M0	Stage IB
Stage IC	T1c	N0	M0	Stage IC
Stage IIA	T2a	N0	M0	Stage IIA
Stage IIB	T2b	N0	M0	Stage IIB
Stage IIIA	T3a	N0	M0	Stage IIIA
Stage IIIB	T3b	N0	M0	Stage IIIB
Stage IIIC	T1	N1	M0	Stage IIIC
	T2	N1	M0	
	T3a	N1	M0	
	T3b	N1	M0	
Stage IVA	T4	Any N	M0	Stage IVA
Stage IVB	Any T	Any N	M1	Stage IVB

The predominant lesion is adnocarcinoma but all histologic types should be reported. However, choriocarcinomas; sarcomas, mixed mesodermal tumors, and carcinosarcomas should be presented separately.

Note: The presence of bullous edema is not sufficient evidence to classify a tumor as T4

FIGURE 9.35 TNM Staging Compared to the Figo system. (From Greene F, Page D, Flemming I, et al, editors, for the American Joint Committee on Cancer: *AJCC cancer staging manual,* ed 6, New York, 2002, Springer.)

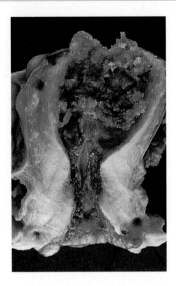

FIGURE 9.36 ENDOMETRIAL ADENOCARCINOMA. Arising from the endometrium in the body of the uterus is a large, polypoid, focally necrotic neoplasm.

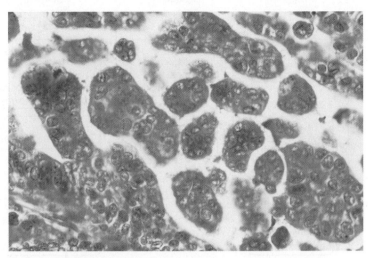

FIGURE 9.38 PAPILLARY SEROUS ADENOCARCINOMA. Histologically and clinically, this rare and virulent form of endometrial cancer resembles its ovarian counterpart; its pattern of transperitoneal spread is also similar.

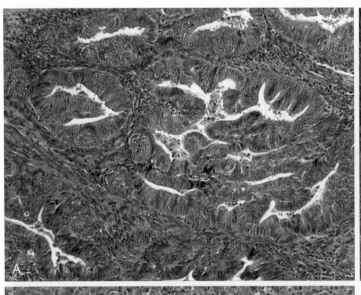

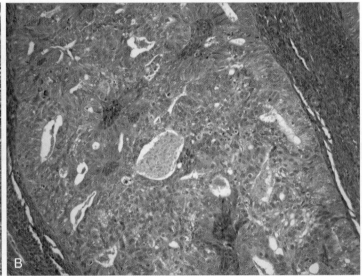

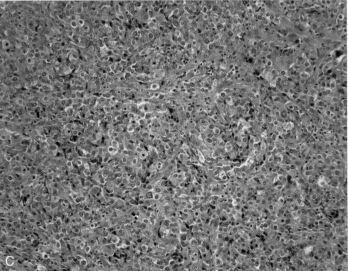

FIGURE 9.37 ENDOMETRIAL ADENOCARCINOMA. (A) In a grade I tumor the glands are well preserved, indicating continuing differentiation, but they have crowded and complex architectural features with supporting stroma that has been crowded out. **(B)** Grade II lesions are marked by piling up and bridging of malignant epithelium within gland spaces, forming cribriform patterns and focally solid areas. Between 5% and 50% of the tumor must have a solid component to diagnose a grade II lesion. **(C)** All organization is lost in grade III tumors, which show solid sheets of cancer cells in >50% of the tumor. Grade is associated with increased depth of invasion, probability of pelvic nodal involvement, a lower likelihood of response to hormonal therapy, and decreased survival.

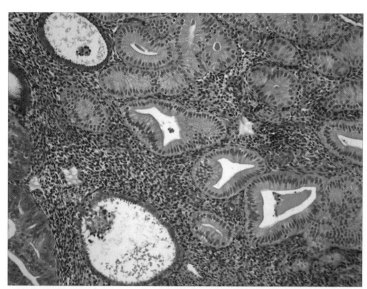

FIGURE 9.39 **ENDOMETRIAL INTRAEPITHELIAL NEOPLASIA (EIN)** Also known as atypical endometrial hyperplasia, diagnostic features of EIN include a gland-to-stroma ratio >50%, cytologic features that differ from the background endometrium, and a size >0.1 cm. EINs (atypical hyperplasias) are considered at high risk for malignant change. Rare benign endometrial glands are seen at the *top* and *bottom* of the image, and a small focus of carcinoma is seen in the *lower left-hand corner*.

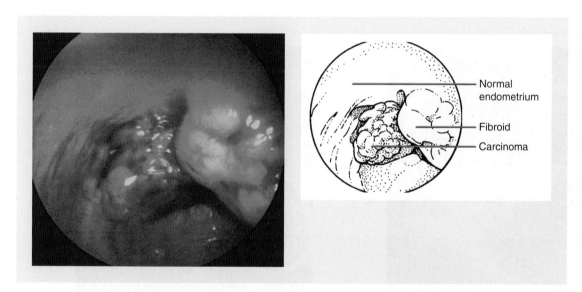

FIGURE 9.40 **STAGE I ENDOMETRIAL CARCINOMA.** A small carcinoma can be seen adjacent to a uterine fibroid in this hysteroscopy photograph. Occasionally, a tumor this small may be missed on curettage.

Normal endometrium
Fibroid
Carcinoma

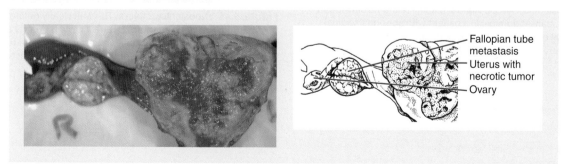

Fallopian tube metastasis
Uterus with necrotic tumor
Ovary

FIGURE 9.41 **STAGE III ENDOMETRIAL CARCINOMA.** This specimen is from a 64-year-old woman with a 1-year history of postmenopausal bleeding. The tumor is ulcerative, deeply invasive, and has spread to the fallopian tube. Pathologic examination showed a poorly differentiated adenocarcinoma. (Courtesy of Howard Goodman, MD, Department of Gynecologic Oncology, Brigham and Women's Hospital, Boston, MA.)

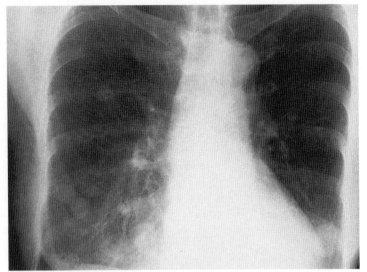

FIGURE 9.42 STAGE IV ENDOMETRIAL CARCINOMA (PULMONARY METASTASES). This 74-year-old woman presented with vaginal bleeding and was found to have a stage IB poorly differentiated adenosquamous carcinoma of the endometrium, which was invasive to one third of the myometrium. One year after surgery the disease recurred with pulmonary nodules. A significant number of patients at recurrence have only distant metastases, the pulmonary parenchyma being the most common site.

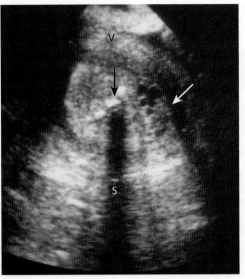

FIGURE 9.44 ENDOMETRIAL CANCER. Coronal real-time ultrasound image through the uterine fundus in the patient in Figure 9.43, using an endovaginal transducer. Note more detailed image of internal structure of the mass, with small areas of calcification (*arrow*) showing acoustic shadow (S), as well as small cystic areas (*arrow*). V, vaginal wall.

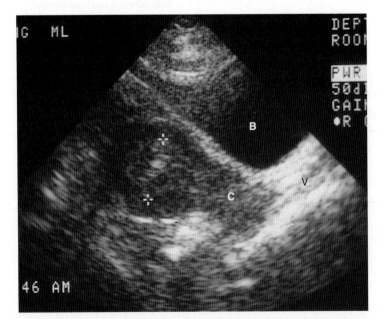

FIGURE 9.43 ENDOMETRIAL CANCER. Sagittal midline real-time ultrasound image of the pelvis, transabdominal in a patient with abnormal vaginal bleeding. No normal endometrium is visible in the fundus, with a heterogeneous central mass present (*between asterisks*). B, bladder; C, cervix; V, vagina.

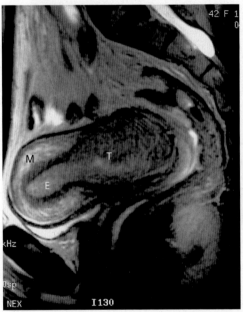

FIGURE 9.45 ENDOMETRIAL CANCER. This MRI clearly defines normal myometrium (M), endometrium (E), and a large tumor (T) arising posteriorly from the uterus. Although MRI gives excellent definition to pelvic tissues, CT scans are better able to differentiate between contrast-filled bowel and nodal disease.

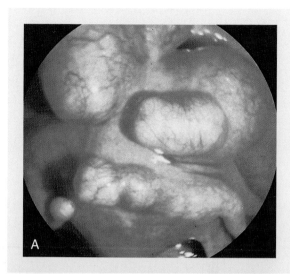

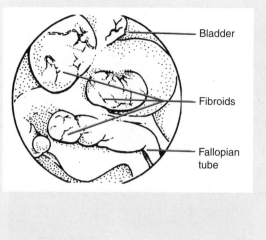

- Bladder
- Fibroids
- Fallopian tube

FIGURE 9.46 LEIOMYOMA. (**A**) This laparoscopic photograph shows multiple intramural/subserosal leiomyomas. (**B**) Similar findings in a different case are seen in this gross photograph of a uterus with multiple intramural and subserosal (pedunculated) fibroids, status post hysterectomy.

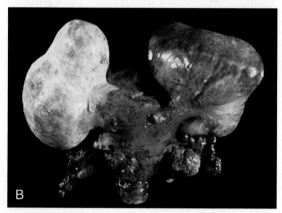

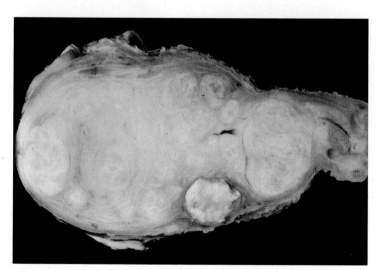

FIGURE 9.47 LEIOMYOMA. This grossly enlarged and distorted uterus has been sectioned to show multiple, well-circumscribed intramural and submucosal tumors displacing and compressing the uterine cavity. The lesions have a typical white/tan whorled appearance without hemorrhage or necrosis. These benign neoplasms of uterine smooth muscle, also known as "fibroids", are very common and typically arise during the reproductive years. They are usually multiple and are thought to be caused by excessive estrogen stimulation; they tend to atrophy after menopause. Various forms of degenerative changes are common, but malignant transformation in a leiomyoma is very rare.

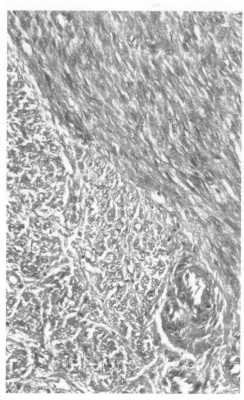

FIGURE 9.48 LEIOMYOMA. The myometrial muscle bundles *above* and to the *right* in this photomicrograph run parallel to the plane of the section. *Below* and to the *left*, the plane of the section cuts across the muscle bundle. These are characteristic features of smooth muscle tumors.

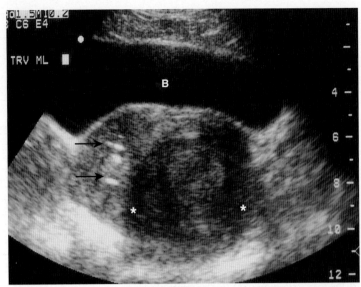

FIGURE 9.49 **Transverse real-time ultrasound image through the uterine fundus in a patient with abdominal pain.** A large hypoechoic mass is seen to the left of the midline (*asterisks*), compatible with a uterine fibroid. Note several portions of an intrauterine device (*arrows*) within the plane of the scan. B, bladder.

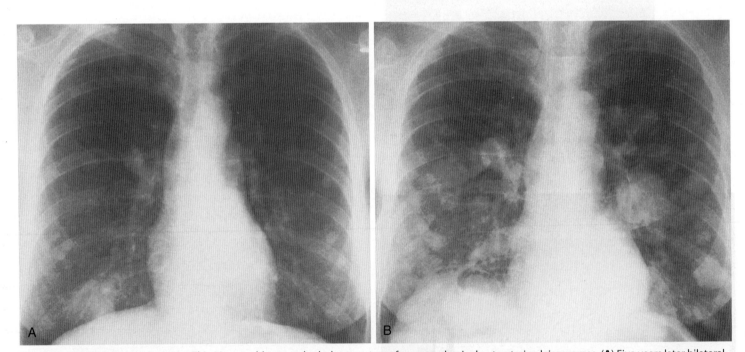

FIGURE 9.50 **Metastatic leiomyoma.** This 39-year-old woman had a hysterectomy for menorrhagia due to uterine leiomyomas. (**A**) Five years later bilateral asymptomatic pulmonary nodules developed. Biopsy showed histologic findings similar to the tumor seen at hysterectomy. (**B**) Over a 6-year interval the size of the lesions slowly increased, still with no major symptoms. This entity has been termed "benign metastasizing leiomyoma" but it undoubtedly represents a very low-grade malignancy.

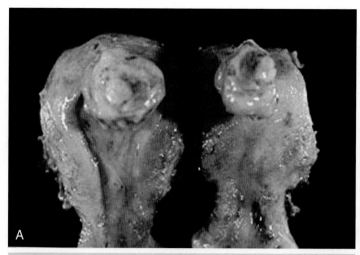

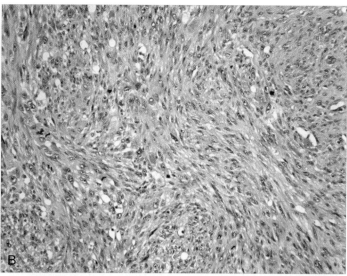

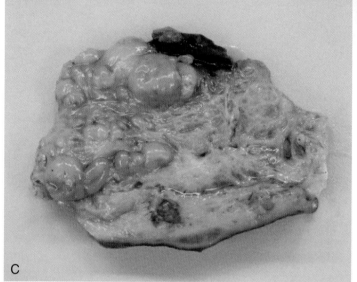

FIGURE 9.51 **LEIOMYOSARCOMA.** (**A**) A tan, polypoid fleshy mass is noted protruding into the lumen of the uterus. This tumor, which arises in the myometrium and is composed of tumor cells with smooth muscle differentiation, lacks the whorled appearance seen in benign leiomyomas and is invariably associated with hemorrhage and necrosis. (**B**) Cytologic atypia (pleomorphism), a brisk mitotic rate, and the presence of necrosis (not seen in this image) clearly identify the malignant nature of this tumor. (**C**) When significant vascular invasion is present it may be seen grossly as tumor plugs protruding through the myometrium ("wormlike" growth pattern, *left lower side of image*; this pattern can also be seen in endometrial stromal sarcomas, see below). Prognosis is related to stage, and the overall 5-year survival rate is about 30%.

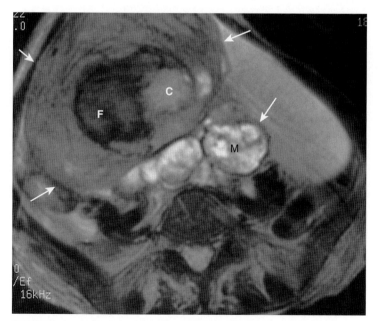

FIGURE 9.52 **UNRESECTABLE LEIOMYOSARCOMA.** This MRI is from a 50-year-old woman who presented with abdominal swelling. The MRI shows a heterogeneous tumor (*arrows*) with areas of solid and cystic (C) tumor, mucin production (M), and fibrosis (F). Whereas CT scan can define a mass, MRI can differentiate some tissue types within a tumor.

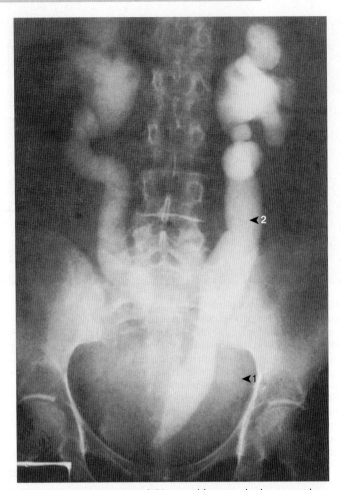

FIGURE 9.53 **LEIOMYOSARCOMA.** A 51-year-old woman had recurrent low-grade uterine leiomyosarcoma. She first presented with a large pelvic mass and was treated surgically. Disease recurred 6 years later and again 3 years afterward, when radiologic evaluation showed a large pelvic mass (*arrowhead 1*) with bilateral hydronephrosis and hydroureters (*arrowhead 2*). Renal function was normal, and the pelvic mass was resected. Chest CT scan showed a single pulmonary nodule, which on resection proved to be a primary, well-differentiated lymphocytic lymphoma.

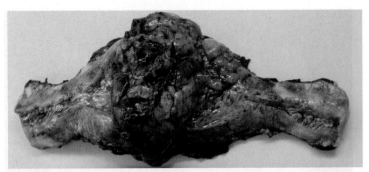

FIGURE 9.54 **CARCINOSARCOMA.** This tumor type was formerly called malignant mixed müllerian tumor. Arising in the uterine fundus is a large, polypoid, hemorrhagic mass with extensive myometrial invasion. These tumors arise most often in the elderly and carry a poor prognosis.

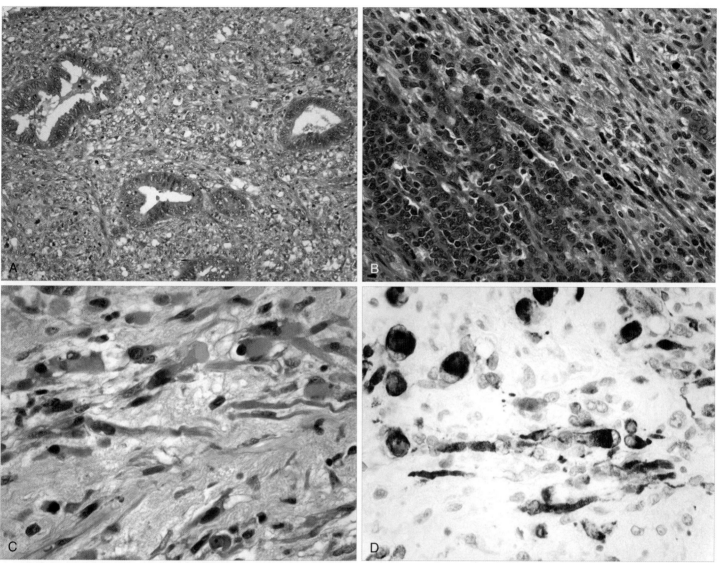

FIGURE 9.55 CARCINOSARCOMA. (A, B) The diagnosis of a carcinosarcoma is based on biphasic morphology, which includes both malignant epithelial and mesenchymal components. The epithelial component usually has endometrioid and/or serous differentiation, and the mesenchymal component is most often sarcoma NOS (not otherwise specified); however, homologous elements (i.e., leiomyosarcoma) can be seen. **(C, D)** The most common heterologous element encountered is rhabdomyosarcoma (skeletal muscle differentiation). Although cross-striations seen by hematoxylin-eosin staining are diagnostic of skeletal muscle differentiation, these can be difficult to identify in some cases, so immunohistochemical stains can be used to confirm (desmin immunostain shown).

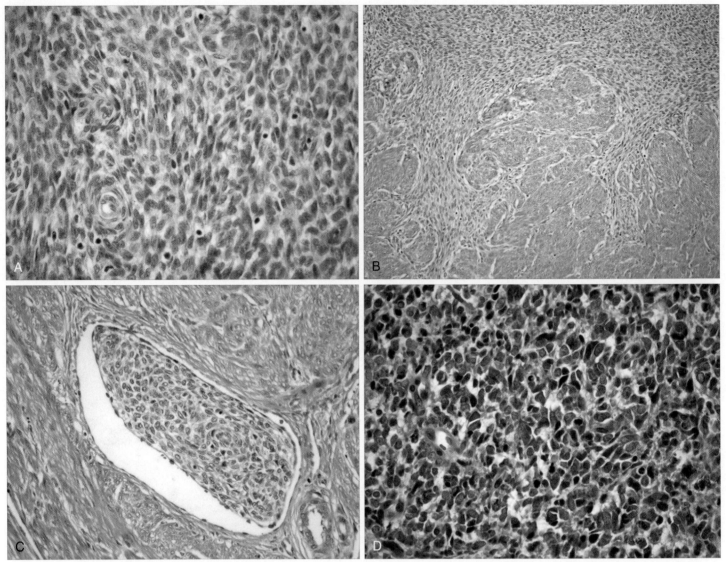

FIGURE 9.56 ENDOMETRIAL STROMAL SARCOMA (ESS). (A) This homologous tumor arises from endometrial mesenchyme, and cytologically it resembles endometrial stroma with bland spindle cells and associated with spiral arterioles. **(B)** Typically, ESSs demonstrate characteristic finger-like projections into the myometrium, and a low mitotic activity (<10 per 10 HPFs); a well-circumscribed single nodule of endometrial stroma is called an "endometrial stromal nodule" and is a benign neoplasm that sometimes is confused with highly cellular leiomyomas. **(C)** It is not infrequent to see vascular invasion in ESS, hence their prior designation of endolymphatic stromal myosis. **(D)** High-grade, undifferentiated spindle cells tumors with increased cytologic atypia, significant necrosis, and numerous mitotic figures, that have also been excluded to be of smooth muscle origin, are called undifferentiated uterine sarcomas; formerly these tumors were called high-grade ESSs, but this term is no longer recognized by the World Health Organization.

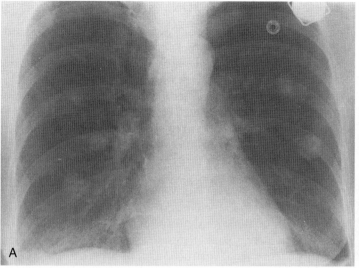
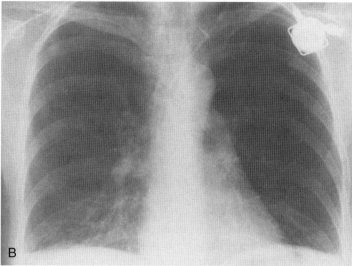

FIGURE 9.57 ENDOMETRIAL STROMAL SARCOMA (ESS). Most ESSs have an indolent clinical course, and many do not recur for 10 years or more. This 37-year-old woman presented with menometrorrhagia and was found at surgery to have a high-grade malignant uterine tumor and a benign Brenner tumor of the ovary. Disease recurred in the abdomen 2 months after surgery, and she was treated with whole-abdominal radiation therapy. (**A**) Pulmonary metastases developed 3 months after completion of radiation therapy, and she was treated with chemotherapy, which resulted (**B**) in complete remission within 2 months. ESS seems to be the most chemoresponsive form of uterine sarcomas.

Cervical Cancer

Cancer of the cervix once accounted for half of the cancer-related deaths in the United States. Although its incidence has decreased, it still accounts for 11,000 cases per year and ~4000 deaths per year (Jemal et al., 2008). This cancer occurs most frequently in the fifth and sixth decades. Risk factors include early age of first intercourse, multiple sexual partners, and history of sexually transmitted diseases. Cervical cancer is thought to arise in preexisting areas of intraepithelial neoplasia over the period of 10–20 years. HPV is the virus implicated in the vast majority of cases of cervical cancer. There are more than 80 types of HPV, but only 25 infect the genital tract; certain types (HPV 16 and 18) are associated with a high risk for development of cervical cancer. HPV vaccines are now in more widespread use against high-risk subtypes.

HISTOLOGY

Cervical squamous intraepithelial lesion (SIL) is divided into low-grade SIL (mild dysplasia, cervical intraepithelial neoplasia—CIN I) and high-grade SIL (severe dysplasia, CIN III); high-grade SIL is the precursor lesion of invasive cervical cancer. It takes years for this orderly progression to occur, and diagnosis by Pap smear and subsequent treatment of these preinvasive lesions has markedly reduced the mortality from invasive cancer.

Squamous cell carcinomas, including small cell variants, constitute ~80% of cervical malignancies and most frequently are found associated with their precursor lesion. Microscopically, carcinomas are characterized by nests, cord, or individual atypical cells that invade through the underlying basement membrane into cervical stroma. Microinvasive cancers infiltrate less than 3 mm and are less frequently associated with metastatic disease. Keratin pearls may be seen, especially

in well-differentiated tumors, but they are absent in poorly differentiated lesions. Poorly differentiated squamous cell carcinomas have dense, hyperchromatic nuclei and frequent mitotic figures. Lymphatic and vascular invasion is found more frequently in poorly differentiated tumors and is associated with nodal involvement and a poorer prognosis. The small cell variant is often associated with a poorly differentiated squamous cell tumor and less commonly presents as a pure neuroendocrine tumor.

Adenocarcinomas are less common than squamous cell tumors, constituting 5% to 20% of cervical neoplasia; however, there seems to be an increase in incidence of these malignancies among younger women. They are more difficult to diagnose by Pap smear or clinical examination, because they are often confined to the endocervix. Grossly, cervical adenocarcinomas may present as a fungating, polypoid mass, but they may also show an endophytic growth pattern that may internally expand the cervix, leading to its having a "barrel shape". Arising from endocervical glands, the tumors are identified by the presence of glands lined by high-columnar and/or mucin-secreting cells, morphologically described as either endocervical or intestinal types. Minimal deviation (also known as adenoma malignum) is a rare variant of adenocarcinoma that morphologically resembles benign glands but characteristically has a deeply invasive, nonlobular growth pattern. Squamous differentiation, which may be malignant (adenosquamous carcinoma) or benign (adenoacanthoma), may also be present within adenocarcinomas, and some reports report that adenosquamous variants have a worse prognosis. Tumors of other cell types are occasionally seen in the cervix, among them clear cell carcinoma, adenoid cystic carcinoma, sarcoma, and melanoma.

STAGING OF CERVICAL CARCINOMA

In the majority of cases, cervical cancers are diagnosed while they are still confined to the cervix either as occult tumors discovered by Pap smear screening (stage IA) or as larger lesions (stage IB). More advanced tumors have spread either to the vagina or to the parametrium (stages II and III); stage IV tumors are defined as involving the bladder or rectum or as having spread to distant sites.

Clinical staging is completed with a pelvic examination under anesthesia as well in some cases magnetic resonance imaging (MRI) or CT of the pelvis and sometimes a positron emission tomography scan. Lymphatic spread is not uncommon, because the cervix is rich in lymphatics; however, the clinical staging system does not include abdominal CT scan or MRI to assess pelvic and para-aortic nodes. Hematogenous spread to the liver, lung, and bone can occur but is usually associated with massive pelvic disease. Whereas the disease is clinically staged, patients may be found at surgery to have more advanced disease. Nodal involvement is common and affects both prognosis and the need for further therapy. Information gained at surgery and from CT or MRI scans is not used for staging, but such information is useful for treatment planning.

CLINICAL MANIFESTATIONS

Because these tumors are usually asymptomatic, in most instances they are discovered at routine pelvic examination and by Pap smear. The Pap test may reveal an entirely unsuspected lesion, in which case colposcopy is performed to view the entire cervix under magnification in the search for changes indicating intraepithelial or invasive neoplasia: white epithelium with vascular punctation or mosaicism or atypical vessels. In addition to obtaining biopsy specimens of abnormal areas, an endocervical curettage is performed.

When cervical tumors progress in size and become symptomatic, the most common complaints are abnormal vaginal bleeding, which can be postcoital, postmenopausal, or intermenstrual, or vaginal discharge, which is often yellow, serosanguineous, and malodorous. Advanced or recurrent disease may present with pelvic pain, tenesmus, bladder irritation, lower extremity edema, renal obstruction, or back pain from retroperitoneal lymph node involvement. Pulmonary or bone metastases may occur late in the course of disease.

FIGURE 9.58 Staging for carcinoma of the cervix uteri (FIGO, 1984).

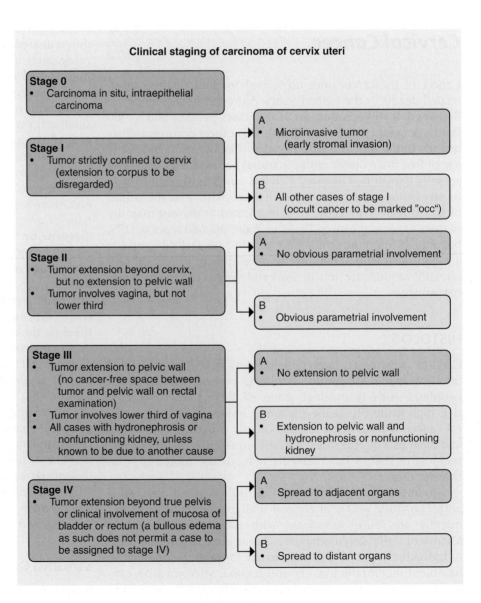

Clinical staging of carcinoma of cervix uteri

Stage 0
- Carcinoma in situ, intraepithelial carcinoma

Stage I
- Tumor strictly confined to cervix (extension to corpus to be disregarded)

A
- Microinvasive tumor (early stromal invasion)

B
- All other cases of stage I (occult cancer to be marked "occ")

Stage II
- Tumor extension beyond cervix, but no extension to pelvic wall
- Tumor involves vagina, but not lower third

A
- No obvious parametrial involvement

B
- Obvious parametrial involvement

Stage III
- Tumor extension to pelvic wall (no cancer-free space between tumor and pelvic wall on rectal examination)
- Tumor involves lower third of vagina
- All cases with hydronephrosis or nonfunctioning kidney, unless known to be due to another cause

A
- No extension to pelvic wall

B
- Extension to pelvic wall and hydronephrosis or nonfunctioning kidney

Stage IV
- Tumor extension beyond true pelvis or clinical involvement of mucosa of bladder or rectum (a bullous edema as such does not permit a case to be assigned to stage IV)

A
- Spread to adjacent organs

B
- Spread to distant organs

AJCC primary	FIGO tumor (T)	
TX	–	Primary tumor cannot be assessed.
T0	–	No evidence of primary tumor
Tis	0	Carcinoma in situ
T1	I	Cervical carcinoma confined to uterus (extension to corpus should be disregarded)
T1a	IA	Invasive carcinoma, diagnosed only by microscopy. All macroscopically visible lesions even with superficial invasion are T1b/IB. Stromal invasion with a maximum depth of 5 mm measured from the base of the epithelium and horizontal spread of 7 mm or less. Vascular space involvement, venous or lymphatic, does not affect classification.
T1a1	IA1	Measured stromal invasion 3 mm or less and 7 mm or less in horizontal spread
T1a2	IA2	Measured stromal invasion more than 3 mm and not more than 5 mm with a horizontal spread of 7 mm or less
T1b	IB	Clearly visible lesion confined to the cervix or microscopic lesion greater than T1a2/IA2
T1b1	IB1	Clearly visible lesion 4 cm or less in greatest dimension
T1b2	IB2	Clearly visible lesion more than 4 cm in greatest dimension
T2	II	Cervical carcinoma invades beyond uterus but not to pelvic wall or to the lower third of vagina
T2a	IIA	Tumor without parametrial invasion
T2b	IIB	Tumor with parametrial invasion
T3	III	Cervical carcinoma extends to the pelvic wall and/or involves lower third of vagina or causes hydronephrosis or non-functioning kidney
T3a	IIIA	Tumor involves lower third of the vagina, no extension to the pelvic wall
T3b	IIIB	Tumor extends to pelvic wall or causes hydronephrosis or nonfunctioning kidney.
T4*	IVA	Tumor invades mucosa of bladder or rectum and/or extends beyond true pelvis.
M1	IVB	Distant metastasis

Regional lymph nodes (N)

Regional lymph nodes include paracervical, parametrial, hypogastric (obturator), common, internal and external iliac, presacral, and sacral.

NX	–	Regional lymph nodes cannot be assessed.
N0	–	No regional lymph node metastasis
N1	–	Regional lymph node metastasis

Distant metastasis (M)

MX	–	Presence of distant metastasis cannot be assessed.
M0	–	No distant metastasis
M1	IVB	Distant metastasis

AJCC, American Joint Committee on Cancer; FIGO, International Federation of Gynecology and Obstetrics. *Presence of bullous edema is not sufficient evidence to classify a tumor T4.

Stage grouping

Stage	Primary tumor	Regional lymph nodes	Distant metastases
0	Tis	N0	M0
IA1	T1a1	N0	M0
IA2	T1a2	N0	M0
IB1	T1b1	N0	M0
IB2	T1b2	N0	M0
IIA	T2a	N0	M0
IIB	T2b	N0	M0
IIIA	T3a	N0	M0
IIIB	T1	N1	M0
	T2	N1	M0
	T3a	N1	M0
	T3b	Any N	M0
IVA	T4	Any N	M0
IVB	Any T	Any N	M1

FIGURE 9.59 Staging of Cervical Cancer. (From Flemming et al., 1997.)

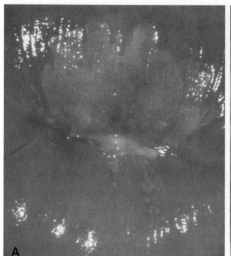
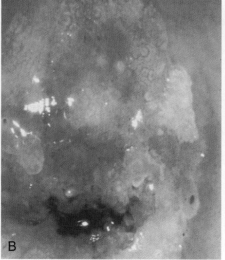
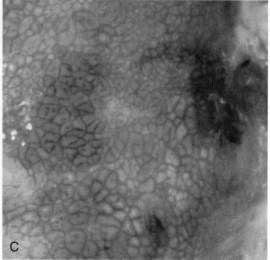

FIGURE 9.60 CERVICAL SQUAMOUS INTRAEPITHELIAL LESION (SIL, CIN). This sequence of photographs, taken through the colposcope, shows progressively more severe examples of SIL. (**A**) Low-grade SIL is marked by mild dysplasia, appearing as a whitened area of epithelium emanating from the transformation zone. (**B**) Early high-grade SIL (moderate dysplasia, CIN II) shows early vascular mosaicism and vessel punctuation findings that are more pronounced (**C**) in advanced high-grade SIL (CIN III, severe dysplasia). Any of these findings on colposcopic examination requires biopsy. (Courtesy of Howard Goodman, MD, Department of Gynecologic Oncology, Brigham and Women's Hospital, Boston, MA.)

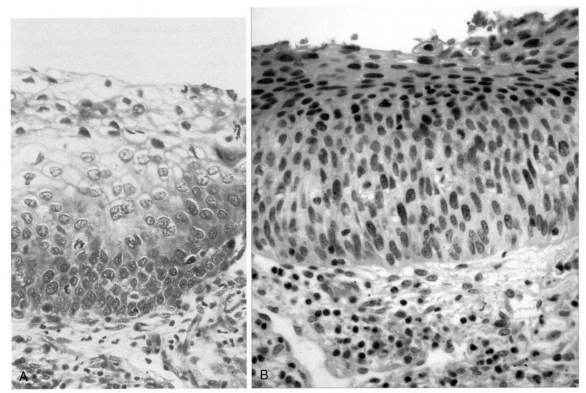

FIGURE 9.61   **CERVICAL SQUAMOUS INTRAEPITHELIAL LESION (SIL).** (**A**) Koilocytosis, multinucleation, hyperchromasia, and nuclear enlargement are present in the upper layers of the epithelium, consistent with a low-grade lesion. (**B**) Full-thickness atypia with absence of normal maturation and atypical parakeratosis is indicative of a high-grade lesion.

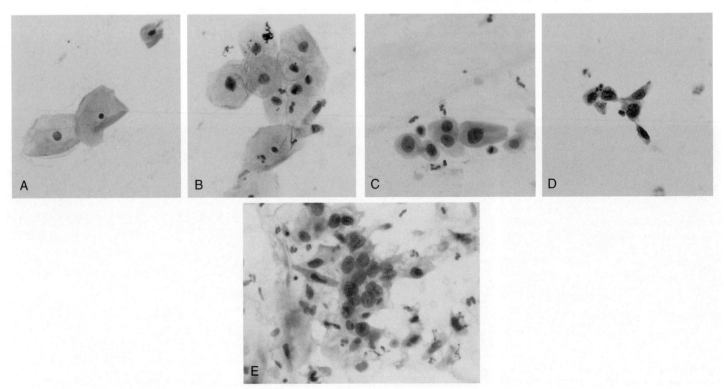

FIGURE 9.62   **CERVICAL SQUAMOUS INTRAEPITHELIAL LESION (SIL).** This series of Pap smears shows progression from normal through invasive carcinoma. (**A**) Two normal squamous cells with small pyknotic nuclei are visible. (**B**) Low-grade SIL (CIN I) is characterized by a slightly higher nucleus-to-cytoplasm ratio. The presence of columnar cells signifies that this is an adequate smear sampling of the endocervix. In high-grade SIL the nucleus-to-cytoplasm ratio is higher than in low-grade SIL. Both moderate dysplasia/CIN II (**C**) and severe dysplasia/CIN III/carcinoma in situ (**D**) are now categorized as high-grade SIL. (**E**) Invasive carcinoma is marked by spindle cells, prominent nucleoli in large nuclei, and extensive acellular necrotic debris in the background. (Courtesy of Edmund Cibas, MD, Department of Pathology, Brigham and Women's Hospital, Boston, MA.)

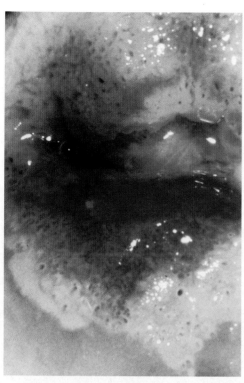

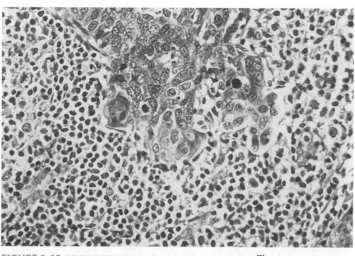

FIGURE 9.65 **MICROINVASIVE SQUAMOUS CELL CARCINOMA.** Three tongues of cells with relative cytoplasmic eosinophilia extend from the overlying basophilic epithelium into the underlying stroma. An intense inflammatory reaction is present. The exact definition of microinvasive carcinoma is controversial, but the inclusion in this category of a tumor such as this, showing less than 1 mm of invasion, no lymphatic or vascular invasion, and no confluence of invasive tongues, cannot be questioned. The risk of nodal involvement in this case is negligible.

FIGURE 9.63 **HIGH-GRADE SQUAMOUS INTRAEPITHELIAL LESION (SIL).** This colposcopic photograph shows extensive areas of white epithelium and punctation. Biopsy revealed an in situ lesion.

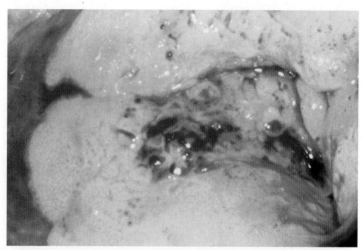

FIGURE 9.66 **SQUAMOUS CELL CARCINOMA.** This colposcopic photograph shows the white epithelium and the grossly atypical vessels and hemorrhage that are characteristic of invasive lesions. (Courtesy of Howard Goodman, MD, Department of Gynecologic Oncology, Brigham and Women's Hospital, Boston MA.)

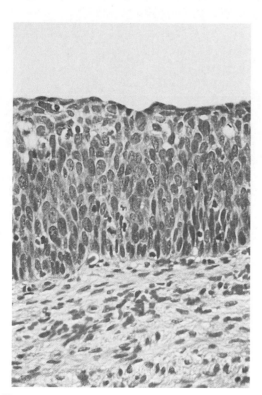

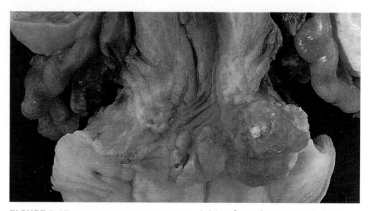

FIGURE 9.64 **HIGH-GRADE SQUAMOUS INTRAEPITHELIAL LESION (SIL).** No squamous cytoplasmic maturation is present except that the topmost cell layer may be flattened, as shown here.

FIGURE 9.67 **SQUAMOUS CELL CARCINOMA.** Arising from the ectocervix is an irregular, fungating, pale neoplasm.

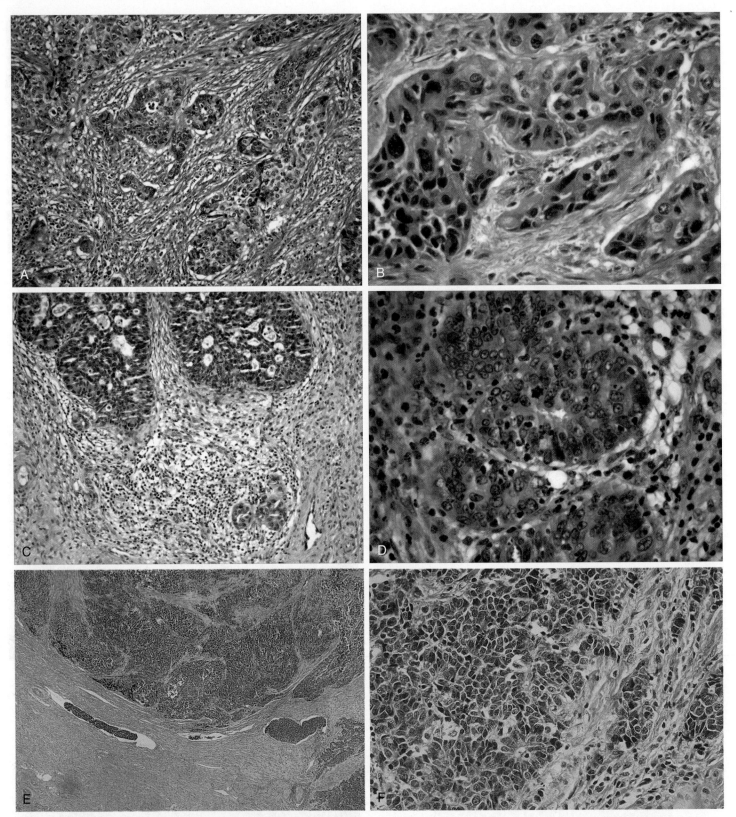

FIGURE 9.68 SQUAMOUS CELL CARCINOMA. (A) Tumor widely infiltrates the cervical stroma. **(B)** This tumor is composed of nests of moderately to poorly differentiated squamous epithelial cells. **(C)** Invasive adenocarcinoma of the cervix (*lower portion* of the image) is frequently seen in association with adenocarcinoma in situ (*top*), but the reverse is not always found. Invasive nests have irregular borders and are associated with a desmoplastic stroma. **(D)** The neoplastic glands in adenocarcinoma have atypical cytologic features and apically located mitotic figures. Occasionally goblet cell differentiation is seen in in situ and/or invasive lesions (not shown). In small cell neuroendocrine carcinoma **(E)** solid nests of hyperchromatic tumor cells infiltrate stroma, and involve lymphatic and vascular channels. **(F)** Tumor cells in small cell neuroendocrine carcinoma have scant cytoplasm and hyperchromatic, molded nuclei.

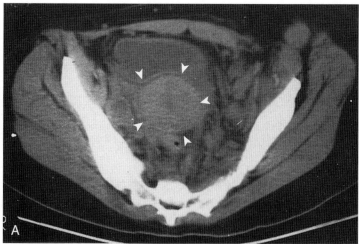 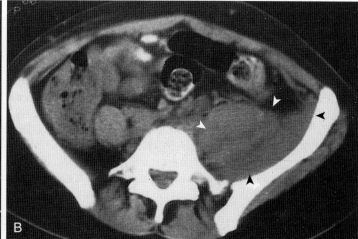

FIGURE 9.69 **STAGE IIIB CERVICAL CARCINOMA.** A 27-year-old woman presented with increased vaginal bleeding, left leg swelling, and abdominal pain. Examination revealed a large, fixed pelvic mass. CT scan evaluation (**A**) confirms the mass (*arrowheads*) and (**B**) shows extension into the left psoas and iliacus muscles (*arrowheads*). She also had hydronephrosis. Pathologic examination showed an adenosquamous carcinoma.

Other Gynecologic Malignancies

VULVAR CARCINOMA

Vulvar carcinoma accounts for approximately 4% of gynecologic malignancies. Whereas preinvasive disease occurs primarily in the premenopausal woman, the median age for invasive vulvar cancer is 60 years. Risk factors include HPV and cigarette smoking. However, it does not appear to be endocrinologically mediated. Vulvar cancer is more common in diabetics and in women with a history of breast, endometrial, or cervical cancer.

Carcinoma in situ (also known as vulvar intraepithelial neoplasia) represents a preinvasive lesion, especially in the elderly and immunosuppressed. The significance of chronic vulvar dystrophy is unknown in that it represents a heterogeneous group of disorders, but in the absence of cellular atypia most cases of chronic vulvar dystrophy will not progress to invasive carcinoma. The most common malignancy of the vulva is a well-differentiated, keratinizing squamous cell carcinoma; however, Paget's disease, melanoma, adenocarcinoma, or basal cell carcinoma are also seen (Hill et al 2008). The staging system for vulvar carcinoma is shown in Figure 9.70.

VAGINAL CARCINOMA

Vaginal carcinoma is usually metastatic from primary tumors of the endometrium, ovary, cervix, breast, or gastrointestinal tract. Additionally, melanoma should always be included in the differential diagnosis when a malignant epithelioid neoplasm involves the vagina. Primary tumors of the vagina are rare, but they may occur in infants (endodermal sinus tumor, embryonal rhabdomyosarcoma), adolescents (clear cell carcinoma), or adults (carcinomas, sarcomas, melanomas). Squamous cell carcinoma, the most common type of malignancy, usually presents late in life with abnormal vaginal discharge or bleeding. Clear cell carcinomas are rare but may occur in approximately 0.1% of women exposed in utero to diethylstilbestrol; the risk for development of these tumors is greatest between the ages of 15 and 25 years. The staging system for vaginal carcinoma is shown in Figures 9.76 and 9.77.

FALLOPIAN TUBE CARCINOMA

Primary fallopian tube carcinoma has traditionally been considered a rare disease, but its incidence is increasing as more women with known *BRCA1* or *BRCA2* mutations undergo prophylactic salpingo-oophorectomy, because ~5% of these women are found to have a microscopic early carcinoma (tubal intraepithelial carcinoma or TIC) within the distal portion of the fallopian tube (fimbria) (Mederios et al 2006; Lee et al 2006; Crum et al 2007). Morphologically, the presence of (at minimum) a small stretch of severely dysplastic cells that are immunoreactive with *TP53* and demonstrate a high proliferation (MIB-1) index is consistent with a TIC (Jarboe et al 2008). An invasive serous carcinoma may be present in association with a TIC but is not required for distant/metastatic disease. Additionally it has been shown in BRCA+ women that approximately 50% of all serous ovarian cancers and a subset of peritoneal carcinomas may arise from the distal fallopian tube (Crum et al 2007; Kindelberger 2007). The clinical course of carcinomas arising from the fallopian tube parallels primary ovarian carcinoma in natural history, pathology, staging, and treatment. Though frequently asymptomatic, it may present with vaginal bleeding or in the same manner as ovarian cancer, with increasing abdominal girth and vague GI complaints. Like ovarian carcinoma, spread is most often peritoneal, but hematogenous dissemination to lung, brain, or pericardium may occur.

PERITONEAL CARCINOMA

Peritoneal carcinoma is a clinical entity that is closely associated with epithelial ovarian cancer and is treated similarly (Barda et al 2004; Fromm et al 1990). The Gynecologic Oncology Group has previously defined peritoneal cancer as involving ovaries normal in size, extra-ovarian involvement greater than ovarian involvement, a predominantly serous histology, and surface involvement less than 5 mm depth and width. Recent and current studies have suggested that at least a subset of peritoneal serous carcinomas may arise from the distal portion (fimbriae) of the fallopian tube (see also "Fallopian Tube Carcinoma," above) (Kindelberger et al 2007; Crum et al 2007).

GESTATIONAL TROPHOBLASTIC NEOPLASIA

This category of gynecologic tumors includes the hydatidiform mole (complete and partial), the invasive mole, choriocarcinoma, placental-site trophoblastic tumor, and epithelioid trophoblastic tumor (Garner et al 2007; Fletmate et al 2006; Feltmate et al 2002; Berkowitz and Goldstein 1995). Molar pregnancies occur with a frequency of 1 in 1500 live births in the United States; in other areas of the world the frequency may be as high as 1 in 120. Although dietary factors have been implicated, the etiology is unknown. Invasive moles or choriocarcinoma develop in ~5% of women with prior complete molar pregnancies; it can usually be cured with a few courses of single-agent chemotherapy, thus preserving fertility. Simple hysterectomy and chemotherapy may be used in women who have completed their childbearing. Choriocarcinoma most commonly follows molar pregnancy but may rarely also complicate an abortion, ectopic pregnancy, or normal delivery. The lung, GI tract, oral cavity, liver, and central nervous system may be sites of metastatic disease. The latter two sites are poor prognostic features, but the majority of these patients may be cured with chemotherapy. Placental-site trophoblastic tumors are more frequently associated with a remote history of pregnancy. The staging system for gestational trophoblastic neoplasms is shown in Figure 9.84.

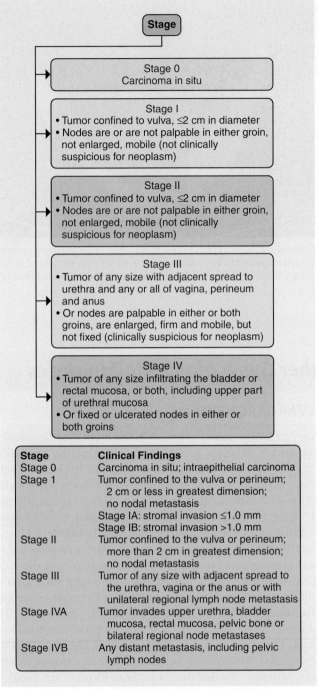

FIGURE 9.70 FIGO staging system for carcinoma of the vulva (1990).

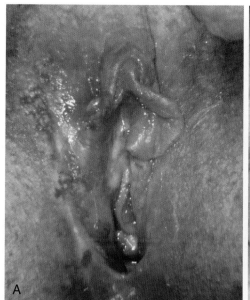

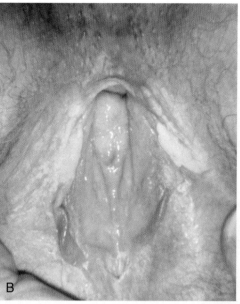

FIGURE 9.71 **CARCINOMA IN SITU.** Clinically, this lesion may present variously. (**A**) In this instance an erythematous patch extends across the midline, whereas in another example (**B**) there is marked whitening of noncontiguous patches of tumor due to hyperkeratosis.

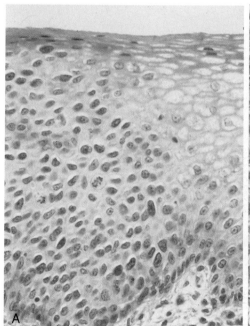

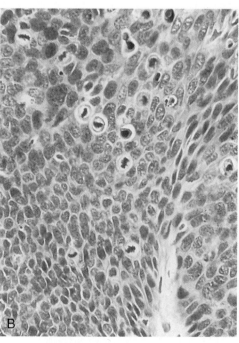

FIGURE 9.72 **CARCINOMA IN SITU.** (**A**) On the *right* side of the field there is normal stratified squamous epithelium, whereas the *left* side is marked by loss of normal cytoplasmic maturation and by cells with enlarged atypical nuclei. (**B**) Multiple atypical mitotic figures, as well as atypical nuclei without degenerative features, are characteristic.

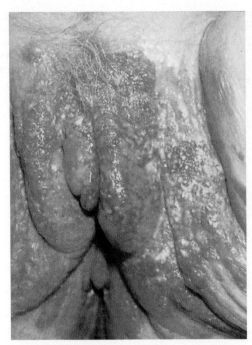

FIGURE 9.73 **PAGET'S DISEASE.** Involvement of the vulva is clinically identical to the far less common penile counterpart of this lesion. Raised erythematous plaques with crusting to excoriation are typical. The clinical circumscription is deceptive, however, because grossly uninvolved margins often contain neoplastic cells. Paget's disease may be associated with invasive adenocarcinoma of the apocrine glands of the vulva or with carcinoma of other organs, most notably the cervix, uterus, breast, and colon.

FIGURE 9.74 **PAGET'S DISEASE.** Basal nests of large, pale cells are found along the basement membrane of the epithelium; between them are less well-differentiated basal cells. Hyperkeratinization also is present. Paget's cells are often seen in rete pegs pushing deep into the dermis. Because of this a more extensive vulvectomy, including epidermis and dermis, is required for treatment. Melanoma in situ has morphologic overlap with Paget's disease and should be excluded when pagetoid cells are present in the epidermis; this can be done with immunostains, because the former is positive for S100 and the latter is positive for keratins CK7 and Cam5.2.

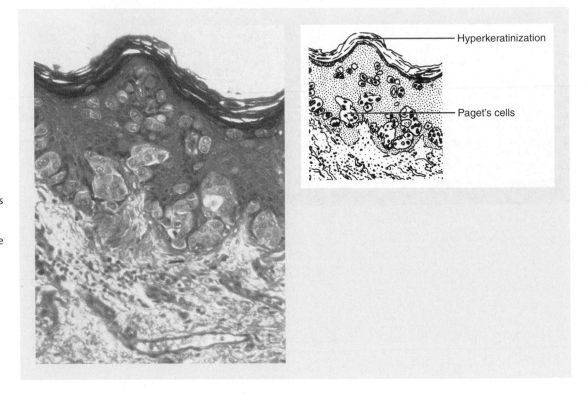

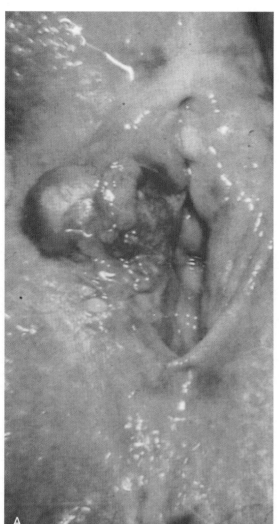

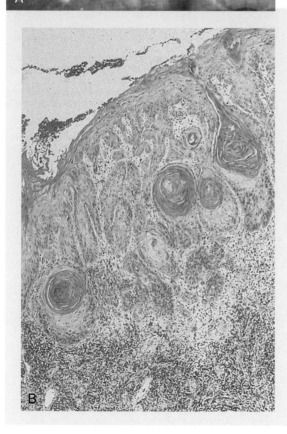

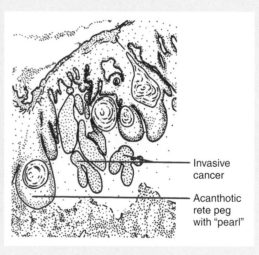

Invasive cancer

Acanthotic rete peg with "pearl"

FIGURE 9.75 SQUAMOUS CELL CARCINOMA. (A) The ulcerative lesion seen here affects a vulva in which many surface structures are inapparent because of atrophic dystrophy. The labia and clitoris are no longer well defined. **(B)** The *left* side of this field shows acanthotic rete pegs that contain prematurely keratinized pearls, but there is no subepithelial infiltration. This is atypical hyperplastic dystrophy. In the *right* side of the field there is infiltration by invasive cancer.

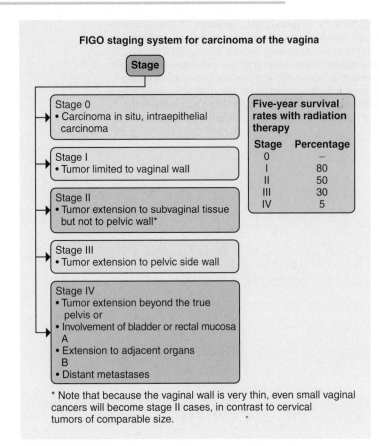

FIGURE 9.76 FIGO staging system for carcinoma of the vagina.

Definition of TNM

Primary tumor (T)*

TNM	FIGO	Definition
TX	–	Primary tumor cannot be assessed.
T0	–	No evidence of primary tumor
T1	I	Carcinoma in situ
T2	II	Tumor confined to the vagina
T3	III	Tumor invades paravaginal tissues but not to the pelvic wall.
T4†	IVA	Tumor extends to the pelvic wall. Tumor invades the mucosa of the bladder or rectum and/or extends beyond the true pelvis.
M1	IVB	Distant metastasis

Regional lymph nodes (N)

NX   Regional lymph nodes cannot be assessed.
N0   No regional lymph node metastasis

Upper two-thirds of the vagina
N1   Pelvic lymph node metastasis

Lower one-third of the vagina
N1   Unilateral inguinal lymph node metastasis
N2   Bilateral inguinal lymph node metastasis

Distant metastasis (M)

TNM	FIGO	Definition
MX	–	Presence of distant metastasis cannot be assessed.
M0	–	No distant metastasis
M1	IVB	Distant metastasis

Stage grouping

AJCC/UICC				FIGO
Stage 0	Tis	N0	M0	Stage 0
Stage I	T1	N0	M0	Stage I
Stage II	T2	N0	M0	Stage II
Stage III	T1	N1	M0	Stage III
	T2	N1	M0	
	T3	N0	M0	
	T3	N1	M0	
Stage IVA	T1	N1	M0	Stage IVA
	T2	N2	M0	
	T3	N2	M0	
	T4	Any N	M0	
Stage IVB	Any T	Any N	M1	Stage IVB

* Squamous cell carcinoma is the most common type of cancer occurring in the vagina, but infrequently an adenocarcinoma may occur in the upper one-third.
† Note: The presence of bullous edema is not sufficient evidence to classify a tumor as T4. If the mucosa is not involved, the tumor is stage III.

FIGURE 9.77 TNM staging compared to the FIGO staging system. (From AJCC: Manual for Staging of Cancer, 4th edn. Lippincott, Philadelphia, 1993.)

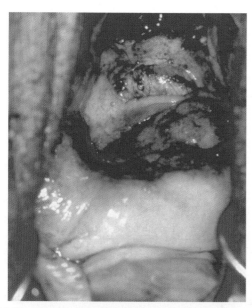

FIGURE 9.78 **VAGINAL CARCINOMA.** The ulceration in the posterior wall of the vagina is an invasive vaginal cancer. Its endophytic growth pattern has resulted in significant penetration of the vaginal wall, although the tumor mass is still small. The cervix is everted and appears inflamed but is uninvolved.

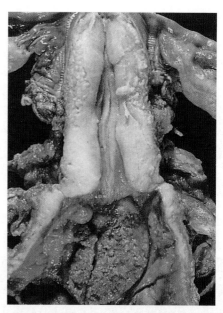

FIGURE 9.80 **SQUAMOUS CELL CARCINOMA.** Arising in the posterior vaginal wall is a raised, irregular neoplasm.

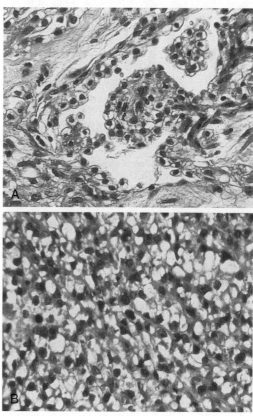

FIGURE 9.81 **CLEAR CELL ADENOCARCINOMA.** (**A**) Clear cells line the glandular spaces and papillae. (**B**) In the other specimen, clear cells with large atypical nuclei form a solid sheet of tumor.

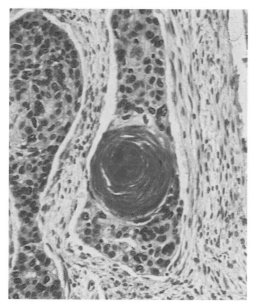

FIGURE 9.79 **SQUAMOUS CELL CARCINOMA.** As is usual with these tumors, keratin pearls are often formed. The degree of histologic differentiation is not a prognostic factor.

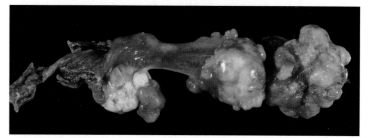

FIGURE 9.82 **FALLOPIAN TUBE CARCINOMA.** A solid, nodular tan fleshy mass is seen at the distal end of the fallopian tube (fimbriae, *right*). Note that the ovary (located more proximally to the *left*, under the fallopian tube) is uninvolved.

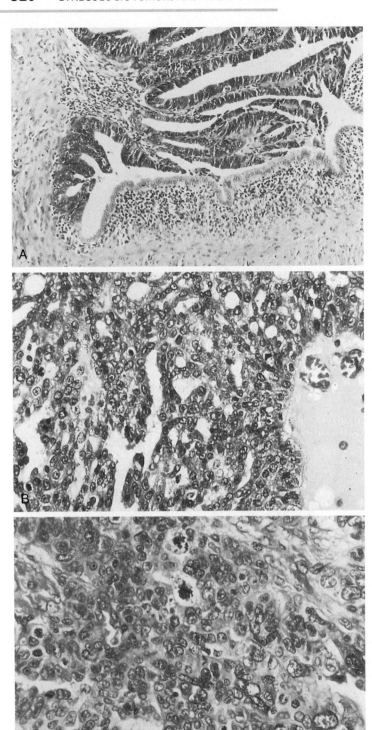

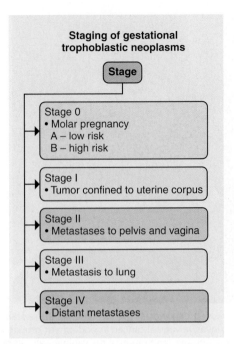

Staging of gestational trophoblastic neoplasms

Stage

Stage 0
• Molar pregnancy
  A – low risk
  B – high risk

Stage I
• Tumor confined to uterine corpus

Stage II
• Metastases to pelvis and vagina

Stage III
• Metastasis to lung

Stage IV
• Distant metastases

FIGURE 9.84 Staging of gestational trophoblastic neoplasms. (Adapted from Goldstein and Berkowitz, 1980.)

FIGURE 9.83 **FALLOPIAN TUBE CARCINOMA.** (**A**) Normal tubal epithelium is seen in the *lower* portion of this field, whereas the remainder contains a serous tubal intraepithelial carcinoma ("STIC") characterized by high-grade nuclei and increased mitotic activity. STICs demonstrate diffuse nuclear immunoreactivity with *TP53* and an increased MIB-1 proliferation index. Mounting evidence suggests that ovarian surface and peritoneal serous carcinoma originate from STICs. Invasive carcinomas of the fallopian tube are characterized by (**B**) papillary-alveolar and (**C**) solid architectures, and can be indistinguishable morphologically from ovarian serous carcinomas.

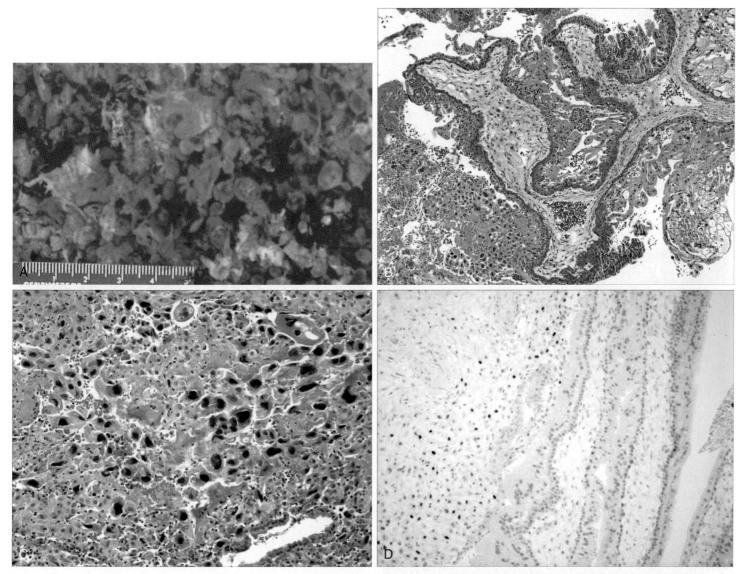

FIGURE 9.85 **COMPLETE HYDATIDIFORM MOLE.** (**A**) Numerous grapelike swellings ("vesicles", molar villi) in placental tissue (both grossly and histologically) are characteristic of second-trimester complete moles; no fetal tissues are present. (**B**) In contrast, first-trimester molar villi ("early complete moles") are characterized by smaller villi with edematous/myxoid stroma, stromal karyorrhexis, and scalloped villi covered by a thick covering of proliferating, markedly atypical trophoblasts. (**C**) Complete moles are also associated with atypical implantation sites. (**D**) An absence of immunostaining for p57 in villous trophoblasts confirms the diagnosis of complete mole (note positive internal control with p57 in maternal decidual cells).

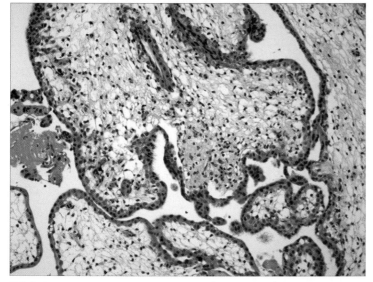

FIGURE 9.86 **PARTIAL HYDATIDIFORM MOLE.** The gestational tissue contains a biphasic population of small, normal-appearing villi and large, edematous cavitated "molar" villi, the latter with irregular shapes ("scalloping"), minimal trophoblast hyperplasia when compared with complete moles and trophoblast inclusions. Fetal parts are present in partial moles and may be present only as nucleated red blood cells.

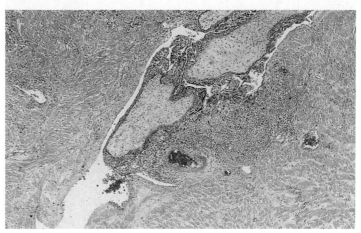

FIGURE 9.87 **INVASIVE MOLE.** Two villi from a complete mole (covered by a thick layer of hyperplastic trophoblast) are present deep within the myometrium in this hysterectomy specimen.

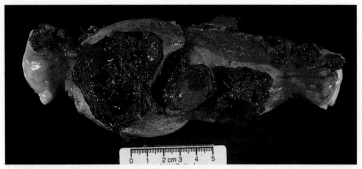

FIGURE 9.88 **POST-GESTATIONAL CHORIOCARCINOMA.** Large hemorrhagic tumor involves endometrium and myometrium.

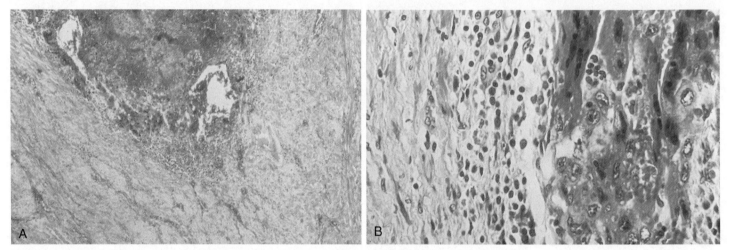

FIGURE 9.89 **CHORIOCARCINOMA OF FUNDUS. (A)** The typical invasive cancer seen here is marked by a large amount of hemorrhage and very little tumor tissue. **(B)** Myometrium on the *left* of this field is being destroyed by a mixture of malignant cytotrophoblasts and syncytiotrophoblasts on the *right*.

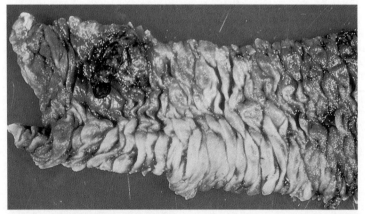

FIGURE 9.90 **INTESTINAL METASTASES.** Bowel metastases from choriocarcinoma are a bad prognostic sign and indicate stage IV disease. They may cause life-threatening hemorrhage and are often treated surgically. (Courtesy of Ross Berkowitz, MD, Department of Gynecologic Oncology, Brigham and Women's Hospital, Boston MA.)

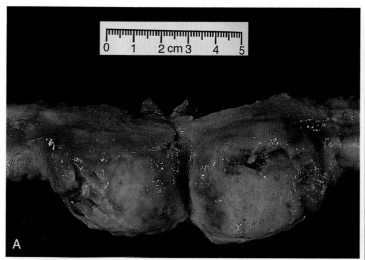

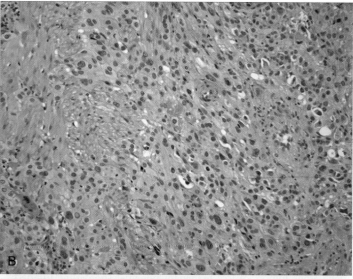

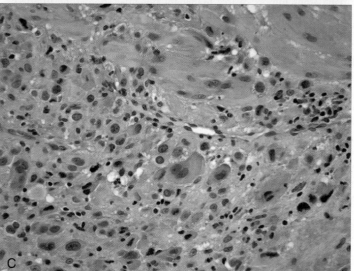

FIGURE 9.91 **PLACENTAL-SITE TROPHOBLASTIC TUMOR. (A)** Myometrium is transmurally replaced by solid tan tumor composed of malignant intermediate trophoblasts. **(B)** Histologically, sheets of monomorphic, single, spindled, and epithelioid cells infiltrate between myometrial fibers. **(C)** Mitotic activity is brisk in this tumor, and the MIB-1 proliferation rate is one prognostic indicator.

References and Suggested Readings

Ayhan A, Guvendag Guven ES, et al.: Recurrence and prognostic factors in borderline ovarian tumors, *Gynecol Oncol* 98(3):439–445, 2005.

Berkowitz RS, Goldstein DP: Gestational trophoblastic disease, *Cancer* 76(10 Suppl):2079–2085, 1995.

Berkowitz RS, Goldstein DP: Current management of gestational trophoblastic diseases, *Gynecol Oncol* 112(3):654–662. Epub 2008 Oct 12.

Carlson JW, Nucci MR, Brodsky J, et al.: Biomarker-assisted diagnosis of ovarian, cervical and pulmonary small cell carcinomas: The role of TTF-1, WT-1 and HPV Analysis, *Histopathol* 51(3):305–313, 2007.

Chang KL, Crabtree GS, Lim-Tan SK, et al.: Primary extrauterine endometrial stromal neoplasms: a clinicopathologic study of 20 cases and a review of the literature, *Int J Gynecol Pathol* 12(4):282–296, 1993.

Crum C.: Contemporary theories in cervical carcinogenesis: the virus, the host and the sterm cell, *Mod Pathol* 13:2451–2459, 2000.

Crum CP, Drapkin R, Kindelberger D, et al.: Lessons from BRCA: the tubal fimbria emerges as an origin for pelvic serous cancer, *Clin Med Res* 5(1):35–44, 2007.

Feltmate CM, Genest DR, et al.: Advances in the understanding of placental site trophoblastic tumor, *J Reprod Med* 47(5):337–341, 2002, Review.

Feltmate CM, Growdon WB, Wolfberg AJ, et al.: Clinical characteristics of persistent gestational trophoblastic neoplasia after partial hydatidiform molar pregnancy, *J Reprod Med* 51(11):902–906, 2006.

Flemming I, Cooper J, Henson D, et al: *AJCC cancer staging manual*, ed 5, Philadelphia, 1997, Lippincott.

Garner EI, Goldstein DP, Feltmate CM, Berkowitz RS: Gestational trophoblastic disease, *Clin Obstet Gynecol* 50(1):112–122, 2007.

Greene FL, Page DL, Fleming ID, et al.: *AJCC cancer staging manual*, ed 6, New York, 2002, Springer.

Irving JA, Alkushi A, Young RH, Clement PB: Cellular fibromas of the ovary: a study of 75 cases including 40 mitotically active tumors emphasizing their distinction from fibrosarcoma, *Am J Surg Pathol* 30(8):929–938, 2006.

Hecht JL, Mutter GL: Molecular and pathologic aspects of endometrial carcinogenesis, *J Clin Oncol* 10, 24(29):4783–4791, 2006.

Hill SJ, Berkowitz R, Granter SR, Hirsch MS: Pagetoid lesions of the vulva: a collision between malignant melanoma and extramammary paget's disease, *Int J Gyn Pathol* 27(2):292–296, 2007.

Hirsch MS, Lee KR: Metastatic tumors to the Ovary. In Crum CP, Lee KR, editors: Diagnostic gynecologic and obsteric pathology, Chap. 31, Philadelphia, 2006, Elsevier Saunders.

Jarboe EA, Folkins AK, Drapkin R, et al.: Tubal and ovarian pathways to pelvic epithelial cancer: a pathological perspective, *Histopathology* 53(2): 127–138, 2008, Epub 2008 Feb 22.

Jarboe E, Folkins A, Nucci MR, et al.: Serous carcinogenesis in the fallopian tube: a descriptive classification, *Int J Gynecol Pathol* 27(1):1–9, 2008.

Jemal A, Siegel R, Ward E, et al: Cancer statistics, *CA Cancer J Clin* 58:71–96, 2008.

Kindelberger DW, Lee Y, Miron A, et al.: Intraepithelial carcinoma of the fimbria and pelvic serous carcinoma: evidence for a causal relationship, *Am J Surg Pathol* 31(2):161–169, 2007.

Lerwill MF, Sung R, Oliva E, et al.: Smooth muscle tumors of the ovary: a clinicopathologic study of 54 cases emphasizing prognostic criteria, histologic variants, and differential diagnosis, *Am J Surg Pathol* 28(11):1436–1451, 2004.

Longacre TA, McKenney JK, Tazelaar HD, et al.: Ovarian serous tumors of low malignant potential (borderline tumors): outcome-based study of 276 patients with long-term (> or = 5-year) follow-up, *Am J Surg Pathol* 29(6):707–723, 2005.

Mayrand M-H, Duarte-Franco E, Rodrigues I, et al.: Human papillomavirus DNA versus Papanicolaou screening tests for cervical cancer, *N Engl J Med* 357:1579–1588, 2007.

McCluggage WG: Ovarian neoplasms composed of small round cells: a review, *Adv Anat Pathol* 11(6):288–296, 2004.

McKenney JK, Balzer BL, Longacre TA: Patterns of stromal invasion in ovarian serous tumors of low malignant potential (borderline tumors): a reevaluation of the concept of stromal microinvasion, *Am J Surg Pathol* 30(10):1209–1221, 2006a.

McKenney JK, Balzer BL, Longacre TA: Lymph node involvement in ovarian serous tumors of low malignant potential (borderline tumors): pathology, prognosis, and proposed classification, *Am J Surg Pathol* 30(5):614–624, 2006b.

Medeiros F, Muto MG, Lee Y, et al.: The tubal fimbria is a preferred site for early adenocarcinoma in women with familial ovarian cancer syndrome, *J Surg Pathol* 30(2):230–236, 2006.

Mutch DG: The new FIGO staging system for cancer of the vulva, cervix, endometrium and sarcomas, *Gynecol Oncol* 115:325–328, 2009, Epub 2009 October 31.

Naucler P, Ryd W, Törnberg S, et al.: Human papillomavirus and Papanicolaou tests to screen for cervical cancer, *N Engl J Med* 357:1589–1597, 2007.

O'Connell JT, Tomlinson JS, Roberts AA, et al.: Pseudomyxoma peritonei is a disease of MUC2-expressing goblet cells, *Am J Pathol* 161(2):551–564, 2002.

Prat J: Serous tumors of the ovary (borderline tumors and carcinomas) with and without micropapillary features, *Int J Gynecol Pathol* 22(1):25–28, 2003.

Prat J, De Nictolis M: Serous borderline tumors of the ovary: a long-term follow-up study of 137 cases, including 18 with a micropapillary pattern and 20 with microinvasion, *Am J Surg Pathol* 26(9):1111–1128, 2002.

Prat J, Ribé A, Gallardo A: Hereditary ovarian cancer, *Hum Pathol* 36(8):861–870, 2005.

Prat J, Gallardo A, Cuatrecasas M, Catasús L: Endometrial carcinoma: pathology and genetics, *Pathology* 39(1):72–87, 2007, Review.

Rollins SE, Young RH, Bell DA: Autoimplants in serous borderline tumors of the ovary: a clinicopathologic study of 30 cases of a process to be distinguished from serous adenocarcinoma, *Am J Surg Pathol* 30(4):457–462, 2006.

Schwartz JK, Siegel BA, Dehadashti F, Grigsby PW: Association of posttherapy positron emission tomography with tumor response and survival in cervical carcinoma, *JAMA* 298:2289–2295, 2007.

Solomon D, Breen N, McNeel T: Cervical cancer screening rates in the United States and the potential impact of implementation of screening guidelines, *CA Cancer J Clin* 57:105–111, 2007.

Ulbright TM: Germ cell tumors of the gonads: a selective review emphasizing problems in differential diagnosis, newly appreciated, and controversial issues, *Mod Pathol* 18(Suppl 2):S61–S79, 2005.

Visintin I, Feng Z, Longton G, et al.: Diagnostic markers for early detection of ovarian cancer, *Clin Cancer Res* 14:1065, 2008.

Young RH: Sex cord-stromal tumors of the ovary and testis: their similarities and differences with consideration of selected problems, *Mod Pathol* 18(Suppl 2):S81–S98, 2005.

Zighelboim I, Goodfellow PJ, Gao F, et al.: Microsatellite instability and epigenetic inactivation of MLH1 and outcome of patients with endometrial carcinomas of the endometrioid type, *J Clin Oncol* 25(15):2042–2048, 2007.

Figure Credits

The following books published by Gower Medical Publishing are sources of figures in the present chapter. The figure numbers given in the listing are those of the figures in the present chapter. The page numbers (or slide numbers) given in parentheses are those of the original publication.

Fletcher CDM, McKee PH: An Atlas of Gross Pathology. Edward Arnold/Gower Medical Publishing, London, 1987: Figs 9.4B (p 74), 9.6 (p 75), 9.9 (p 75) 9.14 (p 76), 9.20A (p 77), 9.22 (p 76), 9.36 (p 80), 9.67 (p 82), 9.80 (p 82).

Fox H, McKee PH, Pugh RCB (eds): Reproductive system. In: Turk JL, Fletcher CDM (eds): RCSI Slide Atlas of Pathology. Gower Medical Publishing, London, 1986: Figs 9.2 (slide 9), 9.47 (slide 41).

Gordon AG, Lewis BV: Gynecological Endoscopy. JB Lippincott/Gower Medical Publishing, Philadelphia/London, 1988: Figs 9.27A (p 6.21), 9.27B (p 6.23), 9.28A (p 6.24), 9.40 (p 9.8), 9.46A (p 6.10).

Price AB, Morson BC, Scheuer PJ (eds): Alimentary system. In Turk JL, Fletcher CDM (eds): RCSE Slide Atlas of Pathology. Gower Medical Publishing, London, 1986: Fig. 9.21A (slide 104).

Weiss MA, Mills SE: Atlas of Genitourinary Tract Disorders. Lippincott/Gower Medical Publishing, Philadelphia/New York, 1988: Fig. 9.73 (p 19.11).

Woodruff JD, Parmley TH: Atlas of Gynecologic Pathology. Lippincott/Gower Medical Publishing, Philadelphia/New York, 1988: Figs 9.5A (p 7.25), 9.5B (p 7.26), 9.10A (p 7.28), 9.12 (p 7.38), 9.15 (p 7.42), 9.17B (p 7.39), 9.18B (p 7.37), 9.20B (p 7.46), 9.21B (p 7.46), 9.37A (p 4.24), 9.38 (p 4.28), 9.48 (p 5.5), 9.52 (p 5.13), 9.61A (p 3.11), 9.64 (p 3.12), 9.65 (3.18), 9.71 (p 1.16), 9.72 (p 1.15), 9.74 (p 1.21), 9.75 (p1.17), 9.76 (p 2.13), 9.78 (p 2.12), 9.79 (p 2.13), 9.81 (p 2.6), 9.83 (6.21), 9.90 (p 8.24), 9.91 (p 8.20).

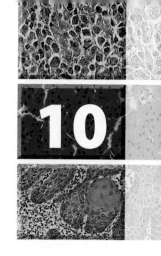

10

Breast Cancer

WENDY Y. CHEN • SUSANA M. CAMPOS • DANIEL F. HAYES

Breast cancer is a major cause of morbidity and mortality across the world. In the United States, each year about 180,000 new cases are diagnosed with more than 40,000 deaths annually (Jemal et al., 2007). It is a highly heterogeneous disease, both pathologically and clinically. Although age is the single most common risk factor for the development of breast cancer in women (see Fig. 10.13), several other important risk factors have also been identified, including a germline mutation (*BRCA1* and *BRCA2*) (Table 10.1), positive family history, prior history of breast cancer, and history of prolonged, uninterrupted menses (early menarche and late first full-term pregnancy) (Table 10.2).

Much progress has been made in the diagnosis and treatment of primary and metastatic breast cancer. The widespread use of routine mammography has led to an increased incidence in the detection of early primary lesions, a factor that has contributed to a significant decrease in mortality (see Figs. 10.38 to 10.41,

Table 10.1		
Estimated Lifetime Incidence of Cancer for *BRCA1/2* Mutation Carriers		
Type of Cancer	***BRCA1* Carrier**	***BRCA2* Carrier**
Breast	40–85	40–85
Ovarian	25–65	15–25
Male breast	5–10	5–10
Prostate	Elevated*	Elevated*
Pancreatic	<10	<10

*Prostate cancer risk is probably elevated, but absolute risk is not known.
Adapted from Table 19.1 in Harris et al., 2004.

10.44). Magnetic resonance imaging (MRI) of the breast may be useful in screening women with a higher lifetime risk of breast cancer, such as those women with a *BRCA1/2* mutation or with a family history strongly suggestive of a hereditary breast/ovarian

Table 10.2				
Selected Breast Cancer Risk Factors				
Risk Factor	**Referent**	**Comparison**	**Approximate Relative Risk**	**Selected References**
Age (years)				
Age at menarche	<12	>14	1.2–1.5	Brinton et al. (1988); Negri et al. (1988); Hunter et al. (1997)
Oral contraceptives	None	Current	1.1–1.2	Romieu et al. (1990); Collaborative Group (1996)
Age at first birth	<20–22	>28–35	1.3–1.8	Trichopoulos et al. (1983); Negri et al. (1988); Hunter et al. (1997)
Breast feeding	None	12 months	0.90	Collaborative Group (2002)
Parity	0	5+	0.6	Negri et al. (1988)
Age at menopause				
Surgical oophorectomy	50+	<40	0.6	Brinton et al. (1988)
Estrogen + progesterone	None	Current use for 5 years	1.2–1.3	Rossouw et al. (2002)
Body mass index				
Premenopausal	<21	>31	0.5–0.7	Ursin et al. (1995); van den Brandt et al. (2000)
Postmenopausal	<21	>28–30	1.2–1.3	van den Brandt et al. (2000)
Physical activity	None	Moderate	0.60–0.90	Thune et al. (1997); McTiernan et al. (2003)
Serum estradiol (postmenopausal)	Lowest quartile	Highest quartile	2	Key et al. (2002)
Mammographic breast density	<25% density	>75% density	4–6	Boyd et al. (1998)
Bone density	Lowest quartile	Highest quartile	2.0–3.5	Cauley et al. (1996); Zhang et al. (1997)
Alcohol consumption	None	3+ drinks per day	1.3–1.4	Smith-Warner et al. (1998); Hamajima et al. (2002)
Benign breast disease (atypical hyperplasia)	No	Yes	2–6	Dupont and Page (1985); Marshall et al. (1997)
Family history of breast cancer in first-degree relative	None	1+	2–4	Collaborative Group (2001)

syndrome (Saslow et al., 2007) (see Fig. 10.7). Moreover, less aggressive, conservative local therapy has been shown to be as effective as mastectomy in prolonging survival, while avoiding the cosmetic disfigurement associated with more extensive surgery. Sentinel node biopsy (see Fig. 10.78) is now routinely being offered to appropriate patients, with a significant decrease in the morbidity associated with the traditional axillary node dissection. Adjuvant systemic therapy, such as chemotherapy and/or hormonal therapy, has also contributed to the prolonged survival of patients with breast cancer (EBCTCG, 2005). The identification of molecular targets such as the overexpression of HER2/neu has allowed biologic therapies directed against the HER2/neu pathway to be considered part of standard treatment in both the adjuvant and metastatic setting for tumors that overexpress HER2/neu (Piccart-Gebhart et al., 2005; Romond et al., 2005).

Incidence

Breast cancer incidence has remained level during the last decade. Breast cancer deaths are decreasing, primarily for white women and younger women. Although white women develop breast cancer more frequently, black women are more likely to die of the disease (Jemal et al., 2007; Smigal et al., 2006) (Fig. 10.8A, B).

Screening

Routine mammographic screening allows better detection of primary breast cancers than physical examination. Mammographic screening has been shown to decrease mortality rates in women 50–69 years of age. A 26% decrease in the relative risk of breast cancer was noted with screening mammography in this group. The role of screening mammography in women 40–49 years of age also appears to be associated with a reduction in breast cancer mortality, but of slightly smaller magnitude (Humphrey et al., 2002; Armstrong et al., 2007). Current imaging modalities include mammography, ultrasound, and, recently, MRI. Only mammography has been demonstrated to be a valuable tool in decreasing mortality.

Over half of all women will develop benign breast lesions. These include macro- and microcysts, adenosis, apocrine changes, intraductal papillomas, fibrosis, fibroadenomas, and epithelial hyperplasias (see Figs. 10.2 to 10.6 and 10.9 to 10.12). Only the latter, however, particularly those showing atypia, are believed to be precursors to the development of malignancy (Dupont et al., 1993; Marshall et al., 1997). Benign lesions may present with pain, tenderness, and nipple discharge, as well as masses and dimpling of the skin. Mammographic changes, such as densities and microcalcifications, may also be noted in benign lesions and at times, may mimic malignancies.

Histology

IN SITU BREAST CANCERS AND NONINVASIVE BREAST CANCER

The enthusiasm for screening has led to the detection of small primary lesions that pose difficult diagnostic dilemmas when breast biopsies reveal premalignant histopathologic findings.

The diagnosis of in situ carcinomas appears to be increasing in frequency. Noninvasive breast cancer includes ductal carcinoma in situ (DCIS) and lobular carcinoma in situ (LCIS). DCIS is described as the proliferation of malignant epithelial cells confined to the mammary ducts without evidence of invasion through the basement membrane (see Figs. 10.14, 10.16 to 10.20, and 10.22) and is considered a precursor lesion. DCIS (also called intraductal carcinoma) is more likely to be localized to a region within one breast. Variants include papillary carcinoma in situ (see Fig. 10.21) which may mimic benign atypical papillomatosis, and comedo carcinoma, which consists of a solid growth of neoplastic cells within the ducts, associated with centrally located necrotic debris (Burstein et al., 2004).

In contrast, LCIS (see Figs. 10.23, 10.24) tends to be diffusely distributed throughout both breasts. LCIS is considered a risk factor for breast cancer and is not a precursor lesion (Page et al., 1991; Chuba et al., 2005).

DCIS is more common than LCIS, representing about 20% of breast cancers diagnosed in the United States (Ernster et al., 2002). Although the prognosis for patients with both types of in situ lesions is excellent, invasive lesions will develop in a certain fraction of patients with in situ carcinomas. Surgery, as either mastectomy or breast-conserving surgery plus adjuvant radiation, has been the treatment of choice for DCIS (Fisher et al., 1993; Julien et al., 2000). Selective estrogen receptor modulators, such as tamoxifen, may further decrease recurrence risk (Fisher et al., 1999). Management options for LCIS include careful observation or bilateral prophylactic simple mastectomy or the use of tamoxifen.

INVASIVE BREAST CANCERS

Over 75% of all infiltrating breast cancers originate in the ductal system (see Figs. 10.1, 10.27 to 10.29; Table 10.3). Several histologic variants of ductal carcinoma have been described. Pure examples of these variants constitute only a small percentage of the total number of cases, but certain features of each may be seen within the main portions of tumors that show the more common presentation designated invasive (or infiltrating) ductal carcinoma. Medullary carcinoma (see Fig. 10.32) is distinguished by poorly differentiated nuclei and infiltration by lymphocytes and plasma cells, whereas tubular carcinomas (see Fig. 10.31) are highly differentiated tumors that are marked, as their name suggests, by tubule formation. In mucinous (or colloid) carcinomas (see Fig. 10.33), nests of neoplastic epithelial

Table 10.3	
Incidence of Histologic Types of Invasive Breast Cancer from SEER*	
Type	**Frequency (%)**
Ductal	75.8
Lobular	8.3
Ductolobular	7.1
Mucinous (colloid)	2.4
Comedocarcinoma	1.6
Inflammatory	1.6
Tubular	1.5
Medullary	1.2
Papillary	<1

*Note: Other miscellaneous tumors (e.g., metaplastic, adenocystic, micropapillary, apocrine, Paget's) were not included in the above list. They compose <5% of invasive breast cancers.

From Li et al. (2005).

cells are surrounded by a mucinous matrix. A few invasive ductal carcinomas exhibit papillary features; hence their designation as papillary carcinomas. Although the above variants may carry a more favorable prognosis than routine infiltrating ductal carcinomas, they are treated similarly, based on stage of disease.

About 5% to 10% of infiltrating cancers arise from the lobules (see Fig. 10.30). Histologically, neoplastic cells of these tumors manifest a distinctive "single file" pattern. The prognosis and treatment of invasive lobular carcinoma are nearly identical to those of the invasive ductal type. However, lobular carcinomas can occasionally metastasize to the serosal surfaces of the abdominal organs, mimicking ovarian cancer (see Fig. 10.8C). Other unusual malignancies can develop in the breast, including apocrine, metaplastic, adenoid cystic, and squamous cell carcinomas. The cell of origin of the latter three has been difficult to determine. Fibroepithelial malignancies, such as cystosarcoma phylloides, are occasionally found in the breast, arising from the mesenchymal stroma (see Fig. 10.34) (Harris et al., 2004).

Diagnosis and Staging of Breast Cancer

Previously, open surgical biopsies were performed for diagnosis of breast cancer (see Fig. 10.68). Now, core needle biopsies are generally performed initially and usually yield sufficient tissue for histologic and immunohistochemical examinations. Needle biopsy can be done with ultrasound or stereotactic guidance (see Fig. 10.8D, E).

After a cancer diagnosis has been established, staging evaluation first begins with a detailed history and physical examination. Particular attention is given to the size, consistency, and fixation of the breast mass, skin changes such as erythema, edema, dimpling, and satellite nodules, as well as nipple changes such as retraction, discharge, and thickening. The status of axillary and infra- and supraclavicular lymph nodes is also evaluated. Chest and abdominal computed tomography (CT) scans and bone scans are performed in patients with node-positive disease and those with localizing symptoms. Head CTs are not routinely done unless patients are experiencing symptoms such as unusual headaches, nausea, cranial nerve deficits, and/or gait disturbances. Determination of biologic tumor markers (e.g., carcinoembryonic antigen [CEA], CA27, CA29) may be useful in patients with metastatic cancer. More recently, positron emission tomography (PET)-CTs have been used for staging and diagnosing recurrences, because they may have higher specificity for metastatic disease than standard CT (Radan et al., 2006) (Fig. 10.8F).

Historically, staging systems were based on the findings of the clinical examination, in particular on the size of the primary lesion and the extent of metastases to regional lymph nodes (see Figs. 10.36 through 10.38). Currently for breast cancer, pathologic findings have become the standard for determination of staging. In particular, lymph nodes may harbor microscopic metastases that would not be clinically or radiographically apparent (see Fig. 10.51). Stage I breast cancers consist of small lesions (<2 cm) with no palpable adenopathy; these account for approximately 60% or more of all newly diagnosed breast cancers. Stage II or III breast cancer has either a larger primary tumor (>2 cm) and/or axillary lymph node involvement. For clinical staging, it is important to determine whether the patient has palpable cervical, supraclavicular, or axillary lymphadenopathy, although these will have to be confirmed by biopsy. The diagnosis of inflammatory breast cancer can be made on pathologic and clinical grounds (e.g., skin edema, erythema, or thickening; see Figs. 10.43 through 10.48). Patients are considered to have stage IV disease if they have any evidence of distant metastases (see Fig. 10.53). Ipsilateral supraclavicular lymphadenopathy is now considered stage IIIC (AJCC, 2002; Harris et al., 2004).

Although even within a stage breast cancer can be heterogeneous, the presence of metastases to axillary lymph nodes (designated pathologic stage II or III) is the single most important prognostic factor in patients with breast cancer. Over 95% of patients with stage I disease are alive 10 years after diagnosis. The overall survival rates at 5 years for patients with stage II and stage III breast cancer are 80% to 90% and 50% to 70%, respectively. Patients with metastatic disease (stage IV) are rarely, if ever, cured, but approximately 20% are still alive 5 years after metastases are detected (see Fig. 10.37).

Primary Treatment

In the late nineteenth century, the technique of mastectomy was pioneered by Halsted and found to improve local control of breast cancer. For the next 50–75 years the concept that breast cancer spread in an orderly fashion from the primary lesion to regional lymph nodes and then to distant organs dominated the treatment of early disease (see Figs. 10.15, 10.16). During this time radical mastectomy (the complete removal of the breast, pectoral muscles, and axillary contents) was the treatment of choice. Subsequent studies have demonstrated that patients treated with less aggressive (modified radical) mastectomies have the same survival as those treated with radical mastectomies. In the last 20 years breast-conserving therapy, in which the initial mass is removed by "lumpectomy" or "quadrantectomy," followed by primary irradiation to the remainder of the breast, has been shown to produce survival rates similar to those seen with treatment by mastectomy. In most cases less aggressive, breast-conserving local therapy provides excellent cosmetic results (see Figs. 10.69, 10.70).

There are also new advances in exploring the axilla for the determination of lymph node involvement. A sentinel axillary lymph node is the first area to receive lymph flow and is usually the first to harbor a metastasis from the breast cancer. In selected patients a sentinel node biopsy serves as a means of avoiding a complete axillary dissection and is the preferred manner to assess disease in the axilla. To localize the sentinel node, surgeons inject one or two markers, blue dye or technetium sulfur colloid–^{99m}Tc, around the tumor or biopsy cavity. The markers are taken up into the lymphatic channels surrounding the tumor site and travel to the nodal basin. In some situations lymphoscintigraphy is performed after the injection to map out the lymphatic drainage pattern. A positive sentinel node requires a full axillary dissection (see Fig. 10.78). If the sentinel node biopsy is negative a full axillary dissection can be spared, eliminating the known potential complications of a dissection such as lymphedema (see Fig. 10.77) (Veronesi et al., 2003).

The completion of breast conservation therapy involves radiation therapy. The whole breast is treated using a pair of tangentially directed fields. The fields are designed to skim along the chest wall and thus irradiate the smallest amount of underlying lung.

At the conclusion of the whole-breast treatment, a boost dose is often given to the tumor bed. Complications of radiation therapy include radiation pneumonitis (see Fig. 10.81). In certain selected patients partial breast irradiation is also being performed, although little long-term data exist to accurately evaluate its equivalence to standard whole-breast irradiation (see Fig. 10.8G).

Such conservative therapy, however, is not appropriate for all patients. Contraindications to breast-conserving surgery include multicentric disease, diffuse malignant microcalcifications, and previous breast radiation therapy. For those who require or prefer mastectomies, remarkable advances have been made in recent years in reconstructive surgery (see Figs. 10.71 through 10.75). Some women will still require radiation therapy after mastectomy, including those with multiple involved lymph nodes or larger primary tumors.

Advances in local therapy have been complemented by the recent demonstration that adjuvant systemic therapy significantly prolongs survival compared with observation alone for certain subgroups of patients. Prognostic factors for stages I–III breast cancer include lymph node status, tumor size, estrogen/progesterone receptor, tumor kinetics, and overexpression/overamplification of *HER2/neu* (Table 10.4).

Metastatic Breast Cancer/Locally Recurrent Disease

Locally recurrent disease is often manifested by subcutaneous nodules or a nodular cutaneous rash along the mastectomy site. Occasionally the subcutaneous nodules become confluent and extend across the chest wall. The confluence is called an "en cuirasse" carcinoma (see Figs. 10.49, 10.50).

Although median survival for metastatic breast cancer is 2–3 years, patients with metastatic breast cancer demonstrate considerable heterogeneity in the clinical course of their disease. Some patients have a rapidly progressing tumor that metastasizes to multiple organs, whereas others have more indolent disease with a small percentage of patients considered "long-term" survivors (>10 years). Survival for patients with metastatic disease varies according to certain prognostic factors: a long, disease-free interval after primary therapy is a more favorable prognostic factor than a short interval; nonvisceral sites of metastases, such as bone, carry a better prognosis than visceral sites; and a

single site of metastasis is more favorable than multiple sites. Estrogen receptor protein (ERP) status of the primary tumor may be a good indicator of prognosis, with positive ERP status more favorable than a negative one. ERP status also predicts response to hormone therapy (see Fig. 10.35).

Breast cancer can recur in almost every tissue and organ in the body. However, common sites of metastases include the ipsilateral chest wall and regional lymph nodes (local-regional recurrence), as well as bone, lung, pleura, liver, gastrointestinal tract, and the central nervous system (see Figs. 10.53 through 10.66). Manifestations of recurrence can vary from asymptomatic findings on physical, serologic, or radiologic examination to symptoms referable to the organ involved (e.g., bone pain, shortness of breath, anorexia, or motor and/or neurologic deficits). Interestingly, tumors that overexpress HER2/neu appear to have a higher rate of brain metastases than HER2/neu-negative cancers (Bendell et al., 2003; Clayton et al., 2004). Although local-regional recurrence can sometimes represent a harbinger for metastatic (stage IV) disease, aggressive multimodality therapy can be associated with long-term disease control. Approximately 5% of newly diagnosed cases present with disseminated metastatic disease.

Until recently, hormonal therapy and chemotherapy have formed the foundation of treatment. Different types of hormonal agents, including SERMs (serum estrogen receptor modulators), SERDs (serum estrogen receptor downregulators), aromatase inhibitors, and luteinizing hormone–releasing hormone agonists, have contributed to the management of women with metastatic hormone-responsive disease. Complications of therapy can lead to myelosuppression, nausea, vomiting, alopecia, neurotoxicity, and integumentary toxicity (see Fig. 10.80). In addition to standard cytotoxic and hormonal therapies, targeted biologic therapies are increasingly used. The most widely used target the HER2/neu pathway and include trastuzumab, a humanized monoclonal antibody to the HER2/neu protein, and lapitinib, an oral dual tyrosine kinase inhibitor of the HER2/neu and epidermal growth factor receptor (EGFR) pathways. HER2/neu is overexpressed in approximately 25% to 30% of breast cancers (see Fig. 10.8H). Several methods of detection of HER2/neu are used. Immunoperoxidase studies use antibodies directed at HER2/neu protein. A more accurate but labor-intensive method looking at the amplification of the gene is fluorescent in situ hybridization (FISH) (see Fig. 10.79). Trastuzumab has been incorporated into the standard treatment in both the adjuvant and metastatic settings for appropriate patients. In addition, agents that target the vascular endothelial growth factor (VEGF) and/or EGFR pathway also appear to have activity in metastatic breast cancer.

Additionally, selective use of surgery or radiation therapy and use of bisphosphonates can provide significant palliation to patients with metastases. Bisphosphonates are routinely used in women with bone metastases to decrease the risk of skeletal complications (Theriault et al., 1999). Monitoring of tumor markers (CEA or CA15-3 or CA27-29) is often helpful in monitoring disease course (see Fig. 10.67). Tumor markers alone, however, should not be the sole determinant of treatment response, because they can transiently increase soon after starting treatment ("flare response") or may be elevated by non-neoplastic causes. In addition, some women with metastatic breast cancer have normal tumor markers.

Table 10.4
Adverse Prognostic Factors in Breast Cancer*

Lymph node status
    Negative < few positive < many positive
Larger tumor size
    Clinical features: fixation; ulceration; inflammation
    High histologic grade
    High nuclear grade
Estrogen-receptor (ER) and progesterone-receptor (PR) content negative
Tumor kinetics
    Thymidine-labeling index; high S-phase fraction
DNA aneuploidy
HER2/neu overexpression/overamplification
Basal phenotype ("triple negative" or ER/PR/HER2/neu-negative)

Adapted from Hayes (1993) and McGuire and Clark (1992).

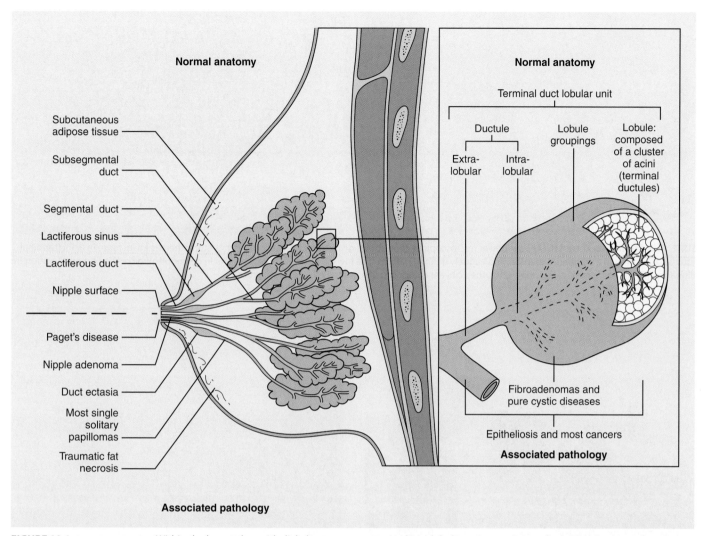

FIGURE 10.1 BREAST ANATOMY. Within the breast the epithelial elements are organized into lobular units consisting of acini that feed into ductules. The latter in turn coalesce into larger ducts that form a reservoir, or lactiferous sinus, proximal to the nipple. These epithelial structures, supported by adipose and fibrous tissue, give rise to more than 95% of breast malignancies.

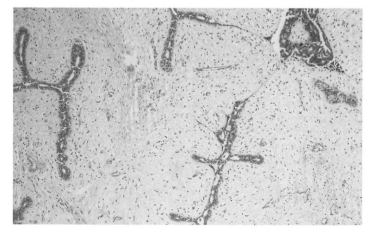

FIGURE 10.2 FIBROADENOMA. The tumor from which this histologic section was taken was a well-circumscribed, discoid mass, clearly demarcated from the surrounding breast tissue. High magnification reveals stroma compressing ducts so that they form slitlike curvilinear spaces. Note the low cellularity of the stroma, an important benign feature.

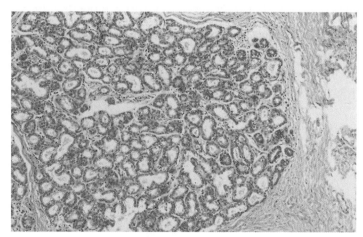

FIGURE 10.3 LACTATING ADENOMA. This well-circumscribed lesion has closely packed acini with prominent epithelial cells marked by large nuclei and abundant, pink, vacuolated cytoplasm. (Courtesy of Dr N. Weidner, Brigham and Women's Hospital, Boston, MA.)

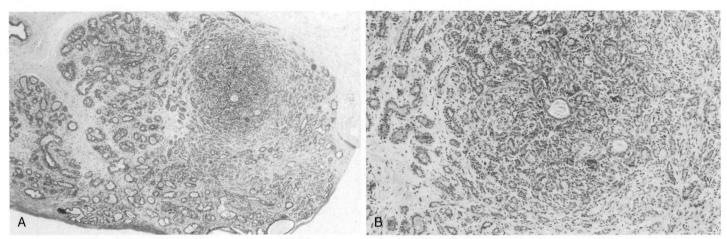

FIGURE 10.4 **SCLEROSING ADENOSIS. (A)** Low-power microscopic section shows distortion of the lobular architecture; there is an increase in acini (terminal ductules), appearing in a whorled, expansile, and vaguely defined pattern. The low-power view is very helpful in distinguishing this benign proliferation from malignancy. **(B)** Higher magnification shows that the acini are composed of a normal two-cell population.

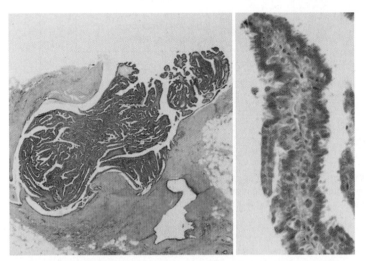

FIGURE 10.5 **PAPILLOMA.** Low-magnification view shows a large duct filled with a papillary proliferation. At higher power (*inset*) a papillary branch can be seen with a normal two-cell population covering a fibrovascular stalk. In this benign tumor the lining epithelial cells can show apocrine changes.

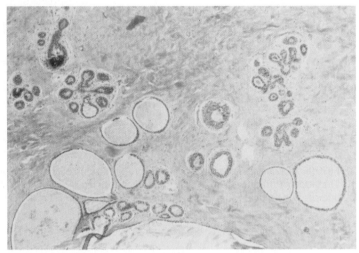

FIGURE 10.6 **FIBROCYSTIC CHANGES.** These benign changes are the most common findings in breast biopsies. They are characterized by dense fibrosis intermixed with cystic areas.

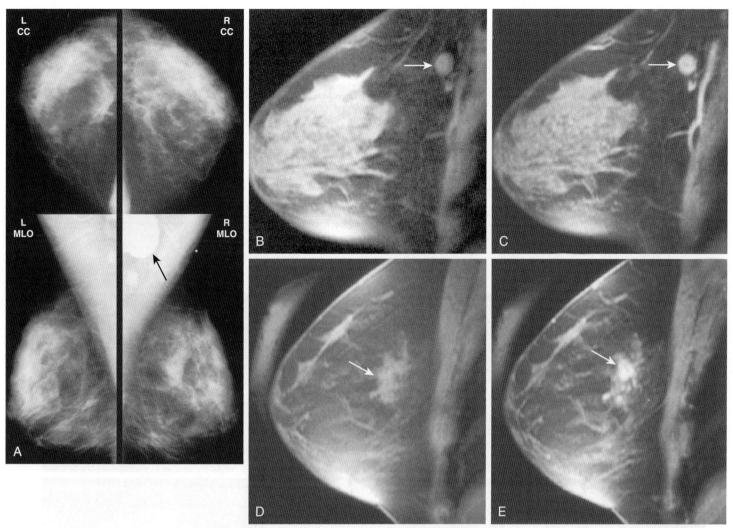

FIGURE 10.7 (A) Bilateral mammograms on a 45-year-old patient with enlarged right axillary nodes (*black arrow*) but no mammographic abnormality within either breast. **(B)** Sagittal MR image of the right breast with fat saturation before administration of gadolinium. A rounded density represents an axillary node (*white arrow*). **(C)** Sagittal MR image at the same location as **B** after administration of gadolinium. Enhancement of the node is evident (*white arrow*). **(D)** Sagittal MR image of the right breast at a level slightly medial to **B** and **C**. A patch of stromal density is evident deep in the breast before contrast administration (*white arrow*). Other retroareolar stromal densities with similar appearance are also present. **(E)** Sagittal MR image of the right breast in the same location as **D**, after administration of gadolinium. The deep stroma is enhancing (*white arrow*) consistent with tumor, while the other stromal densities have not changed, consistent with normal breast tissue.

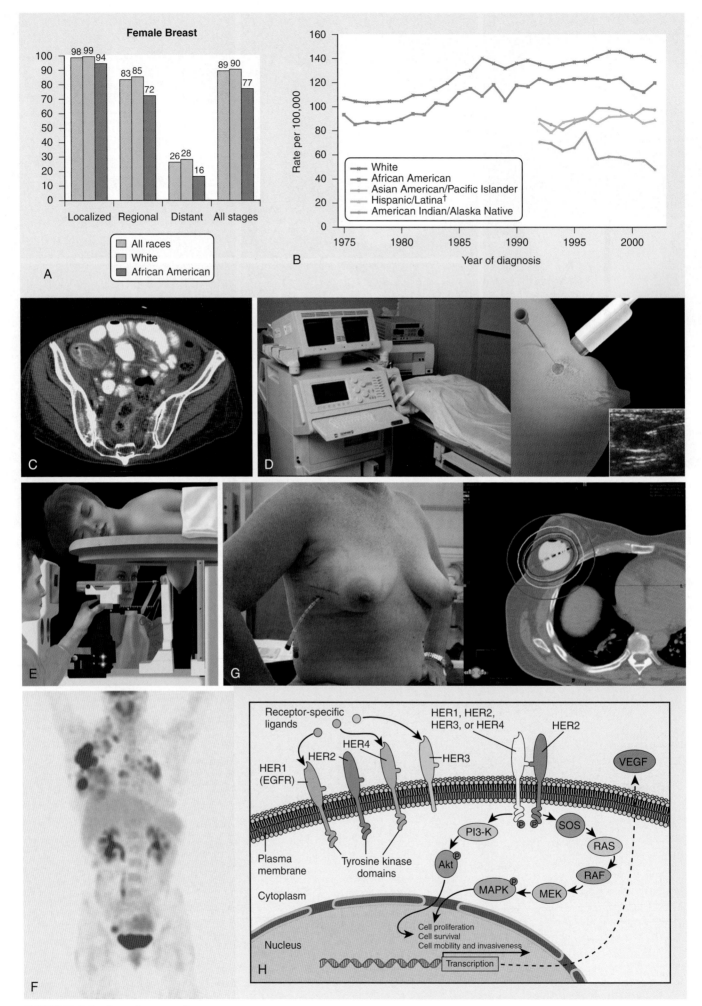

FIGURE 10.8 See legend on opposite page.

FIGURE 10.8 **(A)** Five-year relative survival by race and stage at diagnosis of breast cancer (SEER data, 1996–2002). **(B)** Female breast cancer incidence by race and ethnicity (SEER data). **(C)** When lobular breast cancer metastasizes it can often infiltrate serosal surfaces mimicking ovarian cancer. This patient presented with abdominal bloating, tightness, and narrowing in her stool caliber 9 years after the diagnosis of a stage I breast cancer. Note the diffuse thickening of the rectal and colonic wall, peritoneal carcinomatosis, and ascites. A colonoscopy was performed, and biopsy confirmed diffuse involvement with metastatic adenocarcinoma consistent with a breast primary. On restaging, she was also noted to have multiple osseous metastases. (Image courtesy of Drs. Pamela Dipiro and Wendy Chen, Dana Farber Cancer Institute, Boston, MA.) **(D)** In an ultrasound-guided needle biopsy, the ultrasound probe is used to localize the lesion that was identified either on physical examination or on mammogram. A biopsy needle is passed through the lesion several times to obtain tissue. Compared to a stereotactic biopsy, an ultrasound-guided biopsy is faster and better tolerated by most patients. However, not all lesions may be amenable to an ultrasound-guided biopsy. (Image courtesy of Robyn L. Birdwell, MD, Brigham and Women's Hospital, Boston, MA, and Diagnostic Imaging Breast, Amirsys, Inc., Salt Lake City, UT, 2006.) **(E)** The premise behind stereotactic needle biopsy is that a lesion can be localized in three dimensions by evaluating its changes in position in a series of angled radiographic views. First, a radiograph localizes the suspicious area, then two additional views, angled 15 degrees to either side of the lesion, are obtained. A computer calculates how much the lesion's position appears to have changed on each of the angled views and uses these data to estimate the lesion's location within three-dimensional space. With the advent of digital mammography these images are commonly acquired digitally. (Image courtesy of Robyn L. Birdwell, MD, Brigham and Women's Hospital, Boston, MA, and Diagnostic Imaging Breast, Amirsys, Inc., Salt Lake City, UT, 2006). **(F)** Positron emission tomography (PET) involves injection of a substance labeled with a positron-emitting isotope (commonly, fluorine-18 bound to D-glucose, called FDG for 2-([^{18}F]fluoro-2-deoxy-D-glucose)). Metabolically active cells, especially malignant ones, preferentially take up glucose, and therefore FDG, as compared with non-neoplastic tissue. Sensitivity of PET can vary considerably by tumor type and size. False-positive results can occur in areas of inflammation or infection. Many machines now acquire CT images in tandem with PET images, which can then be fused together to provide anatomic correlation by CT with metabolic activity measurements by PET. This patient presented with palpable axillary adenopathy and a large breast mass with associated erythema, skin edema, and nipple retraction. Note the extremely intense areas of uptake within the right breast and axilla corresponding to the patient's known locally advanced breast cancer. Also note the intense uptake in the right supraclavicular, paratracheal, prevascular, precarinal, and hilar lymph nodes suspicious for metastatic disease. Uptake in the kidney, bladder, and ureters is physiologic and due to FDG excretion. Uptake in the right adnexa and jaw is most likely physiologic and benign. **(G)** Panels 1 and 2: Accelerated partial breast irradiation (APBI) encompasses techniques including intracavitary and interstitial brachytherapy as well as 3D-conformal, intensity-modulated, and intraoperative external-beam radiation therapy. One of the more commonly used brachytherapy methods in the United States, the MammoSite Brachytherapy System (Hologic, Massachusetts) involves insertion of a catheter with a balloon tip into the lumpectomy cavity at the time of surgery or shortly thereafter (panel 1). The balloon is filled with saline and a high-dose-rate radioactive source is introduced twice per day for 5 days by computed axial tomography scan–based treatment planning, permitting a highly conformal dose to be delivered to the first centimeter of remaining breast tissue with optimal sparing of the remaining tissue and other regional organs (panel 2). The balloon catheter is removed upon completion. APBI is an option only for selected patients, mainly older women with smaller, node-negative "low-risk" tumors and with negative margins. (Courtesy of Phillip M. Devlin, MD, Dana Farber/Brigham and Women's Cancer Center, Harvard Medical School, Boston, MA.) **(H)** The HER family of receptors (human epidermal growth factor receptor, also called ErbB) is a group of transmembrane tyrosine kinase receptors that regulate cell growth, survival, and differentiation, via a variety of pathways, including RAS (rat sarcoma), RAF (receptor activation factor), MAPK (mitogen-activated protein kinase), and MEK (mitogen extracellular signal kinase). The tyrosine kinase domains are activated by dimerization. Current therapeutics involve tyrosine kinase inhibitors (e.g., lapatinib) and antibodies directed against the HER2 protein and VEGF (vascular endothelial growth factor)(e.g., trastuzumab and bevacizumab).

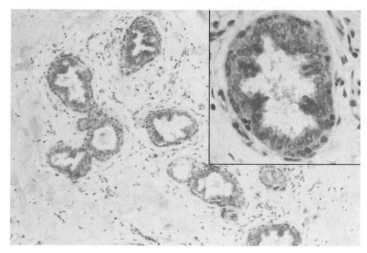

FIGURE 10.9 **EPITHELIAL HYPERPLASIA (MILD).** This lobular unit shows irregular areas of heaped-up cells lining the acini (terminal ductules). At high magnification (*inset*) the epithelial layer of one ductule is three to four cell layers thick, and there is no bridging of cells across the acinar structure.

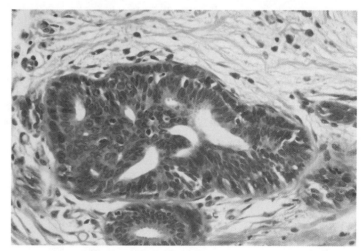

FIGURE 10.10 **EPITHELIAL HYPERPLASIA (MODERATE).** At this stage the acinar structure is distended by hyperplastic cells that frequently bridge the lumen, often filling as much as half of it.

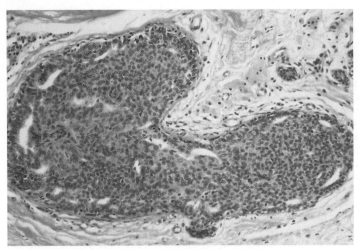

FIGURE 10.11 **EPITHELIAL HYPERPLASIA (FLORID).** Involved spaces show marked distention by hyperplastic cells that occupy the majority of the lumen. Collapsed slitlike spaces are present, frequently at the periphery of the structure. These slits are surrounded by serpentine passages composed of "flowing" cells, which often lack clear cell borders. Moderate and florid hyperplasias imply a slightly higher risk of subsequent invasive carcinoma than mild or no hyperplasia.

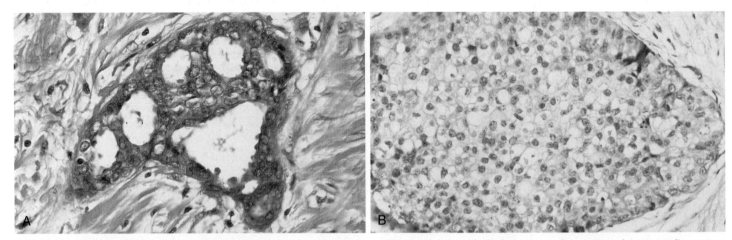

FIGURE 10.12 **EPITHELIAL HYPERPLASIA (ATYPICAL).** **(A)** Atypical cases show a nonuniform population of cells from normochromatic nuclei surrounding spaces that are not quite smooth-lined. It is these features that distinguish atypical epithelial (ductal) hyperplasia from ductal carcinoma in situ, in which smooth, geometric spaces are surrounded by a uniform cell population with hyperchromatic nuclei. **(B)** High magnification shows that these proliferating, relatively nonuniform cells lack the necessary degree of cell-to-cell rigidity. Atypical hyperplasia carries a relatively higher risk of subsequent development of invasive carcinoma than other types. This risk is further elevated in women with a family history of breast cancer in a first-degree relative.

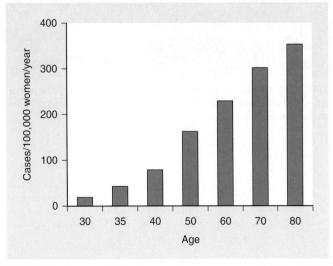

FIGURE 10.13 Age-specific incidence of breast cancer in the United States.

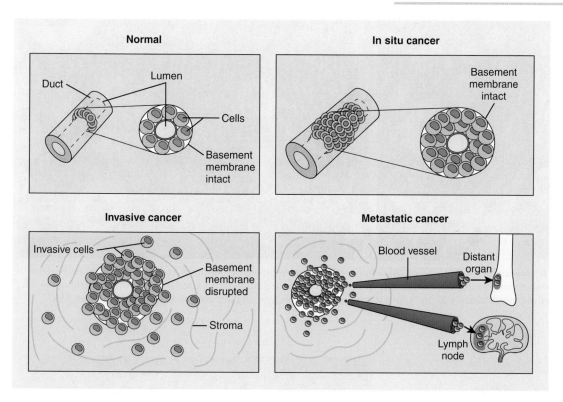

FIGURE 10.14 Timeline of breast cancer suggesting probable heterogeneity. Primary breast cancers begin as single (or more) cells that have lost normal regulation of differentiation and proliferation but remain confined within the basement membrane of the duct or lobule. As these cells go through several doublings, at some point they invade through the basement membrane of the ductule or lobule and ultimately metastasize to distant organs.

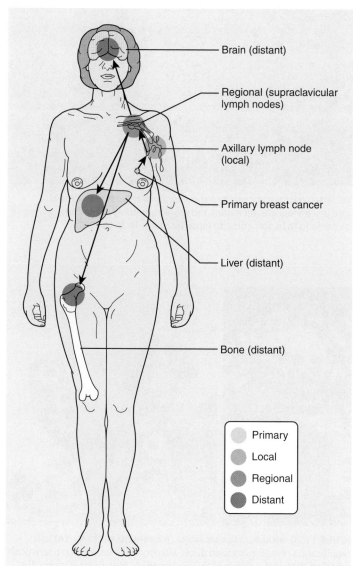

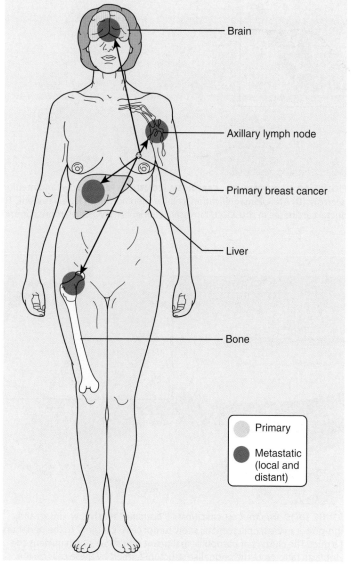

FIGURE 10.15 **HALSTED THEORY OF BREAST CANCER SPREAD.** This theory suggests that breast cancer originates in the breast, eventually spreads to local skin and/or lymph nodes, and then ultimately affects distant organs. This theory maintains that local/regional lymph nodes serve as "barriers" to the spread of metastatic breast cancer. The implication of this theory is that more intensive local therapy should lead to an increased rate of cures.

FIGURE 10.16 **SYSTEMIC THEORY OF BREAST CANCER SPREAD.** This theory suggests that breast cancer becomes metastatic very early in its course, once invasion through the basement membrane of the duct or lobule has occurred. It maintains that local therapy will have few if any long-term effects on survival, because the disease is already systemic at the time of diagnosis.

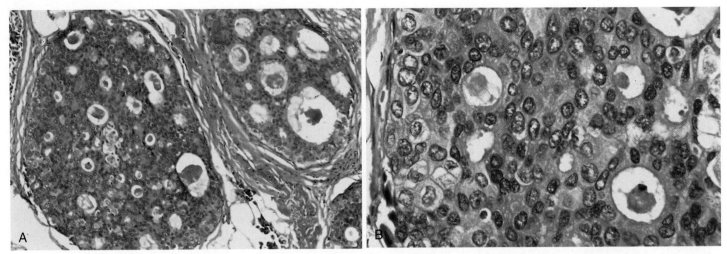

FIGURE 10.17 INTRADUCTAL CARCINOMA (CRIBRIFORM TYPE). (A) Low- and **(B)** high-power photomicrographs demonstrate a cribriform pattern composed of a rather uniform tumor cell population with distinct cytoplasmic borders; the cells are rigidly arranged around crisp, circular holes. With this pattern the risk for the subsequent development of invasive cancer increases 10- to 11-fold. (Courtesy of Dr N. Weidner, Brigham and Women's Hospital, Boston, MA.)

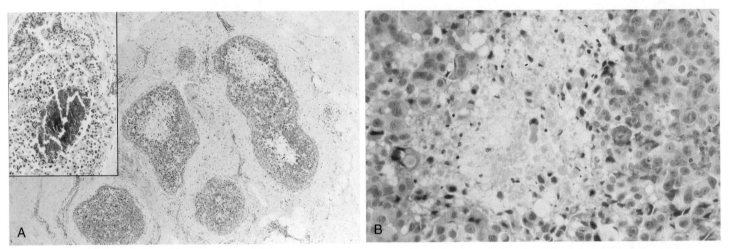

FIGURE 10.18 INTRADUCTAL CARCINOMA (COMEDO TYPE). (A) Low- and medium-power (*inset*) microscopic sections show expanded ducts with central necrosis. **(B)** At high magnification, cellular pleomorphism is also evident. This feature is seen to a greater extent and more commonly in the comedo type of ductal carcinoma in situ. Occult invasive elements may also be more common in the comedo than non-comedo types (see Figs. 10.18 to 10.20).

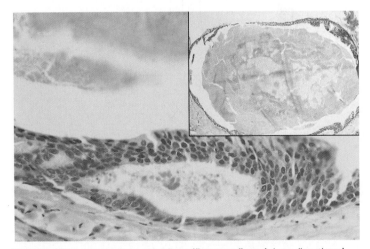

FIGURE 10.19 INTRADUCTAL CARCINOMA ("CLINGING" TYPE). Low- (inset) and high-power microscopic sections show tumor cells "clinging" to the periphery of a duct. The clusters of basophilic malignant cells show a high nucleus-to-cytoplasm ratio. Note the bridgelike structure formed by these cells on the high-power view.

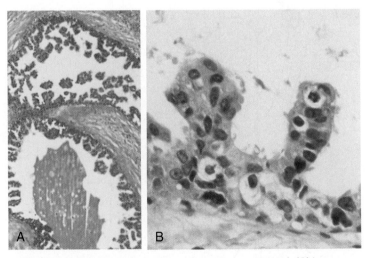

FIGURE 10.20 INTRADUCTAL CARCINOMA (MICROPAPILLARY TYPE). (A) Low magnification reveals expanded ducts with fronds of tumor characteristically extending toward the center of the lumina. **(B)** At high magnification the bulbous fronds typically appear narrow at the base and expanded at the tip. (**A**, Courtesy of Dr N. Weidner, Brigham and Women's Hospital, Boston, MA.)

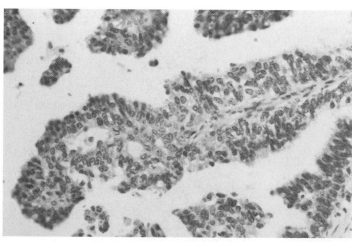

FIGURE 10.21 **PAPILLARY CARCINOMA IN SITU.** The architectural features of this in situ breast cancer are similar to those of a papilloma. The normal two-cell–layer epithelium covering the fibrovascular fronds is replaced by a uniform proliferation of cells with hyperchromatic nuclei.

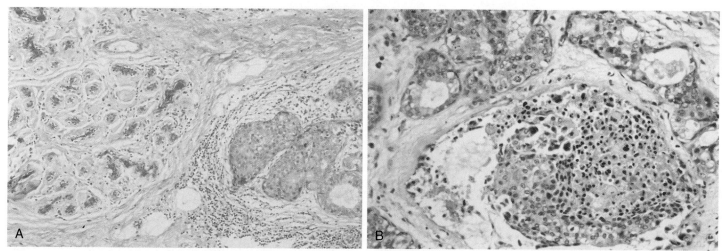

FIGURE 10.22 **INTRADUCTAL CARCINOMA.** **(A)** Microscopic section shows a normal lobular unit on the left and "cancerization of the lobules" on the right, where a ductal carcinoma has extended into the lobules. **(B)** High magnification demonstrates "cancerization of the lobules" in the upper portion of the field, whereas the lower portion reveals a duct that has been expanded by an intraductal carcinoma with foci of necrosis. "Cancerization of the lobules" carries no clinical significance except that it may mimic lobular carcinoma in situ. However, pleomorphism, tubule formation, and necrosis, as seen here, are not encountered in lobular carcinoma.

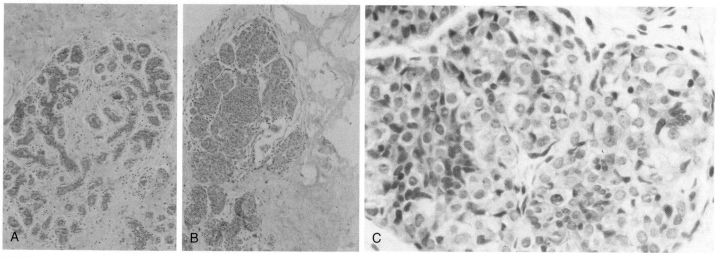

FIGURE 10.23 **LOBULAR CARCINOMA IN SITU.** Low-power photomicrographs show **(A)** the normal architecture of a lobular unit and **(B)** a distended lobular unit showing the typical appearance of LCIS. **(C)** At high magnification the lobular unit is seen to be distended and distorted by characteristically uniform, round tumor cells with bland nuclei. LCIS is usually diffusely dispersed throughout the breast and is often bilateral. Rarely producing a mass or abnormality on mammography, it is commonly discovered coincidentally during a biopsy performed for other suspicious lesions. Women with LCIS have a slightly higher risk of developing invasive cancer, whether ductal or lobular in origin, in their lifetime.

FIGURE 10.24 **LOBULAR CARCINOMA IN SITU.** High-power microscopic section shows clusters of tumor cells spreading along a duct in a "pagetoid" fashion; that is, displacing the normal ductal epithelium toward the lumen, which is lined by attenuated luminal surface cells. This should not be confused with Paget's disease of the breast, a lesion of ductal origin, in which tumor cells extend into the epidermis (see Fig. 10.25).

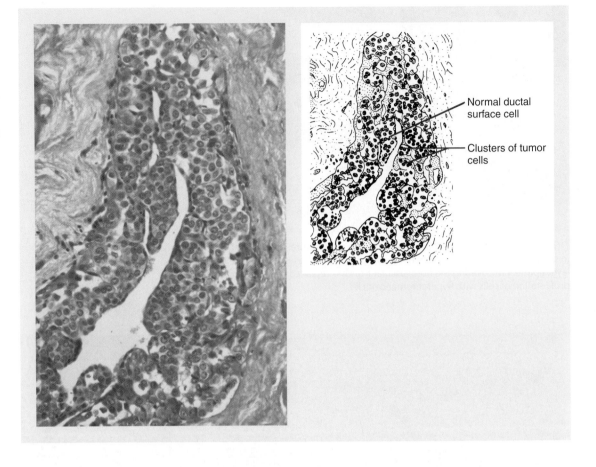

Normal ductal
surface cell

Clusters of tumor
cells

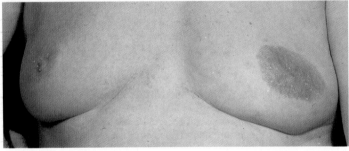

FIGURE 10.25 **PAGET'S DISEASE OF THE BREAST.** In this unique clinical entity, one of the main ducts leading to the nipple becomes engorged with neoplastic cells. Clinically, patients present with an eczematous rash that extends to and involves the areola. This rare condition may or may not be associated with an underlying invasive carcinoma.

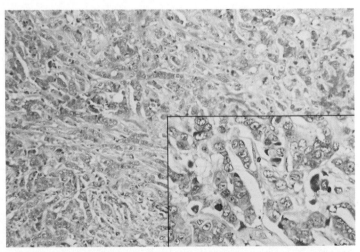

FIGURE 10.27 **INVASIVE DUCTAL CARCINOMA.** Low- and high-power (*inset*) photomicrographs of a poorly differentiated adenocarcinoma show that the stroma is infiltrated by pleomorphic tumor cells showing a high mitotic rate. Note the necrosis and lack of tubule formation.

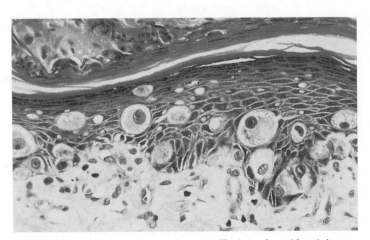

FIGURE 10.26 **PAGET'S DISEASE OF THE BREAST.** The irregular epidermis is infiltrated by characteristic cells with abundant pale-staining granular cytoplasm and large, oval, vesicular nuclei with prominent nucleoli.

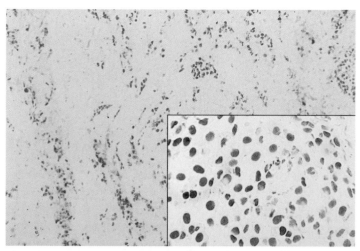

FIGURE 10.28 **INVASIVE DUCTAL CARCINOMA.** Low magnification of a breast biopsy specimen stained for estrogen receptor protein (ERP) using an estrogen receptor immunocytochemical assay (ERICA) shows that most cells are positive (*brown*). ERICA allows for semiquantitation of ERP. High magnification (*inset*) reveals that the antibody is localized to the nuclei (*brown*). (Courtesy of Dr. S.L. Khoury, Brigham and Women's Hospital, Boston, MA.)

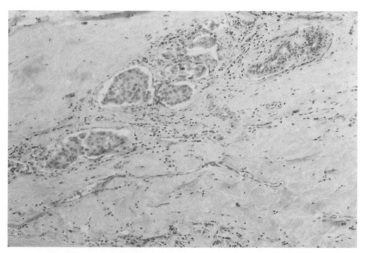

FIGURE 10.29 **INVASIVE DUCTAL CARCINOMA.** Photomicroscopic section of a breast biopsy specimen demonstrates an invasive ductal carcinoma in the lymphatic vessels of the breast parenchyma.

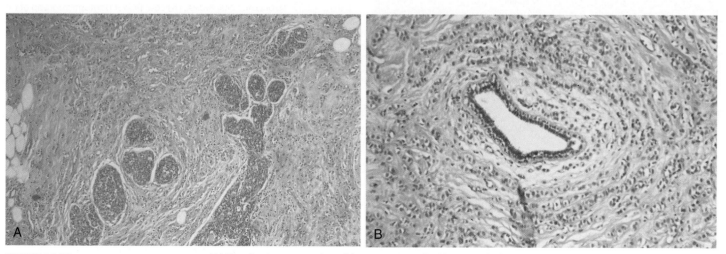

FIGURE 10.30 **INVASIVE LOBULAR CARCINOMA. (A)** The classic presentation of this tumor is marked by a "single-file" pattern of uniform malignant cells infiltrating the stroma. The invasive lesion surrounds foci of in situ tumor. **(B)** Single-file tumor cells surround an involved duct, producing a target-like pattern.

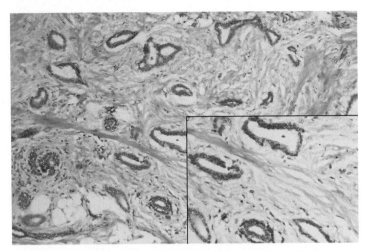

FIGURE 10.31 TUBULAR CARCINOMA. Low- and high-power (*inset*) microscopic sections of this histologic variant of invasive ductal carcinoma show tubular structures infiltrating the stroma. The lumina of the tubules are lined by a single cell layer of well-differentiated cells. This type of breast cancer has a better prognosis than common infiltrating ductal carcinoma.

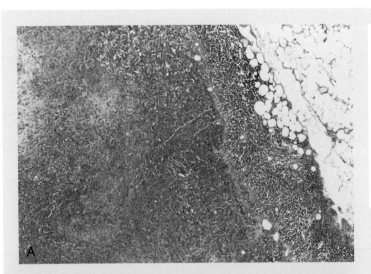

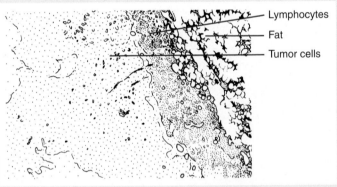

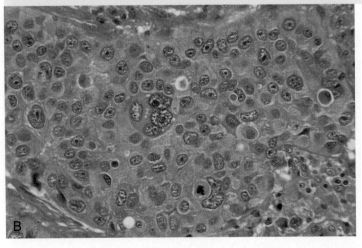

FIGURE 10.32 MEDULLARY CARCINOMA. (A) Low-power photomicrograph of this histologic variant of invasive ductal carcinoma demonstrates its characteristic syncytial growth pattern. The tumor has a smooth, well-circumscribed border and shows a prominent lymphocytic infiltrate. **(B)** At higher magnification, the classic pleomorphic cells with bizarre nuclei are evident. This malignancy has better 5- and 10-year survival rates than common ductal carcinoma. (Courtesy of Dr. N. Weidner, Brigham and Women's Hospital, Boston, MA.)

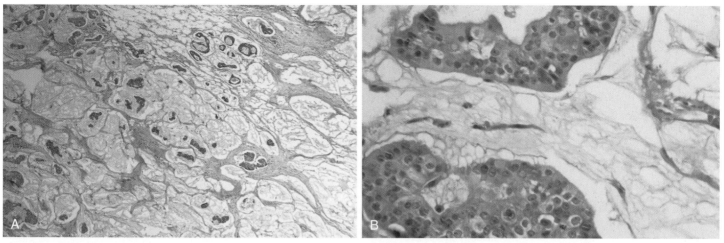

FIGURE 10.33 **MUCINOUS OR COLLOID CARCINOMA. (A)** Low-power microscopic section shows islands of tumor cells within a sea of mucin. **(B)** Higher magnification demonstrates sharply circumscribed tumor aggregates with characteristic smooth borders and a homogeneous cell population. Pure histologic forms of this variant have better prognoses than common ductal carcinoma.

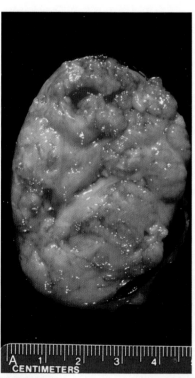

FIGURE 10.34 **CYSTOSARCOMA PHYLLOIDES. (A)** The irregular cut surface of this tumor is marked by clefts that surround glistening gray to yellow islands of tumor intermixed with foci of necrosis (*yellow*). **(B)** Low-magnification study shows the classic leaflike projection of hypercellular stroma into a benign ductal structure. At high magnification **(C)**, hypercellular areas demonstrate osteosarcomatous differentiation with osteoid (*pink*) deposition. Scattered "osteoclast-like" giant cells are also present. Typically, malignant stroma in these tumors appears fibro- or myxoliposarcomatous and less commonly like osteosarcoma, rhabdomyosarcoma, or chondrosarcoma. (Courtesy of Dr. N. Weidner, Brigham and Women's Hospital, Boston, MA.)

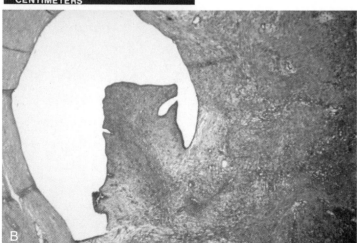

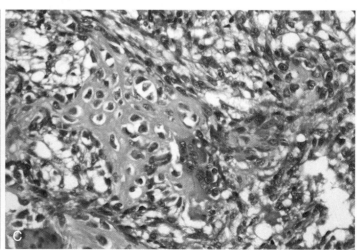

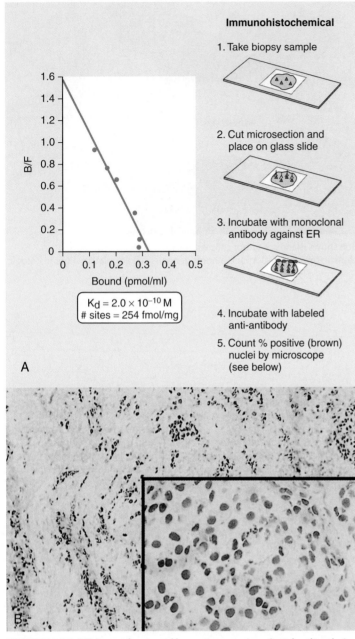

Immunohistochemical

1. Take biopsy sample

2. Cut microsection and place on glass slide

3. Incubate with monoclonal antibody against ER

$K_d = 2.0 \times 10^{-10}$ M
\# sites = 254 fmol/mg

4. Incubate with labeled anti-antibody

5. Count % positive (brown) nuclei by microscope (see below)

A

B

FIGURE 10.35   (A) Assays for steroid hormone receptors. Scatchard analysis of [³H]estradiol binding to estrogen receptor (ER) in human breast cancer cytosol, determined by the multipoint Dextron coated charcoal (DCC) assay. The calculated binding affinity (K_d) and the quantitative receptor content are shown. **(B)** Localization of ERP using the ERICA assay (see Fig. 10.28). In this frozen section of an infiltrating ductal carcinoma, a brown stain in the nucleus defines the presence of ER. Although most cells in this tumor show immunoreactivity, there is heterogeneity in the degree of reactivity among the tumor cells.

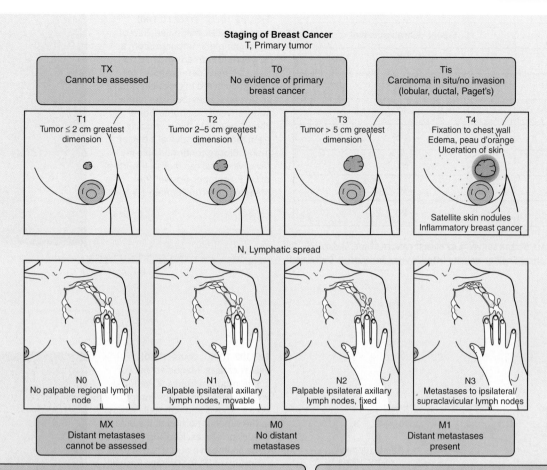

Staging of Breast Cancer
T, Primary tumor

| TX Cannot be assessed | T0 No evidence of primary breast cancer | Tis Carcinoma in situ/no invasion (lobular, ductal, Paget's) |

| T1 Tumor ≤ 2 cm greatest dimension | T2 Tumor 2–5 cm greatest dimension | T3 Tumor > 5 cm greatest dimension | T4 Fixation to chest wall Edema, peau d'orange Ulceration of skin ... Satellite skin nodules Inflammatory breast cancer |

N, Lymphatic spread

| N0 No palpable regional lymph node | N1 Palpable ipsilateral axillary lymph nodes, movable | N2 Palpable ipsilateral axillary lymph nodes, fixed | N3 Metastases to ipsilateral/ supraclavicular lymph nodes |

| MX Distant metastases cannot be assessed | M0 No distant metastases | M1 Distant metastases present |

Staging criteria for breast cancer, TNM classification

Primary tumor (T)

TX — Primary tumor cannot be assessed

T0 — No evidence of primary tumor

Tis — Carcinoma in situ
- Tis (DCIS) — Intraductal carcinoma in situ
- Tis (LCIS) — Lobular carcinoma in situ
- Tis (Paget's) — Paget's disease of the nipple with no tumor; tumor-associated Paget's disease is classified according to the size of the primary tumor

T1 — Tumor 2 cm or less in greatest dimension
- T1mic — Microinvasion 0.1 cm or less in greatest dimension
- T1a — Tumor more than 0.1 cm but not more than 0.5 cm in greatest dimension
- T1b — Tumor more than 0.5 cm but not more than 1 cm in greatest dimension
- T1c — Tumor more than 1 cm but not more than 2 cm in greatest dimension

T2 — Tumor more than 2 cm but not more than 5 cm in greatest dimension

T3 — Tumor more than 5 cm in greatest dimension

T4 — Tumor of any size with direct extension to (a) chest wall or (b) skin, only as described below:
- T4a — Extension to chest wall
- T4b — Edema (including peau d'orange) or ulceration of the breast skin, or satellite skin nodules confined to the same breast
- T4c — Both (T4a and T4b)
- T4d — Inflammatory carcinoma

Note: Dimpling of the skin, nipple retraction, or any other skin change except those described for T4b and T4d may occur in T1–3 tumors without changing the classification.

Regional lymph nodes (N)

NX — Regional lymph nodes cannot be assessed (e.g., previously removed)

N0 — No regional lymph node metastases

N1 — Metastasis to movable ipsilateral axillary lymph node(s)

N2 — Metastasis to ipsilateral axillary lymph node(s) fixed or matted, or in clinically apparent ipsilateral internal mammary nodes in the absence of evident axillary node metastases
- N2a — Metastasis to ipsilateral axillary lymph node(s) fixed to one another (matted) or to other structures
- N2b — Metastasis only in clinically apparent (as detected by imaging studies [excluding lymphoscintigraphy] or by clinical examination or grossly visible pathologically) ipsilateral internal mammary nodes in the absence of evident axillary node metastases

Stage grouping of breast cancer

Stage	T	N	M	5-year overall survival
0	Tis	N0	M0	100
I	T1	N0	M0	100
IIA	T0	N1	M0	92
	T1	N1	M0	
	T2	N0	M0	
IIB	T2	N1	M0	81
	T3	N0	M0	
IIIA	T0	N2	M0	67
	T1	N2	M0	
	T2	N2	M0	
	T3	N1	M0	
	T3	N2	M0	
IIIB	T4	Any N	M0	54
IIIC	Any T	N3	M0	
IV	Any T	Any N	M1	20

FIGURE 10.36 BREAST CANCER STAGING. (From *AJCC Cancer Staging Manual*, 6th ed., 2002.)

Stage	5-year overall survival
0	100
I	100
IIA	92
IIB	81
IIIA	67
IIIB	54
IV	20

FIGURE 10.37 OVERALL 5-YEAR SURVIVAL BY BREAST CANCER STAGE. (Adapted from the American Cancer Society website http://www.cancer.org/). (Accessed 18 September 2007.)

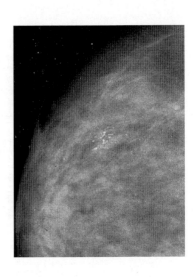

FIGURE 10.39 STAGE I (T1N0) BREAST CANCER. Magnified view of a screening mammogram from a 52-year-old woman who had no palpable mass demonstrates the classic clustered microcalcifications of several shapes and sizes highly suggestive of carcinoma. Some show linear branching, which is even more suggestive of a ductal lesion. Biopsy confirmed an early invasive ductal carcinoma. (Courtesy of Dr. P. Stomper, Roswell Park Memorial Institute, Buffalo, NY.)

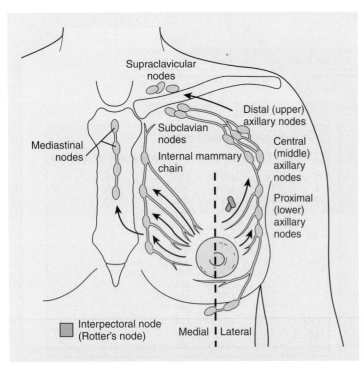

FIGURE 10.38 LYMPHATIC SPREAD OF BREAST CANCER. Lymph node metastases are present at the time of diagnosis in up to 60% of cases. In general, lateral lesions in the breast metastasize to axillary and supraclavicular nodes, whereas medial tumors tend to metastasize to the internal mammary and mediastinal lymph nodes, as well as the supraclavicular nodes. However, lymph node involvement is merely a marker for the probability that the cancer has spread from the breast. A positive finding implies that microdeposits of breast cancer will probably be present in other areas as well.

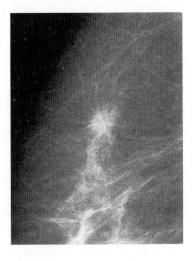

FIGURE 10.40 STAGE (T1N0) BREAST CANCER. Magnified view of a mammogram from a 50-year-old woman with a history of "lumpy" breasts shows a 1.0-cm stellate mass in the superior portion of the breast. The lesion was excised and found to be an invasive ductal carcinoma. (Courtesy of Dr. P. Stomper, Roswell Park Memorial Institute, Buffalo, NY.)

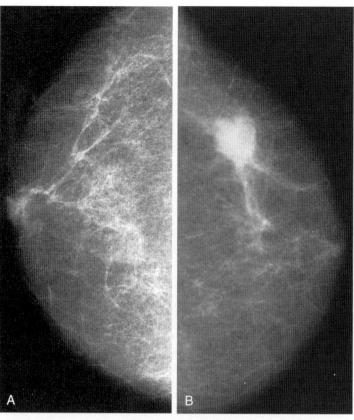

FIGURE 10.41 STAGE IIA (T2N0) BREAST CANCER. This mammogram from a 65-year-old woman shows that the breasts are not too dense; therefore, the 2.5-cm stellate mass in the upper outer quadrant of the right breast was easily palpated. Histologic examination following resection showed an invasive ductal carcinoma.

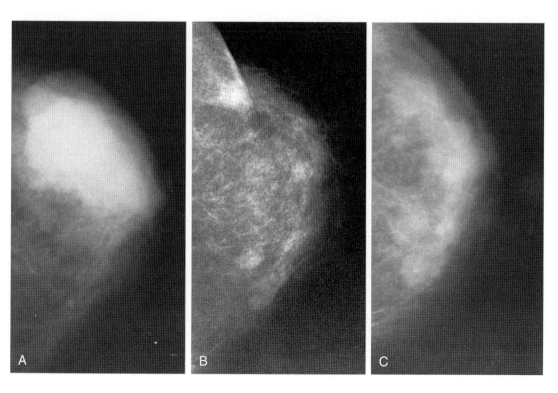

FIGURE 10.42 STAGE IIIB (T4N0) BREAST CANCER. A 45-year-old woman presented with a very large (10 cm) primary tumor. There was an inflammatory component, but a distinct underlying mass was palpable and quite easily detected on the mammogram **(A)**. **(B)** Following chemotherapy and radiation therapy the mass completely disappeared, replaced only by the distortion artifact left by the biopsy. Three months later the tumor recurred within the same breast. **(C)** The mammogram demonstrates multiple nodular tumor masses.

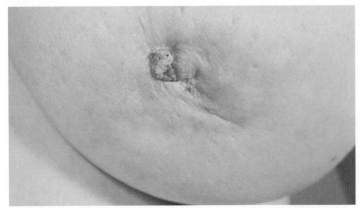

FIGURE 10.43 **STAGE IIIB (T4) BREAST CANCER.** A common presentation at this stage is retraction, dimpling, and thickening of the skin surrounding the nipple. This clinical finding is designated "peau d'orange," a term deriving from the pitting and coloration of the skin that resembles orange peel.

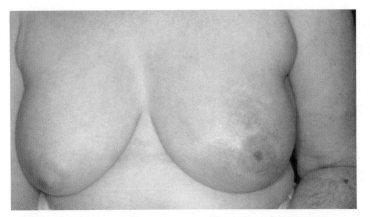

FIGURE 10.44 **STAGE IIB (T4) BREAST CANCER.** Classically, inflammatory breast cancer does not present as a discrete mass but instead as cutaneous erythema with overlying skin warmth, as illustrated in the left breast of this 63-year-old patient.

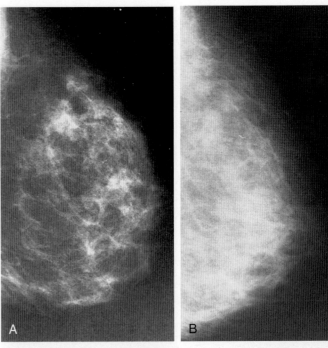

FIGURE 10.45 **STAGE IIB (T4) BREAST CANCER.** Seven months after a normal baseline mammogram **(A)**, a 35-year-old woman developed skin thickening and erythema of the breast. **(B)** At that time her mammogram demonstrated a diffuse increase in density—a characteristic finding in inflammatory breast cancer corresponding to the lack of a distinct mass. Biopsy confirmed the diagnosis of inflammatory breast cancer.

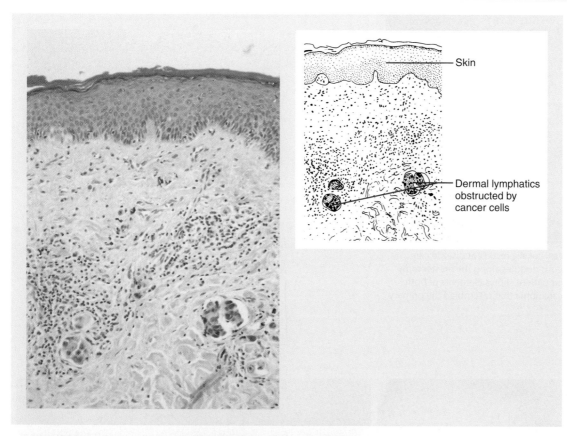

Skin

Dermal lymphatics
obstructed by
cancer cells

FIGURE 10.46 STAGE IIIB (T4) BREAST CANCER. The clinical presentation of inflammatory breast cancer is sufficient to make a diagnosis. Yet pathologic confirmation of invasion of dermal lymphatics by malignant cells, as shown in this photomicrograph, can help distinguish this condition from benign mastitis. Note the absence of skin infiltration by inflammatory cells in cancer. The erythema and warmth observed clinically are due to obstruction of dermal lymphatics and subsequent cutaneous lymphedema.

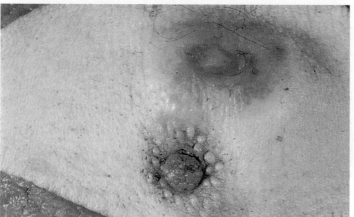

FIGURE 10.47 STAGE IIIB (T4) BREAST CANCER. Advanced primary carcinomas can present with skin ulceration, as shown in this mastectomy specimen, in the area above the nipple, which is raised and ulcerated by an underlying tumor. Biopsy revealed an adenocarcinoma.

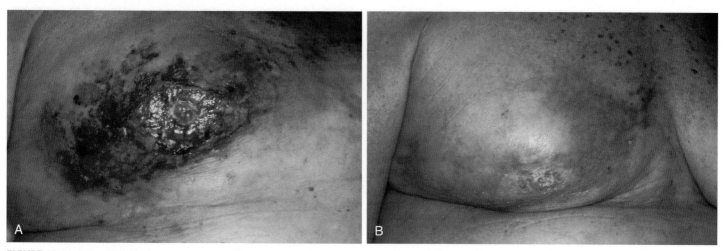

FIGURE 10.48 STAGE IIIB (T4) BREAST CANCER. **(A)** This 66-year-old patient presented with a locally advanced carcinoma that had ulcerated through the skin, causing substantial morbidity. She was treated effectively with chemotherapy, and over 5 months the ulceration decreased as the tumor regressed. **(B)** Ultimately the skin healed completely.

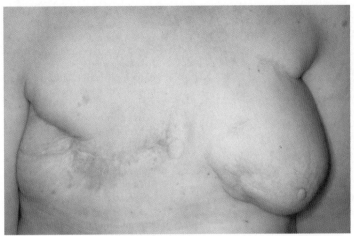

FIGURE 10.49 RECURRENT BREAST CANCER. Locally recurrent disease can often present as very subtle subcutaneous nodules along the mastectomy scar or as a nodular cutaneous rash. This patient shows elements of both presentations. Biopsy revealed adenocarcinoma that resembled the primary carcinoma.

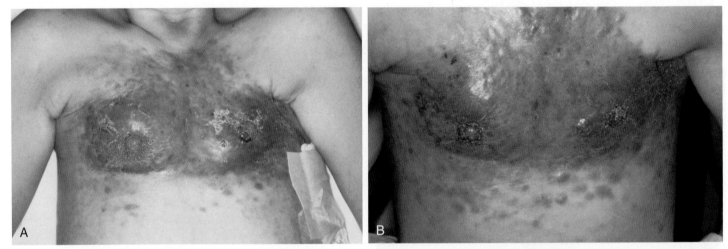

FIGURE 10.50 PROGRESSIVE BREAST CANCER. In a few patients with regional metastases, local problems become the main source of morbidity. Occasionally, as in the case of this 60-year-old patient **(A)**, the subcutaneous nodules become confluent and extend across the chest wall, as well as laterally and posteriorly. This pattern of confluence has been designated an "en cuirasse" carcinoma. Advanced cancer has involved both breasts, resulting in "auto-mastectomies." For most of the course of her illness this patient was plagued by a restriction in pulmonary function due to the bandlike distribution of metastases involving the chest wall. **(B)** Six months later the metastases had progressed despite therapy.

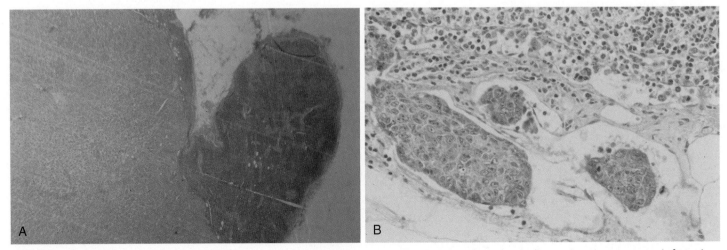

FIGURE 10.51 AXILLARY LYMPH NODE METASTASES. The presence of metastases to the axillary lymph nodes is the single most important prognostic factor in patients with primary breast cancer. **(A)** This lymph node with metastatic breast cancer shows only a small residual area of lymphoid tissue. **(B)** At higher magnification metastatic deposits can be seen in the subcapsular sinus, a common location for metastases.

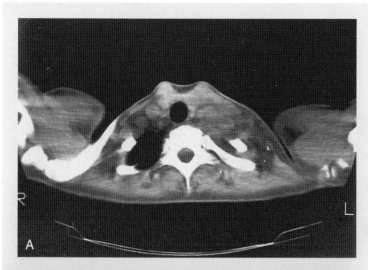

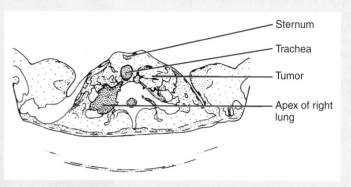

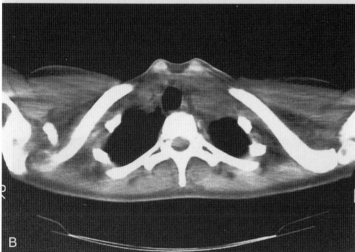

FIGURE 10.52 **SUPRACLAVICULAR/MEDIASTINAL METASTASES.** A 35-year-old woman who had undergone lumpectomy and radiation therapy for stage I breast cancer 2 years previously presented with left-sided Horner's syndrome and was found to have a 1-cm hard, fixed nodule in the left supraclavicular fossa. Her chest film demonstrated a soft tissue mass in the left aortopulmonary window. CT scans of the upper thorax show a soft tissue mass **(A)** filling the left supraclavicular fossa and **(B)** extending interiorly into the left anterior mediastinum. There was no evidence of distant disease. It was of interest that the primary lesion was located in the medial aspect of the left breast, and axillary lymph nodes did not contain cancer. The pattern of recurrence shown here probably represents metastasis to the internal mammary lymph node chain.

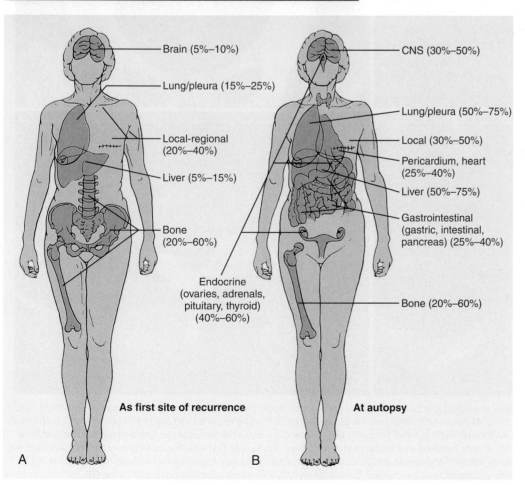

FIGURE 10.53 **FREQUENCY OF BREAST CANCER METASTASES.** The most common first sites of recurrent breast cancer are the chest wall, the regional lymph nodes, and/or bone. Liver, lung, and central nervous system (CNS) are less common sites of recurrence. In patients with well-advanced disease, breast cancer can be found in almost any organ. Autopsy studies show that metastases are most commonly found in the chest wall and in the surrounding lymph nodes, as well as in the bones, liver, lung, pleura, and CNS (brain, spinal cord, meninges). Metastases may also occur in gastrointestinal organs (pancreas, stomach, large and small intestines), endocrine organs (ovaries, adrenals, pituitary, thyroid), and the cardiovascular system (pericardium, endocardium, myocardium).

FIGURE 10.54 BONE METASTASES. Bone is one of the most common sites of metastatic breast disease. Although benign disorders, such as osteoarthritis, osteomyelitis, or benign fractures, can cause a bone scan to be positive, the appearance of multiple "hot spots," especially in the axial and thoracic skeleton, as shown here **(A, B)**, is highly suggestive of metastases.

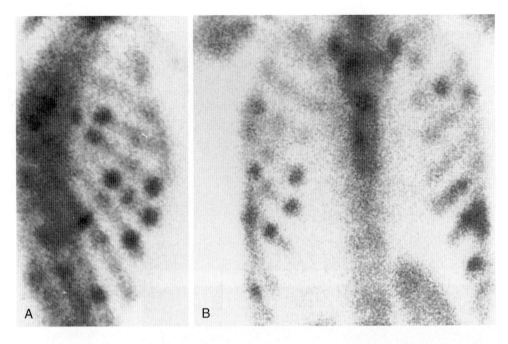

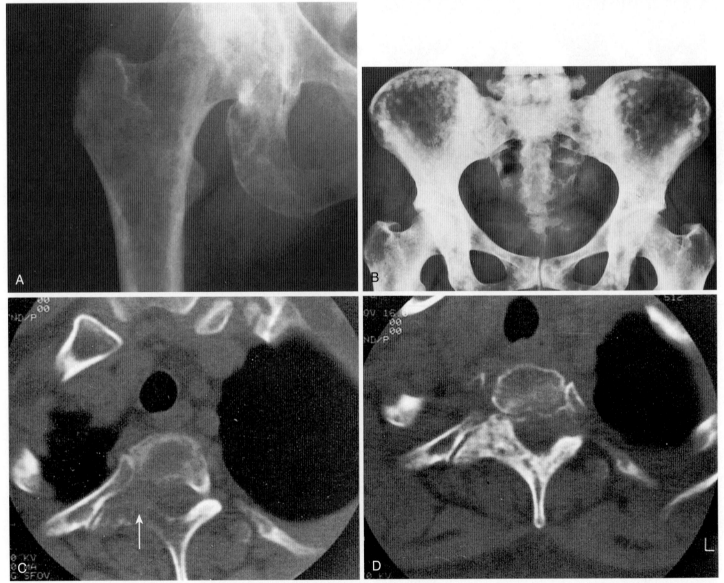

FIGURE 10.55 LYTIC VERSUS BLASTIC BONE METASTASES. In general, lytic bone metastases are more common than osteoblastic lesions, although many patients show mixed lytic lesions with areas of osteoblastic reaction. **(A)** Diffuse lytic lesions can be seen in this patient's right femoral head and ischial pubic ramus. Such lesions weaken the cortex, often resulting in pathologic fracture. **(B)** Radiograph of the pelvis of a 45-year-old woman demonstrates widespread foci of increased bone density representing osteoblastic activity surrounding bone metastases of breast cancer. It is interesting to note that effective therapy may alter the nature of lytic bone metastases, converting them to sclerotic, blastic lesions. For example, the CT scan demonstrated a large lytic region (*arrow*) with destruction of the right pedicle **(C)**. At the same horizontal section following successful radiation therapy, the previously lytic area shows sclerosis and recalcification **(D)**.

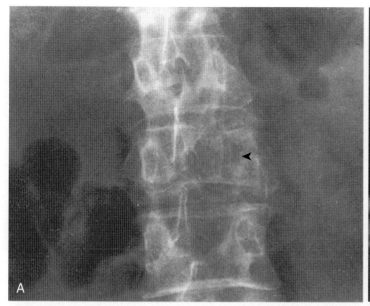

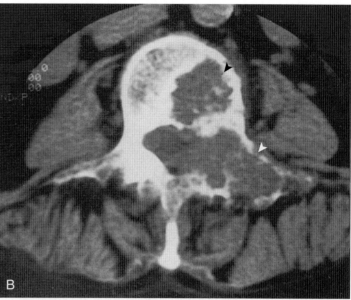

FIGURE 10.56   **VERTEBRAL METASTASES. (A)** Plain film of the lumbar spine demonstrates complete absence of the left pedicle of the L2 vertebra (*arrowhead*). **(B)** On CT scan a large lytic lesion can be seen involving about half of the body of L2, including the left pedicle (*arrowhead*). In addition, a soft tissue mass extends into the spinal canal, compressing the spinal cord. Spinal cord compression is classified as an "oncologic emergency," requiring either immediate decompression or radiation therapy. It can rapidly lead to neurologic deficits and even paraplegia. Although metastases below L2 or L3 may cause significant symptoms, they do not cause spinal cord compression because these sites are at the level of the cauda equina or sacral nerve roots.

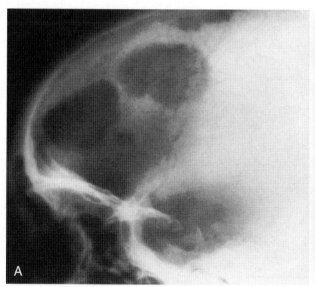

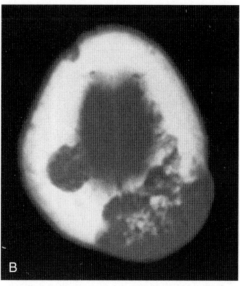

FIGURE 10.57   **SKULL METASTASES.** Breast cancer can metastasize to the skull without involving the brain parenchyma. **(A)** Plain radiograph demonstrates large lytic metastases in the bones of the cranium. **(B)** CT scan of another patient who had a palpable posterior skull metastasis shows a soft tissue mass with extension through the thickness of the bone. Although the brain parenchyma was compressed posteriorly, the patient had no neurologic symptoms.

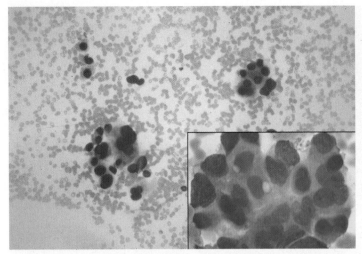

FIGURE 10.58 BONE MARROW METASTASES. Bone marrow metastases may develop with or without lytic or osteoblastic bone lesions. Anemia, leukopenia, thrombocytopenia, or various combinations of these may be the presenting clues to underlying intramedullary metastases. This low-power microscopic section of a bone marrow aspirate shows several clumps of malignant cells. At high power (*inset*) one clump of tumor cells demonstrates the characteristic features of metastatic carcinoma: a syncytial pattern or clumping of cells, the variable size and shape of tumor cells, and a high nucleus-to-cytoplasm ratio. The distinct, rather large, nucleoli seen here may not always be present. (Courtesy of P. Leavitt, Dana-Farber Cancer Institute, Boston, MA.)

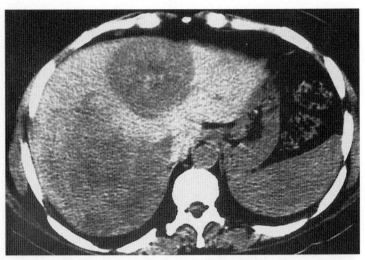

FIGURE 10.59 LIVER METASTASES. Liver metastases of breast cancer are usually suspected in the presence of abnormal liver function tests or elevated circulating tumor markers (e.g., CEA or CA15-3). This CT scan demonstrates two very large metastases.

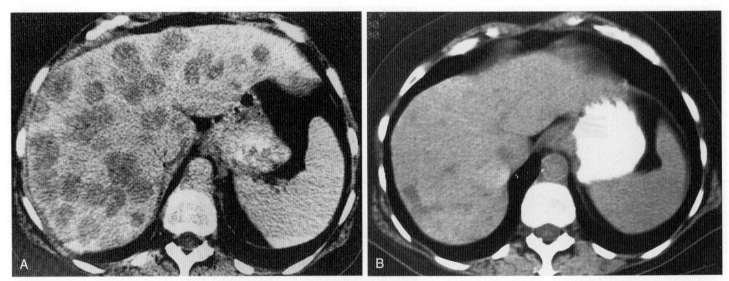

FIGURE 10.60 LIVER METASTASES. (A) CT scan of the abdomen in a 40-year-old patient shows multiple discrete lesions within the liver. **(B)** The response to chemotherapy can be impressive. After three courses of chemotherapy, the improvement in the patient's liver is remarkable.

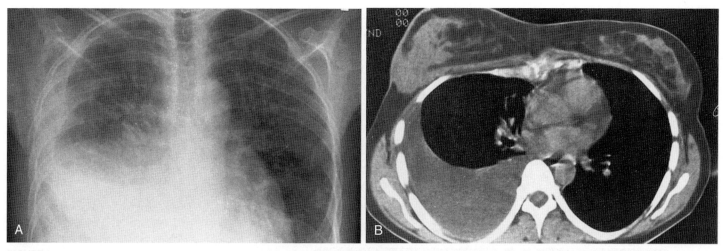

FIGURE 10.61 **INTRATHORACIC METASTASES.** Intrathoracic metastases can be manifested in several ways. Among the more common is malignant pleural effusion, as demonstrated by the large right effusion on this chest film **(A)**; multiple metastatic pulmonary nodules are also evident. **(B)** Chest CT scan confirms the pleural effusion; in addition, the advanced right breast cancer can also be seen.

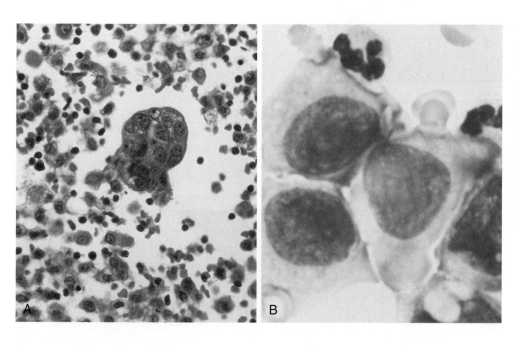

FIGURE 10.62 **MALIGNANT PLEURAL EFFUSION.** Pleural effusions are common in patients with breast cancer as a result of metastatic spread to the pleural surfaces or mediastinum. However, a correct diagnosis may require thoracocentesis with biochemical analysis and cytologic examination of pleural fluid. **(A)** Cytospin preparation from a malignant pleural effusion shows a cluster of highly pleomorphic breast cancer cells with distinct nucleoli. The surrounding cells are all normal mesothelial cells. **(B)** High-power view of a cytocentrifuge smear of pleural fluid shows a clump of large, bizarre, malignant cells with discrete nucleoli. (**A**, Courtesy of Dr. A. Lukacher, Brigham and Women's Hospital, Boston, MA.)

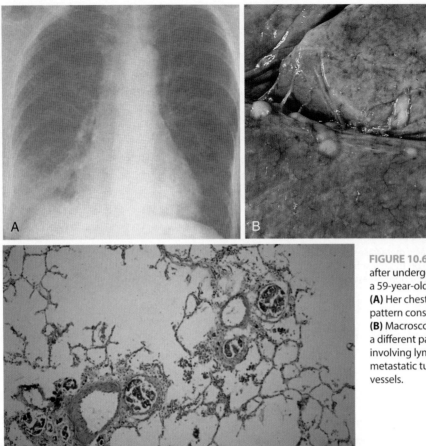

FIGURE 10.63 LYMPHANGITIC METASTASES. Two years after undergoing a left modified radical mastectomy, a 59-year-old patient developed shortness of breath. **(A)** Her chest film shows a diffuse, nodular-interstitial pattern consistent with lymphangitic metastases. **(B)** Macroscopically, lymphangitic metastases (from a different patient) appear as multiple yellow lesions involving lymphatic vessels. **(C)** Microscopically, metastatic tumor cells can be observed filling these vessels.

FIGURE 10.64 BRAIN METASTASES. Breast cancer commonly spreads to the brain, causing neurologic morbidity related to the specific site of involvement. Metastases can be single, multiple, or meningeal. **(A)** CT scan of the brain of a 62-year-old woman, who presented 6 years after having undergone a mastectomy and adjuvant chemotherapy for a stage II breast carcinoma, shows a well-circumscribed, enhancing lesion with surrounding edema in the left temporo-occipital region. She also had pulmonary and hepatic metastases. **(B)** Repeat CT scan taken 3 months after completion of successful radiation therapy reveals that the enhancing lesion is no longer evident and the edema has almost completely resolved. Her symptoms also totally resolved.

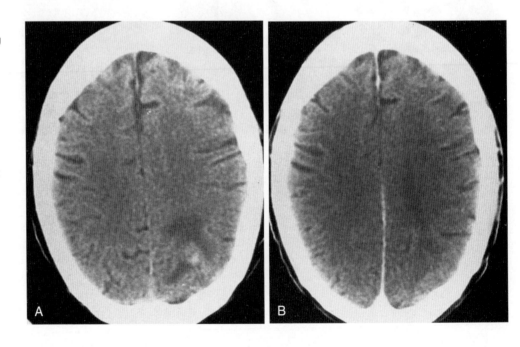

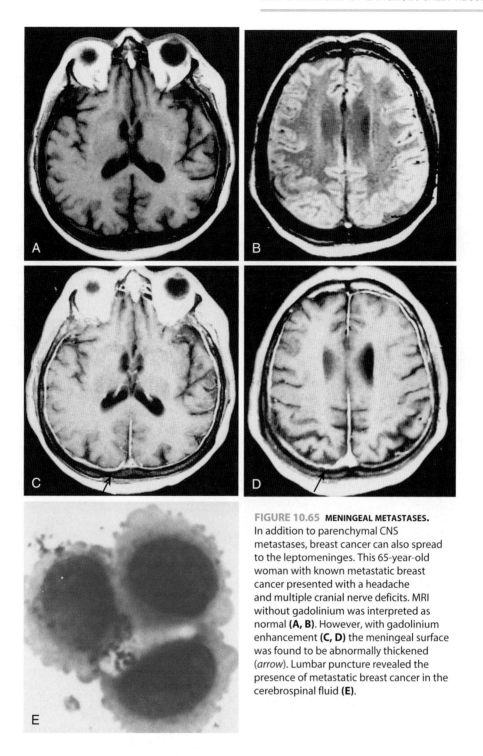

FIGURE 10.65 MENINGEAL METASTASES.
In addition to parenchymal CNS metastases, breast cancer can also spread to the leptomeninges. This 65-year-old woman with known metastatic breast cancer presented with a headache and multiple cranial nerve deficits. MRI without gadolinium was interpreted as normal **(A, B)**. However, with gadolinium enhancement **(C, D)** the meningeal surface was found to be abnormally thickened (*arrow*). Lumbar puncture revealed the presence of metastatic breast cancer in the cerebrospinal fluid **(E)**.

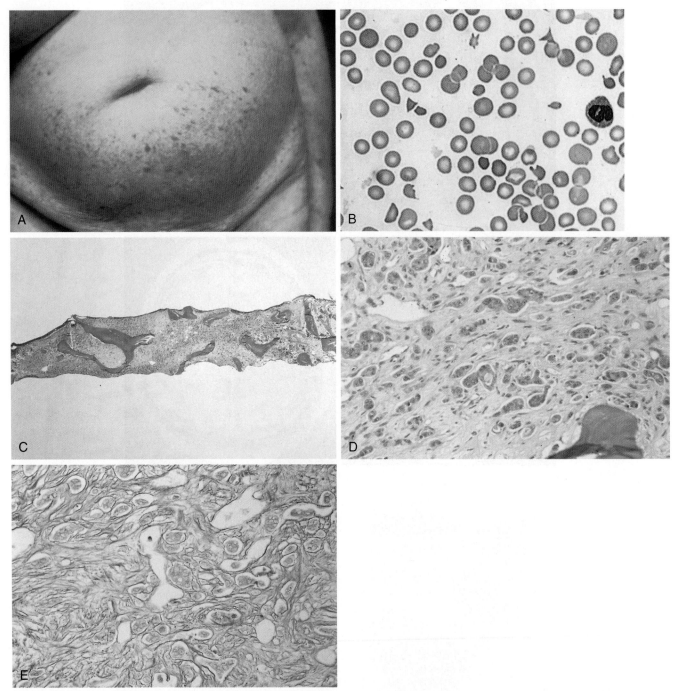

FIGURE 10.66 SIMULTANEOUS METASTASES TO MULTIPLE ORGANS. Occasionally breast cancer metastasizes to multiple organs simultaneously, resulting in complex syndromes that are diagnostically challenging. A 63-year-old patient presented 5 years after a left modified radical mastectomy with complaints of fatigue, malaise, nausea, vomiting, shortness of breath, and multiple areas of bony pain. In addition, she noted bruising, hematuria, and some blood in the stools. Physical examination revealed paleness and multiple petechiae and ecchymoses **(A)**; she also had congestive heart failure and hepatomegaly. CT scan demonstrated diffuse hepatic metastases, and bone scan showed multiple sites of increased uptake. Her chest film was highly suggestive of lymphangitic carcinomatosis. Laboratory evaluation revealed pancytopenia, as well as hepatic and renal insufficiency. **(B)** Evaluation of a peripheral blood smear demonstrates a "red cell fragmentation syndrome" with numerous schistocytes and anisocytosis. Almost no platelets were seen, and the leukocyte count was low. She had microangiopathic hemolytic anemia. **(C)** Bone marrow core biopsy examination reveals almost complete replacement of hematopoietic elements with metastatic breast cancer cells, together with marked fibrosis. **(D)** At higher magnification, nests of tumor cells are seen forming tubular structures within a dense fibrous stroma. **(E)** Silver-stained section shows that the nests of tumor cells are surrounded by reticulin fibers. All the patient's signs and symptoms could be related to widespread metastatic breast cancer.

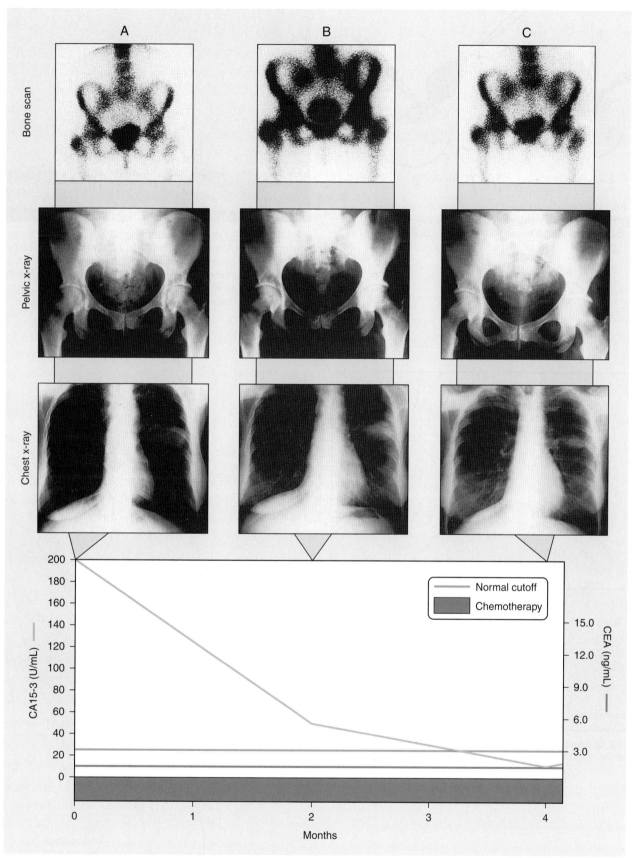

FIGURE 10.67 CIRCULATING TUMOR MARKERS AS MONITORS OF DISEASE COURSE. The preceding figures have illustrated the importance of determining whether a patient is responding to therapy or whether her disease is progressing. History, physical examination, and radiographic tests can be very helpful in determining which of these is occurring. However, circulating tumor markers can also correlate with clinical disease course and can be useful in monitoring patients during therapy. In this figure, a patient with metastatic breast cancer to bone and lung **(A)** was initially treated with chemotherapy. Her symptoms began to resolve during the first 2 months of therapy, but interpretations of her physical examination, chest radiograph, and bone scans were equivocal **(B)**. However, her CA15-3 levels decreased from an initial level of 200 U/mL to 50 U/mL. Her chemotherapy was continued, and by the fourth month of therapy she was found to be responding, as determined by history, bone scan, and chest radiography findings **(C)**. Of note is that the patient's CEA was never elevated and therefore in this patient was of no clinical utility.

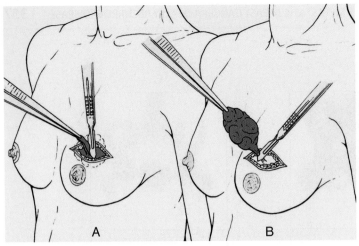

FIGURE 10.68 **(A)** An incisional biopsy makes a definitive diagnosis. **(B)** Excisional biopsies, though diagnostic, can also be therapeutic by eliminating the need for further breast surgery when radiation therapy is performed.

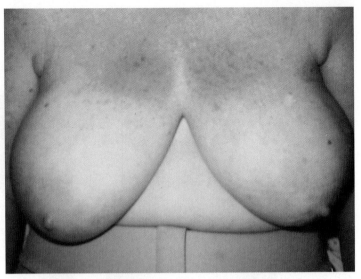

FIGURE 10.70 The cosmetic results of conservative therapy are usually quite satisfactory. This 70-year-old patient had a stage I carcinoma of the left breast that was treated by excisional biopsy and primary irradiation. Although there is some asymmetry of the breast, as well as, on close inspection, some modest skin thickening and retraction due to the therapy, it is very difficult to determine which breast was treated.

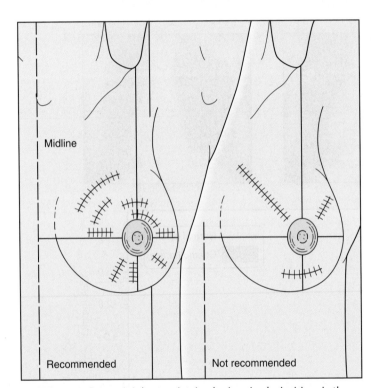

FIGURE 10.69 Cosmesis is best maintained using circular incisions in the upper half of the breast and radial incisions in the lower half of the breast.

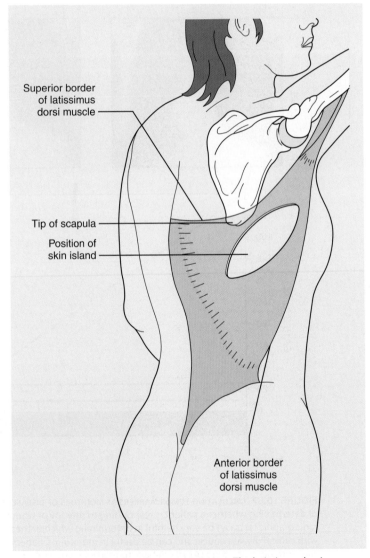

FIGURE 10.71 **BREAST RECONSTRUCTIVE SURGERY.** The latissimus dorsi myocutaneous flap is based on the thoracodorsal artery and vein. This flap is rotated from the back and becomes the breast mound. (From Vasconez et al., 1991.) Alternatively, a transverse rectus abdominis muscle (TRAM) flap can be used, which is advantageous in large-breasted women when additional tissue coverage is needed.

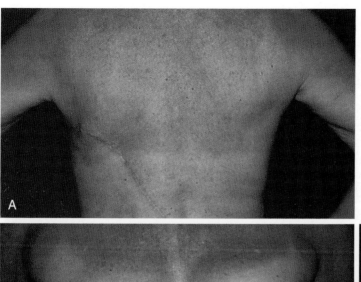

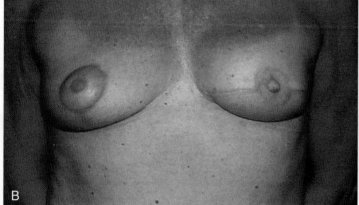

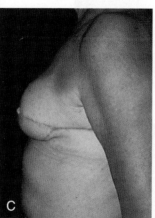

FIGURE 10.72 **(A)** The resultant scar from harvesting a latissimus flap. **(B, C)** The resulting cosmetic effect after reconstruction with a latissimus flap.

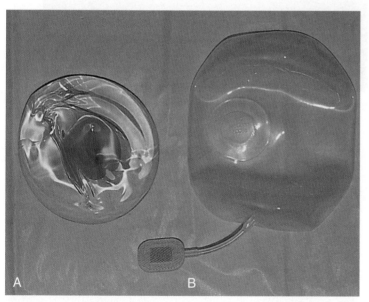

FIGURE 10.73 Silicone implant **(A)** and tissue expander inflated with saline **(B)**.

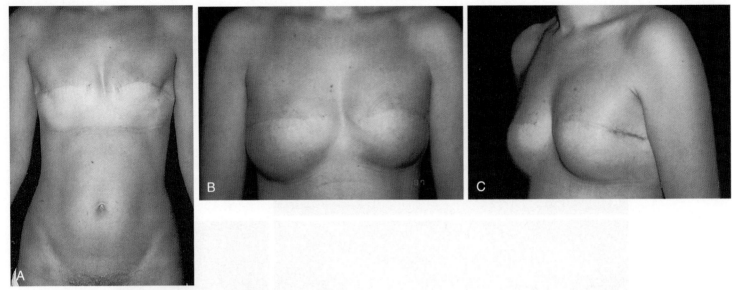

FIGURE 10.74 **(A)** A patient with bilateral mastectomies. **(B, C)** Frontal and side views of the same patient after bilateral silicone implants.

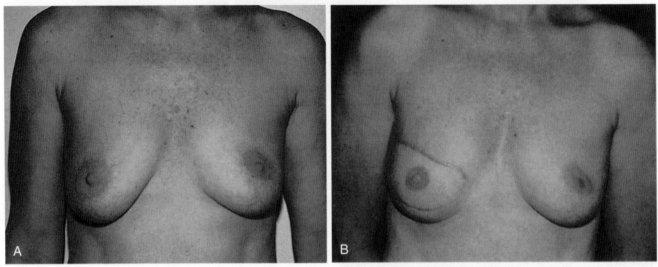

FIGURE 10.75 **(A)** Before mastectomy. **(B)** The same patient after mastectomy and TRAM flap reconstruction.

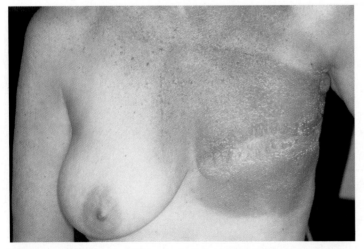

FIGURE 10.76 Stage I and II breast cancer can be treated by conservative therapy or mastectomy. This 46-year-old patient had stage II disease and underwent a left modified radical mastectomy followed by radiation therapy to the chest wall. L-phenylalanine mustard was then administered, resulting in a geometrically shaped area of hyperpigmentation and thickening of the chest wall due to a radiation recall reaction in the skin. Adjuvant radiation to the chest after mastectomy is no longer indicated in most patients. Although it decreases local recurrence, it does not affect survival and may be associated with significant morbidity.

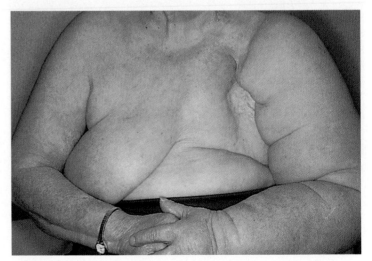

FIGURE 10.77 A 64-year-old patient with significant arm edema after a radical mastectomy, full axillary dissection, and postoperative chest wall and axillary radiation therapy. The patient's left arm is immensely swollen in contrast to her unaffected, normal right arm.

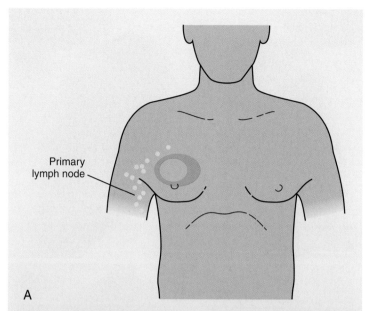

Primary
lymph node

A

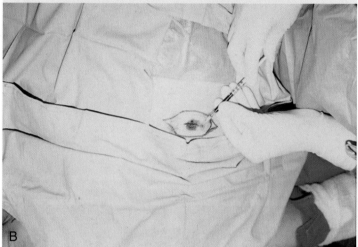

B

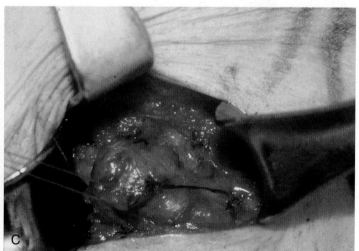

C

FIGURE 10.78 **SENTINEL NODE BIOPSY. (A)** Axillary lymph mapping. **(B)** Injection of blue dye in the tumor cavity. **(C)** Identification of the sentinel node (*follow blue line*).

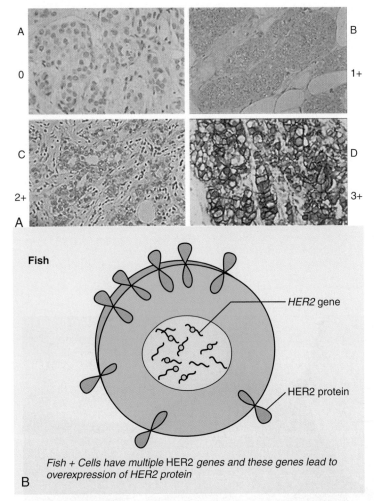

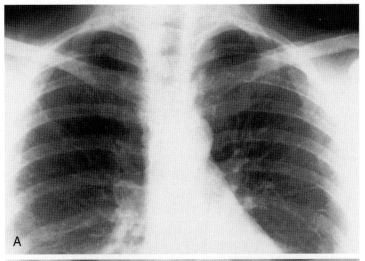

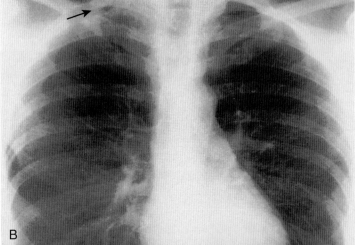

FIGURE 10.79 (A, B) There are two methods to determine *HER2/neu* status of tumors: immunohistochemistry and fluorescent in situ hybridization (FISH). HER2/neu overexpression is assessed by immunohistochemistry and is scored as 0, 1+, 2+, or 3+. Generally HER2/neu 2+ and above are considered positive. HER2/neu overamplification is assessed by FISH.

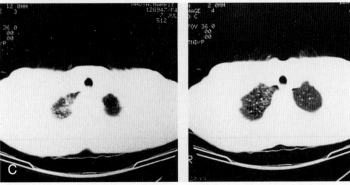

FIGURE 10.81 RADIATION PNEUMONITIS. Radiation therapy can be associated with local tissue damage and toxicity. This patient presented with a T2N3 breast cancer with supraclavicular lymphadenopathy. She was treated by lumpectomy and radiation therapy to the breast, as well as radiation therapy to the supraclavicular fossa. At this time her chest radiograph was normal **(A)**. Two years later the patient presented with a nagging, nonproductive cough and some dyspnea on exertion. A chest radiograph **(B)** demonstrated a nodular, right upper lobe density, and a CT scan **(C)** confirmed the presence of these apical nodules. Bronchoscopic evaluation failed to reveal any endobronchial lesions, and a fine-needle aspiration of this area was also nondiagnostic. Over the next 5 years the patient did not develop any progressive symptoms or signs of malignancy. Therefore, the changes were considered to be secondary to her prior radiation, which included the right pulmonary apex.

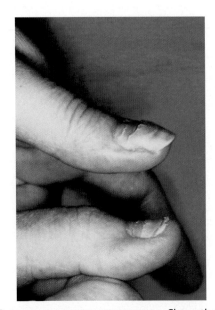

FIGURE 10.80 COMPLICATIONS OF CHEMOTHERAPY. Chemotherapy can also produce integumentary toxicity. This patient had metastatic breast cancer and was treated with high-dose doxorubicin. After her first course she noticed a change in her fingernails. She went on to develop onycholysis and onychomadesis. Although uncommon, this is a potential complication of doxorubicin.

References and Suggested Readings

American Joint Committee on Cancer (AJCC): *AJCC cancer staging manual,* ed 6, New York, 2002, Springer.

Armstrong K, Moye E, Williams S, et al: Screening mammography in women 40 to 49 years of age: a systematic review for the American College of Physicians, *Ann Intern Med* 146:516–526, 2007.

Bendell JC, Domchek SM, Burstein HJ, et al: Central nervous system metastases in women who receive trastuzumab-based therapy for metastatic breast carcinoma, *Cancer* 97:2972–2977, 2003.

Boyd NF, Lockwood GA, Byng JW, et al: Mammographic densities and breast cancer risk, *Cancer Epidemiol Biomarkers Prev* 7:1133–1144, 1998.

Brinton LA, Schairer C, Hoover RN, et al: Menstrual factors and risk of breast cancer, *Cancer Invest* 6:245–254, 1988.

Burstein HJ, Polyak K, Wong JS, et al: Ductal carcinoma in situ of the breast, *N Engl J Med* 350:1430–1441, 2004.

Cauley JA, Lucas FL, Kuller LH, et al: Bone mineral density and risk of breast cancer in older women: the study of osteoporotic fractures. Study of Osteoporotic Fractures Research Group [see comments], *JAMA* 276:1404–1408, 1996.

Chuba PJ, Hamre MR, Yap J, et al: Bilateral risk for subsequent breast cancer after lobular carcinoma-in-situ: analysis of surveillance, epidemiology, and end results data, *J Clin Oncol* 23:5534–5541, 2005.

Clayton AJ, Danson S, Jolly S, et al: Incidence of cerebral metastases in patients treated with trastuzumab for metastatic breast cancer, *Br J Cancer* 91:639–643, 2004.

Collaborative Group on Hormonal Factors in Breast Cancer: Breast cancer and breastfeeding: collaborative reanalysis of individual data from 47 epidemiological studies in 30 countries, including 50,302 women with breast cancer and 96,973 women without the disease, *Lancet* 360:187–195, 2002.

Collaborative Group on Hormonal Factors in Breast Cancer: Breast cancer and hormonal contraceptives: collaborative reanalysis of individual data on 53,297 women with breast cancer and 100,239 women without breast cancer from 54 epidemiological studies, *Lancet* 347:1713–1727, 1996.

Collaborative Group on Hormonal Factors in Breast Cancer: Familial breast cancer: collaborative reanalysis of individual data from 52 epidemiological studies including 58,209 women with breast cancer and 101,986 women without the disease, *Lancet* 358:1389–1399, 2001.

Dupont WD, Page DL: Risk factors for breast cancer in women with proliferative breast disease, *N Engl J Med* 312:146–151, 1985.

Dupont WD, Parl FF, Hartmann WH, et al: Breast cancer risk associated with proliferative breast disease and atypical hyperplasia [see comments], *Cancer* 71:1258–1265, 1993.

Early Breast Cancer Trialists' Collaborative Group (EBCTCG): Effects of chemotherapy and hormonal therapy for early breast cancer on recurrence and 15-year survival: an overview of the randomised trials, *Lancet* 365:1687–1717, 2005.

Ernster VL, Ballard-Barbash R, Barlow WE, et al: Detection of ductal carcinoma in situ in women undergoing screening mammography, *J Natl Cancer Inst* 94:1546–1554, 2002.

Fisher B, Costantino J, Redmond C, et al: Lumpectomy compared with lumpectomy and radiation therapy for the treatment of intraductal breast cancer, *N Engl J Med* 328:1581–1586, 1993.

Fisher B, Dignam J, Wolmark N, et al: Tamoxifen in treatment of intraductal breast cancer: National Surgical Adjuvant Breast and Bowel Project B-24 randomised controlled trial, *Lancet* 353:1993–2000, 1999.

Fisher B, Redmond CK, Fischer ER: Evolution of knowledge related to breast cancer heterogeneity: a 25-year retrospective, *J Clin Oncol* 13:2068–2071, 2008.

Hamajima N, Hirose K, Tajima K, et al: Alcohol, tobacco and breast cancer—collaborative reanalysis of individual data from 53 epidemiological studies, including 58,515 women with breast cancer and 95,067 women without the disease, *Br J Cancer* 87:1234–1245, 2002.

Harris JR, Lippman ME, Morrow M, et al: *Diseases of the breast,* ed 3, Philadelphia, 2004, Lippincott–Williams & Wilkins.

Humphrey LL, Helfand M, Chan BK, et al: Breast cancer screening: a summary of the evidence for the U.S. Preventive Services Task Force, *Ann Intern Med* 137:347–360, 2002.

Hunter DJ, Spiegelman D, Adami HO, et al: Non-dietary factors as risk factors for breast cancer, and as effect modifiers of the association of fat intake and risk of breast cancer, *Cancer Causes Control* 8:49–56, 1997.

Jemal A, Siegel R, Ward E, et al: Cancer statistics, 2007, *CA Cancer J Clin* 57:43–66, 2007.

Julien JP, Bijker N, Fentiman IS, et al: Radiotherapy in breast-conserving treatment for ductal carcinoma in situ: first results of the EORTC randomised phase III trial 10,853. EORTC Breast Cancer Cooperative Group and EORTC Radiotherapy Group, *Lancet* 355:528–533, 2000.

Key T, Appleby P, Barnes I, et al: Endogenous sex hormones and breast cancer in postmenopausal women: reanalysis of nine prospective studies, *J Natl Cancer Inst* 94:606–616, 2002.

Li CI, Uribe DJ, Daling JR: Clinical characteristics of different histologic types of breast cancer, *Br J Cancer* 93:1046–1052, 2005.

Mahoney MC, Bevers T, Linos E, Willett WC: Opportunities and strategies for breast cancer prevention through risk reduction, *CA Cancer J Clin* 58:347–371, 2008.

Marshall LM, Hunter DJ, Connolly JL, et al: Risk of breast cancer associated with atypical hyperplasia of lobular and ductal types, *Cancer Epidemiol Biomarkers Prev* 6:297–301, 1997.

McGuire WL, Clark GM: Prognostic factors and treatment decisions in axillary node-negative breast cancer, *N Engl J Med* 326:1756–1761, 1992.

McTiernan A, Kooperberg C, White E, et al: Recreational physical activity and the risk of breast cancer in postmenopausal women: the Women's Health Initiative Cohort Study, *JAMA* 290:1331–1336, 2003.

Negri E, La Vecchia C, Bruzzi P, et al: Risk factors for breast cancer: pooled results from three Italian case-control studies, *Am J Epidemiol* 128:1207–1215, 1988.

Oeffinger KC, Ford JS, Moskowitz CS, et al: Breast cancer surveillance practices among women previously treated with chest radiation for a childhood cancer, *JAMA* 301:404–414, 2009.

Page DL, Kidd TE Jr, Dupont WD, et al: Lobular neoplasia of the breast: higher risk for subsequent invasive cancer predicted by more extensive disease, *Hum Pathol* 22:1232–1239, 1991.

Piccart-Gebhart MJ, Procter M, Leyland-Jones B, et al: Trastuzumab after adjuvant chemotherapy in HER2-positive breast cancer, *N Engl J Med* 353:1659–1672, 2005.

Radan L, Ben-Haim S, Bar-Shalom R, et al: The role of FDG-PET/CT in suspected recurrence of breast cancer, *Cancer* 107:2545–2551, 2006.

Romieu I, Berlin JA, Colditz G: Oral contraceptives and breast cancer. Review and meta-analysis, *Cancer* 66:2253–2263, 1990.

Romond EH, Perez EA, Bryant J, et al: Trastuzumab plus adjuvant chemotherapy for operable HER2-positive breast cancer, *N Engl J Med* 353:1673–1684, 2005.

Rossouw JE, Anderson GL, Prentice RL, et al: Risks and benefits of estrogen plus progestin in healthy postmenopausal women: principal results from the Women's Health Initiative randomized controlled trial, *JAMA* 288:321–333, 2002.

Saslow D, Boetes C, Burke W, et al: American Cancer Society guidelines for breast screening with MRI as an adjunct to mammography, *CA Cancer J Clin* 57:75–89, 2007.

Sauter G, Lee J, Bartlett JMS, et al: Guidelines for human epidermal growth factor receptor 2 testing: biologic and methodologic considerations, *J Clin Oncol* 27:1323–1333, 2009.

Smigal C, Jemal A, Ward E, et al: Trends in breast cancer by race and ethnicity: update 2006, *CA Cancer J Clin* 56:168–183, 2006.

Smith-Warner SA, Spiegelman D, Yaun SS, et al: Alcohol and breast cancer in women: a pooled analysis of cohort studies, *JAMA* 279:535–540, 1998.

Sotiriou C, Pusztai L: Gene-expression signatures in breast cancer, *N Engl J Med* 360:790–800, 2009.

Theriault RL, Lipton A, Hortobagyi GN, et al: Pamidronate reduces skeletal morbidity in women with advanced breast cancer and lytic bone lesions: a randomized, placebo-controlled trial. Protocol 18 Aredia Breast Cancer Study Group, *J Clin Oncol* 17:846–854, 1999.

Thune I, Brenn T, Lund E, et al: Physical activity and the risk of breast cancer, *N Engl J Med* 336:1269–1275, 1997.

Trichopoulos D, Hsieh CC, MacMahon B, et al: Age at any birth and breast cancer risk, *Int J Cancer* 31:701–704, 1983.

Ursin G, Longnecker MP, Haile RW, et al: A meta-analysis of body mass index and risk of premenopausal breast cancer, *Epidemiology* 6:137–141, 1995.

van den Brandt PA, Spiegelman D, Yaun SS, et al: Pooled analysis of prospective cohort studies on height, weight, and breast cancer risk, *Am J Epidemiol* 152:514–527, 2000.

Vasconez LO, Le Jour H, Gamboa-Bobadilla M: *Atlas of breast reconstruction*, New York, 1991, Gower Medical Publishers.

Veronesi U, Paganelli G, Viale G, et al: A randomized comparison of sentinel-node biopsy with routine axillary dissection in breast cancer, *N Engl J Med* 349:546–553, 2003.

Zhang Y, Kiel DP, Kreger BE, et al: Bone mass and the risk of breast cancer among postmenopausal women, *N Engl J Med* 336:611–617, 1997.

Figure Credits

The following books published by Gower Medical Publishing are sources of figures in the present chapter. The figure numbers given in the listing are those of the figures in the present chapter. The page numbers given in parentheses are those of the original publication.

Besser GM, Cudworth AG: *Clinical endocrinology*. Philadelphia/London, 1987, Lippincott/Gower Medical Publishing: Fig. 10.62A (p. 21.25).

du Vivier A: *Atlas of clinical dermatology*. Edinburgh/London, 1986, Churchill Livingstone/Gower Medical Publishing: Figs. 10.25 (p. 7.12), 10.26 (p. 7.13).

Fletcher CDM, McKee PH: *An atlas of gross pathology*. London, 1987, Edward Arnold/Gower Medical Publishing: Figs. 10.39 (p. 48), 10.48 (p. 47).

Hayes DF, editor: *Atlas of breast cancer*. London, 1993, Mosby Europe: Figs. 10.14 (p. 1.4), 10.15 (p. 1.3), 10.16 (p. 1.3), 10.35 (p. 6.5), 10.40 (p. 12.3), 10.53 (p. 12.6), 10.65 (p. 12.15), 10.67 (p. 12.24), 10.68 (p. 5.4), 10.69 (p. 5.5), 10.71 (p. 5.14), 10.72 (p. 5.14), 10.73 (p. 5.12), 10.74 (p. 5.12), 10.75 (p. 5.17), 10.71 (p. 5.11), 10.80 (p. 12.22), 10.81 (p. 12.22).

Hewitt PE: *Blood diseases (pocket picture guides)*. London, 1985, Gower Medical Publishing: Fig. 10.67A (p. 58).

Hoffbrand AV, Pettit JE: *Clinical haematology illustrated*. Edinburgh/London, 1987, Churchill Livingstone/Gower Medical Publishing: Fig. 10.67B (p. 4.10).

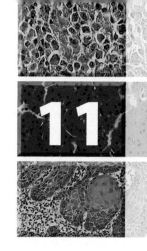

Endocrine Neoplasia

PETER M. SADOW • MARK A. SOCINSKI • FRANCIS D. MOORE, JR.

Endocrine neoplasms are unique among neoplasias of other body systems in that the majority of them have a very benign appearance under the microscope. Additionally, many of these lesions are long-standing and, unless they are hormone-producing or obstructive, with either leading to clinical symptoms, they often are found incidentally. Unfortunately, as is the case for many endocrine neoplasms, the true marker of malignancy is metastasis. However, a good deal of progress has been made in the molecular pathophysiology of endocrine tumors.

Cancer of the Thyroid Gland

Thyroid carcinomas, of all carcinomas, have the highest increase in incidence at 5.3% per year (1995–2004 SEER data) and the second highest increase in U.S. cancer deaths (0.6% per year). In 2007 there were 35,520 expected new cases of thyroid carcinoma, and these changes included a female-to-male incidence of 3:1 and 1:1 female-to-male death rates. Those grim statistics said, the 5-year overall survival rate with thyroid cancer among men and women is over 97%. This high rate of survival may be reflective of early symptoms in truly aggressive lesions or increased diagnosis due to less clear molecular features of malignancy. Cancer of the thyroid gland is a relatively uncommon malignancy, marked by slow growth, delayed symptoms, and a low incidence of morbidity and mortality. In the United States approximately 17,000 new cases are diagnosed each year, and about 1700 deaths occur. The incidence of thyroid cancer in women is twice that in men, with a peak occurring in the third and fourth decades. The prevalence of cancer in a solitary nodule is approximately 1%. The prevalence of microscopic foci of unsuspected thyroid malignancy in multinodular glands is approximately 10% to 15%.

The most well documented risk factor for thyroid cancer is radiation administered during childhood for benign conditions of the head and neck or thymus. The risk seems to be dose-related, with the greatest risk between 2 Gy and 10 Gy. Thyroid cancer is thought to be less common after doses higher than 20 Gy, probably because few cells remain to undergo malignant degeneration after radiation-induced atrophy and fibrosis. However, thyroid cancer cases have been reported within the atypical nodular hyperplasia of the thyroid occurring after radiation for childhood Hodgkin disease or rhabdomyosarcoma

of the neck. Papillary and follicular cancers are most commonly associated with prior radiation exposure. Other less well defined risk factors for thyroid cancer include endemic goiter, high iodine intake, Graves' disease, and Hashimoto's disease (papillary). [131]I therapy for hyperthyroidism does not appear to increase the risk of thyroid cancer. Medullary carcinoma of the thyroid can be sporadic or inherited as an autosomal-dominant trait, either alone or in the context of multiple endocrine neoplasia (MEN) type II. Patients with Hashimoto's thyroiditis also are at increased risk for lymphoma of the thyroid.

HISTOLOGIC SUBTYPES AND FEATURES

Table 11.1 lists the various subtypes of malignant tumors of the thyroid gland.

Papillary Carcinoma

The most common malignancies of the thyroid gland arise within the glandular epithelium, and as such, are adenocarcinoma (carcinomas associated with glandular epithelium). In pathologic diagnoses the "adeno" is typically not used, because inherent carcinomas of the thyroid *gland* are adenocarcinomas.

Papillary thyroid carcinomas (PTCs) occur in highest incidence, and these represent more than 70% of adult thyroid cancers. PTCs most often arise in young adults and show a predilection for females (75%).

Diagnostic pathologic features of PTC include cellular crowding, cleared-out nuclei with dispersed chromatin and occasionally prominent nucleoli ("Orphan Annie eyes"), irregular nuclear borders, loosely assembled, resulting in characteristic nuclear grooves, and intranuclear pseudoinclusions. There are numerous subtypes (variants) of PTC, including classical, follicular, tall

Table 11.1	
Malignant Tumors of the Thyroid Gland	
Epithelial Tumors	**Nonepithelial and Miscellaneous Tumors**
Papillary thyroid carcinoma	Lymphoma
Follicular carcinoma	Sarcoma
Poorly differentiated carcinoma	Metastatic tumor
Undifferentiated (anaplastic) carcinoma	Unclassified malignant neoplasm
Medullary carcinoma	
Squamous cell carcinoma	

cell, diffuse-sclerosing, and solid types, just to name a few of the more commonly encountered variants. These PTC subtypes vary widely in terms of obvious nuclear features and prognoses.

More recently it has become widely recognized through improved imaging modalities that the incidence of thyroid nodules is much greater than the 10% at autopsy often quoted in the literature and texts. Biopsy of these subcentimeter nodules has led to a rapid increase in the diagnosis of PTC. Furthermore, it is unclear that these microscopic, clinically silent nodules would ever progress to lethality. They are pathologically referred to as papillary thyroid microcarcinomas and thought to be of low biologic significance. However, these microscopic foci have been shown to harbor the same genetic alterations as their more lethal relatives, making their true significance unclear. There is some subjectivity, and clinical experience seems to play a role in prognostication. For instance, a microscopic focus of what would be considered to be a higher-grade subtype of PTC, such as tall cell or diffuse sclerosing variant, would probably be regarded to be of greater biologic significance on the basis of the more aggressive clinical course of these carcinomas when they are discovered at larger than 1 cm, the size of tumor considered to be a true pathologic carcinoma by the World Health Organization (WHO) classification system.

Traditionally, involvement of local lymph nodes has been a common finding in PTC, although increased earlier detection has lowered this statistic. The presence of local lymph node metastases, however, does not portend a worse prognosis. Less than 10% of PTCs have metastasized outside the neck region at the time of presentation, the most common sites of metastases being lung and bone. The overall 10-year survival rate is about 93%. Primary treatment is surgery. Adjuvant treatment is often radioactive iodine, imported by thyrocytes via the sodium-iodide symporter, causing local destruction of any thyroglobulin-producing cells (as well as neighboring cells), a method of combating non–hormone-producing cells with clinically local disease. Pretreatment adjuvant therapy with human recombinant thyroid-stimulating hormone (TSH) has been used in some centers to improve uptake of radioactive iodine.

Follicular Carcinoma

Follicular-patterned lesions are a diagnostic conundrum. In that fine-needle aspiration via ultrasound guidance has become the diagnostic modality of choice for primary solitary or multiple large nodules of the thyroid, follicular lesions can present a unique challenge. Among the follicular-patterned lesions are follicular adenoma (FA), follicular carcinoma (FC), PTC (follicular variant), follicular nodules of multinodular goiter, Graves' disease, and Hashimoto's thyroiditis. Although the autoimmune thyroiditides and multinodular goiter can present with follicular-patterned nodules, the real diagnostic dilemma is distinguishing among FA, FC, and sometimes PTC, and this cannot be done without surgical excision.

Diagnostic features of FC essentially include capsular invasion, vascular invasion, and metastasis. Usually the follicular epithelium is very benign-appearing. FAs have well-rounded, dark nuclei with abundant cytoplasm. Lesions can be microfollicular or macrofollicular and may have marked variation in cell size with focal crowding. Compared with the diagnostic features described above for PTC, these benign findings in follicular neoplasms might have otherwise raised alarm. The only way to distinguish FA from FC in lesions with no obvious extrathyroidal extension, vascular invasion, or metastasis is to microscopically visualize the entire lesional capsule to evaluate for capsular invasion, and often take many serial levels through suspicious tissue blocks. Benign adenomatous nodules will not have a capsule but usually maintain a circumscribed architecture. Adenomatous clusters of cells present within the thyroid with infiltrative borders should be scrutinized to rule out that these are metastases from an FC located elsewhere in the gland.

FC represents approximately 25% of thyroid malignancies. Somewhat more common in women, it tends to occur in middle age, with a clinical presentation similar to that of PTC. There are two subtypes of FC, minimally invasive and widely invasive. Minimally invasive carcinoma may often have no overt features of malignancy other than the demonstration of capsular invasion discussed above. Although surgery is usually curative and assertions of "overcalling" of FA as FC (minimally invasive) exist, the propensity for these neoplasms to recur 10–20 years following primary excision warrants regular clinical follow-up. Less common are widely invasive FCs, with a nastier clinical course, often presenting with extensive gross and microscopic disease. As discussed for PTC, FC may respond to radioactive iodine ablation, as a surgical adjuvant or primary treatment in advanced disease. FCs that are oncocytic (former Hürthle cell) in type (large, oxyntic cells on hematoxylin and eosin, and green and gritty on cytologic Papanicolaou stain) are often refractory to iodine treatment. As a result, although the 10-year survival rate for FC is 85%, it is less for oncocytic (Hürthle cell) carcinoma at 75%.

Wider dissemination usually occurs via the hematogenous route, in contrast to the lymphatic spread of PTC. FCs are insidious, as previously mentioned, and bone, lung, and other visceral metastases may not become evident for years.

Poorly Differentiated Thyroid Carcinoma

This entity is somewhat controversial. It is thought to be intermediate prognostically between follicular/papillary carcinomas and undifferentiated carcinomas. These tumors can often be found in association with more well differentiated carcinomas, and conversely, with undifferentiated carcinomas, and they are thought to be part of a spectrum of disease. They are most striking in their insular, solid, or trabecular growth pattern. Necrosis and increased mitoses are also present. A recent consensus conference by a group of experts sought to put together a diagnostic algorithm, but the entity is still evolving.

Undifferentiated (Anaplastic) Carcinoma

Constituting less than 5% of thyroid malignancies, undifferentiated (anaplastic) carcinomas are clinically quite distinct from papillary and follicular carcinomas. They usually present at an older age and are marked by rapid tumor growth and extensive local invasion (often with tracheal stenosis). They may present as large, stony hard masses with little mobility and often a hoarse voice due to recurrent laryngeal nerve palsy. Widespread metastatic disease is a typical finding. They are usually fatal within a year of diagnosis and may originate within long-standing, and neglected, papillary or follicular carcinomas.

Diagnosis of anaplastic carcinoma is often difficult and may require clinical and radiologic correlation. These tumors are histologically diverse, with pleomorphic, spindle cell, and even paucicellular growth patterns. Additionally, the term *undifferentiated* stems from the fact that these tumors often lack not only the histology and appearance of thyroid cells but more importantly, in current laboratories they lack the immunophenotypic markers of thyroid differentiation (thyroglobulin and thyroid transcription factor 1) often used to distinguish conventional thyroid carcinomas. Indeed, there may be a continuum of molecular derangements that lead to their development, involving not only BRAF and RET but further hits in p53 and beta catenin.

Because these tumors are so locally aggressive and destructive and because they are often diagnosed at an advanced stage, conventional treatment modalities, surgery, and radioiodine ablation are generally ineffective. Most treatment centers have used these methods, along with radiation and traditional chemotherapy, largely in a palliative role. As mentioned, patients with this diagnosis largely succumb to disease within weeks to months, with rare patients living for a couple of years. Longer survival is probably associated with misdiagnosis.

Medullary Carcinoma

Medullary thyroid carcinomas (MTCs) arise from parafollicular C cells and account for 5% to 10% of thyroid malignancies. C cells are derived from the neural crest and secrete calcitonin, as well as other polypeptides, such as vasoactive intestinal polypeptide (VIP), carcinoembryonic antigen (CEA), somatostatin, and corticotropin (ACTH). Tumor cells specifically stain with antibodies directed against calcitonin and CEA, but may also show reactivity for neuroendocrine markers such as neuron-specific enolase, synaptophysin, and chromogranin.

MTC usually presents as a solitary solid mass, often with encapsulation. Vascular invasion is common, as is involvement of regional lymph nodes. Severe watery diarrhea, an effect of VIP secretion, is present in some patients. The majority of cases are sporadic and occur in patients over the age of 40; the disease is usually unilateral. This malignancy also occurs as part of the MEN II syndrome, in which case the incidence involves a younger age group and is uniformly bilateral. As a result of routine screening of family members for mutations within the *RET* oncogene and for elevated calcitonin levels, a progressively younger age group with smaller tumors or even preclinical C-cell hyperplasia is now being identified. A non-MEN familial type also exists; it is characteristically bilateral.

STAGING OF THYROID CANCER

The primary determinants of prognosis in thyroid cancer are tumor factors (size, local invasion, lymph node involvement, histology) and host factors (age and gender). In the staging system for thyroid cancers, stage I is marked by confinement of the tumor to the thyroid gland; involvement may be unilateral, bilateral, or multifocal. With stage II disease the tumor is localized to the gland, with movable regional lymph nodes. Direct local invasion or fixed regional nodes mark stage III tumors, and the presence of distant metastases characterizes stage IV lesions.

Additional factors are taken into consideration in determining prognosis. With PTC, presentation at an older age (generally >50 years), tumor size and extent (extrathyroidal extension), cytologic atypia, and lack of differentiation are all unfavorable prognostic factors. FCs that are minimally invasive carry a favorable prognosis. Extension beyond the thyroid, tumor size, and an older age at presentation are likewise unfavorable prognostic features in FC, together with nodal involvement and spread to distant sites. In medullary carcinoma, patients with the sporadic form of the disease usually have a poorer prognosis than those with the familial form, perhaps because of the earlier diagnosis of the latter. Other unfavorable prognostic factors include metastatic disease, tumor size, an older age at diagnosis, male sex, the presence of diarrhea, and rapidly increasing calcitonin levels.

CLINICAL MANIFESTATIONS

Most patients (75%) present with a neck mass. Uncommon manifestations include rapid thyroid enlargement, neck pain, dysphagia, hoarseness, and hyper- or hypothyroidism. The diagnostic approach to the incidentally discovered thyroid nodule is undergoing constant change. Because benign nodules greatly outnumber thyroid cancers, accurate diagnosis is imperative to avoid unnecessary surgery. With the exception of an elevated calcitonin level in medullary carcinoma, the only definitive diagnostic test is biopsy by needle aspiration. Lesions suspicious or diagnostic for malignancy can then be surgically evaluated.

Thyroid scanning is uncertain, because hypofunction is common in benign nodules and only 6% to 20% of "cold" nodules are malignant. Conversely, if a nodule is hyperfunctional (i.e., "hot") on thyroid scan, the likelihood of malignancy is very low but not absent. Because a cystic lesion is less likely to be malignant, ultrasonography has been used to distinguish benign from malignant nodules. Cystic lesions, however, represent only 10% to 25% of thyroid nodules. The cystic nature of the lesion must be confirmed by aspiration and cytologic examination. Because most cysts arise from spontaneous bleeding into small, solid lesions, even a negative cytologic examination does not erase the possibility that a cyst might have been caused by a subcentimeter carcinoma. The prevalence of cancer within a cyst ranges from 0.6% to 2%, the same incidence as in solid nodules overall.

MOLECULAR BIOLOGY

Determination of DNA ploidy status by flow cytometry or growth activity by Ki-67 is not of value in discriminating between FAs and well-differentiated FCs. About 10% to 20% of PTCs are associated with activation of an oncogene named papillary thyroid carcinoma (PTC). PTC is derived from a rearrangement of the *RET* proto-oncogene mapped to chromosome 10q11.2. Sequential dedifferentiation of FCs is associated with overexpression of *TP53* gene mutations and beta catenin mutations (as may be found in poorly differentiated and undifferentiated thyroid cancers). In addition, *RAS* genes are frequently mutated in these tumors. Mutations of mitochondrial DNA are reported in PTC. Some FCs of the thyroid may contain a *PAX-PPARγ* chromosomal translocation, not seen with PTCs or with FAs, although this is not a consistent finding. Patients with familial MTC would be expected to possess a mutation in the *RET* proto-oncogene as is seen in MEN II. These defects occur much less frequently in non-MEN sporadic MTC.

TUMORS OF THE PARATHYROID GLANDS

Parathyroid tumors are most commonly benign and can be identified on the basis of the biochemical abnormality that they induce: hypercalcemia. Parathyroid tissue expresses extracellular calcium receptors. Parathyroid tumors are characterized by deficient expression of these receptors, resulting in impaired calcium regulation. In effect, the tumor senses that the serum ionized calcium concentration is lower than in reality, causing the tumor to secrete parathyroid hormone (PTH) at a physiologically inappropriately elevated level. High levels of PTH unresponsive to physiologic inihibitors result in hypercalcemia, bone demineralization, osteopenia (acutely, osteoporosis if chronic), hypercalciuria, and nephrolithiasis.

The most common parathyroid neoplasm is a solitary adenoma. Adenomas can be located anywhere from the angle of the jaw to the lower mediastinum. However, more than 99% are within the neck and can be identified based on mitochondrial uptake of radiolabeled sestamibi or on gross morphology alone. These cause an indolent disease extending over 5 or more years before detection.

In contrast to parathyroid adenomas, parathyroid carcinomas may cause rapidly progressive hypercalcemia with higher calcium and PTH concentrations than are seen customarily with the diagnosis of hyperparathyroidism. Histologically, these tumors are characterized by large size (>5 g), broad fibrous septae, increased mitotic rate as shown by immunostaining with the monoclonal antibody MIB-1 (MIB-1 proliferative index >10%), vascular invasion, extraparathyroidal extension, and most definitively by metastasis. These carcinomas are quite rare and represent 1% to 2% of cases of hyperparathyroidism. Clinically, they often present with serum PTH levels from hundreds to thousands of picograms per milliliter. Although these tumors are usually hard and fibrotic as compared with the softer nodules of adenoma, grossly, long-standing parathyroid adenomas can become fibrotic with degenerative atypia, and care should be taken before making a diagnosis of carcinoma. The only true marker of malignancy in parathyroid glands is metastasis. However, with several of the above-mentioned features (size, vascular invasion, mitotic index, etc.), the possibility should be communicated for clinical follow-up. Additionally, there have also been non–hormone-producing parathyroid carcinomas, although this is quite rare.

Primary Tumor (T)

Note: All categories may be subdivided: (s) solitary tumor and (m) multifocal tumor (the largest determines the classification).

TX	Primary tumor cannot be assessed
T0	No evidence of primary tumor
T1	Tumor 2 cm or less in greatest dimension limited to the thyroid
T1a	Tumor 1 cm or less, limited to the thyroid
T1b	Tumor more than 1 cm but not more than 2 cm in greatest dimension, limited to the thyroid
T2	Tumor more than 2 cm but not more than 4 cm in greatest dimension limited to the thyroid
T3	Tumor more than 4 cm in greatest dimension limited to the thyroid or any tumor with minimal extrathyroidal extension (e.g., extension to sternothyroid muscle or perithyroidal soft tissues)
T4a	Moderately advanced disease
	Tumor of any size extending beyond the thyroid capsule to invade subcutaneous soft tissues, larynx, trachea, esophagus, or recurrent laryngeal nerve
T4b	Very advanced disease
	Tumor invades prevertebral fascia or encases carotid artery or mediastinal vessels

All anaplastic carcinomas are considered T4 tumors

T4a	Intrathyroidal anaplastic carcinoma
T4b	Anaplastic carcinoma with gross extrathyroidal extension

Regional Lymph Nodes (N)

Regional lymph nodes are the central compartment, lateral cervical, and upper mediastinal lymph nodes.

NX	Regional lymph nodes cannot be assessed
N0	No regional lymph node metastasis
N1	Regional lymph node metastasis
N1a	Metastasis to Level VI (pretracheal, paratracheal, and prelaryngeal/Delphian lymph nodes)
N1b	Metastasis to unilateral, bilateral, or contralateral cervical (Levels I, II, III, IV, or V) or retropharyngeal or superior mediastinal lymph nodes (Level VII)

Distant Metastasis (M)

M0	No distant metastasis
M1	Distant metastasis

ANATOMIC STAGE/PROGNOSTIC GROUPS

Separate stage groupings are recommended for papillary or follicular (differentiated), medullary, and anaplastic (undifferentiated) carcinomas

Papillary or follicular (differentiated)

UNDER 45 YEARS

Stage I	Any T	Any N	M0
Stage II	Any T	Any N	M1

45 YEARS AND OLDER

Stage I	T1	N0	M0
Stage II	T2	N0	M0
Stage III	T3	N0	M0
	T1	N1a	M0
	T2	N1a	M0
	T3	N1a	M0
Stage IVA	T4a	N0	M0
	T4a	N1a	M0
	T1	N1b	M0
	T2	N1b	M0
	T3	N1b	M0
	T4a	N1b	M0
Stage IVB	T4b	Any N	M0
Stage IVC	Any T	Any N	M1

Medullary carcinoma (all age groups)

Stage I	T1	N0	M0
Stage II	T2	N0	M0
	T3	N0	M0
Stage III	T1	N1a	M0
	T2	N1a	M0
	T3	N1a	M0
Stage IVA	T4a	N0	M0
	T4a	N1a	M0
	T1	N1b	M0
	T2	N1b	M0
	T3	N1b	M0
	T4a	N1b	M0
Stage IVB	T4b	Any N	M0
Stage IVC	Any T	Any N	M1

Anaplastic carcinoma

All anaplastic carcinomas are considered Stage IV

Stage IVA	T4a	Any N	M0
Stage IVB	T4b	Any N	M0
Stage IVC	Any T	Any N	M1

FIGURE 11.1 **STAGING OF THYROID CANCERS.** (From Greene FL, Page DL, Fleming ID, et al: *AJCC cancer staging manual*, ed 7, New York, 2009, Springer.)

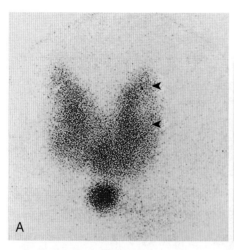

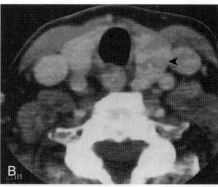

FIGURE 11.2 **PAPILLARY ADENOCARCINOMA.** A 74-year-old woman presented with a thyroid nodule. **(A)** A ^{123}I thyroid scan (*anterior view*) demonstrates a "cold" nodule (*arrowheads*) in the upper portion of the left thyroid lobe. The "hot" spot below the thyroid is a suprasternal marker. **(B)** An axial CT scan demonstrates an irregular density within the left thyroid lobe at the level of the lesion seen on the radionuclide scan. The lesion contains a single area of calcification (*arrowhead*) and is not sharply demarcated from normal thyroid tissue. At operation there proved to be extracapsular extension.

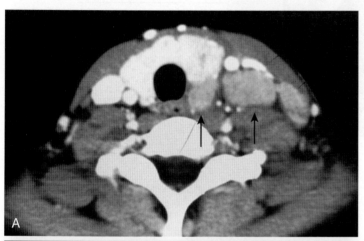

FIGURE 11.3 **METASTATIC PAPILLARY ADENOCARCINOMA.** **(A)** CT scan showing presentation of tumor with involvement of local and regional lymph nodes of neck. *Left arrow* points to paratracheal lymph node involvement. *Right arrow* points to massively enlarged jugular nodes. **(B)** CT scanning showing recurrence of papillary carcinoma after treatment in mediastinal lymph nodes. *Arrow* points to area of involvement, recurrent after mediastinal lymph node dissection on the right. **(C)** Papillary adenocarcinoma may express somatostatin receptors. This is a radiolabeled somatostatin analogue scan of the patient in **B**. *Arrow* points to massive mediastinal involvement.

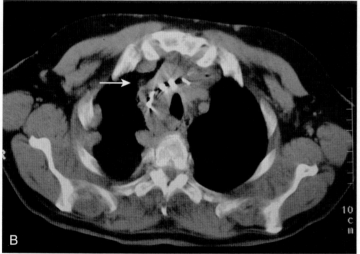

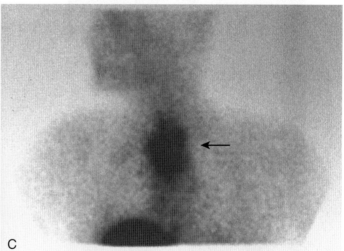

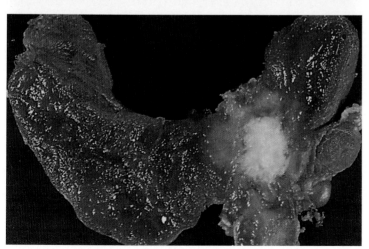

FIGURE 11.4 **PAPILLARY ADENOCARCINOMA.** A pale, irregular neoplasm has arisen in the right lobe of an otherwise normal thyroid gland. A lymph node infiltrated by metastatic tumor is adherent to the lower pole.

FIGURE 11.5 PAPILLARY ADENOCARCINOMA. There is a typical mixture of neoplastic papillae and neoplastic colloid-containing follicles. The diagnosis rests on cytologic, not architectural, features. The nuclei are crowded, are irregular in shape, and appear empty, typically with nuclear membrane folding and nuclear pseudoinclusions.

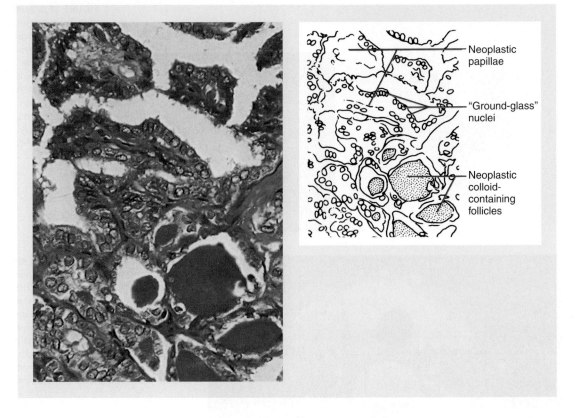

FIGURE 11.6 PAPILLARY ADENOCARCINOMA. Fine-needle aspirate shows a neoplastic tissue fragment with characteristic nuclear features of powdery chromatin, nuclear membrane folds, and macronucleoli.

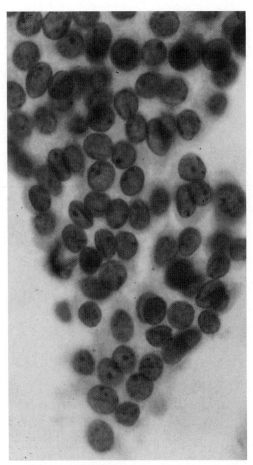

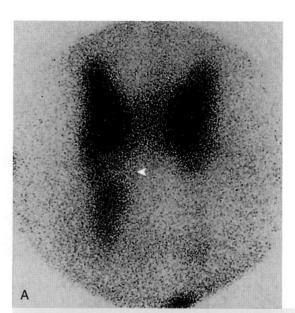

FIGURE 11.7 **FOLLICULAR ADENOMA.** A 51-year-old woman with a history of previous irradiation of the neck had a thyroid scintiscan as a routine follow-up procedure. A mass could not be palpated. **(A)** Pertechnetate scan (*anterior view*) shows a "cold" defect (*arrowhead*) in the medial aspect of the lower portion of the right thyroid lobe. The left lobe is much smaller than the right one. **(B)** High-resolution sagittal sonogram of the right thyroid lobe shows a hypoechoic focus in the posteroinferior region, which corresponds to the "cold" defect seen on the scintiscan. A mound of echogenic tissue projects into the lumen from the posterior wall of the predominantly cystic lesion (measuring 1.01 cm in diameter). Needle aspiration performed under ultrasonic guidance yielded the diagnosis.

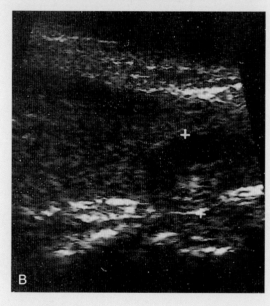

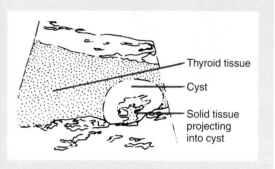

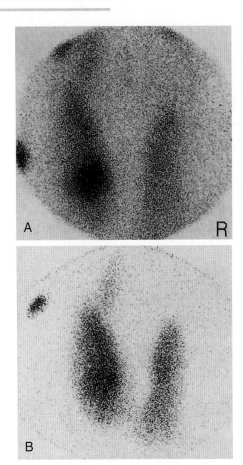

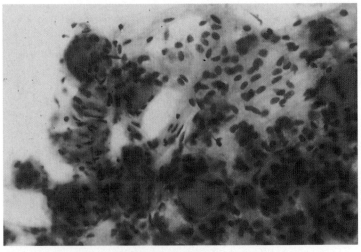

FIGURE 11.10 **FOLLICULAR ADENOCARCINOMA.** Fine-needle aspirate demonstrating neoplastic tissue fragments with a follicular architecture.

FIGURE 11.8 **FOLLICULAR ADENOMA. (A)** Pertechnetate thyroid scan in a 56-year-old man who was found to have a thyroid nodule on routine physical examination shows a "hot" area in the lower portion of the right thyroid lobe. **(B)** ^{123}I scintiscan, obtained to ascertain whether the area represented functioning thyroid tissue, shows no difference in uptake between the nodule and the remainder of the right thyroid lobe, indicating no increase in synthesis of thyroid hormone. The benign nature of the lesion was confirmed at operation.

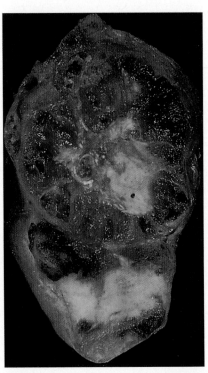

FIGURE 11.9 **FOLLICULAR ADENOCARCINOMA.** Within this lobe of the thyroid, which is distorted by a multinodular goiter, a pale infiltrative neoplasm is visible in the lower pole. Local infiltration and vascular spread are common with this neoplasm.

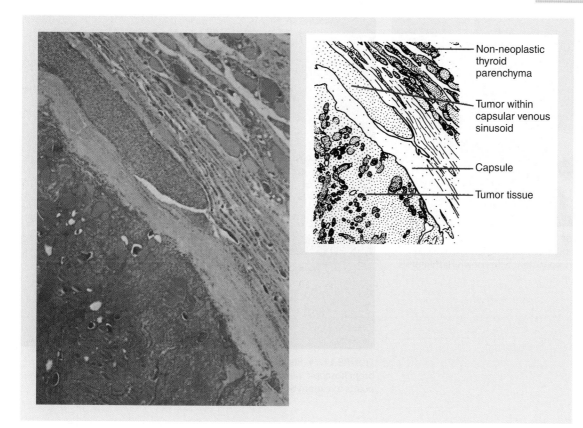

Non-neoplastic thyroid parenchyma

Tumor within capsular venous sinusoid

Capsule

Tumor tissue

FIGURE 11.11 **FOLLICULAR ADENOCARCINOMA.** Neoplastic colloid-containing follicles of various sizes are separated from normal thyroid parenchyma by a thick fibrous capsule in this characteristic histologic section. Note that the lumen of a large venous sinusoid in the capsule is almost filled by a plug of invasive tumor. This feature distinguishes this minimally invasive lesion from a follicular adenoma.

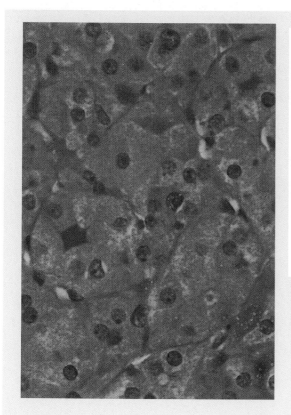

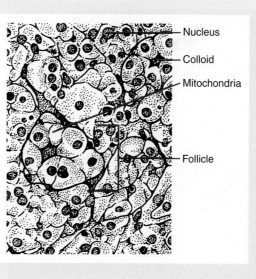

Nucleus

Colloid

Mitochondria

Follicle

FIGURE 11.12 **OXYPHIL FOLLICULAR (HÜRTHLE CELL) ADENOCARCINOMA.** In this variant of follicular carcinoma most neoplastic cells are large, like the polygonal cells seen here, with eosinophilic, granular cytoplasm due to proliferation of mitochondria.

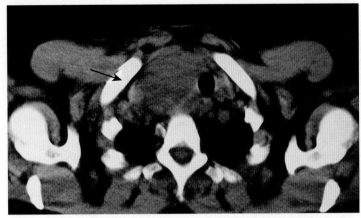

FIGURE 11.13 CT SCAN OF LYMPHOMA OF THYROID. *Arrow* points to lymphomatous mass that is deviating the trachea to the left. Uninvolved thyroid on the left is dense and scarred, consistent with known Hashimoto's disease.

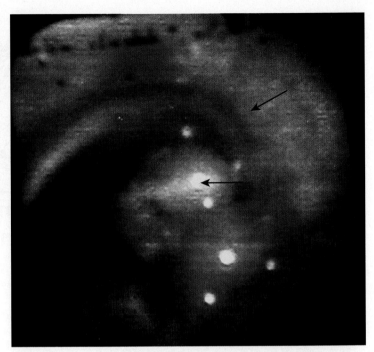

FIGURE 11.14 Recurrent follicular carcinoma invading the trachea, bronchoscopic view. *Outer arrow* points to normal tracheal wall. *Inner arrow* points to exophytic tumor within the tracheal lumen.

FIGURE 11.15 ANAPLASTIC CARCINOMA. Lateral view of the neck shows massive soft tissue swelling with marked anterior displacement of the trachea, which is compressed in its anteroposterior diameter. The displacement is due to gross retrotracheal extension of the thyroid. The malignancy of the lesion was confirmed at operation.

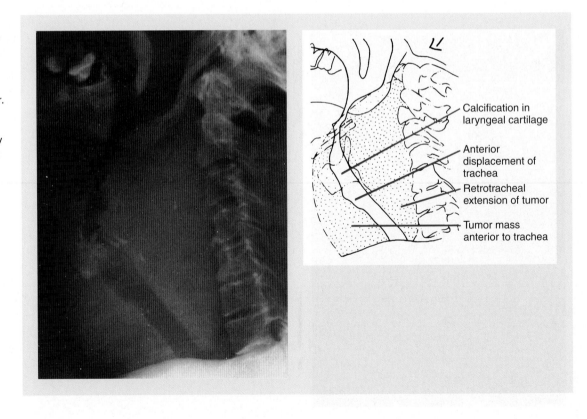

Calcification in laryngeal cartilage

Anterior displacement of trachea

Retrotracheal extension of tumor

Tumor mass anterior to trachea

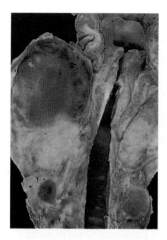

FIGURE 11.16 **ANAPLASTIC CARCINOMA.** This large, pale, and focally hemorrhagic tumor has replaced most of the normal thyroid tissue and has extended directly into adjacent lymph nodes and the tracheal wall. There is an associated florid tracheitis. Extensive local invasion, often with tracheal stenosis, is a common feature of this tumor.

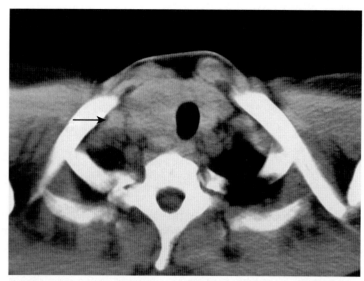

FIGURE 11.19 **CT SCAN OF NECK.** *Arrow* points to metastatic leiomyosarcoma of the thyroid, with tracheal deviation to the left.

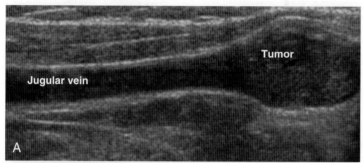

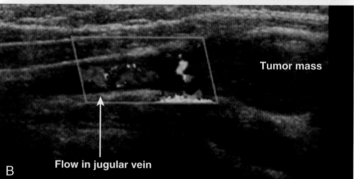

FIGURE 11.17 Ultrasonogram of neck in patient with anaplastic thyroid carcinoma invading the right jugular vein. **(A)** Static image demonstrates the jugular vein with a large tumor thrombus. **(B)** Color Doppler showing blood flow slowed (*blue*) by tumor thrombus.

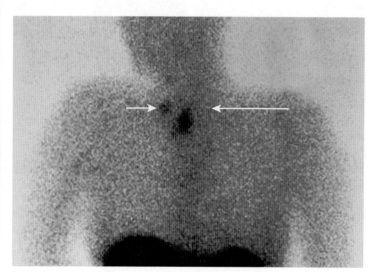

FIGURE 11.20 Medullary carcinomas express somatostatin receptors. This is a scan with radiolabeled somatostatin analogue in a patient with metastatic medullary carcinoma at presentation. *Short arrow* points to an involved jugular lymph node. *Long arrow* points to the primary in the right lower lobe of the thyroid.

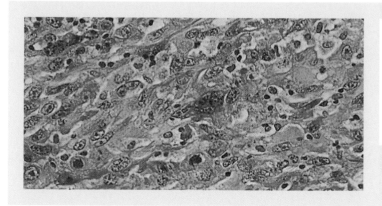

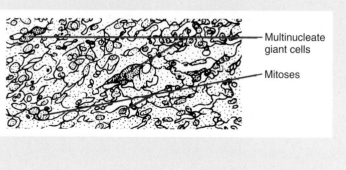

FIGURE 11.18 **ANAPLASTIC CARCINOMA.** Large spindle and giant cells with bizarre nuclei are characteristic of this type of undifferentiated carcinoma. Mitoses are numerous.

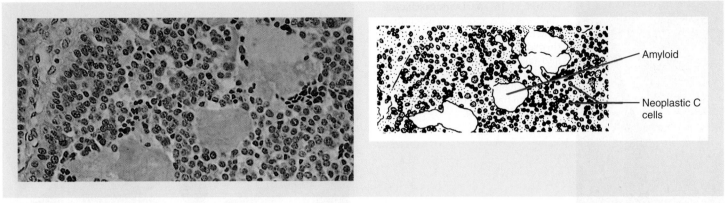

FIGURE 11.21 **MEDULLARY CARCINOMA.** The neoplastic C cells have round nuclei of regular appearance and finely granular cytoplasm. The chromatin appearance is speckled, typical of a neuroendocrine origin. Also present are amorphous intercellular masses of pink (Congo red–positive) amyloid deposits.

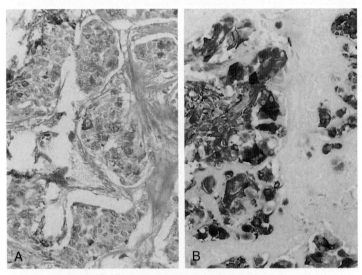

FIGURE 11.22 **MEDULLARY CARCINOMA.** Immunohistochemical stains are useful in the diagnosis of medullary carcinoma. Tumor cells are reactive for neuroendocrine markers such as **(A)** chromogranin and **(B)** calcitonin. Plasma calcitonin and CEA levels may be quite elevated.

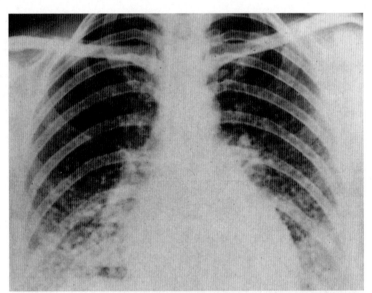

FIGURE 11.24 **PULMONARY METASTASES OF THYROID CANCER.** This posteroanterior chest film shows many small nodular opacities throughout both lungs but most markedly at the bases. A "snowstorm" appearance is characteristic of metastatic thyroid cancer, in this case a papillary carcinoma. Metastatic deposits may remain unchanged over a long period of time because of a very low grade of malignancy.

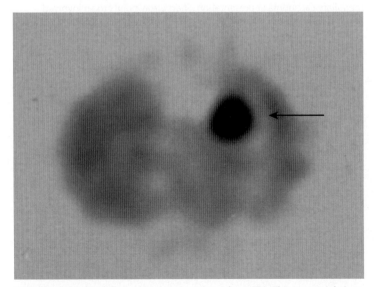

FIGURE 11.23 Medullary carcinomas may produce CEA. This is an axial view of a radiolabeled monoclonal anti-CEA scan in a woman with medullary carcinoma presenting with an enlarged mediastinal lymph node on the left and an occult primary. *Arrow* points to the involved mediastinal lymph node. Scan was obtained after serum CEA was noted to be elevated.

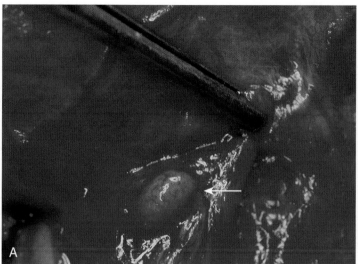
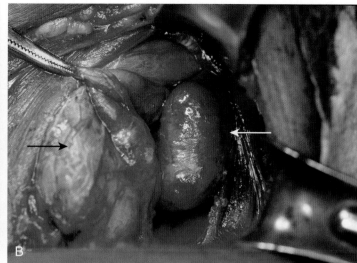

FIGURE 11.25 **GROSS APPEARANCE OF PARATHYROID TUMORS IN SITU. (A)** *Arrow* points to normal parathyroid gland, measuring 3 mm in longitudinal dimension. **(B)** *White arrow* points to a large left upper parathyroid adenoma measuring over 1.5 cm in longitudinal dimension. *Black arrow* points to the normal thyroid gland.

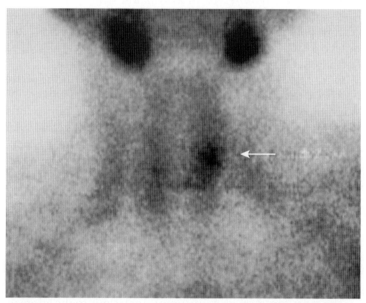

FIGURE 11.26 Anteroposterior view of ^{99m}Tc-2-methoxyisobutylisonitrile (MIBI) scan of the case in Figure 11.25B. *Arrow* points to radiointense focus in left neck. Residual MIBI can be seen in the thyroid in this delayed scan.

Tumors of the Adrenal Gland

The adrenal gland is composed of two defined areas, the adrenal cortex and the adrenal medulla. The outer cortex contains the steroid hormones, glucocorticoids, and mineralocorticoids. Benign tumors of the adrenal cortex are adenomas. These may be discovered incidentally or secondary to hypersecretion of feedback-insensitive hormone-producing cells. Hypersecretion can result in clinical manifestations of Cushing syndrome, Conn syndrome, aldosteronism, and feminization. Although these adenomas have no metastatic potential, their hormone secretion can result in life-threatening metabolic aberrations. Hypersecretion of adrenal cortical hormones may result from a solitary adenoma, multiple adenomas, or nodular hyperplasia, depending upon whether or not this aberration is a result of a primary process or is occurring secondarily as a result of an outside stimulus (Table 11.2).

The incidence of adrenocortical tumors is poorly defined. However, autopsy series suggest that asymptomatic adrenal adenomas are present in 2% of adult patients, in approximately 30% of elderly, obese diabetic patients, and in up to 20% of

Table 11.2

Clinical Manifestations of Functioning Tumors of the Adrenal Cortex

Major Steroid Secreted	Clinical Manifestations
Glucocorticoid	Cushing syndrome (truncal obesity, moon facies, plethora buffalo hump, purple striae, hypertension, psychosis, impaired glucose tolerance, osteoporosis, thinning of the skin) Virilization may also occur.
Mineralocorticoid	Conn syndrome (hypertension and hypokalemic alkalosis) resulting from primary hyperaldosteronism
Androgen	Females: virilization (clitoral hypertrophy, hirsutism, breast atrophy, deepening voice, decreased libido, and oligomenorrhea) Males: precocious puberty
Estrogen	Males: feminization (gynecomastia, testicular atrophy, decreased libido, and impotence) Females: precocious puberty

hypertensive patients. Computed tomography (CT) scans for other conditions identify unsuspected "incidental" adenomas at the same rate. In familial MEN syndromes the autopsy incidence of adrenal adenoma seems to be 33%. About 20% of patients with Cushing syndrome have adrenal tumors, benign tumors being slightly more common than malignant tumors in the adult. An estimated 130 new cases of adrenocortical carcinoma are diagnosed each year in the United States, with the peak incidence occurring in the fourth and fifth decades.

MORPHOLOGY

Grossly benign cortical adenomas are often bright yellow or orange, are well-circumscribed, and range from a couple of millimeters in size to several centimeters. Due to rapid or long-standing growth, adenomas may have variable amounts of hemorrhage, fibrosis, calcification, and/or cystic degeneration. Adrenocortical carcinomas are usually discovered quite late in their clinical course and are usually quite large, often larger than 10 cm in greatest dimension and weighing over 100 g. The reasons for this are that the majority of them do not produce exogenous adrenocortical hormones and therefore do not cause symptoms, growing quite large in the potential space of the retroperitoneum, becoming symptomatic as they invade vessels, metastasize, and become problematic due to mass effect. They are usually larger than 100 g and are often metastatic when diagnosed; they typically show a considerable degree of hemorrhage, necrosis, and calcification. The distinction between benign and malignant tumors is difficult to make on the basis of morphologic characteristics. However, vascular or capsular invasion and distant metastases are certain signs of malignancy, as is gross local invasion at the time of surgical resection. Although extensive necrosis, hemorrhage, numerous mitoses, and cellular and nuclear pleomorphism are more likely to be seen in malignant tumors, these features are not reliable indicators of malignancy.

CLINICAL MANIFESTATIONS

Tumors of the adrenal cortex may be functional or nonfunctional in their ability to synthesize and secrete biologically active steroid molecules. Patients with nonfunctional tumors typically present with manifestations attributable to a large abdominal mass, which is palpable in less than 50% of cases. The most common presentation is on a CT scan for persistent back pain. This is typical of adrenocortical carcinomas, which are inefficient producers of steroids. Patients with functioning tumors present with features attributable to the predominant excess steroid produced. The hypothalamic-pituitary-adrenal axis and the effects of its interaction with exogenous or endogenous steroids or ACTH are shown in Figure 11.27. Also depicted are the effects on this axis of primary pituitary and adrenal tumors, as well as ectopic tumors.

Although in most cases Cushing syndrome has either a primary pituitary or an adrenal etiology, ectopic elaboration of ACTH is also an important cause (see Fig. 11.27). Ectopic secretion of ACTH is usually associated with small cell lung cancer, although other tumors reported to secrete ectopic ACTH include carcinoid tumor, pheochromocytoma, MTC, thymoma, and even pleural-based mesotheliomas. Excess mineralocorticoid secretion is usually caused by benign cortical adenomas and is only rarely observed in association with adrenocortical carcinoma. Syndromes of virilization or feminization and precocious puberty are also seen in primary adrenal enzymatic disorders, as well as in primary hypothalamic, gonadal disorders and adrenal tumors.

Once the diagnosis of excess adrenocortical hormone secretion has been made, attempts at localization are undertaken. CT scanning is useful for localizing adrenal tumors and can exclude local extension from tumors of other abdominal organs. Adrenal hyperplasia is marked by bilateral enlargement, which is usually symmetrical, whereas adrenal tumors are usually unilateral and can be quite massive. Examination of the inferior vena cava by CT scan can document venous invasion in some malignant tumors. Intravenous pyelography and ultrasonography have largely been supplanted by CT. Angiography can be used to map the arterial supply of a tumor and may reveal hepatic metastases. Adrenal venous sampling, often used when radiographic evaluation cannot localize the primary tumor, can accurately localize almost all aldosteronomas.

The most common primary tumors metastatic to the adrenals are lung, breast, gastric, and colorectal tumors and melanoma. Although the involvement is usually unilateral, bilateral metastases sometimes occur. Adrenal insufficiency is uncommon and should be ruled out by an ACTH stimulation test. CT-guided fine-needle aspiration is of value in distinguishing between primary and metastatic tumors.

MOLECULAR BIOLOGY

Establishing a diagnosis of malignancy in adrenocortical tumors is best performed based upon clinical pathologic criteria. Molecular markers are not yet of use in the diagnosis or prognosis of adrenocortical tumors.

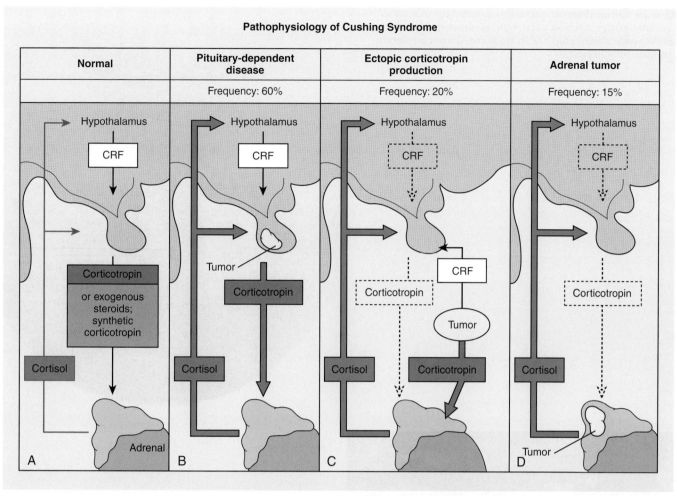

FIGURE 11.27 **PATHOPHYSIOLOGY OF CUSHING SYNDROME. (A)** Cortisol, produced in the adrenals (or by an adrenal tumor), has a negative-feedback effect on corticotropin (ACTH) production. Oral steroids have the same effect. Conversely, ACTH stimulates cortisol production and secretion, as do intramuscular injections of ACTH (as well as pituitary or ectopic tumors). **(B)** In pituitary-dependent Cushing disease, caused by a basophil adenoma, a hypothalamic abnormality, or both, there is excessive production of ACTH. **(C)** Ectopic ACTH production by a tumor leads to enhanced cortisol production. **(D)** Raised cortisol levels are produced by an adrenal tumor. CRF, corticotropin-releasing factor.

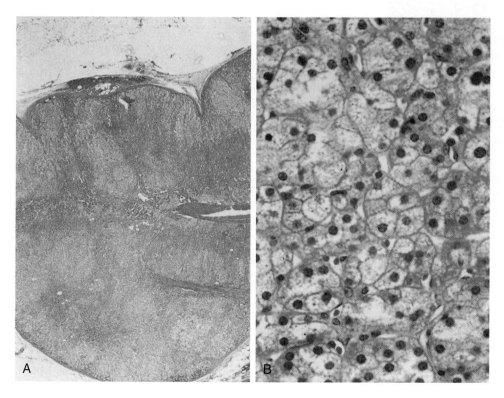

FIGURE 11.28 **ADRENOCORTICAL HYPERPLASIA IN CUSHING SYNDROME. (A)** Low-power microscopic section shows expansion of the fasciculata and reticularis, producing a nodular and diffuse hyperplasia. **(B)** High-power view reveals a bland cytology; cells show small, uniform nuclei and abundant clear cytoplasm.

FIGURE 11.29 Carcinoid tumors can express somatostatin receptors. This is an anteroposterior view of a scan with radiolabeled somatostatin analogue in a patient with ectopic ACTH syndrome. The *arrow* points to an occult bronchial carcinoid.

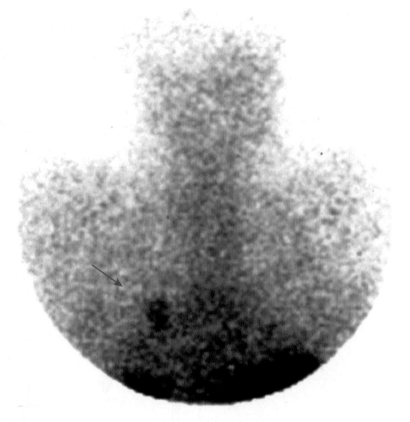

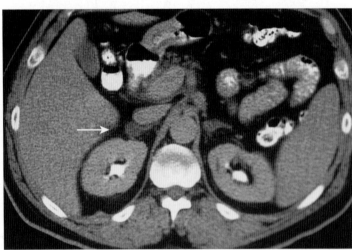

FIGURE 11.30 **ADRENOCORTICAL ADENOMA IN CONN SYNDROME.** CT scan of aldosteronoma in right adrenal gland. *Arrow* points to lesion lying between the right kidney and the vena cava.

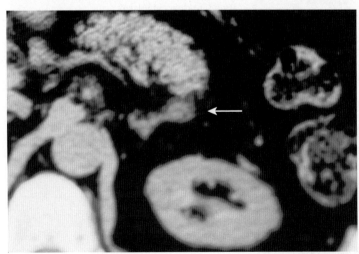

FIGURE 11.31 **ADRENAL CARCINOMA IN CONN SYNDROME.** Magnified CT of aldosteronoma of lateral limb of left adrenal gland. *Arrow* points to lesion immediately behind the pancreatic tail. In each case the aldosteronoma was 1 cm in diameter.

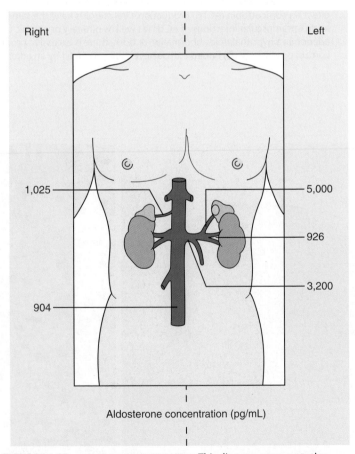

Right   Left

1,025   5,000

                                                                      926

                                                                      3,200

904

Aldosterone concentration (pg/mL)

FIGURE 11.32 **ADRENOCORTICAL ADENOMA.** This diagram represents the results of an adrenal vein catheter study. The concentration of aldosterone (pg/mL) in the right adrenal vein is not significantly different from that found in the inferior vena cava. On the other hand, levels of aldosterone are high in the left adrenal vein. This patient had hypertension and hypokalemia and was subsequently cured after removal of a left adrenal tumor.

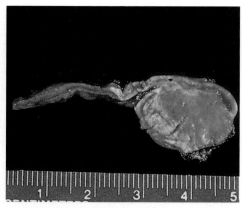

FIGURE 11.33 **ADRENOCORTICAL ADENOMA.** A solitary yellow nodule arises from the thin overlying adrenal gland. The lesion is frequently encapsulated.

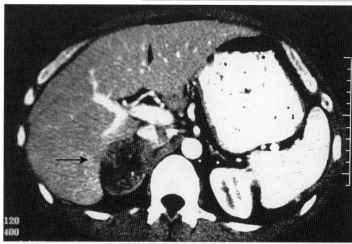

FIGURE 11.36 **ADRENOCORTICAL CARCINOMA.** CT scan of 35-year-old male presenting with gynecomastia and decreased libido. Serum estrogen levels were increased. Resection of the large adrenal mass demonstrated on this CT scan produced instantaneous remission of his clinical syndrome.

FIGURE 11.34 **ADRENOCORTICAL ADENOMA.** Low-power microscopic section shows the adrenal gland at the right overlying adenomatous proliferations.

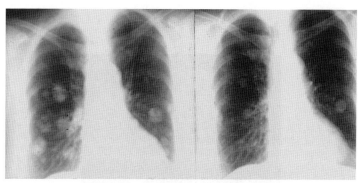

FIGURE 11.37 **METASTATIC ADRENOCORTICAL CARCINOMA.** Chest radiograph along bilateral metastases (*left*). Marked decrease in metastases occurred 6 months after treatment with o,p'DDD (mitotane) (*right*). One year later, all metastases had regressed.

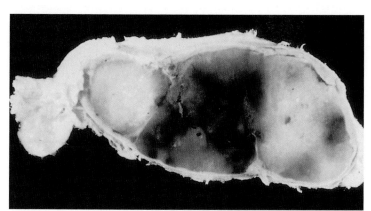

FIGURE 11.35 **ADRENAL MYELOLIPOMA.** This enlarged adrenal gland (measuring 4 × 2 × 2 cm) was an incidental finding at autopsy in a 46-year-old woman. It has been sectioned to show an attenuated rim of adrenal tissue around a well-circumscribed mass of fatty tissue in which there are dark-red hemorrhagic areas, corresponding histologically to myeloid nodules. Adrenal myelolipomas are rare, usually asymptomatic, lesions that may be detected when CT scanning is performed for staging of malignancies. CT scan often shows a low-attenuation area consistent with fat within the enlarged adrenal. Not true neoplasms, myelolipomas are believed to be hamartomatous malformations composed of adipose and hematopoietic tissue. There may be a familial tendency.

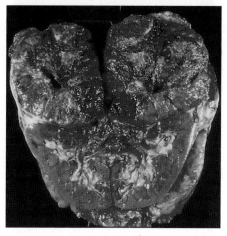

FIGURE 11.38 **ADRENOCORTICAL CARCINOMA.** This tumor consists of a necrotic, hemorrhagic lobular brown mass that compresses the upper pole of the kidney.

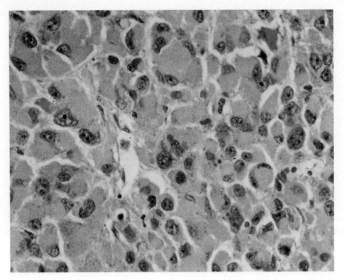

FIGURE 11.39 **ADRENOCORTICAL CARCINOMA.** High-power photomicrograph shows large pleomorphic cells with abundant pink cytoplasm; the eccentric nuclei have prominent nucleoli.

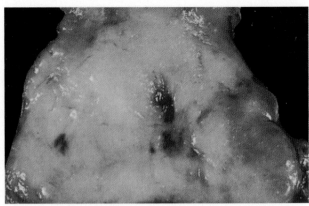

FIGURE 11.41 **ADRENAL LYMPHOMA.** An irregular mass of pale yellowish pink tissue has totally replaced this adrenal gland. Primary lymphoma of the adrenal gland, usually of the non-Hodgkin type, is extremely rare. Even secondary involvement by any histologic type undergoing systemic dissemination is uncommon.

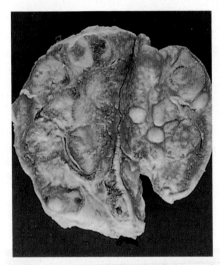

FIGURE 11.40 **METASTATIC CARCINOMA.** This partially bisected adrenal gland is distorted by many nodules of pale secondary tumor, some of which show necrosis or hemorrhage. The patient was a 60-year-old woman with poorly differentiated carcinoma of the lung.

Pheochromocytoma

Pheochromocytoma is a neoplasm of the chromaffin cells of the sympathoadrenal system. It is, by definition, a paraganglioma of the adrenal medulla (see below). It occurs in 0.1% to 1% of hypertensive individuals, with an incidence rate of 0.95 per 100,000 person-years. The peak incidence occurs in the third to fifth decades, without a sex predilection. Although it is typically associated with only a 10% familial etiology, we are increasingly recognizing the genetic linkages in these patients, with identifiable mutations in up to 30% of cases. Many of the familial cases are inherited as an autosomal-dominant trait, either independently or as part of MEN II syndrome (in which case the neoplasm is bilateral in 70% of patients) or familial paragangliomatosis, with mutated SDH (succinate dehydrogenase) genes. Associated heritable disorders include von Recklinghausen's neurofibromatosis, von Hippel-Lindau syndrome, and cerebellar hemangioblastoma.

Pheochromocytomas arise within the adrenal medulla in 90% of cases. Extra-adrenal paragangliomas usually occur intraabdominally within the lower para-aortic sympathetic chains, also called the organs of Zuckerkandl. The tumors range in size from a few grams to 3 kg and are usually encapsulated, highly vascular, and yellowish to reddish brown in color. Hemorrhage or necrosis, or both, is often present. Microscopically, the tumor is composed of clusters of finely granular and basophilic or eosinophilic cells. They are grouped into organized clusters of cells, "zellballen," and they are surrounded by rare, spindled sustentacular cells (positive for S-100 protein by immunohistochemistry). The lesional cells stain for chromogranin and synaptophysin, and in difficult cases, may be distinguished from adrenocortical tumors by negativity for inhibin. In patients with neurofibromatosis a composite tumor may be found, composed of a mixture of pheochromocytoma and ganglioneuroma.

Electron microscopy identifies neuroendocrine granules containing norepinephrine or epinephrine. Only 5% to 10% of cases are malignant, and malignancy can be confirmed only by the presence of direct extension into surrounding structures or distant metastases.

The diagnosis of pheochromocytoma is confirmed by the demonstration of excessive levels of catecholamines or their metabolites in urine or plasma. Measurements of 24-hour urinary catecholamines and their metabolites, vanillylmandelic acid and metanephrines, remain the standard diagnostic tests. Metanephrine measurements are the most sensitive and are considered the best method of screening. One or more of these measurements are positive in 95% of cases. Pharmacologic tests, either provocative or suppressive, are rarely needed to make the diagnosis.

Localization of pheochromocytomas is most often accomplished noninvasively by use of CT or ultrasonography. Abdominal CT is positive in more than 90% of cases and allows localization of extra-adrenal pheochromocytomas. Chest radiographs may detect primary intrathoracic tumors or metastases from a malignant pheochromocytoma. [131I]metaiodobenzyl guanidine (MIBG) scintigraphy has been very useful in localizing tumors. IMBG, an analogue of guanethidine, is taken up by adrenergic storage vesicles. Most pheochromocytomas express receptors for the hormone somatostatin. Thus, imaging with radiolabeled somatostatin analogue (octreotide) has also been useful.

The clinical manifestations of pheochromocytoma are attributable to increased release of catecholamines, mainly epinephrine. Hypertension, either sustained or episodic, is present in the majority of patients, often associated with headache, palpitations, excessive sweating, tremors, nausea/vomiting, and flushing. Hypotension can be seen in some epinephrine-secreting tumors. A normal blood pressure may be associated with dopamine-secreting pheochromocytomas, which are mostly extra-adrenal. Other symptoms include orthostatic hypotension, atrial and ventricular arrhythmias, impaired glucose tolerance, constipation, and symptoms of hypermetabolism such as heat intolerance and weight loss. In several studies, however, a significant proportion (15% to 20%) of pheochromocytomas were clinically unsuspected and diagnosed at autopsy.

Paraganglioma

The paraganglia consist of widely dispersed collections of the neural crest cells that arise in association with segmental or collateral autonomic ganglia throughout the body. The extra-adrenal paraganglionic system is divided into four anatomic groups. Tumors that arise in the branchiomeric or intravagal paraganglia are typically chromaffin-negative and are therefore nonfunctional, whereas tumors in the aorticosympathetic paraganglia have variable chromaffin affinity and functional activity. Viscero-autonomic paraganglia are associated with viscera such as the urinary bladder, gallbladder, and intrathoracic structures.

Carotid body tumors (chemodectoma, non-chromaffin paraganglioma) are the most common of the extra-adrenal paragangliomas. They are highly vascular lesions, usually arising from and adherent to the bifurcation of the common carotid artery. They are inherited as an autosomal-dominant trait. Patients typically present between the ages of 40 and 60 years with a painless, slowly enlarging mass in the upper neck below the angle of the jaw; the mass is bilateral in 2% to 5% of cases. The tumors are rarely functional and must be distinguished from an extra-adrenal paraganglioma arising in the cervical sympathetic chain. Although carotid body tumors are usually benign, in up to 10% of cases they may behave in a malignant fashion, invading locally.

Paragangliomas involving the temporal bone and middle ear (glomus jugulare tumors) constitute the second most common extra-adrenal paragangliomas. They usually occur in middle-aged women, who present with dizziness, tinnitus, and conductive hearing loss. Cranial nerve palsies, seen in 40% of patients, result from tumor extension to the base of the brain. Less than 1% of the tumors are functional.

Vagal paragangliomas (vagal body or glomus vagale tumors) usually arise between the mastoid process and the angle of the jaw in the parapharyngeal space. Patients typically present with necrologic symptoms secondary to cranial nerve palsies (tongue weakness, vocal cord paralysis, hoarseness, and Horner syndrome). Vagal body tumors are more common in women and are multiple in 10% to 15% of cases. They are rarely functional and are often locally invasive, with lymph node metastases.

Mediastinal paragangliomas usually present as asymptomatic anterior or superior mediastinal masses. Posterior mediastinal paragangliomas are less common, typically occur in younger patients, and are more often associated with functional activity. Metastases are seen in up to 10% of patients and locally aggressive disease in 20% to 30%.

Retroperitoneal paragangliomas, which typically arise adjacent to the adrenal glands, manifest in a younger age group (30–40 years) than head and neck paragangliomas. These can also occur at the aortic bifurcation in the organs of Zuckerkandl. Back pain and a palpable mass are the two most common symptoms, although 10% of patients present with metastatic disease. Functional symptoms caused by production of norepinephrine occur in 25% to 60% of patients. The tumors are typically large and chromaffin-positive, and they behave more aggressively than their adrenal counterparts. Metastases occur in 20% to 40% of patients, as compared with only 2% to 10% of patients with adrenal pheochromocytomas.

MOLECULAR BIOLOGY

The importance of molecular studies in paragangliomas is mostly in the context of familial syndromes. There have been no markers of malignancy that have been helpful thus far, although panels, including such markers as stathmin, found to be overexpressed in malignant neoplasms as well as paragangliomas, may be useful. Patients with familial syndromes, particularly with mutations in the *SDHB* gene, are more likely to have malignant disease. Immunohistochemical markers are commercially available to screen excised tumors for changes in *SDH* gene expression. If there is a suspected altered gene locus, either by family history or by tumor expression profile, further genetic workup should be considered—particularly for MEN syndromes, von Hippel Lindau syndrome, or familial paragangliomatosis, for which molecular characterization is more established.

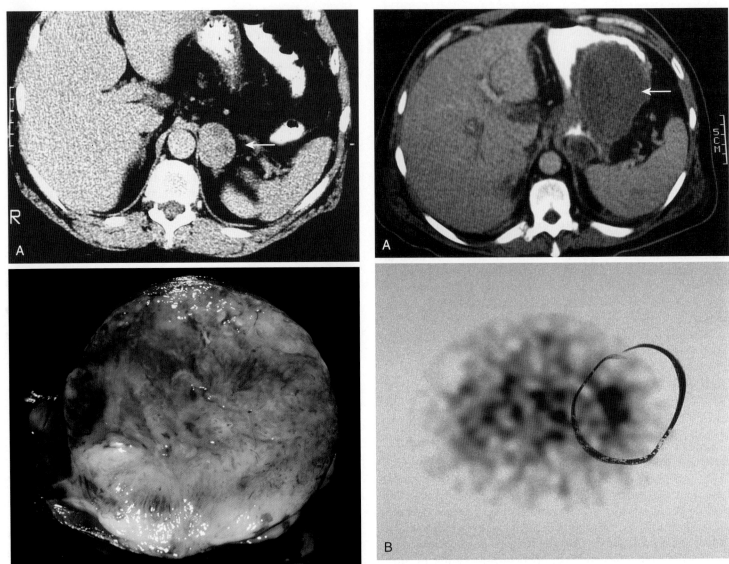

FIGURE 11.42 **PHEOCHROMOCYTOMA. (A)** CT scan of left adrenal pheochromocytoma (*arrow*). Note variegated CT densities within the lesion. **(B)** Operative specimen showing well-encapsulated tumor.

FIGURE 11.43 **CYSTIC PHEOCHROMOCYTOMA. (A)** CT scan showing large retrogastric cystic mass (*arrow*). **(B)** Axial view of MIBG ([^{123}I] metaiodobenzylguanidine) scan showing that functional component (*encircled*) is lateral.

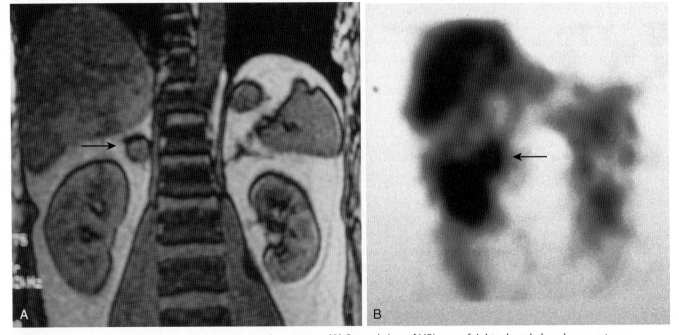

FIGURE 11.44 Pheochromocytomas express somatostatin receptors. **(A)** Coronal view of MRI scan of right adrenal pheochromocytoma. **(B)** Anteroposterior view of radiolabeled somatostatin analogue scan demonstrating right adrenal lesion (*arrow*).

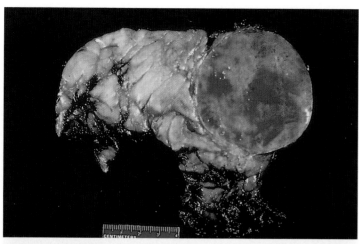

FIGURE 11.45 ADRENAL PHEOCHROMOCYTOMA. A typically well-encapsulated tumor and adjacent fat (*left*) can be seen in this cut section of a right adrenal gland. The brown parenchyma shows areas of hemorrhage.

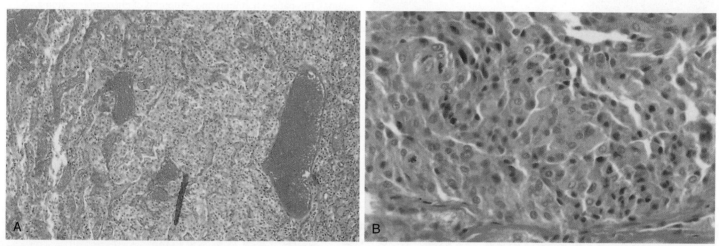

FIGURE 11.46 ADRENAL PHEOCHROMOCYTOMA. (A) Low-power magnification shows nests of tumor cells (zellballen) surrounded by a rich fibrovascular stroma. Dilated capillaries are packed with red blood cells. **(B)** Cells of the nests have abundant pink cytoplasm and uniform, bland nuclei. A wide range of cytologic pleomorphism may be seen.

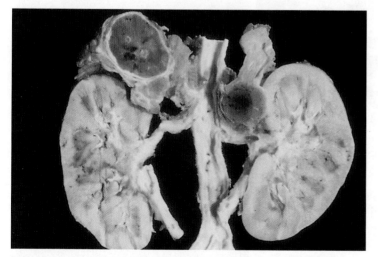

FIGURE 11.47 ADRENAL PHEOCHROMOCYTOMA. This postmortem specimen from an 11-year-old boy consists of both adrenals, with the kidneys, their vessels, and the aorta. In the medulla of each adrenal there is a typically rounded, dark-brown tumor over which is stretched a rim of normal yellow cortical tissue. Note also the atheromatous plaques in the aorta and at the origins of the arteries. The patient presented with a 5-year history of intermittent attacks of acute abdominal pain associated with sweating and tachycardia. He was also found to have florid hypertensive retinopathy, marked but variable hypertension, and left ventricular hypertrophy. He died at laparotomy.

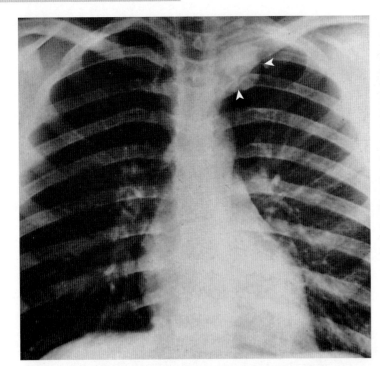

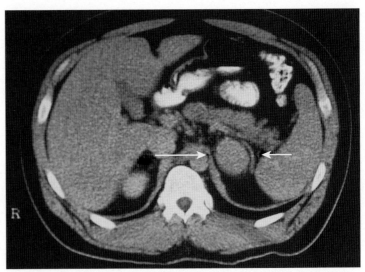

FIGURE 11.49 **PARA-AORTIC PARAGANGLIOMA.** This CT scan demonstrates a 4-cm tumor lying to the left of the aorta just above the kidneys. *Long arrow* points to the tumor. *Short arrow* points to a laterally displaced, normal adrenal. This patient had signs and symptoms of pheochromocytoma. A benign paraganglioma was removed at surgery. If an adrenal tumor is not visible on CT scan in a patient with strong clinical evidence of a pheochromocytoma, it is probable that the tumor lies at an ectopic site along the sympathetic chain. Most such paragangliomas occur in the para-aortic region or around the renal hilum and may be visible on CT. To detect tumors at other ectopic sites or those too small to be seen on CT, venous sampling for catecholamine levels is required.

FIGURE 11.48 **MEDIASTINAL PARAGANGLIOMA.** Posteroanterior chest radiograph shows a mass with a well-defined margin in the left upper paravertebral region (*arrowheads*). The patient complained of occasional headaches and sweating but was normotensive. At operation, however, the blood pressure rose steeply while the tumor was being handled. Although histologic examination revealed what was thought to be a benign lesion, 7 years later the tumor recurred in the chest and metastatic paraganglioma was found on biopsy of a skull lesion.

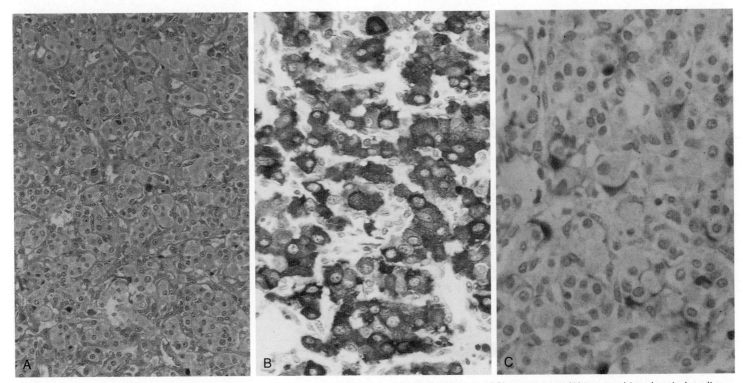

FIGURE 11.50 **CAROTID BODY PARAGANGLIOMA. (A)** Nests of tumor cells (zellballen) with a well-vascularized fibrous stroma. **(B)** Immunohistochemical studies demonstrate strong positive staining for chromogranin by tumor cells. **(C)** Supporting sustentacular cells envelope tumor nests and stain positive for S-100 protein.

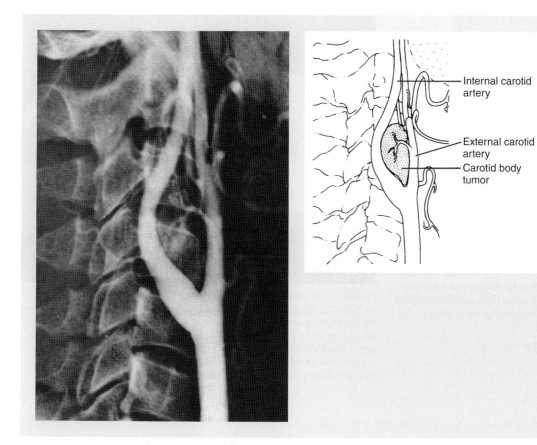

Internal carotid artery

External carotid artery

Carotid body tumor

FIGURE 11.51 **CAROTID BODY TUMOR.** This patient with persistent hypertension after removal of a left adrenal pheochromocytoma had elevated levels of catecholamines in the right side of the neck on venous sampling. Lateral view of a carotid angiogram demonstrates a typical carotid body tumor at the bifurcation of the internal and external carotid arteries; the bifurcation appears to be splayed by the lesion. The blood supply of the tumor arises from the proximal external carotid artery, and a tumor blush is present.

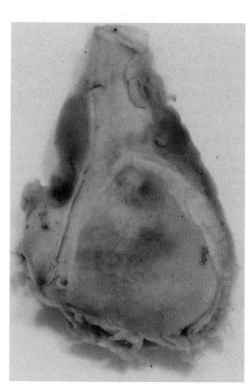

FIGURE 11.52 **CAROTID BODY TUMOR.** A 47-year-old woman had noticed a slow-growing tumor in the right side of the neck for 3 years. At surgery this brownish, encapsulated tumor, measuring 3 cm in maximum diameter, was found to be firmly adherent to a portion of the carotid artery.

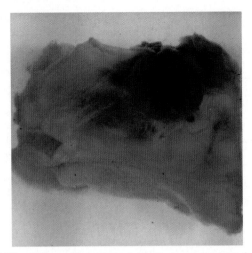

FIGURE 11.53 **GLOMUS JUGULARE TUMOR.** This autopsy specimen is from a 76-year-old woman who died of bronchopneumonia. She had had a middle ear neoplasm, probably a glomus jugulare tumor, for 18 years, and had been treated with radiation therapy alone. A portion of the right petrous temporal bone is shown from which protrudes a small, rounded, pinkish tumor measuring 1 cm in diameter.

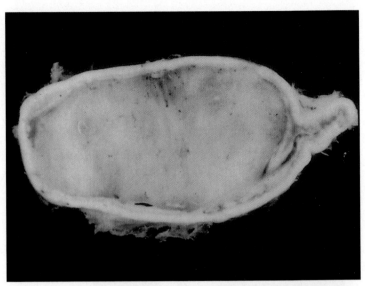

FIGURE 11.54 **ADRENAL GANGLIONEUROMA.** This adrenal gland has been sectioned to show a well-circumscribed, grayish tumor, which was an incidental finding at autopsy of a 55-year-old man who died of bronchopneumonia. Measuring $3 \times 15 \times 1.5$ cm, the tumor has expanded and replaced the medulla and is surrounded by a thin layer of normal cortical tissue. Ganglioneuroma is a benign adrenal medullary tumor derived from the non-chromaffin neural element. It more commonly arises elsewhere in the sympathetic chain.

Tumors of the Pituitary Gland

The pituitary gland is of central importance because of its endocrinologic functions and its anatomic relationships. The hypothalamic-pituitary-adrenal axis regulates the thyroid and adrenal glands as well as gonadal function, growth, and development (see Fig. 11.27). Table 11.3 compares the clinical features of pituitary and ectopic ACTH overproduction. Table 11.4 outlines the properties and biologic actions of the various anterior pituitary hormones. The types of functioning and nonfunctioning pituitary tumors, as well as the parapituitary tumors, that must be considered in the differential diagnosis of sellar and parasellar masses are listed in Table 11.5.

Approximately 10% of symptomatic intracranial neoplasms are pituitary tumors. Asymptomatic adenomas are found at autopsy in 10% to 20% of presumably normal pituitary glands.

Table 11.3

Comparison of the Clinical Features of Pituitary and Ectopic ACTH Overproduction

Features	Pituitary	Ectopic
Age	Usually under 50 years	Usually over 50 years
Sex	Predominantly women	Predominantly men
Anorexia	Rare	Always
Weight loss	Rare: often there is weight gain	Usual
Cushingoid features	Usual	Unusual
Hypertension	Occasional	Usual
Hyperpigmentation	Unusual except after adrenalectomy	Common
Serum potassium	Normal or low (usually 3–4 mmol/L)	Usually low (< 3 mmol/L)

ACTH, adrenocorticotropic hormone.

Table 11.4

Properties and Biologic Actions of Anterior Pituitary Hormones

Hormone	Cell Type	Mean Granule Diameter (nm)*	Biologic Action
Growth hormone (GH)	Acidophil	450	Growth of bone, muscle, cartilage, and connective tissue; elevation of blood glucose
Prolactin (PRL)	Acidophil	550	Promotion of lactation
Follicle-stimulating hormone (FSH)	Basophil	200	Female: maturation of ovarian follicle and promotion of ovarian steroid formation Male: promotion of spermatogenesis
Luteinizing hormone (LH)	Basophil	200	Female: corpus luteum formation Male: testosterone formation by interstitial cells of testis
Thyroid-stimulating hormone (TSH)	Basophil	135	Thyroid growth and hormone synthesis
Corticotropin (adrenocorticotropic hormone; ACTH)	Basophil	360	Adrenocortical growth and steroidogenesis
Melanocyte-stimulating hormone (MSH)	Basophil	360	Skin pigmentation; postulated role in onset of puberty

*Determined by electron-microscopic measurement.

Table 11.5

Pituitary and Parapituitary Tumors

Anterior Pituitary				
Functioning	**Frequency (%)**	**Nonfunctioning***	**Posterior Pituitary**	**Parapituitary**
Prolactin-secreting	24	Adenoma	Ganglioneuroma	Pinealoma (ectopic)
GH-secreting	33	Carcinoma	Astrocytoma (very rare)	Craniopharyngioma
ACTH-secreting	14	Sarcoma		Chordoma
TSH- or gonadotropin-secreting	<1			Optic nerve glioma
				Reticulosis
				Sphenoidal ridge meningioma
				Metastatic deposits (e.g., from breast and lung)

ACTH, adrenocorticotropic hormone; GH, growth hormone; TSH, thyroid-stimulating hormone.
*Nonsecreting tumors represent the remaining 29% of anterior pituitary tumors.

The male-to-female ratio depends on the clinical syndrome produced, with Cushing syndrome and hyperprolactinemia being more common in females. Pituitary adenomas are seen in MEN I and are present in approximately 65% of cases.

HISTOLOGY

The traditional classification of pituitary tumors is based on light-microscopic evaluation of the staining properties of the cell cytoplasm and on electron-microscopic and specific immunohistochemical techniques. The three recognized categories include chromophobe adenomas, which are assumed to be endocrinologically inactive, acidophilic or eosinophilic adenomas, which secrete growth hormone or prolactin, and basophilic adenomas, which secrete ACTH, TSH, follicle-stimulating hormone (FSH), and β-melanocyte-stimulating hormone (β-MSH). The demonstration of hormone-specific granules in tumor cells does not necessarily correlate with secretion or with a clinical endocrinologic syndrome. Normal pituitary parenchyma is arranged in discrete nests, highlighted by reticulin stain. This architecture is disrupted in pituitary neoplasms.

CLINICAL MANIFESTATIONS

The clinical manifestations of pituitary tumors are due to one of three causes: (1) hypersecretion of a specific anterior pituitary hormone, (2) effects of an expanding mass in the sellar region, or (3) symptoms related to a lack of anterior pituitary hormone secretion secondary to a compressive mass. Acromegaly, Cushing disease, and hyperprolactinemic syndrome are the most common clinical signs of hormone-producing pituitary adenomas. Mass-related symptoms are multiple because of the critical location of the pituitary adjacent to many important neural structures (see Fig. 11.55). Optic nerve compression with bilateral visual field loss (bitemporal hemianopsia) is the most common mass effect. Extraocular muscle dysfunction may occur as the result of compression of cranial nerves III, IV, and VI. Headaches, increased intracranial pressure, seizures, and cerebrospinal fluid rhinorrhea may be present. Hypothalamic dysfunction secondary to suprasellar extension of tumor may give rise to diabetes insipidus. Hypopituitarism may be due to either anterior pituitary compression or hypothalamic involvement. Sequential failure of hormone secretion leads initially to loss of gonadotropins and growth hormone. Hypothyroidism or hypoadrenalism appear later as a result of secretory failure of TSH and ACTH, respectively. Nonfunctioning adenomas more commonly produce symptoms secondary to an enlarging mass. Functioning tumors are usually detected earlier because of the clinical syndromes they produce and are more likely to be microadenomas.

Pituitary adenomas are classically divided into either micro- or macroadenomas. Microadenomas are smaller than 10 mm and are usually encapsulated. Because they rarely cause local symptoms, they frequently become clinically suspected secondary to endocrine excess syndromes. Macroadenomas are larger than 10 mm and may be either encapsulated or invasive. These tumors are often characterized by suprasellar extension and are more likely to cause symptoms related to mass effect. Although macroadenomas may show locally aggressive behavior, this does not imply malignancy. Features that may suggest a more aggressive behavior, such as necrosis or vascular invasion, are difficult to assess in the typically fragmented specimens from transsphenoidal resections. The presence of metastatic dissemination allows a clear-cut diagnosis of cancer.

The diagnosis of a pituitary adenoma is accomplished both endocrinologically and radiographically. Magnetic resonance imaging (MRI) is the modality of choice. Initially, all patients with a suspected or documented diagnosis of pituitary tumor should undergo adrenal, gonadal, and thyroid function testing to evaluate the need for hormone replacement therapy. Specific stimulation and suppression tests are performed under certain circumstances for tumor detection, tumor localization, or determination of response to treatment.

MOLECULAR BIOLOGY

Ancillary studies offer little additional prognostic information beyond that gathered from histologic examination. In DNA studies pituitary hyperplasia has been difficult to distinguish from adenomas. There has been no relationship demonstrated between ploidy and clinical behavior, including invasive growth or hormone secretion. Immunohistochemistry can help distinguish the presence of tumor secretagogues, but clinical correlation is needed to relay dysfunction. Generally, an increased MIB-1 proliferative index in pituitary lesions portends more aggressive behavior but does not confer malignancy.

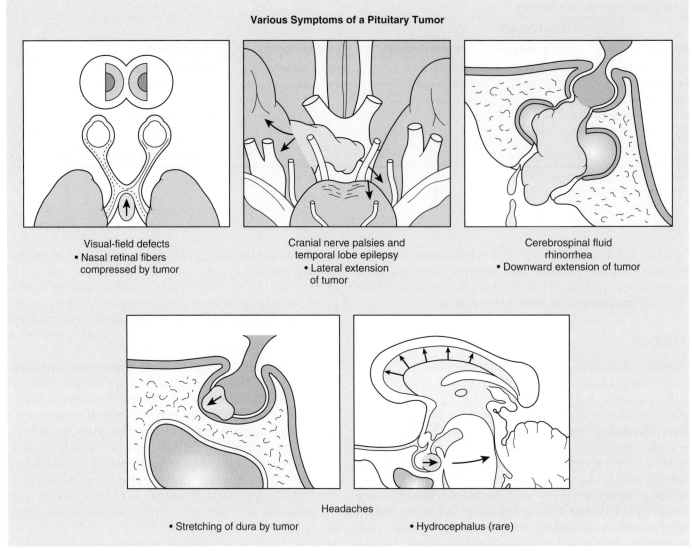

Various Symptoms of a Pituitary Tumor

Visual-field defects
• Nasal retinal fibers compressed by tumor

Cranial nerve palsies and temporal lobe epilepsy
• Lateral extension of tumor

Cerebrospinal fluid rhinorrhea
• Downward extension of tumor

Headaches
• Stretching of dura by tumor

• Hydrocephalus (rare)

FIGURE 11.55 **SYMPTOMS OF PITUITARY TUMORS.** One source of symptoms involves the effects of an expanding mass in the sellar region. Symptoms are usually multiple because of the critical location of the pituitary to many important neural structures.

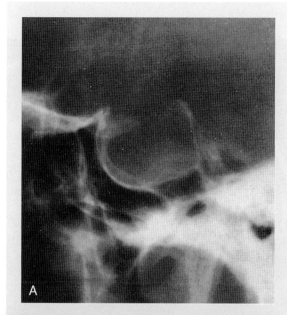

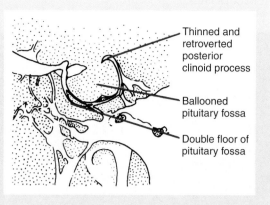

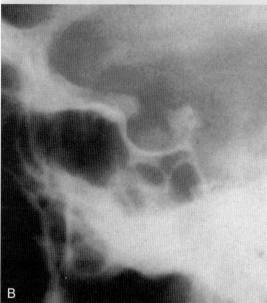

FIGURE 11.56 **PITUITARY TUMOR. (A)** Lateral skull radiograph shows ballooning of the floor of the pituitary fossa due to compression by an enlarging tumor mass. **(B)** The normal appearance of the pituitary fossa is shown for comparison.

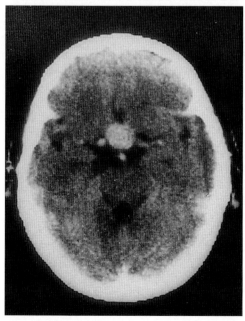

FIGURE 11.57 **CHROMOPHOBE ADENOMA.** Contrast-enhanced CT scan shows a suprasellar mass in a 69-year-old man who complained of difficulty with vision in his left eye for several years. Examination suggested hypopituitarism, which was later confirmed, together with a central defect in the left eye extending temporally and reduced visual acuity. The tumor was resected.

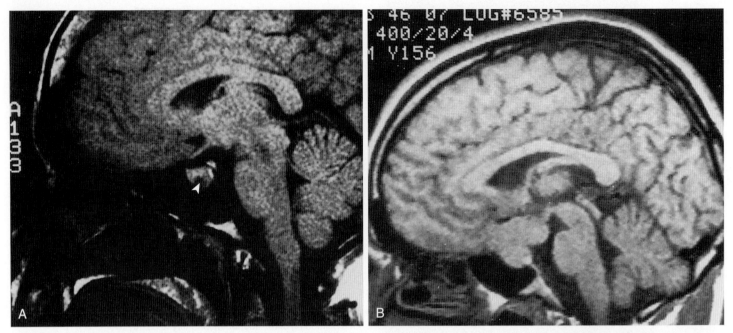

FIGURE 11.58 PITUITARY ADENOMA. (A) T_1-weighted midline sagittal MR image demonstrates a local hypointensity within the pituitary gland, representing a microadenoma (*arrowhead*). (B) A similar scan in another patient shows a large intrasellar mass (macroadenoma) with suprasellar extension.

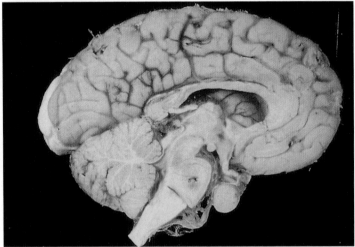

FIGURE 11.59 ACIDOPHILIC ADENOMA. This sagittal section through the brain of a 64-year-old woman shows a well-demarcated, rounded pituitary tumor (1.5 cm in diameter) anterior to the midbrain. The woman presented with a 2-year history of visual disturbance and occipital headaches. She was found to be grossly acromegalic and hyperglycemic. Over the following 2 years she developed severe congestive heart failure, and her persistent hyperglycemia became unresponsive to insulin. Eventually she became comatose and died.

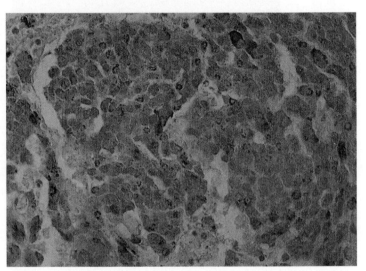

FIGURE 11.61 PROLACTINOMA. Most of the tumor cells contain fine, brown cytoplasmic granules, thus indicating a positive immunoperoxidase reaction with antiprolactin antibody (immunoperoxidase and hematoxylin). (Courtesy of Prof. I. Doniach.)

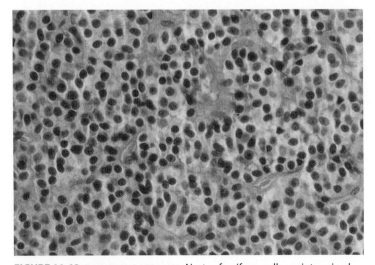

FIGURE 11.60 ACIDOPHILIC ADENOMA. Nests of uniform cells are intermixed with a delicate vascular stroma.

Neuroendocrine Tumors

Neuroendocrine neoplasms occur in every organ of the body, often sharing the common property of the amine precursor uptake and decarboxylation (APUD) reaction. They are a heterogeneous group of tumors, showing either neural differentiation (e.g., neuroblastomas, pheochromocytomas, paragangliomas) and/or epithelial differentiation (e.g., carcinoid tumors and neuroendocrine carcinomas). The epithelial types demonstrate a morphologic and biologic continuum, ranging from the least malignant, cytologically bland carcinoid tumors to the more aggressive, cytologically malignant, undifferentiated neuroendocrine carcinomas. Neuroendocrine carcinomas encompass a large group of tumors, including small and large cell neuroendocrine carcinomas of the lung, as well as neuroendocrine carcinomas of other sites, including the gastrointestinal (GI) tract (pancreas, bowel), prostate, and female genital tract (neuroendocrine tumors of the lung are discussed separately in Chapter 5).

Carcinoid tumors are neoplasms of argentaffin (Kulchitzky) cells, which are characterized by the APUD reaction. In 95% of cases they arise in the GI tract, but they have also been reported in the larynx, lung, bronchus, thymus, esophagus, pancreas, stomach, ovary, testis, and biliary tract. Autopsy series have suggested an incidence of GI carcinoids of approximately 1%, most of which are clinically occult. Within the GI tract the most common site is the appendix, followed by the small bowel and rectum; in fact, carcinoid tumors are the most common neoplasms of the appendix and the second most common tumor of the small bowel. The incidence of malignant carcinoids is approximately 1 in 100,000, with women outnumbering men at a ratio of 1.5:1. Tumors may occur in any age group, but the majority of patients present in the seventh decade.

ETIOLOGY AND CLASSIFICATION

The sites of carcinoid tumors are divided according to their tissue of origin during embryologic development. Foregut carcinoids arise from the oral pharynx to the mid-duodenum; midgut carcinoids originate in the small bowel and proximal colon; and hindgut carcinoids originate in the descending colon and rectum. Foregut and midgut carcinoid tumors are frequently associated with the carcinoid syndrome, whereas hindgut tumors are only infrequently symptomatic. The small bowel is the most common site of origin of clinically significant carcinoids. Tumors smaller than 1 cm are unlikely to metastasize, whereas 80% of tumors larger than 2 cm are associated with metastatic disease, most commonly of liver, lung, and bone.

CLINICAL MANIFESTATIONS

The majority of neuroendocrine tumors are asymptomatic. The classic symptoms associated with the carcinoid syndrome are flushing and diarrhea. For the syndrome to become clinically apparent, metastases to the liver from a bowel primary must be present. In the absence of hepatic metastases the biologically active tumor products are metabolized by the liver and rendered inactive. Exceptions to this are bronchial and ovarian carcinoids, which may manifest the syndrome because of the systemic venous drainage that bypasses the liver. It is estimated that even when liver metastases are present only about half of patients will show the carcinoid syndrome. Of those patients with the carcinoid syndrome up to 50% develop cardiac complications. The average interval between the diagnosis of metastatic carcinoid tumor and the development of clinically apparent heart disease is 5 years. Although usually involvement is limited to the right heart, most often characterized by fibrosis of the right cardiac valves and endocardium, the left heart may be affected, manifesting with mitral valve disease.

Carcinoid tumors secrete a wide variety of endocrinologically active substances, including serotonin, histamine, bradykinin, prostaglandins, and VIP. The predominant substance produced is serotonin, which is derived from tryptophan by hydroxylation followed by a decarboxylation step. The major metabolite of serotonin is 5-hydroxyindoleacetic acid (5-HIAA), which is excreted in the urine. Though not responsible for all the symptoms of the carcinoid syndrome, serotonin is considered to be the probable cause of the diarrhea. The carcinoid flush is caused predominantly by bradykinins. In addition to these substances, carcinoid tumors have been documented to secrete growth hormone, ACTH, and calcitonin.

The symptoms produced by carcinoid tumors may be caused by the primary tumor or by metastases. Because many of these symptoms are nonspecific and are associated with no clearly abnormal physical and radiographic findings, the duration of symptoms before diagnosis averages 2–4 years and may be as long as 20 years. Symptoms characteristic of small bowel carcinoids include abdominal pain, nausea, and vomiting. Intermittent intestinal obstruction may occur as a result of intussusception. The tumors are typically submucosal in location, and the extensive desmoplastic reaction often stimulated by these tumors may lead to bowel obstruction and, rarely, to vascular compromise of the bowel. GI bleeding is unusual.

The diagnosis of functioning carcinoids, with or without the carcinoid syndrome, can be achieved by documenting elevated levels of biologically active substances produced by the tumor. The most useful test is the measurement of 5-HIAA in a 24-hour urine collection. A urine level of 5-HIAA greater than 30 mg per 24 hours confirms the diagnosis. In the rare patient with a foregut carcinoid that lacks the ability to decarboxylate 5-hydroxytryptophan, chromatographic measurement of 5-hydroxytryptophan can be diagnostic. Diagnosis of nonfunctioning carcinoids is more difficult. Abdominal masses are present in only 20% of cases. GI radiographic studies and CT scanning are useful once local symptoms have appeared. Most carcinoid tumors express somatostatin receptors, making imaging with radiolabeled somatostatin analogue a useful localization and staging modality.

MOLECULAR BIOLOGY

Studies investigating DNA content and behavior of carcinoids are infrequent. Aneuploidy does seem to be significantly associated with tumor size, nuclear atypia, and lymph node and vascular involvement; however, these studies are not routinely performed.

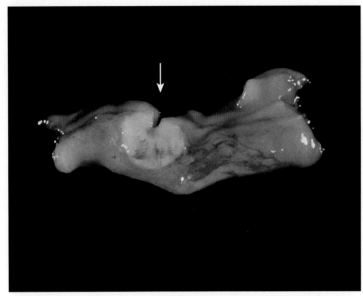

FIGURE 11.62 **CARCINOID TUMOR OF DISTAL ILEUM.** Gross specimen shows thickening, together with angulation and tethering of mucosal folds. A nodular mass has invaded the bowel wall (*arrow*), causing an extensive fibroblastic response.

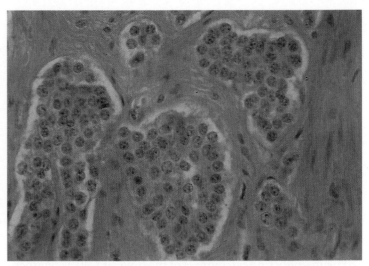

FIGURE 11.63 **CARCINOID TUMOR OF SMALL INTESTINE.** High magnification reveals characteristic solid nests of monomorphic tumor cells with ample cytoplasm. Nuclei are strikingly uniform, and chromatin is deeply stippled.

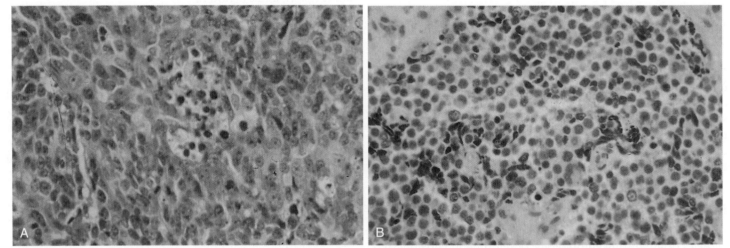

FIGURE 11.64 **NEUROENDOCRINE CARCINOMA. (A)** Tumor cells arranged in nests exhibit scanty cytoplasm and cell pleomorphism. Many mitotic figures and areas of focal necrosis can be seen. **(B)** Tumor cells in this extrapulmonary small cell undifferentiated (oat cell) carcinoma are marked by scanty cytoplasm and lack of a nucleolus. Note the crush artifact.

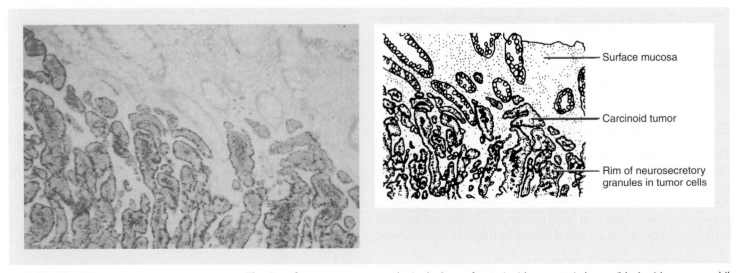

FIGURE 11.65 **CARCINOID TUMOR OF SMALL INTESTINE.** The rims of neurosecretory granules in the base of a carcinoid tumor stain brown/black with an argyrophil stain (Grimelius).

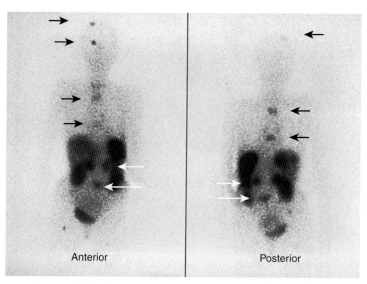

FIGURE 11.66 Carcinoid tumors express somatostatin receptors. Anteroposterior view of radiolabeled somatostatin receptor analogue scan in patient with widely metastatic carcinoid. *White arrows* indicate intra-abdominal disease, of which the lower was the ileal primary. *Black arrows* point to distant metastatic disease.

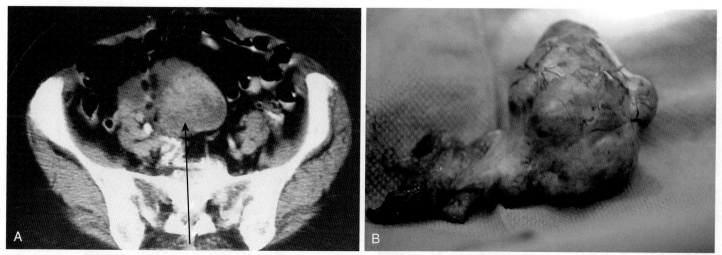

FIGURE 11.67 **OVARIAN CARCINOID. (A)** CT scan of pelvis in older woman with flagrant carcinoid syndrome and tricuspid insufficiency. *Arrow* points to midline mass in low pelvis. **(B)** Operative specimen. There were no liver metastases.

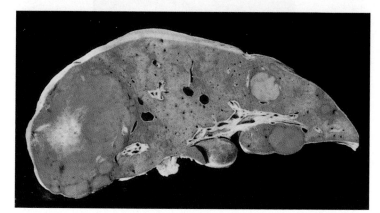

FIGURE 11.68 **LIVER METASTASES.** This liver specimen is from a 66-year-old woman who presented with a 30-month history of facial flushing and recent onset of swelling of the hands and feet and desquamation of the skin. She was found to have hepatomegaly and large amounts of 5-HIAA in the urine. She rapidly developed signs of tricuspid incompetence, jaundice, and ascites and died shortly afterward. At autopsy there were carcinoid tumors in the ileum and within a Meckel's diverticulum, and metastases were present in the liver and lungs. Within the liver are several discrete, rounded secondary deposits of typically yellow-brown metastatic tumor. The largest metastasis shows evidence of necrosis at its center.

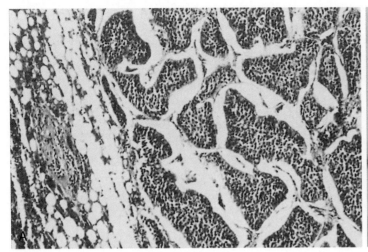

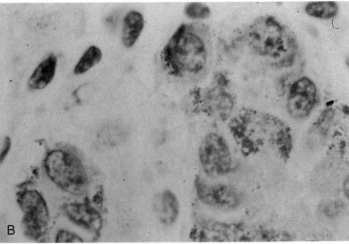

FIGURE 11.69 LIVER METASTASES. (A) This histologic section shows characteristic regular islands of metastatic carcinoid tumor. **(B)** With higher magnification and an alkaline diazo reaction, red-brown neurosecretory granules of a carcinoid tumor can be seen.

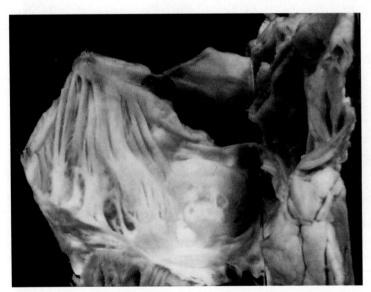

FIGURE 11.70 CARDIAC METASTASES. The right atrium of this postmortem specimen from a 62-year-old man has been opened to show patchy, pale endocardial thickening. The tricuspid valve (*bottom right*) shows similar changes. The patient presented with a 1-year history of intermittent diarrhea and reddish blue discoloration of the face. Examination revealed irregular hepatomegaly and a variable cardiac murmur. Urinary 5-HIAA was grossly elevated, presumably as a result of a small intestinal primary tumor with liver metastases. The patient died 15 months later. (Courtesy of the Gordon Museum, Guy's Hospital Medical School, London, UK.)

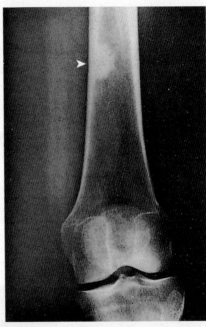

FIGURE 11.71 BONE METASTASIS. Anteroposterior radiograph of the distal femur and knee shows the typical appearance of an intramedullary blastic metastasis (*arrowhead*) from a malignant carcinoid tumor. Lytic metastatic lesions have also been described.

Islet Cell Tumors

The endocrine pancreas contains at least five types of cells, each of which produces its own polypeptide. The clinical manifestations of tumors arising from islet cells, therefore, vary according to the cell of origin (see Table 11.6). Islet cells are believed to be neuroectodermal in origin and are included in the APUD system.

The prevalence and incidence of islet cell tumors are poorly documented. Estimates indicate that 250 new cases are diagnosed each year in the United States, and there seems to be no sex predilection. Islet cell tumors have been identified in up to 1.5% of autopsies and in the majority of cases were not clinically apparent. The peak incidence is seen in the 40- to 60-year age group.

Islet cell tumors of the pancreas may present with excessive hormone production or a mass effect as a result of increasing size. Of the functioning lesions, up to 70% are β-cell tumors that secrete insulin (insulinoma). A further 15% are of α-cell origin (glucagonoma), and γ- and δ-cell tumors (gastrinoma and somatostatinoma, respectively) account for up to 10%. A much smaller group of tumors secretes pancreatic polypeptide or VIP, the latter giving rise to the watery diarrhea, hypokalemia, and achlorhydria (WDHA or Verner-Morrison) syndrome.

Pancreatic islet cell tumors may be multiple and may form part of the MEN I syndrome. They are only rarely malignant. The most common malignant islet cell tumors are of probable γ-cell origin; up to 90% of gastrinomas, for example, are malignant.

Malignancy criteria for pancreatic endocrine neoplasms have been established by the WHO, and much like most endocrine tumors, the true marker of malignancy is metastasis. Those considered to have benign behavior are confined to the pancreas, are nonangioinvasive, show no perineural invasion, are smaller than 2 cm, show fewer than 2 mitoses per 10 high-power fields, and show less than 2% MIB-1 proliferative index (Ki-67). Those considered to be of uncertain malignant behavior are ≥2 cm and show 2–10 mitoses per 10 high-power fields, >2% MIB-1 index, perineural invasion, or vascular invasion. Well-differentiated endocrine carcinomas fit the prior definition and in addition show local invasion or metastasis. Poorly differentiated endocrine carcinomas are high-grade and show ≥10 mitoses per 10 high-power fields as well as meeting the criteria above. Remember, the only true definition of malignancy in endocrine neoplasia is metastasis.

Islet cell tumors often secrete multiple hormones. Immunohistochemistry is useful to assess for the presence of these hormones, but immunoreactivity does not necessarily indicate hormone secretion or malignancy. As tumors grow, the clinical symptoms may change because of alterations in the pattern of hormones they secrete. The clinical syndromes observed may be caused by a benign adenoma, by malignant carcinoma, or sometimes by adenomatous hyperplasia.

Both benign and malignant pancreatic neuroendocrine tumors may show aneuploid DNA patterns. DNA ploidy analyses are unlikely to provide useful prognostic information in these tumors.

Table 11.6

Characteristics of Endocrine Tumors of the Pancreas

Tumor Type	Major Clinical Symptoms	Predominant Hormone	Islet cell Type	Malignant (%)	Localization	Other Clinical Features
Insulinoma	Hypoglycemia (fasting or nocturnal)	Insulin	β	10	Usually pancreatic; rarely extrapancreatic	Catecholamine excess
Glucagonoma	Diabetes mellitus Migratory necrolytic erythema	Glucagon	α	90	Usually pancreatic; rarely extrapancreatic	Panhypoaminoaciduria Thromboembolism Weight loss
Gastrinoma	Recurrent peptic ulcer disease	Gastrin	γ	90	Usually pancreatic but frequently extrapancreatic	Diarrhea/steatorrhea
Somatostatinoma	Diabetes mellitus Diarrhea, steatorrhea	Somatostatin	δ	80	Pancreatic and duodenal	Hypochlorhydria Weight loss Gallbladder disease
VIPoma	Watery diarrhea, hypokalemia, achlorhydria (WDHA syndrome)	Vasoactive intestinal polypeptide (VIP)	δ	50	Usually pancreatic but frequently extrapancreatic	Metabolic acidosis Hyperglycemia Hypercalcemia Flushing
PPoma	Hepatomegaly Abdominal pain	Pancreatic polypeptide (PP)	PP cells	80	Usually pancreatic; rarely extrapancreatic	Occasional watery diarrhea

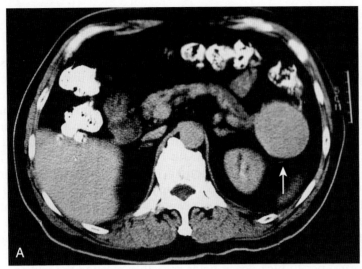
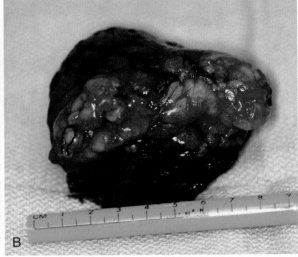

FIGURE 11.72 **INSULINOMA. (A)** This CT scan shows a large mass in the tail of the pancreas in a patient with symptomatic hypoglycemia and elevated insulin levels. **(B)** Operative specimen from same patient. Most insulinomas are smaller than this.

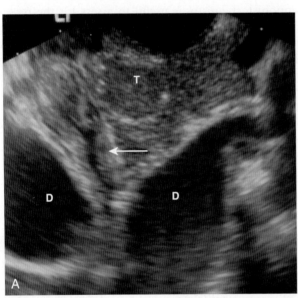
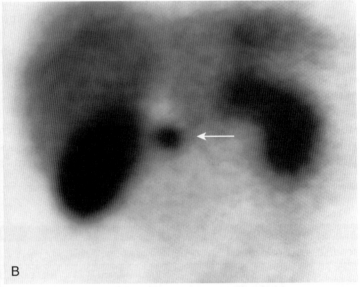

FIGURE 11.73 Insulinomas are well identified by intraoperative ultrasound. Some of these lesions also express somatostatin receptors. **(A)** Intraoperative ultrasonogram of insulinoma of head of pancreas. T, tumor; D, duodenum. The *arrow* points to the distal common duct. **(B)** Anteroposterior view of radiolabeled somatostatin analogue scan from same patient. *Arrow* points to the insulinoma.

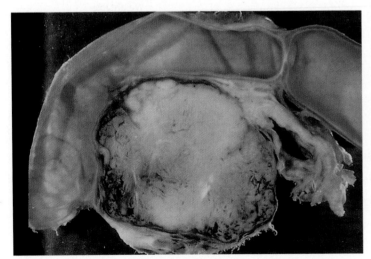
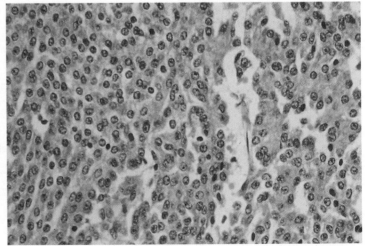

FIGURE 11.74 **ISLET CELL TUMOR.** This specimen, comprising the pyloric canal, proximal duodenum, and head of the pancreas, is from a 35-year-old woman who presented with an 8-month history of backache and intermittent abdominal pain. Following surgery she developed hepatorenal failure and died. The head of the pancreas has been completely replaced by a circumscribed tumor measuring 7 cm in diameter and showing foci of necrosis and hemorrhage. There is no infiltration of the duodenal wall. Note the cystic dilatation of the pancreatic duct in the body of the pancreas (*right*) due to obstruction by tumor.

FIGURE 11.75 **ISLET CELL TUMOR.** High-power photomicrograph shows a solid pattern of tumor cells. Malignant potential cannot be determined solely on the basis of the histopathologic features.

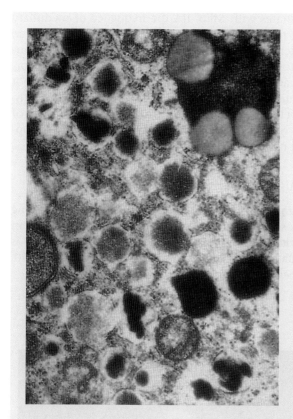

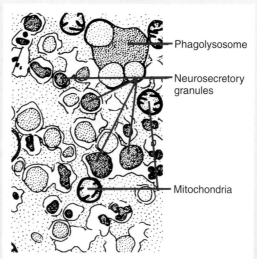

FIGURE 11.76 ISLET CELL TUMOR. Characteristic of a neuroendocrine tumor, the ultrastructure of this pancreatic tumor is marked by numerous neurosecretory granules. Also present is a single granule showing a rectangular crystalline core characteristic of insulin secretion.

Multiple Endocrine Neoplasia Syndrome

Multiple endocrine neoplasia (MEN), a syndrome inherited as an autosomal-dominant trait, is characterized by tumors affecting multiple endocrine glands. Three forms of the syndrome have been identified (MEN I, MEN IIA, and MEN IIB) (see Table 11.7). The individual endocrine neoplasms involved in the syndrome have been discussed in earlier sections.

Table 11.7

Syndromes of Multiple Endocrine Neoplasia

Type	Organ	Neoplasm	Patients Affected (%)
I	Parathyroid	Hyperplasia	90
	Pituitary	Adenoma	65
	Pancreas	Islet cell	75
	Adrenal	Cortical adenoma	Rare
	Thyroid	Adenoma	Rare
	Adipocyte	Lipoma	Rare
	Multiple	Carcinoid	Rare
IIA	Thyroid	Medullary carcinoma	100
	Adrenal	Pheochromocytoma	50
	Parathyroid	Hyperplasia	20
IIB	Thyroid	Medullary carcinoma	75
	Adrenal	Pheochromocytoma	50
	Parathyroid	Hyperplasia	5
	Neuron	Mucosal neuromas; intestinal ganglioneuromas	100

Diagnostic criteria for MEN I are primary hyperparathyroidism (multiglandular hyperplasia and/or adenoma, possibly recurrent), duodenal and/or pancreatic endocrine tumors (functioning [gastrinoma, insulinoma, glucagonoma]; nonfunctioning), anterior pituitary adenoma (growth hormone–secreting, prolactinoma, nonfunctional, or multi-hormone-secreting), adrenocortical tumors, thymic and/or bronchial tube endocrine tumors (foregut carcinoid), and/or a first-degree relative with MEN I according to the above criteria. Approximately 70% of patients have adenomas of two or more systems, and 20% of patients develop adenomas of three or more systems. Parathyroid involvement is manifested as hypercalcemia resulting from parathyroid hyperplasia. The symptoms caused by pituitary adenomas are usually secondary to a mass effect, and only a minority of patients present with acromegaly, Cushing syndrome, or hyperprolactinemia. Pancreatic islet cell tumors in MEN I are often malignant. Cushing syndrome may be due to a pituitary or an adrenal tumor, or to ectopic elaboration of ACTH by an islet cell tumor. Affected individuals may present with simultaneous involvement of multiple endocrine glands, or several glands may become sequentially affected over a period of months to years. Continuing surveillance is necessary to evaluate each patient for new manifestations of the disease. The prevalence in most populations is up to 1:20,000. About 10% of patients have *MEN1* gene mutations arising de novo without prior family history. Mutations have been found in about 5% of patients with sporadic primary hyperparathyroidism, a fairly common disease. Therefore, the true incidence of MEN I may be underestimated.

MEN II is autosomal dominant in its inheritance pattern as a result of germline mutations in the *RET* gene. It is clinically divided into three groups: MEN IIA, MEN IIB, and familial medullary thyroid carcinoma (FMTC).

FMTC is thought to be responsible for up to 25% of all medullary thyroid cancer cases, and medullary carcinomas account for between 5% and 10% of thyroid carcinomas, indicating a fairly high incidence of MEN II.

MEN IIA, also known as Stipple's syndrome, consists of medullary carcinoma of the thyroid, which is usually bilateral, together with often bilateral pheochromocytomas of the adrenal gland in about 50% of patients. The pheochromocytoma is occasionally extra-adrenal. Associated with these in a minority of cases is parathyroid hyperplasia. Symptoms at the initial presentation are usually caused either by medullary carcinoma of the thyroid or by pheochromocytoma; only rarely are symptoms the result of hyperparathyroidism.

MEN IIB shares with MEN IIA the frequency of medullary carcinoma of the thyroid and pheochromocytomas. However, MEN IIB patients also have neuromas of the tongue and ganglioneuromatosis of the intestine. There may be associated corneal changes and a marfanoid body habitus, but these are not pathognomonic. Family members should be screened for serum calcitonin levels or the *RET* proto-oncogene, with the hope of identifying C-cell hyperplasia of the thyroid before the development of overt medullary carcinoma.

MOLECULAR BIOLOGY

MEN I has been localized to the pericentromeric region of the long arm of chromosome 11 and corresponds to mutations in the menin tumor suppressor gene. MEN II syndrome (IIA, IIB, and FMTC) is caused by mutations in the *RET* gene, located on chromosome 10. Mutational analysis can identify carriers of *RET* mutations.

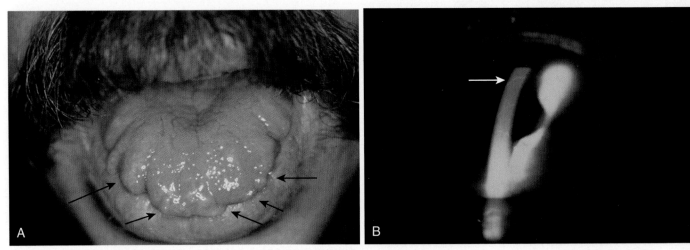

FIGURE 11.77 MEN IIB. (A) In this patient, neuromas of lips and tongue were associated with medullary carcinoma of the thyroid and adrenal pheochromocytomas. **(B)** Prominent corneal nerves were visible with slit lamp examination (*arrow*).

FIGURE 11.78 MEN-IIB. In this patient with thyroid swelling caused by medullary carcinoma, **(A)** the lips are typically swollen and **(B)** there is a marfanoid body habitus. (Courtesy of Mr. K.F. Moos.)

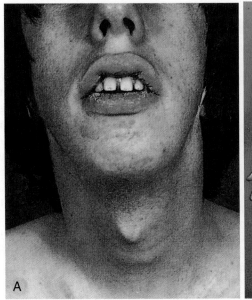
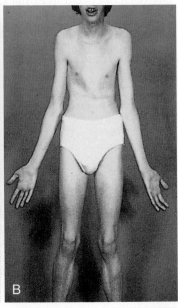

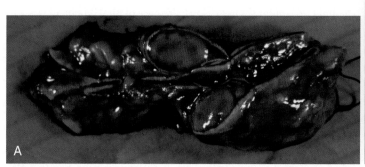
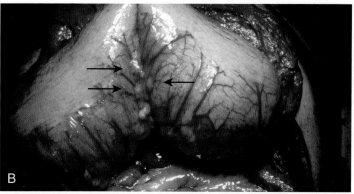

FIGURE 11.79 **MEN IIB. (A)** Operative specimen showing multiple adrenal pheochromocytomas. **(B)** Operative photograph showing neuromas of a megacolon (*arrows*).

References and Suggested Readings

Adler JT, Meyer-Rochow GY, Chen H, et al: Pheochromocytoma: current approaches and future directions, *Oncologist* 13:779–793, 2008.

Benker G, Olbricht T, Reinwein D, et al: Survival rates in patients with differentiated thyroid carcinoma, *Cancer* 65:1517–1520, 1990.

Boggild MD, Jenkinson S, Pistorella M, et al: Molecular genetic studies of sporadic pituitary tumors, *J Clin Endocrinol Metab* 78:387–392, 1994.

Boikos SA, Stratakis CA: Molecular genetics of the camp-dependent protein kinase pathway and of sporadic pituitary tumorigenesis, *Hum Mol Genet* 16(Spec No 1):R80–R87, 2007.

Bystrom C, Larsson C, Blomberg C, et al: Localization of the MEN I gene to a small region within chromosome 11q13 by deletion mapping in tumors, *Proc Natl Acad Sci USA* 87:1968–1972, 1990.

Copeland RM: The incidentally discovered adrenal mass, *Ann Intern Med* 98:940–945, 1983.

DeLellis RA, Lloyd RV, Heitz P, Eng C, editors: *World Health Organization classification of tumours, pathology and genetics of tumors of endocrine organs,* Lyon, 2005, IARC Press.

Dobashi Y, Sugimura H, Sakamoto A, et al: Stepwise participation of p53 gene mutation during dedifferentiation of human thyroid carcinomas, *Diagn Mol Pathol* 3:9–14, 1994.

Eng C, Smith DP, Mulligan LM, et al: A novel point mutation in the tyrosine kinase domain of the RET proto-oncogene in sporadic medullary thyroid carcinoma and in a family with FMTC, *Oncogene* 10:509–513, 1995.

Fernandez-Ranvier GG, Jensen K, Khanafshar E, et al: Nonfunctioning parathyroid carcinoma: case report and review of literature, *Endocr Pract* 13:750–757, 2007.

Friesen SR: Tumors of the endocrine pancreas, *N Engl J Med* 306:508–590, 1982.

Greene FL, Page DL, Fleming ID, et al: *AJCC cancer staging manual,* ed 6, New York, 2002, Springer.

Jhiang SM, Mazzaferri EL: The ret/PTC oncogene in papillary thyroid carcinoma, *J Lab Clin Med* 123:331–337, 1994.

Karagiannis A, Mikhailidis DP, Athyros VG, Harsoulis F: Pheochromocytoma: an update on genetics and management, *Endocr Relat Cancer* 14:935–956, 2007.

Katoh R, Bray CE, Suzuki K, et al: Growth activity in hyperplastic and neoplastic human thyroid determined by an immunohistochemical staining procedure using monoclonal antibody MIB-I, *Human Pathol* 26:139–146, 1995.

Keren DF, Hanson CA, Hurtubise PE: *Flow cytometry and clinical diagnosis,* Chicago, 1994, American Society of Clinical Pathology.

Kifor O, Moore FD Jr, Wang P, et al: Reduced expression of the extracellular Ca^{2+}-sensing receptor in primary and uremic secondary hyperparathyroidism, *J Clin Endocrinol Metab* 81:1598–1606, 1996.

Lack EE: *Pathology of adrenal and extra-adrenal paraganglia: major problems in pathology,* vol 29. Philadelphia, 1994, Saunders.

Lemos MC, Thakker RV: Multiple endocrine neoplasia type 1 (MEN1): analysis of 1336 mutations reported in the first decade following identification of the gene, *Hum Mutat* 29:22–32, 2008.

Lodish MB, Stratakis CA: RET oncogene in MEN2, MEN2B, MTC and other forms of thyroid cancer, *Expert Rev Anticancer Ther* 8:625–632, 2008.

Lumachi F, Basso SM, Basso U: Parathyroid cancer: etiology, clinical presentation and treatment, *Anticancer Res* 26:4803–4807, 2006.

Luton JP, Cerdas S, Billaud L: Clinical features of adrenocortical carcinoma, prognostic factors, and the effects of mitotane therapy, *N Engl J Med* 322:1195–1201, 1990.

Mikhail RA, Moore JB, Reed DN, et al: Malignant retroperitoneal paragangliomas, *J Surg Oncol* 5:1503–1522, 1986.

Min HS, Choe G, Kim SW, et al: S100A4 expression is associated with lymph node metastasis in papillary microcarcinoma of the thyroid, *Mod Pathol* 21:748–755, 2008.

Moertel CA: An odyssey in the land of small tumors, *J Clin Oncol* 5:1503–1522, 1987.

Moran CA, Suster S: Neuroendocrine carcinomas (carcinoid, atypical carcinoid, small cell carcinoma, and large cell neuroendocrine carcinoma): current concepts, *Hematol Oncol Clin North Am* 21:395–407, 2007.

Mulligan LM, Gardner E, Smith BA, et al: Genetic events in tumour initiation and progression in multiple endocrine neoplasia type 2, *Genes Chromosomes Cancer* 6:166–177, 1993.

Nakamura E, Kaelin WG Jr: Recent insights into the molecular pathogenesis of pheochromocytoma and paraganglioma, *Endocr Pathol* 17:97–106, 2006.

Nilsson O, Wangberg B, Kolby L, et al: Expression of transforming growth factor alpha and its receptor in human neuroendocrine tumors, *Int J Cancer* 60:645–651, 1995.

Onitilo AA, Engel JM, Lundgren CI, et al: Simplifying the TNM system for clinical use in differentiated thyroid cancer, *J Clin Oncol* 27:1872–1878, 2009.

Pilato FP, D'Adda T, Banchini E, et al: Nonrandom expression of polypeptide hormones in pancreatic endocrine tumors, *Cancer* 61:1815–1820, 1988.

Pipeleers-Marichal M, Somers G, Willems G, et al: Gastrinomas in the duodenums of patients with multiple endocrine neoplasia type I and Zollinger-Ellison syndrome, *N Engl J Med* 322:723–727, 1990.

Redman BG, Pazdur R, Zingas AP, et al: Prospective evaluation of adrenal insufficiency in patients with adrenal metastasis, *Cancer* 60:103–107, 1987.

Remick SC, Hafez GR, Carbone PP: Extrapulmonary small cell carcinoma: a review of the literature with emphasis on therapy and outcome, *Medicine* 66:457–471, 1987.

de Reyniès A, Assié G, Rickman DS, et al: Gene expression profiling reveals a new classification of adrenocortical tumors and identifies molecular predictors of malignancy and survival, *J Clin Oncol* 27:1108–1115, 2009.

Saad MF, Ordonez NG, Rashid RK, et al: Medullary carcinoma of the thyroid: a study of the clinical features and prognostic factors in 161 patients, *Medicine* 63:319–342, 1984.

Sadow PM, Rumilla KM, Erickson LA, Lloyd RV: Stathmin expression in pheochromocytomas, paragangliomas, and in other endocrine tumors, *Endocr Pathol* 19:97–103, 2008.

Samaan NA, Hickey RC: Adrenal cortical carcinoma, *Semin Oncol* 14:292–296, 1987.

Samaan NA, Hickey RC: Pheochromocytoma, *Semin Oncol* 14:297–305, 1987.

Schlisio S, Kenchappa RS, Vredeveld LC, et al: The kinesin KIF1β acts downstream from egln3 to induce apoptosis and is a potential 1p36 tumor suppressor, *Genes Dev* 22:884–893, 2008.

Simpson WJ, McKinney SE, Carruthers JS, et al: Papillary and follicular thyroid cancer: prognostic factors in 1,578 patients, *Am J Med* 83:479–488, 1989.

Sobol H, Narod SA, Nakamura Y, et al: Screening for multiple endocrine neoplasia type 2a with DNA-polymorphism analysis, *N Engl J Med* 31:996–1000, 1989.

Tischler AS: Molecular and cellular biology of pheochromocytomas and extra-adrenal paragangliomas, *Endocr Pathol* 17:321–328, 2006.

Ugolini C, Giannini R, Lupi C, et al: Presence of BRAF V600E in very early stages of papillary thyroid carcinoma, *Thyroid* 17:381–388, 2007.

Volante M, Collini P, Nikiforov YE, et al: Poorly differentiated thyroid carcinoma: the Turin proposal for the use of uniform diagnostic criteria and an algorithmic diagnostic approach, *Am J Surg Pathol* 31:1256–1264, 2007.

Wolfe MM, Jensen RT: Zollinger-Ellison syndrome, *N Engl J Med* 317:1200–1209, 1987.

Wreesmann VB, Singh B: Clinical impact of molecular analysis on thyroid cancer management, *Surg Oncol Clin North Am* 17:1–35, 2008.

Yeh JJ, Lunetta KL, van Orsouw NJ, et al: Somatic mitochondrial DNA (mtdna) in papillary thyroid carcinomas and differential mtdna sequence variants in malignant and benign thyroid tumors, *Oncogene* 2060:19, 2000.

Figure Credits

The following books published by Gower Medical Publishing are sources of figures and tables in the present chapter. The figure and table numbers given in the listing are those of the figures and tables in the present chapter. The page numbers (or slide numbers) given in parentheses are those of the original publication.

Besser GM, Cudworth AG: *Clinical endocrinology*. Philadelphia/London, 1987, Lippincott/Gower Medical Publishing: Figs. 11.5 (p. 14.4), 11.9 (p. 14.4), 11.10 (p. 14.4), 11.11 (p. 14.5), 11.12 (p. 20.19), 11.14 (p. 14.6), 11.15 (p. 14.6), 11.22 (p. 20.20), 11.28 (p. 9.4), 11.34 (p. 20.10), 11.40 (p. 9.8), 11.42 (p. 20.12), 11.46 (p. 20.13), 11.53 (p. 2.2), 11.54 (p. 2.8), 11.58 (p. 2.3), 11.59 (p. 20.16), 11.62 (p. 20.16), 11.63 (p. 20.11), 11.64 (p. 20.16), 11.71 (p. 20.15), 11.75 (p. 9.7), Table 11.2 (p. 19.5), Table 11.3 (p. 9.4), Table 11.4 (p. 2.9), Table 11.6 (p. 20.15).

Cawson RA, Eveson JW: *Oral pathology and diagnosis*. London, 1987, Heinemann Medical Books/Gower Medical Publishing: Fig. 11.76 (p. 10.13).

Fletcher CDM, McKee PH: *An atlas of gross pathology*. London, 1987, Edward Arnold/Gower Medical Publishing: Figs. 11.4 (p. 57), 11.8 (p. 57), 11.16 (p. 58), 11.38 (p. 60), 11.39 (p. 61).

Kassner EG, editor: *Atlas of radiologic imaging*. Philadelphia/New York, 1989, Lippincott/Gower Medical Publishing: Figs. 11.2 (p. 12.34), 11.3 (p. 12.45), 11.6 (p. 12.33), 11.7 (p. 12.33) 11.35 (p. 8.28).

Perkin GD, Rose FC, Blackwood W, et al: *Atlas of clinical neurology*. Philadelphia/London, 1986, Lippincott/Gower Medical Publishing: Table 11.5 (p. 9.16).

Price AB, Morson BC, Scheuer PJ: Alimentary system. In Turk JL, Fletcher CDM, editors: *RCSE slide atlas of pathology*. London, 1986, Gower Medical Publishing: Fig. 11.63 (slide 323).

Sommers SC: Endocrine system. In Turk JL, Fletcher CDM, editors: *RCSE slide atlas of pathology*. London, 1986, Gower Medical Publishing: Figs. 11.33 (slide 50), 11.45 (slide 44), 11.48 (slide 48) 11.50 (slide 53), 11.51 (slide 55), 11.56 (slide 3), 11.65 (slide 323), 11.70 (slide 56).

Sarcomas of Soft Tissue and Bone and Gastrointestinal Stromal Tumors

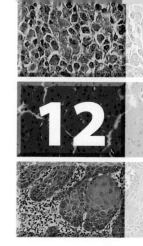

12

SUZANNE GEORGE • JASON L. HORNICK • NANCY E. JOSTE • KAREN H. ANTMAN • GEORGE D. DEMETRI

Sarcomas

Sarcomas are a complex and heterogeneous family of malignancies of mesenchymal origin. As opposed to carcinomas, which represent malignancies of epithelial tissues, sarcomas are neoplastic disorders that differentiate into lineages related to "connective tissues," broadly including bone, fat, stromal supportive cells (such as fibroblasts), cartilage, and blood vessels. The term "sarcoma" is derived from the Greek root *sarc* (flesh) and the suffix *-oma* (tumor). Sarcasm, a flesh-tearing criticism, and sarcophagus, a carrier for a body, are based on the same root.

Though uncommon, sarcomas are highly informative about the mechanisms of human neoplasia. Virtually no class of human solid tumors has yielded as many pathogenetic clues as to specific molecular aberrancies linked to individual tumor subtypes as sarcomas. Tumor-specific chromosomal translocations have been defined for many different types of sarcomas. Identification of these molecular pathways of cancer has had both diagnostic and therapeutic impact. For example, the identity of Ewing sarcoma with primitive neuroectodermal tumor was identified because these entities shared a common cytogenetic abnormality. The best example of the therapeutic impact of this knowledge has been the development of imatinib mesylate (Gleevec; Novartis, Basel, Switzerland) and sunitinib malate (Sutent; Pfizer, New York, NY) as molecularly targeted therapy for gastrointestinal stromal tumors (GISTs), a subtype of sarcoma that was essentially resistant to any systemic therapies before the era of kinase-inhibiting agents such as these. It is hoped that with additional knowledge of oncogenic molecular mechanisms derived from sarcomas, accelerated translation of basic science will allow the development of rational, mechanism-based therapies for many other types of malignancies.

Sarcomas of soft tissue and bone currently represent 1% of adult malignancies but disproportionately affect children, composing 15% of pediatric malignancies. The sex predominantly affected differs considerably among the histologic variants. For example, 70% of patients with Kaposi sarcoma are male, as are 60% of those with liposarcoma and embryonal rhabdomyosarcoma, and 35% with leiomyosarcoma. Sarcomas develop in individuals of all ages. Embryonal rhabdomyosarcoma generally occurs in children and adolescents under 20 years of age; synovial sarcoma, osteosarcoma, alveolar rhabdomyosarcoma, and Ewing sarcoma arise in adolescents and young adults, whereas leiomyosarcoma, chondrosarcoma, and GISTs typically occur in individuals over 50 years of age.

Sarcomas are traditionally classified in two major groupings: those arising in bone or cartilage and those originating in soft tissue. Soft tissue sarcomas can be further subdivided based upon the anatomic site of origin: for example, those that develop in the extremities, retroperitoneum, or visceral organs (such as the gastrointestinal [GI] and gynecologic tracts) (Tables 12.1, 12.2).

SARCOMAS OF BONE AND CARTILAGE

As with any soft tissue mass, tumors of bone may also be benign or malignant. Primary malignant lesions and secondary malignancies (i.e., those arising in association with a prior benign tumor) must be distinguished from metastatic lesions (which are much more common). Each of the structural components of bone may give rise to benign or malignant neoplasms, and it is important to recognize that certain benign lesions have the potential for malignant transformation. Radiographs of a lesion can help in the assessment of whether a lesion is benign or malignant, and in some cases such imaging studies can even suggest the histopathologic subtype of the bone tumor.

Osteosarcoma

Defined as an osteoid-producing primary malignancy of bone, osteosarcoma is the most common primary sarcoma of bone and the second most common primary bone tumor after plasma cell myeloma. It develops in men slightly more frequently than in women, with an incidence ratio of 1.5:1. The distribution by age is bimodal. During adolescence, osteosarcoma arises in areas of rapid growth, for example, around the epiphyses of long bones. In some studies adolescents with this tumor have been found to be taller than age-matched controls. In the second peak in incidence, among older patients, osteosarcoma develops most frequently in areas of prior benign bone lesions or in previously irradiated sites. For example, solitary lesions of osteochondroma rarely give rise to osteosarcoma, but in patients with multiple lesions (enchondromatosis or Ollier disease) osteosarcoma develops more frequently. In 0.2% of patients with Paget's disease, osteosarcoma arises in pagetoid bone. Multicentric tumors have developed in patients with prior chronic radium ingestion, such as watch-dial painters, and occasionally in the absence of any known risk factors, usually in children under age

Table 12.1

American Joint Committee on Cancer (AJCC) Bone, TNM Staging System, 2002

Primary Tumor (T)

TX	Primary tumor cannot be assessed
T0	No evidence of primary tumor
T1	Tumor 8 cm or less in greatest dimension
T2	Tumor more than 8 cm in greatest dimension
T3	Discontinuous tumors in the primary bone site

Regional Lymph Nodes (N)

NX	Regional lymph nodes cannot be assessed
N0	No regional lymph node metastasis
N1	Regional lymph node metastasis

Distant Metastasis (M)

MX	Distant metastasis cannot be assessed
M0	No distant metastasis
M1	Distant metastasis
M1a	Lung
M1b	Other distant sites

Stage Grouping

IA	T1	N0	M0	G1,2	Low grade
IB	T2	N0	M0	G1,2	Low grade
IIA	T1	N0	M0	G3,4	High grade
IIB	T2	N0	M0	G3,4	High grade
III	T3	N0	M0	Any G	
IVA	Any T	N0	M1a	Any G	
IVB	Any T	N1	Any M	Any G	
	Any T	Any N	M1	Any G	

Histologic Grade (G)*

GX	Grade cannot be assessed
G1	Well differentiated–low grade
G2	Moderately differentiated–low grade
G3	Poorly differentiated–high grade
G4	Undifferentiated–high grade

* Ewing sarcoma is classified as grade 4.

Table 12.2

Most Common Bone and Soft Tissue Sarcoma Tumor Types

Sarcoma Type	Frequency (%)
Bone	
Osteosarcoma	45
Chondrosarcoma	22
Ewing sarcoma	13
Chordoma	9
Fibrosarcoma	7
Malignant fibrous histiocytoma	2
Angiosarcoma	1
Other	1
Soft Tissue Sarcomas	
Liposarcoma	25
Well-differentiated (atypical lipomatous tumor) (45)	
Dedifferentiated liposarcoma (15)	
Myxoid (and round cell) liposarcoma (35)	
Pleomorphic liposarcoma (5)	
Leiomyosarcoma	15
Synovial sarcoma	10
Undifferentiated pleomorphic sarcoma ("MFH")	5–10
Malignant peripheral nerve sheath tumor	5–10
Rhabdomyosarcoma	5
Myxofibrosarcoma	5
Other	20

10. Patients with familial retinoblastoma (i.e., those who have inherited deficiencies of the *RB* tumor suppressor gene) have a greatly increased risk of developing osteosarcoma (nearly a 10% lifetime risk, hundreds of times higher than the risk in the general population).

Patients often present with symptoms of bone pain, which may be indolent or of relatively short duration. Alkaline phosphatase levels are generally elevated, except in undifferentiated osteosarcoma, and they have prognostic value; elevated values after amputation herald residual or relapsing disease. (It should be remembered that normal values in children are higher than in adults.)

Characteristic radiographs and computed tomography (CT) scans of primary lesions reveal osteolysis and periosteal new bone formation; later-stage tumors may show cortical destruction and breakthrough into soft tissues. The telangiectatic variant of osteosarcoma is almost entirely lytic. Periosteal elevation results in the classic "Codman triangle" on radiography. Ossification may be slight, moderate, or densely sclerotic. Another pattern of periosteal reaction can be identified by a "sunburst" appearance of ossification. This phenomenon results from newly formed bone spicules oriented at right angles to the cortical soft tissue extension. (In the gross specimens shown among the figures that follow, it is instructive to note the morphology that results in the characteristic radiographic

appearance of osteosarcoma.) In addition to plain radiography, CT examination, including scans of the chest, is essential to evaluate the stage of a lesion; CT scans of the chest help detect pulmonary metastases, the most likely site of disseminated disease. Radionuclide bone scan imaging is useful in the staging evaluation of osteosarcoma. This modality generally reveals intense uptake within the lesion, and may detect skip lesions, metastases, or a multicentric primary tumor. Uptake in the lungs on bone scan may identify early pulmonary lesions. 2-[^{18}F]-fluoro-2-deoxy-D-glucose–positron emission tomography (FDG-PET) scans are being increasingly evaluated as a tool to assess both extent of disease and, possibly, response to therapy.

The demonstration of "malignant osteoid" (i.e., noncalcified bony substance produced by the tumor cells themselves) is required for a histologic diagnosis of osteosarcoma. Based on the predominant cell type, osteosarcomas can be classified into osteoblastic (45% of cases), chondroblastic (27%), anaplastic (17%), fibroblastic (9%), and telangiectatic (1%) variants. Although most reports have shown that histologic subclassification has little prognostic value, histologic grade seems to correlate with tumor behavior.

Juxtacortical (parosteal) osteosarcomas are relatively uncommon (3% to 4%), often low-grade variants that arise equally in either sex. Patients with these tumors are about a decade older than patients with conventional higher-grade types. Gross examination shows bulky tumors that tend to encircle the cortex of bone, generally the distal femur, and less commonly the proximal humerus. The radiologic differential diagnosis includes osteochondroma and myositis ossificans.

Multimodality treatment is the standard approach to management of localized osteosarcoma. Preoperative ("neoadjuvant") and/or postoperative ("adjuvant") chemotherapy for osteosarcoma is now accepted as standard treatment. Histologic evidence of tumor necrosis following preoperative chemotherapy is among the most powerful prognostic factors for survival of patients with osteosarcoma. Doxorubicin and cisplatin are the core agents of adjuvant regimens in osteosarcoma, but ifosfamide and methotrexate may also have useful roles. Although these aggressive combination-chemotherapy regimens can be associated with considerable toxicity, overall survival is significantly improved with chemotherapy when compared with surgical resection alone.

Besides the routine use of chemotherapy in osteosarcoma management, function-sparing surgery has been shown to be equivalent in overall survival when compared to more debilitating amputations, which were the standard of care before the 1970s. Current treatment approaches combine chemotherapy with local resection rather than amputation, with encouraging results in terms of survival rates and the functional status of affected limbs. Intensive chemotherapy with surgical intervention should be considered if metastases develop in the lung. Some patients who present initially with radiographically evident limited metastatic disease in the lung may be cured by resection of both the primary lesion and the pulmonary metastases, combined with systemic chemotherapy.

In sites of prior Paget's disease or irradiation, osteosarcoma seems to be responsive to the usual therapeutic methods. However, because of its more central location and the vascularity of pagetoid bone, curative resection tends to be difficult.

Ewing Sarcoma

Ewing sarcoma is a high-grade small round cell sarcoma of unknown cellular origin. Ewing sarcoma was once considered primarily a bone tumor, but it is increasingly recognized as a primary malignancy of soft tissues as well. Cytogenetically, it is usually characterized by chromosomal translocations involving chromosome 22 (most often an 11;22 translocation, identical to that found in primitive neuroectodermal tumors). The molecular identity of Ewing sarcoma with primitive neuroectodermal tumors has led to a grouping known as the Ewing sarcoma family of tumors based on the molecular pathology; Ewing sarcoma and primitive neuroectodermal tumor are now considered synonymous. Ewing sarcoma accounts for about 10% to 14% of primary malignant bone tumors in whites, but it is rare in blacks. Its incidence peaks between the ages of 10 and 25 years, with a 2:1 male-to-female ratio. Both Ewing sarcoma and osteosarcoma occur primarily in the same sex and age group, but they can be clinically distinguished by other characteristics. The most common sites of occurrence include the femur (27%), pelvis (18%), and tibia or fibula (17%).

Patients with Ewing sarcoma of bone often present with pain and a rapidly enlarging mass and may have fever, leukocytosis, and an elevated erythrocyte sedimentation rate (sometimes mimicking osteomyelitis). Early diagnosis of Ewing sarcoma involving the pelvic bones may be delayed because of poorly localized pain and a clinically inapparent mass. Patients may also have pulmonary symptoms, indicating lung metastases, or spinal cord compression, resulting from metastatic deposits in vertebrae. Radiographically, Ewing sarcoma characteristically presents as a fusiform enlargement of the long bones with central mottling

("cracked ice"), indicating a permeative type of bone destruction, and "onion-skin" layering of the periosteal reaction. Initial diagnostic evaluation should include CT and/or magnetic resonance imaging (MRI) scans of the primary site, as well as imaging of the chest and liver, since those are common sites of disease spread. Additionally, a baseline bone scan should be obtained to rule out occult metastases at diagnosis. Ewing sarcoma can be imaged by FDG-PET scans as well as by labeled octreotide scans, although the value of these more sophisticated imaging studies requires further clarification.

Microscopic examination of biopsy specimens typically reveals cytologically uniform, small, round cells with scant cytoplasm arranged in sheets, bordered by fibrous septae. Immunohistochemical staining for CD99 (O-13) reveals diffuse membranous reactivity. The periodic acid–Schiff stain is positive for glycogen, which can be digested by the diastase reaction. Electron microscopy can confirm the presence of large quantities of glycogen. The latter two features have largely been supplanted by immunohistochemistry. Cytogenetic evaluation, looking for translocations involving the long arm of chromosome 22 (most commonly t(11;22)), or fluorescence in situ hybridization (FISH) evaluation for *EWSR1* rearrangement, is helpful to confirm the diagnosis, particularly in small biopsy specimens or when the histologic and/or clinical features are not typical. FISH can be performed on paraffin-embedded archival material.

Current aggressive multimodality treatment results in long-term disease-free survival in about 70% of children under 16 years of age who present with localized Ewing sarcoma. It is estimated that up to 10% of patients with metastases may also be cured, although this is generally noted in the pediatric population. Metastases most frequently involve the lung, bone, bone marrow, and spinal cord. Survival rates correlate inversely with age: 70% of patients under 10 years of age survive as compared with 46% of those 16 years and older. This may be due in part to differences in the resectability of the disease and a disproportionate finding of unresectable pelvic and proximal sites of disease in adults, or perhaps due to a difference in the ability of older adults to tolerate the high-dose chemotherapy required for adequate treatment.

Chondrosarcomas

Malignant tumors of bone that produce cartilage but no osteoid are defined as chondrosarcomas. They account for 17% to 22% of primary malignant bone tumors and are the second most common bone sarcoma. Their incidence increases steadily with age. Primary lesions occur in previously normal bone, whereas secondary chondrosarcomas arise in prior benign lesions, most frequently enchondromas. Malignant degeneration in multiple enchondromatosis (Ollier disease) is reported in patients with this condition alone or in association with soft tissue hemangiomas (Maffucci disease). Chondrosarcomas in patients with multiple enchondromatosis are generally low-grade. About a tenth of radiation-associated sarcomas are chondrosarcomas, and secondary tumors may also arise in bone affected by Paget's disease. The most common sites of involvement for primary chondrosarcoma are the pelvis (31%), femur (21%), shoulder (13%), ribs (9%), and face (9%). Lesions may be painful, especially if they increase rapidly in size, or they may present as a painless mass.

Radiographically, central chondrosarcomas show fluffy, popcorn-like calcifications. Peripheral tumors, on the other hand, tend to have long, lightly calcified spicules radiating from the cortex to a flattened outer surface, with little evidence of cortical or medullary involvement. A faint Codman triangle may be evident as a result of lifting of the periosteum. Chondrosarcomas tend to take up radionuclides avidly during bone scanning. In their gross aspect, chondrosarcomas have translucent, bluish white, mucoid surfaces; reactive new bone formation is seen in slow-growing lesions, or cortical destruction may be evident, marking high-grade, rapidly enlarging lesions. Its microscopic appearance is characterized by the appearance of cartilage with malignant chondrocytes. Especially in low-grade lesions, the histologic character of a tumor is an unreliable predictor of biologic behavior, since similar lesions may behave differently depending on age, site of origin, lesion size, and particularly radiographic appearance. Rare variants include clear cell chondrosarcoma and mesenchymal chondrosarcoma. The clear cell type, which occurs predominantly in the femoral head or humeral head of adult men, is marked by local recurrences and eventual metastases. Mesenchymal chondrosarcoma is characterized histologically by a small round cell tumor with foci of well-differentiated cartilage. This tumor tends to arise in the ribs, mandible, maxilla, skull, and extraskeletal sites. Extraskeletal myxoid chondrosarcoma (which nearly always arises in deep soft tissue and very rarely in bone), despite its name, is not a chondrosarcoma at all but instead a distinctive myxoid sarcoma of uncertain lineage characterized by translocations involving the *EWS* gene on chromosome 22q.

Because local recurrences generally increase the histopathologic grade of the tumor, and because chondrosarcomas are quite resistant to both radiation therapy and chemotherapy, every effort should be made to resect the primary lesion completely. Thus, expert aggressive resection is indicated, particularly of eminently curable, low-grade chondrosarcomas.

Giant Cell Tumor of Bone

Constituting 5% of primary tumors of bone, giant cell tumor of bone is an unusual lesion that may behave locally in an aggressive manner but has a very low metastatic potential. Incidence of the lesion peaks in the third decade. Fifty-five percent of affected individuals are women. Half of giant cell tumors of bone are located around the knee, arising in the distal femur, patella, or proximal tibia or fibula. Lesions may rarely be associated with areas of active Paget's disease.

Radiographically, giant cell tumors are generally eccentrically situated, epiphyseal lesions having a central lucency and increasing density toward the periphery. No new bone formation is present in actively growing lesions. Grossly, the tumor may appear solid despite a cystic appearance on radiography. Microscopically, it is marked by prominent, multinucleated osteoclast-like giant cells dispersed throughout well-vascularized stromal tumor tissue containing numerous mononuclear cells. The mononuclear cells have nuclei identical to those of the giant cells. Mitotic figures may be present and have no prognostic significance. Although fewer than 10% of these tumors are malignant on first presentation, up to 30% assume a malignant behavior after multiple recurrences.

The prognosis of giant cell tumors is difficult to predict. A recurrence rate of 50% or more has been reported after curettage; most patients require multiple therapeutic interventions before disease is successfully eradicated. Wound implantation may result in recurrences in soft tissue. Sarcomatous transformation is rare and may be related to prior radiation therapy. Case reports of putatively "antiangiogenic" therapy being useful in the management of metastatic, unresectable giant cell tumor of bone suggest that this tumor type may be sensitive to agents such as recombinant human interferon-α, but these anecdotes have not been confirmed in larger trials. The most interesting approach to the management of giant cell tumor of bone involves the monoclonal antibody known as denosuman, which targets the osteoprotegerin/receptor activator of nuclear factor κB (RANK) ligand.

Chordoma

Chordoma, representing 1% of malignant bone tumors, arises from remnants of the embryologic notochord, generally in the cervical or sacral area. The peak incidence is in the fifth to seventh decades. Sacral lesions generally occur in older patients, with a median age of 56 years as compared with 47 years for cervical lesions. Sacral lesions result in pain, usually of over a year's duration before diagnosis; the pain is sometimes referred to the hip or knee. Neurologic bowel or bladder symptoms may be the presenting manifestations. Eighty percent of patients with cranial chordomas report headache. Cranial nerve signs, chiasmal involvement, or endocrine abnormalities may be present. Nasopharyngeal chordomas present as a mass with nasal obstruction before neurologic involvement. Osteolysis of one or more vertebral bodies and a soft tissue mass herald the presence of a sacral chordoma. Cranial chordomas present with destruction of the sella, the clinoid, the clivus, and the apices of the petrous bones. On gross examination, chordomas are lobulated, pseudoencapsulated masses varying in consistency from jelly-like to cartilaginous. Microscopically, the tumor is composed of cords of epithelioid cells with abundant eosinophilic cytoplasm. Intracellular and extracellular mucin production is prominent, and distinctive physaliferous ("bubble") cells are often present. Mitotic figures are uncommon.

Treatment consists of resection and radiation therapy, including promising data using newer radiotherapeutic techniques such as highly focused radiation therapy via proton beam accelerators. Systemic therapy testing the use of tyrosine kinase inhibitors (TKIs) is also being evaluated for unresectable or metastatic disease. Complete resection is seldom possible. Local failure is common, and 5% to 43% of these tumors eventually metastasize. The median survival is about 6 years.

Table 12.3	
Benign Bone Lesions with Potential for Malignant Transformation	
Benign Lesion	**Resultant Malignancy**
Enchondroma: in long or flat bones; in short tubular bones only in Maffucci syndrome or Ollier disease	Chondrosarcoma
Paget's disease	Osteosarcoma
	Unclassified sarcoma (rare)
Neurofibroma: in plexiform neurofibromatosis	Malignant schwannoma

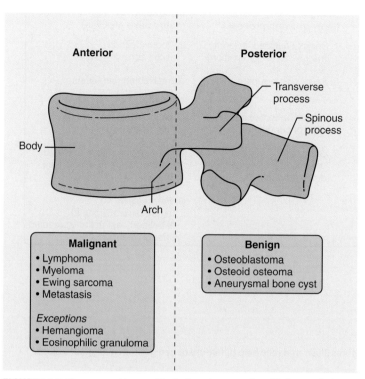

FIGURE 12.1 Tumors and tumor-like lesions in a vertebra. Malignant lesions are seen predominantly in the anterior part of a vertebra (body), whereas benign lesions predominate in the posterior elements (neural arch).

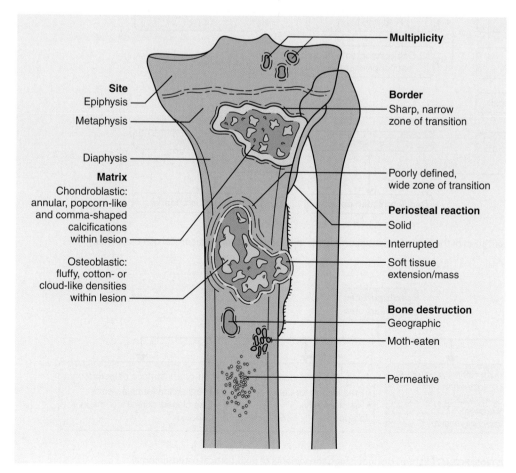

FIGURE 12.2 Radiographic evaluation of tumors and tumor-like lesions of bone. Several features have been identified that help characterize bone tumors and tumor-like lesions. These features include the site of the lesion, its borders and matrix, the presence or absence of soft tissue extension or mass, the type of periosteal reaction (if present), the type of bone destruction, and whether the lesion is singular or multiple.

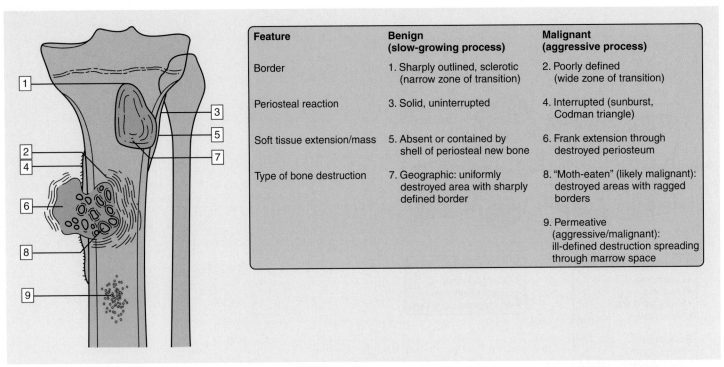

Feature	Benign (slow-growing process)	Malignant (aggressive process)
Border	1. Sharply outlined, sclerotic (narrow zone of transition)	2. Poorly defined (wide zone of transition)
Periosteal reaction	3. Solid, uninterrupted	4. Interrupted (sunburst, Codman triangle)
Soft tissue extension/mass	5. Absent or contained by shell of periosteal new bone	6. Frank extension through destroyed periosteum
Type of bone destruction	7. Geographic: uniformly destroyed area with sharply defined border	8. "Moth-eaten" (likely malignant): destroyed areas with ragged borders
		9. Permeative (aggressive/malignant): ill-defined destruction spreading through marrow space

FIGURE 12.3 **BENIGN VERSUS MALIGNANT BONE LESIONS.** The radiographic features illustrated may help differentiate benign from malignant lesions.

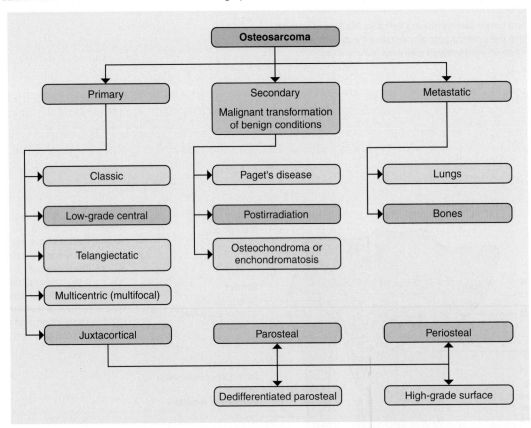

FIGURE 12.4 **OSTEOSARCOMA.** Classification of the type of osteosarcoma, with specific variants of juxtacortical osteosarcoma.

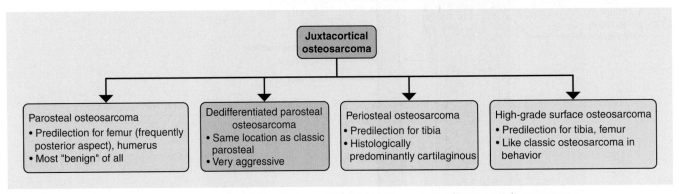

FIGURE 12.5 **JUXTACORTICAL OSTEOSARCOMA.** Features distinguishing the variants of juxtacortical osteosarcoma.

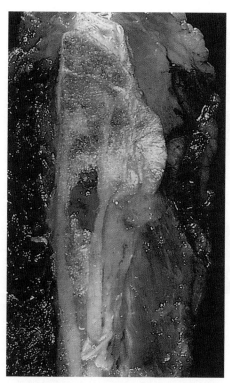

FIGURE 12.6 OSTEOSARCOMA. Longitudinal section through the proximal fibula was made after resection of the bone in a 13-year-old girl. Note the extension of the tumor through the cortex into adjacent soft tissues.

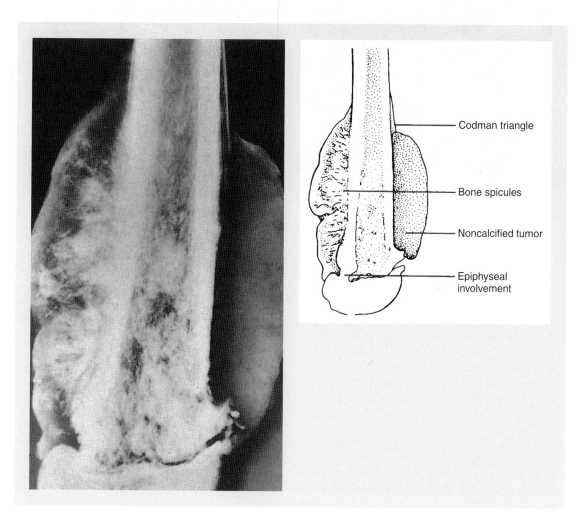

Codman triangle

Bone spicules

Noncalcified tumor

Epiphyseal involvement

FIGURE 12.7 OSTEOSARCOMA. Radiograph of a specimen demonstrates a purely lytic lesion without bone formation, in the anterior part of the tumor. Posteriorly, bone formation has occurred and the newly formed bone spicules are oriented at right angles to the surface of the bone, producing a sunburst pattern. A well-defined Codman triangle is apparent at the upper end of the lesion. Note also the involvement of the epiphysis.

FIGURE 12.8 OSTEOSARCOMA.
A characteristic feature of osteosarcoma is the formation of an abundant mineralized matrix and infiltration of the tumor through the marrow spaces between the existing bone trabeculae. As seen in this photomicrograph, the malignant tumor tissue becomes firmly applied to the surface of the existing bone.

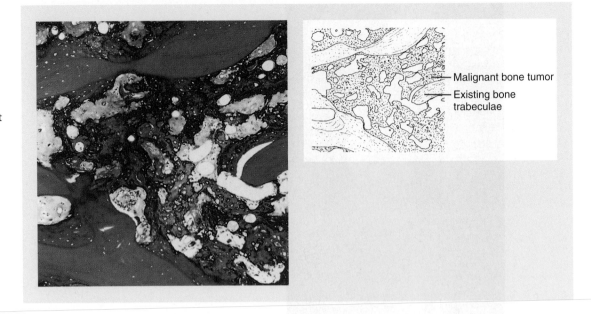

FIGURE 12.9 OSTEOSARCOMA.
Tumor bone has been deposited in a sarcomatous stroma. Note the pleomorphic pattern of malignant cells, many with dark-staining nuclei.

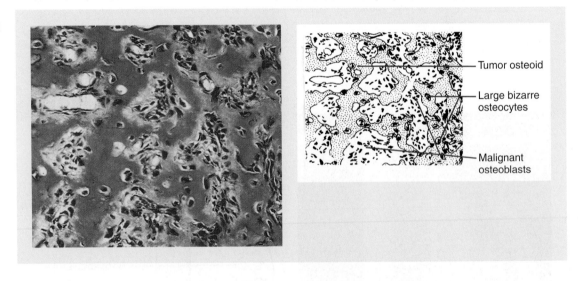

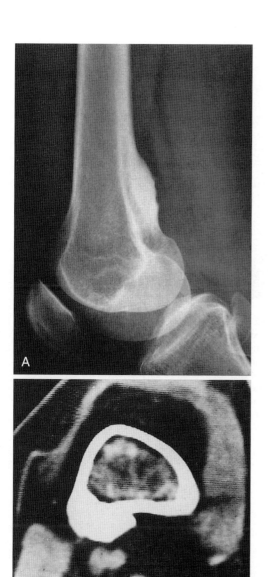

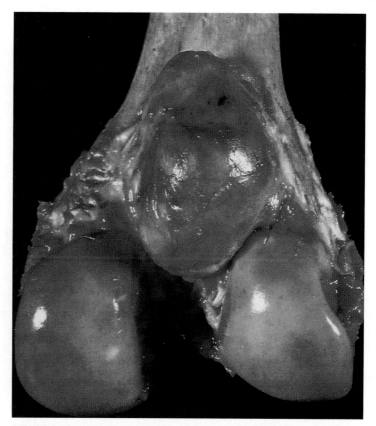

FIGURE 12.11 PAROSTEAL OSTEOSARCOMA. Specimen photograph of the lower end of the femur shows a large mass on the cortex of the bone just above and between the two femoral condyles. This location is typical for parosteal osteosarcoma.

FIGURE 12.10 PAROSTEAL OSTEOSARCOMA. (A) Lateral radiograph of the knee of a 37-year-old woman shows an ossific mass attached to the posterior cortex of the distal femur. Its location and appearance are typical of parosteal osteosarcoma. **(B)** CT section demonstrates lack of invasion of the medullary portion of the bone.

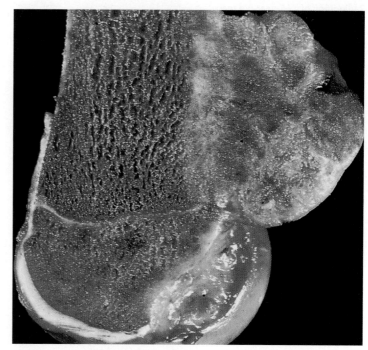

FIGURE 12.12 PAROSTEAL OSTEOSARCOMA. Photograph of a sagittal section through the specimen shown in Figure 12.11 demonstrates that the lesion is well encapsulated and formed of bone-producing tissue. As in the case shown here, parosteal osteosarcoma frequently extends for a short distance through the cortex into the medullary cavity. For this reason, when surgical treatment is planned, medullary extension should be carefully sought and taken into account if local recurrence is to be prevented.

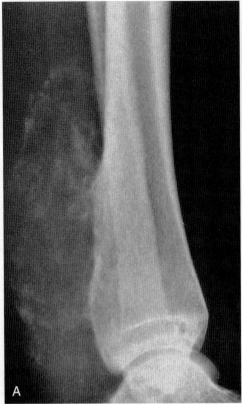

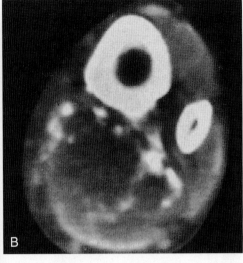

FIGURE 12.13 **HIGH-GRADE SURFACE OSTEOSARCOMA.** (**A**) Lateral view of the lower leg demonstrates a high-grade surface osteosarcoma attached to the posterior cortex of the distal tibia in a 24-year-old man. Ill-defined ossific foci are seen within a large soft tissue mass. (**B**) CT section demonstrates the extent of the lesion. Characteristically, the marrow cavity is not affected.

FIGURE 12.14 **OSTEOSARCOMA ARISING IN PAGET'S DISEASE.** Radiograph of a 65-year-old man who presented with severe pain in the upper right arm shows a large destructive and sclerotic tumor that has developed in the upper end of the humerus, with extension into the soft tissue. The cortex of the bone below the tumor is thickened and indistinct, characteristic of Paget's disease.

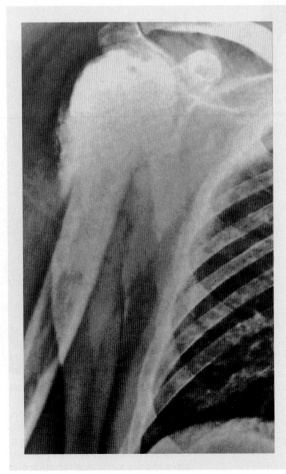

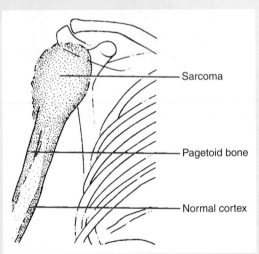

Sarcoma

Pagetoid bone

Normal cortex

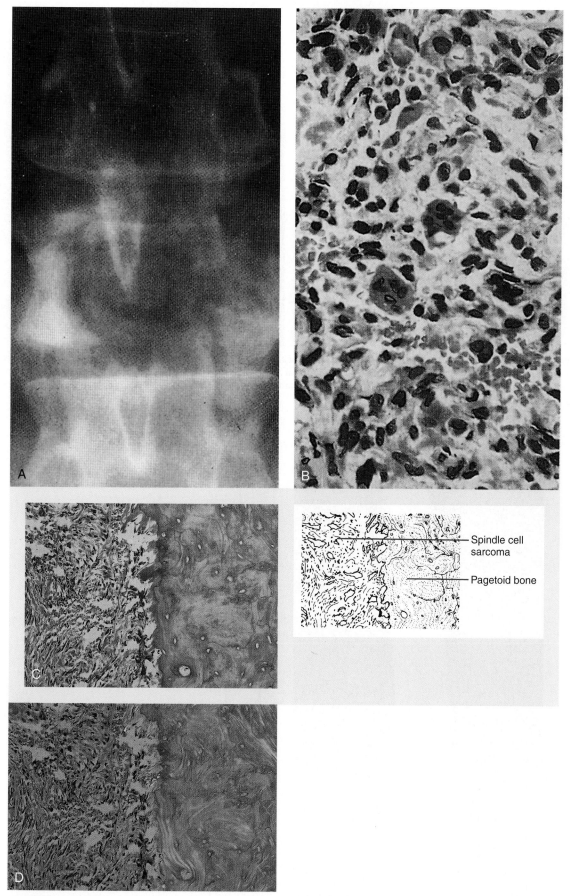

Spindle cell sarcoma

Pagetoid bone

FIGURE 12.15 OSTEOSARCOMA ARISING IN PAGET'S DISEASE. A 58-year-old woman, who 14 years earlier had undergone a hysterectomy for cervical carcinoma, presented with a 2-month history of lower back pain. (**A**) Spiral radiograph of the lumbar spine shows a patchy sclerotic and lytic appearance interpreted to be consistent with metastatic disease. However, there is some widening of the body, which is unusual in metastasis. (**B**) Photomicrograph of a needle biopsy specimen shows an anaplastic tumor with many giant cells, consistent with giant cell–rich osteosarcoma. Foci of bone obtained with this biopsy show the typical mosaic pattern of osteosarcoma arising in Paget's disease. The patient died about 4 months later. Autopsy revealed local extension of the tumor, which involved T12 and L2. Extensive lung metastases had the pattern of osteosarcoma. (**C**) Hematoxylin and eosin–stained section of bone adjacent to the tumor shows an increased number of cement lines within the bone. (**D**) In a polarized section of the same field the disorganized bony architecture is obvious. This case is significant because it demonstrates that even in monostotic Paget's disease, a sarcoma may rarely occur as a complication.

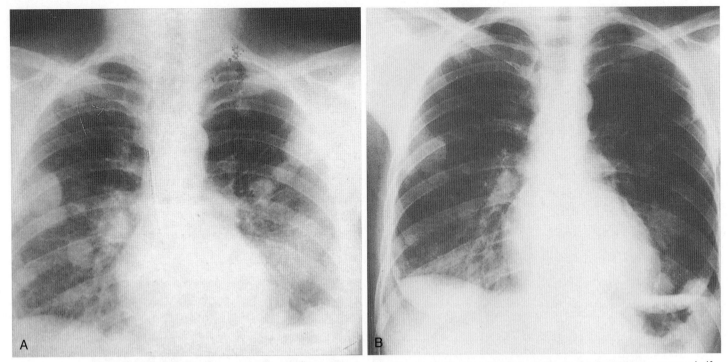

FIGURE 12.16 **"CANNONBALL" LUNG METASTASES OF SARCOMA.** (**A**) The appearance of such metastatic deposits on chest films is characteristic. As many as half of patients who die of metastatic sarcoma have disease confined to the lungs at autopsy. Because metastatic sarcoma is commonly subpleural in location, resection of slow-growing lesions in selected patients results in a 5-year disease-free survival of 15% to 30%. (**B**) In this patient with a leiomyosarcoma, combination chemotherapy has resulted in a partial response.

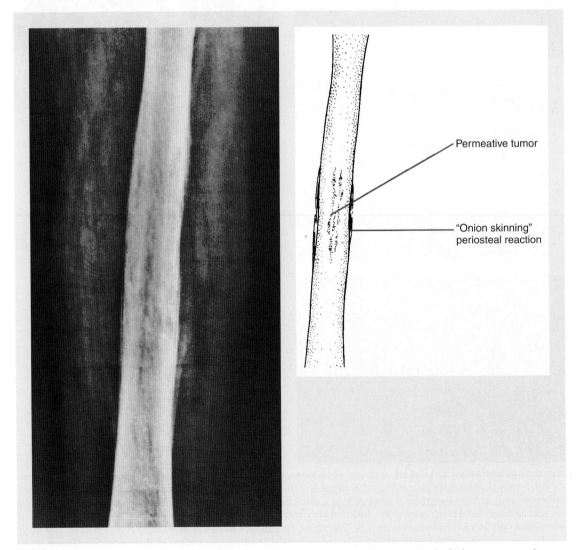

FIGURE 12.17 **EWING SARCOMA.** Radiograph of the femur in a 13-year-old child who complained of pain in the thigh shows an extensive permeative lesion in the midshaft. The overlying periosteum has been elevated and new bone has formed in several layers, giving the periosteum an onion-skin appearance.

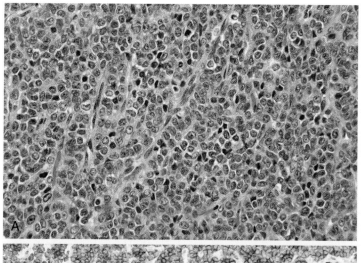

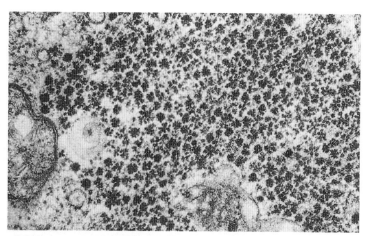

FIGURE 12.19 EWING SARCOMA. Electron photomicrograph of a tumor cell shows packing of the cytoplasm with glycogen granules.

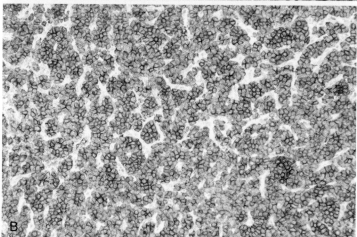

FIGURE 12.18 Ewing sarcoma/primitive neuroectodermal tumor (PNET) is (**A**) a round cell sarcoma composed of sheets of small cells with vesicular nuclei and scant, poorly defined cytoplasm. (**B**) By immunohistochemistry, the tumor cells show characteristic strong, diffuse staining for CD99 (O-13). This expression pattern is helpful to confirm the diagnosis.

FIGURE 12.20 EWING SARCOMA. Characteristic chromosomal rearrangement in Ewing sarcoma.

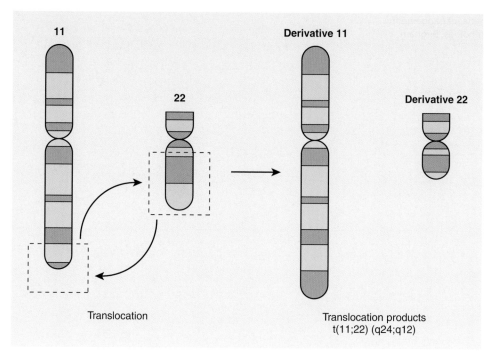

11

22

Derivative 11

Derivative 22

Translocation

Translocation products
t(11;22) (q24;q12)

FIGURE 12.21 Genetic recombination of DNA in Ewing sarcoma: creation of novel fusion transcript.

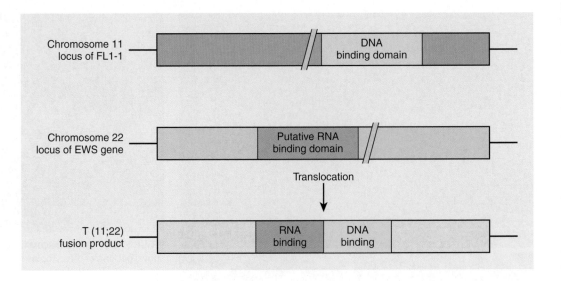

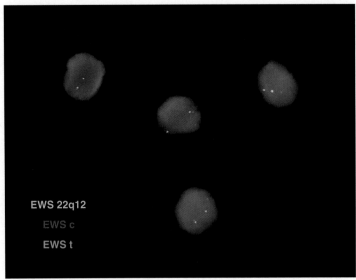

EWS 22q12

EWS c

EWS t

FIGURE 12.22 Fluorescence in situ hybridization (FISH) from a case of Ewing sarcoma using probes directed against the centromeric (c; *red*) and telomeric (t; *green*) sides of the *EWSR1* gene on the long arm of chromosome 22. On the normal chromosome, the two signals are adjacent to one another. The other pair of signals is "split apart" as a result of *EWSR1* gene rearrangement. (Image courtesy of Paola Dal Cin, PhD, Department of Pathology, Brigham and Women's Hospital, Boston, Massachusetts.)

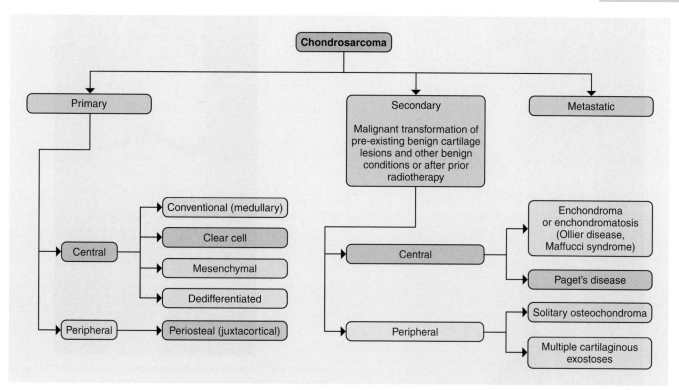

FIGURE 12.23 **CHONDROSARCOMA.** Classification of the types of chondrosarcoma.

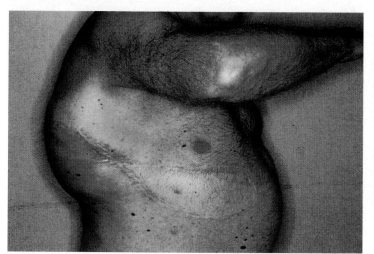

FIGURE 12.24 **CHONDROSARCOMA.** In this 64-year-old man with a long-standing low-grade chondrosarcoma of the chest wall, there is local recurrence despite several radical surgical procedures.

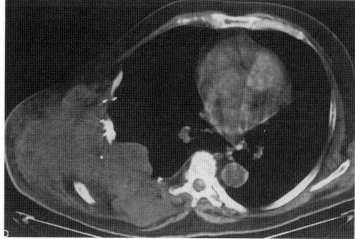

FIGURE 12.25 **CHONDROSARCOMA.** Chest CT scan of the patient shown in Figure 10.27 shows a large, right chest wall mass extending through the ribs and into the pleural space. Surgical clips from previous resections are also seen.

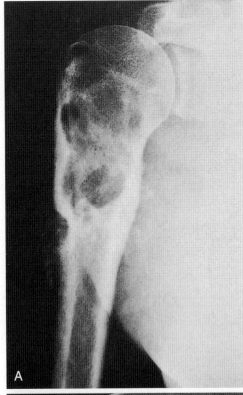

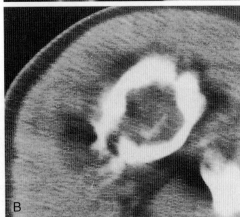

FIGURE 12.26   CHONDROSARCOMA. (A) Anteroposterior plain film of the right proximal humerus of a 62-year-old man is not adequate for demonstrating the soft tissue extension of a chondrosarcoma in the proximal humerus. **(B)** CT section through the lesion demonstrates cortical destruction and an extensive soft tissue mass. Marked irregular destruction, expansion, and cystic areas of the bone are evident.

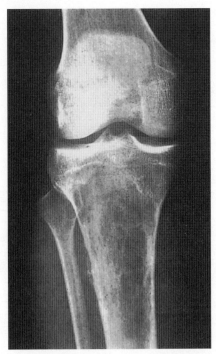

FIGURE 12.27   CHONDROSARCOMA. Radiograph of the knee of a 27-year-old man shows a large, irregular lytic lesion of the proximal tibia.

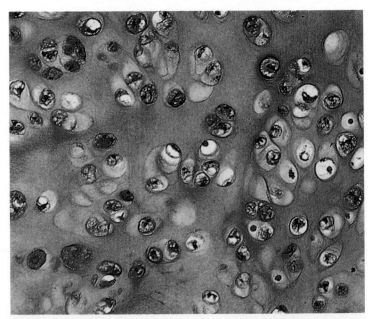

FIGURE 12.28   CHONDROSARCOMA. Photomicrograph shows a moderately cellular tumor composed of chondrocytes separated by abundant chondroid matrix. Cellular pleomorphism and mild nuclear hyperchromatism are evident.

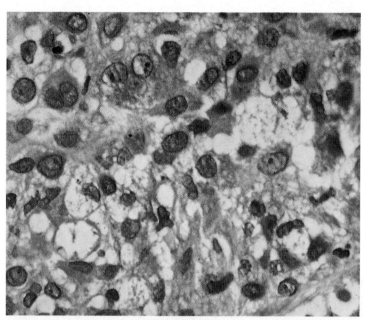

FIGURE 12.29 **CLEAR CELL CHONDROSARCOMA.** Photomicrograph of an area within a tumor shows numerous cells with abundant, clear, vacuolated cytoplasm. Some nuclear variation and occasional giant cells are present.

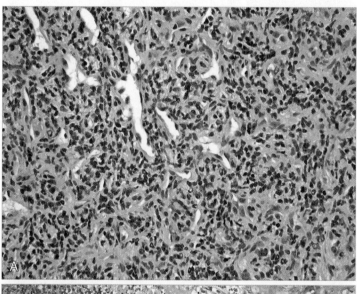

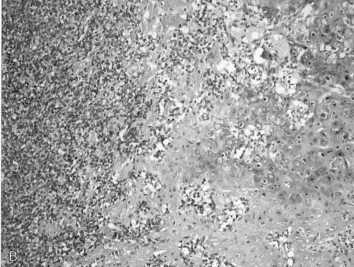

FIGURE 12.30 **MESENCHYMAL CHONDROSARCOMA.** Photomicrographs reveal the typical biphasic pattern of this tumor type. (**A**) Large areas of undifferentiated small round cells, resembling those of Ewing sarcoma, are interspersed between branching "hemangiopericytoma-like" vascular spaces. (**B**) In this histologic image, a focus of bland well-differentiated cartilage can also be seen (*right side of field*).

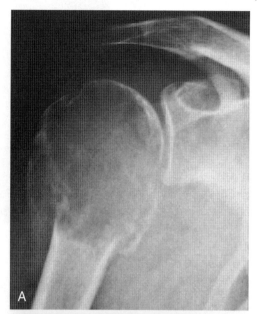

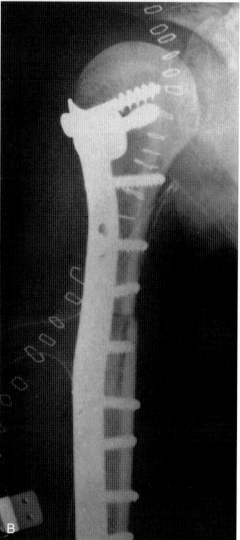

FIGURE 12.31 **GIANT CELL TUMOR OF BONE.** (**A**) Plain film of the shoulder of a 27-year-old woman shows a tumor destroying almost the entire proximal end of the humerus. (**B**) Wide resection was performed, and the humerus was reconstructed by means of allograft.

FIGURE 12.32 GIANT CELL TUMOR OF BONE. Specimen photograph shows the right proximal humerus, which has been sectioned longitudinally, after resection in a 25-year-old man. Note the extension of well-vascularized loculations of tumor outside the bone.

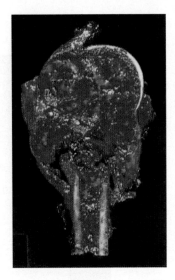

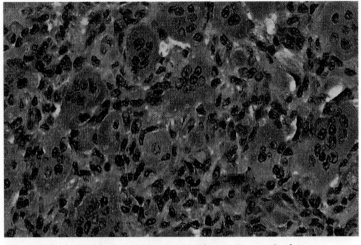

FIGURE 12.33 GIANT CELL TUMOR OF BONE. Photomicrograph of a conventional giant cell tumor demonstrates evenly spaced and crowded giant cells, with intervening polygonal stromal cells.

FIGURE 12.34 ADAMANTINOMA OF DISTAL TIBIA. Adamantinomas typically produce an eccentric, sharply defined osteolytic defect, frequently with infiltration of bone and hemorrhagic and cystic areas. (**A**) Postoperative features related to placement of bone chips after a bone graft. (**B, C**) Histologically, the tumor is composed of epithelial elements within a fibrous stroma. There is extensive diversity of these epithelial elements, with the four major histologic patterns being squamoid, basaloid, tubular, and spindled. These express epithelial antigens (e.g., cytokeratins), which may be critical in recognition of the spindled variants. (**D**) The risk of local recurrence and metastatic disease is significant, with lymph node metastases in approximately 10% of patients. Lung metastases are also common and can occur up to 15 years after diagnosis, necessitating long-term surveillance.

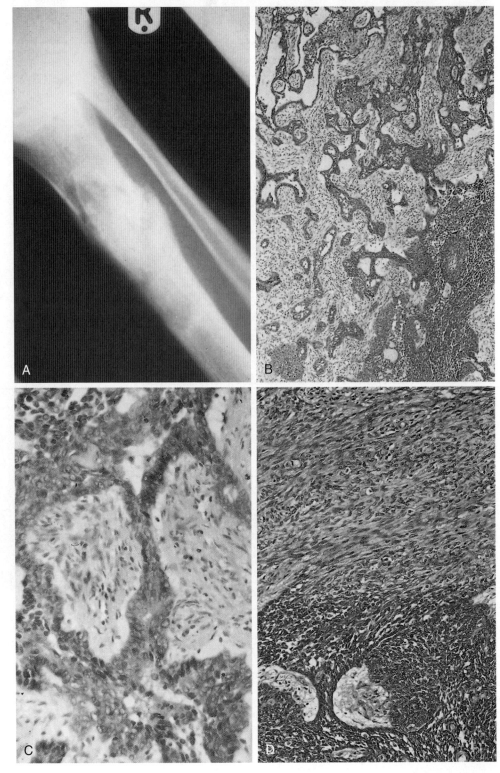

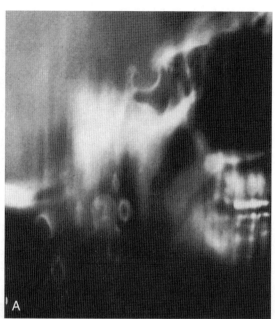

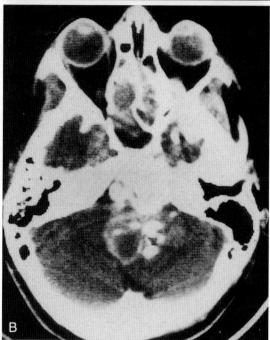

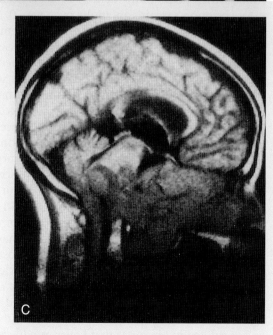

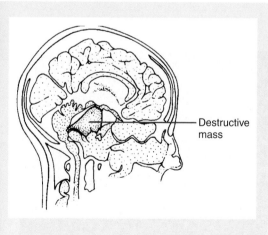

Destructive mass

FIGURE 12.35 **CHORDOMA.** (**A**) Lateral tomogram of the skull of a woman with a chordoma of the clivus that was partially removed 2 years previously shows a large, dense, midline mass. The lesion, which extends anteriorly into the nasopharynx and posteriorly into the posterior fossa, is seen destroying the inferior clivus. (**B**) Contrast-enhanced CT section demonstrates several areas of calcification within the posterior fossa and a large mass occupying the region where the brain stem is normally seen. (**C**) MRI scan shows an enormous mass that fills the nasal cavity and ethmoid sinus anteriorly. It has obliterated the nasopharynx, extending into the hypopharynx. It also extends into the cranial cavity, completely destroying the clivus. It has displaced the brain stem, extending to the fourth ventricle.

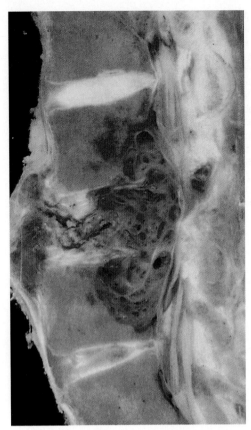

FIGURE 12.36 CHORDOMA. Specimen photograph shows a sagittal section through the lumbar spine of a 70-year-old man who clinically was thought to have metastatic disease. He died with paraplegia and an intractable urinary infection. The specimen shows a destructive hemorrhagic lesion in L3 that involves the bodies of L2 and L4. The lesion has extended posteriorly, compressing the cauda equina. Histologic study revealed a typical chordoma. The lumbar spine is a rare site of involvement for this neoplasm. (Courtesy of the Royal College of Surgeons of England, London, UK.)

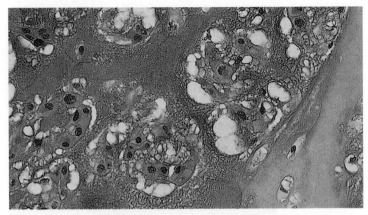

FIGURE 12.38 CHORDOMA. Photomicrograph of the nasopharyngeal mass, resected from the patient shown in Figure 12.35, shows cords of cells with basophilic, round nuclei and abundant, focally vacuolated cytoplasm. The cords are set in a basophilic matrix that is focally vacuolated.

Table 12.4

Osteosarcoma and Ewing Sarcoma: Distinguishing Characteristics

Feature	Osteosarcoma	Ewing Sarcoma
Site of involvement		
Long bone	Metaphysis	Diaphysis
Flat bone	Rare	Common
Medullary cavity	Rare	Common (moth-eaten appearance)
New bone formation	Common	Only secondary
Periosteal reaction	Codman triangle spiculation (sunburst)	Lamellated "onion-skinning"
Soft tissue mass	Less prominent	Large, common
Radiation-associated	Yes	No
Precursor lesions	Yes	No

SARCOMAS OF SOFT TISSUES

Soft tissue sarcomas are a widely heterogeneous family of tumors found in all age groups; they range from orbital rhabdomyosarcoma, which peaks in incidence at 4 years, to liposarcoma, the most common sarcoma in adults over age 50. Forty percent of soft tissue sarcomas develop in the lower extremities, most commonly in the thigh; these tumors may also arise in virtually any site of the body, such as the trunk, head or neck, arm, and retroperitoneum. Patients usually present with a solitary, painless, palpable mass on the extremities or trunk. Intra-abdominal and retroperitoneal primary tumors, when advanced and large, may cause symptoms related to invasion or displacement of organs, weight loss, and pain. The duration of symptoms ranges from a few weeks to decades, with a median of 1–3 months. Soft tissue sarcomas have developed within ports of prior radiation therapy delivered 2–20 years earlier (median about 10 years).

Preoperative evaluation requires CT or MRI scan of the primary lesion to assess the anatomic extent of disease involvement locally. If the lesion abuts bone, MRI may be particularly helpful to determine whether there is periosteal invasion or reaction. Uptake of radionuclide on bone scan is usually not documentation of involvement by tumor but rather indication of a reaction; however, if this is documented at a site distant from the primary, the presence of occult bony metastases should be considered in sarcomas that have a predilection to spread to the bones, such as myxoid liposarcoma, endometrial stromal

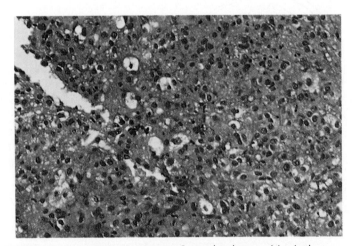

FIGURE 12.37 CHONDROID CHORDOMA. Some chordomas arising in the area of the clivus show a distinctly chondroid appearance, as seen in this photomicrograph. The prognosis for chondroid chordomas in the base of the skull is much better than for tumors in that area that have a conventional pattern. Physaliferous or "bubble" cells, as seen here, are characteristic of chordoma.

sarcoma, and angiosarcoma. Staging is directed at determining whether distant spread of disease has occurred, and this should be performed before starting definitive local therapy. Staging generally requires a CT scan of lungs and liver, the two most common sites of metastasis for soft tissue sarcomas.

The gross appearance of most soft tissue sarcomas is not particularly discriminatory or distinctive. The histopathology, however, varies greatly with the specific subtype of sarcoma, and these distinctions can be subtle. There is no substitute for having pathology reviewed by a pathologist with specialty expertise in the diagnosis of soft tissue sarcomas. Grossly, soft tissue sarcomas are often pseudoencapsulated, fleshy tumors that grow along anatomic tissue planes, thus requiring wide excision beyond the apparent border of the grossly evident disease for local control. However, most soft tissue sarcomas are relatively circumscribed and push aside adjacent structures. Some tumors are characterized by invasion of adjacent organs and prominent areas of necrosis, particularly centrally, as the tumor outgrows its blood supply. Because of microscopic projections of tumor beyond the apparent "capsule," local recurrence follows a "shelling out" procedure in about 80% of cases. Therefore, it is critical to consider a proper surgical repeat resection when a margin-positive "shelling out" surgical procedure had previously been performed.

A summary of the American Joint Cancer Committee (AJCC) staging system for soft tissue sarcomas is shown in Table 12.5. Tumor stage, which is determined by both grade and size, correlates with survival. The 5-year survival rate for soft tissue sarcomas arising in various anatomic locations is similar when it is adjusted for grade. The exceptions to this pattern are intra-abdominal and retroperitoneal primary tumors; these lesions, even if low grade, tend to be large, and at the time of diagnosis they often involve vital organs.

Important new insights continue to be made considering differences between various histopathologic subtypes of soft tissue sarcomas in terms of behavior and specific treatment (van Glabbeke et al., 1999). The goal of treatment of soft tissue sarcomas is to achieve local control and to manage metastases if they develop. In this regard, it is critical to distinguish between clinical scenarios wherein there is some reasonable potential for curative therapy versus those settings in which palliation is the goal. For primary surgical management of sarcomas, wide excision (at least 2 cm of normal tissue) is generally considered optimal, particularly for abdominal or low-grade lesions, to minimize the risks of recurrence due to residual locoregional disease. Limb-sparing surgery, resulting in carefully documented, negative margins pathologically, is preferable if function can be spared. Additional consideration must be given to whether adequate radiation therapy (generally considered high dosing, in the range of 6.6 Gy) is indicated and whether it can be delivered. Radiation therapy may be delivered by the traditional external-beam approach, focused computer-generated fields such as intensity-modulated radiation therapy, or local implants via "brachytherapy," although the latter approach is generally not recommended for low-grade lesions. Careful pathologic examination and documentation of the surgical margins are essential to document adequate resection and to locate any involved margins for further resection.

Adjuvant chemotherapy following complete resection of the primary disease site remains of unclear overall clinical benefit for patients with soft tissue sarcomas. Several well-conducted prospective randomized clinical trials have documented that adjuvant doxorubicin-based chemotherapy improves disease-free

Table 12.5
American Joint Committee on Cancer (AJCC) Soft Tissue Sarcoma, TNM Staging System, 2002

Primary Tumor (T)

TX	Primary tumor cannot be assessed
T0	No evidence of primary tumor
T1	Tumor 5 cm or less in greatest dimension
T1a	Superficial tumor*
T1b	Deep tumor*
T2	Tumor more than 5 cm in greatest dimension
T2a	Superficial tumor
T2b	Deep tumor

Regional Lymph Nodes (N)

NX	Regional lymph nodes cannot be assessed
N0	No regional lymph node metastasis
N1	Regional lymph node metastasis

Distant Metastasis (M)

MX	Distant metastasis cannot be assessed
M0	No distant metastasis
M1	Distant metastasis

Stage Grouping

I	T1a	N0	M0	G1–2	G1	Low
	T1b	N0	M0	G1–2	G1	Low
	T2a	N0	M0	G1–2	G1	Low
	T2b	N0	M0	G1–2	G1	Low
II	T1a	N0	M0	G3–4	G2–3	High
	T1b	N0	M0	G3–4	G2–3	High
	T2a	N0	M0	G3–4	G2–3	High
III	T2b	N0	M0	G3–4	G2–3	High
IV	Any T	N1	M0	Any G	Any G	High or low
	Any T	N0	M1	Any G	Any G	High or low

Histologic Grade (G)†

GX	Grade cannot be assessed
G1	Well differentiated
G2	Moderately differentiated
G3	Poorly differentiated
G4	Poorly differentiated or undifferentiated (four-tiered systems only)

*Superficial tumor is located exclusively above the superficial fascia without invasion of the fascia; deep tumor is located exclusively beneath the superficial fascia, superficial to the fascia with invasion of or through the fascia, or both superficial yet beneath the fascia. Retroperitoneal, mediastinal, and pelvic sarcomas are classified as deep tumors.
†Ewing sarcoma is classified as grade 4.

survival of patients with sarcomas of soft tissues. However, large randomized clinical trials have failed to show an overall survival benefit to adjuvant chemotherapy. These studies tend to be limited by the heterogenous nature of sarcomas and the inclusion of multiple histologic subtypes. Therefore, the risks and potential benefits of adjuvant chemotherapy should be considered and discussed individually with patients based on unique characteristics of presentation, co-morbidities, and risks. Whenever possible, patients should be offered the participation in well-designed clinical investigations to study the impact of adjuvant treatment strategies. Resection of up to six subpleural metastases, especially in patients with relatively slow-growing lesions (doubling time >40 days) and a long disease-free interval (>12 months), may result in long-term disease-free survival in about 20% of patients.

Evolution Away from the Term "Malignant Fibrous Histiocytoma" as a Diagnostic Classification

Characterized as a distinct clinicopathologic entity in 1963, malignant fibrous histiocytoma (MFH) rose to become the most common histologic diagnosis of soft tissue sarcoma in adults in the 1970s. MFH was thought to be derived from cells of fibroblastic origin (based on light microscopy and immunohistochemical staining). It is now clear that a significant subset of what previously would have been called MFH can now be classified under the rubric of other sarcoma terms, using more sophisticated techniques of cytogenetic testing, more appropriate tissue sampling, and immunostaining (Fletcher et al., 2001). The nonspecific morphologic pattern of MFH is also shared by a wide variety of nonmesenchymal poorly differentiated malignant neoplasms (even carcinomas and melanoma). For example, "MFH" of the retroperitoneum can nearly always be found to be dedifferentiated liposarcoma, with the high-grade nonlipogenic elements obscuring (or even replacing) the well-differentiated adipocytic component. Similarly, "inflammatory MFH" is a heterogeneous category, many examples of which are also now recognized to be dedifferentiated liposarcoma. Other forms of MFH can often be reclassified as pleomorphic myogenic sarcomas (e.g., leiomyosarcoma) using newer techniques of immunohistochemical analysis. These various sarcoma types have significant differences in metastatic potential. For example, dedifferentiated liposarcoma has only a 15% to 20% metastatic risk, whereas pleomorphic leiomyosarcoma has a 60% to 70% risk. More than 90% of pleomorphic rhabdomyosarcomas metastasize. Thus, subclassifying pleomorphic sarcomas helps stratify patients to more appropriate therapy or enrollment in subtype-specific clinical trials.

In short, the term MFH is not objectively definable, and therefore, after other diagnostic categories have been excluded, it is preferable to use such designations as "undifferentiated high-grade pleomorphic sarcoma" or "high-grade spindle cell sarcoma, not otherwise specified."

"Fibrosarcomas"

The continuum of neoplasms showing fibroblastic/myofibroblastic differentiation ranges from benign fibromas, such as fibroma of tendon sheath, to locally aggressive lesions of intermediate malignancy, such as desmoid fibromatosis, to sarcomas. In the older literature fibrosarcoma was a common diagnostic category, which was simply based on a histologic pattern. However, large numbers of lesions classified within this category in the past are now classifiable as dedifferentiated liposarcoma, various types of spindle cell sarcomas, sarcomatoid spindle cell carcinomas, malignant peripheral nerve sheath tumors, or even amelanotic melanomas. In addition, specific sarcoma types have emerged within the family of fibroblastic tumors (e.g., low-grade fibromyxoid sarcoma, which harbors a characteristic t(7;16) translocation). A distinctive variant of fibrosarcoma arises in young children (infantile fibrosarcoma, with a t(12;15) translocation), most commonly in the first year of life, although some cases have been congenital; males predominate. Wide excision results in a cure in 80% of very young children. Histologically, uniform fusiform or spindle-shaped cells are characteristic; cell borders are indistinct, and variable mitotic activity, cellularity, and collagen production are present. Interlacing fascicles sometimes form a classic herringbone pattern.

It is important to separate out one entity known as dermatofibrosarcoma protuberans (DFSP). This tumor type affects the skin and subcutaneous tissues and can be cured by appropriate surgical excision with wide margins. DFSP is characterized by a chromosomal translocation involving chromosomes 17 and 22, which causes a fusion of genes encoding the platelet-derived growth factor PDGF B-chain and collagen type I (a-1). This fusion gene leads to uncontrolled production of the PDGF ligand, causing an autocrine loop and altered cell signaling, which contributes to malignant cell proliferation. In addition, recent studies demonstrate that interruption of this signaling by inhibitors of the PDGF pathway (such as imatinib mesylate) may be therapeutically useful in selected cases and has led to regulatory approval of this agent for this clinical indication. Although the incidence of unresectable DFSP is exceedingly low, for such patients a systemic approach using imatinib may be worthwhile.

Myxofibrosarcoma, also formerly known as "myxoid MFH," has, as its name indicates, a prominent myxoid component with branching ("curvilinear") blood vessels, as well as pleomorphic spindle cell elements. Myxofibrosarcoma is the most common sarcoma of the elderly and characteristically arises in the superficial subcutaneous tissues of the extremities. This tumor type is important to recognize, because it has a characteristic insidious, infiltrative pattern of growth along fascial planes (making complete surgical resection difficult) and a high rate of local recurrence. On the other hand, even high-grade myxofibrosarcoma has a lower metastatic potential than most other high-grade pleomorphic sarcomas.

Liposarcomas

Malignant tumors of adipose tissue are the most common soft tissue sarcomas in adults. There is considerable variation in tumor behavior, ranging from low-grade, well-differentiated, and myxoid liposarcomas to high-grade "round cell" and pleomorphic liposarcomas (McCormick et al., 1994). Patients are generally in their sixth decade at diagnosis, with somewhat more than half of liposarcomas affecting men. Most liposarcomas develop in the thigh or retroperitoneum and are solitary, but well-differentiated/dedifferentiated liposarcomas may be apparently multifocal in origin, particularly in the abdominal cavity. They rarely, if ever, arise from benign lipomas. The cytogenetic distinctions between lipomas and the various types of liposarcoma also support different pathogenetic mechanisms between these neoplastic processes. However, certain recent data also point to potential similarities, in certain molecular pathways shared between benign lipomas and well-differentiated liposarcomas (Tallini et al., 1997).

Examination of their gross aspect reveals that liposarcomas are often quite large, with a lobulated surface. On section, the tumors are yellowish white and may have a slimy appearance, particularly in myxoid liposarcomas. Histologically, myxoid liposarcomas are composed of uniform, short spindle cells in a prominent myxoid matrix with branching, thin-walled capillaries and variably prominent univacuolated ("signet-ring cell") or bivacuolated lipoblasts. A poorly differentiated myxoid liposarcoma showing increased cellularity and round cell morphology has an aggressive clinical course, despite a paucity of mitotic activity. Myxoid liposarcomas harbor a characteristic translocation between chromosomes 12 and 16. Well-differentiated liposarcomas may be deceptively similar to lipomas in appearance but show a greater variation in adipocyte size and contain occasional atypical, hyperchromatic stromal cells. Cytogenetics typically reveal abnormal ring chromosomes and giant marker chromosomes with expansion of genetic material derived from chromosome 12q, including the oncogenes *MDM2* and *CDK4*. Recently, antibodies that recognize the protein products of these oncogenes in paraffin-embedded tissue have become available, which can be used to confirm the diagnosis of well-differentiated (or dedifferentiated) liposarcoma by immunohistochemistry. Inflammatory and sclerosing variants have been described. Well-differentiated liposarcomas that arise in somatic soft tissues (e.g., the extremities) are often referred to as "atypical lipomatous tumors" (ALTs; see below) because lesions at these anatomic sites are amenable to surgical cure, in contrast to tumors that arise at intra-abdominal or retroperitoneal sites, which very often recur following radical surgery, albeit commonly 5–10 years or more after surgical resection. It should be emphasized, however, that the designations ALT and well-differentiated liposarcoma are synonymous. Well-differentiated liposarcomas (particularly those arising at central body sites) may contain dedifferentiated areas (which may be composed of sheets of pleomorphic cells or fascicles of spindle cells), often showing abrupt transition between the well-differentiated areas. Unlike well-differentiated liposarcoma (which has no capacity to metastasize), dedifferentiated liposarcoma has a 15% to 20% risk of distant spread, most often to the lungs. Pleomorphic liposarcomas are characterized by the presence of a nondistinctive high-grade pleomorphic or spindle cell sarcoma, with variably prominent pleomorphic lipoblasts. Mitoses are frequent in this form of tumor, and an aggressive clinical course is the rule. Multimodality therapy, including chemotherapy, should be considered for high-grade forms of liposarcoma, since these seem to show sensitivity to chemotherapy in a substantial subset of cases (van Glabbeke et al., 1999).

Dedifferentiated liposarcomas (and rarely well-differentiated liposarcomas) can contain heterologous elements of other differentiation pathways, such as bone (osteosarcoma), smooth muscle (leiomyosarcoma), cartilage (chondrosarcoma), or skeletal muscle (rhabdomyosarcoma). These multicomponent tumors were once termed "malignant mesenchymomas" if they contained three or more different lineages of differentiated mesenchymal tissues. In dedifferentiated liposarcoma the presence of such heterologous elements does not affect survival, nor should it trigger a change in therapy. For example, there is no reason to treat resected dedifferentiated liposarcoma with osteosarcomatous elements with adjuvant chemotherapy, as would be the standard of care for primary high-grade osteosarcomas.

Synovial Sarcoma

Synovial sarcoma is predominantly a tumor of older adolescents and young adults, with a median age of 27 years at diagnosis. It is somewhat more common in men than in women. The tumor was originally named due to a histologic resemblance of some of the tumor cells to tenosynovial tissue and its frequent occurrence around joints, although the tumor does not have any relationship with synovium. Unlike patients with other localized soft tissue sarcomas (who are often asymptomatic at presentation), about half of patients with synovial sarcoma report pain or tenderness. These tumors can arise anywhere in the body and not simply around joint capsules, as was once thought. In particular, it is now recognized that primary pulmonary and pleural synovial sarcomas occur, and this should be considered in the differential diagnosis of difficult-to-classify thoracic malignancies.

Radiographically, about one-third of these tumors contain calcification, from fine stippling to radiopaque masses. Periosteal proliferation or invasion is uncommon. Gross examination reveals that the tumor is usually firmly adherent to surrounding tissues. Histologically, synovial sarcomas can be monophasic or biphasic, with epithelial or spindle cell components, or both. The malignant cells have the potential to differentiate along both mesenchymal and epithelial lineages; both components in biphasic tumors harbor the t(X;18) translocation, which characterizes synovial sarcoma. Synovial sarcomas are high-grade by definition, although there is a "poorly differentiated" variant (which shows round cell morphology and may resemble Ewing sarcoma) that pursues a more aggressive clinical course. Synovial sarcoma is particularly sensitive to combination chemotherapy, and therefore this sensitivity should be considered in developing a comprehensive management plan for any individual patient with this disease (van Glabbeke et al., 1999).

Malignant Peripheral Nerve Sheath Tumor

Malignant peripheral nerve sheath tumors (MPNSTs), also known in the older literature as neurosarcomas or malignant schwannomas, which constitute 5% of soft tissue sarcomas, differ from other sarcomas in that they are of neuroectodermal embryologic origin. Fifty percent of patients with MPNST have type 1 neurofibromatosis (NF1; von Recklinghausen's disease). Of patients with NF1, 80% are male, as compared with 56% of those with sporadic MPNST. The development of pain or the sudden enlargement of a preexisting mass in a patient with NF1 should prompt immediate biopsy to exclude MPNST arising in a preexisting neurofibroma.

MPNSTs may arise as a large fusiform mass within a major nerve, or, more commonly, without an apparent association with a nerve of origin. Most develop in the proximal extremity or trunk, and larger surgical and radiotherapeutic margins are required to ensure local control. Though somewhat similar in histologic appearance to fibroblastic/myofibroblastic sarcomas, MPNSTs show characteristic intratumoral heterogeneity in cellularity, foci of myxoid stroma, and perivascular accentuation, and contain cells with more wavy or buckled nuclear contours.

Angiosarcomas and Other Vascular Sarcomas

Hemangioendothelioma

The term "hemangioendothelioma" is generally applied to a vascular tumor of intermediate malignancy between a benign hemangioma and conventional angiosarcoma. The most common variant of these rare tumors is epithelioid hemangioendothelioma. This relatively rare lesion affects men and women about equally and rarely develops in childhood. The epithelioid variant differs from the benign epithelioid hemangioma in that the epithelioid endothelial cells are arranged in cords and strands, instead of forming vascular channels. Epithelioid hemangioendotheliomas show occasional intracytoplasmic vacuoles (intracellular "lumina"), which may contain erythrocytes. There is little mitotic activity. Metastatic epithelioid hemangioendothelioma can remain remarkably indolent even in the presence of extensive unresectable metastases in liver and/or lung. The utility of chemotherapy or other systemic treatments (such as putatively "antiangiogenic" approaches with agents such as interferon-α) remains unclear, given that this disease can show indolent progression or prolonged periods of stability even without treatment.

Angiosarcomas

Angiosarcomas are malignant lesions of vascular endothelium and vary considerably in histologic differentiation. Described in the older literature under a variety of names, angiosarcomas include tumors previously called hemangiosarcoma and lymphangiosarcoma, since immunoperoxidase stains do not show consistent differences in phenotype to warrant separation. These tumors frequently express the vascular antigen CD34 (an antigen that is shared with hematopoietic stem cells), but the most sensitive immunohistochemical marker is the CD31 antigen.

Of these rare lesions (1% of sarcomas), about one third arise in the skin typically as multicentric scalp lesions in elderly men. A significant subset occur in the skin of the breast of women following radiation therapy for breast cancer. One quarter of these tumors develop in soft tissue sites, and another quarter arise in organs such as the breast, liver, and spleen. Primary angiosarcomas of the breast occur in young and middle-aged women; those of the liver arise in adults and are associated with exposure to thorium dioxide (an outdated reagent used in angiography), arsenic (insecticides), and polyvinyl chloride (plastics). Angiosarcomas represent the most common primary malignant tumors of the heart. As noted above, angiosarcomas also arise in sites of prior radiation therapy (for breast cancer, Hodgkin disease, cervical cancer, and other conditions).

Postmastectomy chronic lymphedema-associated angiosarcoma (Stewart-Treves syndrome) is a comparatively rare complication of radical mastectomy that usually manifests more than 10 years after the development of lymphedema. Although its precise origin is unclear, it is assumed to arise from lymphatics in the arm after dissection of axillary lymph nodes. The prognosis is generally poor; repeated local recurrence and eventual dissemination are the rule.

On gross examination angiosarcomas may appear to be single, but multiple clustered bruises are noted in about half of cases. Tumors infiltrate substantially beyond their apparent gross extent. Microscopically, many moderately to well-differentiated lesions form anastomosing vascular channels. Poorly differentiated angiosarcomas may be difficult to distinguish from carcinomas or other sarcomas. Angiosarcomas that appear deceptively benign under the microscope can be difficult to control locally, in part because of the tendency to be multifocal and in part because of their extensive invasion and high metastatic rate. Histologic grade does not predict clinical behavior, unlike many other subtypes of soft tissue sarcoma. The prognosis is poor overall, especially for advanced disease. Chemotherapy can be effective for palliation of advanced disease, with anthracylines and taxanes demonstrating important activity. A number of continuing trials are evaluating the impact of compounds with antiangiogenic activity in this disease.

Kaposi Sarcoma

This subtype of vascular sarcoma classically presents as multiple blue-red nodules that progress in an indolent manner up the lower legs; it generally occurs in elderly men of Mediterranean origin. A second variant of Kaposi sarcoma occurs in about 0.4% of renal transplant patients; interestingly, this form is also more common in men of Mediterranean extraction. Developing a mean of 16 months after transplantation, Kaposi sarcoma may respond to a decrease in immunosuppressive therapy. A more aggressive endemic form of lymphadenopathic Kaposi sarcoma has been described in Africa, particularly in young children.

A highly aggressive form of Kaposi sarcoma has been associated with human immunodeficiency virus 1–associated acquired immunodeficiency syndrome (AIDS). The lesions involve the mucous membranes of the mouth, stomach, lungs, skin, and lymph nodes. Coexistent opportunistic infections portend a short survival. Lesions progress from flat ("patch-stage") to plaquelike and then nodular lesions that may ulcerate. In the past the fatality of this disease often resulted from uncontrolled disease in the lungs and GI tract. In the era of modern highly effective combination retroviral therapy, this disease has become much less prevalent. Human herpesvirus 8 is important in the pathogenesis of both the human immunodeficiency virus–associated type as well as the sporadic form of Kaposi sarcoma (Landau et al., 2001; Froehner and Wirth, 2001).

Solitary Fibrous Tumor/Hemangiopericytoma

Hemangiopericytoma (HPC) was originally so named because it was thought to arise from vascular pericytes, primarily because of the very prominent vascularity in these lesions. However, it is now known that this tumor type has no relationship to pericytes and instead shows fibroblastic differentiation. The tumors formerly known as HPC are now widely regarded to be indistinguishable from uniformly cellular solitary fibrous tumors (SFTs; first recognized in the pleura but now known to occur at a wide range of anatomic sites). The incidence of SFT/HPC peaks in the fifth decade of life. Thirty-five percent of tumors are found in the thigh and 25% in the retroperitoneum, often in a perirenal location. Hypoglycemia is rare, associated predominantly with large retroperitoneal tumors (due to tumor-derived production of insulin-like growth factor). Intracranial (meningeal) HPC/SFTs (formerly designated angioblastic meningiomas) grow along the sinuses, locally recur, and may metastasize characteristically to bone and intra-abdominal sites, often decades following primary excision.

The histologic appearance of HPC/SFT is marked by a dilated "antler" or "staghorn" configuration of vascular channels lined by a single layer of flattened endothelial cells. It is important to recognize that the "staghorn" vascular channels that have been described in pathology depictions of HPC are not unique to this tumor type; other types of sarcomas, including synovial sarcoma and endometrial stromal sarcoma, can have these same sorts of abnormal tumor-associated vascular patterns.

Leiomyosarcomas

Although leiomyosarcomas show evidence of smooth muscle immunohistochemical staining, the exact cell of origin is not well defined (outside of uterine tumors and those that arise from large blood vessels). Histologically, leiomyosarcomas are composed of fascicles of elongated cells with "cigar-shaped" nuclei and brightly eosinophilic cytoplasm. Immunohistochemistry for smooth muscle actin and desmin are usually extensively positive. As with many other sarcoma subtypes, leiomyosarcomas may occur in a variety of locations, including primary tumors of the uterus, retroperitoneum, extremity, or head and neck. Leiomyosarcomas have also been associated with the wall of large vessels, such as the inferior vena cava or pulmonary artery. Interestingly, sensitivity to chemotherapy seems to vary according to the primary anatomic site of the tumor, suggesting that although these tumors may have a similar pathologic appearance, there is significant biologic variability within this sarcoma subtype. In very general terms, uterine leiomyosarcomas and vascular leiomyosarcomas have been reported to be somewhat more sensitive to chemotherapy than leiomyosarcomas of other anatomic sites. Molecular fingerprints to define these differences in susceptibilities to therapies have not yet been well defined, although cytogenetic studies have shown that leiomyosarcomas have a complex karyotype.

Multiple cutaneous leiomyosarcomas should suggest metastases from an occult retroperitoneal or intra-abdominal primary tumor. It has been observed that children with AIDS have a greatly increased risk of developing smooth muscle tumors, including leiomyomas and leiomyosarcomas. Similarly, an increased risk of such tumors has been observed in chronically immunosuppressed patients following liver transplantation. Recent studies have detected clonal portions of the Epstein-Barr virus genome within the malignant smooth muscle cells, suggesting a potential causative role for Epstein-Barr virus in the etiologic development of these immunosuppression-related tumors.

Endometrial Stromal Sarcomas

Endometrial stromal sarcomas are gynecologic sarcomas for which quite different natural histories can be observed depending on the grade of the tumor. These range from benign endometrial stromal tumors that can mimic leiomyomas, to low-grade endometrial stromal sarcomas, to high-grade ("undifferentiated") uterine sarcomas. A chromosomal translocation between chromosomes 7 and 17 has been identified in low-grade endometrial stromal sarcoma. These tumors can be viewed as stromal proliferations of varying degrees of malignancy: low-grade endometrial stromal sarcomas show an indolent natural history and can often be cured by appropriate surgery alone, whereas the high-grade endometrial stromal sarcomas (now commonly referred to as undifferentiated uterine sarcomas) typically have very aggressive behavior with a predilection to metastasize early and widely. Additionally, the low-grade variant commonly expresses high levels of estrogen and progesterone receptors, which can be therapeutically important, since these tumors can be managed by antiestrogens (e.g., tamoxifen) or progestins (e.g., megasterol acetate). Undifferentiated uterine sarcomas may be transiently responsive to chemotherapy, but resistance develops rapidly and the tumors progress inexorably. These tumors may spread to bony sites.

Rhabdomyosarcomas

These sarcomas, showing skeletal muscle differentiation, include embryonal, alveolar, and pleomorphic variants. Systemic as well as locoregional lymph node metastases are common. The peak incidence for embryonal rhabdomyosarcomas of the orbit occurs at age 4, and for those of the genitourinary tract the peak is in childhood and adolescence. Alveolar rhabdomyosarcomas, which arise most commonly in the extremities of adolescents and young adults, carry a worse prognosis. A cytogenetic feature of alveolar rhabdomyosarcomas is the translocation between the transcription factors FKHR and PAX3 or PAX7, resulting in the characteristic t(2;13) or t(1;13) mutations, respectively. Pleomorphic rhabdomyosarcomas are rare and generally occur in the extremities of older adults.

Without a multimodality approach to treatment, 80% of rhabdomyosarcomas recur systemically. Patients are generally given multiagent chemotherapy in addition to local therapy. Resection is followed by regional radiation therapy. Embryonal rhabdomyosarcomas of the orbit and genitourinary tract are highly sensitive to chemotherapy and radiation therapy. Pleomorphic rhabdomyosarcomas tend to respond poorly to chemotherapy and have a dismal outcome (Table 12.6).

Table 12.6	
Soft Tissue Sarcomas: Distribution of Primary Sites of Occurrence	
Site	**Frequency (%)**
Lower extremity	
Thigh	31
Below knee	10
Trunk	18
Head and neck	15
Retroperitoneum	13
Upper extremity	13

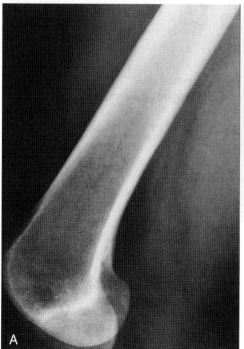

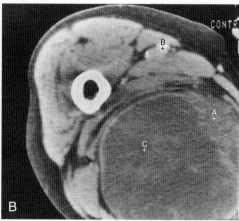

FIGURE 12.39 UNDIFFERENTIATED HIGH-GRADE PLEOMORPHIC SARCOMA. An 86-year-old woman presented with a soft tissue mass on the posteromedial aspect of the right thigh. (**A**) Lateral plain film of the femur demonstrates only a soft tissue prominence posteriorly. (**B**) CT scan shows an axial image of the mass, which is contained by a fibrotic capsule. The overlying skin is not infiltrated. Despite the benign appearance, the mass proved on biopsy to be an undifferentiated high-grade pleomorphic sarcoma.

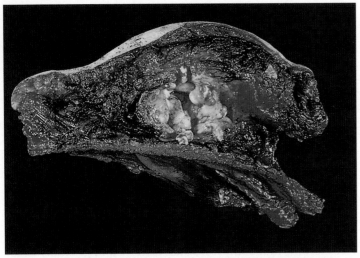

FIGURE 12.40 **UNDIFFERENTIATED HIGH-GRADE PLEOMORPHIC SARCOMA.** This high-grade malignancy was resected from the right upper chest wall of a 60-year-old woman. Note the localized, lobulated, soft tissue mass and adjacent ribs. The black material is India ink used to identify surgical margins.

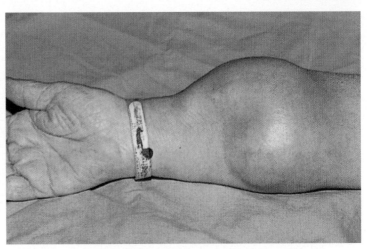

FIGURE 12.43 **LIPOSARCOMA.** This slow-growing tumor of the forearm of a 75-year-old woman was diagnosed as a liposarcoma. Radical resection was carried out with preservation of hand function. Postoperative radiation therapy was also administered. Such patients have a significant chance of remaining disease-free for more than 5 years following local resection, as was the case with this patient.

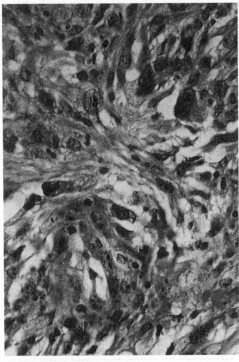

FIGURE 12.41 **UNDIFFERENTIATED HIGH-GRADE PLEOMORPHIC SARCOMA.** Photomicrograph demonstrates a storiform arrangement of spindle cells. The cells show considerable pleomorphism.

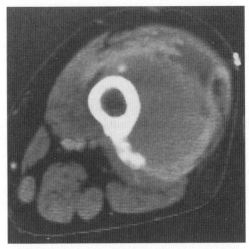

FIGURE 12.44 **LIPOSARCOMA.** CT scan of a 54-year-old man with a slowly enlarging mass on the posterior aspect of the thigh demonstrates a poorly defined soft tissue mass with radiolucent areas and bone formation at the posterior cortex of the femur. Liposarcoma, suggested as a possible diagnosis, was later confirmed on biopsy.

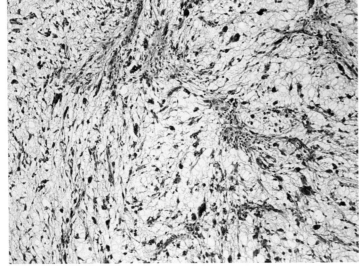

FIGURE 12.42 Myxofibrosarcoma is characterized by scattered pleomorphic cells set in a myxoid stroma with curvilinear blood vessels. Myxofibrosarcoma is the most common sarcoma of the elderly.

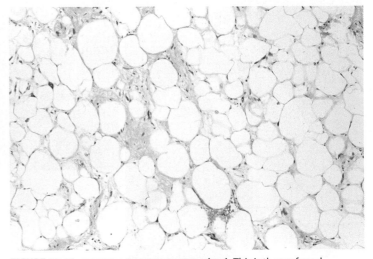

FIGURE 12.45 **ATYPICAL LIPOMATOUS TUMOR (ALT).** This is the preferred terminology for well-differentiated liposarcoma arising in the extremities. Although this tumor type may recur locally, it has no capacity to metastasize. In contrast to the histologic appearances of benign lipomas, ALT shows variation in adipocyte size and occasional atypical hyperchromatic stromal cells.

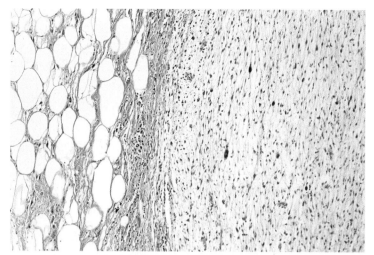

FIGURE 12.46 Dedifferentiated liposarcoma is a histologically nondistinctive sarcoma showing a wide range of appearances. Irrespective of histology, this tumor type has a relatively low (15% to 20%) metastatic potential compared with other types of pleomorphic sarcomas, although the majority of patients with dedifferentiated liposarcoma of the retroperitoneum and intra-abdominal sites eventually succumb to uncontrolled local recurrences. In this example, the dedifferentiated component is composed of elongated spindle cells and occasional pleomorphic cells (*right side of field*). Adjacent areas of well-differentiated liposarcoma (*left side of field*), which is indistinguishable from (and synonymous with) ALT, may coexist.

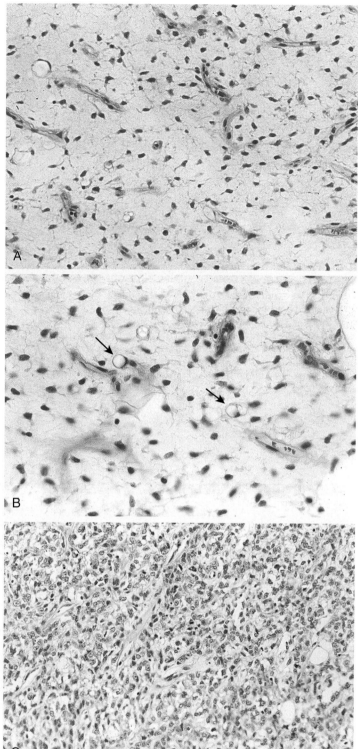

FIGURE 12.47 Myxoid liposarcoma is composed of (**A**) uniform, short spindle cells in a prominent myxoid matrix with branching, thin-walled capillaries. (**B**) Occasional univacuolated or bivacuolated lipoblasts (*arrows*) can be seen. (**C**) High-grade myxoid liposarcoma (sometimes known as "round cell liposarcoma") may be difficult to distinguish from other high-grade sarcomas.

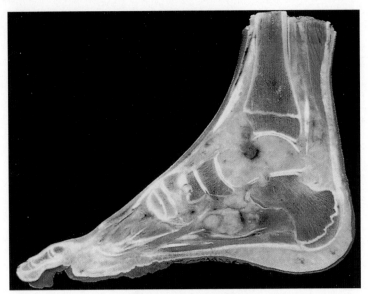

FIGURE 12.48 **SYNOVIAL SARCOMA.** This is an amputation specimen from a 13-year-old boy who reported a painful right ankle for 2½ years. The discomfort had become progressively worse, and swelling had rapidly developed during the previous 6 months. The specimen has been sectioned to show ill-defined, pale tumor masses, which were in continuity in vivo but are now apparent in the sole of the foot, beneath the calcaneal tendon, and on the upper surface of the talus. The tumor has widely invaded bone and soft tissues.

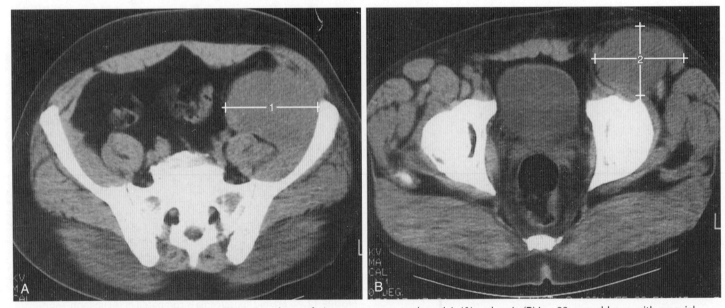

FIGURE 12.49 **SYNOVIAL SARCOMA METASTASES.** CT sections show soft tissue metastases to the pelvis (**A**) and groin (**B**) in a 22-year-old man with synovial sarcoma originating in the thigh.

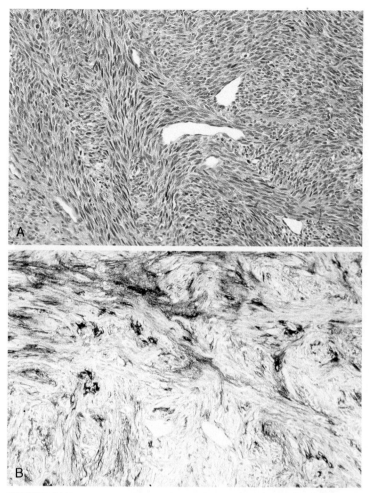

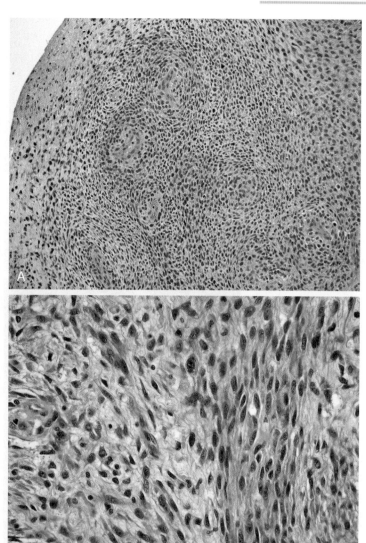

FIGURE 12.50 **SYNOVIAL SARCOMA.** Synovial sarcoma is a relatively common sarcoma whose tissue of origin is unknown. Its name derives from frequent occurrence in para-articular regions and occasional histologic resemblance to synovium. It most commonly occurs in the extremities of adolescents and young adults. Monophasic synovial sarcoma (**A**) is a highly cellular, fascicular spindle cell sarcoma that often shows dilated "hemangiopericytoma-like" blood vessels. This tumor type may be difficult to distinguish from other spindle cell sarcomas. (**B**) By immunohistochemistry, monophasic synovial sarcoma usually shows focal staining for EMA (epithelial membrane antigen; *brown color*). The tumor has a characteristic balanced chromosomal translocation t(X;18) in most cases.

FIGURE 12.52 **MALIGNANT PERIPHERAL NERVE SHEATH TUMOR (MPNST).** (**A**) Typical histologic features include varying cellularity and perivascular accentuation. (**B**) The tumor cells show elongated, tapering nuclei.

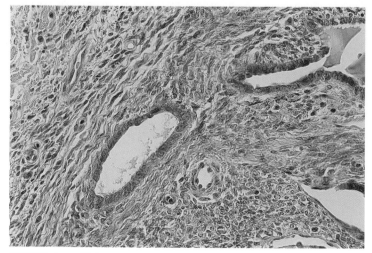

FIGURE 12.51 Biphasic synovial sarcoma shows glandular elements in a background of relatively bland spindle cells and so-called wiry collagen.

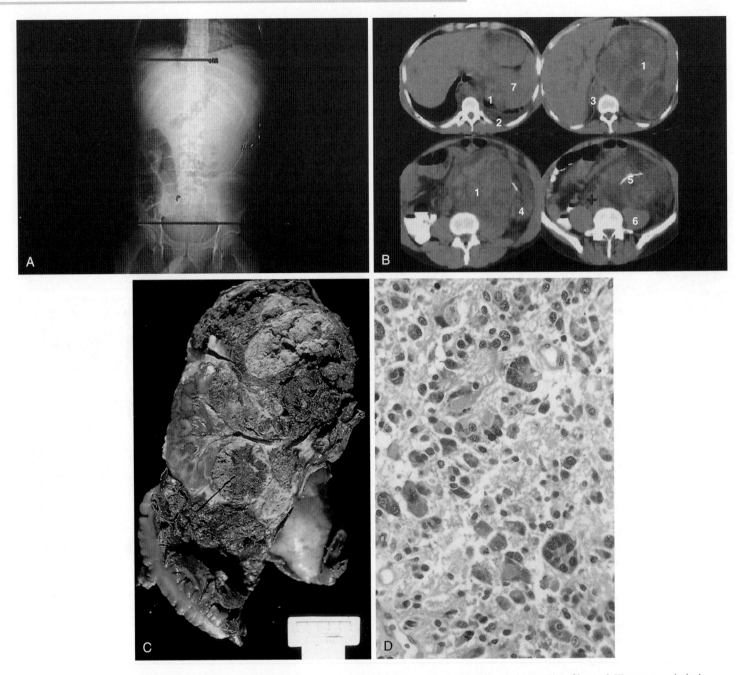

FIGURE 12.53 NEUROBLASTOMA. This neuroblastoma presented in a young man aged 28, with acute abdominal pain. Plain film and CT scan revealed a large retroperitoneal mass. (**A**) Localizing image for CT shows displacement of bowel into the right abdomen. *Black lines* indicate the superior and inferior margins of the large mass. (**B**) CT scan reveals a large heterogeneous tumor mass (1) extending into the lower abdomen. A small left pleural effusion is present (2). A right retrocrural lymph node mass is also evident (3). Lateral displacement of the left kidney is evident (4), with a ureteral stent in place (5). Note compression of the left psoas muscle (6) by the large tumor mass. Spleen (7) is evident in left upper quadrant. (**C**) Needle biopsy revealed a poorly differentiated malignancy, suggestive of sarcoma. Immunoperoxidase studies showed the tumor to be focally positive for chromogranin, synaptophysin, and neurofilament proteins. These results and the neurofibrillary stroma raised the possibility of neuroblastoma. (**D**) The large tumor was resected, and extensive histologic sampling showed some areas with small tumor cells, typical of classic neuroblastoma. The patient continued toward a stable, partial remission.

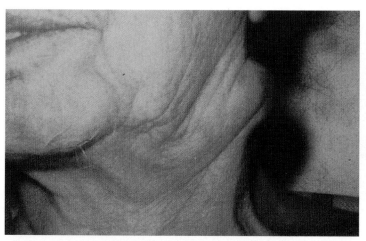

FIGURE 12.54 **ANGIOSARCOMA.** Fatal metastatic disease eventually developed from the angiosarcoma of the left upper neck in this 75-year-old woman.

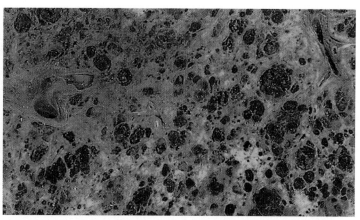

FIGURE 12.56 **HEPATIC ANGIOSARCOMA.** Specimen photograph shows the hepatic parenchyma largely replaced by a diffuse hemorrhagic neoplasm in which multiple small vascular channels are visible.

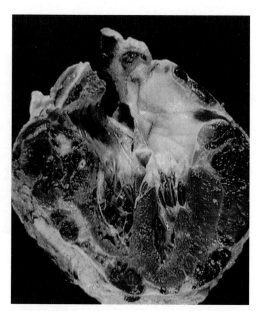

FIGURE 12.55 **MYOCARDIAL ANGIOSARCOMA.** Specimen photograph shows numerous metastases throughout the heart. Angiosarcoma is the most common primary malignancy of the myocardium.

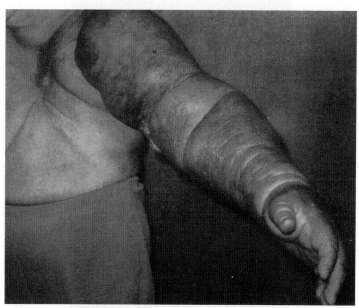

FIGURE 12.57 **POSTMASTECTOMY LYMPHEDEMA-ASSOCIATED ANGIOSARCOMA.** This 65-year-old woman had undergone left radical mastectomy 9 years previously. Massive lymphedema of the left arm had been present since the operation, and in recent months she had noticed the appearance of purplish, ulcerated nodules in the skin of the upper arm. Within 5 months, the entire arm is involved by metastatic disease.

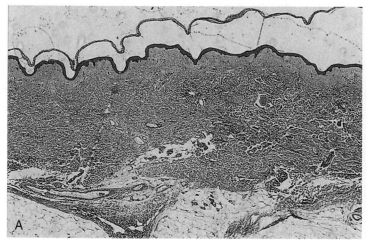
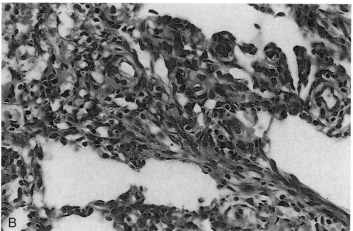

FIGURE 12.58 **ANGIOSARCOMA.** (**A**) Low-power photomicrograph of a skin biopsy from the patient shown in Figure 12.57 shows extensive proliferation of vascular endothelial cells with dissection through dermal collagen. (**B**) Higher-power view shows papillation of cells with hyperchromatic nuclei.

FIGURE 12.59 **RADIATION-ASSOCIATED ANGIOSARCOMA.** (**A**) Multiple small lesions are diagnostic of early angiosarcoma. This 48-year-old woman had a history of Hodgkin disease treated 13 years previously by irradiation. (**B**) The resected tumor shows extension into the subcutaneous tissue.

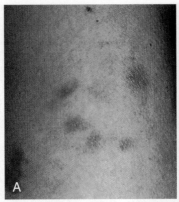

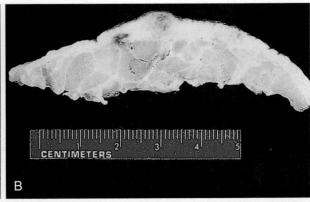

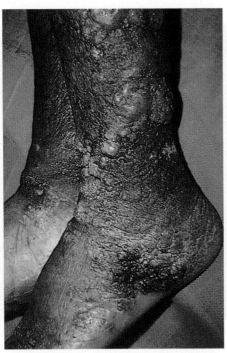

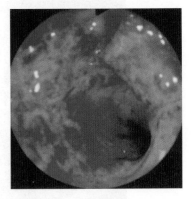

FIGURE 12.62 **KAPOSI SARCOMA.** Endoscopic view shows extensive Kaposi sarcoma of the rectum in an AIDS patient. This is rarely seen.

FIGURE 12.60 **KAPOSI SARCOMA.** Purplish, hyperpigmented plaques and nodules in association with edema of the lower extremities are characteristic cutaneous manifestations of Kaposi sarcoma.

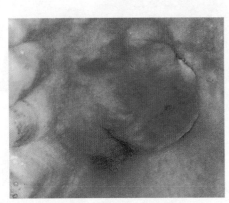

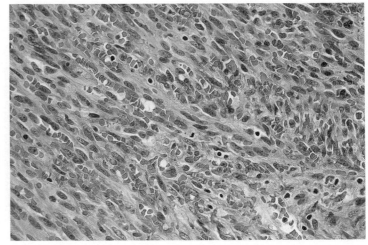

FIGURE 12.61 **KAPOSI SARCOMA.** The palate, lips, and tongue are the most common sites of intraoral involvement. The patient whose palate is shown here was an African with a previous renal transplant.

FIGURE 12.63 Kaposi sarcoma is composed of atypical spindle cells with stromal hemorrhage and scattered chronic inflammatory cells.

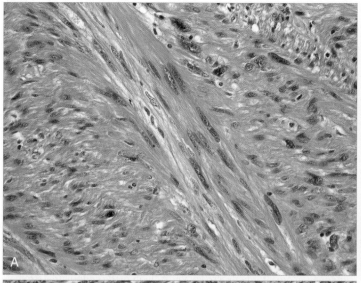

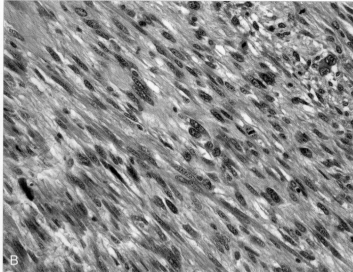

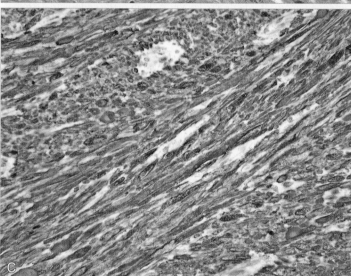

FIGURE 12.64 **LEIOMYOSARCOMA.** (**A**) Low-grade leiomyosarcomas may closely resemble benign leiomyomas, being composed of fascicles of spindle cells with blunt-ended ("cigar-shaped") nuclei and brightly eosinophilic cytoplasm. However, there are enlarged, atypical hyperchromatic nuclei, which would not be seen in benign smooth muscle tumors. (**B**) High-grade leiomyosarcomas show significant nuclear atypia and a high mitotic rate. (**C**) By immunohistochemistry, leiomyosarcomas typically show strong cytoplasmic staining for desmin.

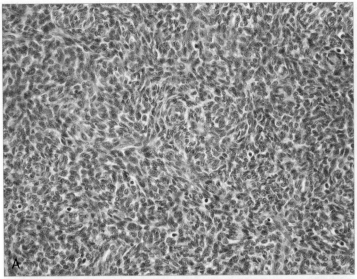

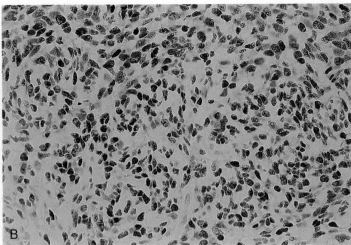

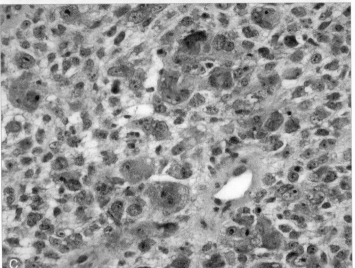

FIGURE 12.65 (A) Low-grade endometrial stromal sarcoma resembles normal endometrial stroma and is composed of uniform ovoid cells with scant cytoplasm and prominent small blood vessels. (B) Immunohistochemical positivity for progesterone receptor is usually present. (C) Undifferentiated uterine sarcoma (formerly also known as "high-grade endometrial stromal sarcoma") is composed of sheets of anaplastic tumor cells. This highly aggressive sarcoma type seems to have no relationship to low-grade endometrial stromal sarcoma.

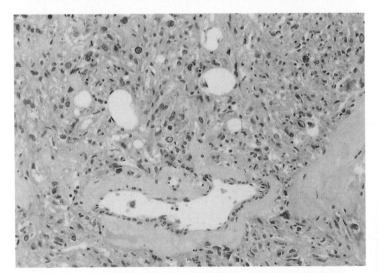

FIGURE 12.66 **ANGIOMYOLIPOMA.** Angiomyolipoma is a hamartomatous lesion that generally arises in one or both kidneys and is associated with tuberous sclerosis. Grossly the tumor is a yellow to gray fatty mass within the renal pelvis. Occasionally, the tumor may become pedunculated, and very large examples may become attached to adjacent diaphragm or liver. Histologically, the tumor is composed of three tissue types in variable proportions: mature adipose tissue with variability in nuclear cytology and cellular size, convoluted thick-walled blood vessels, and irregular bundles of smooth muscle, often with a prominent perivascular arrangement. Angiomyolipoma can occasionally be misinterpreted as a malignant lesion because of striking pleomorphism (as occurred initially in this case) and, rarely, intravascular growth or infiltration of retroperitoneal lymph nodes. Despite these features, the tumor is generally benign. Review of the pathology resulted in a revision of the diagnosis to angiomyolipoma with extensive pleomorphism and, in the example shown, the 56-year-old woman is disease-free following resection of this massive perinephric tumor. This unusual case underscores the critical importance of an experienced pathologist in reviewing the diagnosis.

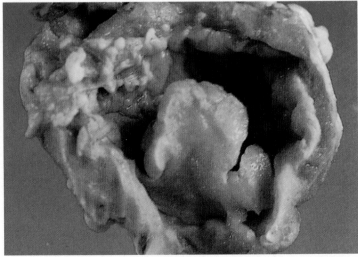

FIGURE 12.67 **BOTRYOID EMBRYONAL RHABDOMYOSARCOMA.** As seen in this bladder specimen in which the walls have been cut away, the botryoid type of embryonal rhabdomyosarcoma produces broad-based, translucent, polypoid masses.

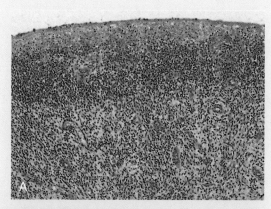

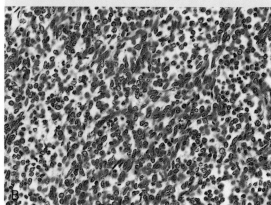

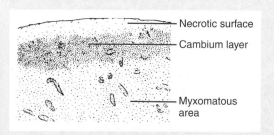

FIGURE 12.68 **BOTRYOID EMBRYONAL RHABDOMYOSARCOMA.**
(**A**) A cambium layer, consisting of a submucosal zone of markedly increased cellularity, is a characteristic feature. (**B**) On high-power view, the lesion is seen to contain primitive, round to oval mesenchymal cells.

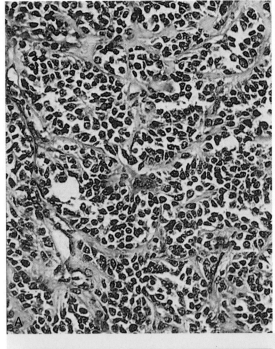

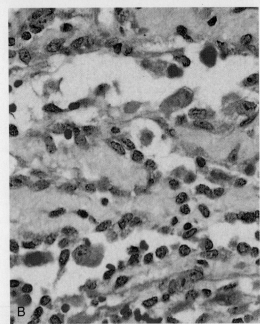

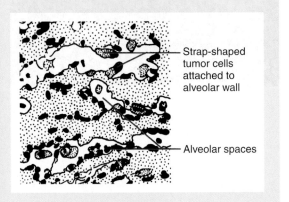

Strap-shaped
tumor cells
attached to
alveolar wall

Alveolar spaces

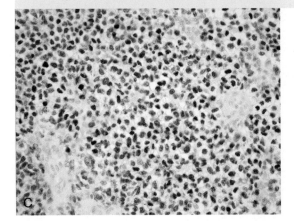

FIGURE 12.69 **ALVEOLAR RHABDOMYOSARCOMA.**
(**A**) Low-power photomicrograph demonstrates fibrous
septae separating slitlike spaces lined by uniform tumor
cells; these can be better appreciated on higher-power
view (**B**). Alveolar rhabdomyosarcoma may also show a
"solid" growth pattern with sheets of round cells.
(**C**) Skeletal muscle differentiation can be confirmed by
immunohistochemical staining for the transcription factor
myogenin (MYOG).

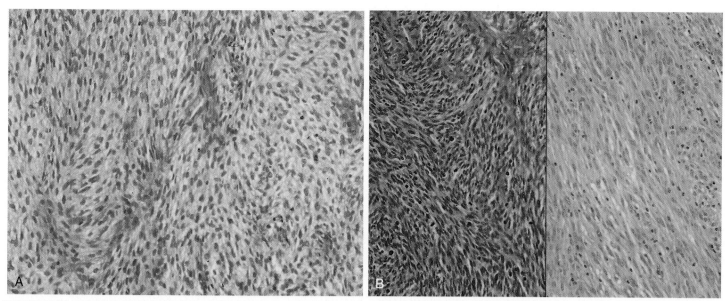

FIGURE 12.70 IMITATORS OF SOFT TISSUE SARCOMAS. The sarcomatoid variant of renal cell carcinoma, an epithelial malignancy, displays extensive spindle cell morphology. This can mislead the unwary toward a misdiagnosis of sarcoma. Note the comparison of sarcomatoid renal cell carcinoma (**A**) with a true sarcoma, a GIST (**B**). Careful pathologic evaluation in conjunction with clinical data and additional studies (e.g., immunocytochemistry, electron microscopy, and cytogenetics) is essential for accurate diagnosis. Pathologists should be consulted before biopsy of such lesions, so that tissue can be handled appropriately. Improper tissue preparation can restrict the array of studies that can be performed and thus limit the ability of the pathologist to arrive at the correct diagnosis.

Table 12.7

Selected Sarcomas with Specific Cytogenetic Abnormalities

Tumor Type	Cytogenetic Aberrancy	Molecular Genetic Abnormality
Alveolar rhabdomyosarcoma	t(2;13) or t(1;13)	*PAX3-FKHR*
Alveolar soft parts sarcoma	t (X;17)	*ASPL-TFE3*
Clear cell sarcoma	t(12;22)	*ATF1-EWSR1*
Desmoplastic small round cell tumor	t(21;22)	*WT1-EWSR1*
Ewing sarcoma/PNET	t(11;22) or others	*FLI1-EWSR1* or *EWS*-other
Extraskeletal myxoid chondrosarcoma	t(9;22)	*TEC-EWSR1*
Low-grade fibromyxoid sarcoma	t(7;16)	*FUS-CREB3L2*
Myxoid/round cell liposarcoma	t(12;16) or t(12;22)	*FUS-CHOP* or *EWSR1-CHOP*
Synovial sarcoma	t(X;18)	*SYT-SSX1* or *SYT-SSX2*

PNET, primitive neuroectodermal tumor.

Gastrointestinal Stromal Tumors

The understanding of GISTs has evolved tremendously since the late 1990s. Understanding of the molecular mechanisms of this disease allowed for rapid application of rationally targeted therapies for patients.

Before the year 2000, the incidence of GIST has been significantly underestimated, with an estimated incidence of 300–500 cases per year. In part, this occurred because there were no clearly defined diagnostic criteria for GIST before the recognition of the aberrant kinase signaling in this disease, and therefore this entity was frequently misclassified as leiomyosarcoma, leiomyoblastoma, or other tumors of the GI tract. However, with the advent of immunohistochemical techniques and the identification of expression of KIT (CD117), it is now estimated that approximately 5000 or more new cases of GIST are diagnosed each year in the United States alone.

A critical understanding of the molecular pathogenesis of GIST came from a study by Hirota et al. in 1998, which first reported activating mutations of the *KIT* proto-oncogene in GISTs. *KIT* (the gene) is transcribed and ultimately translated into the KIT protein, a transmembrane receptor tyrosine kinase. CD117 is an antigenic marker of the KIT protein. In normal physiology the KIT ligand (also known as stem cell factor) binds to the extracellular domain of the KIT protein, resulting in receptor homodimerization and phosphorylation of critical tyrosine residues in the intracellular portion of KIT, thus leading to downstream phosphorylation of intracellular substrates with the net result of cell proliferation and enhanced survival. The vast majority of GISTs (85%) are characterized by gain-of-function mutations in KIT, which lead to constitutive, uncontrolled activation of the receptor signaling cascade and resultant unchecked cell growth. Gain-of-function *KIT* mutations have been identified in several different "hot spots" in the gene, most notably in exon 11 and then in exon 9 and exon 13. Approximately 5% of GISTs harbor mutations in the gene encoding the homologous receptor tyrosine kinase PDGF receptor-α (*PDGFRA*), most in exon 18. Approximately 5% to 10% of GISTs have no identifiable mutation in either the *KIT* or *PDGFRA* gene and are classified as "wild-type" GISTs; nearly all pediatric GISTs are wild type.

Histologically, GISTs are most often composed of spindle cells (70%), but they may also be composed of epithelioid cells (20%) or mixed cells (10%). In contrast to leiomyosarcomas, GISTs contain cells with more palely eosinophilic, fibrillary cytoplasm and indistinct cells, and show relatively uniform, bland cytomorphology. By immunohistochemistry, 95% of GISTs are positive for KIT, which may show a cytoplasmic and/or paranuclear dotlike pattern of staining. Other intra-abdominal spindle cell tumors that may be considered in the differential diagnosis with GIST are negative for KIT. In contrast, immunohistochemical staining for desmin, which is usually positive in leiomyosarcomas, is only rarely positive in GISTs.

EPIDEMIOLOGY

GISTs are known to occur anywhere along the luminal GI tract, with the stomach as the most frequent site (60%), followed by small bowel (30%). GISTs may also occur in association with the rectum or less commonly within the mesentery or peritoneal cavity. Median age at diagnosis is 60, although GISTs occur across the age spectrum. Pediatric GIST is frequently multifocal at presentation. In contrast to GISTs seen in the adult population, mutations in KIT are very uncommon, and it is likely that there are different mechanisms driving the malignant phenotype in pediatric GISTs, which have yet to be defined. Mutations in subunits of the succinate dehydrogenase enzyme have been reported to cause the Carney-Stratakis syndrome, characterized by familial GIST (wild type for *KIT*) and paragangliomas.

TREATMENT AND IMAGING ASSESSMENT

Many localized GISTs will be cured by surgical resection alone; however, even some small tumors with relatively benign histologic features may develop metastasis. A consensus statement was put forth in 2001 to assess risk of metatasis from primary GIST. At that time tumor size and mitotic rate were considered to be the most important predictors of risk of recurrence. This risk assessment has recently been modified to incorporate site of primary tumor (Table 12.8).

Because of the importance of aberrant kinase signaling in this disease, treatment of GIST had been limited to surgical resection, and currently surgical resection remains the standard of care for patients with localized, resectable disease. Initial reports from a recent National Cancer Institute–supported trial have indicated that the use of adjuvant imatinib prolongs disease-free survival in patients with resected solitary GIST, with no overall survival benefit yet observed in short-term follow-up. The benefit seems to be greatest for patients with overall tumor size >10 cm, although detailed subgroup analysis has yet to be presented, including the potential impact of tumor genotype on expected clinical benefit. Additional studies are ongoing worldwide to evaluate in more detail the potential benefit from kinase-inhibiting systemic therapy in addition to surgery for localized GIST.

Table 12.8

Risk Stratification of Primary, Resected Gastrointestinal Stromal Tumor*

| | | Risk of Tumor Recurrence by Tumor Location | |
Mitotic Index	Tumor Size (cm)	Stomach	Small Bowel
<5 per 50 HPFs	<2	Very low	Very low
	>2 ≤ 5	Very low	Low
	>5 < 10	Low	Moderate
	>10	Moderate	High
≥5 per 50 HPFs	≤2	Very low	Moderate
	>2 ≤ 5	Moderate	High
	>5 < 10	High	High
	>10	High	High

*HPFs, high-power fields.
Data are limited for tumors that originate from other anatomic sites. (Modified from Miettinen M, Lasota J: Gastrointestinal stromal tumors: pathology and prognosis at different sites, *Semin Diagn Pathol* 23: 70–83, 2006.)

Patients with advanced, metastatic, or unresectable GIST are now treated with an initial regimen with the selective TKI, imatinib, so as to block the constitutively active KIT or PDGFRA kinases and subsequent downstream signaling. Clinical benefit has been demonstrated in 85% of patients with advanced GIST when treated with imatinib. Resistance may develop, however, after a median of approximately 2 years. The multitargeted TKI, sunitinib, has shown benefit as a second-line therapy for patients after failure of imatinib. Several novel agents are in active clinical investigation for management of GIST that has become resistant to both imatinib and sunitinib.

Inhibition of tumor activity can be seen by FDG-PET scan often within a single day of imatinib dosing. The robust changes seen by PET imaging may lag on CT scan, with patients frequently achieving stable disease by conventional oncologic response criteria (such as RECIST), and it is important to note that benefit may be occurring in the absence of tumor shrinkage as patients with stable disease do as well as patients with bidimensional objective response. Similarly, at the time of outgrowth of resistant GIST clones, some patients may develop increasing nodularity/density within a treated lesion as an early sign of tumor progression. This pattern of activity has been shown to portend treatment failure, although the time course to gross progression may differ greatly between individuals. Patients may also develop unifocal progression due to the development of a secondary KIT resistance mutation in a single lesion, while the remaining lesions remain under good control with TKIs. This pattern is important to recognize, since some patients will do well with local surgical treatment of the progressing lesion and continuation of the same TKI therapy.

Inhibitors of mutant KIT and PDGFR have been the focus of drug development for the treatment of GIST over nearly the past decade. *KIT* and *PDGFR* mutations lead to the activation of many prosurvival pathways. Future directions in the management of GIST will probably focus on inhibition of not only the activating mutation but also inhibition of downstream signaling cascades. In brief, the advances noted in GIST over the past decade are hopefully the paradigm for diagnostic and therapeutic advances that can be made in many other subtypes of sarcomas as well as other more common human malignancies.

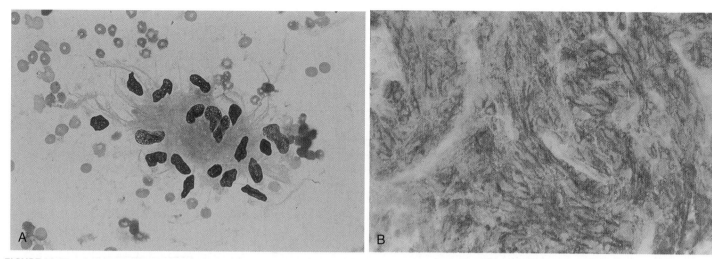

FIGURE 12.71 **GASTROINTESTINAL STROMAL TUMOR.** The characteristic morphologic features of GIST (typically bland spindle cells with abundant delicate cytoplasmic processes) make it possible to make a primary diagnosis by fine-needle aspiration (**A**), when supported by immunohistochemical positivity for c-KIT, performed on cell block tissue (**B**).

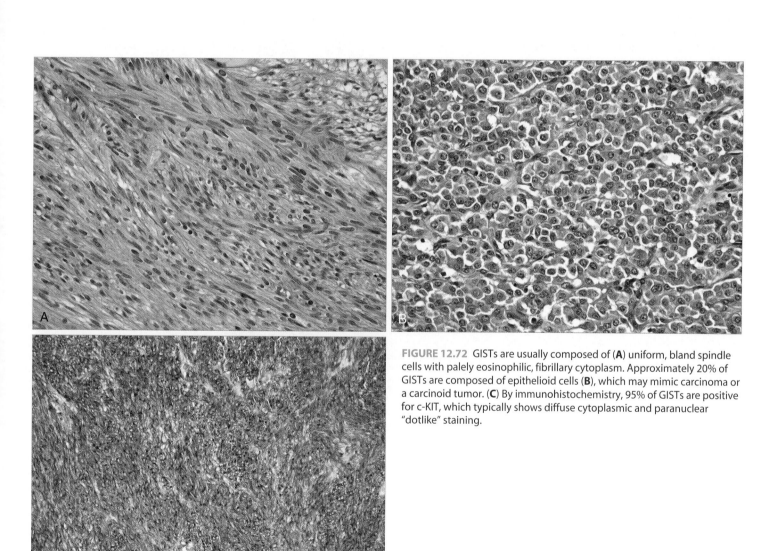

FIGURE 12.72 GISTs are usually composed of (**A**) uniform, bland spindle cells with palely eosinophilic, fibrillary cytoplasm. Approximately 20% of GISTs are composed of epithelioid cells (**B**), which may mimic carcinoma or a carcinoid tumor. (**C**) By immunohistochemistry, 95% of GISTs are positive for c-KIT, which typically shows diffuse cytoplasmic and paranuclear "dotlike" staining.

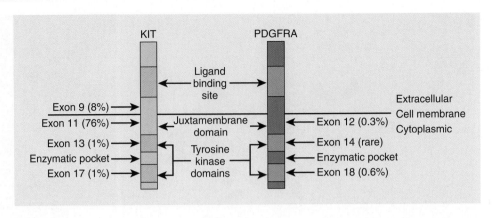

FIGURE 12.73 Distribution of activating mutations in GIST. Activating mutations in GIST occur in the gene encoding the transmembrane tyrosine kinase receptor KIT in the majority of cases. In a smaller number of cases the critical mutation occurs in the PDGFR gene. The mutations are nonrandomly distributed across the receptor, with KIT exon 11 occurring most frequently and KIT exon 9 next most common in frequency.

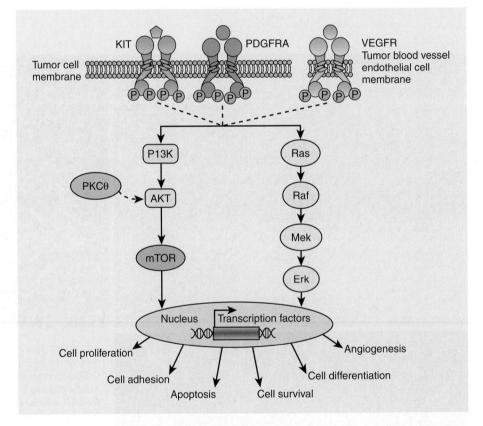

FIGURE 12.74 Activation of the tyrosine kinase KIT or PDGFR leads to downstream phosphorylation and activation of multiple critical signaling pathways that promote cell growth and proliferation. In the majority of GISTs a mutation in KIT or PDGFR leads to constitutive activation and uncontrolled signaling of these pathways. Treatment strategies have involved inhibition of KIT and PDGFR and have been very successful thus far. As resistance develops, newer stratgies are attempting to focus on inhibition of downstream targets.

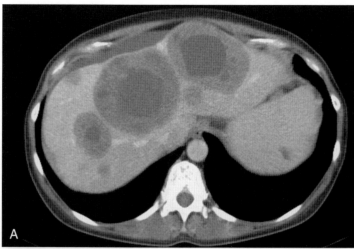

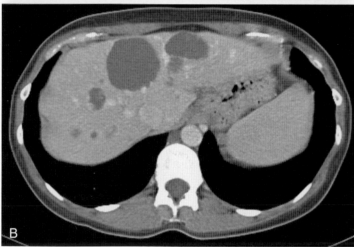

FIGURE 12.75 **CT APPEARANCE OF GIST AND RESPONSE TO IMATINIB. (A)** This CT image demonstrates pretreatment large hepatic metastasis from a primary gastric GIST. The metastases have thick, solid-appearing walls with enhancement, and necrotic centers. **(B)** CT image after 2 months of therapy with imatinib; the tumors became less dense in appearance consistent with tumor response. The tumors are now of low density with a cystic appearance. Although the tumor size did not change significantly, the patient had nearly complete resolution of all tumor-related symptoms and pain.

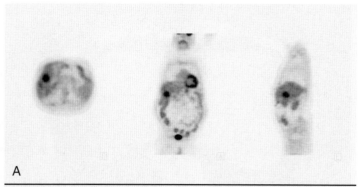

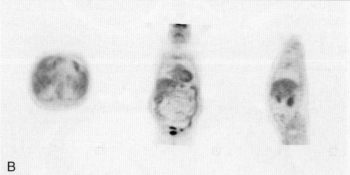

FIGURE 12.76 **FDG-PET RESPONSE TO IMATINIB IN METASTATIC GIST. (A)** FDG-PET images of a patient with a solitary large metastasis in the liver at baseline. **(B)** Follow-up FDG-PET after 1 month of treatment with imatinib shows complete resolution of abnormal FDG uptake consistent with cessation of metabolic tumor activity. Only physiologic uptake remains in the heart, colon, and bladder.

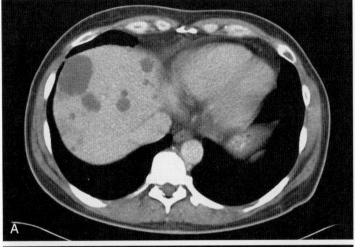

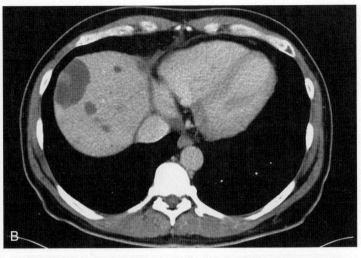

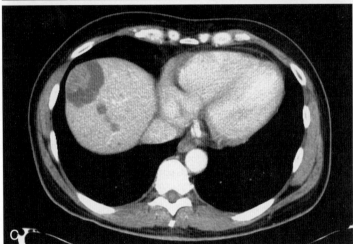

FIGURE 12.77 GIST "NODULE WITHIN A NODULE" PATTERN OF PROGRESSION. (**A**) CT section of liver metastasis in advanced GIST well controlled on imatinib. Tumors are homogeneous and of low density. (**B**) The largest lesion has begun to develop a more solid nodule within the larger mass despite continuing imatinib treatment. (**C**) Follow-up CT imaging 3 months later demonstrates continued increase in the size of the progressing nodule. The overall tumor size remained similar throughout this time period; however, this change in density and CT pattern was consistent with disease progression in this lesion. Molecular analysis of this "nodule within a nodule" pattern of progression has revealed new activating kinase mutations within the progressing nodule that are different from the baseline activating mutation of the patient.

References and Suggested Readings

Akwari OE, Dozois RR, Weiland LH, et al: Leiomyosarcoma of the small and large bowel, *Cancer* 42:1375–1384, 1978.

Antman K, Corson J, Greenberger J, Wilson R: Multi-modality therapy in the management of angiosarcoma of the breast, *Cancer* 50:2000–2003, 1982.

Bramwell VH: Adjuvant chemotherapy for adult soft tissue sarcoma: is there a standard of care? *J Clin Oncol* 19:1235–1237, 2001.

Dahlin D: *Bone tumors: general aspects and data on 6,221 cases*, ed 3, Springfield, IL, 1978, Charles C. Thomas.

Dahlin D, Beabout JW: Dedifferentiation of low-grade chondrosarcomas, *Cancer* 28:461–466, 1971.

Corless CL, Fletcher JA, Heinrich MC: Biology of gastrointestinal stromal tumors, *J Clin Oncol* 22:3813–3825, 2004.

Corless CL, Schroeder A, Griffith D, et al: PDGFRA mutations in gastrointestinal stromal tumors: frequency, spectrum and in vitro sensitivity to imatinib, *J Clin Oncol* 23:5357–5364, 2005.

Delattre O, Zucman J, Melot T, et al: The Ewing family of tumors—a subgroup of small-round cell tumors defined by specific chimeric transcript, *N Engl J Med* 331:294–299, 1994.

Demetri GD, van Oosterom AT, Garrett CR, et al: Efficacy and safety of sunitinib in patients with advanced gastrointestinal stromal tumour after failure of imatinib: a randomised controlled trial, *Lancet* 368:1329–1338, 2006.

Desai J, Shankar S, Heinrich MC, et al: Clonal evolution of resistance to imatinib in patients with metastatic gastrointestinal stromal tumors, *Clin Cancer Res* 13(18 Part 1):5398–5405, 2007.

Enzinger FM, Weiss SW: *Soft tissue tumors*, ed 2, St Louis, 1988, CV Mosby.

Fletcher CD: Soft tissue tumors. In Fletcher CD, et al, editors: *Diagnostic histopathology of tumors*, ed 2, Edinburgh, Churchill Livingstone, pp 1473–1540.

Fletcher CD, Gustafson P, Rydholm A, et al: Clinicopathologic re-evaluation of 100 malignant fibrous histiocytomas: prognostic relevance of subclassification, *J Clin Oncol* 19:3045–3050, 2001.

Frappaz D, Bouffet E, Dolbeau SD, et al: Desmoplastic small round cell tumors of the abdomen, *Cancer* 73:1753–1756, 1994.

Froehner M, Wirth MP: Etiologic factors in soft tissue sarcomas, *Onkologie* 24:139–142, 2001.

Frustaci S, Gherlinzoni F, De Paoli A, et al: Adjuvant chemotherapy for adult soft tissue sarcomas of the extremities and girdles: results of the Italian Randomized Cooperative Trial, *J Clin Oncol* 19:1238–1247, 2001.

Heinrich MC, Corless CL, Demetri GD, et al: Kinase mutations and imatinib response in patients with metastatic gastrointestinal stromal tumor, *J Clin Oncol* 21:4342–4349, 2003.

Heinrich MC, Corless CL, Duensing A, et al: PDGFRA activating mutations in gastrointestinal stromal tumors, *Science* 299:708–710, 2003.

Hirota S, Isozaki K, Moriyama Y, et al: Gain of function mutations of c-kit in human gastrointestinal stromal tumors, *Science* 279:577, 1998.

Ho L, Sugarbaker D, Skarin AT: Malignant mesothelioma. In Ettinger D, editor: *Cancer treatment and research. Part V. Thoracic Oncology*, Boston, 2000, Kluwer Academic Publishers, pp 327–373.

Huvos AG: Ewing's sarcoma. In *Bone tumors: diagnosis, treatment, and prognosis*, Philadelphia, 1979, Saunders, pp 322–344.

Ioachim H, Adsay V, Giancotti F, et al: Kaposi's sarcoma of internal organs, *Cancer* 75:1376–1385, 1995.

Janigan DT, Husain A, Robinson NA: Cardiac angiosarcomas: a review and a case report, *Cancer* 57:852–859, 1986.

Joensuu H, Roberts PJ, Sarlomo-Rikala M, et al: Clinical response induced by the tyrosine kinase inhibitor STI571 in metastatic gastrointestinal stromal tumor expressing a mutant c-kit proto-oncogene, *N Engl J Med* 344:1052–1056, 2001.

Kindblom LG, Remotti HE, Aldenborg F, Meis-Kindblom JM: Gastrointestinal pacemaker cell tumor (GIPACT): gastrointestinal stromal tumors show phenotypic characteristics of the interstitial cells of Cajal, *Am J Pathol* 152:1259–1269, 1998.

Koontz JI, Soreng AL, Nucci M, et al: Frequent fusion of the JAZF1 and JJAZ1 genes in endometrial stromal tumors, *Proc Natl Acad Sci U S A* 98:6348–6353, 2001.

Kruzelock RP, Hansen MF: Molecular genetics and cytogenetics of sarcomas, *Hematol Oncol Clin North Am* 9:513–540, 1995.

Landau HJ, Poiesz BJ, Dube S, et al: Classic Kaposi's sarcoma associated with human herpesvirus 8 infection in a 13-year-old male: a case report, *Clin Cancer Res* 7:2263–2268, 2001.

Lee ES, Locker J, Nalesnk M, et al: The association of Epstein-Barr virus with smooth muscle tumors occurring after organ transplantation, *N Engl J Med* 332:19–25, 1995.

Margue CM, Bernasconi M, Barr FG, Schafer BW: Transcriptional modulation of the anti-apoptotic protein BCL-XL by the paired box transcription factors PAX3 and PAX3/FKHR, *Oncogene* 19:2921–2929, 2000.

Mayer F, Aebert H, Rudert M, et al: Primary malignant sarcomas of the heart and great vessels in adult patients—A single-center experience, *Oncologist* 12:1134–1142, 2007.

McClain KL, Leach CT, Jensen HB, et al: Association of Epstein-Barr virus with leiomyosarcomas in young people with AIDS, *N Engl J Med* 332:12–18, 1995.

McCormick D, Mentzel T, Beham A, Fletcher CD: Dedifferentiated liposarcoma: clinicopathologic analysis of 32 cases suggesting a better prognostic subgroup among pleomorphic sarcomas, *Am J Surg Pathol* 18:1213–1223, 1994.

McWhinney SR, Pasini B, Stratakis CA, for the International Carney Triad and Carney-Stratakis Syndrome Consortium: Familial gastrointestinal stromal tumors and germ-line mutations, *N Engl J Med* 357:10, 2007.

Miettinen M, Lasota J: Gastrointestinal stromal tumors: pathology and prognosis at different sites, *Semin Diagn Pathol* 23:70–83, 2006.

Poon MC, Durant JR, Norgard MJ, et al: Inflammatory fibrous histiocytoma: an important variant of malignant fibrous histiocytoma highly responsive to chemotherapy, *Ann Intern Med* 97:858–863, 1982.

Rubin B: KIT activation is a ubiquitous feature of gastrointestinal stromal tumors, *Cancer Res* 61:8118–8121, 2001.

Russel WO, Cohen J, Enzinger FM, et al: A clinical and pathologic staging system for soft tissue sarcomas, *Cancer* 40:1562–1570, 1977.

Sawyer JR, Tryka AF, Lewis JM: A novel reciprocal chromosome translocation t(11;22) (p13;q12) in an intraabdominal desmoplastic small round-cell tumor, *Am J Surg Pathol* 16:4411–4416, 1992.

Schajowicz F, Sissons H, Sobin L: The World Health Organization's histologic classification of bone tumors, *Cancer* 75:1208–1214, 1995.

Shipley J, Crew J, Guterson B: The molecular biology of soft tissue sarcomas, *Eur J Cancer* 29a:2054–2058, 1993.

Silverberg E, Boring C, Squires T: Cancer statistics, *Cancer* 40:9–28, 1990.

Sjoblom T, Shimizu A, O'Brien KP, et al: Growth inhibition of dermatofibrosarcoma protuberans tumors by the platelet-derived growth factor receptor antagonist STI571 through induction of apoptosis, *Cancer Res* 61:5778–5783, 2001.

Sleijfer S, Wiemer E, Seynaeve C, Verweij J: Improved insight into resistance mechanisms to imatinib in gastrointestinal stromal tumors: a basis for novel approaches and individualization of treatment, *Oncologist* 12:719–726, 2007.

Tallini G, Dal Cin P, Rhoden KJ, et al: Expression of HMGI-C and HMGI(Y) in ordinary lipoma and atypical lipomatous tumors: immunohistochemical reactivity correlates with karyotypic alterations, *Am J Pathol* 151:37–43, 1997.

Tucker MA, Fraumeni JF: Soft tissue. In Schottenfeld D, Fraumeni JF, editors: *Cancer epidemiology*, Philadelphia, 1982, Saunders, pp 827–836.

Tuveson DA, Willis NA, Jacks T, et al: STI571 inactivation of the gastrointestinal stromal tumor c-KIT oncoprotein: biological and clinical implications, *Oncogene* 20:5054–5058, 2001.

van Glabbeke M, van Oosterom AT, Oosterhuis JW, et al: Prognostic factors for the outcome of chemotherapy in advanced soft tissue sarcoma: an analysis of 2,185 patients treated with anthracycline-containing first-line regimens—a European Organization for Research and Treatment of Cancer Soft Tissue and Bone Sarcoma Group Study, *J Clin Oncol* 17:150, 1999.

Verweij J, Casali PG, Zalcberg J, et al: Progression-free survival in gastrointestinal stromal tumours with high-dose imatinib: randomised trial, *Lancet* 364:1127–1134, 2004.

Zagar TM, Triche TJ, Kinsella TJ: Extraosseous Ewing's sarcoma: 25 years later, *J Clin Oncol* 26:4230–4232, 2008.

Figure Credits

The following books published by Gower Medical Publishing are sources of figures in the present chapter. The figure numbers given in the listing are those of the figures given in the present chapter. The page numbers (or slide numbers) given in parentheses are those of the original publication.

Bullough PG, Boachie-Adjei O: *Atlas of spinal diseases.* Philadelphia/New York, 1988, Lippincott/Gower Medical Publishing: Figs. 12.13 (p. 203), 12.26 (p. 196), 12.27 (p. 195), 12.28 (p. 197).

Bullough PG, Vigorita VJ: *Atlas of orthopedic pathology.* Baltimore/New York, 1984, University Park Press/Gower Medical Publishing: Figs. 12.3 (p. 12.8), 12.6 (p. 12.10), 12.7 (p. 12.11), 12.8 (p. 12.11), 12.10 (p. 12.12), 12.14 (p. 13.6), 12.20 (p. 12.20), 12.21 (p. 12.23), Table 12.4 (p. 13.6).

Cawson RA, Eveson JW: *Oral pathology and diagnosis.* London, 1987, Heinemann Medical Books/Gower Medical Publishing: Figs. 12.4 (p. 7.5), 12.33 (p. 10.9), 12.35 (p. 10.8), 12.39 (p. 10.14), 12.49 (p. 7.11), 12.51 (p. 10.20), Table 12.4 (p. 10.8).

Greenspan A: *Orthopedic radiology.* Philadelphia/New York, 1988, Lippincott/Gower Medical Publishing: Figs. 12.5 (p. 16.7), 12.9 (p. 16.9), 12.15 (p. 16.10), 12.17 (p. 16.11), 12.24 (p. 15.18), 12.26 (p. 13.7), 12.34 (p. 13.27), Table 12.3 (pp. 13.14, 13.16, 13.19, 13.21).

Louis MM: *Bone tumor surgery.* Philadelphia/New York, 1988, Lippincott/Gower Medical Publishing: Figs. 12.1 (p. 4.31), 12.21 (p. 4.2), 12.19 (p. 2.14), 12.25 (p. 2.11).

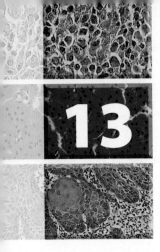

13

Skin Cancer

PHILIP FRIEDLANDER • F. STEPHEN HODI • MICHAEL M. WICK • ELSA F. VELAZQUEZ

Cancer of the skin is the most common human malignancy, and its incidence is rising worldwide. There are approximately 900,000 to 1,200,000 new cases of skin cancer annually in the United States, with melanoma representing about 59,940 cases and about 95% of deaths due to skin cancer (Miller and Weinstock, 1994; Jemal et al., 2007). Although the majority of deaths due to cutaneous cancer are caused by malignant melanoma, nonmelanoma skin cancer is responsible for significant morbidity. Approximately 80% of nonmelanoma skin cancers are basal cell carcinomas, and 20% are squamous cell carcinomas (SCCs) (Alam and Ratner, 2001). SCC is the second most common cancer among whites. Unlike basal cell carcinomas, cutaneous SCCs are associated with a substantial risk of metastasis (Alam and Ratner, 2001). The major factors involved in the development of skin cancer today seem to be a combination of environmental ultraviolet (UV) light exposure and the ability to tan as controlled by genetic differences in skin color. These observations explain the high incidence of skin cancer in fair-skinned individuals and in those living in lower latitudes and higher altitudes. Dark skin is highly protective against the development of skin cancer. Exposure to ionizing radiation, either as part of therapy for a variety of benign disorders or as an occupational risk (e.g., dentists, radiologists), has also been implicated in the development of SCC. Arsenic, which is used in insecticides, has continued to be a significant cause of skin cancer in farmers and industrial workers. Finally, each of these causes may be enhanced by genetic defects in the body's ability to repair DNA and by immunosuppression. Two disorders, xeroderma pigmentosum and basal cell nevus syndrome, are important, genetically transmitted conditions characterized by a much higher than average incidence of skin cancer. Human papillomavirus (HPV), especially in certain sites and in the setting of immunosuppression, has been shown to be implicated in the pathogenesis of SCCs.

Because skin cancer occurs on the body surface, careful inspection is the first step toward early diagnosis. Although each tumor described below demonstrates certain typical features that aid in the diagnosis, any lesion that shows biologic activity—as indicated by change in size, shape, or color—should be considered suspicious. Bleeding and ulceration are generally characteristics of more advanced lesions.

Benign Skin Tumors

Different forms of benign tumors may arise from the skin, reflecting the heterogeneity of resident cell types. It is important to identify these tumors so as to distinguish them from malignancies. Furthermore, it should be noted that many of these benign neoplasms are capable of causing functional disturbances, as well as cosmetic problems.

One of the most common benign tumors of the skin is seborrheic keratosis, which usually affect patients older than 30 years of age (Figs. 13.1 and 13.2). Most people will develop at least one such lesion in their lifetime. Appendage tumors of the skin differentiate toward adnexal structures, including eccrine and apocrine sweat glands, hair follicles, and sebaceous glands. They may be solitary or multiple. Histopathologic examination is necessary for a correct diagnosis and classification of adnexal neoplasms (Fig. 13.3). Other common benign tumors include those of vascular origin (hemangioma and variants), adipose tissue origin (lipoma and variants), fibrohistiocytic tumors (i.e., dermatofibroma), smooth muscle tumors, and neural tumors. Florid reparative processes such as hypertrophic scars and keloids may mimic true tumors (Fig. 13.4). Mastocytosis (mast cell disease) can be classified in cutaneous and systemic variants (Valent et al., 2001). Cutaneous mastocytosis includes mastocytoma (Figs. 13.5 and 13.6), urticaria pigmentosa (Fig. 13.7), and diffuse cutaneous mastocytosis. Cutaneous mastocytosis is frequently a benign condition and especially in children, tends to resolve spontaneously.

Among benign melanocytic neoplasias (nevi), Spitz nevus (spindle and epithelioid nevus) deserves special mention because of its unique characteristics (Figs. 13.8 and 13.9) (Smith, 1987; Spatz and Barnhill, 1999) and the difficulty that it poses to clinicians and pathologists alike when it presents with atypical features. The original name of juvenile melanoma is confusing and should be avoided.

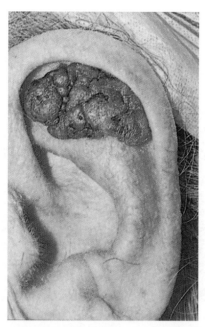

FIGURE 13.1 **SEBORRHEIC KERATOSIS.** A large, dark brown tumor appears to have been "stuck on" the upper portion of the antihelix. Fine cystic inclusions of keratin ("horn cysts") appear as black pits.

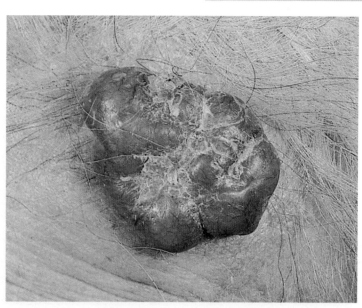

FIGURE 13.3 **CYLINDROMA.** The scalp is a common site for this benign apocrine gland tumor. The nodule has a smooth surface, and telangiectasa may be present.

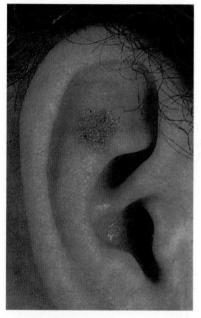

FIGURE 13.2 **SEBORRHEIC KERATOSIS.** A brown, circumscribed lesion is located on the upper portion of the antihelix.

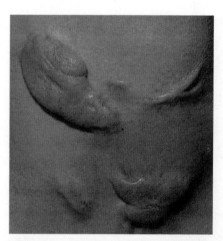

FIGURE 13.4 **KELOIDS.** These tumors represent an abnormal reparative reaction to skin injury. Their frequent extension beyond the original injury distinguishes them from hypertrophic scars, which are confined to the wound margins. Histologically, they are characterized by proliferation of fibroblasts and collagen.

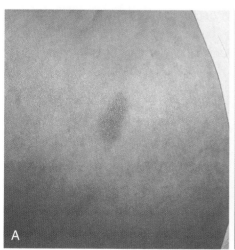

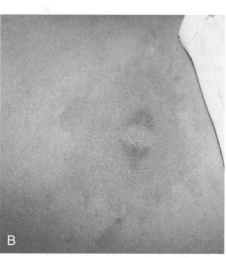

FIGURE 13.5 **MASTOCYTOMA. (A)** Isolated lesions, representing dermal accumulations of mast cells, may be seen in neonates and infants. They are usually skin-colored, slightly indurated, infiltrated plaques 1–2 cm in size. **(B)** The clue to the diagnosis is a wheal-and-flare reaction following slight pressure on the lesions (Darier sign). This response results from the effects on the local vasculature of histamine released from infiltrating mast cells.

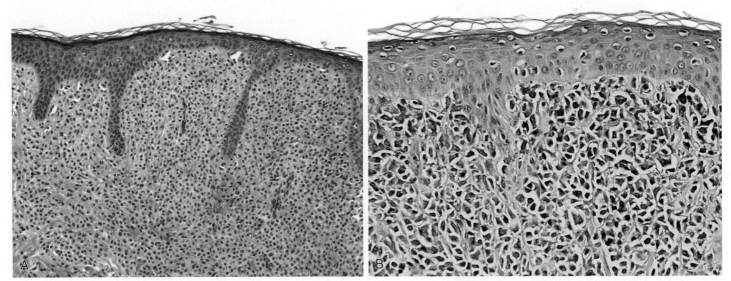

FIGURE 13.6 **MASTOCYTOMA.** Histologically, this lesion is characterized by the presence of numerous monotonous mast cells filling the dermis **(A)**. Scattered eosinophils are often present. **(B)** Positivity of mast cells with chloroacetate esterase stain is shown.

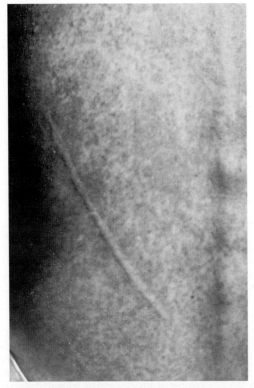

FIGURE 13.7 **URTICARIA PIGMENTOSA IN A 48-YEAR-OLD WOMAN.** There is a generalized hyperpigmented macular skin eruption. A pronounced urticarial reaction (Darier sign) occurred after the skin was stroked with a pointed object. Urticaria pigmentosa in adults is less frequently associated with spontaneous regression and more commonly associated with systemic involvement (particularly bone marrow).

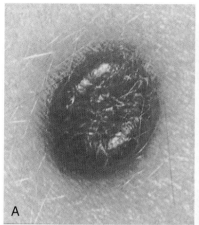
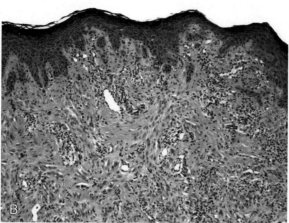

FIGURE 13.8 **SPITZ NEVUS. (A)** This picture illustrates a classical clinical presentation of a well-circumscribed and symmetrical, red to brown papule on the cheek of a young child. **(B)** Histologically, Spitz nevus is characterized by epithelioid and spindle cells with abundant eosinophilic cytoplasm, large vesicular nuclei, and evident nucleoli.

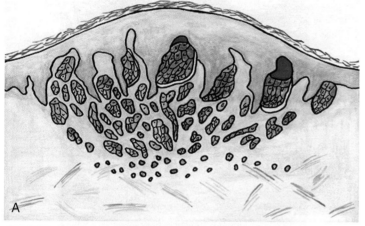
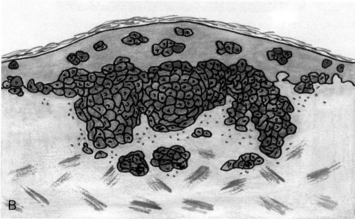

FIGURE 13.9 **SPITZ NEVUS AND MALIGNANT MELANOMA.** Comparative diagram illustrating the most distinctive features. **(A)** Spitz nevus tends to be symmetrical and better circumscribed, without prominent pagetoid spread. Dermal melanocytes in Spitz nevus tend to mature (become smaller) in deeper areas of the lesion. Mitosis may be seen in Spitz nevus; however, they are not atypical and they are not seen at the base of the dermal component. **(B)** Malignant melanoma tends to be asymmetrical with prominent pagetoid spread and lack of maturation. Distinction between the two entities, however, is not always so straightforward, and a gray area of borderline and difficult lesions exists. Spitz nevi are benign lesions more frequently encountered in children. Special caution is recommended with Spitz-like lesions in older adults, since with increasing patient age the likelihood of a Spitz-like lesion representing a melanoma also increases. (Diagram adapted from Smith NP: The pigmented spindle cell tumor of Reed: an underdiagnosed lesion. *Semin Diagn Pathol* 4:75–87; 1987.)

Premalignant Skin Tumors

Actinic keratoses, also called solar keratoses, appear as thin, scaly, red lesions with epidermal hyperplasia and keratinocytic atypia (Figs. 13.10 through 13.15). Although they are allegedly precursors of SCC, most do not proceed to frank malignancy, and conservative treatment is indicated. Because lesions tend to be multifocal and numerous, nonscarring methods of destruction, such as cryosurgery, electrodessication, or topical 5-fluorouracil cream, imiquimod 5% cream, and diclofenac 3% gel, are usually effective alternative therapies. Lesions that persist after treatment should be biopsied to rule out a malignant component. Topical sunscreens and other protective measures against sun exposure seem to be effective in preventing the development of new lesions.

Arsenical keratoses are small, hard, punctate tumors that usually occur on the hands and feet (Fig. 13.16). Increase in depth or diameter and ulceration of the lesions usually indicate progression to SCC.

Xeroderma pigmentosum is an autosomal-recessive disorder characterized by the inability to repair UV light–induced DNA damage and, consequently, a pronounced cutaneous hypersensitivity to the effects of the sun's rays. The disease, which starts in childhood, primarily affects the exposed parts of the body; lesions on the trunk may occur late in the course of the disease (Figs. 13.17 and 13.18). Dryness, desquamation, and freckling are followed first by atrophic and telangiectatic spots, then by verrucous keratotic lesions. The most frequent malignancy is basal cell carcinoma, followed by SCC. Rarely, melanomas or sarcoma may also develop.

Patients with epidermodysplasia verruciformis, a generalized virally induced (HPV 5–associated) dermatosis, are also prone to develop SCCs.

Bowen disease is a term used to describe a characteristic clinical lesion that presents as a well-demarcated, scaly, red plaque and that histologically corresponds to SCC in situ (Figs. 13.19 through 13.22). Usually Bowen disease affects skin unexposed to sunlight. It should be emphasized that the diagnosis of Bowen disease is a clinicopathologic one. Lesions showing similar microscopic changes may not show the classical clinical features of Bowen disease. Some studies have shown an apparent increase in the incidence of visceral cancer in patients with Bowen disease, but others have failed to document such an association. Lesions of Bowen disease seem to be capable of developing into invasive SCC. Removal by simple excision is usually an adequate treatment.

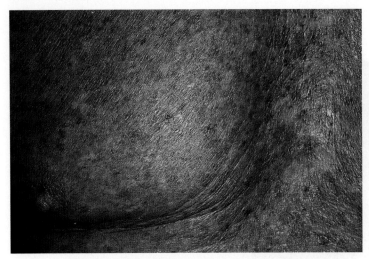

FIGURE 13.10 **SOLAR KERATOSES.** Chronic skin changes on the chest of a 76-year-old man with long-standing sun exposure. There are numerous thin, scaly, erythematous lesions and hyperpigmented areas. Regular use of sunscreens would help to prevent development of these skin changes.

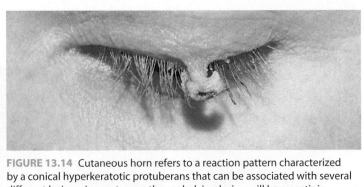

FIGURE 13.14 Cutaneous horn refers to a reaction pattern characterized by a conical hyperkeratotic protuberans that can be associated with several different lesions. In most cases the underlying lesion will be an actinic keratosis. Other lesions that may be associated with a cutaneous horn pattern include verrucae, seborrheic keratosis, and squamous cell carcinoma.

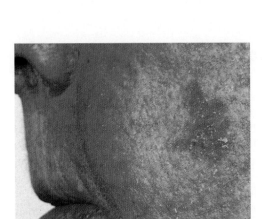

FIGURE 13.11 **SOLAR KERATOSIS.** This tumor appears as either a well-defined, raised red papule or, as shown here, a raised red plaque with an adherent scale.

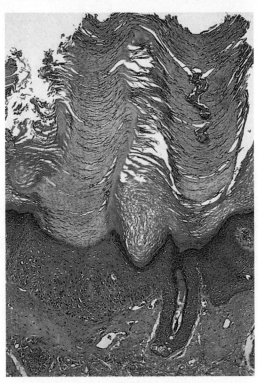

FIGURE 13.15 **SOLAR KERATOSIS.** There are alternating areas of ortho- and parakeratosis. Underneath the parakeratosis, the epidermis shows keratinocytic atypia. The epidermis underneath the areas of orthokeratosis does not show significant pathologic change.

FIGURE 13.12 **SOLAR KERATOSIS.** This patient's scaly plaque **(A)** was treated successfully with 5-fluorouracil cream **(B)**. (Courtesy of St. Mary's Hospital, London, UK.)

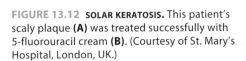

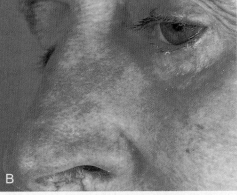

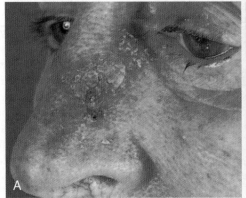

FIGURE 13.13 **SOLAR KERATOSIS. (A)** Ultraviolet light exposure has produced a dry, elevated, white, scaly lesion on the posterior helical rim. **(B)** A solar keratosis arising from the antihelix has produced a small keratin horn.

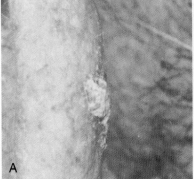

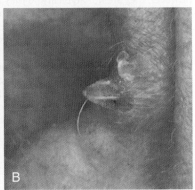

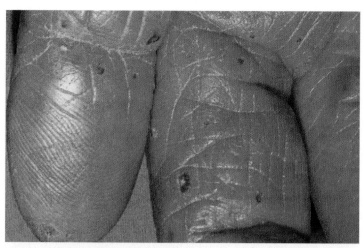

FIGURE 13.16 **ARSENICAL KERATOSIS.** Exposure to arsenic, often as a pesticide, produces keratoses on the palms and fingers.

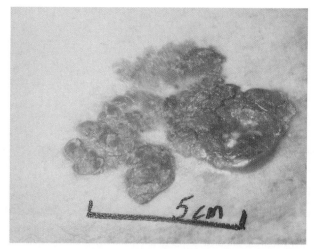

FIGURE 13.19 Bowen disease is characterized by well-defined erythematous scaly plaques histologically representing SCC in situ. In this patient, however, the right side of the lesion has already undergone transformation to invasive SCC.

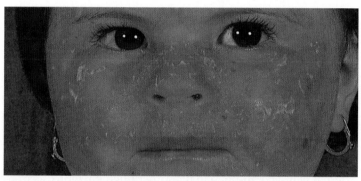

FIGURE 13.17 **XERODERMA PIGMENTOSUM.** Extreme photosensitivity is the feature of this condition. Persistent erythema occurs after seemingly innocent solar exposure. Multiple premalignant keratoses are evident.

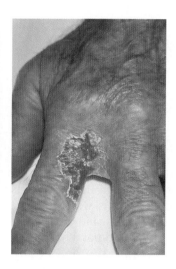

FIGURE 13.20 **BOWEN DISEASE.** Involvement of the hands is quite common and can present diagnostic and therapeutic problems.

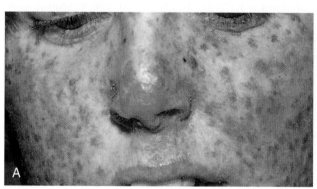

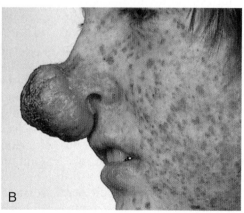

FIGURE 13.18 **XERODERMA PIGMENTOSUM. (A)** After solar exposure, permanent freckling of exposed skin quickly ensues. Malignant change occurs early in life. This patient had her first SCC at the age of 2 years. **(B)** This keratoacanthoma developed when she was 12 years old. The lesion resolved spontaneously.

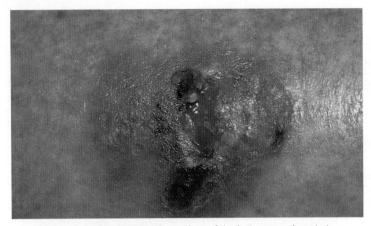

FIGURE 13.21 **BOWEN DISEASE.** The surface of the lesion, seen here in its characteristic presentation as a well-defined, slightly raised, red patch with an adherent scale, may become eroded.

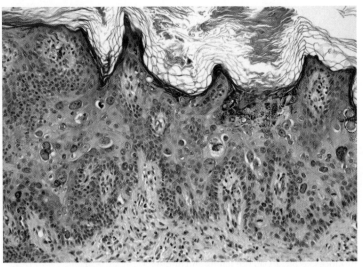

FIGURE 13.22 **BOWEN DISEASE.** There is full-thickness keratinocytic atypia with marked nuclear pleomorphism and numerous mitotic figures. Bowen disease is synonymous with SCC in situ.

Common Skin Cancers

BASAL CELL CARCINOMA

Basal cell carcinoma is the most common malignancy in white people, with an incidence that is increasing worldwide by up to 10% annually. Exposure to UV radiation is the main pathogenetic factor. The most classical clinical presentation is that of a pearly-gray papule or nodule with prominent telangiectasia (Figs. 13.23 through 13.25). Histologically the lesions consist of small, undifferentiated basal cells with minimal nuclear atypia (Fig. 13.26). Several clinical and pathologic variants exist, including nodular, micronodular, superficial, and infiltrative/morpheaform types (Figs. 13.27 and 13.28). The majority of tumors are located on the face, neck, and dorsum of the hands. Superficial variants tend to be located on the trunk. Some basal cell carcinomas may be pigmented and can be clinically confused with melanocytic lesions, especially melanoma (Figs. 13.29 and 13.30). Basal cell carcinomas can be locally destructive, but only exceptional reports of cases with metastatic behavior exist in the literature (Figs. 13.31 through 13.34). The treatment of choice is surgery, but for superficial variants that tend to be broad and multifocal, cryotherapy, photodynamic therapy, and more recently topical treatment with immune response modifiers such as imiquimod have shown to be effective. Infiltrative variants with irregular borders and sometimes perineural invasion are more prone to recur, probably due to insufficient surgery. Recurrent tumors incur serious complications. Treating such lesions in a combined clinic, comprising a dermatologist, a plastic surgeon, and an oncologist, is recommended.

The basal cell nevus syndrome (Gorlin syndrome) refers to an autosomal-dominant disorder characterized by multiple basal cell carcinomas, associated with jaw cysts and skeletal anomalies (Fig. 13.35). Patients have peculiar cutaneous pits in the palms and soles; the pits have histologic features of miniature basal cell carcinomas (Fig. 13.36).

SQUAMOUS CELL CARCINOMA

SCC is the second most frequent cutaneous malignancy (next to basal cell carcinoma) (Alam and Ratner, 2001). Tumors tend to occur in sun-exposed areas such as the face, neck, arms, and hands. The pathogenesis is multifactorial, with chronic actinic damage, particularly, in light-skinned patients, being the most important factor (Figs. 13.37 through 13.40). One of the postulated pathogenetic mechanisms is the induction of *TP53* mutations by UV light (Burnworth et al., 2006). Tumors affecting external genitalia and perianal and periungual regions seem to be HPV-associated in an important percentage of cases. The overall recurrence of SCC seems to be between 3.7% and 10%, and the metastatic rate 5.2% (Fig. 13.41). However, when tumors are located in special sites such as the lip, ear, and anogenital areas, they show a higher rate of recurrence and metastasis. Tumors arising in the setting of inflammatory, scarring, and degenerative processes are also associated with a worse prognosis than those developing in sun-damaged skin (Figs. 13.42 through 13.44). SCCs are usually classified based on a three-grade system as well-differentiated, moderately differentiated, and poorly differentiated tumors. Poorly differentiated tumors tend to have a more aggressive behavior. In addition to the usual classic type, several SCC variants that may show variable clinical behavior have been described (Cassarino et al., 2006). Some of these variants include verrucous carcinoma (Figs. 13.45 and 13.46), carcinoma cuniculatum (Fig. 13.47) (Barreto et al., 2007), warty carcinoma (Fig. 13.48), basaloid carcinoma (Fig. 13.49), sarcomatoid carcinoma (Fig. 13.50A, B), adenoid (acantholytic) carcinoma, angiosarcomatoid (pseudovascular) carcinoma, clear cell carcinoma, mucoepidermoid (adenosquamous cell carcinoma), and lymphoepithelioma-like carcinoma. Independently of the histologic variant and histologic grade and has been shown that depth of invasion and tumor thickness are the most helpful pathologic prognostic parameters (Breuninger et al., 1990). SCCs less than 2 mm thick, which represent a high percentage of tumors, almost never metastasize. The risk of metastasis increases with tumors infiltrating the subcutaneous tissue.

The risk of metastasis for undifferentiated carcinomas greater than 6 mm thick that have infiltrated the musculature, the perichondrium, or the periosteum, however, is quite high. Tumors between 2 and 6 mm thick with moderate differentiation and a depth of invasion that does not extend beyond the subcutis can be classified as low-risk carcinomas. In addition to high histologic grade, infiltration of subcutaneous tissue and deeper structures, and perineural and lymphovascular invasion are also indicators of poor prognosis.

Transplant recipient patients who undergo long-term immunosuppression and patients with other forms of immune suppression are at increased risk for different neoplasms, and in the skin, especially SCC. These tumors tend to affect younger patients and are more frequently located in sun-exposed areas. The lesions tend to be clinically problematic, since they tend to be multiple and arise in a background of dysplastic epidermis (Fig. 13.51). It appears that a good percentage of tumors in this setting may be HPV-related, and in fact it is not unusual to find features suggestive of a viral wart associated with frankly carcinomatous areas (Fig. 13.52). It seems that tumors associated with immunosuppression tend to have a more aggressive behavior with a significant incidence of metastasis and even mortality (Fig. 13.53) (Martinez et al., 2003; Herman et al., 2007).

KERATOACANTHOMA

Keratoacanthoma is a rapidly growing tumor usually affecting sun-exposed skin of elderly patients. The classical presentation is that of a solitary discrete, round to oval, flesh-colored umbilicated nodule with a central keratin-filled crater (Figs. 13.54 and 13.55). Lesions have a rapid clinical evolution and usually regress within 4–6 months (Fig. 13.55). There has been a lot of controversy around this entity concerning whether it represents a benign or a malignant tumor, and multiple clinical and histologic criteria have been proposed to differentiate it from SCC (Fig. 13.56). In unusual cases, however, lesions in the histologic spectrum of typical keratoacanthomas have been shown to follow an aggressive clinical course. Modern immunohistochemical and molecular techniques have not proved to be more useful in this distinction. With all of this controversy, and since there are no clinical or histologic criteria to classify a potential keratoacanthoma as a benign tumor that might spontaneously regress or as a neoplasm with metastatic potential, it seems most appropriate to consider keratoacanthoma as an extremely well-differentiated variant of SCC and to treat it as such (Karaa and Khachemoune, 2007).

MELANOMA

Malignant melanoma is a highly aggressive tumor that arises through genetic alterations within melanocytes. Derived embryologically from the neural crest, melanocytes reside predominantly in the basal layer of the epidermis. They possess a unique biochemical feature, the enzymatic conversion of L-dopa to melanin pigment by tyrosinase. Melanin is transported to surrounding keratinocytes, providing protection against DNA damage triggered by UV radiation. The production of melanin increases in response to UV radiation and to a variety of hormonal agents including melanocyte-stimulating hormone, corticotrophin (Addison disease), and estrogens (increased pigmentation during pregnancy). Melanocyte-stimulating hormone binds to the melanocortin receptor 1 (MC1R) on melanocytes, leading to increased melanin production. A germline polymorphism in the MC1R gene present in people with red hair contributes to reduced receptor activity and an increased lifetime risk for developing melanoma (van der Velden et al., 2001). Chronic low-dose exposure to UV light may induce protection against DNA damage, whereas episodic exposure to high doses of UV light may facilitate DNA damage (Gilchrest et al., 1999).

An estimated 68,720 new cases of malignant melanoma are expected in 2009, with 8650 melanoma-related deaths (Jemal et al, 2009). Fifty-seven percent of cases are estimated to develop in males and 43% in females. In the United States the incidence is approximately 20 per 100,000, having risen from 1975 when it was 8 per 100,000. The incidence varies by region and is highest in California and Florida. The lifetime probability for developing melanoma is 1 in 49 males and 1 in 73 females (Jemal et al, 2007).

The incidence of melanoma has also increased in adolescents. Based on the Surveillance, Epidemiology, and End Results (SEER) database, the incidence of melanoma in children increased approximately 2.9% per year from 1973 through 2001. However, the disease remains relatively rare, with an estimated 475 new cases of melanoma in the United States in 2002 in people younger than 19 years of age and 47 cases in children younger than 10 years. The rarity can result in delayed diagnosis, and younger children are more likely to present with regional or distant metastases (Strouse et al., 2005).

Melanoma and breast cancer are the two malignancies most commonly detected in pregnant women. An estimated incidence of melanoma of up to 5 cases per 100,000 pregnancies has been reported. Melanoma cells can travel across the placenta and deposit in the fetus. Hormonal and immunologic changes may facilitate the development of melanoma during pregnancy (Lens et al., 2004).

Melanoma represents 4% of new cancer diagnoses in men and women. The majority of melanomas are diagnosed as localized disease (80%) and fewer than 20% of cases as regional or distant disease. The 5-year relative survival rate has increased from 82% during the years 1975 to 1977 to 92% from 1996 to 2002. This highlights the importance of early detection. In Australia, where the risk of developing melanoma has been reported as high as 1 in 20, public health initiatives focused on sun protection and early detection have contributed to a leveling off in incidence.

The vast majority of melanomas originate as cutaneous lesions. Less commonly, noncutaneous melanomas arise from melanocytic structures in the eye (uveal and ocular melanoma) or mucosal surfaces including the anal canal, vulva, vagina, mouth, nose, pharynx, sinuses, and esophagus.

Cutaneous melanoma can be classified based upon site of origin and histologic features. Table 13.1 shows the major clinical-histologic types of malignant melanoma. Superficial spreading melanoma is the most common type, representing 70% of cases. It is typified by a radial-growth phase lasting 1–7 years, followed by a vertical-growth phase in which the melanoma becomes increasingly invasive (Figs. 13.61 through 13.64). This emphasizes the importance of early detection of these lesions in determining prognosis. Nodular melanoma arises without a radial-growth phase and therefore often presents as a deeper primary lesion (Figs. 13.65 through 13.68). The sun-induced lentigo maligna melanoma composes 5% to 10% of melanomas and occurs typically on sun-exposed areas such as the cheek of older individuals, arising in a lentigo maligna (Figs. 13.69 through 13.71). Acral lentiginous melanomas are uncommon, develop on palms, soles, and subungual locations, and are not

Table 13.1

Malignant Melanoma: Differential Features of Major Types

Feature	Superficial Spreading	Lentigo Maligna	Nodular
Percentage of all melanomas	70–75	5–10	10–15
Mean age at presentation (years)	47	69	50
Common location	Increased frequency on back of both sexes Increased frequency on lower legs of females	Head, neck, back of hands (90%)	Any site
Duration of radial-growth	Up to a few years	1–7 years (up to 14 years)	Direct tumor invasion postulated, without radial-growth phase
Border of lesion	Raised	Flat	Raised
Histology of adjacent/ surrounding epidermis	Pagetoid distribution of melanocytes in epidermis	Atypical melanocytic hyperplasia at dermal-epidermal junction	No associated in situ component

as closely associated with sun exposure (Figs. 13.72 and 13.73). Desmoplastic or neurotropic melanomas are rare and tend to arise in elderly individuals. They tend to present as deep primary lesions, are frequently amelanotic, with histologic features of spindles and nerve infiltration and frequent local recurrences. Recently considerable progress has been made in the molecular biology and genetic heterogeneity of malignant melanoma (see Fig. 13.57). Approximately 80% of melanomas contain mutations that activate components of the mitogen-activated protein kinase signal transduction (MAPK) pathway. This pathway normally regulates cell growth and survival. Activating mutations are found in two components of the pathway: *N-RAS* and *BRAF*. Through a systematic attempt to sequence the genome in a variety of cancer cell lines, somatic mutations in *BRAF* were detected in 66% of metastatic melanomas. Mutations cluster in the kinase domain, and a nucleotide substitution at codon 600 (V600E) accounts for 80% of the mutations (Davies et al., 2002). Subsequently mutations in *BRAF* were detected in up to 82% of benign nevi, suggesting that the mutation is an early event and not sufficient for malignant transformation. An additional 15% of melanomas contain activating somatic mutations in *N-RAS*, an upstream component of the MAPK pathway. Mutations in *BRAF* and *N-RAS* are almost always mutually exclusive, and therefore more than 80% of melanomas have selected for mutations that activate the MAPK pathway. Inhibition of the MAPK pathway in preclinical models of melanoma demonstrates an inhibitory effect on proliferation and survival (Fecher et al., 2007; Gray-Schopfer et al., 2007).

Genomewide approaches assessing gene copy number, amplifications and deletions in portions of chromosomes, and correlation of histologic features with mutational status of *BRAF* and *N-RAS* have further defined the molecular and genetic heterogeneity of melanoma (Table 13.2; Fig. 13.57). These approaches have demonstrated different patterns of genomic aberration in melanomas arising from chronic sun-exposed, intermittent sun-exposed, acral lentiginous, and mucosal locations. Differentiating melanoma that has developed from chronic as opposed to intermittent sun exposure can be challenging and depends upon the potentially subjective pathologic determination of the presence or absence of solar elastosis in the biopsy specimen (Curtin et al., 2005).

Mucosal and acral melanomas demonstrate more extensive amplification and deletion of chromosomes relative to cutaneous melanomas. Activating mutations in the MAPK pathway are most common in melanoma derived from intermittent sun exposure and are much less common in acral and mucosal melanomas. These mutations are not detected in ocular melanoma.

Activating mutations and amplifications in the *c-KIT* oncogene were recently detected in a subset of melanomas. The *c-KIT* gene encodes a receptor tyrosine kinase bound by ligands including stem cell factor. Activating mutations in *c-KIT* have been detected in other malignancies such as gastrointestinal stromal tumors, where inhibition of *c-KIT* activity has demonstrated significant clinical benefit. In melanoma, mutations seen in *c-KIT* are similar to those in gastrointestinal stromal tumors. Alterations in *c-KIT* expression are present in up to 39%

Table 13.2

Genetic Alterations in Melanoma*

Gene	Characteristics
BRAF	Mutation most frequent in melanoma from intermittent sun-exposed skin
N-RAS	Mutation most frequent in melanoma from intermittent sun-exposed skin Mutually exclusive of *BRAF* mutations
PTEN	Mutation or deletion most common in melanoma from intermittent sun-exposed skin Occurs together with mutant *BRAF* but not mutant *N-RAS*
CCDN1 (cyclin D1)	Increased copy number with highest frequency in melanoma from chronic sun-exposed skin Inversely correlated with mutations in *BRAF*
CDK4	Increased copy number most common in acral and mucosal melanomas
p16	Deletion in 50% of all melanomas Deletion most frequent in acral and mucosal melanomas
C-KIT	Activating point mutations and increased copy number most common in acral, mucosal, and chronic sun-exposed melanomas
Genome-wide chromosomal gains and deletions	Highest frequency in acral and mucosal melanomas

*Recent advances in molecular biology and genetics further defined the molecular heterogeneity of melanoma and localized genes to the pathogenesis of melanoma. Mucosal, acral, chronic sun-exposed, and intermittent sun-exposed melanomas can be categorized by differences in genetic alterations (Curtin JA, Fridlyard J, Kagesnita T, et al: Distinct sets of genetic alterations in melanoma, *N Engl J Med* 353:2135–2147, 2005).

of mucosal, acral, and chronic sun-derived melanomas but are infrequent in the setting of intermittent sun exposure. The clinical significance of these mutations is currently unclear but is under active investigation (Curtin et al., 2006).

Major risk factors for the development of malignant melanoma are genetic and sun exposure history. First-degree relatives with a history of melanoma, significant intermittent sun exposure, and sun exposure in early adulthood have been determined to be particularly important prognostic factors. Phenotypes of blue eyes, blond or red hair, and tendency to freckle or burn increase the risk of developing melanoma. Approximately 10% of patients with melanoma have a family history of melanoma, and specific inherited susceptibility genes have been identified (Bishop et al., 2007). The dysplastic nevus syndrome refers to individuals with atypical moles or nevi, marked by irregularities in outline and pigmentation, who are at increased risk for developing melanoma (Figs. 13.93 and 13.94). The nevi may be acquired or may occur in a familial melanoma syndrome. The benign lesions tend to be larger and more numerous than common moles and occur in sun-shielded areas such as the scalp and the bathing suit area. The risk of developing melanoma is up to 60%, and these patients should be followed closely by a dermatologist. The malignant potential of an isolated dysplastic nevus is less well established and complicated by lack of concordance among pathologists in the identification of dysplasia. However, people with multiple dysplastic nevi and a family history of more than one first-degree family member having melanoma have a lifetime risk for developing melanoma nearing 100%. In addition, congenital nevi have the potential to develop into malignant melanoma(Fig. 13.92).

Favorable prognostic factors include female gender and location of the primary lesion on an extremity. The most important factors involved in determining the overall prognosis of a patient with malignant melanoma are the depth of the primary lesion and lymph node status. Level of invasion may be determined anatomically by the Clark technique or micrometrically by the Breslow technique (Fig. 13.59). The more useful measure is the Breslow technique, since it is not dependent on histologic interpretation. Depth of invasion is classified as thin (<1 mm), intermediate (1.01–3.99 mm), and deep (>4 mm). As the depth of the primary lesion increases, the risk of recurrence becomes greater. Other favorable prognostic factors include the absence of ulceration or mitoses in the primary lesion.

The involvement of lymph nodes is the strongest negative prognostic factor. The risk of recurrence increases with the number of lymph nodes involved. Macroscopic as opposed to microscopic lymph node involvement further increases the risk.

Features that characterize early melanoma have been quantified in an effort to increase early diagnosis. The average size of a level II lesion is 17×15 mm as compared with 28×23 mm for level V lesions. In the majority of patients with early lesions, an increase in size and a darkening in color are present. Changes such as nodularity, ulceration, or bleeding correspond to the development of histologically poorer prognoses. Other adverse prognostic features include advanced age, male gender, head and neck primary sites, increased mitotic rate, lack of inflammatory lymphoid infiltrate below the primary lesion, and satellite or in-transit lesions.

Through a series of phenotypic changes melanocytes progress toward malignant transformation. Normal melanocytes proliferate, creating a benign nevus. Either within a benign nevus or at a new anatomic location aberrant growth can develop. The dysplastic or atypical nevus is characterized by discontiguous cytologic atypia. The nevus can display irregular shape, multivariate color, asymmetry, and increased diameter. In radial–growth–phase melanoma the melanocytes display contiguous cellular atypia and proliferate within the epidermis, and a few cells may invade the superficial dermis. In the vertical-growth phase the malignant cells invade the dermis and sometimes the subcutaneous tissue. Melanoma can disseminate through both the lymphatic and the vascular systems. Dissemination along draining dermal lymphatic pathways can lead to the development of local and regional melanoma deposits termed satellite and in-transit metastases. Regional involvement also includes the spread of melanoma to lymph node basins draining from the site of the primary lesion. Hematogenous or distant lymphatic spread signifies dissemination of the melanoma (Miller and Mihm, 2006).

In the American Joint Committee on Cancer (AJCC) staging system melanoma is categorized into four stages (Fig. 13.60). An increase in stage predicts a poorer prognosis. Stage I and II melanomas display no clinically detectable tumor outside of the primary lesion. These primary lesions are classified as either stage I or II based on Breslow thickness and the presence or absence of ulceration. In stage III melanoma local-regional tumor deposits are detectable in the draining dermal lymphatics or lymph node basins. Disseminated hematogenous or lymphatic spread defines stage IV melanoma.

Evaluation of a suspicious pigmented lesion includes a full-thickness excisional biopsy with 1- to 3-mm margins. Shave biopsies should be avoided. If melanoma is detected, then a wide local excision should be performed with appropriate margins for the depth of the primary. Recommended margins are 0.5 cm for in situ melanoma, 1 cm for lesions less than 1 mm deep, 1–2 cm for lesions 1.01-2 mm deep, and at least 2 cm for lesions deeper than 2.01 mm. The wide excision decreases risk for local recurrence and allows for additional assessment of microscopic satellite deposits of tumor.

The lack of efficacy for elective lymph node dissections led to the development of a technique to identify and biopsy the sentinel, or first draining, lymph node from the region of skin. The procedure involves injection of a blue dye and intraoperative lymphoscintigraphy with radiolabeled technetium-99 dextran or sulfur colloid in the region of the primary site before the wide excision. The accuracy of this procedure to detect true sentinel lymph nodes greatly decreases if wide excision is performed first.

In patients with a primary melanoma of intermediate thickness the incidence of micrometastases in the sentinel lymph node is approximately 16%. A study suggests that patients in this intermediate thickness group (1.2 to 3.5 mm thick melanomas) who undergo a sentinel lymph node procedure followed by (if melanoma is present in the sentinel node) complete lymph node dissection have statistically significant improvement in 5-year disease-free survival rates when compared with patients who are observed and do not undergo lymph node sampling at the time of diagnosis (78% vs 73%). However, five-year melanoma-specific survival rates were similar in the two groups. The risk for nodal relapse in the observed patients is 15.6%, similar to the 16% incidence of melanoma detected using a sentinel lymph node procedure. However, when observed patients develop lymph node recurrence they have an increased mean number of lymph nodes involved (3.3 versus 1.4). Among this subset of patients with intermediate thick primary melanomas and sentinel node metastases, the 5-year survival rate seems to be increased in those undergoing immediate lymphadenectomy as opposed to those with expectant observation of the lymph node basin (Morton et al., 2006).

When melanoma is detected in the sentinel lymph node, the risk of detecting involved nonsentinel nodes by complete lymphadenectomy is approximately 20%. The location of melanoma deposits within the sentinel node may predict the risk of nonsentinel node involvement. When confined to the subcapsular component of the lymph node (as opposed to involving the parenchyma of the node), the likelihood of nonsentinel nodal involvement is lower (Dewar et al., 2004).

Patients with deep primaries (>4 mm) and/or lymph node involvement have significant risk for developing disseminated disease by hematogenous spread. Adjuvant chemotherapy has not revealed significant efficacy. Positive results from randomized prospective trials of high-dose interferon alfa-2b in the adjuvant setting have led to U.S. Food and Drug Administration approval for this subgroup of patients. Investigational approaches include an array of vaccine-based strategies with the goal of educating the immune system to detect and control micrometastatic disease. These approaches remain experimental and unproven in terms of survival benefit.

The most common sites of metastases for patients with stage IV disease are the brain, lung, and liver, but virtually any area can be involved (Figs. 13.74 through 13.91). The histologic findings of metastatic melanoma vary considerably, from heavily pigmented cells to poorly differentiated amelanotic cells that may mimic lymphoma, carcinoma, or sarcoma. Some patients may have no history of a primary skin lesion or may have had a melanoma removed many years earlier. The prognosis for a patient with metastatic melanoma is in general poor. Patients with metastatic disease limited to the lungs, soft tissue, lymph nodes, and skin have a slightly better prognosis than patients with disease elsewhere, such as in the liver or brain. Increased lactate dehydrogenase levels in the blood also confer a worse prognosis in patients with stage IV disease. In-transit metastases frequently present a problem of local control of the disease. If in-transit disease is limited to a limb, success for local control has occurred with various limb perfusion or infusion strategies that include the use of hyperthermia with infusions of chemotherapy with response rates greater than 50%.

Once melanoma metastasizes to distant sites it is difficult to treat and almost always fatal. Although recent technologic advances such as positron emission tomography scanning improve the ability for detection, early detection of metastatic disease has not been demonstrated to improve patient outcome significantly. Melanoma is typically a relatively chemoresistant and radioresistant disease. Treatment of stage IV disease is palliative, and no systemic therapy has demonstrated significant overall survival benefit. Standard systemic approaches to systemic therapy include chemotherapy and immunotherapy. The most active chemotherapeutic compound is dacarbazine, having response rates less than 20%. Responses tend to be nondurable, and complete responses are rare. Other compounds with activity in melanoma include taxanes, platinum compounds, nitrosureas, and vinca alkaloids. Cytokines such as interferon and interleukin-2 have been widely used for the treatment of metastatic melanoma, with response rates of 20% or less. Combining standard dacarbazine with other chemotherapies or immunotherapies (biochemotherapy) increases the response rate but also increases toxicity, and the increased activity does not translate into improvements in overall survival.

Given the poor prognosis for patients who develop metastatic melanoma and the limited efficacy of standard systemic approaches, experimental therapies are being investigated. Approaches under active investigation include agents that inhibit components of the MAPK pathway (over 80% activating mutation rate) and antiangiogenesis agents. Melanomas tend to have a rich vasculature.

Another focus of investigation has been the use of immunotherapies. The basis of such investigation centers on an understanding of the role the immune system can play in responding to melanoma and the observation that melanoma on rare occasion can undergo spontaneous regression. Technical advances in biochemistry and molecular biology have led to the discovery of numerous melanoma rejection antigens, and over 60 cell surface antigens have been identified (see Fig. 13.58). Vaccination strategies include the use of specific targeted antigens or manipulated whole-tumor cells. Targeted antigens are of a variety of categories, the most studied including the melanoma differentiation antigens and a number of oncofetal proteins. Several of these targets have epitopes restricted to human leukocyte antigen-A02 and therefore limit clinical trial participation to those patients who possess that haplotype. Whole cell–based vaccines can use allogeneic vaccines prepared from established cell lines or autologous vaccines. These vaccines include cell lysates or genetically modified cells. All of the vaccine-based approaches are investigational and should be administered as part of a clinical investigation.

Advances in understanding the regulation of T cells have led to the development of treatment strategies that inhibit the suppression of T cells. For optimal T-cell activation the interaction of co-stimulatory signals is necessary in conjunction with the binding of the T-cell receptor to antigen within major histocompatibility complex molecules on the antigen-presenting cell (APC). One such co-stimulatory interaction is between CD28 on the surface of the T cell and the B7 family on the APC. In activated T cells the expression of CTLA4 protein on the cell surface increases. CTLA4 competes with CD28 for binding to the B7 family, leading to suppression of T-cell activity. Antibodies that inhibit CTLA4 have been developed and have demonstrated promise in trials for stage IV patients. These advances in our understanding of immunoregulation and of the molecular heterogeneity of melanoma permit translational research to be applied not only for the diagnosis of melanoma but also for the development of novel therapeutic strategies.

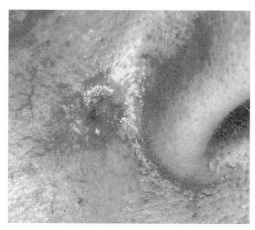

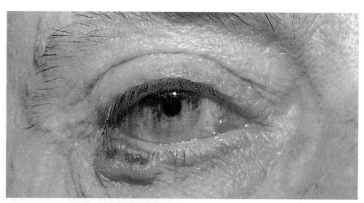

FIGURE 13.23 BASAL CELL CARCINOMA. This early lesion is beginning to show the translucent, pearly appearance typical of these nodules as they begin to undergo central ulceration.

FIGURE 13.25 BASAL CELL CARCINOMA. This is the most common malignant tumor of the eyelid and usually occurs either on the lower eyelid or at the medial canthus. This is an example of a relatively benign type of basal cell carcinoma with a classic pearly margin laced with blood vessels and a shallow ulcerated base at the center.

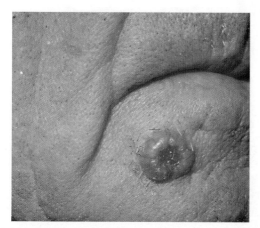

FIGURE 13.24 BASAL CELL CARCINOMA. A typical lesion, with a rolled edge, appears on this patient's chin. Small vessels sweep over the edge, and the center is ulcerated.

FIGURE 13.26 BASAL CELL CARCINOMA. (A) Low-power photomicrograph shows dermal aggregates of small basaloid cells. **(B)** Higher-power view illustrating the peripheral palisading of basaloid cells.

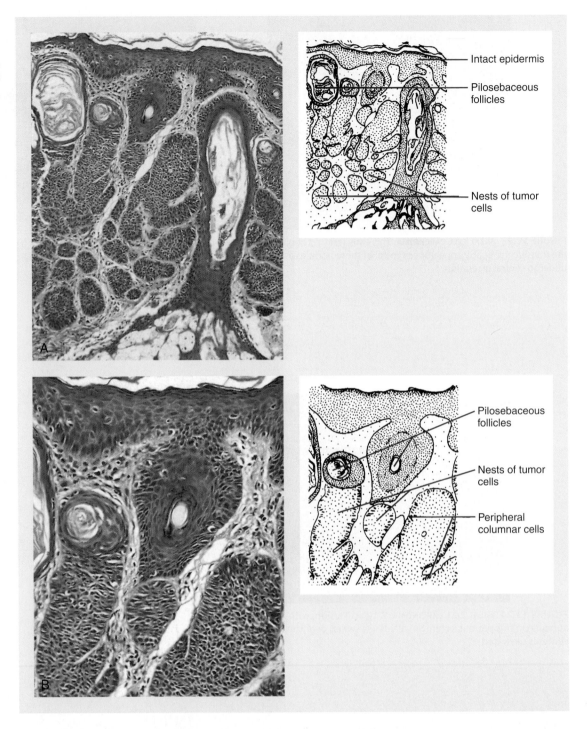

FIGURE 13.26 labels: Intact epidermis; Pilosebaceous follicles; Nests of tumor cells; Pilosebaceous follicles; Nests of tumor cells; Peripheral columnar cells

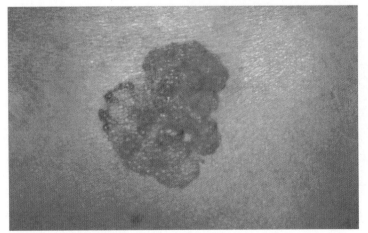

FIGURE 13.27 SUPERFICIAL BASAL CELL CARCINOMA. This variant of basal cell carcinoma presents as a plaque with a rolled, pearly margin. It is a less aggressive version of the ulcerative type of basal cell tumor.

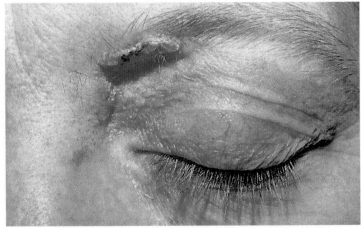

FIGURE 13.28 MORPHEAFORM OR INFILTRATIVE BASAL CELL CARCINOMA. This is a more locally aggressive variant characterized by infiltrative, less clearly defined borders and sometimes perineural invasion. A wider surgical excision is required to prevent recurrence.

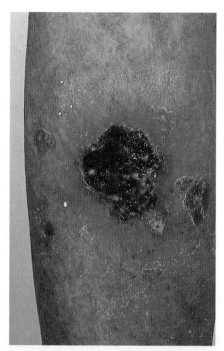

FIGURE 13.29 **PIGMENTED BASAL CELL CARCINOMA.** This subtype of basal cell tumor is similar in presentation to the nodular-ulcerative type except that the margin of the ulcer is rolled and pigmented. The clinical significance of this variant is that it may be mistaken for malignant melanoma. This lesion occurred on the leg, an unusual site.

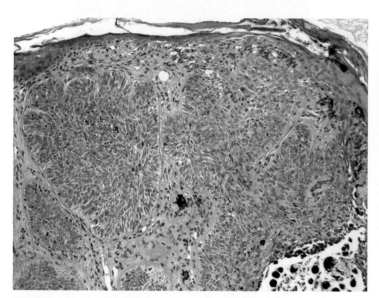

FIGURE 13.30 **PIGMENTED BASAL CELL CARCINOMA.** Histologically, this lesion shows features of a nodular basal cell carcinoma. The neoplastic cells, however, contain melanin in their cytoplasm. Melanin is also seen within melanophages in the dermis.

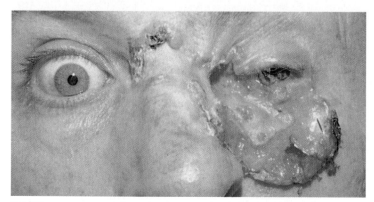

FIGURE 13.31 **BASAL CELL CARCINOMA.** These tumors spread by direct extension and may be highly invasive, although they rarely metastasize. In this example an extensive basal cell carcinoma has spread to involve surrounding structures.

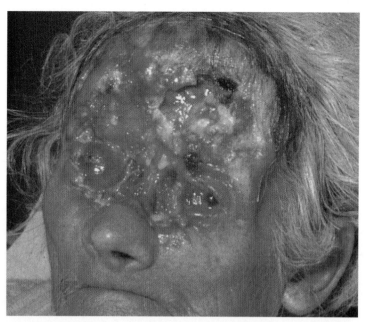

FIGURE 13.32 **BASAL CELL CARCINOMA.** If neglected the tumor grows inexorably, causing marked destruction of normal structures. (Courtesy of Dr. D.E. Sharvill, Canterbury, UK.)

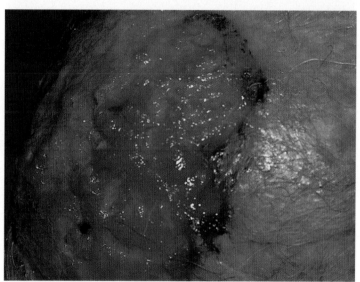

FIGURE 13.33 **RADIATION-INDUCED BASAL CELL CARCINOMA.** A tumor developed on this patient's scalp 60 years after she underwent irradiation for tinea capitis as a child. She had chronic alopecia following the overirradiation. The lesion was successfully excised. (Courtesy of J.P. Bennett.)

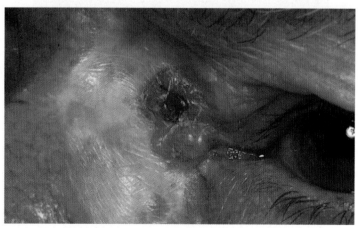

FIGURE 13.34 **RECURRENT BASAL CELL CARCINOMA.** This tumor has recurred on the area of a skin graft used to repair the site of a previously excised lesion. This is more frequently seen with infiltrative/morpheaform variants, advanced/large lesions, and multifocal tumors.

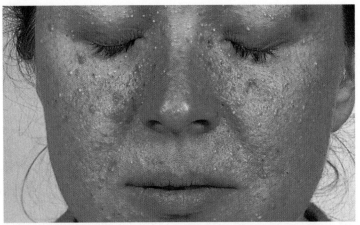

FIGURE 13.35 **BASAL CELL–NEVUS SYNDROME.** In this autosomal-dominant disorder, multiple basal cell carcinomas develop from childhood onward, as shown in this patient. (Courtesy of Dr. A.C. Pembroke.)

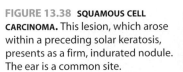
FIGURE 13.38 **SQUAMOUS CELL CARCINOMA.** This lesion, which arose within a preceding solar keratosis, presents as a firm, indurated nodule. The ear is a common site.

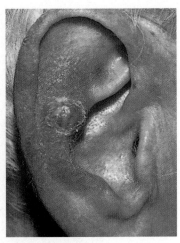

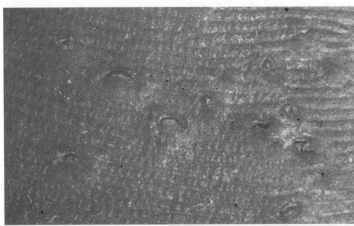

FIGURE 13.36 **BASAL CELL–NEVUS SYNDROME.** Tiny pits on the palms, as shown in this low-power magnified view, are characteristic features of the condition. (Courtesy of Dr. Eugene van Scott, Skin and Cancer Hospital, Philadelphia, PA.)

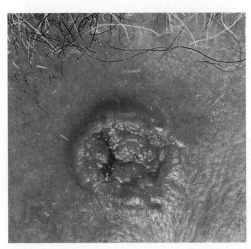

FIGURE 13.39 **SQUAMOUS CELL CARCINOMA.** The lesion may also present as an ulcer having a raised, firm, indurated margin.

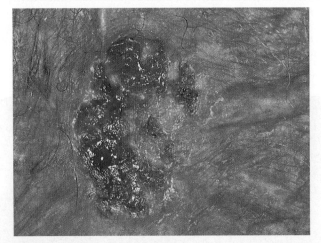

FIGURE 13.37 **SQUAMOUS CELL CARCINOMA.** The back of the hand is a common site for SCC. This ulcerated lesion consists of a purulent base surrounded by a firm, everted, and irregular margin. Note the surrounding atrophic, sun-damaged skin.

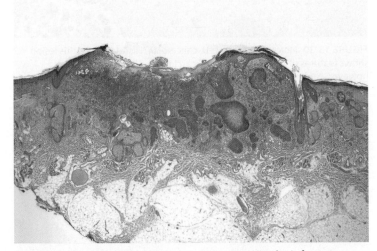

FIGURE 13.40 **INVASIVE SQUAMOUS CELL CARCINOMA.** Histologic features. This is a classical example of an invasive SCC of the usual type arising in sun-damaged skin showing actinic keratosis. Emanating from a dysplastic epidermis and infiltrating the reticular dermis, there are aggregates of neoplastic keratinocytes. The subcutaneous tissue is not affected, and this is important because the invasion of the subcutaneous tissue would have been an adverse prognostic factor.

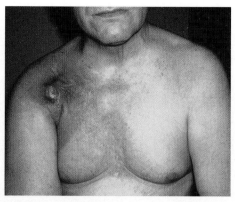

FIGURE 13.41 **SQUAMOUS CELL CARCINOMA.** Spread of metastases to the right anterior shoulder from a primary SCC of the hand. There is extensive involvement of the axilla causing lymphatic obstruction and arm edema. Note ulceration of the tumor. Skin hyperemia is secondary to radiation therapy. In some patients metastases can develop in the lung, bone, liver, and other sites.

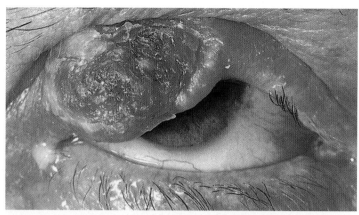

FIGURE 13.44 **SQUAMOUS CELL CARCINOMA IN XERODERMA PIGMENTOSUM.** Development of a squamous cell cancer in the rare syndrome of xeroderma pigmentosum is especially common. The lesion may arise de novo or from a preexisting senile keratosis or keratoacanthoma and is relatively more common in sun-exposed areas. Characteristically, this lesion has an everted edge and is irregular in shape.

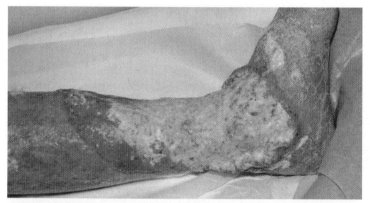

FIGURE 13.42 **SQUAMOUS CELL CARCINOMA.** Arising in an area of chronic ulceration, this large lesion, showing a purulent base and indurated margin, had been misdiagnosed as a benign varicose ulcer.

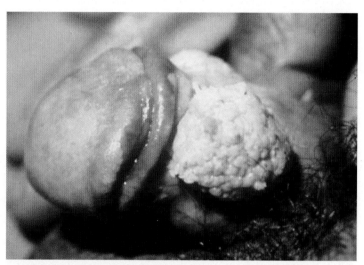

FIGURE 13.45 **VERRUCOUS CARCINOMA.** Clinical picture illustrating two separate verrucous carcinomas of the foreskin arising in a background of long-standing lichen sclerosis.

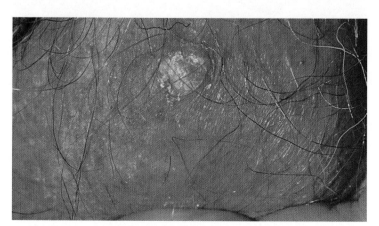

FIGURE 13.43 **TREATMENT-INDUCED SQUAMOUS CELL CARCINOMA.** This early-stage lesion of the scrotum developed after a decade of nitrogen mustard therapy for mycosis fungoides. Topical nitrogen mustard and psoralen + UV A therapy for this disorder are known cutaneous carcinogens. (Courtesy of Dr. Eugene van Scott, Skin and Cancer Hospital, Philadelphia, PA.)

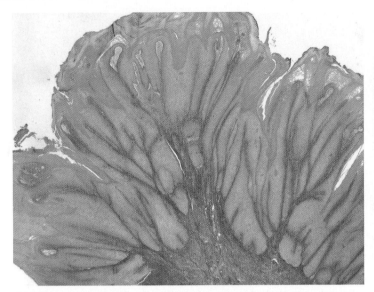

FIGURE 13.46 VERRUCOUS CARCINOMA. Histologically, verrucous carcinoma is characterized by papillary surface and bulbous deep borders. It is an extremely well differentiated tumor without koilocytosis. Between the papillae there is a characteristic piling up of keratin. Pure verrucous carcinomas (not associated with higher-grade areas or infiltrative borders) have an excellent prognosis. Hybrid or mixed verrucous carcinomas are associated with a worse prognosis.

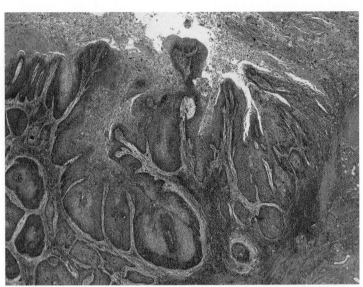

FIGURE 13.48 Warty carcinoma is an HPV-related tumor usually affecting genital/perianal areas. The lesion has some features of condyloma but architectural (infiltrative borders) and cytologic (nuclear pleomorphism) features of carcinoma. There is marked koilocytosis throughout the neoplasm. This tumor should be distinguished from verrucous carcinoma. Warty carcinoma is associated with local-regional metastasis in approximately a fourth of the cases.

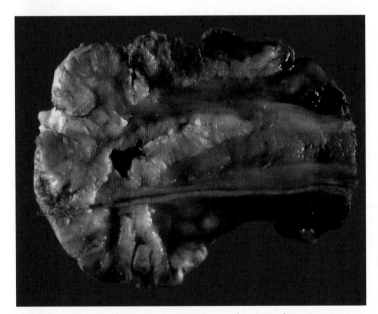

FIGURE 13.47 CARCINOMA CUNICULATUM. Unusual variant of verrucous carcinoma showing deep tumoral invaginations simulating rabbit's burrows. The picture shows a cut section of a partial penectomy specimen with carcinoma cuniculatum.

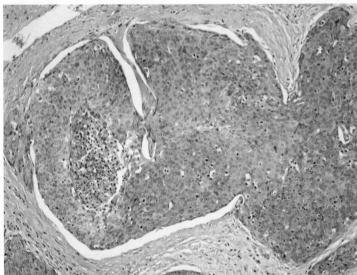

FIGURE 13.49 BASALOID CARCINOMA. Aggressive HPV-related variant of SCC usually affecting genital/perianal areas. The lesion is characterized by aggregates of poorly differentiated basaloid cells with prominent apoptosis and numerous mitoses. Central areas of comedonecrosis and vascular and perineural invasion are common findings in this lesion. It should be distinguished from basal cell carcinomas; the latter are highly unusual in mucosal genital areas.

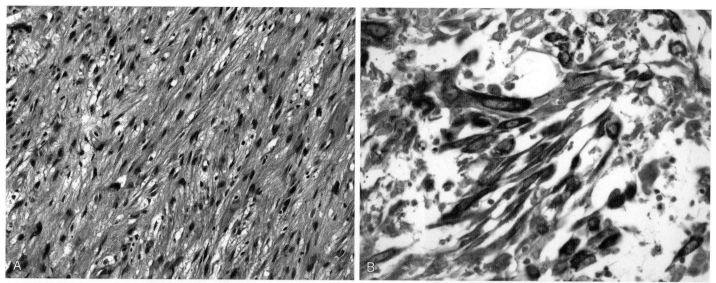

FIGURE 13.50 SARCOMATOID SQUAMOUS CELL CARCINOMA. Not infrequently, squamous cell carcinomas are predominantly composed of spindle cells **(A)**. Immunohistochemical studies are necessary to confirm the epithelial nature of these lesions and differentiate them from spindle cell melanomas, atypical fibroxanthomas, and sarcomas. **(B)** Expression of cytokeratin 34Beta12 by the tumor cells in this example of sarcomatoid carcinoma.

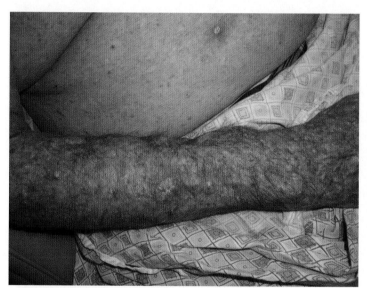

FIGURE 13.51 Arm of a man who had received a kidney transplant more then 30 years earlier. There is a background of actinic keratosis and several invasive SCCs. In transplant recipient patients the risk for developing cutaneous squamous cell carcinoma is related to the duration and level of immunosuppression. (Courtesy of Dr. Danielle Miller, Department of Dermatology, Brigham and Women's Hospital, Boston, MA.)

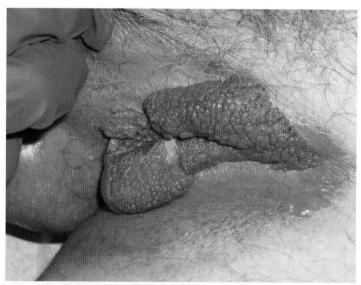

FIGURE 13.52 PATIENT WITH HEART TRANSPLANT. There is an SCC with "warty features" of the left groin. (Courtesy of Dr. Danielle Miller, Department of Dermatology, Brigham and Women's Hospital, Boston, MA.)

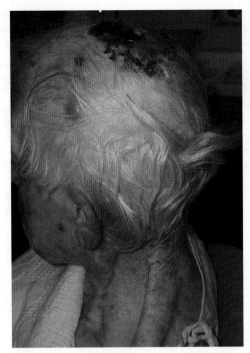

FIGURE 13.53 Elderly patient who had a history of significant sun exposure throughout his life with an SCC of the scalp associated with in-transit metastasis. (Courtesy of Dr. Danielle Miller, Department of Dermatology, Brigham and Women's Hospital, Boston, MA.)

FIGURE 13.54 KERATOACAN-THOMA. (A) A small, early keratocanthoma has arisen on a sun-exposed portion of the ear. Cuplike hyperplastic epithelium can be seen around the base, and the central crater is granular and friable. **(B)** A larger, more mature keratoacanthoma, also in the conchal bowl, shows a central crater filled with keratinous material and a deep surrounding cuff of hyperplastic epithelium.

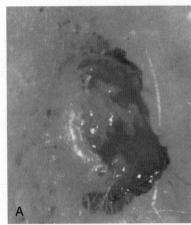

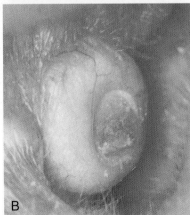

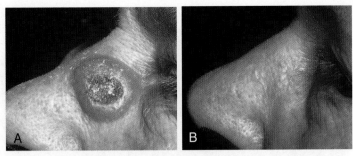

FIGURE 13.55 KERATOACANTHOMA. (A) The hallmark of this tumor is rapid growth up to several centimeters and then gradual involution over a period of months. The lesion illustrated in **(A)** spontaneously regressed as shown in **(B)**.

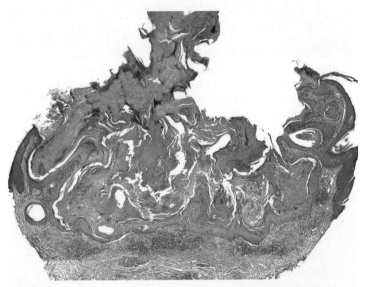

FIGURE 13.56 Keratoacanthoma is a symmetrical, crateriform, exo- and endophytic complex lesion containing a central keratin-filled crater and bulbous lobules of extremely well differentiated squamous cells. The presence of marked nuclear pleomorphism and/or jagged infiltrative borders would strongly argue against a diagnosis of keratoacanthoma. A diagnosis of keratoacanthoma should never be provided in partial biopsies. A diagnosis of keratoacanthoma should only be made in the right clinical setting and when the entire lesion is available for histologic evaluation.

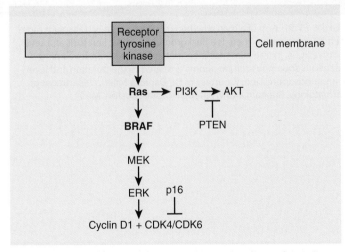

FIGURE 13.57 Dysregulation of signal transduction signaling pathways in melanoma: The MAPK and phosphatidylinositol 3-kinase (PI3K)—AKT signal transduction pathways regulate melanocyte proliferation and survival. More than 80% of melanomas contain mutations that activate components of the MAPK pathway (*N-RAS* and *BRAF*). Other abnormalities seen in melanoma include deletion of *p16* and *PTEN* and increased expression of cyclin D1 and CDK4.

Cancer-testis antigens (CT antigens): MAGE, BAGE, and GAGE gene families
Several members in each family; resemble oncofetal proteins; found normally in testis and placenta

Melanocyte lineage proteins/normal differentiation antigens
Abundant proteins function in melanin production
Tyrosinase
Gp75
Gp100
Melan-A/MART1
Tyrosinase-related protein 2 (TRP2)

Tumor-specific antigens
Subtle mutations of normal cellular proteins: e.g., e of coding region mutations
Cyclin-dependent kinase-4
B-catenin
BRAF with mutation V600E

Other mutated peptides
Activated as a result of cellular transformation
Mutated introns
p15

Candidate antigens identified by monoclonal antibodies
Melanoma gangliosides (GM2, GD2, GM3, and GD3)

A

Vaccine class	Type of vaccine	Examples
Allogeneic tumor	Whole cell Tumor cell lysate Virus oncolysate Shed antigen	Canvaxin Melacine Vaccinia virus Byrstryn virus
Autologous tumor	Granulocyte-macrophage colony-stimulating factor (GM-CSF) secreting Coupled to hapten	GVAX MVAX
Defined tumor antigen	Peptide Ganglioside DNA vaccine Pulsed dendritic cell	Differentiation antigens Cancer-testis antigens GM2-ganglioside GP100

B

FIGURE 13.58 IMMUNE TARGETING OF MELANOMA. (A) Examples of identified melanoma antigens. Melanoma rejection antigens have been identified as target T cells. This list continues to expand both in numbers within groups as well as in new categories of antigenic targets. **(B)** Examples of vaccine-based therapeutic approaches in melanoma.

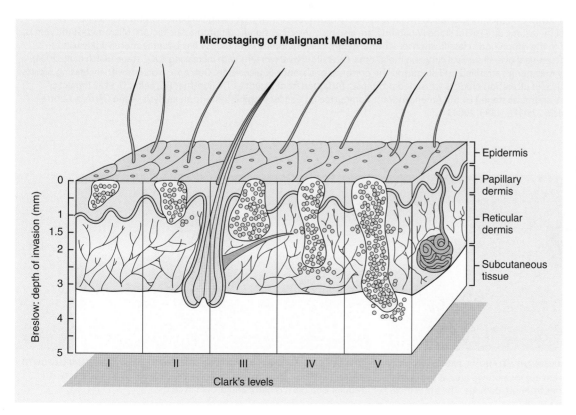

Microstaging of Malignant Melanoma

FIGURE 13.59 MALIGNANT MELANOMA. This diagram represents the combined microstaging techniques of Clark and Breslow. The Clark system of levels of invasion is based on anatomy, whereas the Breslow technique relies on the depth of invasion (in millimeters) from the granular layer of epidermis to the deepest tumor cell. (Adapted from Goldsmith HS: Melanoma: an overview, *CA Cancer J Clin* 29: 194–215, 1979.)

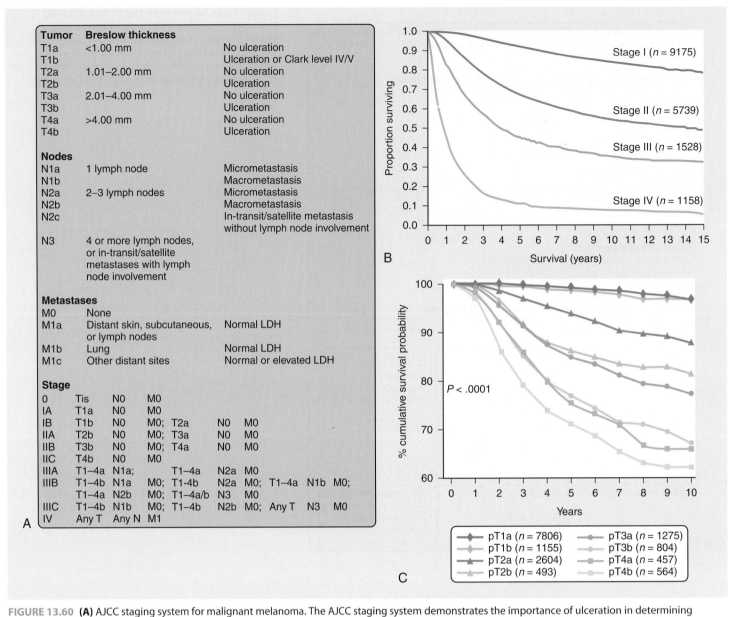

Tumor	Breslow thickness	
T1a	<1.00 mm	No ulceration
T1b		Ulceration or Clark level IV/V
T2a	1.01–2.00 mm	No ulceration
T2b		Ulceration
T3a	2.01–4.00 mm	No ulceration
T3b		Ulceration
T4a	>4.00 mm	No ulceration
T4b		Ulceration

Nodes		
N1a	1 lymph node	Micrometastasis
N1b		Macrometastasis
N2a	2–3 lymph nodes	Micrometastasis
N2b		Macrometastasis
N2c		In-transit/satellite metastasis without lymph node involvement
N3	4 or more lymph nodes, or in-transit/satellite metastases with lymph node involvement	

Metastases		
M0	None	
M1a	Distant skin, subcutaneous, or lymph nodes	Normal LDH
M1b	Lung	Normal LDH
M1c	Other distant sites	Normal or elevated LDH

Stage									
0	Tis	N0	M0						
IA	T1a	N0	M0						
IB	T1b	N0	M0;	T2a	N0	M0			
IIA	T2b	N0	M0;	T3a	N0	M0			
IIB	T3b	N0	M0;	T4a	N0	M0			
IIC	T4b	N0	M0						
IIIA	T1–4a	N1a;		T1–4a	N2a	M0			
IIIB	T1–4b	N1a	M0;	T1–4b	N2a	M0;	T1–4a	N1b	M0;
	T1–4a	N2b	M0;	T1–4a/b	N3	M0			
IIIC	T1–4b	N1b	M0;	T1–4b	N2b	M0;	Any T	N3	M0
IV	Any T	Any N	M1						

A

B

C

FIGURE 13.60 (A) AJCC staging system for malignant melanoma. The AJCC staging system demonstrates the importance of ulceration in determining prognosis, principally upstaging patients with evidence for ulceration. The number of lymph nodes involved for stage III patients, and the lactate dehydrogenase (LDH) levels and sites of metastatic disease for stage IV patients, are also recognized as significant prognostic factors. Micrometastatic versus macrometastatic disease is recognized in the lymph node classification as sentinel lymph node mapping with biopsy has become more widely used. (Adapted from Balch et al., 2001.) **(B)** Fifteen-year overall survival curves in melanoma. Overall survival worsens with increasing AJCC stage (Balch et al., 2004). **(C)** Survival estimates of 15,158 primary melanomas stratified by T stage and the presence or absence of ulceration. Outcome worsens with increasing Breslow thickness. For a given T stage the presence of ulceration predicts worsened prognosis. (Adapted from Eigentler TK, Buettner PG, Leiter U, et al: Impact of ulceration in stages I to III cutaneous melanoma as staged by the American Joint Committee on Cancer Staging System: an analysis of the German Central Malignant Melanoma Registry, *J Clin Oncol* 22:4376–4383, 2004.)

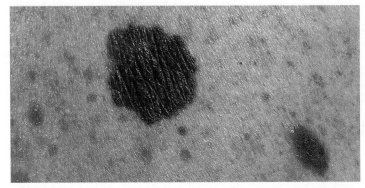

FIGURE 13.61 SUPERFICIAL SPREADING MALIGNANT MELANOMA, RADIAL-GROWTH PHASE. The lesion is almost totally black except for a brown area at the upper left edge. Note the surrounding lentigines from sun damage. The other mole is benign.

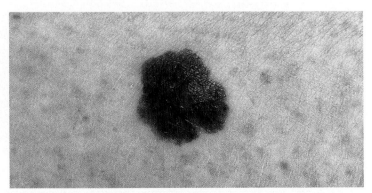

FIGURE 13.62 SUPERFICIAL SPREADING MALIGNANT MELANOMA, RADIAL-GROWTH PHASE. This lesion appears as a slightly raised plaque with a characteristic irregular outline. It is black and brown in color.

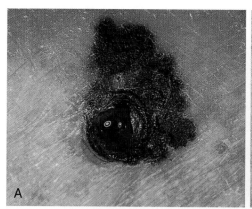

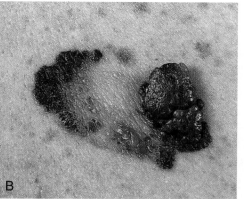

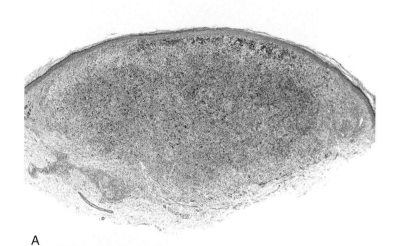

FIGURE 13.63 **SUPERFICIAL SPREADING MALIGNANT MELANOMA, VERTICAL-GROWTH PHASE.** The radial-growth phase of a lesion is ultimately followed by vertical growth and deep invasion with formation of a nodule **(A)**. **(B)** Another example of a vertical-growth–phase melanoma with areas of regression (*white, gray, and red foci*).

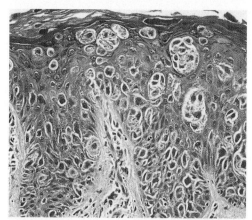

FIGURE 13.64 **SUPERFICIAL SPREADING MALIGNANT MELANOMA.** Clusters of "pagetoid" melanocytes are present at all layers of the epidermis.

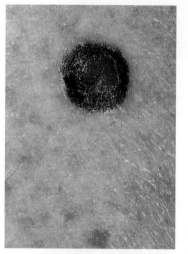

FIGURE 13.65 **NODULAR MALIGNANT MELANOMA.** This variant of malignant melanoma lacks a horizontal-growth phase. The lesion grows vertically from the beginning, and invasion produces a nodule. Note the surrounding lentigines.

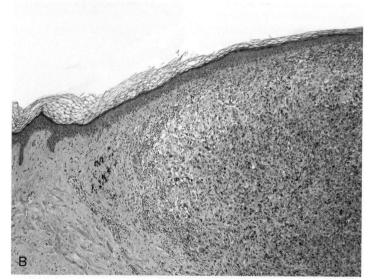

FIGURE 13.67 **NODULAR MALIGNANT MELANOMA.** Histologically, the nodular type of malignant melanoma is predominantly composed of a dermal component in vertical-growth phase. There is no evidence of a preceding radial-growth phase. The low-power view **(A)** illustrates a sharply circumscribed nodule of melanoma within the dermis. The higher-power view **(B)** shows absence of a melanoma in situ component in the adjacent epidermis. Note the presence of solar elastosis in the dermis.

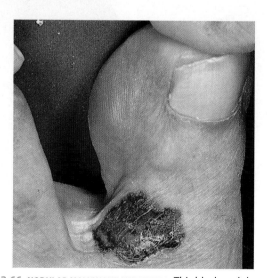

FIGURE 13.66 **NODULAR MALIGNANT MELANOMA.** This black nodule represents the classic conception of a malignant melanoma. The prognosis for these lesions is poor.

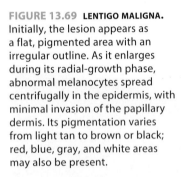

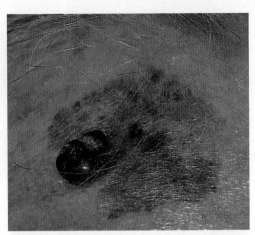

FIGURE 13.71 **LENTIGO MALIGNA MELANOMA, VERTICAL-GROWTH PHASE.** In time, the radial-growth phase is followed by a vertical-growth phase; at this stage the lesion thickens and becomes nodular.

FIGURE 13.68 **AMELANOTIC MALIGNANT MELANOMA.** Rarely, a lesion presents with no apparent visible pigmentation, as in the case of this plum-colored nodule on the sole of a foot. These lesions show aggressive behavior, evolving quickly and penetrating deeply.

FIGURE 13.69 **LENTIGO MALIGNA.** Initially, the lesion appears as a flat, pigmented area with an irregular outline. As it enlarges during its radial-growth phase, abnormal melanocytes spread centrifugally in the epidermis, with minimal invasion of the papillary dermis. Its pigmentation varies from light tan to brown or black; red, blue, gray, and white areas may also be present.

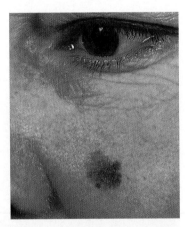

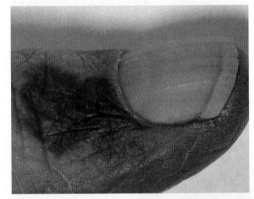

FIGURE 13.72 **ACRAL LENTIGINOUS MALIGNANT MELANOMA.** Clinically, this lesion appears similar to lentigo maligna, but it shows much more aggressive biologic behavior. It grows quickly, becoming raised and subsequently nodular, an indication of a vertical-growth phase. (Courtesy of Dr A.C. Pembroke.)

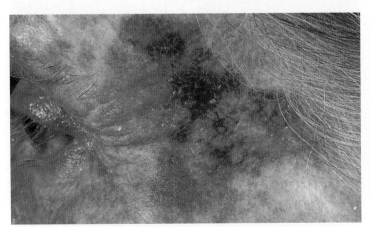

FIGURE 13.70 **LENTIGO MALIGNA.** Typical of the radial-growth phase, this lesion is made up of various colors and has an irregular, indented margin. Like many such tumors, it grew slowly and attained a large size before presentation.

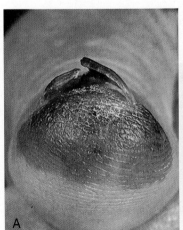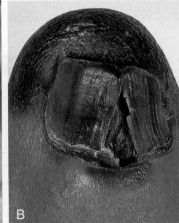

FIGURE 13.73 **ACRAL LENTIGINOUS MALIGNANT MELANOMA. (A, B)** This lesion arising from the nailbed has an irregular outline; its colors vary from black to gray and blue. As it invades, the lesion distorts and splits the nailplate. (Courtesy of Dr A.C. Pembroke.)

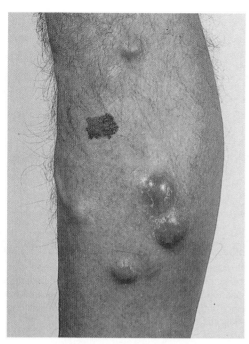

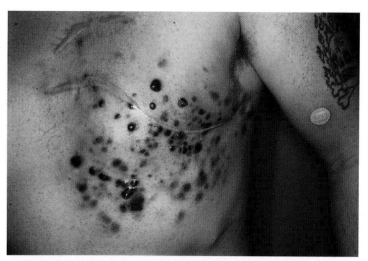

FIGURE 13.76 Thirty-year-old man with numerous regional cutaneous metastases. In some patients localized areas of metastases cluster together. Eventually, however, metastases occur at distant sites.

FIGURE 13.74 **METASTATIC MALIGNANT MELANOMA.** Hard flesh- and plum-colored tumors have spread from this man's neglected primary lesion. The leg is a common site for malignant melanoma.

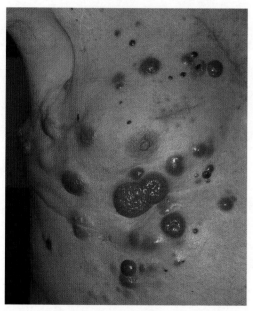

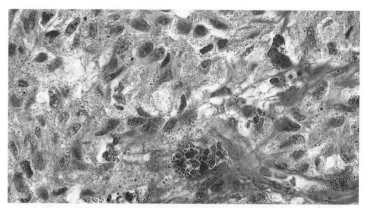

FIGURE 13.77 **METASTATIC MALIGNANT MELANOMA, PIGMENTED.** Tumor tissue is characterized by increased numbers of atypical melanocytes showing pleomorphism and prominent chromatin clumping. Fine particles of melanin can be seen throughout the cytoplasm.

FIGURE 13.75 **METASTATIC MELANOMA.** Regional chest lesions in an 85-year-old man that developed several years after removal of the primary. Note lesions of variable size and appearance. Visceral metastases eventually occurred.

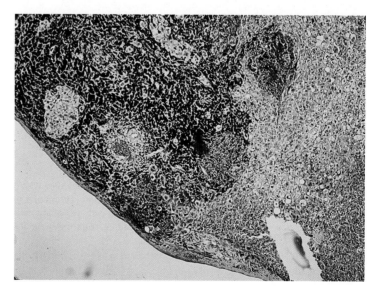

FIGURE 13.78 **METASTATIC MALIGNANT MELANOMA TO A LYMPH NODE.** Low-power view of lymph node metastasis shows numerous heavily pigmented tumor cells as well as areas of amelanotic poorly differentiated malignant cells.

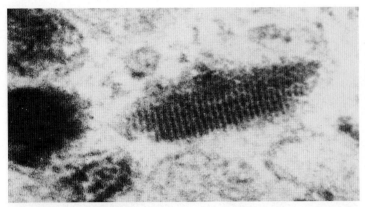

FIGURE 13.79 **MALIGNANT MELANOMA.** Electron micrograph of a melanosome shows the typical oval structure of these tyrosinase-containing granules. This partially developed melanosome demonstrates the lamellated internal structure, which is obscured by pigment production in mature granules.

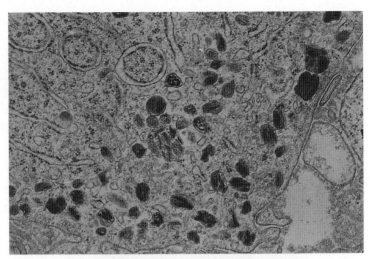

FIGURE 13.80 **MALIGNANT MELANOMA.** Electron micrograph shows prominent, characteristic dense-core granules. In some patients with amelanotic melanoma presenting with metastases from an unknown primary site, the presence of these granules will help to confirm a diagnosis of malignant melanoma.

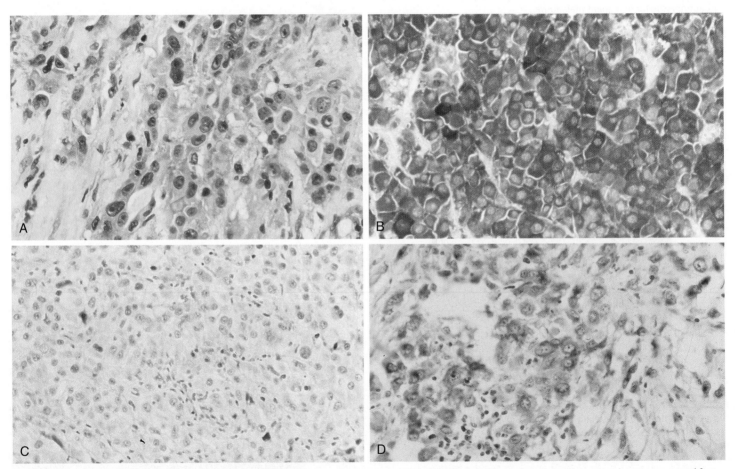

FIGURE 13.81 **METASTATIC AMELANOTIC MELANOMA.** A 60-year-old man, who 6 years previously had a level III amelanotic malignant melanoma removed from his back, presented with cervical adenopathy. **(A)** Microscopic section of a lymph node biopsy specimen shows an undifferentiated epithelioid malignancy. **(B)** Positive S-100 immunoperoxidase stain is consistent with malignant melanoma; a negative keratin stain **(C)** rules out an epithelial neoplasm. **(D)** Positive immunoperoxidase staining with HMB-45 is also positive, confirming the diagnosis of melanoma.

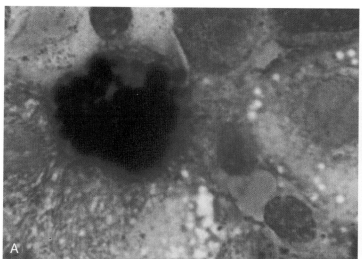
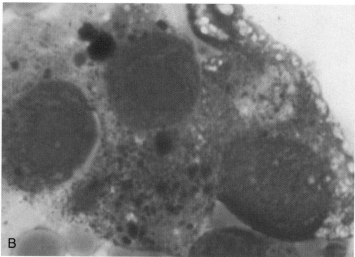

FIGURE 13.82 **METASTATIC MELANOMA TO THE BONE MARROW.** A 26-year-old man presented with level IV cutaneous melanoma involving the mid-back. He also had mild anemia. Bone marrow shows infiltration by clumps of large malignant cells with abundant basophilic cytoplasm, immature nuclei, and very prominent nucleoli. Large clumps of extracellular melanin are noted **(A)**. In addition, melanin granules (*dark bluish-green in color*) are noted in the cytoplasm of many individual melanoma cells **(B)** (×1000, Wright-Giemsa stain).

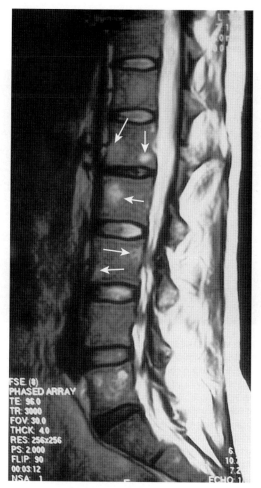

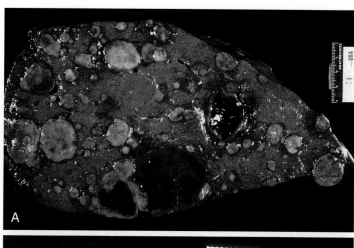
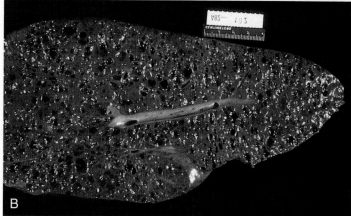

FIGURE 13.83 **METASTATIC MALIGNANT MELANOMA TO THE BONE.** A 38-year-old woman with previous resection of a level III cutaneous melanoma developed subsequent metastases to the brain and liver. Because of mild back pain, magnetic resonance imaging of the spine was carried out. Sagittal T_2-weighted image of the lumbar spine reveals multiple foci of increased signal (*arrows*) consistent with metastases.

FIGURE 13.84 **METASTATIC MALIGNANT MELANOMA TO THE LIVER.** Metastases frequently occur to the liver. Two major patterns are noted, including large nodular deposits with hemorrhage, as well as pigment production **(A)** and a diffuse process with smaller-size metastases **(B)**. In the the latter case the liver weighed 4060 g and contained numerous small, cystic metastases that were filled with blood.

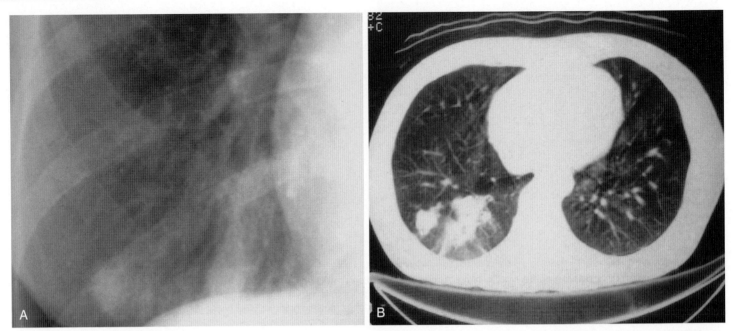

FIGURE 13.85 **METASTATIC MALIGNANT MELANOMA TO THE LUNG.** In some patients metastatic disease to the lung may stimulate primary lung cancer. **(A)** Plain radiograph of the right lower lung of this 40-year-old patient, with previous resection of a cutaneous melanoma, reveals nodular infiltrate. **(B)** Computed tomography (CT) scan reveals the prominent localized metastases in the right lower lung.

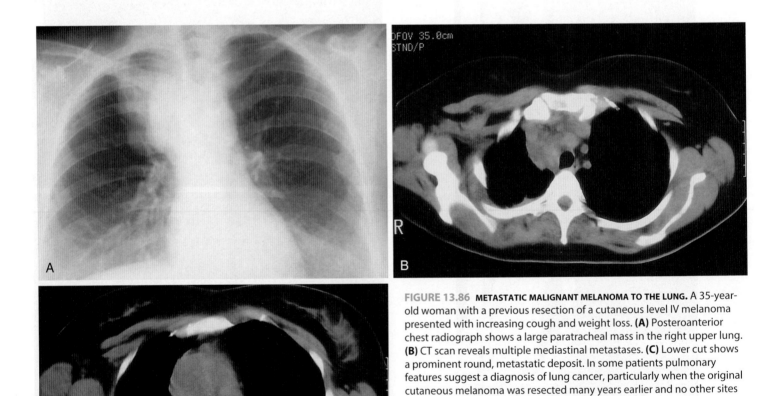

FIGURE 13.86 **METASTATIC MALIGNANT MELANOMA TO THE LUNG.** A 35-year-old woman with a previous resection of a cutaneous level IV melanoma presented with increasing cough and weight loss. **(A)** Posteroanterior chest radiograph shows a large paratracheal mass in the right upper lung. **(B)** CT scan reveals multiple mediastinal metastases. **(C)** Lower cut shows a prominent round, metastatic deposit. In some patients pulmonary features suggest a diagnosis of lung cancer, particularly when the original cutaneous melanoma was resected many years earlier and no other sites of metastases are initially identified. The diagnosis is further confounded when the late metastases are amelanotic.

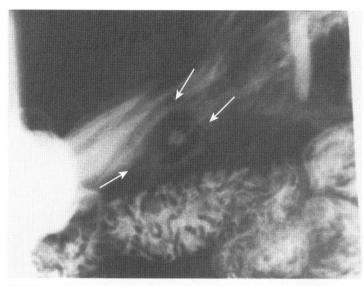

FIGURE 13.87 **METASTATIC MELANOMA.** Typical "target lesion" noted in the stomach wall of this 50-year-old man with prior resection of a level IV cutaneous lesion, who recently presented with anemia due to gastric bleeding. The "target" appearance is due to central necrosis and ulceration of the metastatic tumor masses.

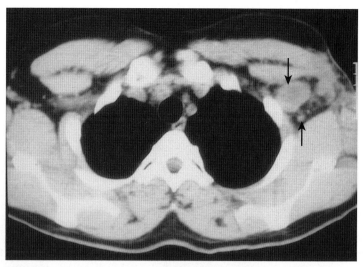

FIGURE 13.89 **METASTATIC MELANOMA TO LYMPH NODE.** In this 40-year-old man with metastatic malignant melanoma, CT scan of the chest shows an enlarged left axillary lymph node (*arrows*).

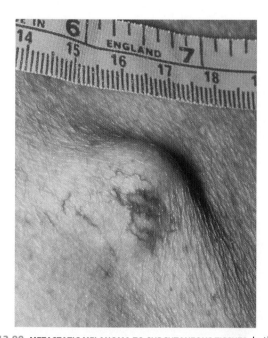

FIGURE 13.88 **METASTATIC MELANOMA TO SUBCUTANEOUS TISSUES.** In this 60-year-old man the first evidence of metastatic malignant melanoma was the rapid growth of a subcutaneous nodule on his mid-back.

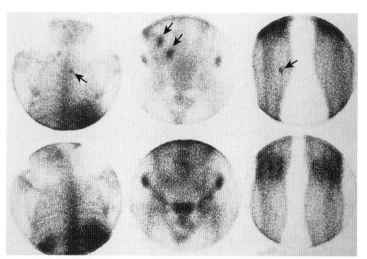

FIGURE 13.90 **METASTATIC MELANOMA TO SOFT TISSUES.** Gallium-67 scanning will often reveal palpable as well as nonpalpable early metastases to soft tissues, as illustrated in this 60-year-old patient. The scan at 72 hours shows increased uptake in paraspinal tissues (*upper left*), iliac lymph nodes (*upper center*), and medial calf (*upper right*). The following scan, repeated 6 weeks later after multidrug chemotherapy, shows no significant uptake, corresponding to a clinical remission. The hot spots in the lower middle view represent normal marrow, bladder, and rectal sites due to a higher count rate, which accentuates the images.

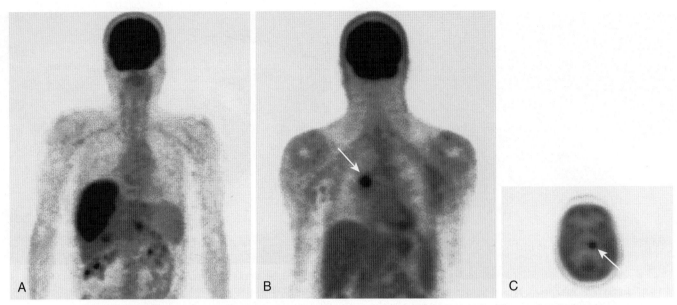

FIGURE 13.91 **POSITRON EMISSION TOMOGRAPHY SCANNING IN MELANOMA. (A)** Seventy-year-old patient with a history of ocular melanoma demonstrates ¹⁸F-FDG-glucose uptake in multiple liver metastases, including a dominant right hepatic lobe mass. **(B)** Fifty-six-year-old patient with a history of stage III malignant melanoma demonstrates uptake in a hilar mass (*arrow*) that was not significant on CT scan. **(C)** Same patient as in **(B)** demonstrates an asymptomatic mass in the brain (*arrow*) that was subsequently confirmed by head magnetic resonance imaging. (Courtesy of Drs. Milos Janicek and Annick van den Abbeele, Dana-Farber Cancer Institute, Boston, MA.)

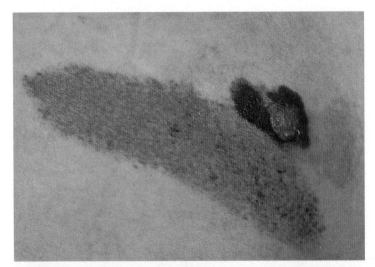

FIGURE 13.92 **MALIGNANT MELANOMA.** In the exceptional case, as shown here, malignant melanoma develops in a large melanocytic nevus that has been present from birth.

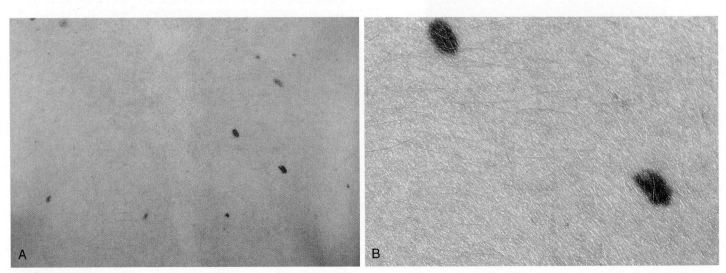

FIGURE 13.93 **DYSPLASTIC NEVUS SYNDROME. (A)** Photograph of the back of a 15-year-old girl who had a family history of malignant melanoma shows numerous atypical nevi. **(B)** Of the two moles shown on this close-up view, the one on the right with an irregular margin proved to be malignant.

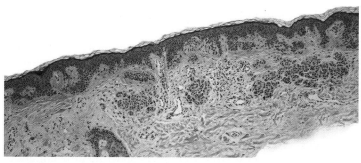

FIGURE 13.94 DYSPLASTIC NEVUS. Histologically, a dysplastic nevus is characterized by a basilar proliferation of melanocytes showing bridging of rete ridges by confluence of melanocyte nests. In compound lesions the junctional component extends at least three rete ridges beyond a dermal component (shoulder). There are also lamellar fibrosis, telangiectasia, and lymphocytic infiltrates in the papillary dermis. Most dysplastic nevi show some degree of cytologic atypia, which tends to be discontinuous and random.

Miscellaneous Skin Cancers

Cutaneous T-cell lymphomas (CTCLs) are malignancies of the skin derived from peripheral T lymphocytes (Table 13.3) (Girardi et al., 2004). Mycosis fungoides—which is characterized by scaly flat patches that progress to plaques, tumors, and ulcers—is the most common type. Mycosis fungoides and Sézary syndrome represent approximately 65% of the cases of CTCLs (Olsen et al., 2007) (Figs. 13.95 through 13.104). Both are characterized by a monoclonal proliferation of predominantly CD4$^+$/CD45R0$^+$ helper T cells and the loss of mature T-cell antigens in the skin and other involved organs. Sézary syndrome is currently defined by the International Society of Cutaneous Lymphomas (ISCL) as a distinctive erythrodermic CTCL (albeit potentially lacking the diagnostic histologic features in the skin) with hematologic evidence of leukemic involvement. In some instances the diagnosis of mycosis fungoides can be rendered with confidence on a skin biopsy specimen based on typical light microscopic changes, that is, marked epidermotropism of cytologically atypical T lymphocytes without significant spongiosis, clusters of these cells in the epidermis (Pautrier microabscesses), or a bandlike infiltrate containing abnormal lymphocytes in the upper dermis usually associated with papillary dermal fibrosis (Olsen et al., 2007) (Figs. 13.98 and 13.99). However, a definitive histopathologic diagnosis by light microscopy alone may be difficult to make in early mycosis fungoides. The ISCL recently proposed a diagnostic algorithm for early mycosis fungoides (Olsen et al., 2007). Multiple skin biopsies may be necessary to establish a firm diagnosis. Molecular studies (T-cell rearrangement) showing clonality aid to confirm the diagnosis. For patients who present with tumors, it is important to differentiate tumor-stage mycosis fungoides from non-mycosis fungoides subtypes of CTCL. The classification and staging of mycosis fungoides and Sézary syndrome have been recently revised by ISCL/EORTC (Olsen et al., 2007). This revised classification no longer includes the former category T0 for "clinical and histopathological suspicious lesions." Current practice is to apply clinical staging to cases in which the diagnosis of CTCL has been established. T1 rating is defined by papules, patches, and/or plaques covering less than 10% of the skin surface. When they cover more than 10% of the skin surface the stage would be T2. One or more tumors qualify for T3. T4 is characterized by confluent erythema covering more than 80% of the body surface. Regional lymph node involvement and visceral dissemination occur in advanced disease. In the revised staging system N0 or not clinically abnormal peripheral lymph nodes require no biopsy. Only abnormal peripheral lymph nodes such as those such 1.5 cm or larger or any palpable lymph node (regardless of size) that is firm, irregular, clustered, or fixed have to be biopsied. N1 refers to lymph nodes showing dermatopathic lymphadenopathy and N2 to early involvement by mycosis fungoides. N3 can be subdivided into two grades according to the presence of partial or complete lymph node effacement by mycosis fungoides. Patients with no visceral organ involvement are rated as M0 and those with visceral involvement as M1 (the organ involved should be specified). Blood involvement in mycosis fungoides is classified as B0 when less than 5% of peripheral blood lymphocytes are atypical and as B1 when more than 5% of peripheral lymphocytes are atypical. However, if there are more than 1000/μL Sézary cells and/or presence of a clonal rearrangement of the TCR in the blood, criteria are met for B2. Blood involvement has independent prognostic significance. Survival rates decrease with advancing stages of disease.

Table 13.3		
Classification of Cutaneous T-Cell Lymphomas		
Type of Disease	**European Organization for Research and Treatment of Cancer Classification**	**World Health Organization Classification**
Indolent	Mycosis fungoides Mycosis fungoides and follicular mucinosis Pagetoid reticulosis Large–cell cutaneous T-cell lymphoma, CD30-positive Anaplastic Immunoblastic Pleomorphic Lymphomatoid papulosis	Mycosis fungoides Mycosis fungoides–associated follicular mucinosis Pagetoid reticulosis Primary cutaneous anaplastic large–cell lymphoma Lymphomatoid papulosis
Aggressive	Sézary syndrome Large–cell cutaneous T-cell lymphoma, CD30-negative Immunoblastic Pleomorphic	Sézary syndrome Peripheral T-cell lymphoma (not otherwise specified)
Provisional	Granulomatous slack skin Cutaneous T-cell lymphoma, pleomorphic, small to medium size Subcutaneous panniculitis-like T-cell lymphoma	Granulomatous slack skin Peripheral T-cell lymphoma (not otherwise specified) Subcutaneous panniculitis-like T-cell lymphoma

From Girardi M, Heald PW, Wilson LD: The pathogenesis of mycosis fungoides. *N Engl J Med* 350:1978–1988;2004.

Kaposi sarcoma is a malignancy of the vascular endothelium that occurs in elderly men (classic Kaposi sarcoma), African natives, organ-transplanted patients, and patients with acquired immunodeficiency syndrome. The disease shows diverse clinical and histopathologic manifestations and may be difficult to diagnose in early stages. Typical established cutaneous lesions are reddish to purplish brown nodules affecting the lower extremities (Figs. 13.105 and 13.106). The course of classic Kaposi sarcoma is usually prolonged. Elderly patients may die of intercurrent disease. In other patients, widespread visceral involvement may be found. The most commonly involved organs include the lymph nodes and gastrointestinal tract. Indicators of poor prognosis are immunosuppression and age over 50. African cases tend to behave more aggressively. An important and relatively recent discovery is the presence of herpesvirus (HHV-8) in almost all cases of Kaposi sarcoma (human immunodeficiency virus–related, classic, iatrogenic, or endemic) (Viejo-Borbolla and Ottinger, 2004). The presence of HHV-8 can now be detected by immunohistochemical techniques in tissue sections. Microscopically, the most typical feature of Kaposi sarcoma is the presence of spindle cells forming slits containing red blood cells (Fig. 13.107).

Merkel cell (neuroendocrine) carcinoma is a rare but highly aggressive epithelial malignancy of the skin (Bayrou et al., 1991). It occurs mainly in adults and elderly persons. The face and extremities are the most common locations (Figs. 13.108 and 13.109). Histologically, it should be distinguished from lymphomas, small cell melanoma, and metastatic tumors including small cell (oat cell) carcinoma of the lung (Fig. 13.110). Immunohistochemical studies are helpful in achieving the correct diagnosis (Fig. 13.111) (Byrd et al., 2000). Ultrastructurally, Merkel cells show neurosecretory-type granules. Regional nodal and distant metastases such as to the lungs, liver, and bones are commonly associated with Merkel cell carcinoma. Local-regional recurrence carries an ominous prognostic significance. Sentinel node biopsies seem to be of importance to correctly stage patients (Gupta et al., 2006).

Malignant counterparts of adnexal tumors (with follicular, sweat gland, and sebaceous gland differentiation) can also be seen. Sebaceous carcinoma is rare but important to recognize, because especially those tumors located in the eyelid, caruncles, and orbit tend to have an aggressive behavior (Figs. 13.112 and 13.113). Primary mucinous carcinomas of the skin are exceptional tumors often appearing on the scalp of elderly patients. Some cases have been found to show eccrine and others apocrine differentiation. They show identical features to mucinous breast carcinoma and should be distinguished from metastasis (Fig. 13.114).

Mammary Paget's disease of the nipple and areola is an uncommon neoplastic condition, almost always associated with breast carcinoma. The underlying breast cancer may be in situ or invasive. The condition is usually unilateral and characterized by red, weeping, scaly plaques that may mimic psoriasis or eczema. Extramammary Paget's disease is a rare condition that usually presents in areas rich in apocrine sweat glands. It usually affects elderly patients, and it is more frequently seen in women. The most commonly affected sites include the perineal region and vulva (Fig. 13.115). In the majority of cases the lesion is confined to the epidermis. Although the association is less common, patients with extramammary Paget's disease should also be screened for an underlying malignancy (Lloyd and Flanagan, 2000).

It is important to remember that in some cases malignant skin tumors may represent metastasis from other sites (Spenser and Helm, 1987). It is crucial to recognize such tumors as metastases and differentiate them from primary skin cancers. The most common origin of cutaneous metastasis in male patients includes the lung followed by the large intestine (Fig. 13.116). In women, the most common source of skin metastasis is the breast.

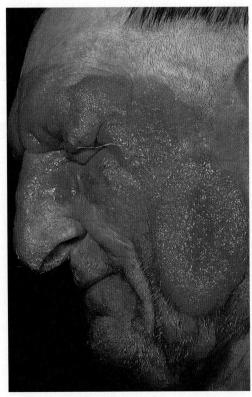

FIGURE 13.95 **MYCOSIS FUNGOIDES.** In a late stage of the disease, lesions develop into mushroom-like tumors on the skin.

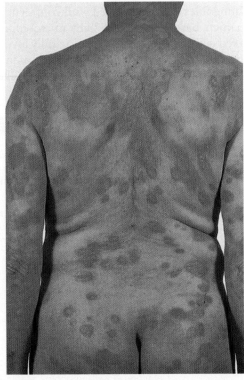

FIGURE 13.96 **MYCOSIS FUNGOIDES.** Although these widespread lesions mimic psoriasis in their patch or premycotic stage, they are asymmetrical, an unusual finding in psoriasis. Skin biopsy confirmed the diagnosis of mycosis fungoides. (Courtesy of Dr. A.C. Pembroke.)

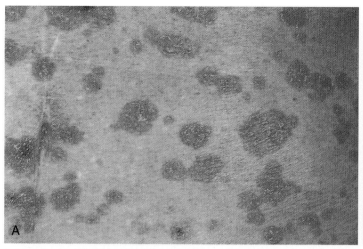

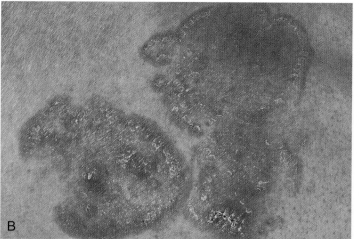

FIGURE 13.97 **MYCOSIS FUNGOIDES. (A)** The pink, scaly patches may occur in various shapes and sizes. This early-stage disease is sometimes called "parapsoriasis en plaque." **(B)** The borders of the eruptions may be quite bizarre.

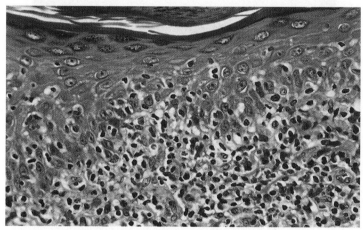

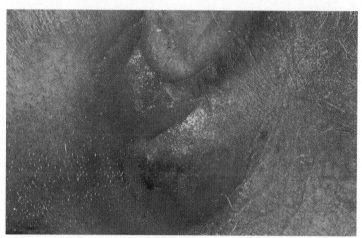

FIGURE 13.98 **MYCOSIS FUNGOIDES.** This more advanced patch-stage lesion shows parakeratosis, orthohyperkeratosis, and acanthosis. The epidermis and dermis are diffusely infiltrated by large numbers of cells with highly irregular cerebriform and dark-staining nuclei (mycosis cells).

FIGURE 13.100 **MYCOSIS FUNGOIDES.** As the disease progresses, plaques develop into tumorous masses, as seen in this large nodular lesion. This patient had widespread infiltrated plaques elsewhere. (Courtesy of Dr. A.C. Pembroke.)

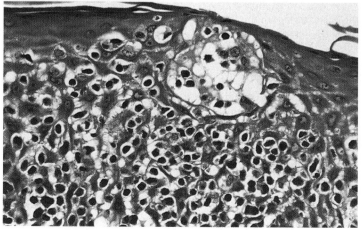

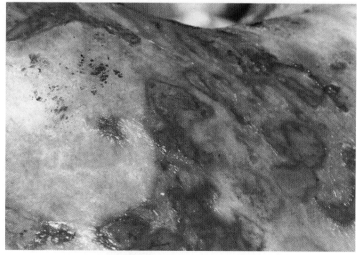

FIGURE 13.99 **MYCOSIS FUNGOIDES.** Photomicrograph of a plaque-stage lesion shows a characteristic Pautrier microabscess situated just below the stratum corneum.

FIGURE 13.101 **MYCOSIS FUNGOIDES.** Very occasionally, ulcerative lesions develop in the late stage of the disease.

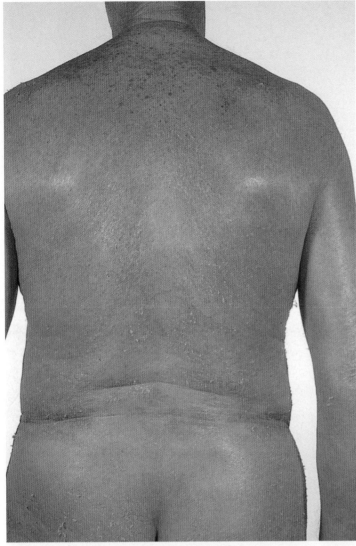

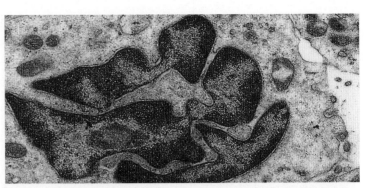

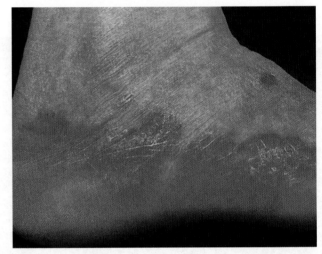

FIGURE 13.104 SÉZARY SYNDROME/MYCOSIS FUNGOIDES. Electron micrograph shows the characteristic appearance of the nucleus of a mycosis/Sézary cell. The T lymphocyte shows abundant cytoplasm and a centrally located, irregular, highly convoluted nucleus with a peripheral chromatin distribution.

FIGURE 13.102 SÉZARY SYNDROME. Clinically, this condition is an erythroderma or exfoliative dermatitis marked by a universal redness of the skin with associated scaling. This patient had a white blood count of 90,000 cells/μL with 70% Sézary cells (see Fig. 13.98).

FIGURE 13.105 KAPOSI SARCOMA. Purple plaques and nodules, particularly on the lower legs and feet, are characteristic of this vascular malignancy. (Courtesy of Dr. Neil Smith, Institute of Dermatology, London, UK.)

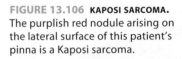

FIGURE 13.106 KAPOSI SARCOMA. The purplish red nodule arising on the lateral surface of this patient's pinna is a Kaposi sarcoma.

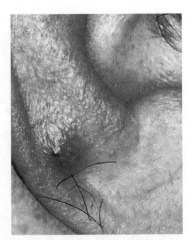

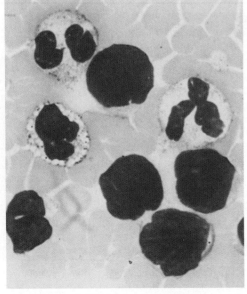

FIGURE 13.103 SÉZARY SYNDROME/MYCOSIS FUNGOIDES. The cerebriform, hyperchromatic nuclei of mycosis/Sézary cells are evident in this peripheral blood smear. Such cells are present in abundance in the peripheral blood in Sézary syndrome, but they are seen in smaller numbers in some patients with mycosis fungoides.

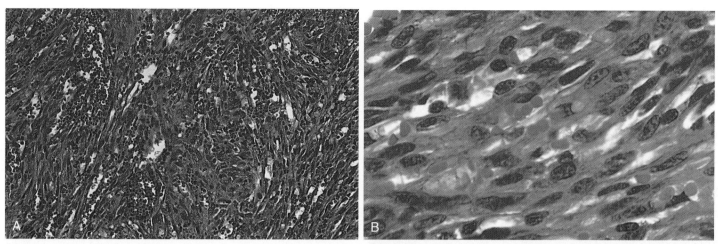

FIGURE 13.107 KAPOSI SARCOMA. Microscopically, the most typical feature of Kaposi sarcoma is the presence of spindle cells forming slits containing red blood cells **(A)**. Admixed in this lesion are inflammatory cells including numerous plasma cells and abundant hemosiderin. Higher-power view **(B)** illustrating the relatively uniform spindle cells, slitlike spaces containing erythrocytes, and characteristic hyaline globules of variable size, probably representing degenerated red blood cells.

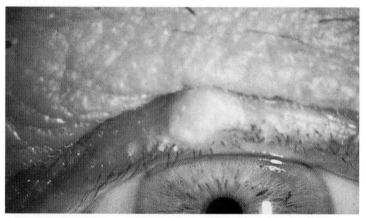

FIGURE 13.108 MERKEL CELL TUMOR. Clinically the lesion presents as a firm, raised, painless nodule as shown here in the middle portion of the upper eyelid. The slowly enlarging tumor may be violaceous; ulceration is rare.

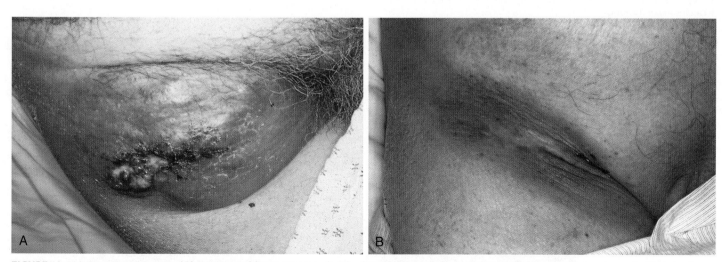

FIGURE 13.109 MERKEL CELL TUMOR. (A) A 65-year-old man presented with a large, ulcerative skin lesion in the right groin. Biopsy showed a Merkel cell tumor. **(B)** Combination chemotherapy resulted in a marked regression of the malignancy. Follow-up surgical resection and postoperative radiation therapy were carried out, and the patient remained disease-free 4 years later. Merkel cell tumors may be confused with other "small blue cell" tumors such as small cell (oat cell) lung cancer. Widespread dissemination may occur in all of these highly malignant tumors, including metatases to the brain, skin, bone, and bone marrow.

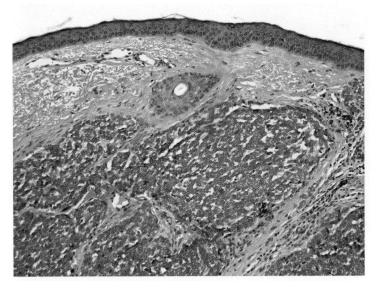

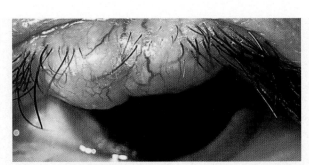

FIGURE 13.112 **SEBACEOUS CARCINOMA.** The clinical appearance of this lesion simulates that of a large chalazion. It presents as a steadily enlarging, nonulcerated nodule of the upper eyelid. Note the characteristic loss of hair over the lesion.

FIGURE 13.110 **MERKEL CELL CARCINOMA.** Typical microscopic appearance showing aggregates of small round blue cells within the dermis.

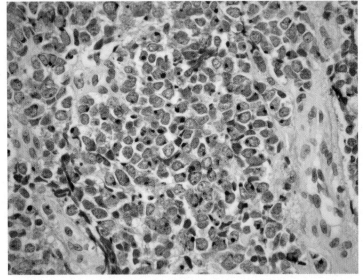

FIGURE 13.111 **MERKEL CELL CARCINOMA. CHARACTERISTIC DOTLIKE EXPRESSION OF CYTOKERATIN 20.** In addition to cytokeratin 20, Merkel cell carcinoma is usually positive with CAM 5.2, chromogranin, and synaptophysin. Cytokeratin 7 and thyroid transcription factor 1, which are typically negative, aid in distinguishing primary lesions from cutaneous metastasis from small cell carcinoma of the lung.

FIGURE 13.113 **SEBACEOUS CARCINOMA. (A)** Low-power view illustrating lobular and infiltrative aggregates of basaloid cells with central necrosis. It is important to distinguish this tumor from basal cell carcinomas and SCCs. **(B)** Higher-power view highlights the presence of sebaceous differentiation and numerous mitotic figures. **(C)** Frozen tissues can be stained with oil-red-O to demonstrate the presence of lipids. **(D)** Large, single, pale tumoral cells may be seen throughout the epidermis (pagetoid spread).

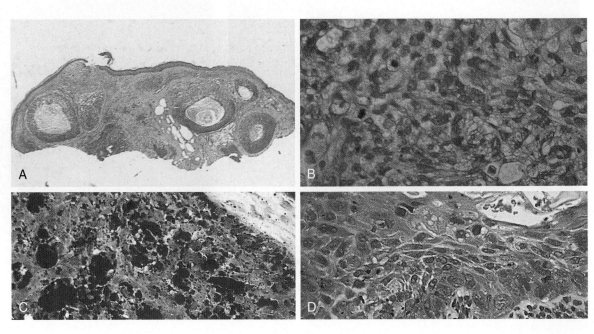

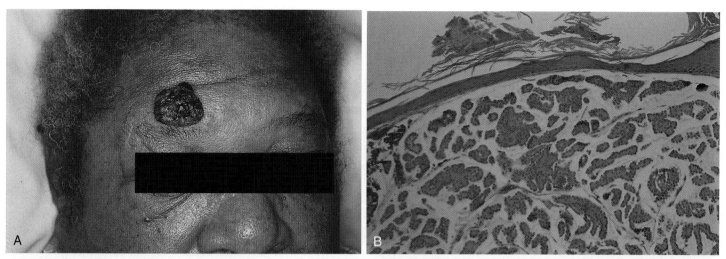

FIGURE 13.114 **PRIMARY MUCINOUS CARCINOMA OF THE SKIN. (A)** Note pigmented, protuberant localized lesion in a 69-year-old black male, of about 1 year's duration. **(B)** Low-power view shows a pseudoglandular pattern with islands of solid tumor. This uncommon tumor is a histologic subtype of sweat gland (eccrine) carcinoma. It may be confused with metastatic adenocarcinoma to the skin. It has a low malignant potential with a long indolent clinical course (Bellezza G, Sidoni A, Bucciarelli E: Primary mucinous carcinoma of the skin, *AM J Dermatopathol* 22:166–170, 2000).

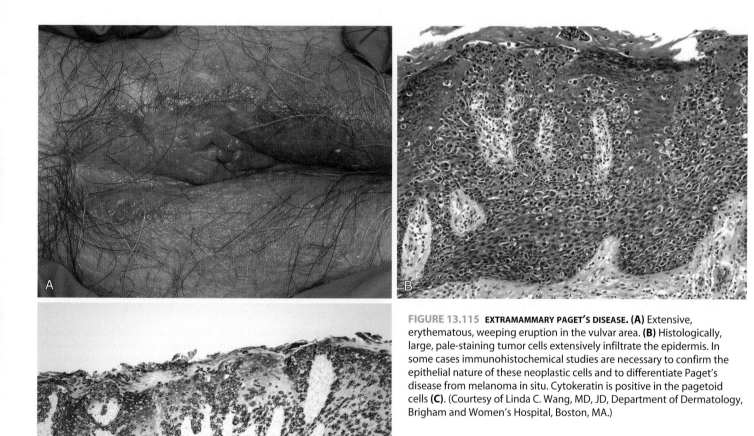

FIGURE 13.115 **EXTRAMAMMARY PAGET'S DISEASE. (A)** Extensive, erythematous, weeping eruption in the vulvar area. **(B)** Histologically, large, pale-staining tumor cells extensively infiltrate the epidermis. In some cases immunohistochemical studies are necessary to confirm the epithelial nature of these neoplastic cells and to differentiate Paget's disease from melanoma in situ. Cytokeratin is positive in the pagetoid cells **(C)**. (Courtesy of Linda C. Wang, MD, JD, Department of Dermatology, Brigham and Women's Hospital, Boston, MA.)

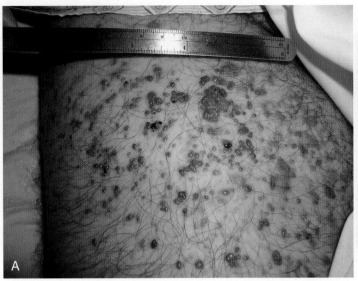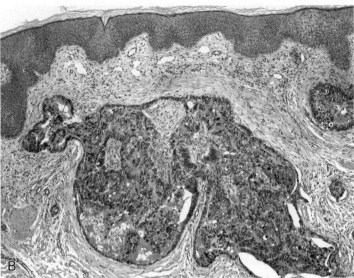

FIGURE 13.116 CUTANEOUS METASTASIS FROM COLORECTAL ADENOCARCINOMA. (A) Numerous red metastatic nodules are seen in the inner thigh of this patient with a history of colorectal carcinoma. (Courtesy of Dr. Danielle Miller, Department of Dermatology, Brigham and Women's Hospital, Boston, MA.) **(B)** Histologically there are foci of adenocarcinoma in the dermis with no connection to the epidermis.

References and Suggested Readings

Alam M, Ratner D: Cutaneous squamous-cell carcinoma, *N Engl J Med* 344:975–983, 2001.

Bakalian S, Marshall J-C, Logan P, et al: Molecular pathways mediating liver metastasis in patients with uveal melanoma, *Clin Cancer Res* 14:951–956, 2008.

Balch CM, Buzaid AC, Soong SJ, et al: Final version of the American Joint Committee on Cancer staging system for cutaneous melanoma, *J Clin Oncol* 19:3635–3648, 2001.

Balch CM, Soong SJ, Atkins MB, et al: An evidence-based staging system for cutaneous melanoma, *CA Cancer J Clin* 54:131–149, 2004. quiz 182–184.

Barreto JE, Velazquez EF, Ayala E, et al: Carcinoma cuniculatum: a distinctive variant of penile squamous cell carcinoma, *Am J Surg Pathol* 31:71–75, 2007.

Bayrou O, Avril MF, Charpentier P, et al: Primary neuroendocrine carcinoma of the skin. Clinicopathologic study of 18 cases, *J Am Acad Dermatol* 24:198–207, 1991.

Bellezza G, Sidoni A, Bucciarelli E: Primary mucinous carcinoma of the skin, *Am J Dermatopathol* 22:166–170, 2000.

Bishop JN, Harland M, Randerson-Moor J, et al: Management of familial melanoma, *Lancet Oncol* 8:46–54, 2007.

Breuninger H, Black B, et al: Microstaging of squamous cell carcinomas, *Am J Clin Pathol* 94:624–627, 1990.

Burnworth B, Arendt S,Muffler S, et al: The multi-step process of human skin carcinogenesis: a role for p53, cyclin D1, hTERT, p16, and TSP-1, *Eur J Cell Biol* 86:763–780, 2007.

Byrd-Gloster AL, Khoor A, Glass LF, et al: Differential expression of thyroid transcription factor 1 in small cell lung carcinoma and Merkel cell tumor, *Hum Pathol* 31:58–62, 2000.

Cassarino DS, Derienzo DP, Barr RJ, et al: Cutaneous squamous cell carcinoma: a comprehensive clinicopathologic classification. Part one, *J Cutan Pathol* 33:191–206, 2006.

Curtin JA, Busam K, Pinkel D, et al: Somatic activation of KIT in distinct subtypes of melanoma, *J Clin Oncol* 24:4340–4346, 2006.

Curtin JA, Fridlyand J, Kageshita T, et al: Distinct sets of genetic alterations in melanoma, *N Engl J Med* 353:2135–2147, 2005.

Davies H, Bignell GR, Cox C, et al: Mutations of the BRAF gene in human cancer, *Nature* 417:949–954, 2002.

Dewar DJ, Newell B, Green MA, et al: The microanatomic location of metastatic melanoma in sentinel lymph nodes predicts nonsentinel lymph node involvement, *J Clin Oncol* 22:3345–3349, 2004.

Eigentler TK, Buettner PG, Leiter U, et al: Impact of ulceration in stages I to III cutaneous melanoma as staged by the American Joint Committee on Cancer Staging System: an analysis of the German Central Malignant Melanoma Registry, *J Clin Oncol* 22:4376–4383, 2004.

Fecher LA, Cummings SD, Keefe MJ, et al: Toward a molecular classification of melanoma, *J Clin Oncol* 25:1606–1620, 2007.

Gilchrest BA, Eller MS, Geller AC, et al: The pathogenesis of melanoma induced by ultraviolet radiation, *N Engl J Med* 340:1341–1348, 1999.

Girardi M, Heald PW, Wilson LD: The pathogenesis of mycosis fungoides, *N Engl J Med* 350:1978–1988, 2004.

Goldsmith HS: Melanoma: an overview, *CA Cancer J Clin* 29:194–215, 1979.

Gray-Schopfer V, Wellbrock C, Marais R, et al: Melanoma biology and new targeted therapy, *Nature* 445:851–857, 2007.

Gupta SG, Wang LC, Peñas PF, et al: Sentinel lymph node biopsy for evaluation and treatment of patients with Merkel cell carcinoma: the Dana-Farber experience and meta-analysis of the literature, *Arch Dermatol* 142:685–690, 2006.

Herman S, Rogers HD, Ratner D, et al: Immunosuppression and squamous cell carcinoma: a focus on solid organ transplant recipients, *Skinmed* 6:234–238, 2007.

Jemal A, Siegel R, Ward E, et al: Cancer statistics, 2009, *CA Cancer J Clin* 59:225–249, 2009.

Karaa A, Khachemoune A: Keratoacanthoma: a tumor in search of a classification, *Int J Dermatol* 46:671–678, 2007.

Lange JR, Palis BE, Chang DC, et al: Melanoma in children and teenagers: an analysis of patients from the National Cancer Data Base, *J Clin Oncol* 25:1363–1368, 2007.

Lens MB, Rosdahl I, Ahlbom A, et al: Effect of pregnancy on survival in women with cutaneous malignant melanoma, *J Clin Oncol* 22:4369–4375, 2004.

Lloyd J, Flanagan AM: Mammary and extramammary Paget's disease, *J Clin Pathol* 53:742–749, 2000.

Martinez JC, Otley CC, et al: Transplant-skin cancer collaborative: defining the clinical course of metastatic skin cancer in organ transplant recipients: a multicenter collaborative study, *Arch Dermatol* 139:301–306, 2003.

Miller AJ, Mihm MC Jr: Melanoma. *N Engl J Med* 355:51–65, 2006.

Miller DL, Weinstock MA: Nonmelanoma skin cancer in the United States: incidence, *J Am Acad Dermatol* 30(5 Pt 1):774–778, 1994.

Morton DL, Thompson JF, Cochran AJ, et al: Sentinel-node biopsy or nodal observation in melanoma, *N Engl J Med* 355:1307–1317, 2006.

Olsen E, Vonderheid E, Pimpinelli N, et al: Revisions to the staging and classification of mycosis fungoides and Sezary syndrome: a proposal of the International Society for Cutaneous Lymphomas (ISCL) and the cutaneous lymphoma task force of the European Organization of Research and Treatment of Cancer (EORTC), *Blood* 110:1713–1722, 2007.

The Rockville Merkel Cell Carcinoma Group: Merkel cell carcinoma: recent progress and current priorities on etiology, pathogenesis, and clinical management, *J Clin Oncol* 27:4021–4026, 2009.

Sabel MS, Wong SL: Review of evidence-based support for pretreatment imaging in melanoma, *JNCCN* 7:281–289, 2009.

Savas S, Liu G: Studying genetic variations in cancer prognosis (and risk): a primer for clinicians, *Oncologist* 14:657–666, 2009.

Sekulic A, Haluska P, Miller AJ ,et al: Malignant melanoma in the 21st century: the emerging molecular landscape, *Mayo Clin Proc* 83:825–846, 2008.

Smith NP: The pigmented spindle cell tumor of Reed: an underdiagnosed lesion, *Semin Diagn Pathol* 4:75–87, 1987.

Spatz A, Barnhill RL: The Spitz tumor 50 years later: revisiting a landmark contribution and unresolved controversy, *J Am Acad Dermatol* 40:223–228, 1999.

Spenser PS, Helm TN: Skin metastasis in cancer patients, *Cutis* 39:119–121, 1987.

Strouse JJ, Fears TR, Tucker MA, et al: Pediatric melanoma: risk factor and survival analysis of the surveillance, epidemiology and end results database, *J Clin Oncol* 23:4735–4741, 2005.

Thiers BH, Sahn RE: Callen JP: Cutaneous manifestations of internal malignancy, *CA Cancer J Clin* 59:73–98, 2009.

Valent P, Horny H-P, Escribano L, et al: Diagnostic criteria and classification of mastocytosis: a consensus proposal, *Leuk Res* 25:603–625, 2001.

van der Velden PA, Sandkuijl LA, Bergman W, et al: Melanocortin-1 receptor variant R151C modifies melanoma risk in Dutch families with melanoma, *Am J Hum Genet* 69:774–779, 2001.

Viejo-Borbolla A, Ottinger M: Human herpesvirus 8: biology and role in the pathogenesis of Kaposi's sarcoma and other AIDS-related malignancies, *Curr HIV/AIDS Rep* 1:5–11, 2004.

Zhan FQ, Packianathan VS, Zeitouni NC: Merkel cell carcinoma: a review of current advances, *JNCCN* 7:333–339, 2009.

Figure Credits

The following books published by Gower Medical Publishing are sources of figures in the present chapter. The figure numbers given in the listing are those of the figures in the present chapter. The page numbers given in parentheses are those of the original publication.

Cawson RA, Eveson JW: *Oral pathology and diagnosis.* London, 1987, Heinemann Medical Books/Gower Medical Publishing: Figs. 13.23 (p. 13.16), 13.26 (p. 13.16).

du Vivier A: *Atlas of clinical dermatology.* Edinburgh/London, 1986. Churchill Livingstone/Gower Medical Publishing: Figs. 13.8 (p. 5.18), 13.3 (p. 6.16), 13.11 (p. 7.4), 13.12 (p. 7.5), 13.16 (p. 7.23), 13.17 (p. 7.34), 13.18 (p. 7.34), 13.21 (p. 7.9), 13.32 (p. 7.20), 13.27 (p. 7.22), 13.29 (p. 7.21), 13.33 (p. 7.35), 13.34 (p. 7.36), 13.35 (p. 7.24), 13.36 (p. 7.24), 13.37 (p. 7.15), 13.38 (p. 7.14), 13.39 (p. 7.14), 13.42 (p. 19.8) 13.43 (p. 8.11), 13.61 (p. 7.29), 13.62 (p. 7.29), 13.63 (p. 7.30), 13.64 (p. 7.30), 13.69 (p. 7.28), 13.70 (p. 7.28), 13.71 (p. 7.28), 13.79 (p. 1.5), 13.65 (p. 7.32), 13.66 (p. 7.32), 13.68 (p. 7.32), 13.72 (p. 7.31), 13.73 (p. 7.31), 13.74 (p. 7.30), 13.92 (p. 7.26), 13.93 (p. 7.27), 13.95 (p. 8.2), 13.96 (p. 8.2), 13.97 (p. 8.3), 13.98 (p. 8.8), 13.99 (p. 8.9), 13.100 (p. 8.6), 13.101 (p. 8.6), 13.102 (p. 8.12), 13.103 (p. 8.12), 13.104 (p. 8.7).

Hawke M, Jahn AF: *Diseases of the ear: clinical and pathologic aspects.* Philadelphia/New York, 1987, Lea & Febiger/Gower Medical Publishing: Figs. 13.1 (p. 1.45), 13.2 (p. 1.45), 13.54 (p. 1.44), 13.4 (p. 1.47), 13.15 (p. 1.47), 13.63 (p. 1.57), 13.106 (p. 1.58), 13.107 (p. 1.59).

Sharvill DE: *Skin diseases (pocket picture guides to clinical medicine).* Baltimore/New York, 1984, Williams and Wilkins/Gower Medical Publishing: Figs. 13.55 (p. 54), 13.19 (p. 52), 13.20 (p. 53), 13.24 (p. 57).

Spalton DJ, Hitchings RA, Hunter PA: *Atlas of clinical ophthalmology.* Philadelphia/London, 1984, Lippincott/Gower Medical Publishing: Figs 13.14 (p. 2.9), 13.25 (p. 2.12), 13.26 (p. 2.13), 13.28 (p. 2.13), 13.44 (p. 2.14).

Yanoff M, Fine BS: *Ocular pathology.* Philadelphia/New York, 1988, Lippincott/Gower Medical Publishing: Figs. 13.112 (p. 67), 13.113 (p. 67), 13.108 (p. 68).

Zitelli BJ, Davis HW (eds): *Atlas of pediatric physical diagnosis.* St. Louis, New York, 1987, CV Mosby/Gower Medical Publishing: Figs. 13.4 (p. 8.22), 13.5 (p. 8.22).

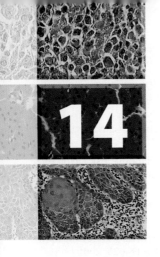

14 Neoplasms of the Central Nervous System

ELIZABETH A. MAHER • ANN C. MCKEE

The Central Brain Tumor Registry of the United States (CBTRUS) estimated 51,410 new cases of malignant and non-malignant brain tumors in 2007. Among children the incidence is 4.5 cases per 100,000 person-years. Among adults malignant tumors are estimated at 7.3 per 100,000 person-years and nonmalignant tumors at 9.2 cases per 100,000 person-years. An early peak in incidence starts at birth and extends to 4 years of age; after age 24 a gradual rise in incidence occurs, leading to a second peak at 50–79 years. For 2008 the SEER Cancer Statistics Review estimates that cancers of the brain and nervous system will account for 1.5% of all new cancer cases and 2.3% of cancer deaths annually (SEER 1975–2005). The relative risk of central nervous system (CNS) malignancy is 1.38 male to female, 3.18 elderly to young adult, and 1.86 Caucasian to African-American. In children, CNS tumors are the most common solid neoplasms and are the second leading cause of cancer deaths in patients younger than 15 years of age (SEER 1975–2005). The American Cancer Society estimates that in 2009 there will be 12,010 new cases of men with brain cancers with 7330 deaths and 10,060 new cases of women with brain cancer with 5590 deaths (Jemal et al., 2009).

The fourth edition of the World Health Organization (WHO) classification of primary brain tumors (Louis et al., 2007) is presented in Figure 14.1. All but the least common primary and secondary neoplasms of the CNS are reviewed in this chapter. Gliomas account for 36% of all primary brain tumors and 81% of malignant tumors (CBTRUS). Among these glioblastoma is the most common, accounting for at least 50% of cases. Meningiomas account for 32.1%, and pituitary tumors, nerve sheath tumors, lymphomas, medulloblastomas, and craniopharyngiomas range from 0.8% to 9%. Spinal cord neoplasms account for fewer than 15% of CNS tumors, and 10% of these represent spinal metastases from a primary intracranial tumor. Of all primary tumors of the spinal cord, schwannomas and meningiomas each account for 30%, ependymomas 13%, sarcomas 12%, astrocytomas 7%, and chordomas 4%. The distribution of CNS tumors varies with age: 90% of adult brain tumors are supratentorial, whereas 70% of childhood brain tumors arise in the posterior fossa. The distribution and differential diagnoses of CNS tumors are given in Figure 14.2 and Table 14.1. Pituitary tumors, which represent between 5% and 15% of all brain tumors, are discussed in Chapter 7.

The biologic potential of CNS neoplasms depends largely on three factors: (1) the histology and degree of malignancy (grade) of the tumor; (2) the anatomic compartments involved (cerebral hemisphere, basal ganglia, posterior fossa, brain stem, third ventricle, visual system, spinal cord, etc.); and (3) the spatial delimitation of the tumor (e.g., diffuse, circumscribed, multifocal). CNS tumors of low histologic grade may have as poor a prognosis as high-grade malignancies if they are considered surgically unresectable—because they show a diffusely infiltrating growth pattern, because they involve a critical anatomic structure, or because they are technically unapproachable by surgery.

There has been an increase in the incidence of primary malignant brain tumors over the past 25 years, with rates increasing at approximately 1.2% per year, particularly among the elderly. This increase does not seem to be related to an increase in lifespan over this same period of analysis. Although there have been significant improvements in diagnostic capabilities over the past 25 years, there is growing concern that the increase in incidence reflects exposure to an unrecognized environmental toxin. The only known environmental risk for malignant brain tumors is irradiation to the brain in childhood, usually as part of treatment for leukemia (Neglia et al., 1991) or fungal infection of the scalp (Ron et al., 1988). Large epidemiologic studies have not identified absolute environmental risks, but there have been trends toward increased risks from vinyl chloride, pesticides, or fungicides, chemicals used in the rubber industry, and electronic and electrical equipment (Thomas et al., 1987). In addition, it was reported in 2005 that Gulf War veterans exposed to sarin nerve gas have a 2.5-fold increase in fatal brain tumors when compared with unexposed veterans in the same theater of operations (Bullman et al., 2005).

Despite the recent heightened concern that the low-level radiation associated with cellular telephone use poses an increased risk for the development of brain tumors, a meta-analysis of nine case-control studies containing 5259 cases of primary brain tumors and 12,074 controls did not detect an overall risk (OR 0.90, 95% confidence interval [CI] 0.81–0.99). However, more than 10 years of use had an OR of 1.25 (95% CI 1.01–1.54) (Kan et al., 2007), suggesting that longer-term follow-up may be necessary to adequately evaluate risk.

There are well-recognized associations between malignant brain tumors and familial syndromes of germline mutations, although these account for only a small proportion of total cases (Bondy et al., 1993). Patients with Li-Fraumeni syndrome carry a germline mutation in *TP53* and develop a variety of tumors, including those of bone, breast, blood, adrenal cortex, and brain. The majority of brain tumors are gliomas, predominantly low grade, and occasional glioblastomas. Less common

Table 14.1

Distribution and Differential Diagnosis of Tumors of the Central Nervous System

Region	Adult Tumors		Childhood and Adolescent Tumors	
Cerebral hemisphere	Astrocytoma Anaplastic astrocytoma Glioblastoma Meningioma	Metastatic carcinoma Oligodendroglioma Ependymoma Lymphoma Sarcoma	Astrocytoma Anaplastic astrocytoma Ependymoma	Oligodendroglioma Embryonal tumor Ganglion cell tumor
Lateral ventricle	Ependymoma Meningioma Subependymoma	Choroid plexus papilloma	Ependymoma Choroid plexus papilloma	Subependymal giant cell astrocytoma
Third ventricle	Colloid cyst	Ependymoma	Ependydoma	Choroid plexus papilloma
Peri-third ventricular region	Astrocytoma Anaplastic astrocytoma	Oligodendroglioma Ependymoma Pilocytic astrocytoma Glioblastoma	Pilocytic astrocytoma Astrocytoma	
Pineal region	Germ cell tumor Pineal parenchymal tumor	Glioma	Germ cell tumor	Pineal parenchymal tumor
Optic chiasm and nerve	Meningioma	Astrocytoma	Astrocytoma	
Pituitary and sellar region	Pituitary adenoma Craniopharyngioma	Meningioma Germ cell neoplasms	Craniopharyngioma Germ cell neoplasms	Pituitary adenoma
Corpus callosum	Astrocytoma Anaplastic astrocytoma	Glioblastoma Oligodendroglioma Lipoma	Astrocytoma Anaplastic astrocytoma	Oligodendroglioma Lipoma
Brain stem	Astrocytoma Anaplastic astrocytoma	Glioblastoma	Astrocytoma Anaplastic astrocytoma	Glioblastoma
Cerebellopontine angle	Schwannoma Meningioma Epidermoid cyst	Choroid plexus papilloma	Ependymoma	
Cerebellum	Hemangioblastoma Metastatic carcinomas	Astrocytoma Medulloblastoma	Medulloblastoma	Dermoid cyst Astrocytoma
Fourth ventricle	Ependymoma Subependymoma	Choroid plexus papilloma	Ependymoma	Choroid plexus papilloma
Region of foramen magnum	Meningioma	Schwannoma		
Spinal region	Ependymoma Astrocytoma Hemangioblastoma Meningioma	Schwannoma Neurofibroma Paraganglioma	Ependymoma	Astrocytoma

familial syndromes include neurofibromatosis type 1 (NF1), linked to a gene on chromosome 17, which is associated with nerve sheath tumors, astrocytomas, and meningiomas in 5% to 10% of patients. Patients with neurofibromatosis type 2 (NF2) carry a genetic mutation on chromosome 22 that predisposes to schwannomas and meningiomas of the cranial nerves and spinal nerve roots, as well as astrocytomas in rare cases (Louis et al., 1995). Tuberous sclerosis, associated with two distinct inherited loci, 9q34 (*TSC1*) and 16p13 (*TSC2*), predisposes to subependymal giant cell astrocytomas and subcortical glioneuronal hamartomas in addition to a wide variety of non-CNS tumors. Turcot's syndrome, familial intestinal polyposis, results from a mutation of 5q21 (*ANAPC1*) and predisposes to medulloblastoma. Other patients with this syndrome have

lesions in 3p21 (*MLH1*) or 7p22 (*GPSM2*), both associated with glioblastoma at low frequency. Medulloblastoma is also associated with Gorlin syndrome, resulting from a mutation of 9q31 (*PTCH1*). In some instances primary brain neoplasms constitute an essential feature of the familial syndrome, as for example cerebellar hemangioblastoma in von Hippel-Lindau syndrome, which results from a lesion in the *VHL* gene (3p25).

Sporadic mutations seem to play a major role in the genesis and maintenance of brain tumors, although how the genetic pathways govern the biologic behavior of the tumors is largely unknown. The data are perhaps strongest for gliomas, wherein mutations in cell cycle control and receptor tyrosine kinase pathways are common (see below).

Tumors of neuroepithelial tissue

Astrocytic tumors
Diffuse astrocytoma
- Variants: Fibrillary
  - Protoplasmic
  - Gemistocytic

Anaplastic astrocytoma
Glioblastoma
- Variants: Giant cell glioblastoma
  - Gliosarcoma
  - Gliomatosis cerebri

Pilocytic astrocytoma
Pilomyxoid astrocytoma
Pleomorphic xanthoastrocytoma
Subependymal giant cell astrocytoma

Oligodendroglial tumors
Oligodendroglioma
Anaplastic oligodendroglioma

Ependymal tumors
Ependymoma
- Variants: Cellular
  - Papillary
  - Clear cell
  - Tanycytic

Anaplastic ependymoma
Myxopapillary ependymoma
Subependymoma

Mixed gliomas
Oligoastrocytoma
Anaplastic oligoastrocytoma

Choroid plexus tumors
Choroid plexus papilloma
Atypical choroid plexus papilloma
Choroid plexus carcinoma

Glial tumors of uncertain origin
Astroblastoma
Choroid glioma of third ventricle
Angiocentric glioma

Neuronal and mixed neuronal-glial tumors
Gangliocytoma
Ganglioglioma
Anaplastic ganglioglioma
Central neurocytoma
Dysplastic gangliocytoma of cerebellum (Lhermitte-Duclos)
Desmoplastic infantile ganglioglioma/astrocytoma
Dysembryoplastic neuroepithelial tumor
Paraganglioma of filum terminale
Extraventricular neurocytoma
Cerebellar liponeurocytoma
Papillary glioneuronal tumor
Rosette-forming glioneuronal tumor of fourth ventricle

Neuroblastic tumors
Olfactory neuroblastoma (esthesioneuroblastoma)
Olfactory neuroepithelioma
Neuroblastomas of adrenal gland and sympathetic nervous system

Pineal parenchymal tumors
Pineocytoma
Pineoblastoma
Pineal parenchymal tumor of intermediate differentiation
Papillary tumor of pineal region

Embryonal tumors
Medulloepithelioma
- Variants: Neuroblastoma
  - Ganglioneuroblastoma
  - Ependymoblastoma

Primitive neuroectodermal tumors (PNETs)

Medulloblastoma
- Variants: Medullomyoblastoma
  - Melanotic medulloblastoma
  - Large cell medulloblastoma

Medulloblastoma with extensive nodularity
Anaplastic medulloblastoma
Desmoplastic medulloblastoma

Tumors of cranial and spinal nerves

Schwannoma (neurilemmoma, neurinoma)
Neurofibroma
- Plexiform

Perineuroma
- Intraneural perineuroma
- Soft tissue perineuroma

Malignant peripheral nerve sheath tumor (MPNST)
Neurogenic sarcoma
Anaplastic neurofibroma, "malignant schwannoma"
- Variants: Epithelioid MPNST with divergent mesenchymal and/or epithelial differentiation
  - Melanotic
  - Melanotic psammomatous

Tumors of meninges

Tumors of meningothelial cells
Meningioma
- Variants: Meningothelial
  - Fibrous (fibroblastic)
  - Transitional
  - Psammomatous
  - Angiomatous
  - Microcystic
  - Secretory
  - Clear cell
  - Choroid
  - Lymphoplasmacyte-rich
  - Metaplastic
  - Atypical meningioma
  - Papillary meningioma
  - Anaplastic meningioma
  - Rhabdoid

Mesenchymal, nonmeningothelial tumors
Benign neoplasms
Osteocartilaginous tumors
Lipoma
Fibrous histiocytoma
Others

Malignant neoplasms
Hemangiopericytoma
Chondrosarcoma
- Variant: Mesenchymal chondrosarcoma
  - Malignant fibrous histiocytoma
  - Rhabdomyosarcoma
  - Meningeal sarcomatosis
  - Others

Primary melanocytic lesions
Diffuse melanocytosis
Melanocytoma
Malignant melanoma
Meningeal melanomatosis

Tumors of uncertain histogenesis
Hemangioblastoma (capillary hemangioblastoma)

Lymphomas and hematopoietic neoplasms
Malignant lymphomas
Plasmacytoma
Granulocytic sarcoma

Germ cell tumors
Germinoma

Embryonal carcinoma
Yolk sac tumor (endodermal sinus tumor)
Choriocarcinoma
Teratoma
- Variants: Immature
  - Mature
  - Teratoma with malignant transformation

Mixed germ cell tumors

Cysts and tumor-like lesions
Rathke cleft cyst
Epidermoid cyst
Dermoid cyst
Colloid cyst of third ventricle
Enterogenous cyst
Neuroglial cyst
Granular cell tumor (choristoma, pituicytoma)
Hypothalamic neuronal hamartoma
Nasal glial heterotopia
Plasma cell granuloma

Tumors of sellar region
Pituitary adenoma
Pituitary carcinoma
Craniopharyngioma
- Variants: Adamantinomatous papilary
  - Pituicytoma
  - Spindle cell oncocytoma of adenohypophysis

Local extensions from regional tumors
Paraganglioma
Chordoma
Chondroma
Chondrosarcoma
Carcinoma

Unclassified tumors
Metastatic tumors
To skull and vertebral column:
Carcinomas: Lung
- Breast
- Kidney
- Skin (malignant melanoma)
- Thyroid
- Nasopharynx and nasal sinuses
- Prostate

Neuroblastoma (children)
Multiple myeloma
Sarcomas
Lymphoma

To meninges:
Lymphoma
Leukemias
Carcinomas: Breast
- Lung
- Stomach
- Other

Malignant melanoma

To brain and spinal cord:
Carcinomas: Lung (35%)
- Breast (20%)
- Skin (melanoma) (10%)
- Kidney (renal cell carcinoma) (10%)
- Gastrointestinal tract (5%)
- Thyroid
- Choriocarcinoma
- Rarely: Prostate
  - Ovary
  - Bladder
  - Thymus

Sarcomas (rare)

Partially adapted from Kleihues and Cavenee (2000), Burger et al. (1991), and Louis et al. (2007).

FIGURE 14.1 Primary and metastatic neoplasms of the CNS.

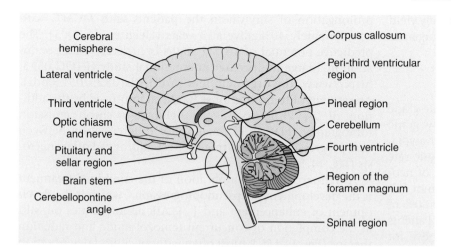

FIGURE 14.2 Distribution of tumors of the CNS.

Primary Neoplasms of the Central Nervous System

TUMORS OF NEUROEPITHELIAL TISSUE

In the adult, over 60% of all primary CNS tumors are gliomas. In children gliomas constitute 80% to 90% of all CNS neoplasms. Gliomas have been defined pathologically as tumors that display histologic, immunohistochemical, and ultrastructural evidence of glial differentiation. They are classified according to their differentiation lineage (i.e., astrocytic, oligodendroglial, or ependymal cells) and further subdivided by tumor grade (Louis et al., 2007); see below.

Astrocytic Tumors

Astrocytoma

Astrocytomas range in incidence from five to seven new cases per 100,000 population per year and are predominantly diffusely infiltrating tumors. Although they can arise anywhere in the CNS, they preferentially develop in the cerebral hemispheres. Three histologic types are recognized: fibrillary, gemistocytic, and protoplasmic. Of these, fibrillary astrocytoma is by far the most common and protoplasmic astrocytoma the most unusual. Astrocytomas are graded on a scale of I–IV according to their degree of malignancy as judged by various histologic features (see below). Unlike other solid tumors, gliomas do not metastasize outside the CNS, and thus tumor grade is the primary determinant of clinical outcome. Grade I tumors are biologically benign and can be surgically cured if deemed resectable at the time of diagnosis. Grades II–IV tumors are diffusely infiltrating tumors and are incurable with current therapies. They differ in their aggressiveness, with grade II tumors, referred to as low-grade gliomas, often following long clinical courses (see below) and grade III tumors initially responding well to chemotherapy and radiation therapy but usually progressing to death within 3 years. Grade IV tumors (glioblastoma) have a median survival of 14.6 months when treated with the standard regimen of concurrent temozolomide and radiation therapy followed by 6–12 months of adjuvant temozolomide (Stupp et al., 2005). A subset of patients seems to have prolonged survival with this regimen, although the determinants of the response have not yet been elucidated. Seventy percent of grade II gliomas

in adults transform into grade III and IV tumors within 5–10 years of diagnosis and then behave clinically like the higher-grade tumors.

The diffuse gliomas are classified histologically as astrocytomas, oligodendrogliomas, or tumors with morphologic features of both astrocytes and oligodendrocytes, termed oligoastrocytomas. Astrocytic tumors are subsequently graded as pilocytic astrocytoma, grade I; astrocytoma, grade II; anaplastic astrocytoma, grade III; and glioblastoma, grade IV. Oligodendrogliomas and oligoastrocytomas are subsequently graded as grade II or anaplastic, grade III. Such grading is related to the presence of histologic features of malignancy, such as high cellularity, cellular pleomorphism, mitotic activity, microvascular proliferation, and necrosis (Fig. 14.3).

Diffuse, Low-Grade Astrocytoma (WHO Grade II/IV)

The clinical hallmarks of low-grade astrocytomas are low mitotic rate, ability to migrate long distances away from the original site of tumor development, and high propensity to progress to a higher-grade tumor after a long latency. These are tumors primarily of young adults, with peak age of incidence at 34 years, and often present initially with seizures. The tumor cells are well differentiated, show robust glial marker immunoreactivity, and are not associated with neovascularization or cellular necrosis. Magnetic resonance imaging (MRI) often demonstrates a diffuse large mass that is hypointense on T_1-weighted imaging and does not enhance following administration of gadolinium. Whereas the reported median survival approaches 10 years, approximately 70% of patients transform to high-grade astrocytomas within 5 years of initial diagnosis (see Fig. 14.5A and B), the remaining 30% die of infiltrating low-grade tumor. Surgical resection is the primary modality of treatment. Although radiation therapy is associated with prolongation of progression-free survival, there is no increase in overall survival when compared to surgery alone. Chemotherapy, utilizing BCNU (carmustine) or temozolomide, has not been shown to prolong either progression-free survival or overall survival. The basic strategy is to follow patients with serial MRI scans and start radiation therapy, with or without chemotherapy, at the time of progression or transformation to high-grade tumor. Mutational analysis of these tumors has identified two common genetic lesions: p53 loss-of-function mutations (Chung et al., 1991; von Deimling et al., 1992) and platelet-derived growth factor ligand and receptor overexpression (Heldin and Westermark, 1990; Claesson-Welsh, 1994). Whole-genome high-resolution-array comparative hybridization has identified additional copy number gains and losses

(E. Maher, unpublished observations) and may ultimately yield insights into genes and pathways governing tumor maintenance and the transition to high-grade astrocytoma.

Anaplastic Astrocytoma (WHO Grade III/IV)

Anaplastic astrocytomas, also referred to as intermediate-grade astrocytomas, may arise de novo or develop from low-grade lesions. They are characterized histologically by nuclear atypia, increased cellularity, and a significant increase in mitotic rate over that seen in low-grade lesions without induction of neo-vascularization. MRI demonstrates enhancement of tumor following administration of gadolinium in approximately 80% of cases (Fig. 14.8). The median age at diagnosis is 41 years. Patients present with symptoms similar to those described above for patients with low-grade astrocytomas. Survival is significantly shorter than with low-grade astrocytomas, ranging from 3 to 4 years. Treatment consists of surgery, external-beam irradiation, and chemotherapy using temozolomide. Genetic mutations associated with anaplastic astrocytomas include allelic losses on chromosome 9p or 13q, and, less frequently, by 12q amplification. Notably, these mutations are mutually exclusive events (Ueki et al., 1996) and are key components of the retinoblastoma pathway governing cell cycle progression.

Glioblastoma Multiforme (WHO Grade IV/IV)

Two glioblastoma subtypes have been identified clinically (Kleihues and Cavenee, 2000) (Fig. 14.11). "Primary glioblastoma" typically presents in older patients as an aggressive, highly invasive tumor, usually without any evidence of prior clinical disease. "Secondary glioblastoma" has a very different clinical history. It is usually observed in younger patients who initially present with a low-grade astrocytoma that transforms into glioblastoma within 5–10 years of the initial diagnosis, regardless of prior therapy. Despite their distinctive clinical courses, they arrive at an indistinguishable clinical and pathologic endpoint characterized by widespread invasion and resistance to therapy. MRI is characterized by a diffuse enhancing mass, often with areas of necrosis. As such, tumors are managed as if they are one disease entity. However, global genomic analysis of these two glioblastoma subgroups showed wide-scale differences in their genomes that were previously unappreciated. Secondary glioblastoma was further classified into two distinct molecular subclasses, one characterized by multiple regions of loss and the other characterized by gain of chromosome 7 (without EGFR amplification) and several regions of gain and loss. Primary glioblastoma was characterized by the classic findings of EGFR amplification, and by chromosome 9p21 and chromosome 10 loss (Maher et al., 2006). Ongoing studies are directed at functional characterization of the unique genes and pathways in the molecular subclasses.

The treatment of glioblastoma has evolved over the past several years with the demonstration that treatment with temozolomide, an oral alkylating agent, when given concurrently with radiation therapy as initial therapy after surgical resection or debulking and as adjuvant therapy for six cycles, improved overall survival from 12.1 to 14.6 months and 2-year survival from 10.4% to 26.5% when compared with surgery followed by radiation therapy alone (Stupp et al., 2005). Correlation of methylation status of MGMT, a gene that repairs DNA after alkylation, with survival in patients treated with combined temozolomide and radiation therapy demonstrated marked prolongation of survival in the patients with MGMT, with approximately 40% alive at 3 years (Heigi et al., 2005). The predictive potential of MGMT status is currently under evaluation in a large multicenter international study (RTOG 0525; http://www.rtog.org/members/protocols/0525/0525.pdf). Assessment of tumor response has been improved by the addition of 2-[^{18}F]-fluoro-2-deoxy-D-glucose–positron emission tomography (FDG-PET) imaging for differentiation between true progression and treatment effect and/or radiation necrosis (Fig. 14.16A and B).

A well-recognized complication of the combined treatment is the development of "pseudoprogression," which is the development of enhancement and T$_2$/FLAIR abnormalities on MRI at the completion of concurrent temozolomide and radiation therapy (Fig. 14.16C), most often without clinical deterioration (Brandsma et al., 2008). Despite MRI findings that are often indistinguishable from true progression, FDG-PET shows no uptake, the imaging abnormalities resolve over 2–6 months, and the patients may have long disease-free intervals (Fig. 14.16D). Patients who have undergone reoperation seem to consistently have necrosis without clear evidence of recurrent tumor. The pathobiology (reviewed in Brandsma et al., 2008) seems to be consistent with treatment-related exaggerated local tissue reaction with an inflammatory component, edema, and abnormal vessel permeability leading to increased contrast enhancement. In severe cases this can lead to treatment-related necrosis. The condition may be self-limiting or require prolonged steroid administration and, in severe cases, reoperation.

Gliosarcoma

Gliosarcoma is a variant of glioblastoma characterized by the presence of both glial and sarcomatous elements. The origins of this tumor are unknown, although it has been speculated that it represents malignant transformation of a neural stem cell or glial progenitor that retained the ability to differentiate into both glial and mesenchymal lineages. Gliosarcomas carry the same prognosis as glioblastomas, and the general approach to treatment is the same as that described above for glioblastoma.

Pilocytic Astrocytoma (WHO Grade I/IV)

These tumors of childhood and adolescence differ from the diffuse astrocytomas previously discussed in that they are relatively well circumscribed and of low grade with little potential for malignant transformation. They are uncommon in the cerebral hemispheres and show geographic preferences for the region of the third ventricle, optic chiasm, and thalamus. Surgical resection is associated with long-term survival. Pilocytic astrocytomas are not associated with TP53 mutations, suggesting a different genetic basis for these low-grade tumors.

Pleomorphic Xanthoastrocytoma

These rare tumors occur most often in the temporal or parietal lobe of young people (third or fourth decade) with a history of epilepsy. Usually there is prominent leptomeningeal involvement; underlying cyst formation with mural nodules is also typical. These tumors are typically densely cellular and cytologically pleomorphic. However, mitoses are rare and necrosis is absent. The tumor is notable because it has a favorable prognosis yet bears superficial resemblance to a giant cell glioblastoma or malignant fibrous histiocytoma. Some tumors may eventually develop malignant transformation.

Subependymal Giant Cell Astrocytoma

Though characteristically associated with tuberous sclerosis, subependymal giant cell astrocytoma occasionally occurs in the absence of the disease. It usually arises from the wall of the lateral ventricle and presents as an intraventricular mass obstructing the foramen of Monro. The clinical signs are commonly those of obstructive hydrocephalus. Subependymal astrocytomas are low-grade tumors, with essentially no tendency for malignant transformation.

Astrocytoma: Sites of Preference

OPTIC NERVE AND CHIASMAL ASTROCYTOMA

Representing 1% of intracranial neoplasms in adults and 5% of intracranial tumors in children younger than 10 years old, optic nerve and chiasmal astrocytomas most commonly (≈70%) arise in the first decade. The most frequent symptom is visual loss, which may be pronounced. Bilateral optic astrocytomas may arise in association with von Recklinghausen's neurofibromatosis, more often affecting the chiasm than the optic nerves. Although malignant transformation is rare, it occurs more frequently in adults with chiasmal lesions. Treatment is surgical; however, 20% of optic nerve tumors and 33% of optic chiasm tumors recur. The 20-year survival rate for optic nerve astrocytomas is 85%, as compared with 50% for optic chiasm tumors. The tumor grows by local extension, and chiasmal tumors frequently extend into the third ventricle or the optic tract. The histology is that of a pilocytic astrocytoma.

ASTROCYTOMA OF THE THIRD VENTRICULAR REGION

Both pilocytic astrocytomas and diffuse astrocytomas may be found in this site, most commonly in children. Although such tumors are benign and slow growing, their deep location limits surgical resection. The clinical signs are usually those of obstructive hydrocephalus.

BRAINSTEM ASTROCYTOMA

Most commonly occurring in children, this tumor usually presents as a diffuse astrocytoma originating in the pons. As with astrocytomas of the third ventricle, surgical resection is hindered by the deep location and infiltrating character of this tumor. Malignant transformation is frequent and may occur early in the disease course. The clinical signs include symptoms of brain stem dysfunction and cranial nerve palsies. Obstructive hydrocephalus occurs late in the course as a result of obstruction of the fourth ventricle. The prognosis depends on tumor grade; 30% of patients with well-differentiated astrocytomas survive for 15 years. Patients with high-grade astrocytomas have a typical survival time of less than 1 year. Occasionally brain stem astrocytomas are of the discrete pilocytic type, which is associated with prolonged survival.

CEREBELLAR ASTROCYTOMA

Accounting for 5% of all brain gliomas and 15% of all intracranial tumors of children and adolescents, cerebellar astrocytomas may be either diffuse (15%) or, more commonly, pilocytic (85%). The presenting signs are usually those of cerebellar dysfunction and hydrocephalus resulting from obstruction of the fourth ventricle. Surgical resection, even if partial, is associated with long-term survival. Malignant transformation and cerebrospinal dissemination are rare.

SPINAL CORD ASTROCYTOMA

Representing approximately 13% of all neoplasms affecting the spinal cord, these tumors commonly appear as fusiform enlargements affecting the thoracic and cervical segments. Diffuse low-grade fibrillary astrocytoma is the usual histologic type, although high-grade astrocytomas may occur. As many as 40% of these tumors are associated with proximal or distal syringomyelia. The prognosis is related to tumor grade. Mean survival time for patients with well-differentiated tumors may be as long as 8 years, whereas with high-grade lesions it may be as short as 6 months. Death is usually the result of intercurrent infection or medullary extension of the tumor.

Oligodendroglial Tumors

Oligodendroglioma

Constituting 4% of all CNS neoplasms and 5% to 19% of all gliomas, oligodendroglioma is predominantly a tumor of the middle decades, with a peak incidence between 35 and 40 years, although it occasionally arises in younger persons. Considered to be tumors of the white matter, they have geographic predilections based largely on the amount of white matter in a given location. Sites of preference include the frontal, parietal, and temporal lobes of the cerebral hemispheres, as well as the thalamus, particularly in the younger age groups. They occur rarely in the spinal cord and extremely rarely in the cerebellum. The clinical evolution may be prolonged and is frequently characterized by a long history of seizures. Calcification in these tumors is common, detectable radiographically in 40% of cases and histologically in 90%. Although previously graded like astrocytomas, the most recent WHO classification no longer recognizes glioblastoma as a grade of oligodendrogliomas. Thus, these tumors are grade II or maximum III, even when necrosis and neovascularization are present. This change reflects the clear difference in biologic behavior of the highest-grade tumor when compared to glioblastomas of astrocytic origin. The high-grade oligodendrogliomas are often exquisitely sensitive to the standard glioma treatments, PCV (combination therapy with procarbazine, CCNU [lomustine], and vincristine) or temozolamide (see response demonstrated in Fig. 14.22 after five cycles of chemotherapy), and median survival is often significantly longer than in patients with anaplastic astrocytomas. Genetic analysis of these tumors demonstrates a high incidence of mutations in 1p and 19q. Although the specific genes mutated in these tumors have not yet been identified, they are likely to be involved in conferring the chemosensitivity of these tumors.

Mixed Glioma (Oligoastrocytoma)

Mixed gliomas are tumors that clearly demonstrate both malignant oligodendrocytes and astrocytes. Similar to gliosarcoma, the origin of these tumors is unknown. They may represent malignant transformation of a neural stem cell or early glial progenitor. The molecular genetics are less clear than for pure oligodendrocytes; some have the characteristic 1p and 19q deletions, whereas most have a genetic profile similar to anaplastic astrocytomas. Treatment is similar to anaplastic astrocytomas, although prognosis may vary depending on the genetic profile of the tumor.

EPENDYMAL TUMORS

Ependymoma

Ependymomas represent approximately 3% to 9% of all neuroepithelial tumors. They are primarily tumors of childhood and adolescence, with peak incidence occurring between 10 and 15 years. They represent 6% to 12% of all intracranial tumors in childhood and a striking 30% in children under 3 years of age. The tumors can occur at any site along the ventricular system and spinal canal but are predominantly found in the fourth ventricle and spinal cord. Embryologically the ependyma is related to astrocytes and oligodendroglia, a glial heritage that is often expressed when the cells are neoplastically transformed. Characteristically, ependymomas are benign, slow-growing neoplasms; anaplastic transformation may occur, especially focally, but transformation to overt glioblastoma is rare. Because of its predominantly intraventricular location, symptoms are most often secondary to obstruction of cerebrospinal fluid (CSF) flow and resultant hydrocephalus. Tumors of the spinal cord are associated with symptoms related to the site of disease occurrence. The prognosis of ependymoma depends largely on the anatomic site of origin and the histologic grade. Long-term survivals tend to be the exception. Even benign-appearing tumors show a tendency to recur locally and metastasize via the subarachnoid space. Treatment is surgical resection, most often only partial, and radiation therapy.

Myxopapillary Ependymoma

These tumors represent a special variant of ependymoma found almost exclusively in the region of the filum terminale, although occasionally they have been found higher in the spinal cord or, rarely, in the brain. They may occur at any age, but most arise in the fourth decade. Myxopapillary ependymomas characteristically form a sausage-shaped mass in the lumbosacral region, displacing spinal nerve roots of the cauda equina. Their biologic behavior is usually benign, but because of their location they are often associated with significant compression-induced paralysis. Treatment consists of local excision, which must often be only partial because of the tumor's location; approximately 20% recur even after complete initial resection. Metastases infiltrating the CSF and extradural space may occur, but transformation to anaplastic variants is extremely rare.

Subependymoma

This slow-growing, benign variant of ependymoma consists of proliferating ependyma and astrocytes. Seventy-five percent of these tumors are infratentorial, arising on ependymal surfaces. They are commonly found along the fourth ventricle, the walls of the lateral ventricles, the septum pellucidum, and the cerebellopontine angle. They are often an incidental finding at autopsy, particularly in the middle-aged and elderly. Symptomatic tumors may arise at any age, most commonly in the fourth decade, and show a male predominance. The clinical signs are usually those of hydrocephalus resulting from blockage of CSF flow through the ventricles. Treatment is surgical, and the prognosis depends entirely on the tumor's location and resectability.

Choroid Plexus Tumors

Choroid Plexus Papilloma

Choroid plexus papillomas occur most frequently in the first decade of life, accounting for 10% to 20% of intracranial neoplasms in children; they are occasionally congenital. The lateral ventricle and third ventricle are the favored sites in children; the rare adult neoplasm favors the fourth ventricle. Symptoms are usually caused by hydrocephalus, which may result from mechanical obstruction to CSF flow or overproduction of CSF by the tumor. Although they are benign neoplasms and can be cured by surgery, they have a tendency to disseminate widely via the CSF, particularly after surgical intervention.

Choroid Plexus Carcinoma

This malignant tumor is distinguishable from choroid plexus papilloma on the basis of local brain invasion, a solid pattern of growth and cytologic features of anaplasia, including necrosis and mitoses. Choroid plexus carcinoma almost always occurs in patients under the age of 10, grows more rapidly than choroid plexus papillomas, and has a 5-year survival rate of approximately 40%. In older individuals it should be distinguished from the much more common metastatic papillary adenocarcinoma.

NEUROEPITHELIAL TUMORS OF UNCERTAIN ORIGIN

Gliomatosis Cerebri

This extreme form of diffuse astrocytoma in adults is characterized by widely infiltrating anaplastic glia, although the cell of origin is unknown. It typically presents in the second or third decade and diffusely enlarges the cerebral hemispheres, brain stem, and/or cerebellum. There is often expansion of compact fiber pathways, such as the optic nerves, corpus callosum, fornices, or cerebral peduncles. Its distinct clinical behavior is probably related to the overall very poor prognosis.

NEURONAL AND MIXED NEURONAL-GLIAL TUMORS

Gangliocytoma and Ganglioglioma

Gangliogliomas are distinguished from gangliocytomas (ganglioneuromas) by the presence of glial elements in gangliogliomas. Both tumors show a geographic predilection for the temporal lobes in children and young adults, and seizures are thus the most common presenting symptoms. However, these tumors occur in all brain regions, including the frontal lobes, third ventricle, and hypothalamus. They carry an excellent prognosis following surgical resection, although transformation of the glial elements in gangliogliomas can occur that then carry a less favorable prognosis.

Central Neurocytoma

The central neurocytoma is typically a tumor of young adults, in whom a discrete, often partially calcified mass intrudes into the lateral ventricle near the foramen of Monro. Symptoms are often related to increased intracranial pressure rather than focal neurologic deficits. Surgery may be curative if complete resection is achieved.

Paraganglioma

Paragangliomas are tumors derived from neural crest cells, the most common type of which is the pheochromocytoma. The designation also includes tumors of the carotid body, glomus jugulare, glomus tympanicum, filum terminale, vagus nerve, orbit, and duodenum. Certain of these tumors show a predilection for middle-aged women, such as the jugulotympanic paraganglioma, which usually arises from the lateral portion of the temporal bone, and the vagal body paraganglioma, which often presents as a mass in the neck or at the skull base beneath the jugular foramen. Clinically, these tumors manifest with signs of cranial nerve palsies. In the case of paragangliomas involving the cauda equina, which tend to be sausage-shaped intradural tumors, symptoms include lower back pain, sensorimotor deficits, and incontinence. Carotid body tumors present as painless masses of the skull base, where they may produce cranial nerve palsies, a palpable thrill, and an audible bruit. The incidence of carotid body tumors is markedly increased in regions of high altitude, possibly as a result of hypoxia-induced hyperplasia. An autosomal-dominant pattern of inheritance for these tumors has been recognized, and familial tumors may be bilateral. Most paragangliomas are benign and carry a favorable postoperative prognosis, although recurrences are not uncommon. Approximately 5% of these tumors are malignant and may invade tissue locally or metastasize to lymph nodes, lung, or bone marrow.

Olfactory Neuroblastoma (Esthesioneuroblastoma)

This rare neoplasm arises high in the nasal cavity from neurosensory receptor cells or basilar cells in the olfactory mucosa. The age distribution is bimodal, one peak occurring in adolescence and young adulthood and the second peak occurring in late middle age. Olfactory neuroblastomas are slow-growing but aggressive, locally invasive tumors that may invade the nasal sinuses, nasopharynx, palate, orbit, cribriform plate, and brain. Metastases to the CSF, lymph nodes, and viscera may occur. There seem to be several types of esthesioneuroblastomas, one with classic features of neuroblastoma, the type most likely to occur in young patients, and the other with characteristics of neuroendocrine carcinoma, more common in older patients. The importance of initial gross total surgical excision has been emphasized. Because the tumor is highly radiosensitive, radiation therapy is often indicated. The 10-year survival rate has been reported as 77% for patients with neuroendocrine carcinoma and 67% for those with neuroblastoma.

PINEAL PARENCHYMAL TUMORS

Pineocytoma and Pineoblastoma

These uncommon tumors, derived from pineal parenchymal cells, are divided into two types: the pineocytoma, originating from mature cells, and the pineoblastoma, derived from more primitive pineal cells. Pineocytoma, which may occur at any age, is typically well circumscribed, slow growing, and noninvasive, and it rarely metastasizes via the CSF. Its highly malignant anaplastic counterpart, the pineoblastoma, occurs primarily in children and frequently metastasizes via the CSF. Because pineocytomas tend to be less radiosensitive than pineoblastomas, their treatment usually includes surgical resection. Mean survival time is approximately 5 years for pineocytoma, whereas it is less than 2 years for pineoblastoma.

EMBRYONAL TUMORS

Medulloepithelioma

Believed to arise from the primitive medullary plate and neural tube, these rare, highly malignant tumors occur early in life, most frequently between the ages of 6 months and 5 years. The preferred geographic location is periventricular in the cerebral hemispheres; tumors are often deeply situated and lie near the midline. These tumors can also arise in the cauda equina, presacral area, outside the CNS along nerve trunks, and in the eye. Radical surgical removal, followed by extensive neuraxial irradiation, is the treatment of choice, given the highly primitive and malignant character of these tumors. Mortality is high, and extracranial metastases may occur.

Neuroblastoma (Cerebral)

Derived from ganglion cell precursors, central neuroblastomas are rare tumors, occurring most frequently in children in the first decade of life. They are frequently situated deep in the cerebrum, forming a well-defined mass. Approximately 50% disseminate via CSF pathways, and distant metastases may occur. Treatment consists of radical surgical excision followed by radiation therapy, in that the primitive character of these lesions suggests some degree of sensitivity to radiation therapy. The 5-year postoperative survival rate is approximately 30%.

Ependymoblastoma

Although their histologic designation is somewhat controversial, ependymoblastomas are distinguished from ependymomas by their highly malignant biologic behavior and the frequency of focal microscopic invasion and leptomeningeal involvement. They are rare tumors affecting predominantly the cerebral hemispheres of neonates and young children. They are generally large and supratentorial, closely approximated to the ventricles. They have a propensity for CSF seeding, rapid local growth, and extraneural and extracranial metastases.

PRIMITIVE NEUROECTODERMAL TUMORS

Medulloblastoma

These embryonic cerebellar tumors are believed to originate from remnants of the fetal external granular cell layer of the cerebellum. Overall, they account for less than 0.5% of intracranial primitive neuroectodermal tumors, but in children they represent 25% of intracranial tumors. Most arise in patients younger than 25 years of age, although occasionally they occur as late as the fifth decade and have a male predominance (65%).

Medulloblastomas arise in the cerebellum, particularly favoring the midline in early life, whereas in later life tumors tend to arise in the lateral hemispheres. The clinical signs are usually those of cerebellar dysfunction and increased intracranial pressure due to obstruction of the fourth ventricle. Medulloblastomas frequently infiltrate the subarachnoid space early and extensively and metastasize widely via CSF pathways. Systemic metastases to bone and lymph nodes may occur, although the lung characteristically remains free of metastatic deposits. Since these tumors are extremely radiosensitive, the treatment of choice is radiation therapy of the entire neuraxis, usually in combination with surgical extirpation. The 5-year survival rate ranges from 40% to 80%. Variants of medulloblastoma include medullomyoblastoma, containing myoblasts or myocytes, and melanotic medulloblastoma, containing melanosomes and premelanosomes.

Grade I/IV:

Pilocytic astrocytoma

Elongated, bipolar astrocytes
Rosenthal fibers

Grade II/IV:

Well-differentiated, low-grade astrocytoma

Mild hypercellularity
One histologic criterion:
        nuclear atypia
No mitoses
No vascular proliferation
No necrosis

Grade III/IV:

Anaplastic astrocytoma

Increased cellularity
Two histologic criteria:
        usually nuclear atypia and
        mitotic activity

Grade IV/IV:

Glioblastoma multiforme

Densely cellular tumor with at least three criteria:
        nuclear atypia
        endothelial proliferation and/or
        necrosis

FIGURE 14.3 Histologic grading of astrocytomas.

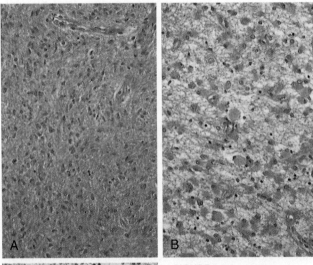

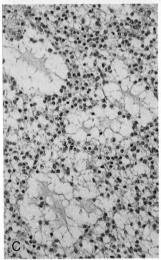

FIGURE 14.4 **DIFFUSE ASTROCYTOMA.** The three common types of diffuse astrocytoma are **(A)** fibrillary, composed of tightly interlacing bundles of small, spindle-shaped cells amid a predominantly fibrillar matrix; **(B)** gemistocytic, containing plump cells with distinct, round, pink cytoplasm arranged on a more delicately interlacing fibrillar matrix; and **(C)** protoplasmic, composed of small, round, regular cells with indistinct cytoplasmic boundaries arranged on a loosely fibrillar stroma.

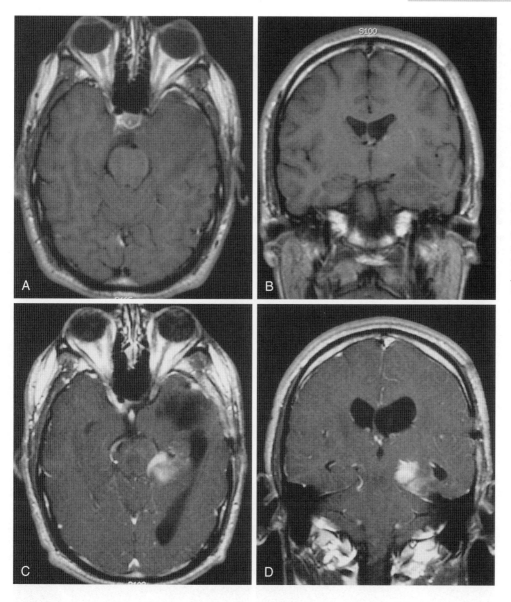

FIGURE 14.5 **DIFFUSE LOW-GRADE ASTROCYTOMA.**
(A) Axial T_1-weighted MR image after gadolinium administration. A large left temporal tumor is present without any abnormal enhancement. The tumor is evident through its obliteration of normal sulci and gyri. **(B)** Coronal T_1-weighted MR image after gadolinium enhancement. The tumor is slightly heterogeneous in signal but shows no abnormal enhancement. It extends into the deep temporal structures. **(C)** Axial T_1-weighted MR image after gadolinium enhancement. Recurrent tumor is seen in the deep temporal region abutting the brain stem. The temporal and occipital horns of the left lateral ventricle (v) are dilated because of ex vacuuo changes related to intervening treatment. **(D)** Coronal T_1-weighted MR image after gadolinium administration. Enhancing tumor extends into the deep temporal structures just above the tentorium. Dilatation of the left lateral ventricle (v) is present.

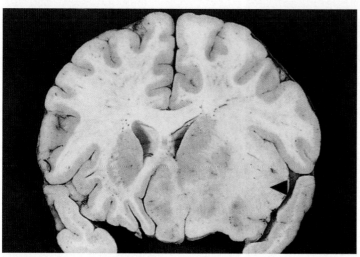

FIGURE 14.6 **DIFFUSE, LOW-GRADE ASTROCYTOMA (GRADE II/IV).** Coronal section shows a tumor diffusely infiltrating the right frontal lobe. Gross determination of the tumor's boundaries is almost impossible, but the tumor is evident as an ill-defined area of enlargement , with loss of distinction between the gray and white matter.

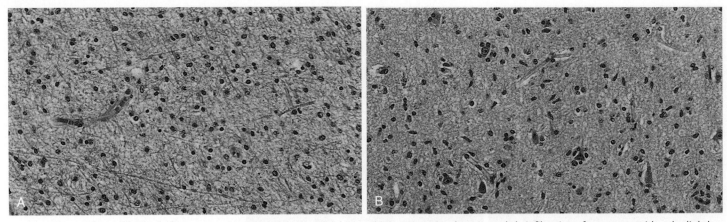

FIGURE 14.7 DIFFUSE, LOW-GRADE ASTROCYTOMA (GRADE II/IV). In the **(A)** white and **(B)** gray matter there is a subtle infiltration of astrocytes with only slightly irregular features. In the gray matter the neoplastic astrocytes cluster around neurons. This feature, termed satellitosis, is not seen in reactive astrocytes.

FIGURE 14.8 **ANAPLASTIC ASTROCYTOMA (GRADE III/IV).** **(A)** Axial T_2-weighted image at the level of the upper portion of the lateral ventricles. A large cystic tumor is present on the left, with relatively little surrounding edema. The tumor shifts the midline to the right. **(B)** Axial T_1-weighted image after gadolinium administration at a level just above the lateral ventricles. Two adjacent cystic components are present, along with some nodular enhancing solid tumor. **(C)** Coronal T_1-weighted image after gadolinium administration. A focal linear area of enhancing tumor is present between adjacent cystic components. **(D)** Coronal T_1-weighted MR image after gadolinium administration just posterior to the level shown in **(C)**. Solid tumor is again seen adjacent to cystic components. The tumor compresses and displaces the left lateral ventricle downward.

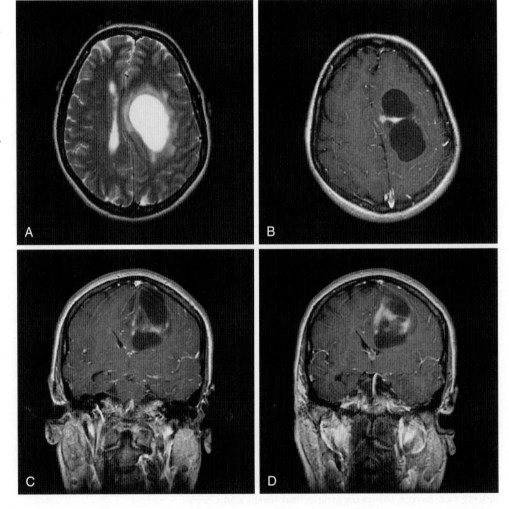

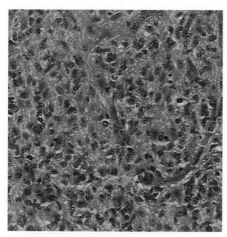

FIGURE 14.9 **ANAPLASTIC ASTROCYTOMA (GRADE III/IV).** Microscopy reveals a densely cellular tumor with a high degree of cellular pleomorphism and increased mitotic activity. This tumor is distinguished from glioblastoma multiforme by the conspicuous absence of two other criteria of malignancy: necrosis and endothelial proliferation. However, its high cellularity and pleomorphism raise suspicion that a larger sample size might have included areas showing features of greater malignancy.

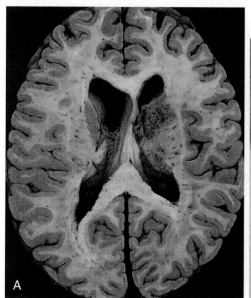
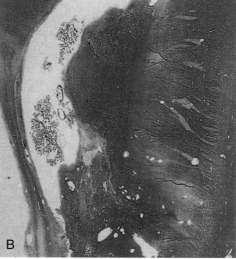

FIGURE 14.10 **ANAPLASTIC ASTROCYTOMA (GRADE III/IV). (A)** Arising in the right basal ganglia, this tumor has caused enlargement of the caudate nucleus with hemorrhage, disruption of the ventricular ependyma, and extension into the ventricular space. **(B)** These features are further emphasized in this histologic section taken from the involved area. Note the high cellularity of the tumor.

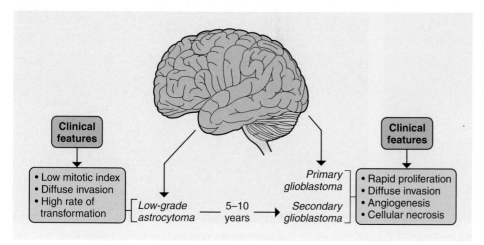

FIGURE 14.11 **TWO PATHWAYS TO GLIOBLASTOMA.** Glioblastoma can develop over 5–10 years from a low-grade astrocytoma (secondary glioblastoma), or it can be the initial pathology at diagnosis (primary glioblastoma). The clinical features of glioblastoma are the same regardless of clinical route. (Reproduced with permission from Maher E, Furnari FB, Bachoo RM, et al: Malignant glioma: genetics and biology of a grave matter. *Genes Dev* 15: 1311–1333, 2001.)

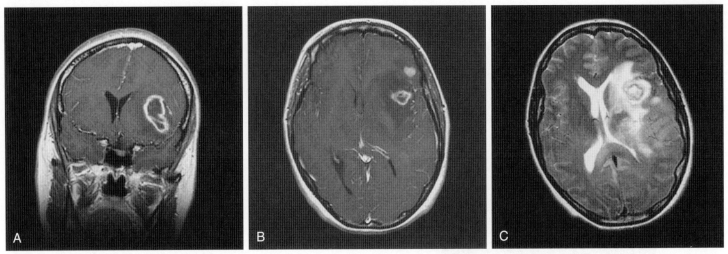

FIGURE 14.12 GLIOBLASTOMA MULTIFORME (GRADE IV/IV). (A) Coronal T_1-weighted MR image after gadolinium administration. An irregular mass is present in the left frontal region with central necrosis and surrounding rim of abnormal enhancement. The mass compresses and displaces the left lateral ventricle. (B) Axial T_1-weighted MR image after gadolinium administration. The mass is seen in the left frontal region with a solid nodular component as well as a larger necrotic mass. (C) Axial T_2-weighted MR image. The rounded tumor mass in the left frontal region is seen, with extensive surrounding vasogenic edema extending along white matter tracts.

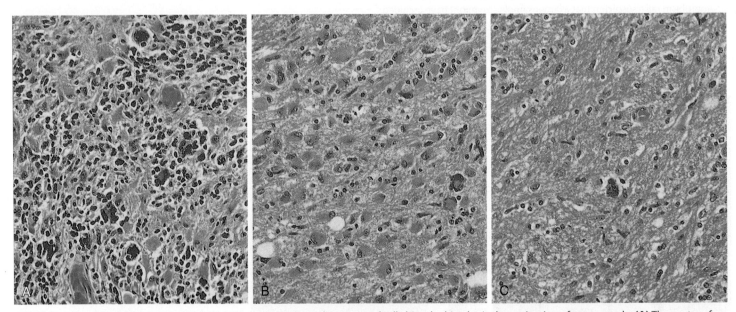

FIGURE 14.13 GLIOBLASTOMA (GRADE IV/IV). Variations in tumor sampling can markedly bias the histologic determination of tumor grade. (A) The center of the tumor is densely populated with highly pleomorphic neoplastic cells, including giant cells, gemistocytic astrocytes, and small anaplastic cells. Also typical are mitotic activity, proliferation of blood vessel endothelium, and zones of necrosis. The cell nuclei tend to line up at the periphery of the necrotic area, a feature termed "pseudopalisading." A biopsy from this area would result in the diagnosis of glioblastoma multiforme. (B) Other areas are characterized by gemistocytic astrocytes only. Sampling from this area would be interpreted as gemistocytic astrocytoma, grade II. (C) At the periphery of the tumor there is only a mild increase in fibrillary astrocytes with rare, bizarre astrocytes. Biopsy from this area would also yield a diagnosis of astrocytoma, grade II.

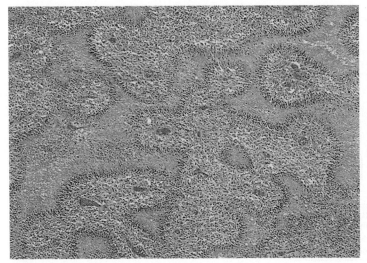

FIGURE 14.14 GLIOBLASTOMA MULTIFORME. Pseudopalisading around areas of necrosis may be a dominant feature. Zones of necrosis appear as serpiginous, cell-free, pink areas.

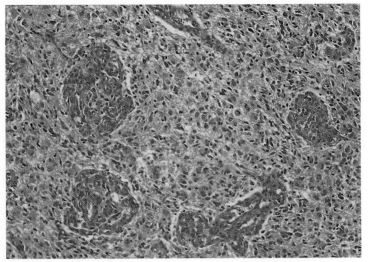

FIGURE 14.15 GLIOBLASTOMA MULTIFORME. Endothelial proliferation may reach marked proportions with the formation of tangled clusters of neovascular channels, occasionally referred to as "glomeruloid" blood vessels because of their resemblance to renal glomeruli.

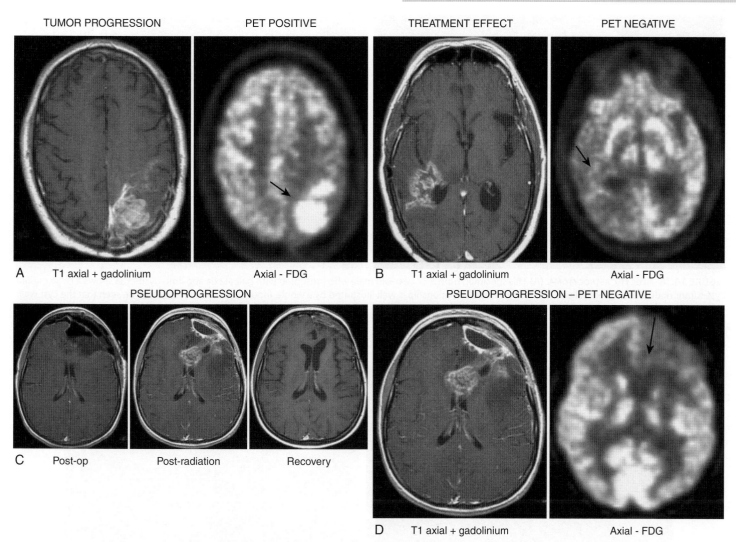

| TUMOR PROGRESSION | PET POSITIVE | TREATMENT EFFECT | PET NEGATIVE |

A   T1 axial + gadolinium   Axial - FDG   B   T1 axial + gadolinium   Axial - FDG

PSEUDOPROGRESSION   PSEUDOPROGRESSION – PET NEGATIVE

C   Post-op   Post-radiation   Recovery

D   T1 axial + gadolinium   Axial - FDG

FIGURE 14.16 Assessment of tumor response has been improved by the addition of FDG-PET imaging for differentiation between true progression and treatment effect **(A)** and/or radiation necrosis **(B)**. **(C)** A well-recognized complication of the combined treatment is the development of "pseudoprogression," which is the development of enhancement and T_2/FLAIR abnormalities on MRI at the completion of concurrent temozolomide and radiation therapy. **(D)** The imaging abnormalities resolve over 2–6 months, and the patients may have long disease-free intervals.

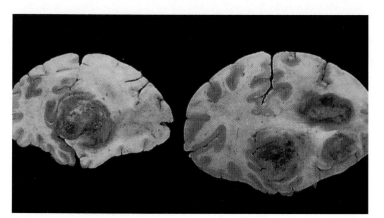

FIGURE 14.17 ASTROCYTOMA. Multifocal malignant transformation occurring within an astrocytoma may simulate a metastatic neoplasm, as illustrated here, with three apparently discrete tumor masses within the right frontal lobe.

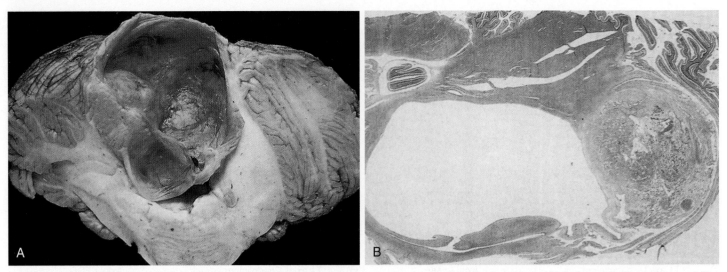

FIGURE 14.18 PILOCYTIC ASTROCYTOMA. (A) This specimen from a 37-year-old male who presented with gait ataxia and limb dysmetria shows a large midline cyst-tumor nodule of the cerebellum. **(B)** The cyst-nodule relationship is well illustrated by a whole-mount section in which it can be seen that the cyst wall is composed of compressed white matter, not tumor.

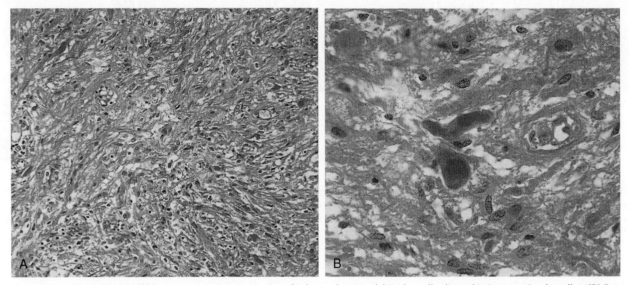

FIGURE 14.19 PILOCYTIC ASTROCYTOMA. (A) Low-power microscopic view discloses elongated, bipolar cells aligned in intersecting bundles. **(B)** Sausage-shaped, brightly eosinophilic fibers, known as Rosenthal fibers, are very characteristic of pilocytic astrocytomas and other low-grade, slowly progressing gliomas.

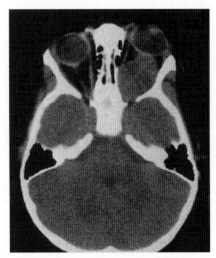

FIGURE 14.20 OPTIC NERVE ASTROCYTOMA. Computed tomography (CT) scan of a 2-year-old girl with proptosis shows a large pilocytic tumor surrounding and involving the right optic nerve.

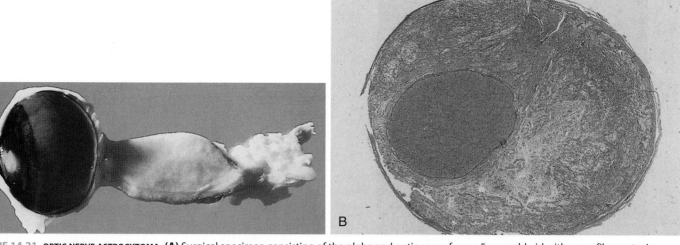

FIGURE 14.21 **OPTIC NERVE ASTROCYTOMA. (A)** Surgical specimen consisting of the globe and optic nerve from a 5-year-old girl with neurofibromatosis shows the tumor as a fusiform enlargement of the nerve. **(B)** On cross-sectional view this optic nerve shows only modest enlargement, but there is marked infiltration of the surrounding subarachnoid space by tumor.

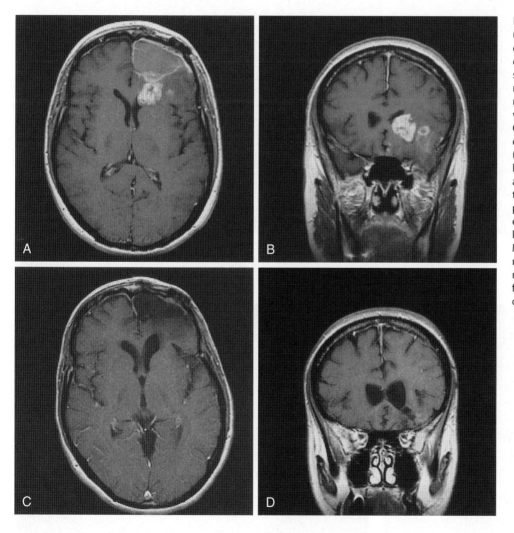

FIGURE 14.22 **ANAPLASTIC OLIGODENDROGLIOMA.**
(A) Axial T_1-weighted MR image after gadolinium enhancement. The patient has undergone a left craniotomy with a postoperative cavity with some peripheral rim enhancement probably representing surgical change. There is also nodular enhancement abutting the left lateral ventricle compatible with residual tumor. **(B)** Coronal T_1-weighted MR image after gadolinium enhancement. Multifocal tumor is evident (*arrows*) encroaching on and displacing the left lateral ventricle. **(C)** Axial T_1-weighted MR image after gadolinium enhancement. This study after treatment shows complete resolution of the prior enhancing periventricular mass. There is ex vacuuo dilatation of the frontal horn of the left lateral ventricle. **(D)** Coronal T_1-weighted MR image after gadolinium enhancement. No residual enhancing tumor is visible, and there are now only low signal areas probably representing fluid as well as mild dilatation of the frontal horn of the left lateral ventricle.

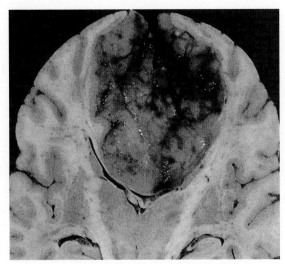

FIGURE 14.23 **OLIGODENDROGLIOMA.** This specimen from a 42-year-old man shows a massive bifrontal, relatively circumscribed tumor.

FIGURE 14.24 **OLIGODENDROGLIOMA. (A)** Microscopic section from the periphery of the tumor shown in Figure 14.22 reveals the neoplastic oligodendrocytes as uniform cells with small, round nuclei and a characteristic perinuclear halo ("fried egg" cells). Satellitosis of the neoplastic cells around neurons is also a characteristic feature of this tumor. **(B)** A section from the center of the tumor demonstrates a monotonous cellular pattern and delicate vasculature. Blood vessels often form fine, straight lines that intersect each other at right angles.

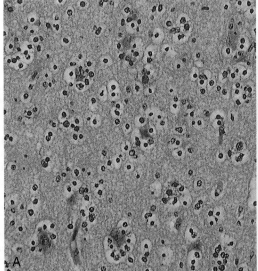

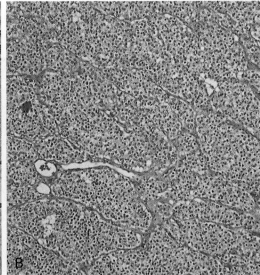

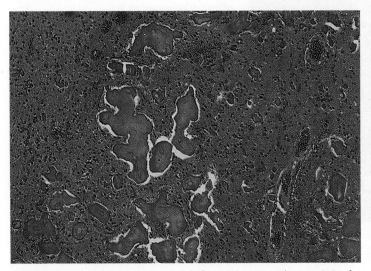

FIGURE 14.25 **OLIGODENDROGLIOMA.** Calcifications are very characteristic of this tumor and are often most pronounced at the periphery of the neoplasm.

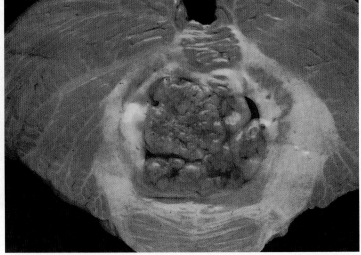

FIGURE 14.26 **EPENDYMOMA.** This specimen from a 42-year-old woman shows a tumor arising from the floor of the fourth ventricle, filling and expanding the ventricle and compressing the underlying pons. The lobulated gross appearance of the tumor is characteristic.

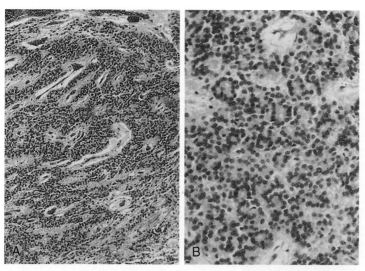

FIGURE 14.27 EPENDYMOMA. **(A)** The low-power microscopic pattern of this tumor is often quite characteristic. Note the striking pattern of pseudorosettes and tubules. The perivascular pseudorosettes appear as a maze of tubules when sectioned longitudinally to the blood vessel. **(B)** A typically cellular tumor is composed of uniform cells with regular, round nuclei arranged in pseudorosettes.

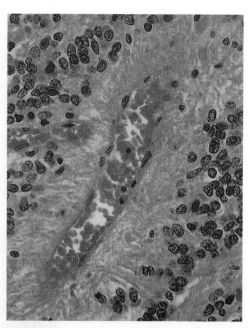

FIGURE 14.28 EPENDYMOMA. High-power photomicrograph of a pseudorosette shows that it is composed of cells aligned around a blood vessel with their processes toward the lumen of the vessel.

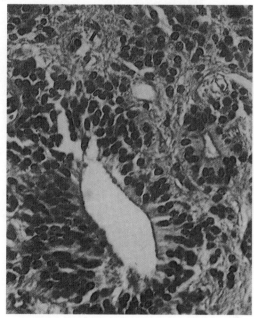

FIGURE 14.29 EPENDYMOMA. True rosettes are also a feature of ependymomas, though they are less common than pseudorosettes. A true rosette consists of cells aligned around a central lumen that does not contain a blood vessel.

FIGURE 14.30 **MYXOPAPILLARY EPENDYMOMA.** (A) This spinal cord specimen was resected from a 15-year-old boy who experienced rapid onset of lower-limb paraplegia and incontinence. The red-brown tumor appears deeply vascular. (B) Microscopically, it is composed of cuboidal or columnar cells arranged in a papillary fashion around a fibrovascular stalk. Abundant mucin accumulation may be present, either in the neoplastic cells or in the associated connective tissue.

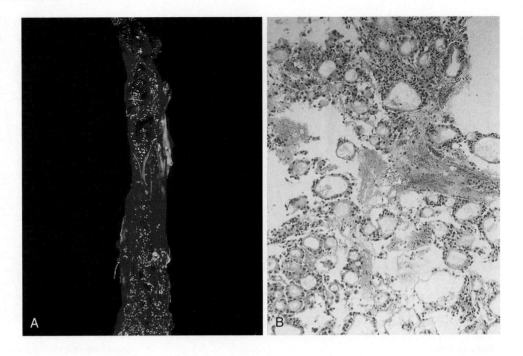

FIGURE 14.31 **CHOROID PLEXUS PAPILLOMA.** (A) In this specimen from a 10-year-old boy, a discrete, irregular papillary mass is confined to the left posterior horn. There is massive dilatation of the entire ventricular system, with marked compression of the surrounding cerebral tissue. (B) A tumor involving the fourth ventricle has expanded and severely compressed the medulla. Although this pattern of growth may compromise surgical resection, it should not be confused with parenchymal invasion. Note the vascular nature of the tumor; these tumors have a tendency toward spontaneous hemorrhage.

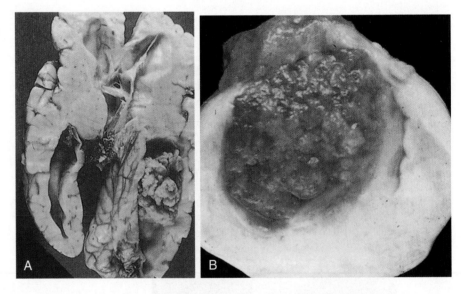

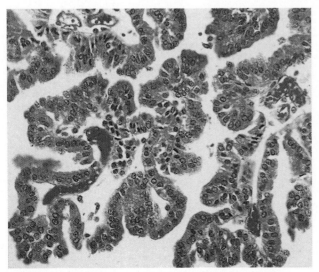

FIGURE 14.32 **CHOROID PLEXUS PAPILLOMA.** The microscopic appearance of this tumor closely resembles that of normal choroid plexus.

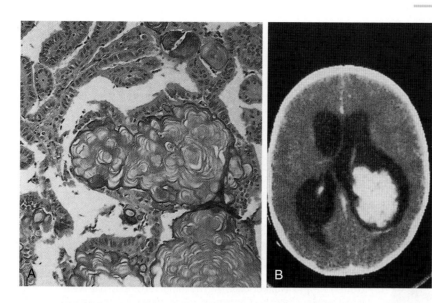

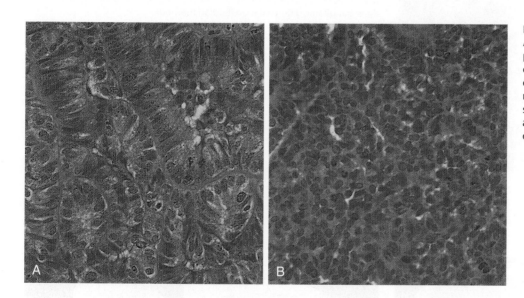

FIGURE 14.33 **CHOROID PLEXUS PAPILLOMA. (A)** Calcification is common both in normal, aging choroid plexus and in choroid plexus papillomas, and is associated with **(B)** hyperdensity on CT scan.

FIGURE 14.34 **CHOROID PLEXUS CARCINOMA.** A spectrum of morphologic atypia links choroid plexus papilloma with the rare choroid plexus carcinoma. **(A)** A low-grade malignancy is characterized by piling up of epithelium and mitotic activity. **(B)** At the opposite end of the spectrum, this anaplastic example demonstrates an absence of the orderly architectural features of a papilloma.

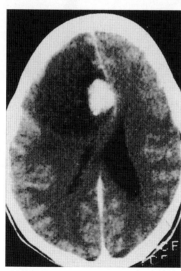

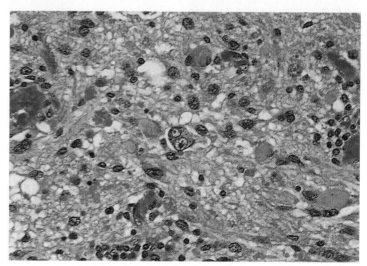

FIGURE 14.35 **GANGLIOGLIOMA.** The CT appearance of gangliogliomas and ganglioneuromas is characteristic; foci of calcification and small cysts are common. Occasionally the tumor consists of a single large cyst with a single calcified mural nodule, as illustrated here.

FIGURE 14.36 **GANGLIOGLIOMA.** The key histologic feature is the presence of neoplastic ganglion cells like the binucleate cell in the center of this field. The primary differential distinction is from infiltrative glioma with entrapment of normal neuron.

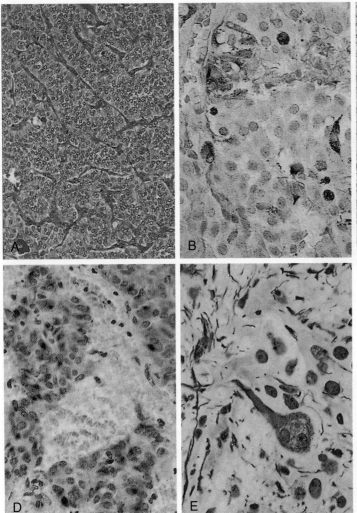

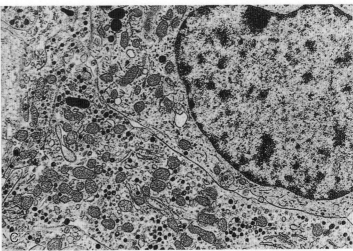

FIGURE 14.37 **PARAGANGLIOMA. (A)** The tumor is composed of well-defined lobules (Zellballen) of regular, round, clear cells intersected by thin-walled capillaries. A diffuse pattern may also be seen. **(B)** Tumor cells are argyrophilic (Grimelius method). **(C)** Electron microscopy reveals cytoplasmic neurosecretory granules. Immunostaining techniques are positive for both **(D)** neurofilament protein and (not shown) neuron-specific enolase. **(E)** Approximately half of tumors of the filum terminale show ganglionic differentiation (Bodian method).

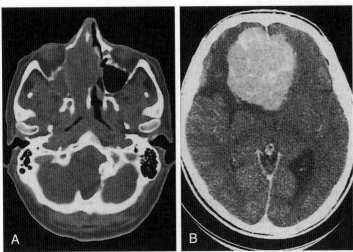

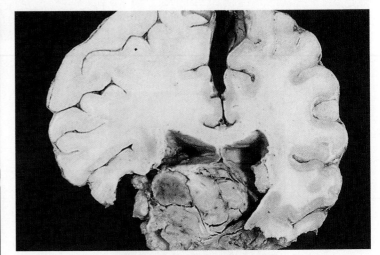

FIGURE 14.38 **OLFACTORY NEUROBLASTOMA (ESTHESIONEUROBLASTOMA). (A)** CT scan in a 19-year-old boy shows a mass filling the left nasal cavity. **(B)** In the case of a 15-year-old girl, a large tumor mass is apparent at the base of the left frontal lobe; it extends across the midline and is associated with surrounding edema. These tumors may grow either downward to fill the nasal cavity or upward through the cribriform plate to enter the cranial vault (Mills et al., 1985).

FIGURE 14.39 **OLFACTORY NEUROBLASTOMA (ESTHESIONEUROBLASTOMA).** Autopsy specimen shows a tumor mass that has destroyed and replaced a large proportion of the base of the anterior brain.

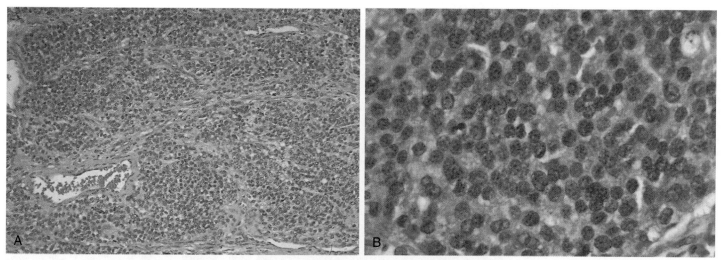

FIGURE 14.40 **OLFACTORY NEUROBLASTOMA (ESTHESIONEUROBLASTOMA). (A)** In a typical neuroendocrine-type esthesioneuroblastoma, low-power microscopy reveals rather monotonous-looking cells arranged in lobules on a delicate fibrovascular stroma. **(B)** With high magnification there may be no particular pattern. Some esthesioneuroblastomas contain true Homer Wright rosettes, and axons may be demonstrable with special stains. Electron microscopy may be required to identify this tumor and to distinguish it from other small, round cell tumors (Schochet et al., 1975).

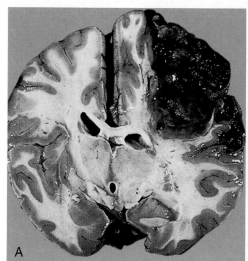

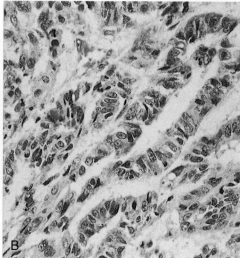

FIGURE 14.41 **MEDULLOEPITHELIOMA. (A)** Like most embryonal tumors, this left frontal neoplasm arising in a 5-year-old girl is solid and discrete, with a soft, grayish pink, highly necrotic appearance. **(B)** The distinctive microscopic features consist of a papillary or tubular arrangement of columnar cells.

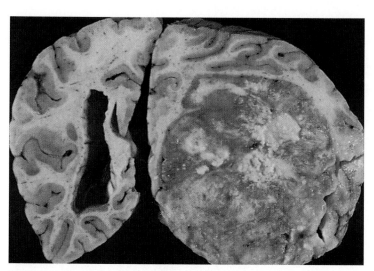

FIGURE 14.42 **CEREBRAL NEUROBLASTOMA.** This large central tumor in a 10-year-old boy is commonly well demarcated from the surrounding tissue.

FIGURE 14.43 CEREBRAL NEUROBLASTOMA.
(A) Neuroblastomas consist of a fairly uniform population of cells frequently arranged in Homer Wright rosettes. Desmoplasia may also be a feature. (B) Special stain for neuritic processes highlights the immature axons (frozen Bielschowsky method). Neuroblastomas in tissue culture form similar neuritic processes. Occasionally tumors show the formation of mature neurons (not shown).

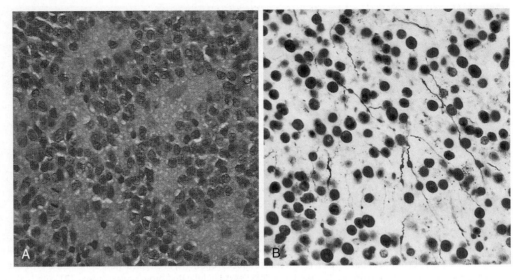

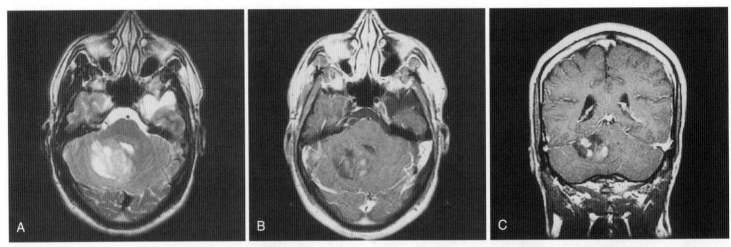

FIGURE 14.44 MEDULLOBLASTOMA. (A) Axial T$_2$-weighted MR image at the level of the fourth ventricle. A large heterogeneous mass is present in the right cerebellum that compresses and displaces the fourth ventricles (*arrow*). **(B)** Axial T$_1$-weighted MR image after gadolinium administration at the same level, showing some nodular enhancement of the tumor. **(C)** Coronal T$_1$-weighted MR image after gadolinium administration at a level posterior to the brain stem. The tumor abuts the tentorium and again shows heterogeneous enhancement.

FIGURE 14.45 MEDULLOBLASTOMA.
Spinal arachnoid spread of tumor may entirely encase and deform the cord and produce **(A)** studding of the caudal nerve roots. **(B)** Malignant cells are often readily identified on CSF examination.

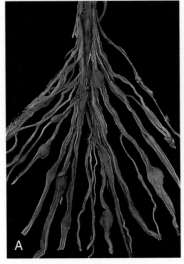

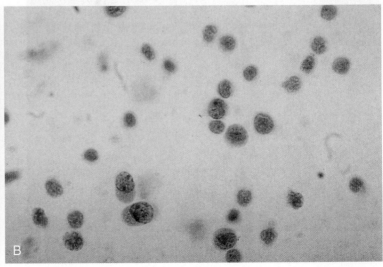

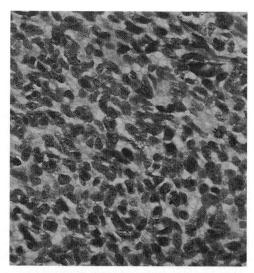

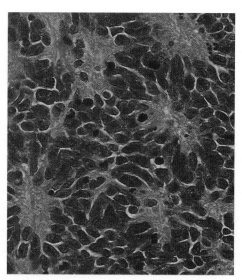

FIGURE 14.46   MEDULLOBLASTOMA. The tumor is highly cellular and composed of dark-staining, ovoid cells with hyperchromatic nuclei and ill-defined cytoplasmic outlines; there is no definite architectural arrangement.

FIGURE 14.47   MEDULLOBLASTOMA. In approximately one third of cases, characteristic Homer Wright rosettes are found, with nuclei arranged radially around a delicately fibrillated, eosinophilic center. Pseudorosettes, marked by a perivascular arrangement of tumor cells, may also occur.

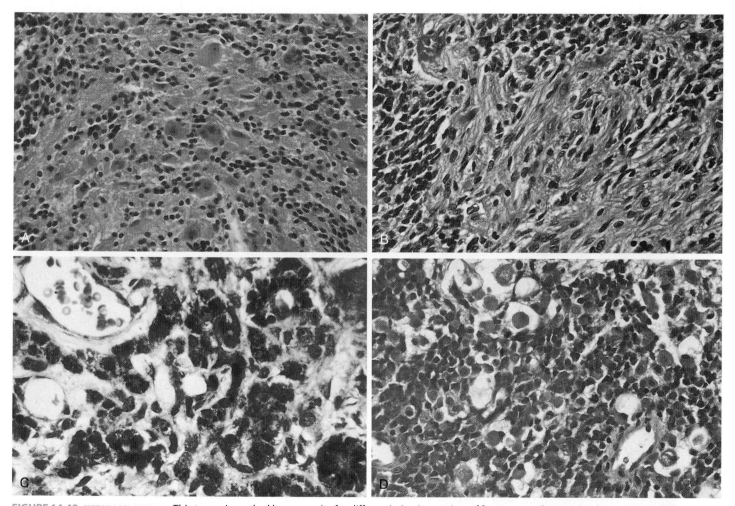

FIGURE 14.48   MEDULLOBLASTOMA. This tumor is marked by a capacity for differentiation in a variety of forms, as can be seen by the presence of **(A)** neurons, **(B)** glial cells, **(C)** pigmented neuroepithelium, and, in rare cases, **(D)** striated muscle.

Tumors of Cranial and Spinal Nerves

SCHWANNOMA

Constituting 5% to 10% of all intracranial tumors, schwannomas are usually solitary tumors discovered in the middle and later decades of life. Schwannomas presenting at an early age and/or bilaterally are seen in association with neurofibromatosis. The lesions are firm, encapsulated, slow growing, and benign. Schwannomas show a marked predilection for sensory nerves. In the cranial cavity they principally involve cranial nerve VIII (particularly the vestibular component) and, far less commonly, cranial nerves V, IX, and X. Clinical symptoms of auditory and/or cerebellar dysfunction are common. Intraspinal schwannomas, representing 30% of these tumors, most often involve the lumbar segment and give rise to signs of local root irritation and spinal cord compression. Both intradural and extradural growth is observed, and large lesions may traverse and expand the intervertebral foramina, resulting in a dumbbell-shaped lesion. Schwannomas are treated surgically and may recur if resection is not complete. Malignant transformation is rare.

NEUROFIBROMA

Variants: Circumscribed (Solitary) and Plexiform

Like schwannomas, neurofibromas are tumors of Schwann cells and can be distinguished by their morphology. Intraneural neurofibromas diffusely transform a nerve segment and its branches (the "plexiform" variant) and only infrequently produce an isolated lesion involving one nerve fascicle (the "circumscribed" or "solitary" variant). It is the plexiform variety that is pathognomonic of neurofibromatosis, whereas solitary neurofibromas infrequently share this association. Neurofibromas may be found along cranial or spinal nerve roots and ganglia, major nerves of the trunk and limbs, including the sympathetic system and subcutaneous branches, and along visceral sympathetic plexuses. Symptoms are related to compression of surrounding structures by tumor. Treatment is surgical, but resection almost invariably sacrifices the involved nerve because neurofibromas infiltrate the nerve directly. Partial resection may result in recurrence.

As discussed above, patients with neurofibromatosis type 2 (NF2) are predisposed to schwannomas and meningiomas of the cranial nerves and spinal nerve roots, whereas patients with neurofibromatosis type 1 (NF1) are susceptible to peripheral neurofibromas. The *NF1* gene has been mapped to chromosome 17, and recently the *NF2* gene was mapped to chromosome 22. Alterations in the *NF1* gene may also be associated with pilocytic astrocytomas.

Malignant Peripheral Nerve Sheath Tumors

Malignant peripheral nerve sheath tumors arise by malignant transformation of a neurofibroma, usually plexiform, or arise de novo in a normal nerve sheath. Malignant peripheral nerve sheath tumors are highly malignant tumors that infiltrate locally and commonly metastasize to distant sites. The tumors occur primarily in adults, in whom they present as painful, rapidly enlarging masses that favor the trunk, neck, and proximal limbs, and only rarely affect cranial nerves. Treatment is usually surgical; the prognosis is directly related to tumor size. Fewer than 20% of patients survive 5 years.

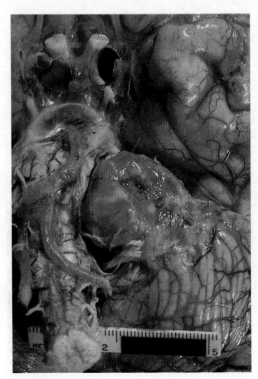

FIGURE 14.49 SCHWANNOMA (ACOUSTIC NEUROMA). A large, discrete tumor nodule, arising from the left eighth cranial nerve, obscures the underlying seventh and eighth cranial nerves and causes lateral compression of the pons and medulla.

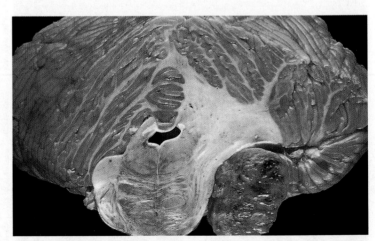

FIGURE 14.50 SCHWANNOMA (ACOUSTIC NEUROMA). This horizontal section through the pons and cerebellum demonstrates the usual gross appearance of a schwannoma. The tumor is well circumscribed, mottled red-yellow in color, and most commonly originates on the vestibular portion of the eighth cranial nerve.

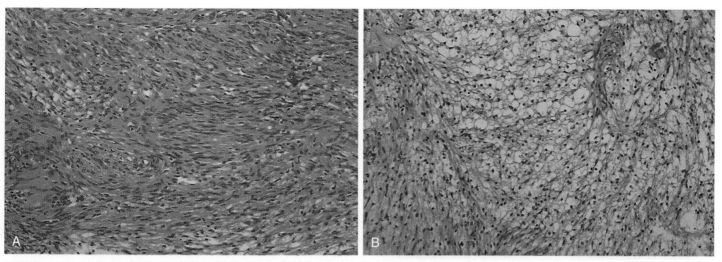

FIGURE 14.51 **SCHWANNOMA (ACOUSTIC NEUROMA).** Microscopic features include **(A)** compact areas composed of densely interlacing bundles of spindle-shaped cells (Antoni A pattern) and **(B)** more loosely arranged round-to-ovoid cells with pale cytoplasm (Antoni B pattern).

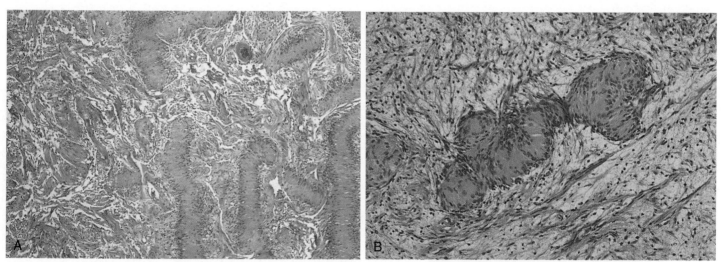

FIGURE 14.52 **SCHWANNOMA. (A)** Palisading, or lining up of nuclei, may be a striking feature, particularly in spinal schwannomas. **(B)** If the palisading forms are pronounced, the term "Verocay body" is commonly applied.

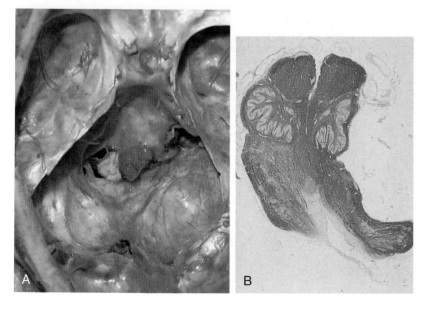

FIGURE 14.53 **GLOMUS JUGULARE TUMOR. (A)** A tumor of the skull base compresses the high cervical spinal cord and medulla (seen in cross-section). **(B)** This whole-mount transverse section reveals the degree of medullary deformity.

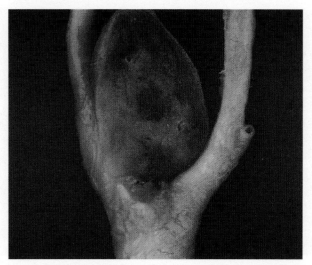

FIGURE 14.54 **CAROTID BODY TUMOR.** A globoid, encapsulated carotid body ganglioglioma overlies the bifurcation of the common carotid artery.

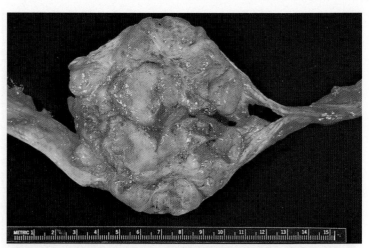

FIGURE 14.56 **MALIGNANT PERIPHERAL NERVE SHEATH TUMOR.** In this cross-section of a tumor arising in the sciatic nerve, its origin from the nerve can clearly be seen, a helpful feature in the diagnosis. The tumor is typically encapsulated and on cross-section appears more vascular and variegated than a benign neurofibroma.

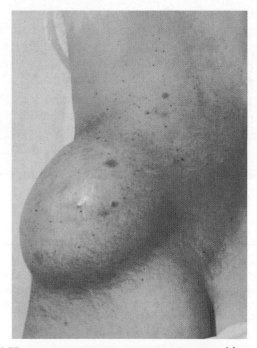

FIGURE 14.55 **MALIGNANT PERIPHERAL NERVE SHEATH TUMOR.** A large tumor has arisen in the left flank of a 28-year-old woman with neurofibromatosis. Note the extensive café-au-lait patch surrounding the tumor.

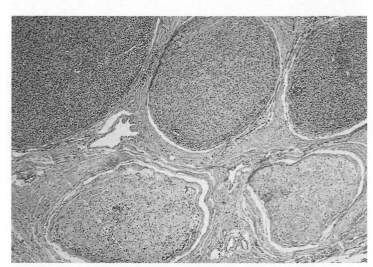

FIGURE 14.57 **MALIGNANT PERIPHERAL NERVE SHEATH TUMOR.** Tumor involves three of the five nerve fascicles shown here, as evidenced by their increased cellularity; there is no obvious deformity of the nerve structure. Surgical resection margins must be evaluated with great care because of such insidious intraneural growth.

Tumors of the Meninges

TUMORS OF MENINGOTHELIAL CELLS

Meningioma

Meningiomas constitute 15% of intracranial and 25% to 32% of intraspinal tumors in adults; they are uncommon in children. There is a striking female preponderance, especially among intraspinal tumors, believed to be related to a stimulatory effect of female hormones. Approximately 90% of meningiomas are supratentorial, favoring such sites as the parasagittal region, falx cerebri, cerebral convexities, olfactory groove, sphenoid ridge, and tuberculum sellae. Infratentorial meningiomas frequently are attached to the tentorium cerebelli or the foramen magnum. Meningiomas are commonly divided into descriptive subtypes on the basis of their histologic appearance: meningothelial, fibrous (fibroblastic), transitional (mixed), psammomatous, angiomatous, microcystic, secretory, clear cell, chordoid, lymphoplasmacyte-rich, and metaplastic meningioma. With rare exceptions, the biologic behavior does not vary among these subtypes. All are slow-growing neoplasms that usually only displace normal structures. Occasionally, they invade the cerebral parenchyma by finger-like processes, and they commonly invade dura, bone, and soft tissues. In rare instances penetration of the facial sinuses presents as a nasal polyp. Hyperostosis of overlying bone is a frequently encountered radiologic sign, whose presence does not necessarily indicate bone invasion.

Atypical and Anaplastic (Malignant) Meningioma

Atypical and malignant tumors are associated with a high recurrence rate. Atypical features in meningiomas include high cellularity, lack of lobularity or a "sheeting" pattern of growth, prominent nucleoli, mitotic figures, and focal necrosis. The necrosis may be accompanied by pseudopalisading. Invasion of brain and/or metastases, either to the CNS or extracranially, signify frank malignancy.

Papillary Meningioma

This subtype of meningioma is of special interest because of its locally aggressive nature, its tendency for late distant metastases, and its occurrence in children and young adults.

MESENCHYMAL, NONMENINGOTHELIAL TUMORS

Malignant Neoplasms

HEMANGIOPERICYTOMA ("ANGIOBLASTIC MENINGIOMA")

Although this tumor was previously considered an usual and highly malignant form of meningioma, the "angioblastic meningioma," the WHO classification clearly designates this entity as a mesenchymal tumor of nonmeningeal origin. Intracranial meningeal hemangiopericytomas, like their somatic soft tissue counterpart, are highly vascular tumors with the capability of rapid growth, and all have a marked tendency for systemic metastasis. Meningeal hemangiopericytomas may occur at any age, but there is a marked increase in incidence in the fourth to sixth decades. Their geographic sites of origin are similar to those of meningiomas. Treatment consists of surgical resection and adjuvant radiation therapy, but in 75% of cases tumors recur despite therapy. The diagnosis is often suspected angiographically.

Sarcomas

A wide variety of sarcomas affect the CNS; most are highly malignant and all are unusual. Fibrosarcomas and malignant fibrous histiocytomas (fibrous histiocytic sarcomas) grow both inside and outside the dura, but despite their fairly circumscribed appearance, they tend to infiltrate the brain parenchyma. Some of these tumors arise as complications of high-dose radiation therapy after a long latent interval. They must be distinguished from anaplastic meningiomas and gliosarcomas. Meningeal sarcomatosis, a rapidly fatal disorder, is a diffuse sarcoma of the leptomeninges, occurring in young or middle-aged patients. Rhabdomyosarcomas may occur as the dominant feature of teratomas or in conjunction with medulloblastomas; they may also arise de novo in the leptomeninges. Chondrosarcomas may affect the clivus, sella, nasopharynx, or vertebrae. Patients range in age from 20 to 60 years, and the tumors are seen more commonly in males. Osteosarcomas very rarely occur in the skull, and only exceptionally is the skull the site of metastases from osteosarcomas elsewhere in the skeleton.

TUMORS OF UNCERTAIN HISTOGENESIS

Hemangioblastoma (Capillary Hemangioblastoma)

Hemangioblastomas constitute 1.2% of all intracranial neoplasms. Most arise in the third to fifth decade with a twofold male preponderance. Sites of preference, in descending order of frequency, are the cerebellar vermis and hemispheres, the roof of the fourth ventricle (area postrema), the spinal cord, and occasionally the cerebral hemispheres, where they tend to be meningeal rather than intraparenchymal. This tumor has a tendency to form large cysts, and multiplicity is common. The clinical signs are frequently those of cerebellar dysfunction and obstructive hydrocephalus. Approximately 10% of hemangioblastomas occur in association with von Hippel-Lindau disease, a term reserved for hereditary forms of cerebellar hemangioblastoma in combination with angiomas of the retina, hypernephromas, and cysts of the pancreas and kidney. Hemangioblastomas are benign brain tumors, although they may infiltrate the brain parenchyma. Malignant transformation and metastasis have not been recorded. Treatment is surgical resection, which usually results in cure unless a second tumor has been overlooked or the cyst is opened at surgery. Approximately 10% to 20% secrete erythropoietin and thus give rise to polycythemia.

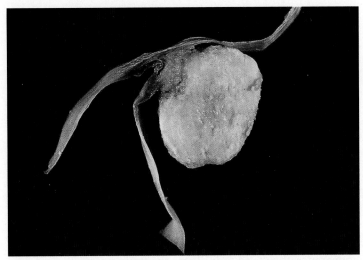

FIGURE 14.58 MENINGIOMA. In this parasagittal tumor the sagittal sinus is involved, a feature that affects resectability and results in increased incidence of recurrence of meningiomas at this site.

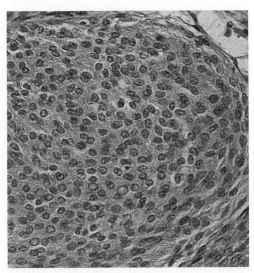

FIGURE 14.60 MENINGIOTHELIOMATOUS MENINGIOMA. These tumors are characterized by lobules of uniform, oval epithelioid cells with typical intranuclear haloes.

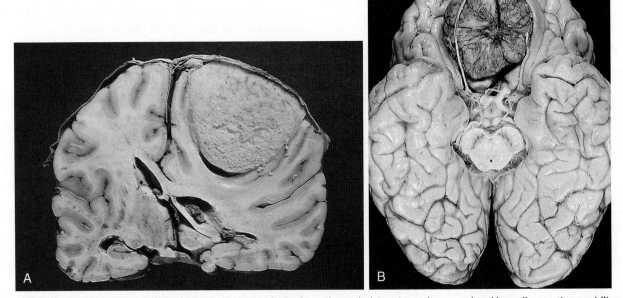

FIGURE 14.59 MENINGIOMA. (A) A large convexity meningioma severely displaces the underlying tissue downward and laterally, creating a midline shift and marked ventricular compression. **(B)** An olfactory groove meningioma bows the olfactory nerves and splays the frontal lobes.

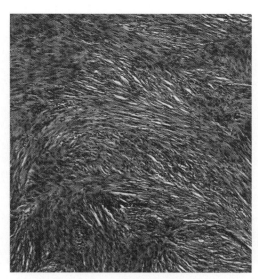

FIGURE 14.61 **FIBROUS (FIBROBLASTIC) MENINGIOMA.** This variant of meningioma is marked by collections of spindle-shaped cells (bearing some resemblance to fibroblasts) arranged in a dense network of intersecting bundles.

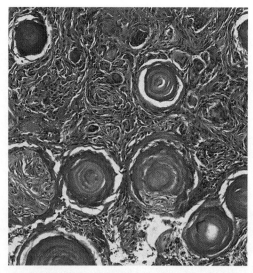

FIGURE 14.64 **PSAMMOMATOUS MENINGIOMA.** These tumors contain rounded microcalcifications that often center on the meningeal whorls. The psammoma bodies arise extracellularly, originating within the matrix produced by the tumor cells.

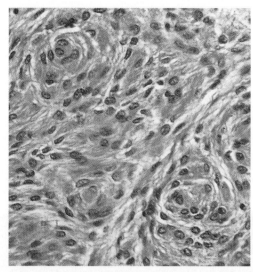

FIGURE 14.62 **TRANSITIONAL (MIXED) MENINGIOMA.** Meningotheliomatous and fibrous features intermix in this histologic subtype of meningioma. The whorled architecture is a common finding.

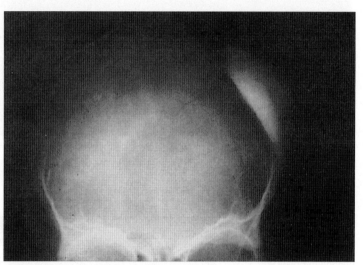

FIGURE 14.65 **MENINGIOMA.** Focal hypertrophy of the overlying skull is frequently a valuable radiologic sign, suggesting the presence of a meningioma. Usually a reactive process, osseous hypertrophy may also be caused by meningiomatous invasion of bone, as demonstrated in this radiograph.

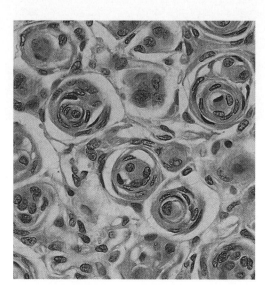

FIGURE 14.63 **MENINGIOMA.** Whorl formation is often a valuable diagnostic feature. The whorls may be quite prominent, with cells tightly wrapping around one another in an "onion-skin" pattern.

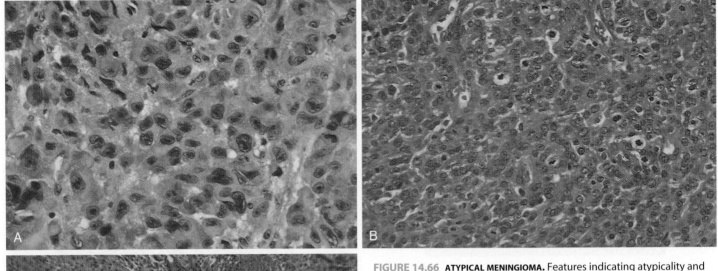

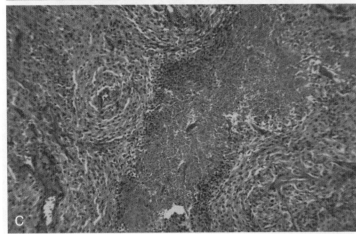

FIGURE 14.66   ATYPICAL MENINGIOMA. Features indicating atypicality and potential malignant behavior are: **(A)** prominence of nucleoli, **(B)** mitotic figures with high cell density and a sheetlike growth pattern, and **(C)** necrosis, occasionally with pseudopalisading.

FIGURE 14.67   MALIGNANT MENINGIOMA. The determination of frank malignancy rests on demonstration of invasion into adjacent brain parenchyma, a feature that can be identified grossly **(A, B)** as well as microscopically **(C).**

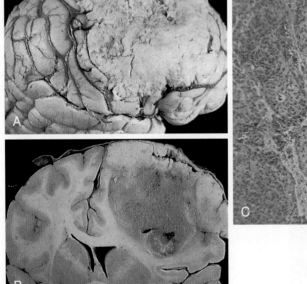

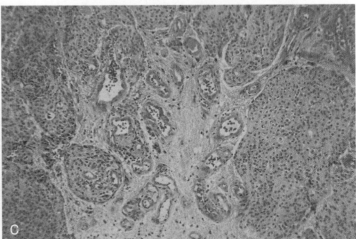

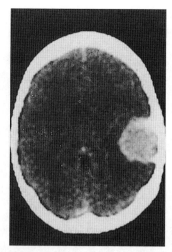

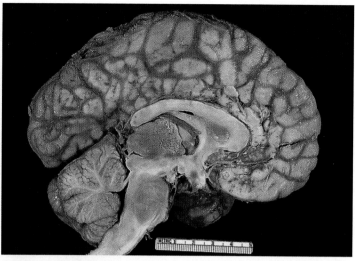

FIGURE 14.68 **MALIGNANT FIBROUS HISTIOCYTOMA.** CT scan in a 16-year-old girl shows a discrete, enhancing tumor based in the dura.

FIGURE 14.70 **RHABDOMYOSARCOMA.** In this specimen from a child, the tumor involves the pineal region and is associated with diffuse leptomeningeal seeding.

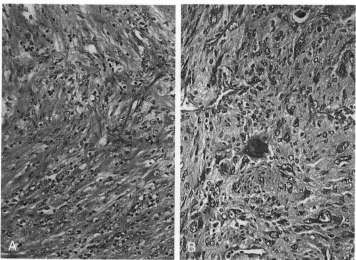

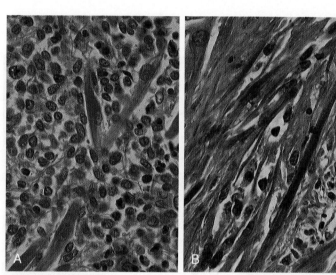

FIGURE 14.69 **MALIGNANT FIBROUS HISTIOCYTOMA. (A)** Its microscopic appearance is marked by spindle-shaped and plump cells arranged in fascicles. Inflammatory cells are occasionally present. **(B)** In rare instances giant cells and mitoses are observed in addition to bizarre, spindle-shaped cells. Such lesions must be distinguished from giant cell astrocytoma secondarily involving the meninges.

FIGURE 14.71 **RHABDOMYOSARCOMA. (A)** The tumor is composed of small, poorly differentiated, round cells intermingled with elongated, eosinophilic muscle fibers. **(B)** On phosphotungstic acid–hematoxylin stain, the myoblasts show cytoplasmic cross-striations. Microscopic sampling of such neoplasms is necessary to exclude the presence of coexisting germ cell tumor components.

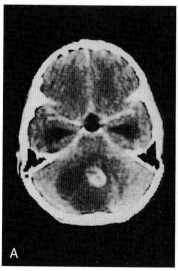

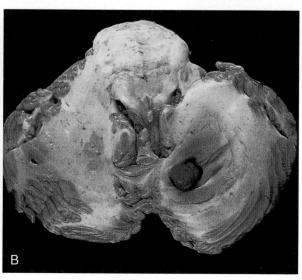

FIGURE 14.72 **HEMANGIOBLASTOMA. (A)** CT scan of a 35-year-old male reveals an enhancing cystic lesion of the cerebellum with a central tumor nodule, features characteristic of hemangioblastoma. **(B)** Gross specimen confirms a central, vascular tumor nodule surrounded by cystic, gliotic, and darkly discolored cerebellar white matter.

FIGURE 14.73 **HEMANGIOBLASTOMA. (A)** Its histologic appearance is marked by large, oval, often foamy cells amid a dense network of thin-walled, closely packed blood vessels. **(B)** Occasionally clusters of immature red blood cells are seen, indirect evidence of the known capacity of hemangioblastomas to secrete erythropoietin (extramedullary erythropoiesis).

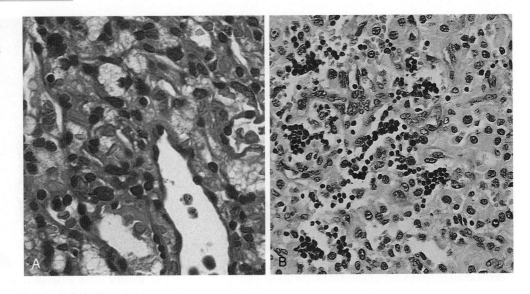

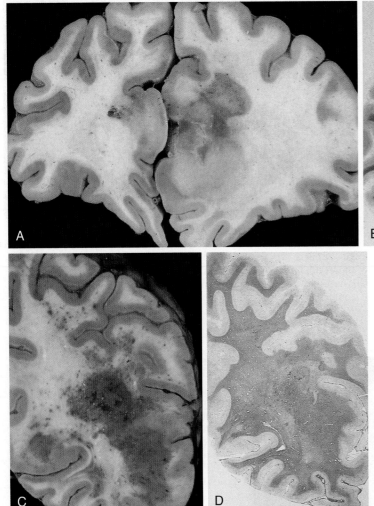

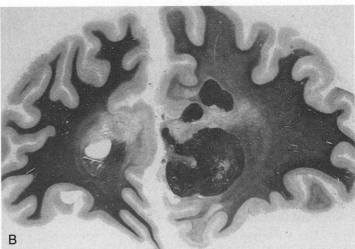

FIGURE 14.74 **PRIMARY CEREBRAL LYMPHOMA. (A)** A reasonably circumscribed mass of white tumor tissue lies within the paramedian right frontal lobe. The deeply staining lymphomatous masses are more easily visualized on the corresponding whole-mount section **(B)**. The pale areas surrounding the tumor nodules represent edema. **(C)**, **(D)** The lesion may be more diffuse, like that shown here in the right posterior temporoparietal lobe; no discrete mass is evident.

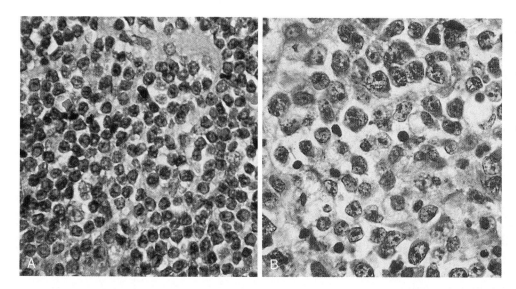

FIGURE 14.75 **PRIMARY CEREBRAL LYMPHOMA.** The histologic appearance is variable, ranging from **(A)** small cell tumors to **(B)** the more common large cell, immunoblastic type. Monotypic immunoreactivity for immunoglobulin components is typical of B-cell lymphoma. (See also Chapter 16, "Hodgkin Disease and Non-Hodgkin Lymphomas," and Chapter 19, "AIDS-Associated Malignancies.")

CNS LYMPHOMA

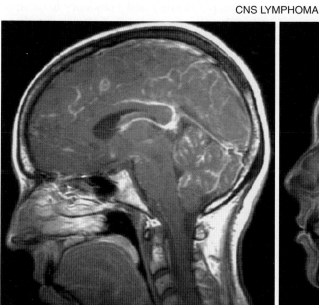

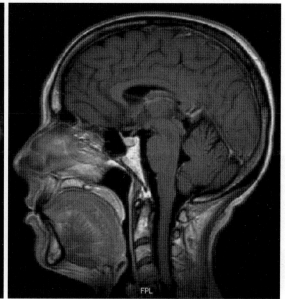

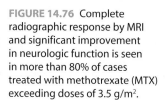

At diagnosis   2 cycles of high-dose MTX

FIGURE 14.76 Complete radiographic response by MRI and significant improvement in neurologic function is seen in more than 80% of cases treated with methotrexate (MTX) exceeding doses of 3.5 g/m².

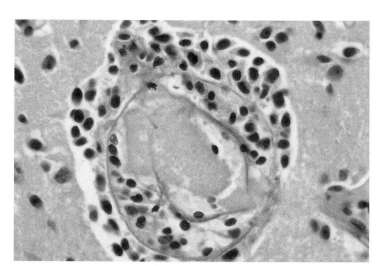

FIGURE 14.77 **PRIMARY CEREBRAL LYMPHOMA.** The growth pattern is typically perivascular. Neoplastic lymphocytes not only surround small blood vessels but also penetrate the vascular wall.

Lymphomas and Hematopoietic Neoplasms

Malignant Lymphoma

Primary CNS non-Hodgkin lymphomas have become increasingly common over the last 10 years with the advent of the acquired immunodeficiency syndrome (AIDS) epidemic. They represent approximately 2% of all intracranial tumors and show a marked male predominance. All immunosuppressed patients, including post-transplantation and AIDS patients, are particularly vulnerable. The tumors tend to be supratentorial, most commonly deeply situated and midline. The majority are B-cell neoplasms, although T-cell forms have been reported. The tumors may be multiple; they may form a discrete mass, or they may infiltrate diffusely by expanding existing structures without destroying their gross architecture. Although cerebral lymphomas are extremely sensitive to radiation therapy and steroids, overall median survival time ranges from 2 to 4 years with the addition of high-dose methotrexate. Complete radiographic response by MRI and significant improvement in neurologic function is seen in more than 80% of cases treated with methotrexate exceeding doses of 3.5 g/m^2 (Fig. 14.76). In the setting of immunosuppression the responses are less common and of shorter duration, and survival time is considerably shorter.

Germ Cell Tumors

Germinoma

Germinomas, which are derived from developmental germ cell rests, represent 0.5% to 0.7% of brain tumors, with a slightly higher incidence among Asian peoples. The pineal region is the most common site of occurrence, and men represent 70% to 90% of cases, as is true of most tumors of the pineal region. Germinomas may show a circumscribed or an infiltrative growth pattern. They may disseminate via the CSF and occasionally via the bloodstream to extracranial sites, including lungs, lymph nodes, and liver. These tumors are extremely radiosensitive; the 5-year survival rate following surgery and postoperative radiation may be as high as 80%.

Teratoma

Accounting for 0.2% to 0.9% of all brain tumors, teratomas show a marked male preponderance and a tendency to occur in the first two decades. They are most typically found in the pineal and sellar regions. Classically they are composed of three germinal layers. The majority are benign and slow growing, although instances of malignant change and CSF seeding have been described. Teratomas tend to be well circumscribed, and surgical resection is often associated with an excellent prognosis.

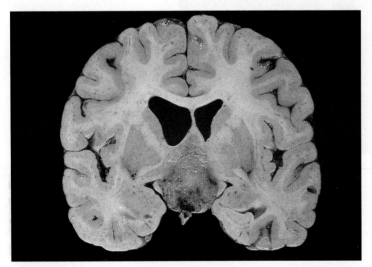

FIGURE 14.78 GERMINOMA. This coronal section shows a lesion of the hypothalamic region that, together with the pineal region, constitute the primary sites of occurrence.

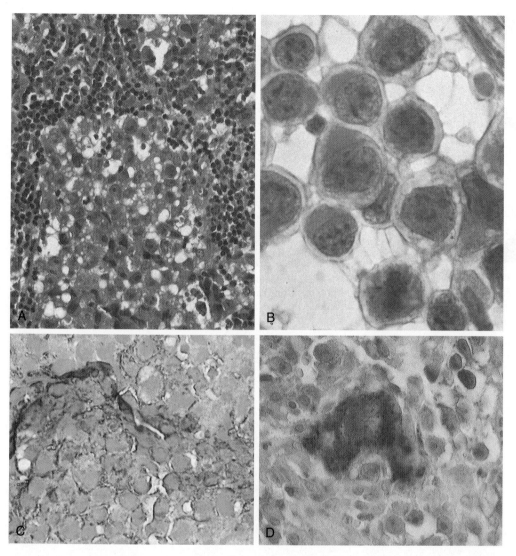

FIGURE 14.79 **GERMINOMA. (A)** Two distinct cell populations are present: one is of small lymphocytes and the other of large, spheroidal cells, each with a prominent central nucleus containing distinct nucleoli and vesiculated nucleoplasm. Granuloma formation is infrequent, unlike the situation with gonadal tumors. **(B)** Touch preparation demonstrates common cytologic features of tumor cells, including a high nucleus-to-cytoplasm ratio, round nuclei, and somewhat elongated nucleoli. Immunostaining techniques reveal the presence of **(C)** placental alkaline phosphatase within tumor cells, as well as **(D)** occasional syncytiotrophoblastic giant cells reactive for human chorionic gonadotrophin (HCG). Carrying no prognostic significance, the latter finding may be associated with elevated levels of HCG in CSF and blood.

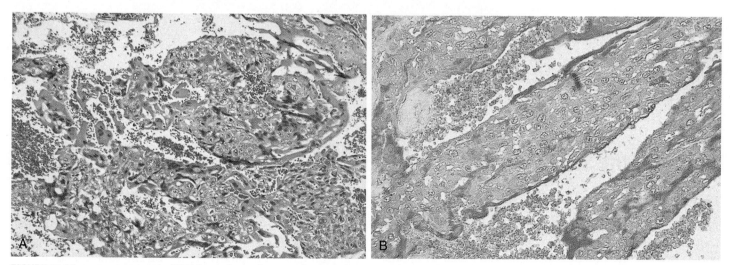

FIGURE 14.80 **CHORIOCARCINOMA. (A)** This rare form of germ cell tumor shows a tendency to hemorrhage, as seen microscopically in this tumor arising in the pineal region in a 12-year-old girl, who had a sudden intracranial hemorrhage and died on the same day. The tumor consists of multinucleate syncytiotrophoblastic and cytotrophoblastic cells arranged in a bilayer fashion, often surrounding vascular spaces. **(B)** Immunostaining reveals HCG reactivity in the syncytiotrophoblasts.

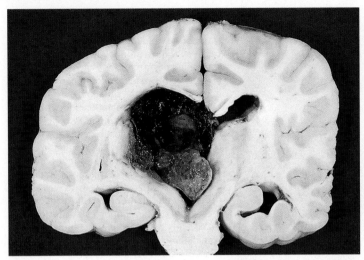

FIGURE 14.81 **IMMATURE TERATOMA.** This specimen from a 12-year-old boy shows a tumor projecting anteriorly from the pineal region. Intraventricular hemorrhage occurred postoperatively.

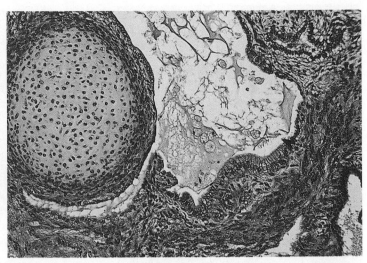

FIGURE 14.82 **IMMATURE TERATOMA.** Resembling fetal tissue, the constituents of this tumor include cartilage on the left and mucin-producing columnar epithelium in the center, together with a spindle cell stroma.

FIGURE 14.83 **MATURE TERATOMA. (A, B)** Unlike its immature counterpart, this tumor resembles benign adult tissue, showing mature hyaline cartilage, respiratory epithelium, and a loose, fibrous stroma. Mature teratomas are far less common than immature teratomas.

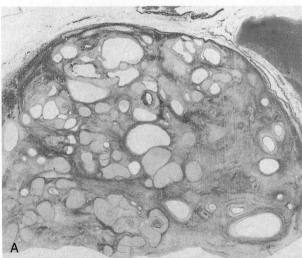
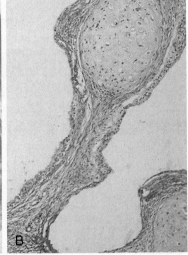

Tumors of the Sellar Region

Craniopharyngioma

Craniopharyngiomas are tumors of children and adolescents in whom they constitute 2% to 3% of all intracranial neoplasms. Two distinct varieties exist: the classic adamantinomatous craniopharyngioma and a less common form, the papillary craniopharyngioma. The majority of these tumors of maldevelopmental origin are found above the sella, although a few arise in the sella itself. They grow slowly, compressing neighboring tissue and frequently affecting the pituitary, optic chiasm, and their ventricle. The adamantinomatous craniopharyngioma usually presents with disturbances of the hypothalamic-pituitary axis, visual symptoms, and hydrocephalus as a result of obstructed CSF flow. Most adamantinomatous craniopharyngiomas are sufficiently calcified to be visualized on skull radiographs. Combined radiotherapy and surgical resection is the recommended treatment; however, recurrences are frequent (up to 40% of cases), particularly in the pediatric age group. The papillary craniopharyngioma, on the other hand, is often solid rather than cystic and infrequently calcified. In addition, the tumor seems to arise in the third ventricle and usually does not affect the sella. The prognosis of patients with the papillary craniopharyngioma is better than with the adamantinomatous tumor, as the papillary variety is more discrete and less infiltrative.

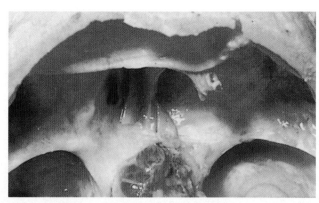

FIGURE 14.84 **CYSTIC CRANIOPHARYNGIOMA.** Usually partially solid and partially cystic, these tumors often contain a dark, oily fluid that has been likened to machine oil. This specimen shows a small cystic lesion in the suprasellar region.

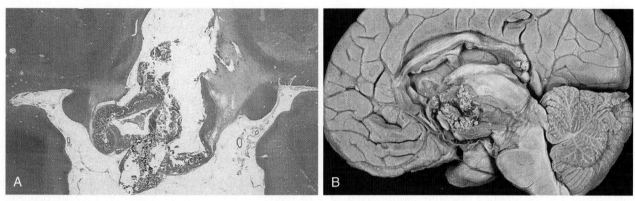

FIGURE 14.85 **CYSTIC CRANIOPHARYNGIOMA.** The tumor may grow, extending into the third ventricle, as seen **(A)** in this coronal-section photomicrograph and **(B)** in this midsagittal section, where a massive tumor fills the third ventricle.

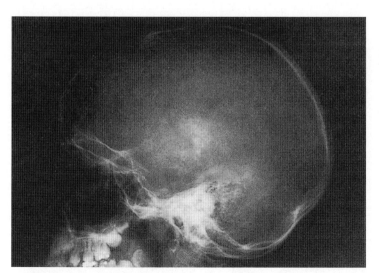

FIGURE 14.86 **CYSTIC CRANIOPHARYNGIOMA.** Lateral skull radiograph demonstrates the radial calcifications of a large, suprasellar tumor.

FIGURE 14.87 CRANIOPHARYNGIOMA. (A) The tumor is composed of a complex arrangement of columnar epithelium and prominent cystic spaces. **(B)** In many areas the epithelium is squamous and arranged in whorls with keratin pearl formation. Craniopharyngiomas have irregular contours and often show finger-like extensions into the surrounding brain, thus evoking intense gliosis.

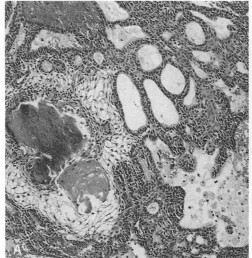
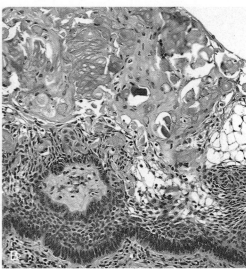

Local Extension from Regional Tumors

Chordoma

Representing approximately 0.2% of all brain tumors, chordomas are most commonly encountered in the fourth to sixth decades; there is a slight male preponderance. Derived from notochordal rests, they tend to be midline tumors of the skull base. The sella and clivus are the predominant cranial sites, from which these tumors may expand into the foramen magnum, nasopharynx, or optic chiasm, with considerable bone erosion and destruction. Spinal column tumors favor the dens of the axis and the sacrococcygeal region. Complete surgical resection is usually not feasible, and metastases to lungs, lymph nodes, bone, and skin may occur, particularly in sacrococcygeal chordomas. The survival time for cranial chordomas averages from 2 to 3 years and from 6 to 7 years for sacrococcygeal tumors.

Chondroma

Chondromas constitute less than 1% of all brain tumors. They commonly arise in the dura of the skull base but may arise in dura over the cerebral convexities or spinal cord, in the sinuses, or, rarely, in the choroid plexus. They are typically benign and slow growing. Treatment is surgical, which may be difficult because of the tumors' tendency to invade bone, a typical feature not considered a sign of malignant potential. Metastatic deposits represent 40% of all CNS tumors; they are commonly multiple. The most common carcinomas metastasizing to the CNS are those of the lung, breast, skin (melanoma), kidney (renal cell carcinoma), gastrointestinal tract, and thyroid. Perhaps as a result of prolonged survival, the incidence of cerebral metastases in patients with sarcomas has increased in the past decade.

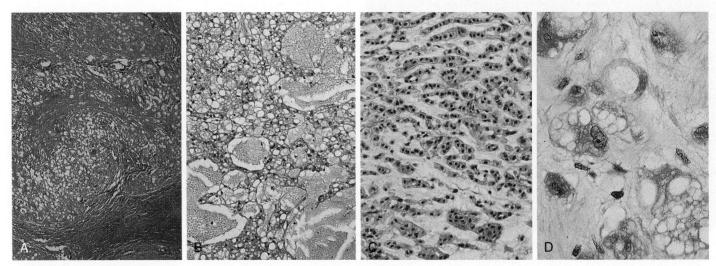

FIGURE 14.88 CHORDOMA. The spectrum of microscopic features of this tumor include **(A)** a lobular growth pattern, **(B)** pools of mucin among cells with abundant, foamy vacuoles, **(C)** elongated cords of pale, eosinophilic cells with regular cytologic features, and **(D)** large, physaliphorous ("bubbly") cells. Partial cartilaginous differentiation marks a "chondroid" chordoma (not shown), a variant associated with a more favorable prognosis.

Metastatic Tumors

SITES OF PREFERENCE

Skull and Epidura

Metastatic tumor deposits in the skull and vertebrae may penetrate and destroy bone and dura. They may extend into the epidural or subarachnoid space, compressing adjacent neural tissue.

Dural Tumors

Tumors with a tendency toward dural metastasis include those of the breast and prostate, as well as lymphomas and peripheral neuroblastoma. Prostatic carcinoma is unusual in that it favors dural metastasis to the exclusion of parenchymal invasion. Dural metastases often evoke an intense desmoplastic reaction, which may give the false impression of a meningioma on radiographic studies. Dural metastases may form either discrete, nodular masses or a thick lining of tumor on the inner aspect of the dura.

Leptomeninges

Leptomeningeal metastasis or meningeal carcinomatosis refers to diffuse involvement of the subarachnoid space by metastatic tumor and is often accompanied by perivascular infiltration of adjacent brain. Clinical signs include cranial and spinal nerve dysfunction, meningismus, and headache. Diagnosis is made by demonstration of tumor cells in the CSF. Adenocarcinomas of the lung, ovary, and stomach are the tumors most frequently associated with leptomeningeal spread.

Parenchyma

Metastases to the brain and spinal cord are proportional to the volume of the structures. Parenchymal metastases tend to be multiple and well circumscribed. Metastases from small cell (oat cell) carcinoma of the lung, choriocarcinoma, and melanoma have a tendency to hemorrhage spontaneously. Other tumor types, such as renal cell carcinoma, may undergo cystic degeneration.

SYSTEMIC LYMPHOMA INVOLVING THE CNS

Most systemic lymphomas that involve the CNS are hematogenous metastases or direct extensions of systemic tumors. Metastases may involve the dura, leptomeninges, or parenchyma, often in combination.

NON-HODGKIN LYMPHOMA

Lymphomatous leptomeningitis, both cerebral and spinal, is the most common pattern of neoplastic infiltration in non-Hodgkin lymphomas. Subarachnoid infiltration is often associated with perivascular and subependymal infiltration of the parenchyma, as well as the spinal and cranial nerve roots. The optic chiasm, tuber cinereum, and hypothalamus are the regions most frequently involved. The incidence of subarachnoid and parenchymal invasion of the CNS in non-Hodgkin lymphoma is relatively high, with reported frequency varying between 6% and 29%. Large cell lymphomas (diffuse and immunoblastic), followed closely by small cell lymphomas (undifferentiated and poorly differentiated lymphocytic), are the most common types of lymphoma that spread to the CNS. Nodular or follicular lymphomas do not involve the CNS unless they have progressed to a diffuse pattern.

Dural infiltration by non-Hodgkin lymphomas is also common. The spinal axis is affected more frequently than the cranial cavity. Clinical signs may result from direct spinal cord compression or ischemia secondary to involvement of the spinal radicular arteries. If the dural deposits remain relatively restricted, they may be amenable to surgical removal. Most spinal epidural lymphomas are of the diffuse, small cell type, which have a relatively favorable prognosis because of their low grade of malignancy and their responsiveness to irradiation.

HODGKIN DISEASE

Secondary intracranial Hodgkin disease is a rare event, with an incidence of approximately 0.5%. Metastases may be dural, in which case they are usually associated with involvement of adjacent bone, or subdural, often forming lobulated masses simulating a meningioma. Leptomeningeal infiltration occurs infrequently, and intracerebral parenchymal involvement is rare.

Intraspinal epidural masses arising as extensions of adjacent bony or soft tissue deposits are the most common form of metastatic disease. The thoracic segment is most frequently affected, followed by the lumbar and cervical regions.

LEUKEMIA

The incidence of leukemic involvement of the CNS has dropped dramatically over the past 10 years, largely as a result of more intensive modalities of treatment. Recent figures indicate that 20% show intraparenchymal involvement. Acute leukemias have a greater tendency to involve the CNS than chronic leukemias, with acute lymphoblastic leukemia having a greater propensity than acute myeloblastic disease. Both children and adults are prone to this complication. Leukemic involvement of the CNS usually takes two forms: (1) diffuse leptomeningeal infiltration, often in combination with cranial and spinal nerve root invasion, and focal intraparenchymal and microscopic dural infiltration; and (2) massive hemorrhagic stasis and impaction of leukemic cells in blood vessels with resultant destruction of the vessel wall, hemorrhage, and infarction of the central white matter. Epidural, subdural, or intracerebral solid tumor deposits (myeloblastomas or "chloromas") originating from the skull or spine have become extremely rare in recent years. Intracranial hemorrhage, either intracerebral or subarachnoid, is a frequent terminal event, accounting for death in 20% of cases. Fatal intracerebral hemorrhages are associated with intracerebral leukostasis and the development of leukemic nodules; the critical leukocyte count is approximately 100,000 leukocytes/mm^3. Fatal subarachnoid hemorrhages are not associated with blast crises and seem to be related to thrombocytopenia.

Skull and epidura
Dura
Leptomeninges
Parenchyma

FIGURE 14.89 CNS sites of preference of metastatic tumors.

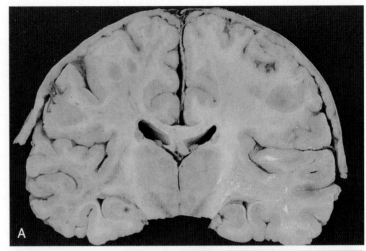

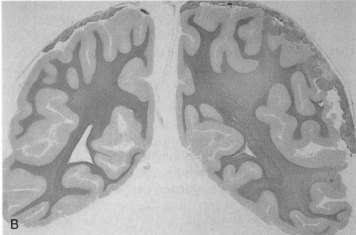

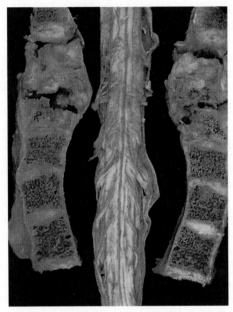

FIGURE 14.90 **METASTATIC LUNG ADENOCARCINOMA.** Osseous metastases have expanded and destroyed several cervical vertebrae, with consequent flattening and distortion of the spinal cord. The subdural space was free of tumor.

FIGURE 14.91 **METASTATIC BREAST CARCINOMA.** **(A)** Coronal section of a brain and dura shows diffuse subdural involvement by metastatic deposits. The dura is uniformly and symmetrically thickened. **(B)** Corresponding whole-mount section shows focal, direct extension of tumor into the right parietal cortex and subcortical white matter, with resultant edema evidenced by pallor of the white matter.

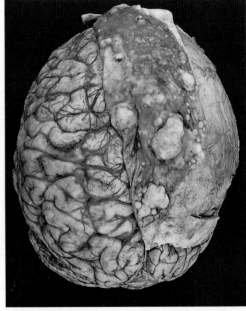

FIGURE 14.92 **METASTATIC BREAST CARCINOMA.** The dura of this specimen has been reflected to reveal multiple subdural metastatic deposits. Note the lack of discernible infiltration of the subjacent brain by tumor.

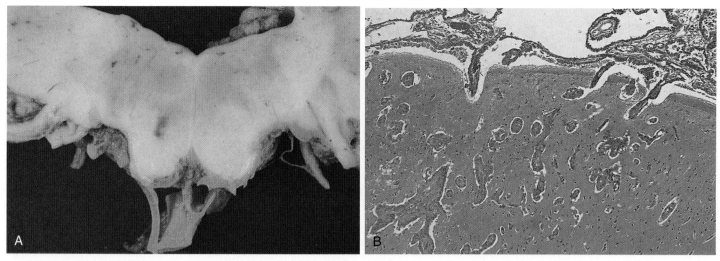

FIGURE 14.93 **METASTATIC LUNG ADENOCARCINOMA. (A)** Leptomeningeal infiltration in this specimen is diffuse, appearing as a glassy coat. **(B)** Microscopically, in addition to infiltration of the leptomeninges, tumor extension into the cerebral cortex via perivascular (Virchow-Robin) spaces is evident.

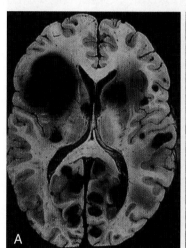
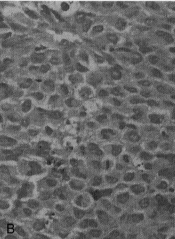
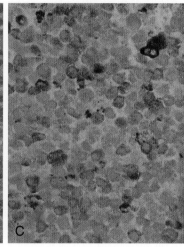

FIGURE 14.94 **METASTATIC MALIGNANT MELANOMA. (A)** Deeply pigmented, hemorrhagic metastases are characteristic. Melanin may be absent or **(B)** very sparse by H&E staining but **(C)** is usually visible on special (Fontana) stain.

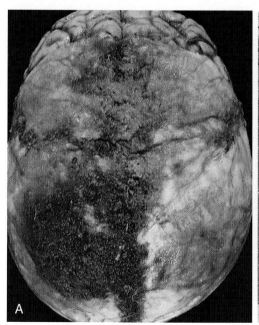
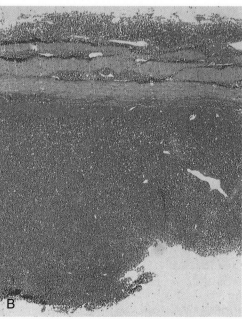

FIGURE 14.95 **SYSTEMIC NON-HODGKIN LYMPHOMA INVOLVING THE CNS. (A)** This specimen shows diffuse, granular, hemorrhagic epidural and subdural tumor deposits. **(B)** On microscopy there is extensive infiltration of the dura, together with a large, subdural accumulation of tumor. Morphologic and immunophenotypic studies were diagnostic of a B-large cell lymphoma.

FIGURE 14.96 SYSTEMIC NON-HODGKIN LYMPHOMA INVOLVING THE CNS. Cross-sectional photomicrograph of lumbar spinal cord shows dense subdural and epidural tumor deposits and spinal root infiltration. There is also mild dorsolateral cord compression.

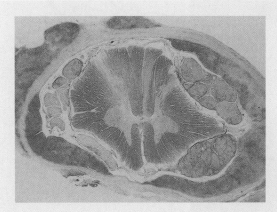

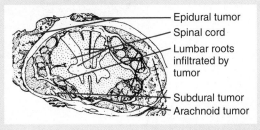

- Epidural tumor
- Spinal cord
- Lumbar roots infiltrated by tumor
- Subdural tumor
- Arachnoid tumor

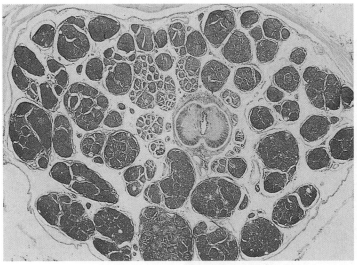

FIGURE 14.97 SECONDARY LEUKEMIC INVOLVEMENT OF CNS. Cross-sectional micrograph of the sacral spinal cord and cauda equina nerve roots in a 4-year-old girl with acute lymphoblastic leukemia shows dense infiltration of nerve roots by deep blue–staining leukemic cells.

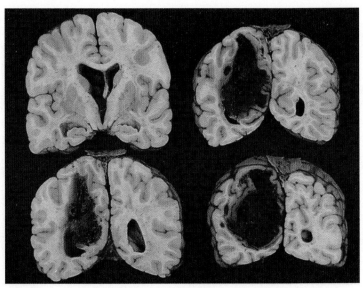

FIGURE 14.99 SECONDARY LEUKEMIC INVOLVEMENT OF CNS. These coronal sections of the brain of a 20-year-old man with acute myeloblastic leukemia show a large left posterior cerebral hemorrhage. Intracerebral hemorrhage is a frequent complication of nonlymphocytic forms of leukemia, perhaps secondary to associated thrombocytopenia.

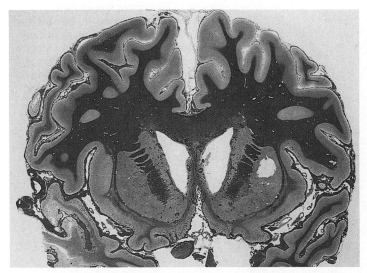

FIGURE 14.98 SECONDARY LEUKEMIC INVOLVEMENT OF CNS. Whole-mount coronal section from a 10-year-old boy with acute lymphoblastic leukemia demonstrates thick, subarachnoid accumulations of leukemic cells, which encase the entire neuraxis.

References and Suggested Readings

Alexander E, Moriarty T, Davis R, et al: Stereotactic radiosurgery for the definitive noninvasive treatment of brain metastases, *J Natl Cancer Inst* 86:34–40, 1995.

Ashley Hill D, Pfeifer J, Marley E, et al: WT1 staining reliably differentiates desmoplastic small round cell tumor from Ewing sarcoma/primitive neuroectodermal tumor: an immunohistochemical and molecular diagnostic study, *Am J Clin Pathol* 114:345–353, 2000.

Bondy M, Wiencke J, Wrensch M, Kyritis AP: Genetics of primary brain tumors: a review, *J Neurooncol* 18:69–81, 1993.

Brandsma D, Stalpers L, Taal W, et al: Clinical features, mechanisms, and management of pseudoprogression in malignant gliomas, *Lancet Oncol* 9:453–461, 2008.

Bruner JM: Neuropathology of malignant gliomas, *Semin Oncol* 21:126–138, 1994.

Bullman NM, Mahan CM, Kang HK, et al: Mortality in US Army Gulf War veterans exposed to 1991 Khamisiyah chemical munitions destruction, *Am J Public Health* 95:1382–1388, 2005.

Burger PC, Scheithauer BW, Vogel FS: *Surgical pathology of the nervous system and its coverings*, ed 3, New York, 1991, Churchill Livingstone.

Central Brain Tumor Registry United States (CBTRUS): 2007–2008. Available from: http://www.cbtrus.org/.

Chung R, Whaley J, Kley N, et al: *TP53* gene mutations and 17p deletions in human astrocytomas, *Genes Chromosomes Cancer* 3:323–331, 1991.

Claesson-Welsh L: Platelet-derived growth factor receptor signals, *J Biol Chem* 269:32023–32026, 1994.

The European Chromosome 16 Tuberous Sclerosis Consortium: Identification and characterization of the tuberous sclerosis gene on chromosome 16, *Cell* 75:1305–1315, 1993.

Ganju V, Jenkins RB, O'Fallon JR, et al: Prognostic factors in gliomas, *Cancer* 74:920–927, 1994.

Greig NH, Ries LG, Yancik R, Rapoport SI: Increasing annual incidence of primary malignant brain tumors in the elderly, *J Natl Cancer Inst* 82:1621–1624, 1990.

Harkin JC, Reed RJ: Tumors of the peripheral nervous system. In *Atlas of tumor pathology*, 2nd ser., fasc. 3. Washington, DC, 1969, Armed Forces Institute of Pathology.

Heigi ME, Diserens AC, Gorlia T, et al: MGMT gene silencing and benefit from temozolomide in glioblastoma, *N Engl J Med* 352:997–1003, 2005.

Heldin CH, Westermark B: Platelet-derived growth factor: mechanism of action and possible in vivo function, *Cell Regul* 1:555–566, 1990.

Henske EP, Ozelius L, Gusella JF, et al: A high resolution linkage map of human 9q34.1, *Genomics* 17:587–591, 1993.

Inskip PD, Tarone RE, Hatch EE, et al: Cellular telephone use and brain tumors, *N Engl J Med* 344:79–86, 2001.

Jemal A, Siegel R, Ward E, et al: Cancer statistics, 2009, *CA Cancer J Clin* 59:225–249, 2009.

Kan P, Simonsen SE, Lyon JL, et al: Cellular phone use and brain tumor: a meta-analysis, *J Neurooncol* 86:71–78, 2007.

Keeps JJ: Pleomorphic xanthoastrocytoma: the birth of a diagnosis and concept, *Br Pathol* 3:269–274, 1993.

Kleihues P, Cavenee WK: *World Health Organization classification of tumours of the nervous system*, Lyon, 2000, IARC/WHO.

Kurpad SN, Wikstrand CJ, Bigner DD: Immunobiology of malignant astrocytomas, *Semin Oncol* 21:149–161, 1994.

LeBihan D, Jezzard P, Haxby J, et al: Functional magnetic resonancy imaging of the brain, *Ann Intern Med* 122:296–303, 1995.

Louis DN: The p53 gene and protein in human brain tumors, *J Neuropathol Exp Neurol* 53:11–21, 1994.

Louis DN, Ohgaki H, Wiestler OD, et al, editors: *WHO classification of tumors of the central nervous system*, Lyon, 2007, IARC.

Louis DN, Ramesh V, Gusella JF: Neuropathology and molecular genetics of neurofibromatosis 2 and related tumors, *Brain Pathol* 5:163–172, 1995.

Louis DN, von Deimling A, Chung RY, et al: Comparative study on p53 gene and protein alteration in human astrocytomas, *J Neuropathol Exp Neurol* 52:31–38, 1993.

Lucas DR, Bentley G, Dan ME, et al: Ewing sarcoma vs lymphoblastic lymphoma: a comparative immunohistochemical study, *Am J Clin Pathol* 115:11–17, 2001.

Maher E, Brennan C, Wen P, et al: Marked genomic differences characterize primary and secondary glioblastoma subtypes and identify two distinct molecular and clinical secondary glioblastoma entities, *Cancer Res* 66:11502–11513, 2006.

Maher E, Fine HA: Primary CNS lymphoma, *Semin Oncol* 26:346–356, 1999.

Maher E, Furnari FB, Bachoo RM, et al: Malignant glioma: genetics and biology of a grave matter, *Genes Dev* 15:1311–1333, 2001.

Mills SE, Frierson HF Jr: Olfactory neuroblastoma: a clinicopathological study of 21 cases, *Am J Surg Pathol* 9:317–327, 1985.

Neglia JP, Meadows AT, Robison LL, et al: Second neoplasms after acute lymphoblastic leukemia in childhood, *N Engl J Med* 325:1330–1336, 1991.

Okazaki H, Scheithauer BW: *Atlas of neuropathology*, New York/Philadelphia, 1988, Lippincott/Gower Medical Publishing.

Ron E, Modan B, Boice JD, et al: Tumors of the brain and nervous system and radiotherapy in childhood, *N Engl J Med* 319:1033–1039, 1988.

Rubinstein LJ: Tumors of the central nervous system. In *Atlas of tumor pathology*, 2nd ser., fasc. 6. Washington, DC, 1972, Armed Forces Institute of Pathology.

Russell DS, Rubinstein LJ: *Pathology of tumors of the nervous system*, ed 5, Baltimore, 1989, Williams and Wilkins.

Sanai N, Alvarez-Buylla A, Berger MS: Neural stem cells and the origin of gliomas, *N Engl J Med* 353:811–822, 2005.

Schochet SS Jr, Peters B, O'Neal J, et al: Intracranial esthesioneuroblastoma: a light and electron microscopic study, *Acta Neuropathol (Berl)* 31:181–189, 1975.

Smith J, Tachibana I, Passe S, et al: PTEN mutation, EGFR amplification and outcome in patients with anaplastic astrocytoma and glioblastoma multiforme, *J Natl Cancer Inst* 93:1246–1256, 2001.

Stuart ET, Kioussi C, Aguzzi A, et al: PAX5 expression correlates with increasing malignancy in human astrocytomas, *Clin Cancer Res* 1:207–214, 1995.

Stupp R, Mason WP, van den Bent MJ, et al: Radiotherapy plus concomitant and adjuvant temozolomide for glioblastoma, *N Engl J Med* 325:987–996, 2005.

Thomas TL, Stewart PA, Stemhagen A, et al: Risk of astrocytic brain tumors associated with occupational chemical exposures: a case-control study, *Scand J Work Environ Health* 13:417–423, 1987.

Ueki K, Ono Y, Henson JW, et al: CDKN2/p16 or RB alterations occur in the majority of glioblastomas and are inversely correlated, *Cancer Res* 56:150–153, 1996.

von Deimling A, Eibl RH, Ohgaki H, et al: p53 mutations are associated with 17p allelic loss in grade II and grade III astrocytoma, *Cancer Res* 52:2987–2990, 1992.

Watkins D, Rouleau GA: Genetics, prognosis and therapy of central nervous system tumors. *Cancer Detection Prev* 18:139–144, 1994.

Wen PY, Kesari S: Malignant gliomas in adults, *N Engl J Med* 359:492–507, 2008.

Wong AJ, Zoltick PW, Moscatello DK: The molecular biology and molecular genetics of astrocytic neoplasms, *Semin Oncol* 21:139–148, 1994.

Zulch KJ: *Brain tumors*, ed 3, New York, 1986, Springer-Verlag.

Figure Credits

The following books published by Gower Medical Publishing are sources of figures in the present chapter. The figure numbers given in the listing are those of the figures in the present chapter. The page numbers given in parentheses are those of the original publication.

Hawke M, Jahn AF: *Diseases of the ear: clinical and pathologic aspects.* New York/Philadelphia, 1987: Lea and Febiger/Gower Medical Publishing Fig. 14.80 (p. 5.42).

Okazaki H, Scheithauer BW: *Atlas of neuropathology.* New York/Philadelphia, 1988: Lippincott/Gower Medical Publishing Figs. 14.2 (p. 60), 14.3 (p. 62), 14.4 (p. 65), 14.6 (p. 65), 14.7 (p. 65), 14.9 (p. 75), 14.10 (p. 67), 14.13 (p. 69), 14.14 (p. 69), 14.15 (p. 70), 14.17 (p. 86), 14.18 (p. 77), 14.19 (p. 82), 14.20 (p. 82), 14.21 (p. 89), 14.23 (p. 90), 14.24 (p. 91), 14.25 (p. 93), 14.27 (p. 93), 14.28 (p. 94), 14.30 (p. 103), 14.31 (p. 103), 14.32 (p. 109), 14.33 (p. 113), 14.34 (p. 114), 14.35 (p. 110), 14.36 (p. 111), 14.37A, B (p. 111), 14.37C, D (p. 112), 14.38 (p. 114), 14.39 (p. 115), 14.40 (p. 116), 14.41 (p. 116), 14.42 (p. 116), 14.43 (p. 121), 14.45 (p. 126), 14.46 (p. 126), 14.47 (p. 130), 14.48 (p. 130), 14.49 (p. 131), 14.50 (p. 131), 14.51 (p. 131), 14.52 (p. 133), 14.53A, B (p. 134), 14.54 (p. 135), 14.55 (p. 98), 14.56 (p. 99), 14.57 (p. 99), 14.58 (p. 99), 14.59 (p. 139), 14.60 (p. 141), 14.61 (p. 148), 14.62 (p. 149), 14.64 (p. 142), 14.65 (p. 142), 14.66 (p. 143), 14.67 (p. 143), 14.68 (p. 146), 14.69 (p. 151), 14.71A, B (p. 151), 14.71C, D (p. 152), 14.70 (p. 154), 14.72 (p. 154), 14.73 (p. 155), 14.74 (p. 156), 14.75 (p. 157), 14.77 (p. 157), 14.78 (p. 157), 14.79 (p. 158), 14.81 (p. 183), 14.82 (p. 184), 14.83 (p. 184), 14.84 (p. 198), 14.85 (p. 199), 14.88A–D (p. 198), 14.87 (p. 192), 14.86 (p. 192), 14.89 (p. 193), 14.91 (p. 165), 14.92 (p. 167), 14.93 (p. 167), 14.94 (p. 169), 14.95 (p. 171), 14.96 (p. 174), 14.97 (p. 177), 14.98 (p. 178), 14.99 (p. 178).

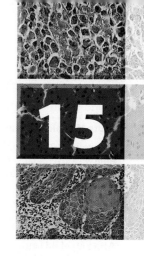

Acute and Chronic Leukemias

MARTHA WADLEIGH • DAVID M. DORFMAN • ARTHUR T. SKARIN

Acute Leukemias

Acute leukemias are neoplastic disorders marked by uncontrolled proliferation of hematopoietic cells, with a predominance of immature lymphoid or myeloid cells, in the bone marrow and peripheral blood. Although leukemic cells do not divide more rapidly than normal marrow cells, they possess a growth advantage because the blasts fail to differentiate in response to normal hormonal signals and cellular interactions. The malignant cells eventually replace the marrow and invade other tissues and organs, leading to manifestations of the disease. Production of normal erythrocytes, granulocytes, and megakaryocytes is diminished, resulting in anemia, infection, and hemorrhage.

Approximately 18,000 cases of acute leukemia occur in the United States each year. The incidence increases with age. About 80% of leukemic children have acute lymphoblastic leukemia (ALL), the most common childhood malignant neoplasm, whereas 80% of adults with leukemia have acute myeloid leukemia (AML). The known etiologies include chromosomal damage from ionizing radiation or from chemicals (e.g., benzene and alkylating agents used in therapy), congenital disease (e.g., Down syndrome), chronic bone marrow diseases (e.g., myelodysplasia), congenital predisposition (e.g., identical twins with leukemia), and congenital immunodeficiency syndromes (e.g., ataxia-telangiectasia).

MORPHOLOGY AND BIOLOGY

Acute leukemias—defined as 20% or more blasts in blood or bone marrow under the World Health Organization (WHO) criteria—are classified according to the predominant neoplastic cell line and thus may be designated as lymphoblastic or myeloid. The WHO classification takes into account cytogenetic and molecular findings in addition to morphologic and histochemical criteria (see Tables 15.1 and 15.4). About 70% to 80% of cases can be classified on the basis of morphology alone, whereas an additional 10% to 15% of cases require histochemical determinations for specific diagnosis. In approximately 10% of cases, surface marker and cytogenetic studies are necessary for accurate classification, particularly in the "undifferentiated" acute leukemias. Use of monoclonal antibodies has revealed that about 20% of cases of ALL are of T-cell origin; most of the remainder are of B-cell or pre-B cell origin (see Table 15.3).

Development of colony assays and new monoclonal antibodies has led to a clearer understanding of normal myeloid ontogeny. The patterns of expression of a variety of antigens during normal myeloid differentiation have been established. Immunophenotyping techniques have demonstrated that some cases of acute "undifferentiated" leukemia, or those considered on the basis of morphology to be ALL, show myeloid markers. Improvement of cytogenetic studies by the use of new banding techniques has revealed that almost all acute leukemias are characterized by chromosomal abnormalities, ranging from hypoploidy to polyploidy. Significant cytogenetic defects that have prognostic importance (e.g., are seen only with certain subgroups) have been identified, involving the ALLs as well as the AMLs. Genetic abnormalities in the acute leukemias can affect genes that encode proteins involved in signal transduction, transcription regulation, cellular differentiation, and apoptosis, as well as tumor suppression (antioncogenes).

In about 10% of adults with ALL, cytogenetic studies will show the presence of the Philadelphia chromosome (t(9;22)(q34;q11)), and the incidence increases with age. These Ph-positive patients tend to be older (median age 46 years vs 35 years) and to have a lower incidence of anemia and a higher incidence of leukocytosis than Ph-negative patients (Preti et al., 1994). Ph-positive ALL patients are also likely to have FAB-L2 morphology (see Table 15.1), to be common ALL antigen-positive (CALLA-CD10-positive) and CD34-positive, and to have a worse prognosis than Ph-negative ALL cases. In a few patients with ALL and AML who are Ph-negative, molecular studies (e.g., polymerase chain reaction) will reveal the presence of BCR-ABL transcripts diagnostic of the Ph-chromosome abnormality not otherwise detected because of insufficient metaphases (Kantarjian et al., 1994).

CLINICAL MANIFESTATIONS

Patients can present with a variety of clinical manifestations, which correlate with the degree of marrow and other organ involvement. Among the more common symptoms are fatigue, bruisability, oral lesions, fever, and infection. Perirectal infections are particularly frequent in AML, and skin and gum infiltrates are seen mainly in AMLs. Joint swelling and bone pain with rheumatic symptoms occur commonly in ALL, which may also present as a meningitis-like syndrome. Diffuse lymphadenopathy and hepatosplenomegaly are more common in ALL (50% of cases) than in AML.

Table 15.I

World Health Organization (WHO) Classification of Acute Leukemias

Acute Myeloid Leukemia with Recurrent Genetic Abnormalities

AML with t(8;21)(q22;q22); *RUNX1-RUNX1T1*
AML with inv(16)(p13.1q22) or t(16;16)(p13.1;q22) *CBFB-MYH 11*
APL with t(15;17)(q22;q12); *PML-RARA*
AML with t(9;11)(p22;q23); *MLLT3-MLL*
AML with t(6;9)(p23;q34); *DEK-NUP214*
AML with inv(3)(q21;q26.2) or t(3;3)(q21;q26.2); *RPN1-EVI1*
AML (megakaryoblastic) with t(1;22)(p12;q13); *RBM15-MKL1*

Acute Myeloid Leukemia with Myelodysplasia-Related Changes
Therapy-Related Myeloid Neoplasms
Acute Myeloid Leukemia, not Otherwise Specified

AML with minimal differentiation
AML without maturation
AML with maturation
Acute myelomonocytic leukemia
Acute monoblastic/monocytic keukemia
Acute erythroid leukemias
　Pure erythroid leukemia (DiGuglielmo's)
　Erythroleukemia, erythroid/myeloid
Acute megakaryoblastic leukemia
Acute basophilic leukemia
Acute panmyeloisis with myelofibrosis

Myeloid Sarcoma
Myeloid Proliferations Related to Down Syndrome

Transient abnormal myelopoiesis
Myeloid leukemia associated with Down Syndrome

Acute Leukemias of Ambiguous Lineage

Acute undifferentiated leukemia
Mixed phenotype acute leukemia with t(9;22)(q34;q11.2); *BCR-ABL1*
Mixed phenotype acute leukemia with t(v;11q23); *MLL* rearranged
Mixed phenotype acute leukemia, T/myeloid, NOS

Precursor Lymphoid Neoplasms

B lymphoblastic leukemia/lymphoma, not otherwise specified

B Lymphoblastic Leukemia/Lymphoma with Recurrent Genetic Abnormalities

B lymphoblastic leukemia/lymphoma with t(9;22)(q34;q11.2); *BCR-ABL1*
B lymphoblastic leukemia/lymphoma with t(v;11q23); *MLL* rearranged
B lymphoblastic leukemia/lymphoma with t(12;21)(p13;q22); *TEL-AML1 (ETV6-RUNX1)*
B lymphoblastic leukemia/lymphoma with hyperdiploidy
B lymphoblastic leukemia/lymphoma with hypodipoidy (hypodiploid ALL)
B lymphoblastic leukemia/lymphoma with t(5;14)(q31;q32); *IL3-IGH*
B lymphoblastic leukemia/lymphoma with t(1;19)(q23;p13.3); *E2A-PBX1 (TCF3-PBX1)*

T Lymphoblastic Leukemia/Lymphoma

In patients with AML, unusual masses in soft tissues, nodal sites, or other areas may appear, representing collections of extramedullary immature myeloid cells. These lesions may precede overt marrow and peripheral blood invasion (and thus the diagnosis of AML) and may be mistaken for lymphoma or metastatic carcinoma. When they are localized these extramedullary leukemic infiltrates have been called myeloblastomas; the older term, granulocytic sarcoma, is inappropriate. Another term, chloroma, has been used when the tumor appears green, because of the presence in the leukemic

Table 15.2

Morphologic Criteria for Lymphoblastic Leukemic Cells

Cytologic Features	L1 (Small Cell)	L2 (Large and Small Cell)	L3 (Burkitt Cell Type)
Cell size	Predominance of small cells	Large; heterogeneous in size	Medium; homogeneous
Nuclear chromatin	Homogeneous in any one case	Variable; heterogeneous in any one case	Finely stippled; homogeneous
Nuclear shape	Regular; occasional clefting or indentation	Irregular; clefting and indentation common	Regular; oval to round
Nucleoli	Not visible or small, inconspicuous	One or more present; often large	Prominent; one or more vesicular
Amount of cytoplasm	Scanty	Variable; often moderately abundant	Small to moderate
Basophilia of cytoplasm	Slight or moderate; rarely intense	Variable; deep in some cases	Very deep
Cytoplasmic vacuolation	Variable	Variable	Often prominent

Table 15.3

Immunologic Classification of Acute Lymphoblastic Leukemias (ALL)*

Subtype/Translocation	Molecular Alteration	Frequency (%)	FAB type	HLA-DR	CALLA	CD19/CD20	c	sIg	T cell	TdT
B-precursor ALL[†]			L1, L2	+	+/−	+−/+−	+	−	−	+
t(12;21)(p13;q22)	TEL-AML1	20–25								
t(1;19)(q23;p13.3)	E2A-PBX1	5–6								
t(17;19)(q22;p13.3)	E2A-HLF	<1								
t(9;22)(q34;q11)	BCR-ABL	4								
t(4;11)(q21;q23)	MLL-AF4	4								
Other 11q23	Other MLL fusions	1								
t(5;14)(q31;q32)	IL-3 dysregulation	<1								
B-cell ALL		2	L3	+	+	+/+	−	+	−	−
t(8;14)(q24;q32)	MYC dysregulation									
t(2;8)(q12;q24)										
t(8;22)(q24;q11)										
T-cell ALL		8	L1, L2	−	−/−	−/−	−	−	+	+
t(1;14)(p32;q11)	TAL1 dysregulation									
t(1;7)(p32;q35)	TAL1 dysregulation									
t(7;9)(q34;q32)	TAL2 dysregulation									
t(7;19)(q34;p13)	LYL1 dysregulation									
t(10;14)(p24;q11)	HOX11 dysregulation									
t(7;10)(p35;q24)	HOX11 dysregulation									
t(11;14)(p15;q11)	LMO1 dysregulation									
t(7;11)(q35;p13)	LMO2 dysregulation									
t(11;14)(p13;q11)	LMO2 dysregulation									
t(1;7)(p34;q34)	LCK dysregulation									
t(7;9)(q34;q34)	TAN1 dysregulation									

*In children. Data from Pui et al. (1993).

[†]Additional cytogenetic abnormalities include hyperdiploidy with >50 chromosomes (favorable prognostic factor), hyperdiploidy with 47–50 chromosomes, and hypodiploidy (unfavorable prognostic factor). The presence of t(9;22) or T(4;11) is associated with a poor prognosis as well.

C, cytoplasmic immunoglobulin; CALLA, common ALL antigen (CD10); CD19, B4 antigen; CD20, B1 antigen; HLA-DR, also 1a antigen; IL-3, interleukin-3; sIg, surface immunoglobulin (IgM); T cell, markers include CD7 and CD2; TdT, terminal deoxynucleotidyl transferase.

About 80% of children have non-T cell ALL (early pre-B and pre-B cell types) derived from early B-cell progeny. In adults, 20% of leukemias are pre-B cell ALL, expressing HLA-DR (Ia), CD19 (B4), CD10 (CALLA), and CD20 (B1) antigens; expression of sIg marks B-cell acute leukemia (FAB type L3), which is also called Burkitt type. T-cell acute leukemias are heterogeneous, but most express early-stage-I thymocyte markers. TdT is also positive in T-cell ALL, as well as in some non-B cell types. Cytogenetic abnormalities include the Ph chromosome in some cases of undifferentiated or common ALL and t(8;14) and t(8;22) in B-cell ALL. Compared with other types, B- and T-cell ALLs are high-risk leukemias, although modern intensive therapy has improved the prognosis.

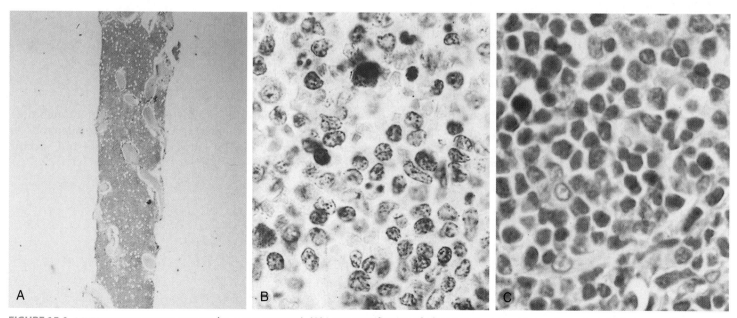

FIGURE 15.1 **ACUTE LYMPHOBLASTIC LEUKEMIA (L1, T-CELL SUBTYPE).** **(A)** Low magnification of a bone marrow core biopsy shows a markedly hypercellular marrow (Giemsa stain). **(B)** At high magnification convoluted lymphoblasts can be seen; the small to intermediate-size cells show a characteristic irregular or cerebriform nuclear outline, finely dispersed chromatin, and scant cytoplasm. The nucleolus is typically indistinct (Giemsa stain). **(C)** Lymphoblasts stain positively with H&E. Immunophenotyping showed positivity for CD5 (T1), CD4 (T4), CD8 (T8), and CD2 (T11).

Table 15.4

Classification of Acute Myeloid Leukemias*

Subtype	FAB type	Frequency (%)[†]	Morphology	MP	SE	NSE	Immune Markers	Cytogenetic Abnormalities[‡]	Genes Involved
Acute myeloblastic leukemia with minimal differentiation	M0	3	Rare granules; no Auer rods	–	–	–	CD11, CD13, CD33 HLA-DR	inv (3q26), t(3;3)	EVII
Acute myeloblastic leukemia without maturation	M1	15–20	A few azurophilic granules or Auer rods	+[§]	+/–	–	CD11, CD13, CD33 HLA-DR	t(9;22) +8 t(v;11) –7e–5 or 5q	
Acute myeloid leukemia with maturation	M2	25–30	Some maturation beyond promyelocytes; Auer rods	++	++	–	CD11, CD13, CD33 HLA-DR	t(8;21)[¶] t(9;22), t(6;9) +8 –7e–5 or –5q	AMLI-ETO DEK-CAN
Acute promyelocytic leukemia	M3	5–10	Hypergranular promyelocytes; multiple Auer rods	+++	+++	–	CD11, CD13, CD33	t(915;17) t(11;17) t(5;17)	PML-RAR PLZF-RAR NPM-RAR
Acute myelomonocytic leukemia	M4	20	≥20% monocytes; monocytoid cells in blood; Auer rods	++	++	++	CD11, CD13, CD14, CD33 HLA-DR	11q23 inv (3q26), t(3;3) EVI t(6;9) +8–7–5[††] or 5q	MLL DEK-CAN
	M4**	5–10	Eosinophilia; early eosinophils with large purple granules	++	++	++	CD2, CD13, CD14, CD33 HLA-DR	inv(16)[¶], del(16) (q22) t(16;16)d	CBF-MYHII
	M5						CD11, CD13, CD14, CD33 HLA-DR		
Acute monocytic leukemia		2–9	Monoblastic (M5A) Promonocytic (M5B), no Auer rods	–	–	+++		11q23 t(8;16)	
Erythroleukemia	M6	3–5	Predominance of erythroblasts; dyserythropoiesis; Auer rods in myeloblasts	+	–	–		+8 +8 –7[††]	MLL MOZ-CBP
Acute megakaryoleukemia	M7	3–12	"Dry" aspirate; biopsy specimen with blasts and dysplastic megakaryocytes; no Auer rods	–	–	–	CD33, glycophorin A CD33, CD41, CD61 HLA-DR	–5 or 5q t(1;22) –7[††] –5 or 5q	

*Findings may be somewhat variable.
[‡]Complex chromosome defects may be seen in M0, M1, M2, M4–M7.
[¶]Associated with a more favorable prognosis.
**Eosinophilic variant of M4.
[††]Associated with a less favorable prognosis.
[§]More than 3% blasts positive.
MP, myeloperoxidase; NSE, nonspecific esterase (naphthylbutyrate); SE, specific esterase (chloracetate); –, negative; +/–, equivocal; +, positive, ++, moderately positive; +++, very positive.

cells of enzymes capable of metabolizing heme products; the green color rapidly disappears after oxidation on exposure to air. Myeloblastomas can occur anywhere, but the most common sites are soft tissues, skin, periosteum, bone, and lymph nodes. Diagnosis can be rapidly established on a touch prep stained with Wright-Giemsa and examined for Auer rods or azurophilic granules. The latter are peroxidase- and specific esterase–positive.

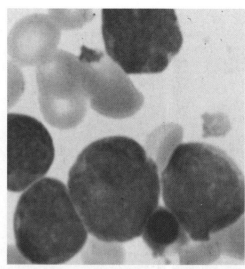

FIGURE 15.2 **ACUTE LYMPHOBLASTIC LEUKEMIA (L1, T-CELL SUBTYPE).** High-power view of a bone marrow aspirate reveals small lymphoblasts with scanty cytoplasm and indistinct nucleoli. The nuclear contours in many of the cells are convoluted or cerebriform.

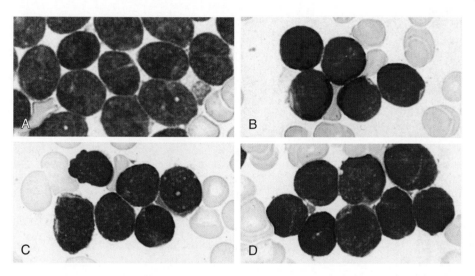

FIGURE 15.3 **ACUTE LYMPHOBLASTIC LEUKEMIA (L1, CALLA [CD10]-POSITIVE PRE-B SUBTYPE). (A–D)** Lymphoblasts are rather small and uniform, with scanty cytoplasm and rounded or cleft nuclei, which may have one indistinct nucleolus.

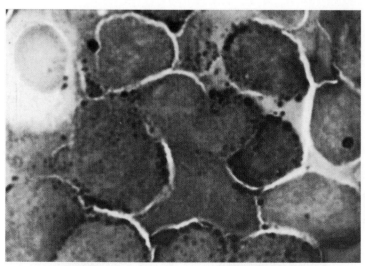

FIGURE 15.4 **ACUTE LYMPHOBLASTIC LEUKEMIA (L1, CALLA [CD10]-POSITIVE PRE-B CELL SUBTYPE).** This bone marrow aspirate shows cells with numerous coarse cytoplasmic granules or blocks staining positive with periodic acid–Schiff (PAS). Seen in about 80% of cases, these findings are diagnostic of ALL. By contrast, myeloblasts may have small, fine-staining granules.

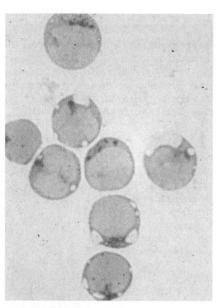

FIGURE 15.5 **ACUTE LYMPHOBLASTIC LEUKEMIA (L1, T-CELL SUBTYPE).** Red staining of the cytoplasm in this bone marrow aspirate, with marked coloration of the Golgi zone adjacent to or indented into the nucleus, supports a diagnosis of T-cell ALL. However, this occurs in only 50% to 75% of cases (acid phosphatase stain).

FIGURE 15.6 **ACUTE LYMPHOBLASTIC LEUKEMIA (L1, T-CELL SUBTYPE).** Indirect immunofluorescence microscopy of bone marrow aspirates demonstrates **(A)** red-staining cell membrane T antigen and **(B)** green-staining nuclear terminal deoxynucleotidyl transferase (TdT). (Courtesy of Prof. G. Janossy.)

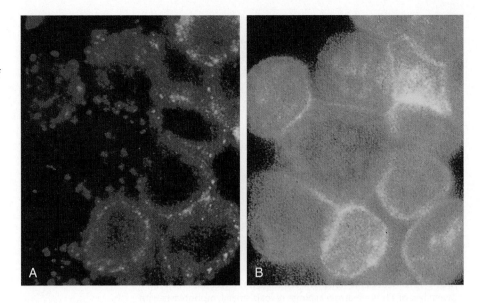

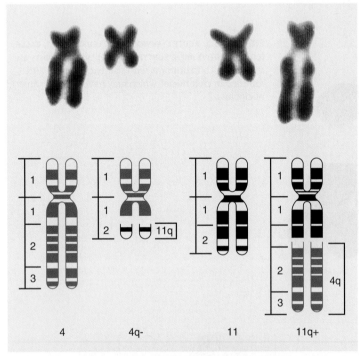

FIGURE 15.7 **ACUTE LYMPHOBLASTIC LEUKEMIA (L1 SUBTYPE).** This partial karyotype of G-banded chromosomes 4 and 11 (above) was obtained from a patient with blasts of "null" phenotype (TdT-positive, CALLA (CD10)-negative). The translocated chromosomes are on the right in each pair. The corresponding diagrams (below) represent a systematized description of the structural aberration. (Courtesy of Dr L.M. Secker-Walker.)

FIGURE 15.8 **ACUTE LYMPHOBLASTIC LEUKEMIA (L2 SUBTYPE). (A–C)** Blast cells in these peripheral blood smears vary considerably in size and amount of cytoplasm; the nucleus-to-cytoplasm ratio is rarely as high as in the L1 subtype. The nuclei are of various shapes and often contain multiple nucleoli.

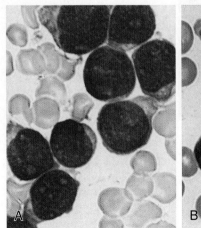
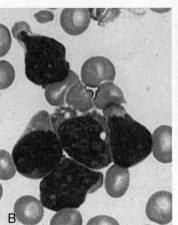
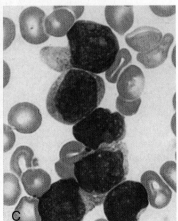

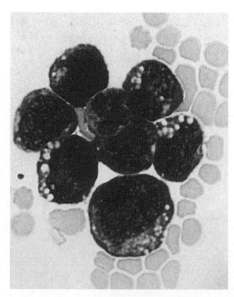

FIGURE 15.9 **ACUTE LYMPHOBLASTIC LEUKEMIA (L3 SUBTYPE).** The deeply staining blue cytoplasm of these blast cells contains many small, perinuclear vacuoles; prominent nucleoli are commonly seen. This appearance is associated with B-cell ALL. Identical cells are seen in Burkitt small noncleaved cell leukemia/lymphoma.

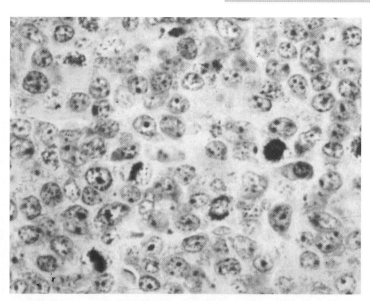

FIGURE 15.11 **ACUTE LYMPHOBLASTIC LEUKEMIA (L3 SUBTYPE).** Bone marrow core biopsy of a markedly hypercellular marrow containing small to intermediate-size cells with one or more distinct nucleoli. Multiple mitotic figures are seen (Giemsa stain).

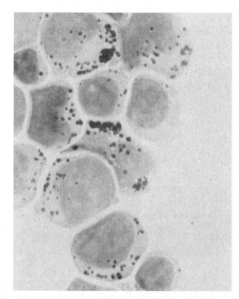

FIGURE 15.10 **ACUTE LYMPHOBLASTIC LEUKEMIA (L3 SUBTYPE).** Bone marrow aspirate stained with oil red-O shows prominent cytoplasmic lipid collections corresponding to some of the vacuoles shown by Romanowsky staining (see Fig. 15.9).

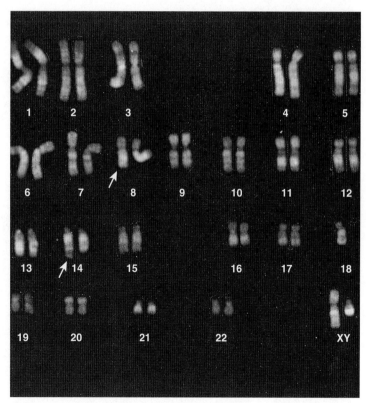

FIGURE 15.12 **ACUTE LYMPHOBLASTIC LEUKEMIA (L3, BURKITT LEUKEMIA/LYMPHOMA).** This Q-banded karyotype shows 46; X,Y, t(8;14) (q24;q23). (Courtesy of Ramana Tantravahi, PhD, Dana-Farber Cancer Institute, Boston, MA.)

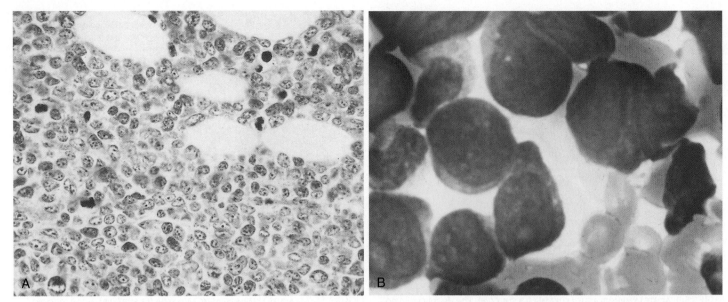

FIGURE 15.13 **ACUTE MYELOBLASTIC LEUKEMIA (M0 SUBTYPE). (A)** Hypercellular bone marrow biopsy composed of myeloblasts with minimal differentiation. The blasts were negative for Auer rods and histochemical markers of AML, but were positive for myeloid differentiation markers (CD13, CD33) by flow-cytometric examination (Giemsa stain). **(B)** Bone marrow aspiration smear from same case showing blasts with prominent nucleoli and basophilic cytoplasm without any granules (×1000; Wright-Giemsa stain).

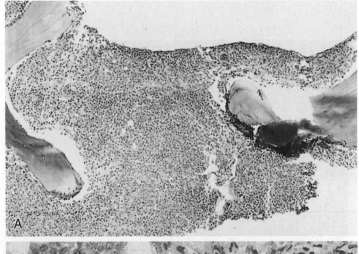

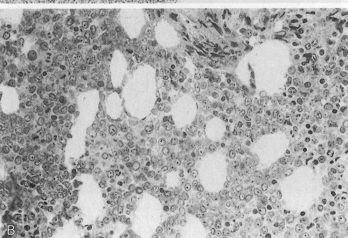

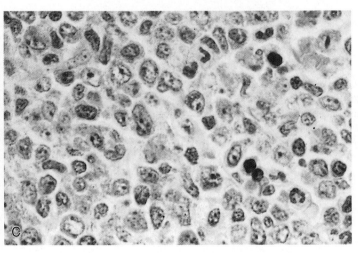

FIGURE 15.14 **ACUTE MYELOBLASTIC LEUKEMIA (M1 SUBTYPE). (A)** Acute leukemia is marked by replacement of the normal bone marrow by blasts. In this instance the cellularity is 99%, whereas normal cellularity is about 50%, with fat representing the remaining 50%. Rare cases of "hypocellular" AML have been described in which the background fat is normal or increased. **(B, C)** At higher magnification, characteristic myeloblasts can be seen showing predominantly round nuclear outlines, distinct nucleoli (often centrally located), and a moderate amount of cytoplasm. Distinct red-pink cytoplasmic granules are occasionally noted (Giemsa stain).

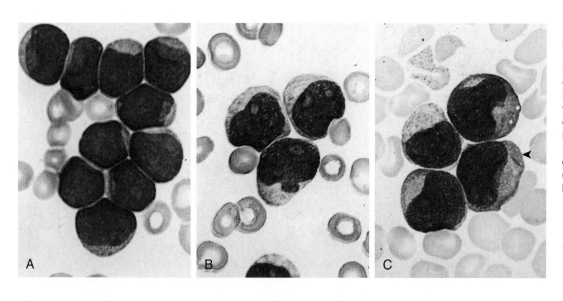

FIGURE 15.15 **ACUTE MYELOBLASTIC LEUKEMIA (M1 SUBTYPE).** These bone marrow aspirates show blasts with large, often irregular nuclei having one or more nucleoli. **(A, B)** Typical type 1 blasts contain loose, open chromatin with distinct nucleoli and immature cytoplasm without granules. **(C)** Type II blasts are similar but contain up to 15 delicate cytoplasmic azurophilic granules and an occasional Auer rod (*arrowhead*). At least 3% of cells stain by Sudan black or myeloperoxidase.

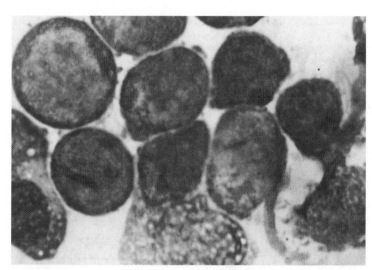

FIGURE 15.16 **ACUTE MYELOBLASTIC LEUKEMIA (M1 SUBTYPE).** Peroxidase staining (Kaplan method) of a bone marrow aspirate shows many Auer rods and early azurophilic granules (golden color) in myeloblasts.

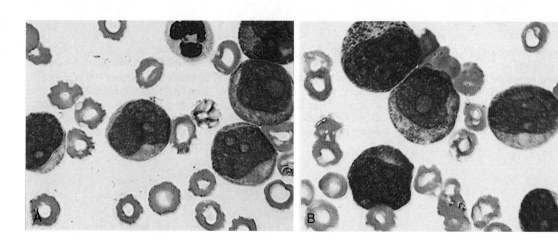

FIGURE 15.17 **ACUTE MYELOBLASTIC LEUKEMIA WITH MATURATION (M2 SUBTYPE). (A, B)** Type III blasts, which predominate in this subtype, have relatively numerous azurophilic granules but still lack a Golgi area. Auer rods may be present. A characteristic t(8;21) chromosomal abnormality is usually present (see Fig. 15.18).

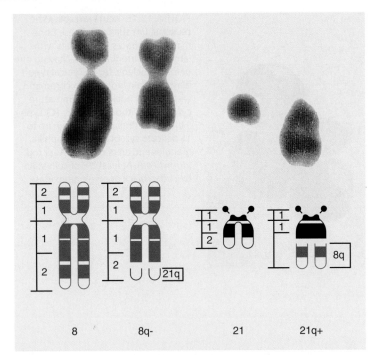

FIGURE 15.18 **ACUTE MYELOBLASTIC LEUKEMIA WITH MATURATION (M2 SUBTYPE).** A partial karyotype of G-banded chromosomes 8 and 21 is shown *above*. The translocated chromosomes are on the *right* in each pair. The corresponding diagrams *below* represent a systematized description of the structural aberration. (Courtesy of Dr L.M. Secker-Walker.)

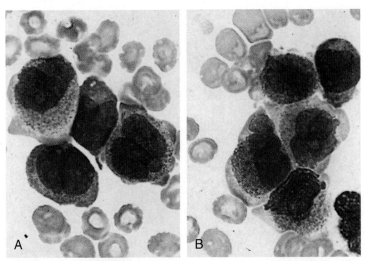

FIGURE 15.20 **ACUTE PROMYELOCYTIC LEUKEMIA (M3 SUBTYPE, MICROGRANULAR VARIANT).** The usually bilobar cells contain many small, azurophilic granules. In some cases the cells resemble monocytes ("pseudomonocytic leukemia"), but peroxidase and specific esterase stains are strongly positive, confirming a diagnosis of M3 AML. Nonspecific esterase is negative.

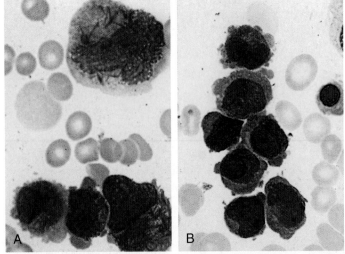

FIGURE 15.19 **ACUTE PROMYELOCYTIC LEUKEMIA (M3 SUBTYPE). (A, B)** Promyelocytes contain coarse, azurophilic granules and Auer rods, which stain similarly to the granules. The nuclei have one or two nucleoli. A prominent Golgi area is noted in most cells. This subtype is associated with chromosomal rearrangement t(15;17) (see Fig. 15.22). A serious complication of M3 AML is bleeding due in part to release of tissue factors from the blasts, leading to disseminated intravascular coagulation.

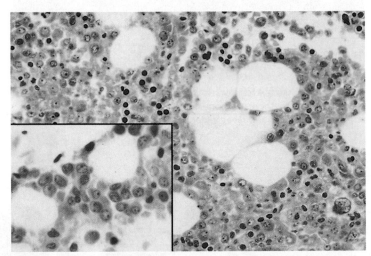

FIGURE 15.21 **ACUTE PROMYELOCYTIC LEUKEMIA (M3 SUBTYPE).** High-power photomicrograph of a bone marrow core biopsy shows abundant promyelocytes intermixed with occasional erythroid elements and megakaryocytes. (*Inset*) Characteristically, promyelocytes show abundant pink cytoplasm and an eccentric nucleus. Diagnostic Auer rods may occasionally be seen.

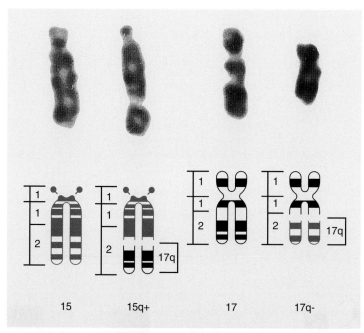

FIGURE 15.22 **ACUTE PROMYELOCYTIC LEUKEMIA (M3 SUBTYPE).** A partial karyotype of G-banded chromosomes 15 and 17 is shown (*above*). The translocated chromosomes are on the *right* in each pair. The corresponding diagrams (*below*) represent a systematized description of the structural aberration that fuses the *PML* gene on chromosome 15 with the retinoic acid receptor-α on chromosome 17, resulting in a fusion protein involved in leukemogenesis. (Courtesy of Dr. L.M. Secker-Walker.)

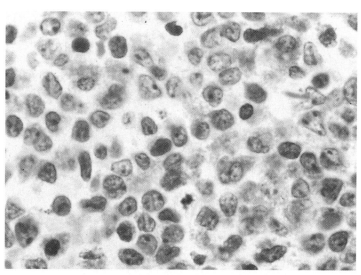

FIGURE 15.24 **ACUTE MYELOMONOCYTIC LEUKEMIA (M4 SUBTYPE).** High magnification of a bone marrow core biopsy shows many blasts with irregular, folded nuclear outlines and some with pink-red cytoplasmic granules. Histochemical staining is necessary for definitive diagnosis.

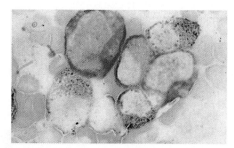

FIGURE 15.25 **ACUTE MYELOMONOCYTIC LEUKEMIA (M4 SUBTYPE).** Histochemical staining of a bone marrow aspirate shows a deep red-orange staining of monoblast cytoplasm by nonspecific esterase and blue staining of myeloblast cytoplasm by chloracetate (specific esterase).

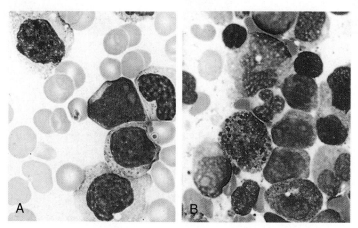

FIGURE 15.23 **ACUTE MYELOMONOCYTIC LEUKEMIA (M4 SUBTYPE). (A)** Blast cells contain cytoplasmic granules (myeloblasts and promyelocytes) or pale cytoplasm with occasional vacuoles and granules, as well as folded or rounded nuclei (monoblasts). **(B)** Eosinophils with basophilic granules are present. Specific cytogenetic abnormalities (inv(16) or t(16;16)) are associated with the presence of abnormal or dysplastic eosinophils in M4 AML. Eosinophils may be greatly increased. (**A**, Courtesy of Dr. M. Bilter; **B**, courtesy of Prof. J. Rowley.)

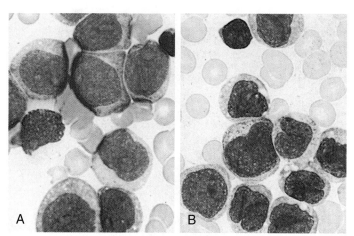

FIGURE 15.26 **ACUTE MONOCYTIC LEUKEMIA (M5A AND M5B SUBTYPES). (A)** Blast cells of the M5A (monoblastic) variant have pale-blue cytoplasm or perinuclear "haloes," prominent nucleoli, and cytoplasmic vacuoles, but only occasional granules. **(B)** The usually centrally placed nuclei are folded, rounded, or kidney-shaped in the M5B (promonocytic) type, which is marked by more differentiated promonocytes that often contain fine granules.

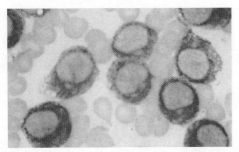

FIGURE 15.27 **ACUTE MONOCYTIC LEUKEMIA (M5A SUBTYPE).** Histochemical staining of a bone marrow aspirate shows deep red-orange monoblast cytoplasm by nonspecific esterase.

FIGURE 15.28 **ERYTHROLEUKEMIA (M6 SUBTYPE). (A–C)** Erythroblasts predominate in these high-power views of a bone marrow aspirate, and many dyserythropoietic features are evident, such as multinucleate cells, vacuolated cytoplasm, abnormal mitoses, and megaloblastic nuclei. Myeloblasts are often present and may predominate in end-stage disease. Di Guglielmo's syndrome refers to different phases of this disease: erythroleukemia, erythremic myelosis, and acute myeloblastic leukemia.

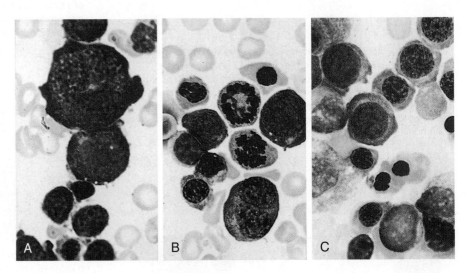

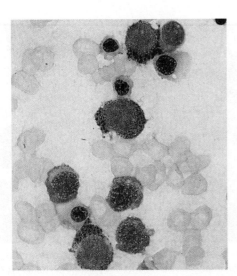

FIGURE 15.29 **ERYTHROLEUKEMIA (M6 SUBTYPE).** The cytoplasm of some erythroblasts in this bone marrow aspirate shows block-positive red staining by PAS.

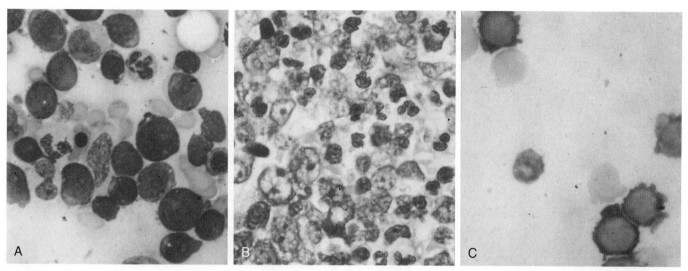

FIGURE 15.30 **ACUTE MEGAKARYOCYTIC LEUKEMIA (M7 SUBTYPE). (A)** The blasts are large to medium-sized, and many cells have distinct nucleoli. The cytoplasm shows pseudopod-like margins, an appearance associated with but not confined to this subtype. **(B)** Appearance of bone marrow biopsy from a patient with acute megakaryocytic leukemia with numerous blast forms present in the marrow (Giemsa stain). **(C)** The blasts are PAS-positive but peroxidase-stain negative. Immunohistochemical stain for glycoprotein IIIa (CD61) is diagnostically positive in this case.

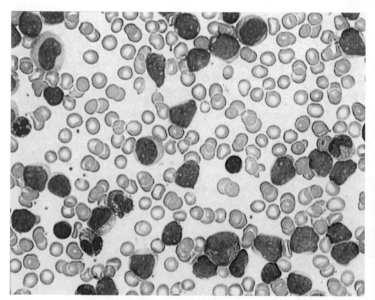

FIGURE 15.31 **ACUTE LEUKEMIA (MIXED-CELL TYPE).** Bone marrow aspirate shows blasts of various sizes and morphologies. Some possess scanty cytoplasm without granules (lymphoblastic), whereas others, usually large blasts, show eccentric nuclei, substantial cytoplasm, and granules (myeloblastic). Histochemical stains and cell surface markers will clarify the diagnosis (see Table 15.3, Fig. 15.2). Very rarely the blasts may express both lymphoid and myeloid markers, e.g., CALLA (CD10), CD19 (B4), MY7 (CD13), and MY9 (CD33).

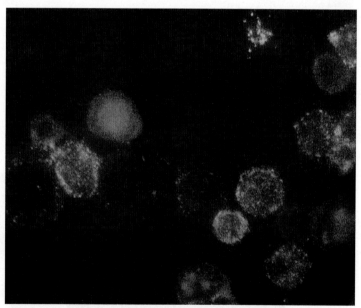

FIGURE 15.32 **ACUTE LEUKEMIA (MIXED-CELL TYPE).** Indirect immunofluorescence microscopy of a bone marrow aspirate shows one population of cells (lymphoblasts) to have nuclear TdT (green), whereas another population (myeloblasts) has myeloid surface antigen (yellow-orange). Mixed-lineage leukemias (biphenotypic) are unusual, but recent studies using monoclonal antibodies directed toward myeloid-associated cell surface antigens have demonstrated two populations of blasts in up to 20% of cases. This has been confirmed by immunoglobulin and T-cell receptor gene rearrangement studies. The choice of therapy may be affected by the finding of biphenotypic acute leukemia. (Courtesy of Prof. G. Janossy.)

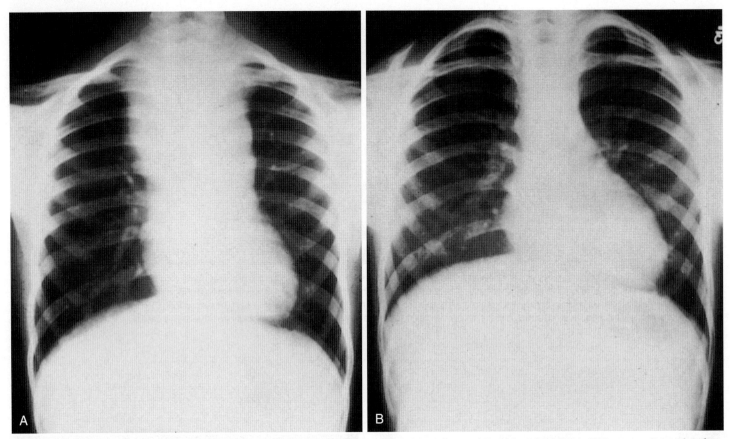

FIGURE 15.33 **MEDIASTINAL INVOLVEMENT. (A)** A mediastinal mass is clearly seen on this chest radiograph in a case of T-cell ALL. **(B)** Repeat radiography after 2 weeks of therapy with vincristine and prednisolone shows a rapid response, with shrinkage of the mass. Further intensive therapy is required, including CNS prophylaxis.

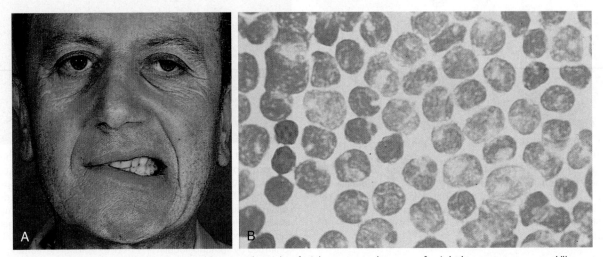

FIGURE 15.34 **MENINGEAL INFILTRATION. (A)** This 59-year-old man with ALL has facial asymmetry because of a right lower motor neuron VII nerve palsy resulting from leukemic infiltration of the CNS. **(B)** Stained centrifuge sample of cerebrospinal fluid shows L1-type lymphoid blast cells in a case of meningeal leukemia. CNS leukemia is uncommon in AML. **(A,** Courtesy of Dr. H.G. Prentice.)

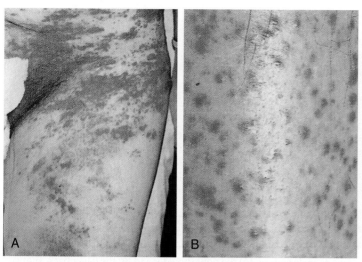

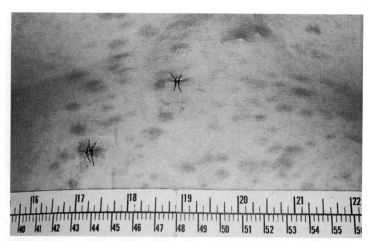

FIGURE 15.35 **CUTANEOUS MANIFESTATIONS. (A)** Marked ecchymoses, petechial hemorrhages, and bruises involve the groin and thigh in this patient with AML. **(B)** Petechial hemorrhages, seen here covering the leg, represent the most common cutaneous presentation of acute leukemia; they are due to severe thrombocytopenia.

FIGURE 15.37 **CUTANEOUS MANIFESTATIONS.** A 35-year-old woman with previous AML developed extensive skin lesions on the anterior chest as the first evidence of relapse. Biopsy showed infiltration of the dermis by monoblasts. Leukemic skin infiltrates can occur in any type of AML but are especially common in the M4 and M5 subtypes. They may be flat or raised, solitary or multiple.

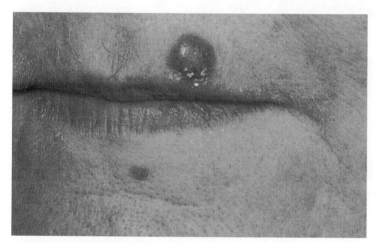

FIGURE 15.36 **LEUKEMIA CUTIS.** Firm, red-purple papules or nodules occasionally occur in AML, especially on the face. Skin involvement is rare in ALL.

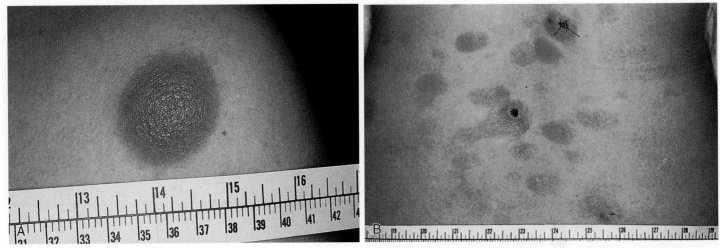

FIGURE 15.38 **CUTANEOUS MANIFESTATIONS.** A 23-year-old woman with AML developed skin lesions on **(A)** the right shoulder and **(B)** the lower back. The lesions regressed after 2 weeks' chemotherapy.

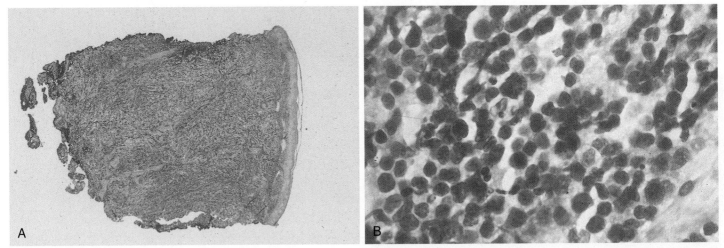

FIGURE 15.39 **(A)** Histologic section (low power) from a patient with leukemia cutis, showing diffuse infiltration of the dermis and subcutaneous tissue. **(B)** High-power view shows immature myeloid cells, including numerous blast forms (H&E). (Courtesy of Dr. S. Granter.)

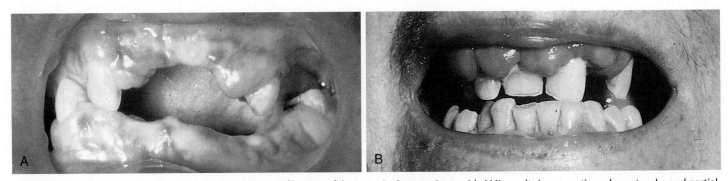

FIGURE 15.40 **INTRAORAL MANIFESTATIONS. (A, B)** Leukemic infiltration of the gums in these patients with AML results in severe tissue hypertrophy and partial covering of the teeth.

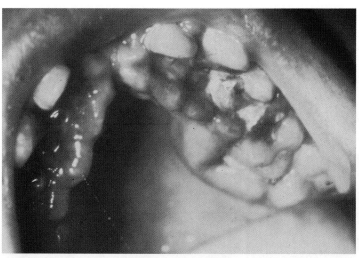

FIGURE 15.41 **INTRAORAL MANIFESTATIONS.** Gingival hypertrophy most often occurs when there is a monoblastic element in AML. It is not seen in edentulous patients. This patient had AML.

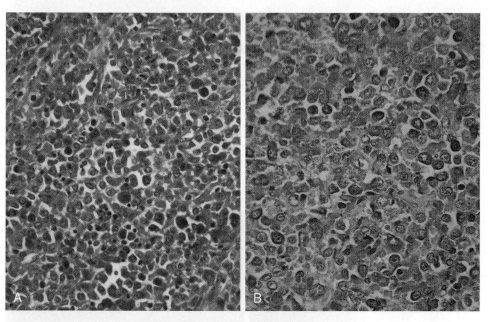

FIGURE 15.42 **MYELOBLASTOMA (GRANULOCYTIC SARCOMA).** A destructive maxillary tumor was the presenting symptom in an apparently healthy 20-year-old man. **(A)** The cellular picture is pleomorphic, but the eosinophilia of the myeloblasts is conspicuous even at low magnification. **(B)** Positive eosinophilic staining of myeloid cells is confirmed by the naphthol AS-D-chloracetate esterase reaction. Other confirmatory studies include a positive lysozyme stain and a positive myeloperoxidase stain of a touch prep.

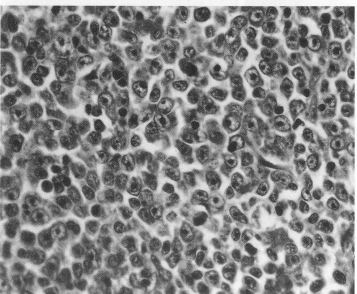

FIGURE 15.43 **MYELOBLASTOMA PRESENTING IN A LYMPH NODE.** In this 30-year-old man who presented with cervical lymphadenopathy, nodal architecture was effaced by homogeneous myeloblasts with large, round nuclei with prominent central nucleoli. The differential diagnosis includes non-Hodgkin lymphoma, large cell, immunoblastic type. The infiltrate was reactive for myeloperoxidase and chloracetate esterase, confirming a diagnosis of extramedullary acute myeloblastic leukemia.

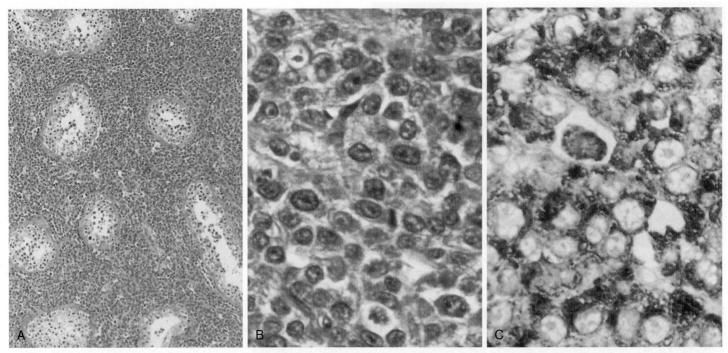

FIGURE 15.44 **MYELOBLASTOMA (GRANULOCYTIC SARCOMA).** A 37-year-old man underwent orchidectomy for a testicular mass believed to represent primary testicular carcinoma. **(A)** Histologic examination, however, reveals AML, as evidenced by the dense leukemic infiltrate enveloping the intact seminiferous tubules. **(B)** High magnification shows that the tumor is composed of cells with predominantly round nuclear outlines and distinct nucleoli. **(C)** Immunoperoxidase staining for lysozyme is strongly reactive.

FIGURE 15.45 **ACUTE FEBRILE NEUTROPHILIC DERMATOSIS (SWEET'S SYNDROME). (A, B)** These patients with AML developed fever and multiple cutaneous, tender, red plaquelike lesions on the face, arms, and hands. Skin biopsy showed a dense nodular and patchy dermal infiltrate composed primarily of mature neutrophils. There was marked edema of the papillary dermis, but the epidermis was essentially normal. There was eventual total resolution of the lesions following corticosteroid treatment. Sweet's syndrome occurs in association with AML and may predate the diagnosis of acute leukemia. It is also associated with chronic myeloproliferative disorders and miscellaneous malignancies, or it may be idiopathic. The differential diagnosis includes pyoderma. The lesions may involve the mucous membranes or cause pulmonary infiltrates; systemic symptoms may also occur. The etiology remains obscure.

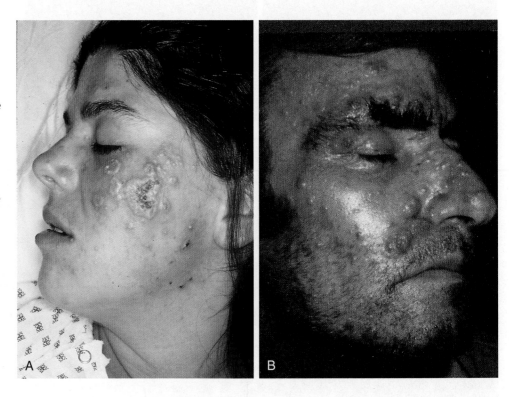

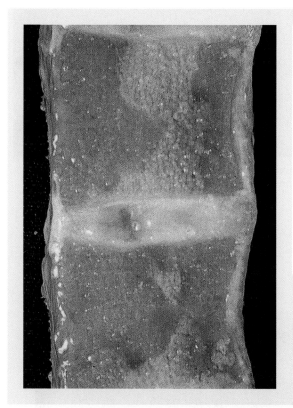

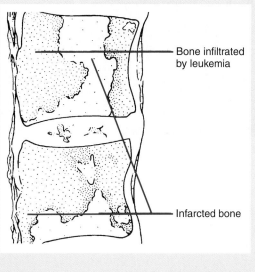

FIGURE 15.46 **VERTEBRAL INFILTRATION.** This sagittal section through the spine is from a child who died of acute leukemia. Areas of necrosis within the vertebral bodies are marked by yellow opacification of the bone and marrow, which are surrounded by a thin rim of hyperemic tissue. Viable bone marrow has a fleshy tan color, reflecting leukemic infiltration.

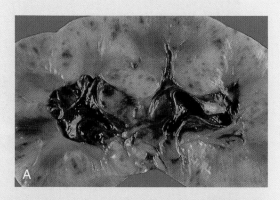

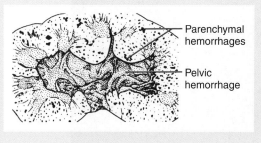

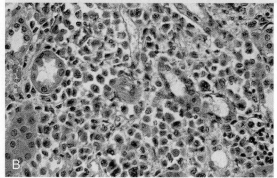

FIGURE 15.47 **KIDNEY INVOLVEMENT. (A)** Leukemic infiltrates in this case of AML are diffusely present throughout the cortex of the kidney. Parenchymal and pelvic mucosal hemorrhages are secondary to severe thrombocytopenia. **(B)** Microscopically, many myeloblasts are seen in the interstitial infiltrates.

FIGURE 15.48 **OPHTHALMIC INVOLVEMENT. (A)** This patient with AML presented with a large infiltrate of leukemic cells positioned nasally within the conjunctiva of the right eye; this clinical picture is characteristic. Lesions such as this appear quite similar to those caused by benign lymphoid hyperplasia or amyloidosis. **(B)** Biopsy of the lesion reveals myeloblasts.

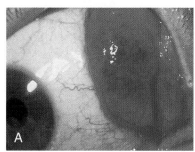

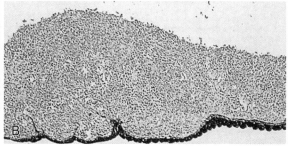

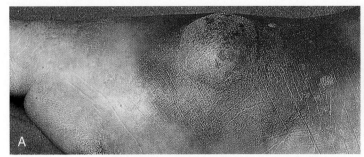

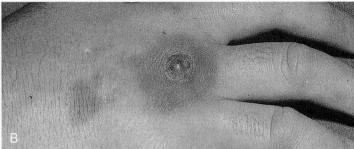

FIGURE 15.49 **COMPLICATIONS OF ACUTE LEUKEMIA.** **(A)** A purplish black bullous lesion with surrounding erythema in this patient with AML is caused by *Pseudomonas pyocyanea* infection of the foot. **(B)** A similar but less marked infection is present on the back of the hand.

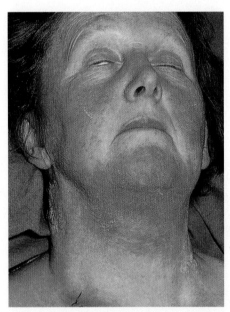

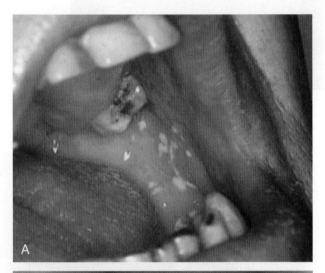

FIGURE 15.50 **COMPLICATIONS OF ACUTE LEUKEMIA.** Spreading cellulitis of the neck and chin in this woman with AML results from mixed streptococcal and candidal infection, previous chemotherapy, and prolonged periods of neutropenia.

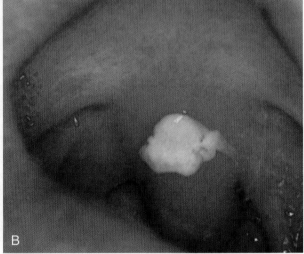

FIGURE 15.51 **COMPLICATIONS OF ACUTE LEUKEMIA.** Plaques of *Candida albicans* are present on **(A)** the buccal mucosa and **(B)** the soft palate in a patient with AML.

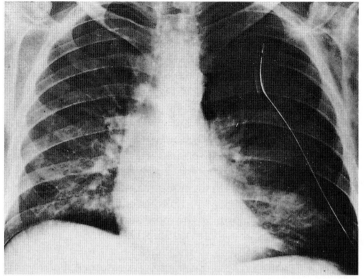

FIGURE 15.52 **COMPLICATIONS OF ACUTE LEUKEMIA.** Chest radiograph of a patient with ALL shows consolidation spreading bilaterally from the hilar regions ("bat-wing" shadowing) due to infection with *Pneumocystis carinii*.

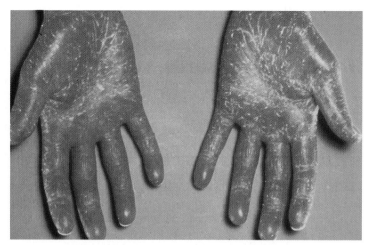

FIGURE 15.53 **COMPLICATIONS OF THERAPY OF ACUTE LEUKEMIA.** Graft-versus-host disease is a major cause of morbidity and mortality following allogenic bone marrow transplantation. It manifests as abnormalities of the skin, liver, and gut. Skin involvement ranges from mild erythema to papulosquamous eruptions and desquamation, and is often most marked on the palms and soles.

Diseases	Blood Findings	Bone Marrow Findings
Refractory cytopenias with unilineage dysplasia (RCUID) Refractory anemia (RA); Refractory neutropenia (RN); Refractory thrombocytopenia (RT)	Unicytopenia or bicytopina* No rare or rare blasts (<1%)†	Unilineage dysplasia ≥10% of the cells in one myeloid lineage <5% blasts <15% of erythroid precursors are ring sideroblasts
Refractory anemia with ring sideroblasts (RARS)	Anemia No blasts	≥15% of erythroid precursors are ring sideroblasts Erythroid dysplasia only <5% blasts
Refractory cytopenia with multilineage dysplasia (RCMD)	Cytopenia(s) No rare or rare blasts (<1%)† No Auer rods <11×10⁹/L monocytes	Dysplasia in ≥10% of the cells in ≥ two myeloid lineages (neutrophil and/or erythroid precursors and/or megakaryocytes) <5% blasts in marrow No Auer rods ±15% ring sideroblasts
Refractory anemia with excess blasts-1 (RAEB-1)	Cytopenia(s) <5% blasts† No Auer rods <1×10⁹/L monocytes	Unilineage or multilineage dysplasia 5%–9% blasts† No Auer rods
Refractory anemia with excels blasts-2 (RAEB-2)	Cytopenia(s) 5–19% blasts Auer rods±‡ <1×10⁹/L monocytes	Unilineage or multilineage dysplasia 10%–19% blasts Auer rods ±‡
Myelodysplastic syndrome – unclassified (MDS-U)	Cytopenias ≤1% blasts†	Unequivocal dysplasia in less than 10% of cells in one or more myeloid cell lines when accompanied by a cytogenetic abnormality considered as presumptive evidence for diagnosis of <5% blasts
MDS associated with isolated del(5q)	Anemia Usually normal or increased platelet count No or rare blasts (<1%)	Normal to increased megakaryocytes with hypolobated nuclei <5% blasts Isolated del(5q) cytogenetic abnormality No Auer rods

*Bicytopenia may occasionally be observed. Cases with pancytopenia should be classified as MDS-U.

†If the marrow myeloblast percentage is <5% but there are 2%–4% myeloblasts in the blood, the diagnostic classification is RAEB-1. Cases of RCUD and RCMD with 1% myeloblasts in the blood should be classified as MDS, U.

‡Cases with Auer rods and <5% myeloblasts in the blood and <10% in the marrow should be classified as RAEB-2.

FIGURE 15.54 WHO classification of the myelodysplastic syndromes with peripheral blood and bone marrow findings.

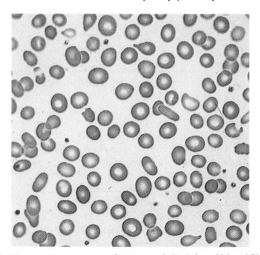

FIGURE 15.55 **REFRACTORY ANEMIA (MDS TYPE I).** Peripheral blood film shows marked anisocytosis and poikilocytosis.

Hematologic Disorders with a Tendency to Leukemic Transformation

MYELODYSPLASTIC SYNDROMES

The myelodysplastic syndromes (MDSs) are a group of disorders that primarily occur in the elderly, who present with an anemia that proves refractory to treatment, with progressive neutropenia and thrombocytopenia, or with various combinations of these. In the past these syndromes, particularly those with normal numbers of blasts (<5%) in the marrow, have been referred to as "preleukemia." To varying degrees there is a tendency to progression to acute leukemia, ranging from progression in approximately 10% of cases of refractory anemia and refractory anemia with ringed sideroblasts to progression in more than 40% of cases of refractory anemia with excess blasts.

Classification and Cytogenetics

Given the variable presentation and prognosis of these disorders, various classification schemes have been devised to better divide and define these disorders. According to the French-American-British (FAB) classification scheme, the MDSs have been classified into five subgroups, which have been modified by the WHO into seven subgroups (see Fig. 15.54). The blood film abnormalities in each subgroup are highly variable, although general features include macrocytic red cells, qualitative granulocytic and monocytic changes, and giant platelets. Whereas patients with refractory anemia may show no gross changes in blood morphology, patients with refractory anemia with ringed sideroblasts frequently show a dimorphic red cell population. Leukoerythroblastic changes are common in patients with refractory anemia with excess blasts. "Chronic myelomonocytic leukemia," a diagnostic entity included with the MDSs by the FAB classification scheme, is marked by abnormal myelomonocytic cells and monocytosis of more than 1.0×10^9 cells/L, with or without splenomegaly, and is considered separately by the WHO classification. A former category, RAEB-T, is no longer an entity under the WHO classification and is considered a progression to AML.

The bone marrow in the MDSs is typically hypercellular and shows morphologic abnormalities, often in all three series of hematopoietic cells. Cytogenetic abnormalities are common, particularly in secondary MDS (related to prior radiation therapy or therapy with alkylating agents) (Table 15.5). They include –5 or –5q, –7 or –7q, –20 or –20q, +8 and –9q. Patients with complex cytogenetic abnormalities (the most common chromosomal abnormality observed) or –7 or –7q typically have an aggressive clinical course. There is usually evidence of dyserythropoiesis with nuclear atypia, some megaloblastosis, and ringed sideroblasts. In some cases reticulin is increased, whereas occasional cases are hypocellular. Granulocytic abnormalities include hypogranular or agranular myelocytes, metamyelocytes and neutrophils, pseudo-Pelger-Huët cells, and hypersegmented or polypoid neutrophils. Megakaryocyte abnormalities include small mononuclear or binuclear forms or large megakaryocytes with multiple, round nuclei and large granules in the cytoplasm. In the more advanced MDSs the blast cell population is also increased, but by definition these cells constitute less than 20% of the marrow cell total. When the level of blast cells exceeds this figure, it is assumed that a transformation to AML has occurred.

Clinical Manifestations and Prognosis

Clinically, patients present with symptoms related to bone marrow failure, with frequent episodes of infection and with bleeding abnormalities. These complications of severe neutropenia or thrombocytopenia result in death in many patients, but in others the disease progresses to frank AML. Typically, the liver, spleen, and lymph nodes are not enlarged. Gum hypertrophy and skin deposits do not usually occur. The prognosis is variable, and prognostic schemes have been devised. The most widely accepted and adopted has identified cytogenetics, the number of cell lines affected, and the number of blasts in the bone marrow to be important predictors of prognosis (see Table 15.6).

POLYCYTHEMIA VERA AND MYELOFIBROSIS

Transformation is generally accepted as part of the natural history of the myeloproliferative syndrome. Polycythemia vera undergoes transformation to myelofibrosis in approximately 10% of cases and to acute leukemia, usually AML, in about half that number. There is a similar incidence of leukemia in patients treated with ^{32}P or chemotherapy. Myelofibrosis undergoes leukemic transformation in 20% of patients. Survival after the transition to leukemia in either condition is brief.

Table 15.6	
International Prognostic Scoring System for Myelodysplastic Syndrome	
Overall Score*	**Median Survival (Years)**
Low (0)	5.7
Intermediate	
1 (0.5 or 1.0)	3.5
2 (1.5 or 2.0)	1.2
High (≥2.5)	0.4

*The overall score is the sum of the scores for bone marrow blasts, karyotype, and cytopenias. The percentage of blasts is scored as follows: <5%, 0; 5% to 10%, 0.5; 11% to 20%, 1.5; 21% to 30%, 2.0. Cytogenetic features associated with a good prognosis (normal karyotype, Y–, 5q–, or 20q–) are scored as 0; those associated with a poor prognosis (abnormal chromosome 7 or three or more abnormalities) are scored as 1.0; and all other cytogenetic abnormalities, which are associated with an intermediate prognosis, are scored as 0.5. A score of 0 is assigned if the patient has no cytopenia or only one type, and a score of 0.5 is assigned if the patient has two or three types of cytopenia. The various types of cytopenia are defined as follows: hemoglobin, <10 cells/dL, absolute neutrophil count, <1500 cells/mm³, and platelet count, <100,000 cells/mm³.

Adapted from Greenberg P , Cox C, LeBeau MM, et al: International Scoring System for evaluating prognosis in myelodysplastic syndromes, *Blood* 89:2079–2088, 1997.

Table 15.5	
Common Cytogenic Abnormalities in Myelodysplastic Syndrome	
Abnormality	**Incidence (%)**
Loss of all or part of chromosome 5	13
Loss of all or part of chromosome 7	5
Trisomy 8	5
del 17p	<1
del 20q	2
Loss of X or Y chromosome	2

Adapted from Greenberg P , Cox C, LeBeau MM, et al: International Scoring System for evaluating prognosis in myelodysplastic syndromes, *Blood* 89:2079–2088, 1997.

ACUTE MYELOFIBROSIS

Patients with this syndrome present acutely with symptoms due to anemia, neutropenia, or thrombocytopenia. Peripheral blood examination reveals leukoerythroblastic changes, and needle biopsy of bone marrow shows evidence of myelofibrosis; attempts at marrow aspiration are usually unsuccessful. In typical cases the features of the blast cells indicate that a transformation to the megakaryoblastic variant (M7) or AML has occurred; transformation to lymphoma has also been reported. Other diagnostic possibilities include agnogenic myeloid metaplasia in acute transformation and AML other than M7 with fibrosis. The majority of patients do not have gross splenomegaly. This acute syndrome has a poor prognosis (see "Chronic Leukemias").

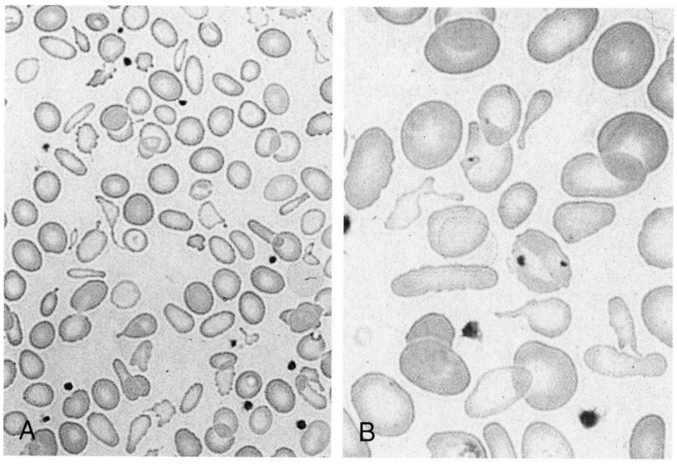

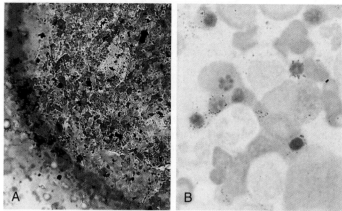

FIGURE 15.59 **ACQUIRED SIDEROBLASTIC ANEMIA (MDS TYPE II).** Bone marrow fragment shows **(A)** increased iron stores and **(B)** pathologic ring sideroblasts at higher magnification (Perls' stain).

FIGURE 15.56 **ACQUIRED SIDEROBLASTIC ANEMIA (MDS TYPE II). (A)** Peripheral blood film shows marked red cell anisocytosis and poikilocytosis. Although the majority of cells are markedly hypochromic, a second population of cells is normochromic. **(B)** At higher magnification the central red cell shows two small basophilic inclusions (Pappenheimer bodies). Perls' staining demonstrated that similar inclusions were Prussian blue–positive (siderotic granules). These granules are far more numerous after splenectomy.

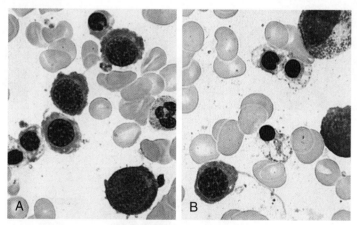

FIGURE 15.57 **ACQUIRED SIDEROBLASTIC ANEMIA (MDS TYPE II).** Bone marrow aspiration smear shows marked, defective hemoglobinization **(A)** and vacuolation **(B)** in later-stage polychromatic and pyknotic erythroblasts.

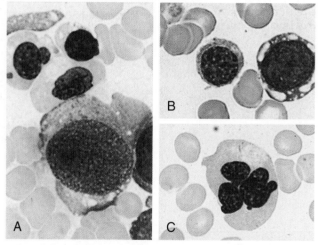

FIGURE 15.60 **REFRACTORY ANEMIA WITH EXCESS BLASTS (MDS TYPE II).** Bone marrow aspirate shows **(A)** abnormal proerythroblasts and megaloblast-like changes and **(B)** prominent cytoplasmic vacuolation in the basophilic erythroblasts **(C),** evidence of dyserythropoiesis.

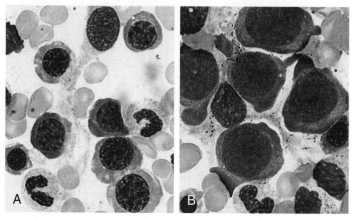

FIGURE 15.58 **ACQUIRED SIDEROBLASTIC ANEMIA (MDS TYPE II).** Bone marrow aspiration smear shows erythroblasts with **(A)** vacuolation of cytoplasm in later cells, mild megaloblastic features, and **(B)** a prominent group of proerythroblasts.

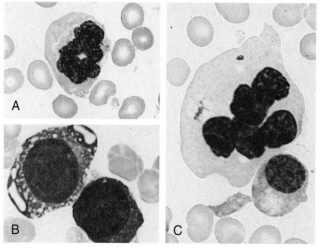

FIGURE 15.61 **REFRACTORY ANEMIA WITH EXCESS BLASTS (MDS TYPE III). (A–C)** Bone marrow aspirate shows three examples of polypoid multinucleate polychromatic erythroblasts, further evidence of gross dyserythropoiesis.

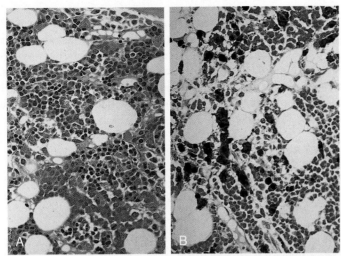

FIGURE 15.62 **REFRACTORY ANEMIA WITH EXCESS BLASTS.** Needle biopsy specimens show **(A)** clusters of blast forms and prominent hemosiderin-laden macrophages, and **(B)** a gross increase in reticuloendothelial iron stores, confirmed by Perls' staining.

FIGURE 15.63 **REFRACTORY ANEMIA WITH EXCESS BLASTS.** Bone marrow aspirates show disturbed granulopoiesis with **(A)** agranular promyelocytes and **(B)** agranular neutrophils and abnormal myelomonocytic cells. Some cells ("paramyeloid" cells) are difficult to classify as monocytic or granulocytic.

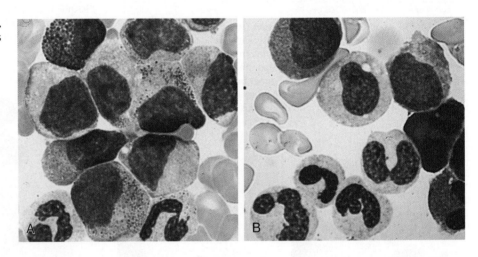

FIGURE 15.64 **REFRACTORY ANEMIA WITH EXCESS BLASTS.** Bone marrow aspirates show **(A)** an atypical megakaryoblast and **(B, C)** atypical mononuclear megakaryocytes, all of which show evidence of cytoplasmic maturation and granulation.

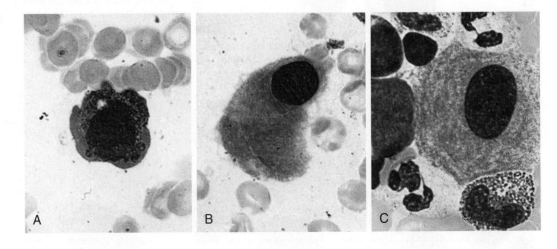

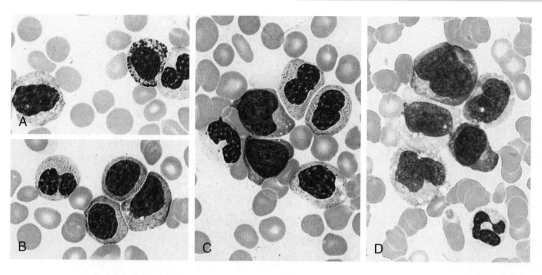

FIGURE 15.65 **CHRONIC MYELOMONOCYTIC LEUKEMIA (MDS TYPE IV). (A–C)** In these peripheral blood films showing white cells there are many atypical myelo-monocytic cells and pseudo-Pelger neutrophils, some of which are agranular. **(D)** The majority of cells shown here are more monocytoid; the neutrophil is agranular.

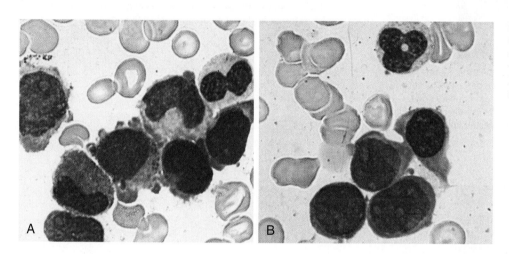

FIGURE 15.66 **REFRACTORY ANEMIA WITH EXCESS BLASTS IN TRANSFORMATION.** Bone marrow aspirates show increased numbers of blast cells **(B)**, some of which have atypical features. Blast cells constituted 23% of total marrow cells. Agranular neutrophils and myelomonocytic cells are also evident **(A)**.

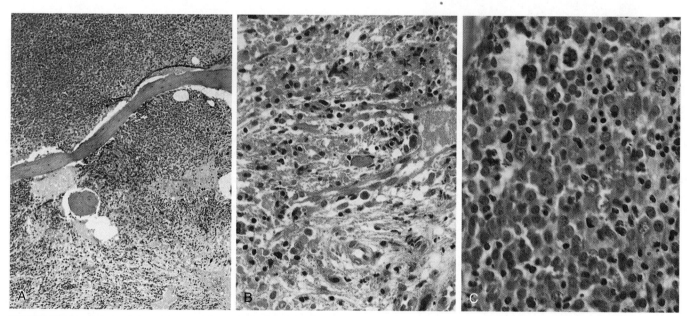

FIGURE 15.67 **MYELOFIBROSIS TRANSFORMED TO ACUTE LEUKEMIA. (A)** Low magnification of needle biopsy specimen shows areas in the *lower portion* of the field that are consistent with myelofibrosis, but the intertrabecular space in the *upper part* of the field contains sheets of closely packed mononuclear cells without obvious stromal connective tissue. **(B)** High-power view of the lower area shows isolated hematopoietic cells surrounded by a loose, fibrous connective tissue. **(C)** Primitive myeloid blast cells and promyelocytes predominate in this high-magnification view of the upper area. After a 9-year history of myelofibrosis this patient presented with fever and bronchopneumonia. About 10% of patients with myelofibrosis (agnogenic or postpolycythemia) eventually develop acute myeloblastic leukemia.

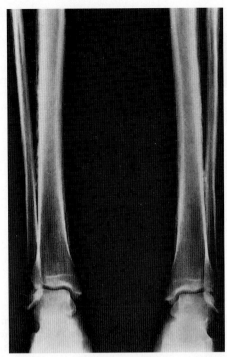

FIGURE 15.68 **MYELOFIBROSIS TRANSFORMED TO ACUTE LEUKEMIA.** Radiograph of the lower legs of a middle-aged man shows extensive periosteal elevation due to infiltration by myeloid blast cells from underlying medullary bone. Although the medullary cavities of these bones in adults usually contain only fat, there may be extension of hematopoietic tissue to distal skeletal tissues in long-standing myeloproliferative disease.

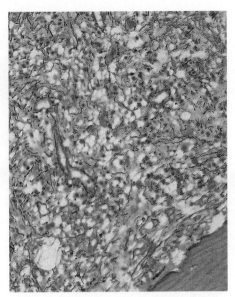

FIGURE 15.70 **ACUTE MYELOFIBROSIS.** Bone needle biopsy specimen with silver staining shows a marked increase in reticulin fiber density.

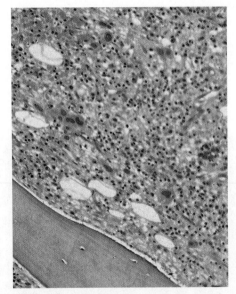

FIGURE 15.69 **ACUTE MYELOFIBROSIS.** Bone needle biopsy shows abnormal hematopoietic tissue with predominant mononuclear cells, isolated megakaroycytes, and abundant fibrous stroma.

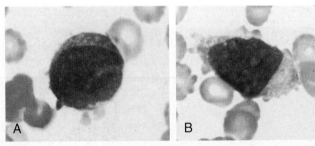

FIGURE 15.71 **ACUTE MYELOFIBROSIS. (A, B)** Peripheral blood films show blast cells that are somewhat larger than classic myeloblasts and have irregular cytoplasmic borders. Electron microscopic studies and detection of factor VIIIR:AG in their cytoplasm, using monoclonal antibodies, confirmed that they were megakaryoblasts. A diagnosis of M7 AML requires more than 20% blasts in the peripheral blood and/or bone marrow.

Chronic Leukemias

CHRONIC LYMPHOCYTIC LEUKEMIA

Chronic lymphocytic leukemia (CLL) is a malignant hematologic disorder characterized by a persistent absolute increase in mature-appearing lymphocytes in the peripheral blood and bone marrow. In the majority of cases surface marker studies have shown that the cells are a monoclonal population of immature B lymphocytes possessing low-density surface immunoglobulin (Table 15.9); in about 5% to 10% of patients, CLL is of T-cell origin. The disease is rare in individuals younger than 30 years of age, increasing in incidence with each decade. The average patient age is about 65 years, and CLL is more common in men than in women. About 6000 new cases occur in the United States each year, with an annual incidence of 2.6 cases per 100,000 people.

Staging of CLL is carried out by the Rai or International Workshop system, based on blood counts, lymphadenopathy,

Table 15.7

The Rai Staging System for Chronic Lymphocytic Leukemia

Stage	Features	Median Survival (Years)
0	Lymphocytosis in blood and marrow	12.5
I	Lymphocytosis with lymphadenopathy	8.4
II	Lymphocytosis with splenomegaly	5.9
III	Lymphocytosis with anemia	1.6
IV	Lymphocytosis with thrombocytopenia	1.6

Table 15.8

International Workshop Staging Classification of Chronic Lymphocytic Leukemia

Stage	Features	Median Survival (Years)
A	Lymphocytosis with clinical involvement of <3 lymph node groups No anemia or thrombocytopenia	>10
B	>3 Lymph node groups involved	5
C	Anemia or thrombocytopenia regardless of number of lymph node groups involved	2

and splenomegaly (Tables 15.7 and 15.8). The survival time varies widely, ranging from less than 2 years to more than 10 years.

In about 20% of patients CLL is an incidental finding on routine blood counts, at which time the physical examination may be otherwise normal. A small number of patients have a prolonged, asymptomatic course, without significant change in the lymphocytosis. Cytogenetic studies have demonstrated trisomy 12 as well as structural abnormalities of 13q, 14q, 6q, and 11 in a significant number of CLL patients, with an associated poor prognosis. As the disease progresses, symmetrical lymphadenopathy develops, accompanied by hepatosplenomegaly and variable degrees of anemia and thrombocytopenia. Symptoms include weight loss, fatigue, fever, and recurrent infections. Immunologic abnormalities appear, such as hypogammaglobulinemia, development of monoclonal proteins, "warm" autoimmune hemolytic anemia (10% of cases), and, in a small number of cases, autoimmune thrombocytopenia.

From 1% to 10% of patients develop transition to a diffuse large cell lymphoma or immunoblastic sarcoma (Richter syndrome) during the clinical course of CLL. The patients usually have active or advanced CLL, although some have been in remission (Robertson et al., 1993). The transition is heralded by sudden clinical deterioration, with increasing adenopathy, extranodal disease, systemic symptoms, elevated lactate dehydrogenase, and a monoclonal gammopathy. Immunoglobulin gene rearrangement and light-chain isotype analysis support a common origin for the malignant cells of both diseases in most cases. Prognosis is poor with Richter syndrome; median survival is only 5 months, despite multidrug therapy.

Prolymphocytic Leukemia

This variant of CLL usually occurs in the elderly and is associated with marked splenomegaly, absolute lymphocytosis (usually $>100 \times 10^9$ lymphocytes/L), and minimal lymph node enlargement. Peripheral blood films reveal larger lymphocytes than are found in classic CLL. In the majority of patients surface marker studies indicate a B-cell origin of prolymphocytes, but occasionally patients have a T-cell variant of this disease and concomitantly a less predictable prognosis.

Large Granular Lymphocytic Leukemia

Clonal diseases of large granular lymphocytes (LGLs) are either of T-cell origin (T-LGL leukemia) or of natural killer (NK)-cell origin (NK-LGL leukemia). T-LGL leukemia is associated with neutropenia and consequent recurrent bacterial infections and may also be associated with rheumatoid arthritis, resembling Felty syndrome, with the triad of arthritis, neutropenia, and splenomegaly. The majority of patients have a chronic disease course, with major complications secondary to neutropenia. Neoplastic cells are typically CD3-, CD8-, CD16-, and CD57-positive and show T-cell receptor gene rearrangements. NK-LGL leukemia typically has an acute clinical course, with pancytopenia, massive hepatosplenomegaly, and systemic illness. Neoplastic cells are typically CD3-, CD8-, and CD57-negative, and CD16- and CD56-positive, without T-cell receptor gene rearrangements. In both types of LGL leukemia the cause is unknown.

Table 15.9

Immunologic Classification of Chronic Lymphocytic Leukemias

	Study	B Cell (CLL)	B Cell (PLL)	Hairy Cell Leukemia	T-Cell CLL/PLL
Surface antigens	sIg	± (IgM ± IgD)	++ (IgM ± IgD)	+ (IgM or IgG or IgA)	–
	MRBC rosettes	++	±	±	–
	SRBC rosettes	–	–	–	+
	HLA-DR (Ia)	+	+	+	–
	CD19	+	+	+	–
	CD20	+	+	+	–
	CD5	+	–/+	–	–
	CD2	–	–	–	+
	CD3	–	–	–	+
	FMC7	–	+	±	–
	DBA.44 & CD103	–	–	+	–
Gene rearrangement	IgH	+	+	+	–
	TCRβ	–	–	–	+

CLL, chronic lymphocytic leukemia; DBA.44, a monoclonal antibody highly sensitive for neoplastic cells of hairy cell leukemia; FMC7, a cell membrane antigen occurring on late B lymphocytes; IgH, immunoglobulin heavy chain; MRBC, mouse red blood cell; PLL, prolymphocytic leukemia; sIg, surface immunoglobulin; SRBC, sheep red blood cell; TCRβ, T-cell receptor β-chain; ++, strongly positive; ±, equivocal; –, negative.

Hairy Cell Leukemia

This rare disorder, also known as leukemic reticuloendotheliosis, is characterized by pancytopenia, massive splenomegaly, and accumulation in peripheral blood of lymphoid-appearing cells with "hairy" cytoplasmic projections. In many patients the marrow is difficult to aspirate ("dry tap") because of myelofibrosis and infiltration by hairy cells. The characteristic cells are almost always of B-cell origin and coexpress CD11c, CD25, and CD103. New purine analogues are extremely effective for the treatment of hairy cell leukemias.

CHRONIC MYELOGENOUS LEUKEMIA

Chronic myelogenous leukemia (CML), also called chronic granulocytic leukemia, is a clonal myeloproliferative disorder arising from neoplastic proliferation at the level of the pluripotential stem cell. In most patients (90%) normal marrow is replaced by cells with an abnormal G-group chromosome, the Ph chromosome. About 4000–5000 new cases are diagnosed in the United States each year. Although CML can occur at any age, it is rare in childhood and peaks in the mid-fifth decade.

The Ph-chromosome abnormality results from a reciprocal translocation involving the long arm of chromosome 9 band q34 and chromosome 22 band q11 (Fig. 15.100). The cellular oncogene *ABL*, which encodes a tyrosine protein kinase, is translocated to a specific breakpoint cluster region (*BCR*) of chromosome 22. Part of the *BCR* gene (the 5′ end) remains on chromosome 22, the 3′ end moving to chromosome 9 together with the oncogene *c-SIS* (which encodes a protein with close homology to one of the two subunits of platelet-derived growth factor). As a result of the translocation onto chromosome 22, a chimeric oncogene is formed that produces a *BCR/ABL* messenger RNA (mRNA) encoding a 210-kDa fusion protein that transforms normal hematopoietic cells (Fig. 15.101). Clonal proliferation of these abnormal cells leads to progressive expansion of the total burden of granulocytes. The Ph chromosome is present in granulocytic, erythroid, and megakaryocytic precursor cells, but not in fibroblasts. It has also been demonstrated in B and T lymphocytes (e.g., in leukemic transformation) and has been observed in cases of de novo ALL. CML in some patients is diagnosed incidentally after a routine blood count. The white blood cell (WBC) count progressively rises, reaching levels of 50×10^9 to 500×10^9 per liter, and a complete spectrum of granulocytic cells is seen in the blood smear. The bone marrow is hypercellular, with a predominating granulocyte population.

The symptoms of CML are related to hypermetabolism and include anorexia, lassitude, weight loss, and night sweats. Splenomegaly, often massive, is common. As the spleen enlarges, symptoms of compression may develop, such as early satiety and peripheral leg edema. Splenic infarcts may occur, causing splenic pain referred to the left shoulder.

An accelerated phase known as "CML crisis" is characterized by the appearance of new symptoms, similar to those mentioned above, with a rapid rise in WBC count. Approximately 70% to 80% of patients undergo blastic transformation, with the presence of 20% blasts in the peripheral blood or bone marrow, which is associated with rapid clinical deterioration and progressive bone marrow failure. Infiltration of the skin and other nonhematopoietic tissues may occur. The transformation may be myeloblastic, lymphoblastic, mixed, or, rarely, monoblastic or erythroblastic.

About 5% to 10% of patients have a variant of CML (Ph-negative) that is associated with fewer myelocytes, more monocytoid cells, and atypical neutrophils in the peripheral blood. Severe anemia and thrombocytopenia are more frequent than in classic CML. Although the Ph chromosome is not found in these patients, in one third of cases the chimeric *BCR/ABL* mRNA is produced and can be demonstrated with molecular diagnostic methods. As a group, patients with true Ph-negative CML are elderly, have a less favorable prognosis, and present with leukocytosis and multilineage dysplasia that evolves into acute leukemia in 30% to 40% of patients. Another Ph-negative variant occurs in children, referred to as juvenile myelomonocytic leukemia, and is often accompanied by marked lymphadenopathy and eczematoid rashes. As in the adult form, there are morphologic differences from classic CML.

Recently, imatinib mesylate (Gleevec; Novartis, Basel, Switzerland), an oral selective tyrosine kinase inhibitor, has been developed as targeted therapy for CML. It has demonstrated hematologic, cytogenetic, and molecular remission rates in newly diagnosed chronic-phase CML with relatively few side effects. More importantly, it represents one of the first successfully molecularly targeted therapies. Newer-generation oral tyrosine kinase inhibitors, dasatinib and nolotinib, have demonstrated efficacy in imatinib resistance, although none of these agents inhibits the *BCR-ABL* mutation T315I.

World Health Organization classification of neoplastic disease
of the chronic lymphoid leukemias (proposed)

B-cell neoplasms

B-cell chronic lymphocytic leukemia/small lymphocytic lymphoma
B-cell prolymphocytic leukemia
Hairy cell leukemia

T-cell neoplasms

T-cell prolymphocytic leukemia
T-cell large granular lymphocytic leukemia

FIGURE 15.72 WHO classification of neoplastic diseases of the chronic lymphoid leukemias (proposed). (Adapted from Harris NL, Jaffe ES, Diebold J, et al: World Health Organization classification of neoplastic diseases of the hematopoietic and lymphoid tissues: report of the clinical advisory committee meeting—Airlie House, Virginia, November 1997, *J Clin Oncol* 7:3835–3849,1999.)

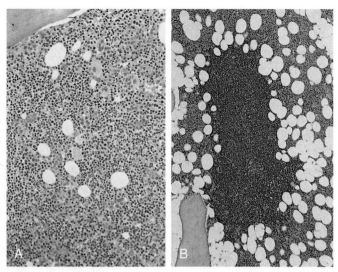

FIGURE 15.75 **CHRONIC LYMPHOCYTIC LEUKEMIA.** Bone needle biopsy samples show **(A)** a marked, diffuse increase in marrow lymphocytes, which are closely packed and have small dense nuclei. **(B)** In a different patient there is a nodular pattern of lymphocyte accumulation.

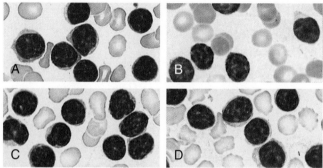

FIGURE 15.73 **CHRONIC LYMPHOCYTIC LEUKEMIA. (A–D)** Lymphocytes in the peripheral blood of four different patients show a thin rim of cytoplasm, condensed coarse chromatin, and only rare nucleoli.

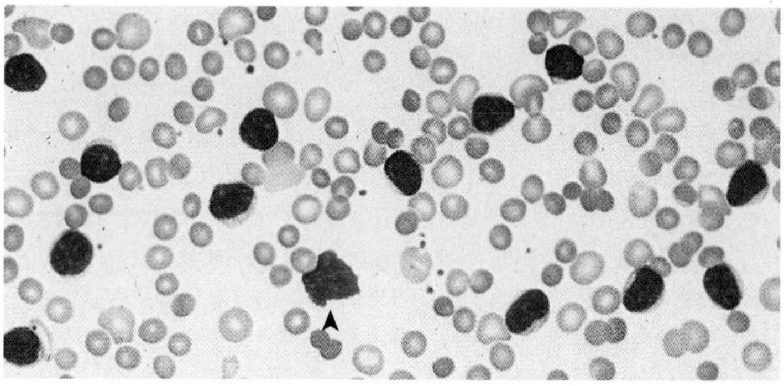

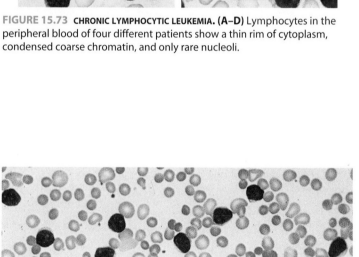

FIGURE 15.74 **CHRONIC LYMPHOCYTIC LEUKEMIA WITH AUTOIMMUNE HEMOLYTIC ANEMIA.** Peripheral blood film shows increased numbers of lymphocytes, red cell spherocytosis, and polychromasia. The direct Coombs test was strongly positive with IgG on the cell surfaces. Note the "smudge" cell (*arrowhead*), which is often seen in CLL.

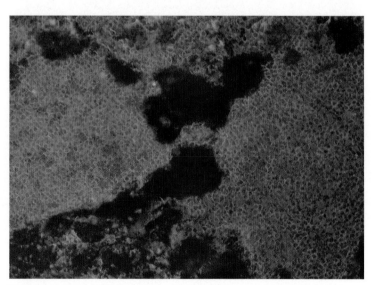

FIGURE 15.76 **CHRONIC LYMPHOCYTIC LEUKEMIA.** Two neoplastic lymphoid nodules in this bone marrow biopsy contain predominantly B cells that react positively for IgM (green fluorescein staining). Many reactive T cells are identified by a monoclonal antibody to the CD5 (T1) antigen (red rhodamine staining). (Courtesy of Dr. G. Pizzolo and Dr. M. Chilosi.)

FIGURE 15.77 **LYMPH NODE INVOLVEMENT.**
(A) High magnification of a lymph node biopsy specimen from a patient with CLL shows small, well-differentiated lymphocytes with scanty cytoplasm. **(B)** Touch prep reveals typical small lymphocytes with condensed nuclear chromatin and a rim of cytoplasm (Wright-Giemsa stain). Immunoperoxidase staining (not shown) for IgM was weakly positive; it was also positive for both CD20 (B1) and CD5 (T1), which is characteristic for CLL.

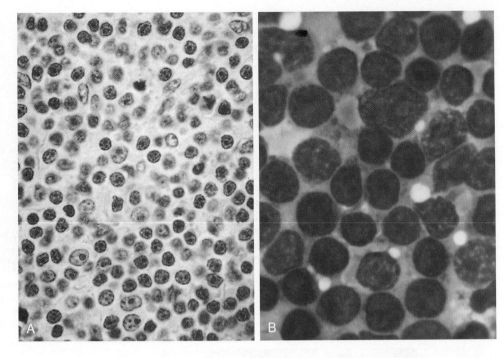

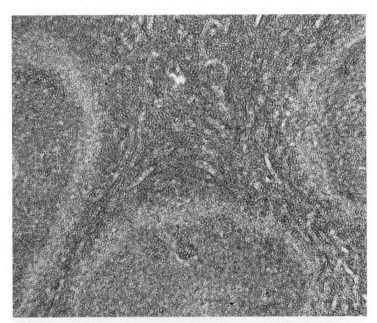

FIGURE 15.78 **SPLENIC INVOLVEMENT.** Histologic section of spleen from a patient with CLL and secondary autoimmune hemolytic anemia shows expansion of lymphoid tissue in the periarterial sheaths of the white pulp and obvious red cell entrapment in the reticuloendothelial cords and splenic sinuses.

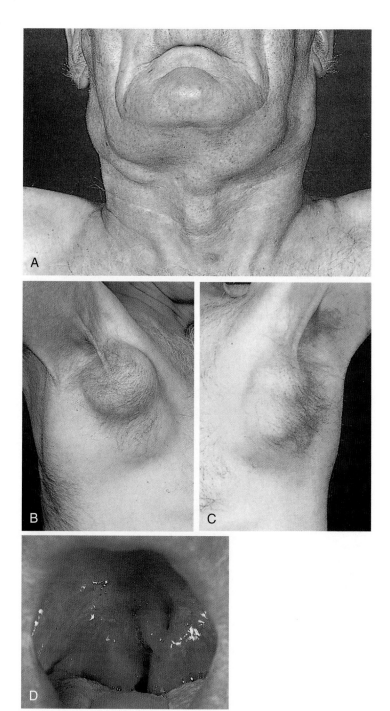

FIGURE 15.79 LYMPHADENOPATHY. This 65-year-old man with CLL presented with bilateral **(A)** cervical and **(B, C)** axillary lymphadenopathy, as well as **(D)** massive enlargement of the pharyngeal tonsils.

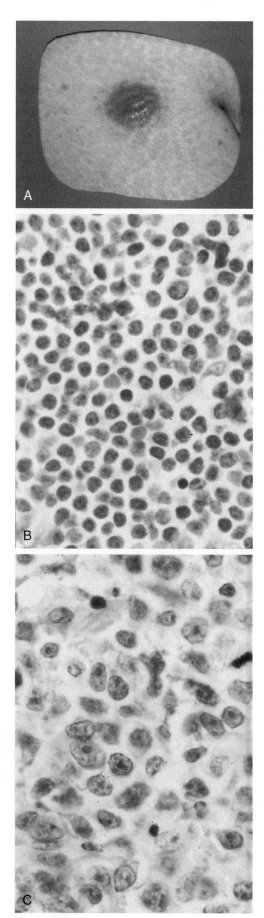

FIGURE 15.80 TRANSFORMATION TO LARGE CELL LYMPHOMA (RICHTER SYNDROME). A 78-year-old woman who had stable CLL of 3 years' duration developed new subcutaneous masses on the trunk along with generalized adenopathy, weight loss, and fatigue. **(A)** This 3-cm by 3-cm abdominal wall tumor mass appears fixed, raised, and reddish tan. Biopsy showed a B-immunoblastic-type, diffuse large cell lymphoma. **(B)** The small cells of CLL contrast sharply with **(C)** the large, irregular, malignant lymphoid cells of diffuse large cell lymphoma. Richter syndrome, originally described in 1928, was thought to represent a new malignancy (reticulum cell sarcoma) arising in a patient with CLL. Immunophenotyping and gene arrangement studies, however, typically reveal identical lineage consistent with clonal progression to an activated, aggressive lymphoma cell line.

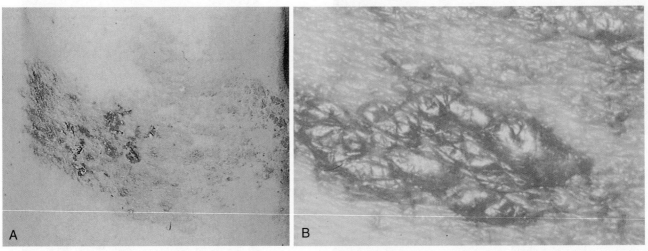

FIGURE 15.81 COMPLICATIONS OF CHRONIC LYMPHOCYTIC LEUKEMIA. (A) The posterior right lateral flank of this 68-year-old woman with CLL is extensively affected with a herpes zoster infection. **(B)** The eruption is typically vesicular with an erythematous base.

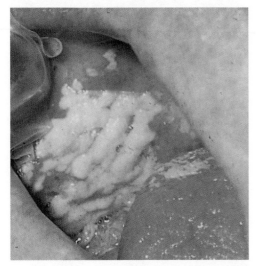

FIGURE 15.82 COMPLICATIONS OF CHRONIC LYMPHOCYTIC LEUKEMIA. Extensive *Candida albicans* infection involves the buccal mucosa of a 73-year-old woman.

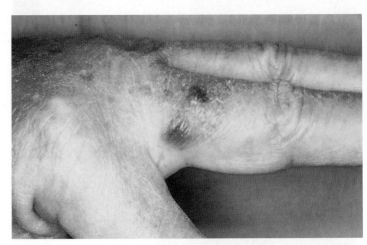

FIGURE 15.83 COMPLICATIONS OF CHRONIC LYMPHOCYTIC LEUKEMIA. Hypersensitivity to insect bites occasionally occurs, as noted on the middle finger of this 66-year-old man 10 days after mosquito bites. The hemorrhagic lesions are generally quite painful and may become infected. The hypersensitivity reaction, which is poorly understood, is related in part to underlying immune abnormalities.

FIGURE 15.84 CUTANEOUS INVOLVEMENT.
(A) This 75-year-old man with T-cell CLL developed edema of the face and ears, along with generalized adenopathy and edema. Note the marked erythema and thickening of the ears. **(B)** Skin biopsy revealed infiltration of the dermis by small, well-differentiated lymphocytes. Although skin lesions may be seen in patients with B-cell CLL, they are more common in the T-cell type, which usually has a more aggressive clinical course.

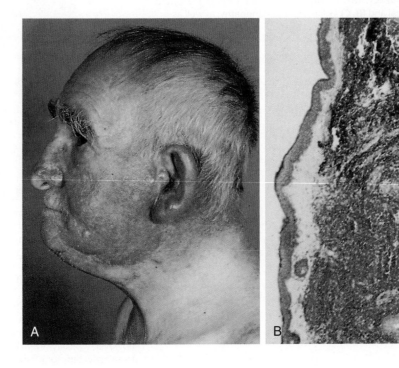

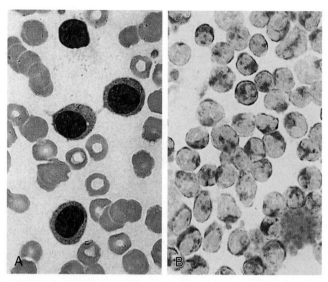

FIGURE 15.85 **CHRONIC LYMPHOCYTIC LEUKEMIA (T-CELL TYPE).** Peripheral blood films show **(A)** abnormal lymphocytes in which nuclear "convolutions" are occasionally seen and **(B)** characteristic "clump" positivity in the Golgi zone on acid-phosphatase staining. The clinical course is usually more rapid, compared with B-cell CLL.

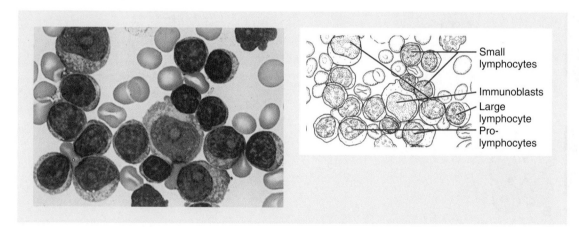

FIGURE 15.86 **TRANSFORMATION TO PROLYMPHOCYTIC LEUKEMIA.** Peripheral blood film from a patient with CLL with prolymphocytoid transformation shows B lymphocytes at various stages of development. (Courtesy of Dr. J.V. Melo.)

Small lymphocytes

Immunoblasts

Large lymphocyte

Pro-lymphocytes

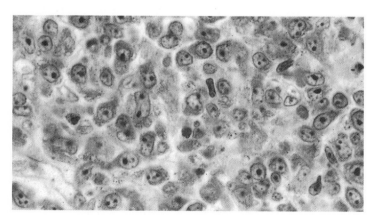

FIGURE 15.87 **PROLYMPHOCYTIC LEUKEMIA.** Bone marrow biopsy shows a diffuse infiltrate composed predominantly of lymphoid cells larger than those seen in CLL, with round nuclei and prominent central nucleoli (Giemsa stain).

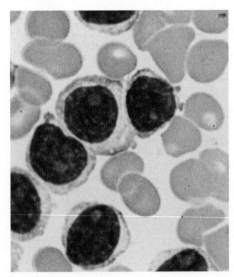

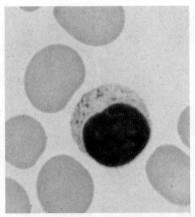

FIGURE 15.88 **PROLYMPHOCYTIC LEUKEMIA (B-CELL TYPE).** Peripheral blood film shows prolymphocytes with prominent, central nucleoli and an abundance of pale cytoplasm. A high density of surface immunoglobulin confirmed their B-cell nature. (Courtesy of Dr. D. Catovsky.)

FIGURE 15.90 **LGL LEUKEMIA.** Peripheral blood film shows a large lymphocyte with many coarse, azurophilic cytoplasmic granules (LGL). Immunologic marker studies demonstrated that the cells were positive for surface antigens CD8 (T8) and CD3 (T3), as well as for NK-cell markers. The patient had rheumatoid arthritis, splenomegaly, chronic neutropenia, and lymphocytosis. LGL leukemias represent a heterogeneous group of lymphoproliferative disorders including at least three distinct clinical syndromes that can present with acute or chronic manifestations (Loughran, 1993).

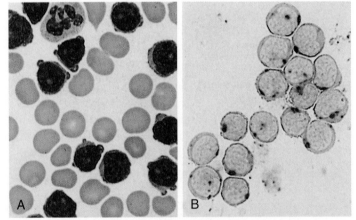

FIGURE 15.89 **PROLYMPHOCYTIC LEUKEMIA (T-CELL TYPE). (A)** Peripheral blood film shows prolymphocytes and a single neutrophil. Cell marker studies revealed positive reactions with anti-T-cell antisera and an absence of surface immunoglobulin. The majority of cases of T-cell prolymphocytic leukemia show structural abnormalities of chromosome 14, most commonly inv(14). **(B)** The cells show "clump" positivity with acid-phosphatase staining. (Courtesy of Dr. D. Catovsky.)

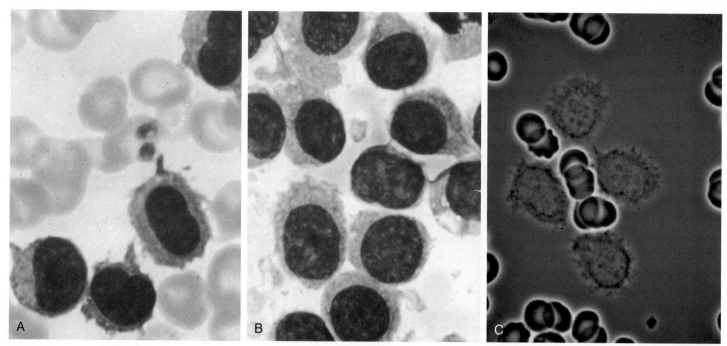

FIGURE 15.91 **HAIRY CELL LEUKEMIA.** A 58-year-old man presented with fatigue, weight loss, and abdominal distention. Evaluation shows pancytopenia, and **(A)** this peripheral blood film demonstrates characteristic lymphoid cells with fine hairlike cytoplasmic projections. Some cells have an ovoid or kidney-shaped nucleus, and small nucleoli may be seen. Bone marrow aspiration was "dry," but **(B)** the marrow biopsy sample shows infiltration by hairy cells, some with abundant cytoplasm (Wright-Giemsa stain). **(C)** Phase-contrast microscopy of a drop of peripheral blood diluted with saline markedly demonstrates the cells' hairy projections. Immunophenotyping in this case showed positivity for IgM, HLA-DR (Ia), CD20 (B1), CD19 (B4), CD22 (B3), CD11c, CD25 (IL2R), and PCA-1.

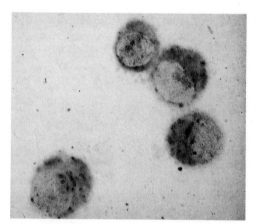

FIGURE 15.92 **HAIRY CELL LEUKEMIA.** Typically, hairy cells show a strongly positive cytochemical reaction to tartaric acid–resistant acid phosphatase. Alphanaphthyl butyrate esterase staining (not shown) is also positive in these cells, which often exhibit a fine, granular, crescentic positive accumulation at one side of the nucleus.

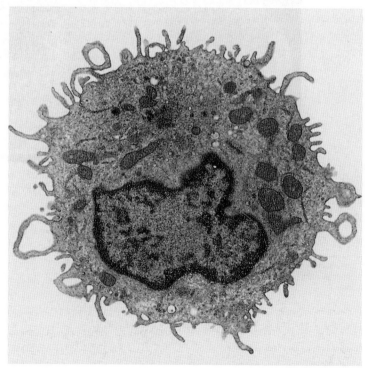

FIGURE 15.93 **HAIRY CELL LEUKEMIA.** Typical ultrastructural features of the hairy cell are its abundant cytoplasm, low nucleus-to-cytoplasm ratio, and the cytoplasmic projections or villi giving it a "hairy" appearance (×9200). (Courtesy of Mrs. D. Robinson and Dr. D. Catovsky.)

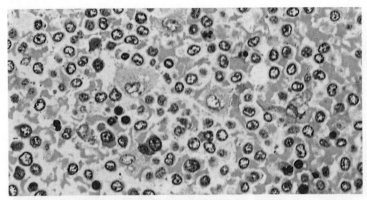

FIGURE 15.94 HAIRY CELL LEUKEMIA. Needle biopsy specimen of bone marrow shows extensive replacement of normal hematopoietic tissue by discrete mononuclear hairy cells. The nuclei are typically surrounded by a clear zone of cytoplasm (methacrylate section).

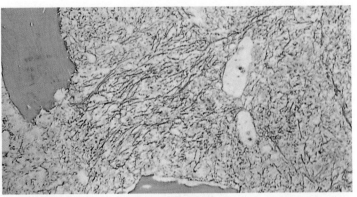

FIGURE 15.95 HAIRY CELL LEUKEMIA. Needle biopsy specimen of bone marrow shows increased fiber density and thickness in the reticulin fiber pattern (silver impregnation technique).

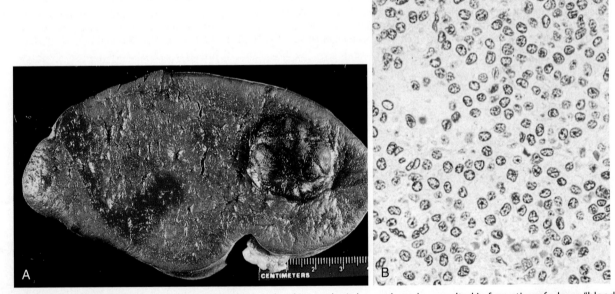

FIGURE 15.96 SPLENIC INVOLVEMENT IN HAIRY CELL LEUKEMIA. (A) Localized intrasplenic hemorrhage has resulted in formation of a large "blood lake." **(B)** Microscopic section of spleen reveals the characteristic spacing of individual, uniform mononuclear cells with reniform nuclei, indistinct nucleoli, finely stippled chromatin, and abundant, pale cytoplasm.

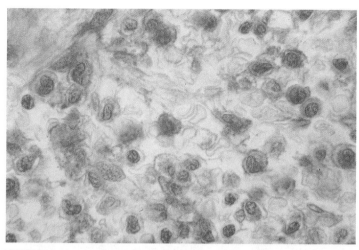

FIGURE 15.97 **HAIRY CELL LEUKEMIA.** Neoplastic cells are reactive with monoclonal antibody DBA.44, which is highly sensitive for hairy cells, outlines their cytoplasmic projections, and is capable of detecting minimal bone marrow involvement.

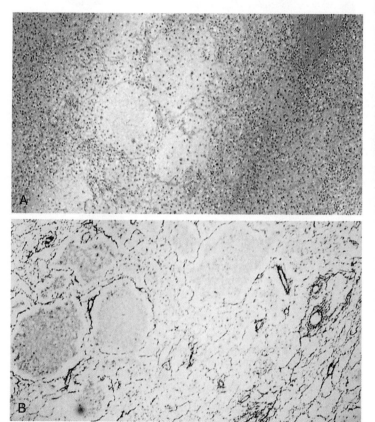

FIGURE 15.98 **SPLENIC INVOLVEMENT IN HAIRY CELL LEUKEMIA. (A)** Hairy cells have infiltrated the reticuloendothelial cords and sinuses. Many blood "lakes" are seen in the *center* of the field. **(B)** Silver impregnation technique shows more clearly the reticulin fiber pattern outlining the abnormal venous "lakes." The presence of these structures may explain the extensive splenic red cell pooling that occurs in this disease.

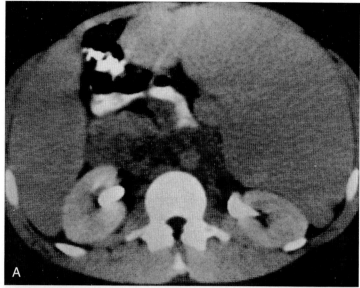

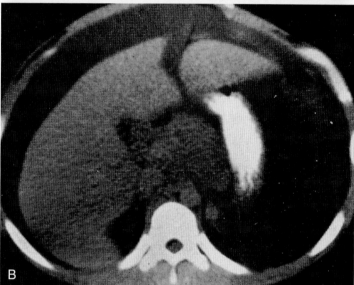

FIGURE 15.99 **SPLENIC INVOLVEMENT IN HAIRY CELL LEUKEMIA. (A)** Abdominal computed tomography scan shows massive splenomegaly displacing the stomach and bowel medially. No retroperitoneal lymphadenopathy is present. **(B)** Follow-up scan 2 years after splenectomy reveals ascites and enlarged retroperitoneal nodes. The ascitic fluid was positive for hairy cells, which is an unusual feature.

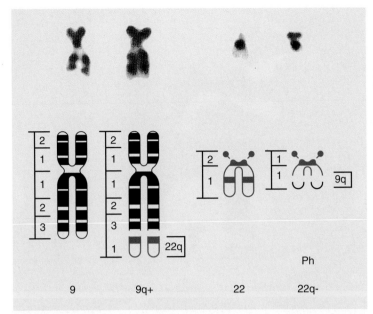

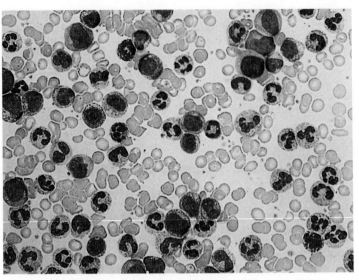

FIGURE 15.102 **CHRONIC MYELOGENOUS LEUKEMIA.** Peripheral blood film shows cells at all stages of granulopoietic development.

FIGURE 15.100 **CHRONIC MYELOGENOUS LEUKEMIA.** The translocated chromosomes are on the *right* in each pair shown in this partial karyotype of G-banded chromosomes 9 and 22 (*above*). The corresponding diagrams (*below*) represent a systematized description of the structural aberration. Ph, Philadelphia chromosome. (Courtesy of Dr. L.M. Secker-Walker.)

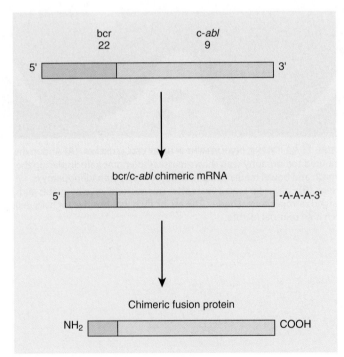

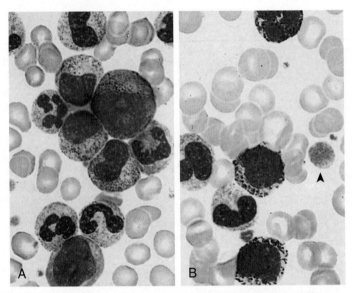

FIGURE 15.103 **CHRONIC MYELOGENOUS LEUKEMIA.** Peripheral blood films show **(A)** a myeloblast, promyelocytes, myelocytes, metamyelocytes, and band and segmented neutrophils, as well as **(B)** basophils and a giant platelet (*arrowhead*).

FIGURE 15.101 **CHRONIC MYELOGENOUS LEUKEMIA.** Chimeric *BCR/ABL* mRNA is encoded partly by the breakpoint cluster region (bcr) of chromosome 22 and partly by the *ABL* oncogene translocated from chromosome 9 to 22.

WHO Classification of myeloproliferative and myelodysplastic/myeloproliferative neoplasms

Myeloproliferative neoplasms (MPNs)

Chronic myelogenous leukemia, BCR-ABL1 positive (CML)
    Chronic neutrophilic leukemia (CNL)
    Polycythemia vera (PV)
    Primary myelofibrosis (PMF)
    Essential thrombocythemia (ET)
    Chronic eosinophilic leukaemia, NOS (CEL, NOS)
    Mastocytosis
    Myeloproliferative neoplasm, unclassifiable (MPN<U)

Myelodysplastic/myeloproliferative neoplasms (MDS/MPN)
    Chronic myelomonocytic leukemia
    Atypical chronic myeloid leukemia, *BCR-ABL1*-negative
    Juvenile myelomonocytic leukemia
    Myelodysplastic/myeloproliferative neoplasm, unclassifiable

---

Provisional entity: refractory cytopenia with ring sideroblasts and thrombocytosis
(Adapted from Swerdlow et al, 2009)

FIGURE 15.104 WHO classification of myeloproliferative and myelodysplastic/myeloproliferative diseases.

Characteristics of patient with chronic myeloid leukemia at presentation

Clinical findings*

Fatigue, anorexia, weight loss
Splenomegaly
Hepatomegaly

Peripheral blood findings

Elevated white cell count (usually >25,000/mm³)
Elevated platelet count in 30%–50% of cases
Basophilia
Reduced leukocyte alkaline phosphatase activity
All stages of granulocyte differentiation visible on peripheral smear

Bone marrow findings

Hypercellularity, reduced fat content
Increased ratio of myeloid cells to erythroid cells
Increased numbers of megakaryocytes
Blasts and promyelocytes constitute less than 10% of all cells

*Approximately 40% of patients are asymptomatic.

FIGURE 15.105 Characteristics of patients with chronic myeloid leukemia at presentation. (Adapted from Sawyers, 1999.)

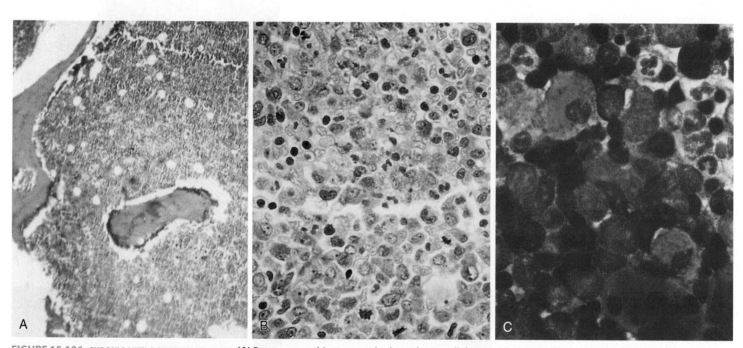

FIGURE 15.106 **CHRONIC MYELOGENOUS LEUKEMIA. (A)** Bone marrow biopsy sample shows hypercellularity with about 10% residual fat. **(B)** At higher magnification, packed marrow shows increased myeloid elements ranging from blasts to mature forms. There are increased numbers of eosinophilic myeloid forms (Giemsa stain). **(C)** Occasional "sea-blue" histiocytes are noted with Wright-Giemsa stain; these represent benign reactive storage cells attracted by the increased cellular debris.

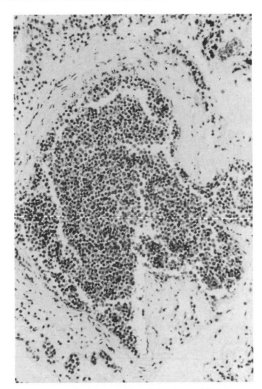

FIGURE 15.107 PULMONARY INVOLVEMENT (LEUKOSTASIS). In some patients with accelerated CML or blastic transformation, dyspnea may occur as a result of pulmonary leukostasis, as noted in this vessel obstructed by excess myeloid cells. Chest radiography often reveals bilateral infiltrates. Leukostasis may also occur in cerebral vessels, yielding a clinical picture resembling a stroke. Some patients with AML, especially M4 and M5 subtypes, also develop leukostasis with or without hemorrhage, particularly when the WBC count is >100,000 cells/μL. The syndrome is very rare in ALL and CLL.

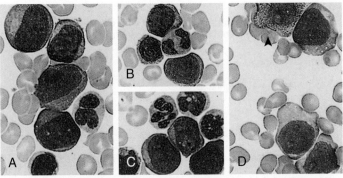

FIGURE 15.108 BLAST CELL TRANSFORMATION (ACCELERATED CML). (A-D) Peripheral blood films at high magnification show many myeloblasts, atypical neutrophils, and an abnormal promyelocyte (*arrowhead*).

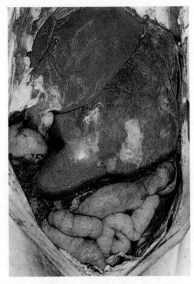

FIGURE 15.109 SPLENIC INVOLVEMENT. The abdominal contents at autopsy of a 54-year-old man are dominated by a grossly enlarged spleen that extends toward the right iliac fossa. The central, pale area covered by fibrinous exudate overlies an extensive splenic infarct. The liver is moderately enlarged.

FIGURE 15.110 OPHTHALMIC INVOLVEMENT (HYPERVISCOSITY SYNDROME). (A) The ocular fundus shows distended retinal veins and deep retinal hemorrhages at the macula. **(B)** There are also prominent leukemic infiltrates fringed by areas of retinal hemorrhage.

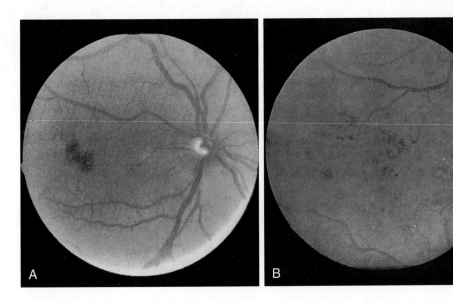

 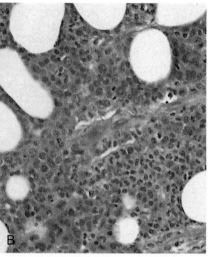

FIGURE 15.111 CUTANEOUS INVOLVEMENT. (A) Nodular leukemic infiltrates are present in the skin over the anterior surface of the tibia in a 48-year-old woman with blast cell transformation. **(B)** Histologic section of skin reveals infiltration by myeloblasts and other early myeloid cells.

References and Suggested Readings

Brunning RD, McKenna RW: Tumors of the bone marrow. In Brunning RD, McKenna RW, editors: *Atlas of tumor pathology*, 3rd ser., fasc. 9, Washington, DC, 1994, Armed Forces Institute of Pathology.

Bullinger L, Rucker FG, Kurz S, et al: Gene-expression profiling identifies distinct subclasses of core binding factor acute myeloid leukemia, *Blood* 110:1291–1300, 2007.

Calabretta B, Perrotti D: The biology of CML blast crisis, *Blood* 103:4010–4022, 2004.

Carey JL, Hanson CA: Flow cytometric analysis of leukemia and lymphoma. In Keren DF, Hanson CA, Hurtubise PE, editors: *Flow cytometry and clinical diagnosis*, Chicago, 1994, American Society of Clinical Pathologists, pp 197–308.

Chiorazzi N, Rai KR, Ferrarini M: Chronic lymphocytic leukemia, *N Engl J Med* 352:804–815, 2005.

Cooper PH, Innes DJ, Greer KE: Acute febrile neutrophilic dermatosis (Sweet's syndrome) and myeloproliferative disorders, *Cancer* 51:1518–1526, 1983.

Cortes JE, Talpaz M, O'Brien S, et al: Staging of chronic myeloid leukemia in the imatinib era, *Cancer* 106:1306–1315, 2006.

Creutzig U, Ritter J, Budde M, et al: Early deaths due to hemorrhage and leukostasis in childhood acute myelogenous leukemia, *Cancer* 60:3071–3079, 1987.

Davey FR, Abraham N, Brunetto VL, et al: Morphologic characteristics of erythro-leukemia (acute myeloid leukemia: FAB-M6), *Am J Hematol* 49:29–38, 1995.

Druker BJ, Guilhot F, O'Brian S, et al: Five-year follow-up of patients receiving imatinib for chronic myeloid leukemia, *N Engl J Med* 355:2408–2417, 2006.

Ebert BL, Golub TR: Genomic approaches to hematologic malignancies, *Blood* 104:923–932, 2004.

Freedman AS, Boyd AW, Bieber FR: Normal cellular counterparts of B cell chronic lymphocytic leukemia, *Blood* 70:418–427, 1987.

Gidron A, Tallman MS: 2-CdA in the treatment of hairy cell leukemia: a review of long-term follow-up, *Leuk Lymphoma* 47:2301–2307, 2006.

Goldman JM, Druker BJ: Chronic myeloid leukemia; current treatment options, *Blood* 98:2039–2042, 2001.

Goldman JM, Melo JV: Chronic myeloid leukemia—advances in biology and new approaches to treatment, *N Engl J Med* 349:1451–1464, 2003.

Greenberg P, Cox C, LeBeau MM, et al: International scoring system for evaluating prognosis in myelodysplastic syndromes, *Blood* 89:2079–2088, 1997.

Griffin JD, Nadler LM: Immunobiology of chronic leukemias. In Wiernik PH, Canellos GP, Kyle RA, et al, editors: *Neoplastic diseases of the blood*, ed 2, New York, 1991, Churchill Livingstone, pp 39–60.

Harris NL, Jaffe ES, Diebold J, et al: World Health Organization classification of neoplastic diseases of the hematopoietic and lymphoid tissues:

report of the clinical advisory committee meeting—Airlie House, Virginia, November 1997, *J Clin Oncol* 17:3835–3849, 1999.

Hounieu H, Chittal SM, Al Saati T: Hairy cell leukemia: diagnosis of bone marrow involvement in paraffin-embedded sections with monoclonal antibody DBA.44, *Am J Clin Pathol* 98:26–33, 1992.

Jemal A, Siegel R, Ward E, et al: Cancer statistics, 2007, *CA Cancer J Clin* 57:43–66, 2007.

Juliusson G, Liliemark J: Purine analogues: rationale for development, mechanisms of action, and pharmacokinetics in hairy cell leukemia, *Hematol Oncol Clinic North Am* 20:1087–1097, 2006.

Kantarjian HM, Dixon D, Keating MJ, et al: Characteristics of accelerated disease in chronic myelogenous leukemia, *Cancer* 61:1441–1446, 1988.

Kantarjian HM, Hirsch-Ginsberg C, Yee G, et al: Mixed lineage leukemia revisited: acute lymphocytic leukemia with myeloperoxidase-positive blasts by electron microscopy, *Blood* 76:808–813, 1990.

Kantarjian H, Talpaz M, Estey E, et al: What is the contribution of molecular studies to the diagnosis of BCR-ABL-positive disease in adult acute leukemia, *Am J Med* 96:133–138, 1994.

Kantarjian H, Talpaz M, Giles F, et al: New insights into the pathophysiology of chronic myeloid leukemia and imatinib resistance, *Ann Intern Med* 145:913–923, 2006.

Kreil S, Pfirrmann M, Haferlach C, et al: Heterogeneous prognostic impact of derivative chromosome 9 deletions in chronic myelogenous leukemia, *Blood* 110:1283–1290, 2007.

Larson RA, Williams SF, LeBeau MM, et al: Acute myelomonocytic leukemia with abnormal eosinophils and inv (16) or t (16;16) has a favorable prognosis, *Blood* 68:1242–1249, 1986.

Loughran TP: Clonal diseases of large granular lymphocytes, *Blood* 82:1–14, 1993.

Lowenberg B, Downing JR, Burnett A: Acute myeloid leukemia, *N Engl J Med* 341:1051–1062, 1999.

Malcovati L, Giovanni Della Porta M, Pascutto C, et al: Prognostic factors and life expectancy in myelodysplasia syndromes classified according to WHO criteria: a basis for clinical decision making, *J Clin Oncol* 23:7594–7603, 2005.

Melnick A, Licht JD: Deconstructing a disease: RARalpha, its fusion partners, and their roles in the pathogenesis of acute promyelocytic leukemia, *Blood* 93:3167–3215, 1999.

Montillo M, Hamblin T, Hallek M: Chronic lymphocytic leukemia: novel prognostic factors and their relevance for risk-adapted therapeutic strategies, *Haematologica* 90:391–399, 2005.

Moorman AV, Harrison CJ, Buck GAN, et al: Karyotype is an independent prognostic factor in adult acute lymphoblastic leukemia (ALL): analysis of cytogenetic data from patients treated on the Medical Research Council (MRC) UKALLXII/Eastern Cooperative Oncologic Group (ECOG) 2993 trial, *Blood* 109:3189–3197, 2007.

Myers TJ, Cole SR, Klatsky AU, et al: Respiratory failure due to pulmonary leukostasis following chemotherapy of acute nonlymphocytic leukemia, *Cancer* 51:1808–1813, 1983.

Nowakowski GS, Hoyer JD, Shanafelt TD, et al: Using smudge cells on routine blood smears to predict clinical outcome in chronic lymphocytic leukemia: a universally available prognostic test, *Mayo Clin Proc* 82:449–453, 2007.

O'Hare T, Eide CA, Deininger MWN, et al: BCR-ABL kinase domain mutations, drug resistance, and the road to a cure for chronic myeloid leukemia, *Blood* 110:2242–2249, 2007.

Preti HA, O'Brien S, Giralt S, et al: Philadelphia-chromosome-positive adult acute lymphocytic leukemia: characteristics, treatment results, and prognosis in 41 patients, *Am J Med* 97:60–65, 1994.

Pui C-H, Behm FG, Crist WM: Clinical and biologic relevance of immunologic marker studies in childhood acute lymphoblastic leukemia, *Blood* 82:343–362, 1993.

Pui CH, Relling MV, Downing JR: Acute lymphoblastic leukemia, *N Engl J Med* 350:1535–1548, 2004.

Robak T, Jamroziak K, Gora-Tybor J, et al: Cladribine in a weekly versus daily schedule for untreated active hairy cell leukemia: final report from the Polish Adult Leukemia Group (PALG) of a prospective, randomized, multicenter trial, *Blood* 109:3672–3675, 2007.

Robertson LE, Pugh W, O'Brien S, et al: Richter's syndrome: a report of 39 patients, *J Clin Oncol* 11:1985–1989, 1993.

Rosenfeld C, Lista A: A hypothesis for the pathogenesis of myelodysplastic syndromes: implications for new techniques, *Leukemia* 14:2–8, 2000.

Rowley JD: Chromosome abnormalities in leukemia, *J Clin Oncol* 6:194–202, 1988.

Rozman C, Montserrat E: Chronic lymphocytic leukemia, *N Engl J Med* 333:1052–1057, 1995.

Rubnitz JE, Look AT: Molecular genetics of childhood leukemias, *J Pediatr Hematol Oncol* 20:1–11, 1998.

Savin A, Piro L: Newer purine analogues for the treatment of hairy-cell leukemia, *N Engl J Med* 330:691–697, 1994.

Sawyers CL: Chronic myeloid leukemia, *N Engl J Med* 340:1330–1340, 1999.

Schlenk RF, Döhner K, Krauter J, et al: Mutations and treatment outcome in cytogenetically normal acute myeloid leukemia, *N Engl J Med* 358:1909–1918, 2008.

Semenzato G, Zambello R, Starkebaum G, et al: The lymphoproliferative disease of granular lymphocytes: updated criteria for diagnosis, *Blood* 89:256–260, 1997.

Shanafelt TD, Geyer SM, Kay NE: Prognosis at diagnosis: integrating molecular biologic insights into clinical practice for patients with CLL, *Blood* 103:1202–1210, 2004.

Skarin AT: Pathology and morphology of chronic leukemias and related disorders. In Wiernik PH, Canellos GP, Kyle RA, et al, editors: *Neoplastic diseases of the blood*, ed 2, New York, 1991, Churchill Livingstone, pp 15–38.

Swerdlow SH, Campo E, Harris NL, et al: WHO Classification of tumours of haematopoietic and lymphoid tissues, 4th ed, IARC: Lyon, 2008.

Tefferi A: Myelofibrosis with myeloid metaplasia, *N Engl J Med* 342:1255–1265, 2000.

Traweek A: Immunophenotypic analysis of acute leukemia, *Am J Clin Pathol* 99:504–512, 1993.

Vannucchi AM, Guglielmelli P, Tefferi A: Advances in understanding and management of myeloproliferative neoplasms, *CA Cancer J Clin* 59:171–191, 2009.

Vardiman JW, Harris NL, Brunning RD: The World Health Organization (WHO) classification of the myeloid neoplasms, *Blood* 100:2292–2302, 2002.

Waldmann T: Human T-cell lymphotropic virus Type I-associated adult T-cell leukemia, *JAMA* 273:735–737, 1995.

Wanko SO, de Castro C: Hairy cell leukemia: An elusive but treatable disease, *Oncologist* 11:780–789, 2006.

Yee KW, O'Brien SM: Chronic lymphocytic leukemia: diagnosis and treatment, *Mayo Clin Proc* 81:1105–1129, 2006.

Figure Credits

The following books published by Gower Medical Publishing are sources of figures in the present chapter. The figure numbers given in the listing are those of the figures in the present chapter. The page numbers given in parentheses are those of the original publication.

Bullough PG, Boachie-Adjei O: *Atlas of spinal diseases*. Philadelphia/New York, 1988, Lippincott/Gower Medical Publishing: Fig. 15.46 (p. 203).

Cawson RA, Eveson JW: *Oral pathology and diagnosis*. London, 1987, Heinemann Medical Books/Gower Medical Publishing: Fig. 15.42 (p. 18.8).

du Vivier A: *Atlas of clinical dermatology*. Edinburgh/London, 1986, Churchill Livingstone/Gower Medical Publishing: Fig. 15.36 (p. 8.16).

Hewitt PE: *Blood diseases (pocket picture guides)*. London, 1985, Gower Medical Publishing: Figs. 15.33 (p. 21), 15.34B (p. 22), 15.53 (p. 27), 15.81B (p. 39).

Hoffbrand AV, Pettit JE: *Clinical haematology illustrated*. Edinburgh/London, 1987, Churchill Livingstone/Gower Medical Publishing: Figs. 15.3 (p. 8.9), 15.4 (p. 8.11), 15.5 (p. 8.11), 15.6 (p. 8.12), 15.7 (p. 8.16), 15.8 (p. 8.9), 15.9 (p. 8.10), 15.10 (p. 8.11), 15.15 (p. 8.7), 15.17 (p. 8.7), 15.18 (p. 8.16), 15.19 (p. 8.8), 15.20 (p. 8.8), 15.21 (p. 8.16), 15.23 (p. 8.8), 15.25 (p. 8.11), 15.26 (p. 8.8), 15.27 (p. 8.11), 15.28 (p. 8.9), 15.29 (p. 8.11), 15.30 (p. 8.9), 15.31 (p. 8.13), 15.32 (p. 8.13), 15.34 (p. 8.6), 15.35 (p. 8.5), 15.40 (p. 8.5), 15.49 (p. 8.2), 15.50 (p. 8.3), 15.51 (p. 8.5), 15.52 (p. 8.5), 15.56 (p. 9.12), 15.57 (p. 9.13), 15.58 (p. 9.13), 15.59 (p. 9.13), 15.60 (9.13), 15.61 (p. 9.13), 15.62 (p. 9.13), 15.63 (p. 9.14), 15.64 (p. 9.14), 15.65 (p. 9.12), 15.66 (p. 9.14), 15.67 (p. 12.11), 15.68 (p. 12.11), 15.69 (p. 12.11), 15.70 (p. 12.11), 15.71 (p. 12.12), 15.73 (p. 9.3), 15.74 (p. 9.3), 15.75 (p. 9.4), 15.76 (p. 9.4), 15.78 (p. 9.4), 15.79 (p. 9.2), 15.81A (p. 9.3), 15.82 (p. 9.3), 15.85 (p. 9.5), 15.86 (p. 1.24), 15.88 (p. 9.5), 15.89 (p. 9.5), 15.90 (p. 9.5), 15.92 (p. 9.6), 15.93 (p. 9.6), 15.94 (p. 9.7), 15.95 (p. 9.7), 15.98 (p. 9.7), 15.100 (p. 9.8), 15.102 (p. 9.9), 15.103 (p. 9.9), 15.108 (p. 9.10), 15.109 (p. 9.8), 15.110 (p. 9.8), 15.111 (p. 9.10).

Weiss MA, Mills SE: *Atlas of genitourinary tract disorders*. Philadelphia/New York, 1988, Lippincott/Gower Medical Publishing: Fig. 15.47 (p. 11.57).

Yanoff M, Fine BS: *Ocular pathology*. Philadelphia/New York, 1988, Lippincott/Gower Medical Publishing: Fig. 15.48 (p. 116).

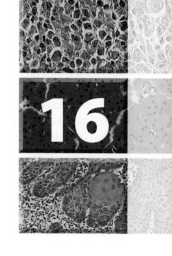

Hodgkin Disease and Non-Hodgkin Lymphomas

16

ERIC JACOBSEN • DAVID M. DORFMAN • ARTHUR T. SKARIN

Hodgkin Disease

About 7400 new cases of Hodgkin disease are diagnosed in the United States each year, with a slightly higher incidence in men. A bimodal age distribution is observed in the Western world, with peaks at 30 and 70 years of age. In Japan, however, this disease is less common in young adults. A bimodal distribution is not seen in underdeveloped countries, suggesting that Hodgkin disease is an uncommon, late complication of a common childhood infection. However, the cause is unknown.

CLASSIFICATION AND IMMUNOBIOLOGY

The histologic features of Hodgkin disease vary widely and may not exhibit the classic criteria for malignancy. Moreover, in about 10% to 15% of cases, recognition of the disorder and its distinction from benign and other malignant lymphoproliferative disorders is difficult. In these cases surface marker studies may be extremely important, and accurate diagnosis may depend on the availability of fresh tissue for evaluation by an experienced hematopathologist.

The first histopathologic classification of Hodgkin disease was established in 1966 by an international conference in Rye, New York, and consists of four subtypes. The subtypes are still included in the new World Health Organization (WHO) classification (see Fig. 16.1). The majority of cells composing a tumor mass appear to be benign or reactive and include lymphocytes, eosinophils, granulocytes, plasma cells, fibroblasts, and mononuclear cells. The pathognomonic finding for the diagnosis is the Reed-Sternberg cell in the appropriate immunoreactive background.

Molecular biologic analysis of micromanipulated Reed-Sternberg cells supports the B lymphocyte as the cell of origin. It is noteworthy that cells morphologically indistinguishable from Reed-Sternberg cells have been found in other hematologic disorders, both benign (e.g., infectious mononucleosis) and malignant (e.g., angioimmunoblastic T-cell lymphoma). Surface marker studies are useful in the differential diagnosis. The immunophenotype of the typical Reed-Sternberg cell is positive for Ki-1 (CD30), CD15 (Leu-M1), HLA-DR, and CD25 (interleukin-2 [IL-2] receptor); it is negative for leukocyte common antigen (LCA) (CD45) and is usually negative for T-cell and B-cell antigens, as well for most monocyte, macrophage, and histiocyte antigens. An exception is lymphocyte-predominant Hodgkin disease in which Reed-Sternberg cells have the immunophenotype of B cells.

The Reed-Sternberg cell is known to secrete a number of cytokines, including interleukin-1 (IL-1), IL-5, IL-6, IL-9, tumor necrosis factor-α, macrophage colony-stimulating factor, and transforming growth factor-β. These cytokines may attract the mixed inflammatory cell infiltrate seen in Hodgkin disease, result in the characteristic fibrosis seen in the nodular sclerosis subtype, and contribute to the immunosuppression that may occur in Hodgkin disease. Epstein-Barr virus (EBV) has been associated with a significant percentage of cases of Hodgkin disease, particularly the mixed-cellularity type, by a number of investigational methods.

CLINICAL EVALUATION AND STAGING

Evaluation of a patient includes a detailed history and physical examination, complete blood cell count with differential, blood chemistries, chest radiograph, computed tomography (CT) scan of the chest, abdomen, and pelvis, and bone marrow aspiration and biopsy. Historically, gallium-67 citrate scanning, using a dose of 10 nCi, with delayed views up to 72 and 96 hours if necessary, could reveal clinically inapparent sites. In addition, gallium scans were useful in the differential diagnosis of residual masses and in following the response to therapy. Increasingly, gallium scanning has been replaced by positron emission tomography (PET). PET is more sensitive than gallium scanning, and the whole study can be accomplished in a matter of hours without the inconvenience of bringing the patient back to the radiology suite for delayed images on subsequent days. As with gallium scans, PET may be useful in evaluating residual masses after chemotherapy, with residual activity on PET scan suggesting residual disease. Staging laparotomy and lymphangiography are of historical interest but have been rendered obsolete by modern imaging techniques and the routine use of chemotherapy as part of the treatment regimen.

In most cases, Hodgkin disease tends to progress in an orderly fashion from one lymph node–bearing area to the next. The results of the staging workup are a part of the Ann Arbor staging system (Fig. 16.13). The mainstay of treatment is chemotherapy. Historically, many patients were treated with radiation therapy alone, but outcomes are generally better when chemotherapy is added. Only rare patients with limited stage I disease or patients who are too elderly or infirm to tolerate chemotherapy are treated with radiation alone. Whether or not radiation is added to chemotherapy depends on the stage of disease, the bulk of disease, and the chemotherapy regimen chosen, among other factors.

CLINICAL MANIFESTATIONS

Most patients present with localized disease. Lymph node enlargement may wax and wane for unknown reasons, although "spontaneous" remissions are rare. About 20% to 30% of cases have B symptoms (fever of >38°C, unexplained weight loss of >10% of body weight in 6 months, and/or night sweats); however, only 5% to 10% of patients present with extranodal sites of disease, including lung, liver, and bone marrow. The latter presentation is more often seen in patients over 60 years of age.

Of note, nodular lymphocyte-predominant Hodgkin disease seems to behave differently than classical Hodgkin disease and more like an indolent lymphoma. For instance, late relapses, even 20 or more years after therapy, and subsequent development of non-Hodgkin lymphoma are much more common with nodular lymphocyte-predominant Hodgkin disease than with classical Hodgkin disease. Whether nodular lymphocyte-predominant Hodgkin disease should be treated differently than classical Hodgkin disease remains a source of controversy.

Hodgkin lymphoma (Hodgkin disease)
Nodular lymphocyte-predominant Hodgkin lymphoma (5%)
Classical Hodgkin lymphoma (95%)
Hodgkin lymphoma, nodular sclerosis (grades I and II)
Classical Hodgkin lymphoma. Lymphocyte rich
Hodgkin lymphoma. Mixed cellularity
Hodgkin lymphoma. Lymphocytic depletion (includes most Hodgkin-like anaplastic large-cell lymphomas)

FIGURE 16.1 **HISTOLOGIC CLASSIFICATION OF HODGKIN DISEASE.** The original classification developed by Jackson and Parker in 1944 was modified by Lukes and colleagues in 1966 into a clinically useful system and simplified in the same year by the Rye classification. This was later modified in the Revised European-American Classification of Lymphoid Neoplasms (REAL) and the current WHO classification listed here (Harris et al., 1999).

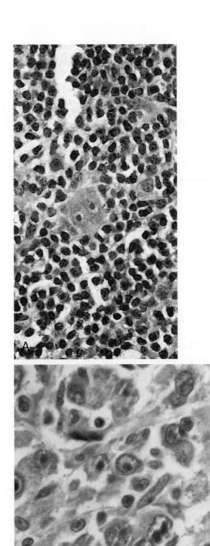

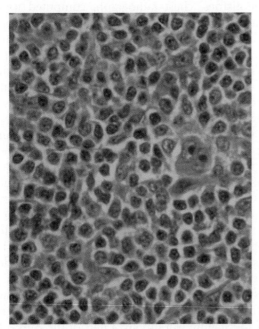

FIGURE 16.2 **HODGKIN DISEASE (LYMPHOCYTE-PREDOMINANT TYPE).** A rare, diagnostic Reed-Sternberg cell is seen *(center)* in a "sea" of lymphocytes. Optimal cytologic detail is obtained by use of B5 fixative, which also preserves cell antigens very well for subsequent immunoperoxidase studies using monoclonal antibodies (MAbs).

FIGURE 16.3 **HODGKIN DISEASE. (A)** Lymph node biopsy specimen shows a single Reed-Sternberg cell surrounded by lymphocytes and other mononuclear cells in lymphocyte-predominant disease. **(B)** In lymphocyte-depleted disease, large numbers of Reed-Sternberg cells and mononuclear variants can typically be seen, but only small numbers of lymphocytes are present.

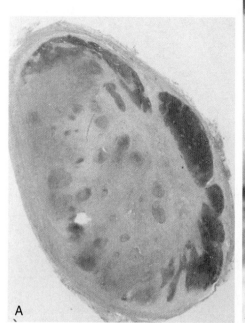

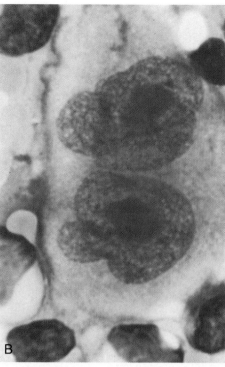

FIGURE 16.4 **HODGKIN DISEASE (NODULAR-SCLEROSIS TYPE). (A)** Low magnification of a lymph node shows aggregates of tumor cells (*blue areas*) surrounded by sclerosing fibrous bands (*eosinophilic or pink areas*). **(B)** Lymph node touch prep reveals a classic Reed-Sternberg cell with a bilobed nucleus and large, round, inclusion-like nucleoli.

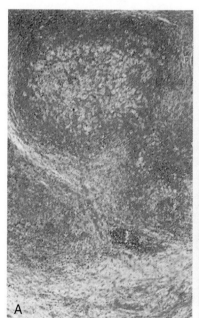

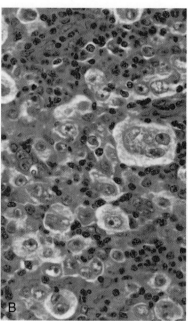

FIGURE 16.5 **HODGKIN DISEASE (NODULAR-SCLEROSIS TYPE). (A)** Gross capsular thickening and fibrous tissue bands divide this lymph node into discrete nodules containing foci of pale "lacunar" cells. **(B)** At high magnification, characteristic "lacunar" cell variants of Reed-Sternberg cells show haloes, representing shrinking of the cells' abundant pale cytoplasm during fixation in formalin.

FIGURE 16.6 **HODGKIN DISEASE (NODULAR-SCLEROSIS TYPE).** **(A)** This lymphoid tumor nodule is surrounded by characteristic sclerosing bands of collagen that are birefringent with polarized light. **(B)** Nodular-sclerosis Hodgkin disease is the only type that is more common in women than men.

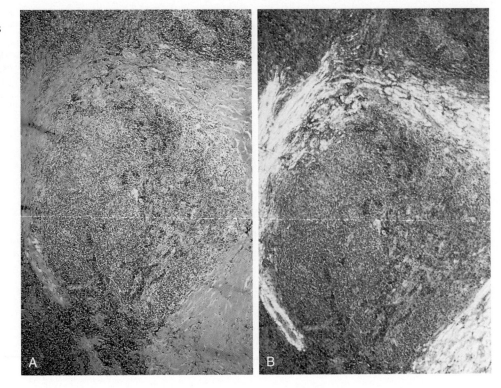

FIGURE 16.7 **HODGKIN DISEASE.** High-power photomicrograph demonstrates a binucleate Reed-Sternberg cell showing prominent inclusion-like eosinophilic nucleoli giving it an "owl's eye" appearance.

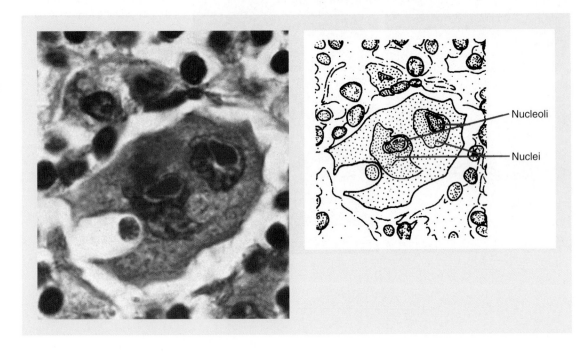

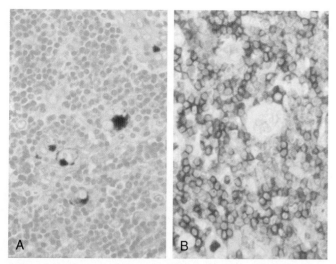

FIGURE 16.8 Hodgkin disease immunoperoxidase staining of Reed-Sternberg cells and variants reveals **(A)** their characteristic immunoreactivity for CD15 (Leu-M1) in a perinuclear localization pattern and **(B)** a lack of reactivity for LCA (CD45); note the strong reactivity of the surrounding lymphocytes. CD15 (Leu-M1) also stains some nonlymphoid tumors (e.g., various adenocarcinomas and papillary thyroid cancer), as well as some NHLs.

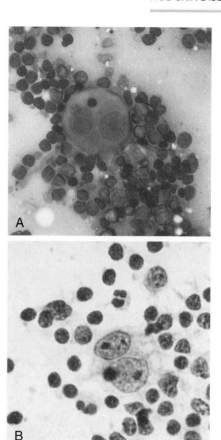

FIGURE 16.10 **HODGKIN DISEASE.** Fine-needle aspiration biopsy specimens of involved lymph nodes demonstrate Reed-Sternberg cells stained **(A)** by May-Grünwald-Giemsa and **(B)** Papanicolaou techniques.

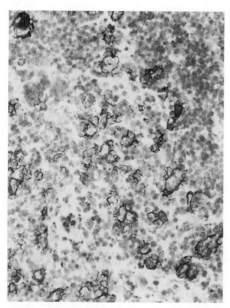

FIGURE 16.9 **HODGKIN DISEASE.** Lymph node biopsy specimen shows a positive reaction for the MAb specific to Ki-1 (CD30), which reacts particularly, but not exclusively, with Reed-Sternberg cells (alkaline phosphatase–anti-alkaline phosphatase). (Courtesy of Prof. H. Stein.)

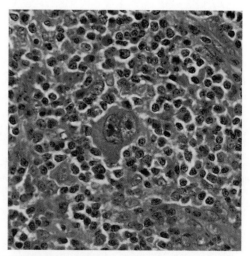

FIGURE 16.11 **HODGKIN DISEASE (MIXED-CELLULARITY TYPE).** The histopathologic features characteristically seen in this type include abundant and readily identifiable Reed-Sternberg cells and variants, which are easily seen in most low-power microscope fields; in this instance, a conspicuous Reed-Sternberg cell is present, showing mirror-image nuclei and prominent nucleoli. This type is also marked by a mixed cellular background—in this case containing sheets of lymphocytes, plasma cells, and eosinophils—and the absence of sclerosing fibrosis.

FIGURE 16.12 HODGKIN DISEASE. Marrow biopsy specimen shows **(A)** Hodgkin tissue replacing normal hematopoietic elements in the *lower right field*. **(B)** On higher-power view, there is extensive replacement of hematopoietic tissue by atypical mononuclear cells in the *center* and *lower fields*. Note the Reed-Sternberg cell (*arrowhead*).

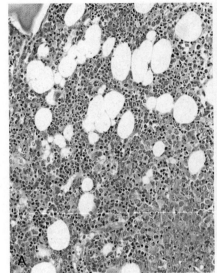
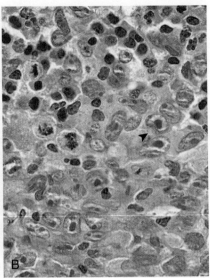

Ann Arbor Staging System for Hodgkin Disease and Non-Hodgkin Lymphomas

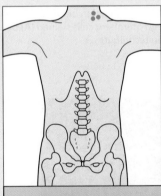
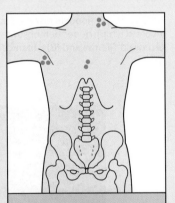
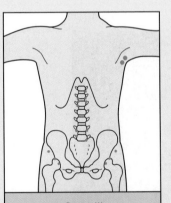
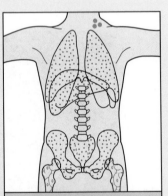

Stage I

- Involvement of single lymph node region
- Or involvement of single extralymphatic site (stage I$_E$)

Stage II

- Involvement of ≥2 lymph node regions on same side of diaphragm
- May include localized extralymphatic involvement on same side of diaphragm (stage II$_E$)

Stage III

- Involvement of lymph node regions on both sides of diaphragm
- May include involvement of spleen (stage III$_S$) or localized extranodal disease (stage III$_E$) or both (III$_{E+S}$)

For Hodgkin disease:

III$_1$
- Disease limited to upper abdomen—spleen, splenic hilar, celiac, or porta hepatis nodes

III$_2$
- Disease limited to lower abdomen—periaortic, pelvic, or inguinal nodes

Stage IV

- Disseminated (multifocal) extralymphatic disease involving one or more organs (e.g., liver, bone marrow, lung, skin), +/– associated lymph node involvement
- Or isolated extralymphatic disease with distant (non-regional) lymph node involvement

FIGURE 16.13   ANN ARBOR STAGING OF HODGKIN DISEASE AND NON-HODGKIN LYMPHOMAS. Lymph node involvement in one area is designated as stage I disease. Involvement of two or more areas confined to one side of the diaphragm constitutes stage II disease. In stage III disease, lymph node areas above and below the diaphragm are affected. The spleen may be involved (stage III$_S$), and this often precedes widespread hematogenous dissemination. In Hodgkin disease, stage III is subdivided into stage III$_1$, for disease limited to the upper abdomen (spleen, and splenic hilar, celiac, or porta hepatis nodes), and III$_2$, for disease involving the lower abdomen (periaortic, pelvic, or inguinal nodes). Stage IV is marked by diffuse extralymphatic disease that may affect, for example, the liver, bone marrow, lungs, and skin. A subscript E in stages I, II, and III disease indicates localized extranodal extension from a nodal mass, and designation of a stage as either A or B indicates the absence (A) or presence (B) of unexplained weight loss >10% of body weight in the preceding 6 months and/or fever of >38°C and/or night sweats.

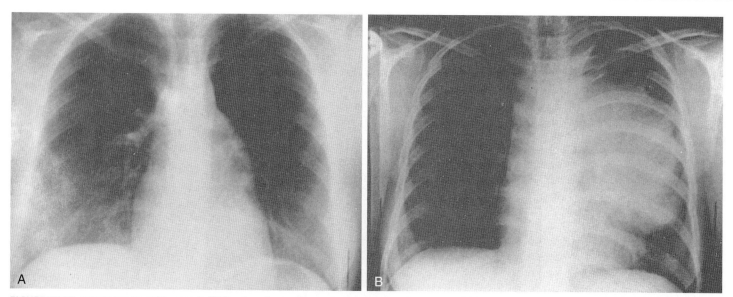

FIGURE 16.14 **HODGKIN DISEASE (STAGE IA$_E$). (A)** Routine chest radiograph of a 24-year-old woman, which was originally read as normal, shows mediastinal widening in the left parahilar region. **(B)** Two years later a huge mass extends to the lateral chest wall, a classic example of the natural history of untreated Hodgkin disease. The patient was cured with chemotherapy and radiation therapy.

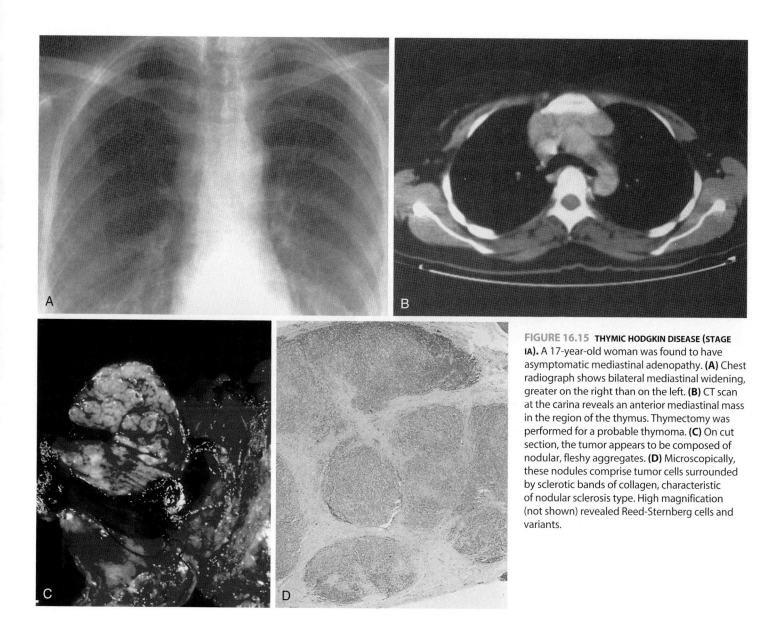

FIGURE 16.15 **THYMIC HODGKIN DISEASE (STAGE IA).** A 17-year-old woman was found to have asymptomatic mediastinal adenopathy. **(A)** Chest radiograph shows bilateral mediastinal widening, greater on the right than on the left. **(B)** CT scan at the carina reveals an anterior mediastinal mass in the region of the thymus. Thymectomy was performed for a probable thymoma. **(C)** On cut section, the tumor appears to be composed of nodular, fleshy aggregates. **(D)** Microscopically, these nodules comprise tumor cells surrounded by sclerotic bands of collagen, characteristic of nodular sclerosis type. High magnification (not shown) revealed Reed-Sternberg cells and variants.

FIGURE 16.16 HODGKIN DISEASE (STAGE IIA$_E$). Endobronchial disease, shown here affecting the left lower bronchus (photographed through a rigid bronchoscope for clarity), is unusual, and patients often present with hemoptysis. (This view is oriented for a bronchoscopist standing in front of the patient.) (Courtesy of Dr. P. Stradling.)

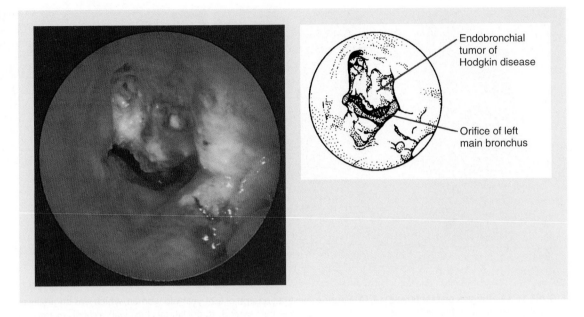

Endobronchial tumor of Hodgkin disease

Orifice of left main bronchus

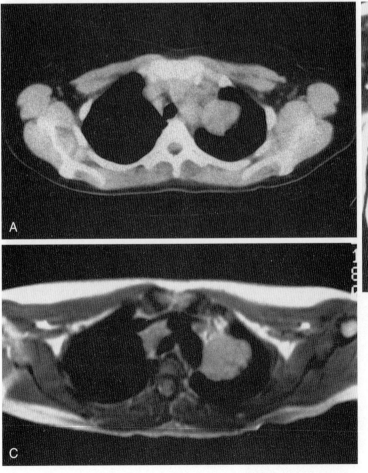

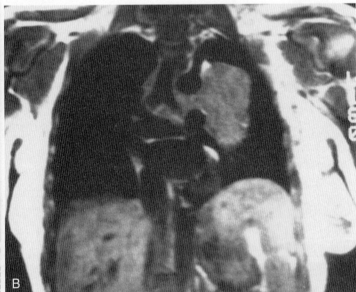

FIGURE 16.17 HODGKIN DISEASE (STAGE IIA). A 19-year-old woman presented with cervical adenopathy. Chest radiography showed a predominantly left-sided mediastinal mass, which appears well delineated **(A)** on CT scan. There is no parenchymal extension. **(B)** T$_1$-weighted magnetic resonance (MR) scan clearly shows the extent of disease in the coronal plane. The mass has the same intensity as muscle. **(C)** T$_2$-weighted image in the axial plane reveals the mass to be almost as intense as fat. This change from lower (muscle) to higher (fat) intensity in the shift from T$_1$- to T$_2$-weighted imaging indicates an active tumor.

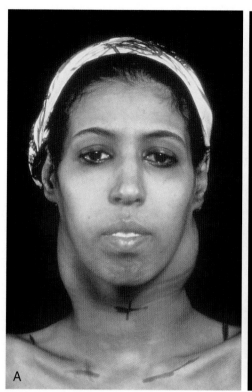
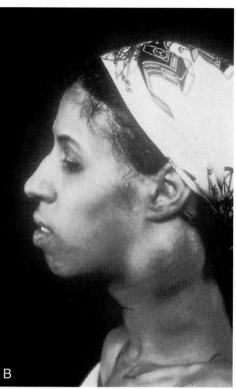

FIGURE 16.18 **HODGKIN DISEASE (STAGE IIA). (A, B)** Marked enlargement of cervical lymph nodes is present in this patient. It is usually painless and may be confined to only one area or may affect two or more areas. A scar from a previous biopsy can be seen on the lateral view.

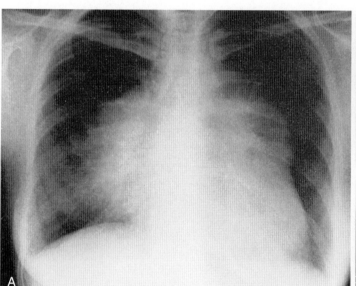
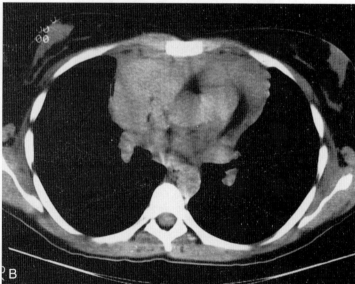
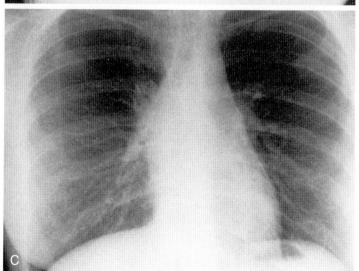

FIGURE 16.19 **HODGKIN DISEASE (STAGE IIA).** A 21-year-old woman presented with cough and chest discomfort. **(A)** Chest film and **(B)** CT scan show bulky mediastinal adenopathy. **(C)** Chest film after treatment shows that the mediastinum is almost normal. Residual widening in the aortopulmonary window is a common finding after treatment and does not necessarily indicate residual tumor. Gallium-67 citrate scan is usually negative unless lymphoma persists.

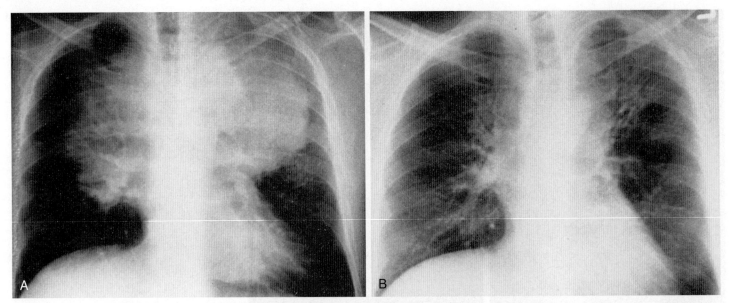

FIGURE 16.20   **HODGKIN DISEASE (STAGE II$_E$). (A)** Chest radiograph of a 30-year-old man who presented with cough and dyspnea shows extensive bilateral, bulky, mediastinal adenopathy with extension into the pulmonary parenchyma of the right lung. **(B)** Marked reduction in tumor mass is noted after combined chemotherapy and radiation therapy.

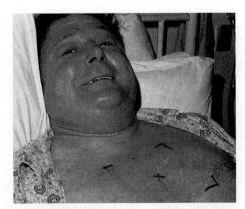

FIGURE 16.21   **HODGKIN DISEASE (STAGE II).** Cyanosis and edema of the face, neck, and upper trunk are due to superior vena cava obstruction caused by mediastinal node involvement (see Fig. 5.49). The skin markings over the anterior chest indicate the field of radiation therapy.

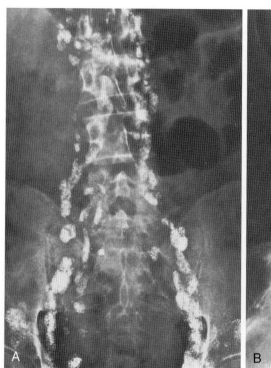
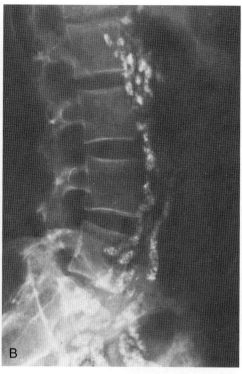

FIGURE 16.22 HODGKIN DISEASE (STAGE IIIA$_2$).
(A, B) Positive nodal-phase lymphangiogram of a 35-year-old man demonstrates enlargement of all the iliac and para-aortic nodes. More important is the alteration in the normal architecture of the nodes, with many small filling defects and a generalized "foamy" appearance. These findings are typical of lymphomatous involvement, confirmed in this case at laparotomy. Lymphangiography has been essentially replaced by CT scanning and in many cases by gallium-67 or PET scanning, which require less time, are highly accurate, and are also useful for follow-up evaluation for residual disease even in normal-sized nodes (see Chapter 2).

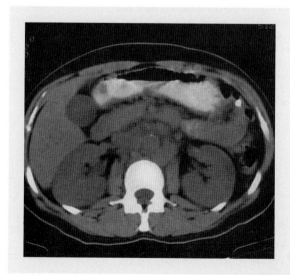
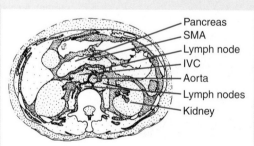

FIGURE 16.23 HODGKIN DISEASE (STAGE IIIB$_2$). A 32-year-old woman presented with fever and night sweats and was found to have left cervical adenopathy. Biopsy showed nodular sclerosis–type Hodgkin disease. This CT scan of the abdomen demonstrates retroperitoneal adenopathy at the level of the renal hilum. Calcification in the wall of the aorta can also be noted. Gallium-67 citrate scan of the abdomen (not shown) was positive in the retroperitoneum, correlating with the CT scan abnormalities. IVC, inferior vena cava.

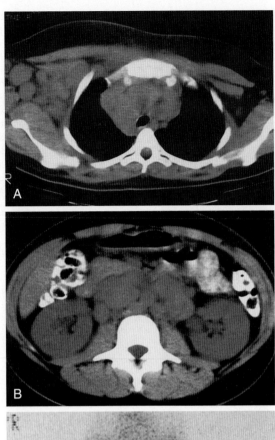

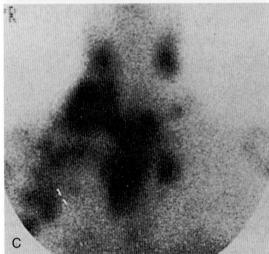

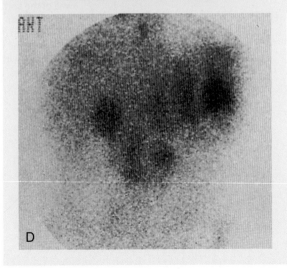

FIGURE 16.24 **HODGKIN DISEASE (STAGE IIIA₂).** A 24-year-old woman presented with cervical and axillary adenopathy. **(A)** CT scan of the chest shows mediastinal disease and also bulky right axillary adenopathy. **(B)** Retroperitoneal adenopathy and a mass at the porta hepatis were also present. An abdominal CT scan (not shown) revealed an enlarged spleen with a heterogeneous texture, consistent with involvement by Hodgkin disease. Images from a gallium-67 citrate scan show uptake **(C)** in the neck bilaterally, right axilla, and mediastinum, and **(D)** in the porta hepatis and spleen. Retroperitoneal and pelvic lymph nodes (not shown) also demonstrated increased uptake. Biopsy revealed the nodular-sclerosis type of Hodgkin disease.

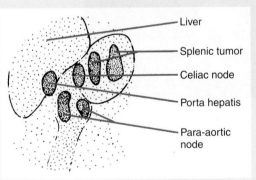

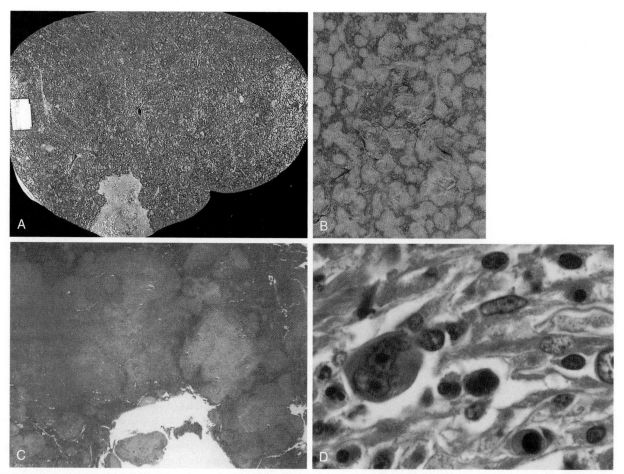

FIGURE 16.25 HODGKIN DISEASE (STAGE III$_S$). (A) Cross-section of a spleen removed at laparotomy shows a single large Hodgkin deposit adjacent to the capsule. Many focal grayish yellow areas, up to 4 mm in diameter, are also scattered throughout the tissue. **(B)** Higher magnification reveals the classic appearance of the spleen in Hodgkin disease (so-called salami spleen), although almost any macroscopic distribution may be seen, as in non-Hodgkin lymphomas. **(C)** The white pulp is expanded and replaced by innumerable irregular, pale deposits of tumor. **(D)** These deposits contain a mixed inflammatory cell infiltrate as well as characteristic Reed-Sternberg cells and variants.

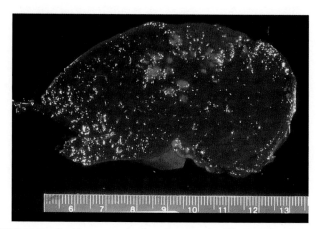

FIGURE 16.26 Another example of a spleen involved by Hodgkin disease, removed during a staging laparotomy. The scattered macroscopic nodules seen were not detected by a prior CT scan (not shown).

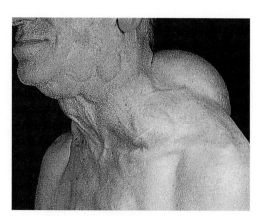

FIGURE 16.27 HODGKIN DISEASE (STAGE IV). Massive cervical and suboccipital lymphadenopathy is seen in a 73-year-old man who presented with stage IV$_B$ disease.

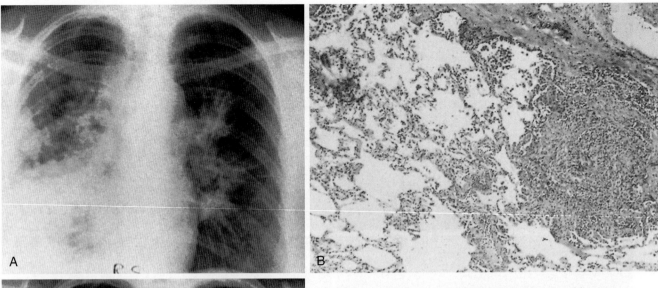

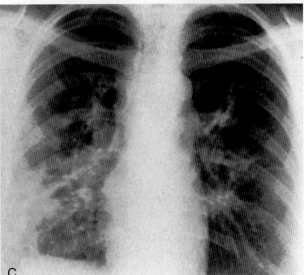

FIGURE 16.28 **HODGKIN DISEASE (STAGE IVB).** A 25-year-old woman presented with weight loss, fever, and night sweats and was found to have cervical and axillary adenopathy. **(A)** Chest radiograph shows bilateral pulmonary infiltrates, consistent with involvement with Hodgkin disease. **(B)** Lung biopsy confirms earlier lymph node biopsy findings, which were positive for Hodgkin disease, mixed-cellularity type. CT scan (not shown) demonstrated hepatosplenomegaly. She was treated with chemotherapy and showed a clinically complete response. **(C)** Chest radiograph demonstrates residual pulmonary scarring 2 months later. A new mediastinal mass developed 3 years afterward and responded to radiation therapy. Seven years later, because of fever and anemia, a bone marrow biopsy was obtained, showing involvement by Hodgkin disease. Once again she responded to chemotherapy but died 6 years later from recurrent Hodgkin disease. Although most relapses occur within 4 years of therapy, rare late relapses beyond 10 years have been reported, as in this patient who died 16 years after the initial diagnosis.

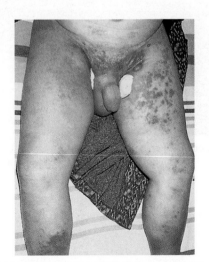

FIGURE 16.29 **HODGKIN DISEASE (STAGE IV).** Gross edema of the legs, genitals, and lower abdominal wall (with umbilical herniation) is due to lymphatic obstruction resulting from extensive involvement of the inguinal and pelvic lymph nodes. There is a staphylococcal infection in the skin folds of the groins.

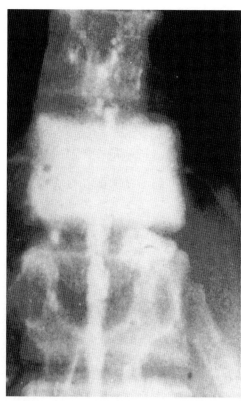

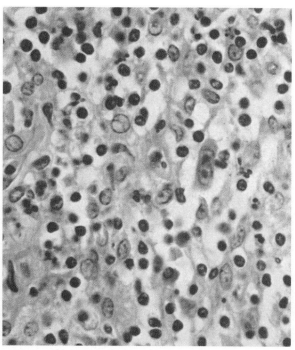

FIGURE 16.31 **HODGKIN DISEASE (STAGE IV).** Photomicrograph of an area of Hodgkin disease in bone shows a fibrous stroma with a mixed cellular infiltrate of small round cells, larger histiocytes, and a diagnostic Reed-Sternberg cell near the center.

FIGURE 16.30 **HODGKIN DISEASE (STAGE IV).** This radiograph of the thoracic spine in a 35-year-old man who presented with vague back pain shows a single, dense, sclerotic ("ivory") vertebra, which on biopsy proved to be involved by Hodgkin disease. Bone involvement manifests with considerable marrow fibrosis and reactive bone formation, which may be extensive enough to obscure the lymphomatous tissue.

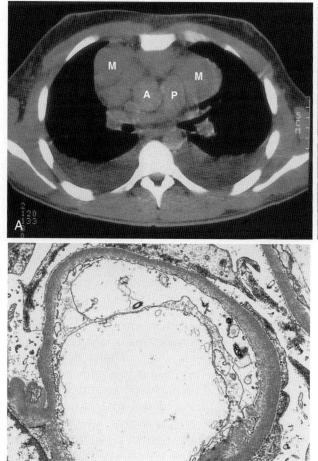

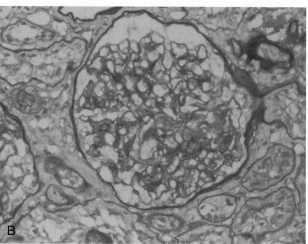

FIGURE 16.32 **HODGKIN DISEASE (NEPHROTIC SYNDROME).** An 18-year-old man presented with classic features of nephrotic syndrome including facial edema, ascites, and peripheral edema. Cervical adenopathy was present, and lymph node biopsy showed nodular sclerosis–type Hodgkin disease. **(A)** Axial CT image at the level of the main pulmonary artery, without intravenous contrast, shows a large, lobular mass (M) extending to the right and left of the great vessels anteriorly. Bilateral pleural effusions (*arrows*) are present. A, ascending aorta; P, main pulmonary artery. **(B)** Renal biopsy shows glomeruli with open capillary loops and thin, delicate basement membranes (light microscopy, high power). **(C)** Electron microscopy reveals extensive effacement of podocyte foot processes diagnostic of minimal-change disease (lipoid nephrosis). Nephrotic syndrome associated with Hodgkin disease is rare, with under 50 reported cases. Pathogenesis of nephrotic syndrome is unknown but includes immune complex deposition, abnormalities of T-cell function, viral antigens, tumor antigens, and fetal antigen expression (Dabbs et al., 1986). (**C**, Courtesy of Dr. F.S. Lee and Dr. A. Krishnan.)

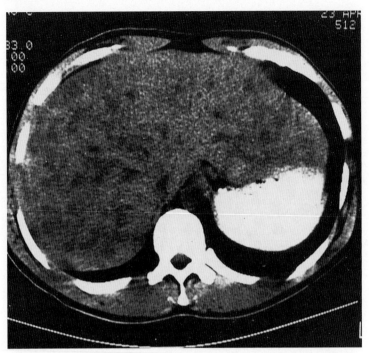

FIGURE 16.33 HODGKIN DISEASE (RELAPSE). A 26-year-old man presented with stage IA disease (mixed-cellularity type) and was treated by radiation therapy. Relapse occurred at multiple nodal sites within 2 years, followed 3 years later by liver involvement, as seen in this non–contrast-enhanced CT scan. The liver shows diffuse areas of low attenuation, consistent with infiltration by Hodgkin disease.

FIGURE 16.34 HODGKIN DISEASE (RELAPSE). Depressed cell-mediated immunity in Hodgkin disease is associated with an increased incidence of infections, particularly herpes zoster, as seen here represented by **(A)** a vesicular cutaneous eruption of the neck and **(B)** an atypical herpetic eruption on the palmar surface of the hand in a patient who relapsed after primary radiation therapy. Lymphopenia, particularly with depression of the CD4/CD8 T-cell ratio secondary to radiation therapy, may further contribute to increased infections.

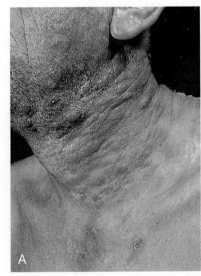

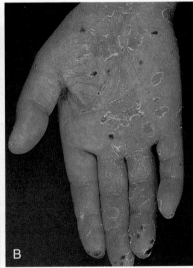

Non-Hodgkin Lymphoma

Non-Hodgkin lymphomas (NHLs) are a diverse group of malignancies of the lymphoreticular system that have heterogeneous histopathologic, immunologic, cytogenetic, and clinical characteristics. About 55,000 new cases are diagnosed in the United States each year, and the incidence is rising. Although the disease can appear at any age, the median age is 67 years and the incidence increases with age. Indolent NHLs are particularly rare in children. NHL is slightly more prevalent in men than in women. Although the etiology is unknown, malignant lymphomas are more common in patients with immune deficiency syndromes (e.g., acquired hypogammaglobulinemia), autoimmune disorders (e.g., rheumatoid arthritis), immunosuppressive states (e.g., renal transplants), chronic hepatitis B and C, and AIDS. In AIDS patients, for example, 5% to 10% develop intermediate- to high-grade B-cell NHLs, and these are included as part of the Centers for Disease Control and Prevention (CDC) AIDS diagnosis criteria. EBV has been observed in a significant percentage of AIDS-associated lymphomas and seems to have an etiologic role in their pathogenesis (see Chapter 19). The African form of Burkitt lymphoma is associated with EBV infection as well. A form of aggressive T-cell leukemia-lymphoma associated with human T-cell lymphoma-leukemia virus (HTLV-1) infection has been reported in southern Japan, the Caribbean, and the southeastern United States. Genetic factors may also predispose to lymphomas, as evidenced by cases in patients with chromosomal disorders (e.g., ataxia-telangiectasia) and those with immunodeficiency disorders other than AIDS.

CLASSIFICATION AND IMMUNOBIOLOGY

Histopathologic classifications and frequency of NHL subsets are shown in Figure 16.35 and Tables 16.1 and 16.8. The "working formulation" classification (see Fig. 16.35), devised by an international panel of clinicians and pathologists sponsored by the National Cancer Institute (NCI), retained the relevant features of the previous Rappaport system and divided lymphomas into 10 separate subgroups (A to J) and three major prognostic categories. These classification schemes have been replaced by the WHO classification of lymphoid neoplasms based on morphologic, immunophenotypic, and cytogenetic features (Harris et al., 1999). Broadly the WHO classification identifies two subsets of lymphoid neoplasms: B-cell and T/NK (natural killer)-cell neoplasms. The B and T/NK subgroups are then further subclassified as precursor or mature neoplasms. Clinically, the histologies can be considered in three broad categories—indolent, aggressive, and highly aggressive—based upon the natural history of the disease.

A considerable understanding of the immunology of lymphomas has been achieved by the availability of specific monoclonal antibodies (MAbs) directed against cell surface antigens (see Figs. 16.37 and 16.38 and Table 16.5). It has been found that the malignant cells of most lymphomas have normal cell counterparts. By use of an extensive panel of MAbs, about 90% of lymphomas can be identified as B-cell lymphomas and 10% as T-cell lymphomas. With modern immunohistochemical and genetic techniques, what were once thought to be true "histiocytic" lymphomas are now recognized as B- or T-cell neoplasms in most cases or true histiocytic disorders such as histiocytic sarcoma in others.

Most lymphomas express LCA (CD45), which is detectable by immunoperoxidase staining using MAbs specific to LCA; LCA staining is very useful because it is immunoreactive (positive) even in poorly differentiated lymphomas that might otherwise be mistaken for carcinoma, sarcoma, or melanoma, all of which are LCA-negative. Furthermore, LCA staining can be performed on formalin- and B5-fixed tissues. (The latter is preferred because of better histologic detail, particularly of the cell nucleus.) Cell lineage as determined by the use of MAbs usually requires fresh tissue. The monoclonality of B-cell lymphomas can be confirmed by immunoperoxidase staining for one class of immunoglobulin light chain or by immunoglobulin gene rearrangement studies. T-cell lymphomas, on the other hand, do not express cell surface immunoglobulins, but many show clonal loss of expression of pan–T-cell antigens, which can be tested using MAbs. Gene rearrangement studies of the T-cell receptor may also be used to determine monoclonality, although lack of monoclonality does not exclude the diagnosis of lymphoma. Lymphomas of T-cell lineage can also be identified by the formation of so-called "rosettes" on reaction with sheep erythrocytes. T-cell phenotyping is carried out by reaction with available MAbs (see Fig. 16.38).

Many chromosomal, molecular, and genetic defects have been detected in various lymphomas. These are described in the section on lymphoma subsets (see below). A better understanding of the biology of lymphomas allows for clarification of the pathogenesis and also for future novel therapeutic approaches.

Amplification of DNA can now be performed on small amounts of tissue by the polymerase chain reaction technique, thus allowing for detection of abnormal clones (i.e., monoclonal population of malignant cells). The method is extremely sensitive and may detect residual tumor or early disease relapse.

Histologic Subtypes

Immunophenotypic and other classification markers are noted in Figures 16.37 to 16.40 and Table 16.5.

B-Cell Non-Hodgkin Lymphomas

B-CELL CHRONIC LYMPHOCYTIC LEUKEMIA/SMALL LYMPHOCYTIC LYMPHOMA

This subtype of NHL is a generally indolent lymphoma with a favorable prognosis. The tumor is characterized by a diffuse pattern of growth with effacement of nodal architecture by round lymphocytes of small to medium size. Mitotic figures are rare. In a minority of cases there may be plasmacytic differentiation with associated macroglobulinemia. Small lymphocytic lymphoma (SLL) and chronic lymphocytic leukemia (CLL) probably represent different clinical manifestations of the same disease process, the former marked mainly by adenopathy and the latter by lymphocytosis involving the bone marrow and peripheral blood.

Until recently, identifying cytogenetic abnormalities in SLL/CLL cells was difficult. With modern cytogenetic techniques and fluorescence in situ hybridization, however, chromosomal abnormalities can be detected in 70% to 80% of SLL/CLL cells (Sanchez et al., 2007). These abnormalities can give insight into the pathogenesis of the disease and are also useful in predicting clinical behavior. Deletion of 17p and 11q seem to predict more aggressive disease, whereas deletion of 13q predicts a more indolent course. Normal cytogenetics and trisomy 12 predict an intermediate course. Other factors, such as increased expression of CD38, increased expression of ZAP-70 (Del Giudice et al., 2005), deletion of the p53 gene, and an unmutated immunoglobulin heavy-chain gene also can predict a more aggressive clinical course (Oscier et al., 2002). None of these markers, however, is perfect, and the interplay of the various prognostic markers is complex. Thus, the clinical management of the patient is still dictated by the behavior of the disease and the presence or absence of disease-related side effects.

LYMPHOPLASMACYTIC LYMPHOMA

Lymphoplasmacytic lymphoma (LPL) is a rare B-cell neoplasm composed of a diffuse proliferation of small B lymphocytes, plasmacytoid lymphocytes, and plasma cells. Frequently the disease is associated with an IgM monoclonal gammopathy. The combination of lymphoplasmacytic lymphoma with an IgM monoclonal gammopathy is termed Waldenstrom's macroglobulinemia. Accumulation of IgM in the cytoplasm of LPL cells results in characteristic Dutcher bodies. LPL is generally an indolent disease, although high levels of IgM can cause hyperviscosity syndrome resulting in headache, epistaxis, visual changes, and coma necessitating plasmapheresis to remove the antibody and chemotherapy to debulk the disease and decrease antibody production.

MANTLE CELL LYMPHOMA

Mantle cell lymphoma is uncommon, accounting for only 3% to 4% of all cases of NHL. It is composed of small lymphocytes with intermediate-sized nuclei. The lymphoma appears to arise from B lymphocytes found in the mantle zone of lymphoid follicles. The histologic pattern of mantle cell lymphoma may be nodular, with neoplastic cells surrounding residual germinal centers (mantle zone pattern), or diffuse. Seventy percent or more of cases show a t(11;14) chromosomal translocation involving the BCL1 locus on chromosome 11, resulting in overexpression of the PRAD1 gene, the product of which, cyclin D1, is involved in cell cycle regulation. Also, over 70% of cases will show nuclear staining for cyclin D1. Expression of cyclin D1 can occur even in cases with no detectable t(11;14). Mantle cell lymphoma typically pursues an aggressive course with a median survival of 3–4 years, although rare cases do behave in an indolent fashion similar to CLL/SLL. The blastoid variant in particular can be very aggressive and can present with spontaneous splenic rupture. Mantle cell lymphoma has a predilection for the gastrointestinal (GI) tract with involvement in 15% to 30% of cases.

FOLLICULAR LYMPHOMA

Follicular lymphoma is the second most common B-cell NHL, accounting for approximately 35% of all cases. Follicular lymphoma is composed of both small centrocytes (cleaved follicle center cells) and large centroblasts (noncleaved follicle center cells). Follicular lymphoma is assigned a grade based upon the percentage of centroblasts present. Follicular lymphoma is classified as grade I when there are 5 or fewer centroblasts per high-power field (HPF), grade II when there are 6 to 15 centroblasts per HPF, and grade III when there are more than 15 centroblasts per HPF.

Most cases of follicular lymphoma exhibit a t(14;18) chromosomal translocation, which results in deregulation of expression of the BCL2 proto-oncogene on chromosome 18. This gene blocks programmed cell death (apoptosis), and its overexpression results in prolongation of the lifespan of involved cells, contributing to the pathogenesis of lymphoma. Of note, approximately 20% of diffuse large B-cell NHLs show the t(14;18) translocation, and therefore this translocation is not pathognomonic of follicular lymphoma.

MARGINAL ZONE LYMPHOMA (NODAL AND EXTRANODAL)

This low-grade B-cell NHL tends to involve lymph node sinuses and interfollicular zones and to surround follicles in a marginal zone pattern. Monocytoid B cells have small nuclei with irregular outlines and fairly abundant pale cytoplasm and may involve bone marrow and extranodal sites such as the salivary gland, with an indolent clinical course. The normal cellular counterpart of marginal zone lymphomas may be the marginal zone cells in the spleen. Though similar in appearance to hairy cell leukemia cells, marginal zone B-cell neoplasms are CD103-negative, whereas hairy cells are usually CD103-positive.

There are several important subtypes of marginal zone lymphoma. One is splenic marginal zone lymphoma with villous lymphocytes. Patients tend to present with left upper quadrant pain and early satiety from splenomegaly. Bone marrow involvement is common, but these patients tend to have comparatively little lymph node involvement. Splenectomy is often an effective palliative therapy and can result in regression of disease in other sites. Chemotherapy or immunotherapy is sometimes needed, although the disease tends to be indolent. Splenic marginal zone lymphoma with villous lymphocytes is associated with infection with viral hepatitis, and treating the hepatitis can lead to improvement in or resolution of the lymphoma.

Extranodal marginal zone lymphoma, also known as MALToma because it involves mucosa-associated lymphoid tissue, can occur at any number of mucosal sites and is notable for its association with certain underlying medical conditions. A common site of involvement is the stomach, where there is a strong association with Helicobacter pylori infection. This is discussed in more detail below. Extranodal marginal zone lymphomas of the eye have been associated with Sjögren syndrome and infection with certain strains of Chlamydia, whereas marginal zone lymphomas of the skin have been associated with infection with certain Borrelia species. Although there are reports of antibiotics being effective in treating marginal zone lymphomas occurring in these sites, the data are not as compelling as they are in gastric extranodal marginal zone lymphoma.

DIFFUSE LARGE B-CELL LYMPHOMA

Diffuse large B-cell lymphoma (DLBCL) is the most common NHL, accounting for approximately 40% of all cases of NHL. DLBCL follows an aggressive clinical course, and patients frequently present with rapidly enlarging lymphadenopathy and/or B symptoms such as fever, night sweats, and unintentional weight loss. The tumor is composed of large cells with prominent nucleoli. Notably, benign, reactive histiocytes are present in many cases of DLBCL.

There are several morphologic variants of DLBCL including the immunoblastic and centroblastic variants, although none of the variants have meaningful prognostic or treatment implications. T-cell/histiocyte-rich DLBCL can be easily confused with T-cell NHL or even Hodgkin disease. The distinction is important, since Hodgkin disease and T-cell NHL are treated much differently than DLBCL. This variant often presents in younger patients with disproportionate involvement of the bone marrow, spleen, and liver. At one time, T-cell/histiocyte-rich DLBCL was thought to have a worse prognosis than other DLBCLs, but when controlling for the International Prognostic Index (IPI) this no longer seems to be the case. The anaplastic variant of DLBCL can express CD30 and can also be easily confused with Hodgkin disease, especially since Hodgkin disease can express B-cell markers. Anaplastic DLBCL can also be confused with T/null anaplastic large cell lymphoma, another CD30$^+$ neoplasm, although the two entities can easily be distinguished based upon CD20 staining and the lack of anaplastic lymphoma kinase (ALK) in anaplastic DLBCL.

Modern methods of treatment and the addition of MAbs to conventional chemotherapy have markedly improved the rate of survival of patients with these tumors, with approximately 50% to 60% of cases cured at present.

MEDIASTINAL DIFFUSE LARGE B-CELL LYMPHOMA

This variant in DLBCL presents with bulky mediastinal lymphadenopathy, often with relatively little disease in other areas. Mediastinal DLBCL tends to present in young patients with a slight female predominance and can mimic Hodgkin disease clinically and morphologically. Superior vena cava (SVC) syndrome is a common presentation. Although the disease has a tendency to relapse in unusual extranodal sites such as the kidney, GI tract, and ovaries, it does have a favorable prognosis when treated with combination chemotherapy often in conjunction with radiation.

FOLLICULAR LYMPHOMA, GRADE III

Grade III follicular lymphoma (>15 centroblasts/HPF) is classified as an aggressive lymphoma, since its behavior and treatment mirror that of DLBCL.

BURKITT LYMPHOMA AND BURKITT-LIKE LYMPHOMA

Small non–cleaved cell lymphomas have a characteristic cytogenetic finding, t(8;14), which occurs in about 80% of cases of Burkitt type. The c-MYC proto-oncogene on chromosome 8, thought to have a role in repressing differentiation and stimulating proliferation of cells, becomes constitutively expressed when it relocates to the immunoglobulin heavy-chain locus on chromosome 14, with reciprocal relocation of the heavy-chain gene locus to the c-MYC locus on chromosome 8. Variant translocations t(2;8) and t(8;22) involving immunoglobulin light-chain loci can be detected in the remaining 20% of cases. Classic Burkitt lymphoma is marked by small to medium-sized malignant cells having one to several distinct nucleoli, basophilic cytoplasm, and characteristic vacuoles. It is most commonly seen in pediatric patients. In Africa, patients classically present with large tumor masses of the maxilla or mandible, whereas in the United States a rapidly expanding abdominal mass is the usual presentation, occasionally accompanied by central nervous system (CNS) or bone marrow involvement.

Burkitt-like lymphoma exhibits greater cell pleomorphism than classic Burkitt lymphoma. It is composed of small to intermediate-sized immature lymphoid cells with basophilic cytoplasm and several distinct nucleoli. In patients who have undergone treatment for Hodgkin disease and in those with AIDS, this is the most common type of lymphoma occurring as a complicating factor. Unlike Burkitt lymphomas, c-MYC gene rearrangements usually do not occur in this subtype. Both Burkitt lymphoma and Burkitt-like lymphoma have a proliferation fraction (e.g., based on Ki-67 staining) close to 100%.

PRECURSOR B-LYMPHOBLASTIC LEUKEMIA/LYMPHOMA

More common in children than adults, this disease is morphologically identical to B-cell acute lymphoblastic leukemia, and the distinction between the two is arbitrary. Lymphadenopathy is common, as is skin involvement. This disease is associated with t(9;22), which becomes progressively more common with increasing age of incidence and which is associated with a poor prognosis.

T-Cell Non-Hodgkin Lymphomas

Anaplastic Large Cell Lymphoma, T/Null Type

This distinct clinicopathologic entity, usually T-cell or null cell in phenotype, expresses CD30 (Ki-1) and, in the systemic form, is associated with a t(2;5) chromosome translocation and expression of the ALK protein. Cases of anaplastic large cell lymphoma, T/null type (ALCL) with a cutaneous presentation may be a different entity, inasmuch as they lack the t(2;5) mutation and ALK protein expression and have a clinically indolent course. It is of interest to note that the Ki-1 (CD30) antigen is also expressed on Reed-Sternberg cells in Hodgkin disease, as well as on activated B and T cells. The classic-type ALCL is characterized by a preferential perifollicular involvement of the lymph node, with sinusoidal and subcapsular infiltration. Two peaks in the age distribution have been observed—a large peak in the second to third decades and a smaller peak in the sixth to seventh decades. The disease is rapidly progressive and usually involves lymph nodes, skin, and visceral sites. ALCL may be confused with metastatic carcinoma or Hodgkin disease. The differential diagnosis, using MAbs, of several entities with similar clinical presentations is shown in Table 16.9.

PERIPHERAL T-CELL LYMPHOMA, NOT OTHERWISE SPECIFIED

This is the most common subtype of T-cell lymphoma. The tumor may express CD2, CD3, CD5, and/or CD7. CD4 is more commonly expressed than CD8. There is no characteristic cytogenetic finding, although cytogenetic abnormalities involving chromosomes 7 and 14 are common. Treatment is with combination chemotherapy as with aggressive B-cell lymphomas, although the long-term survival rate is lower.

ANGIOIMMUNOBLASTIC T-CELL LYMPHOMA

This lymphoma typically presents in older patients with a rapid onset of B symptoms (fever, night sweats, weight loss) along with a skin rash. There is a high incidence of extranodal involvement including the liver, spleen, and bone marrow. There is some heterogeneity in the disease course, however, with some patients having very indolent disease and occasionally spontaneous remissions. Concomitant immunologic problems are common, resulting in the angioimmunoblastic lymphoma with dysproteinemia syndrome with polyclonal gammopathy and such problems as autoimmune arthritis or autoimmune hemolytic anemia with a positive Coombs test. In most patients this disease is rapidly fatal, with a median survival of 12–18 months.

EXTRANODAL NK/T-CELL LYMPHOMA, NASAL TYPE

Formerly known by the less appealing "lethal midline granuloma" and also angiocentric lymphoma, this disease is most common in Asian males and is usually EBV-positive. The tumor cells often express the NK-cell marker CD56 in addition to T-cell markers. The outcome for localized disease is quite good with radiation therapy alone, but patients with disseminated disease often respond poorly to chemotherapy.

ENTEROPATHY-TYPE T-CELL LYMPHOMA

This type of T-cell lymphoma is almost always seen in the setting of celiac sprue, although the tumor cells themselves have no characteristic cytogenetic or molecular abnormality. Enteropathy-type T-cell lymphoma can present as an initial manifestation of sprue but more typically presents in patients with long-standing noncompliance with a gluten-free diet or as a sudden worsening of previously well-controlled celiac sprue. Following a gluten-free diet is extremely effective in preventing the disease but not in treating it. This is a very aggressive entity with few long-term survivors even with aggressive combination chemotherapy. Intestinal perforation and/or obstruction are common, especially in advanced disease.

SUBCUTANEOUS PANNLITIS-LIKEICU T-CELL LYMPHOMA

This is a rare lymphoma that often presents with multiple subcutaneous nodules. Since the initial course can be indolent, the disease is often misdiagnosed as benign panniculitis. Unfortunately, the disease almost invariably becomes rapidly progressive and in its later stages does not respond well to chemotherapy. For some unknown reason there is a high incidence of hemophagocytic syndrome associated with this type of T-cell lymphoma.

HEPATOSPLENIC GAMMA DELTA T-CELL LYMPHOMA

This extremely rare disease typically presents with rapid onset of hepatosplenomegaly in young males. Bone marrow involvement is common, but lymphadenopathy is generally not prominent. The neoplastic cells express the usual T-cell antigens but not the alpha beta T-cell receptor that predominates in most other forms of T-cell lymphoma. Hepatosplenic gamma delta T-cell lymphoma is extremely aggressive, and few patients survive even with aggressive chemotherapy and/or hematopoietic stem cell transplantation. A rare alpha beta variant also exists.

PRECURSOR T-LYMPHOBLASTIC LEUKEMIA/LYMPHOMA

Common in children, particularly boys, and in young adults, precursor T-lymphoblastic lymphoma is a high-grade, immature T-cell lymphoma that is usually associated with a prominent mediastinal mass and often with SVC syndrome. It is the counterpart of childhood T-cell acute lymphoblastic leukemia, and patients in both groups are at high risk for CNS involvement. Morphologically, the malignant cells are small and uniform in appearance, showing scanty cytoplasm and indistinct nucleoli. Characteristic nuclear convolutions are usually present; mitoses are frequent.

ADULT T-CELL LYMPHOMA-LEUKEMIA

This unusual T-cell malignancy is composed of neoplastic lymphoid cells of various sizes, having irregular nuclei, some containing nucleoli, often with marked convolutions of the nuclear contours. Lymph node biopsy characteristically shows a leukemic pattern of infiltration. Seen predominantly in Japan and in blacks of the West Indies, the Caribbean nations, and the southeastern United States, adult T-cell lymphoma-leukemia (ATLL) typically shows rapid progression, with early involvement of lymph nodes, skin, bone, blood, and bone marrow. Hypercalcemia often develops. The lung, liver, GI tract, and CNS may also be involved. The disease is caused by a C-type RNA retrovirus known as HTLV-1, infection with which often occurs many decades before the development of ATLL.

MISCELLANEOUS LYMPHOMAS

Extranodal Lymphomas

NHLs often secondarily invade visceral sites, resulting in stage IV disease. Primary involvement of extranodal sites is less common, occurring in up to 25% of cases. Extranodal lymphomas may arise in almost any site, particularly the skin, thyroid, orbit, Waldeyer's ring, CNS, lung, GI tract, reproductive organs, breast, stomach, and kidneys. The vast majority of these cases respond to combination chemotherapy, with or without local radiation therapy.

Lymphoma of the Breast

Primary lymphomas of the breast, which are rare, may present as an expanding breast mass, clinically simulating breast carcinoma. Therefore, biopsy specimens must be carefully examined, with the use of surface marker studies when possible, to avoid an unnecessary mastectomy. Most lymphomas of the breast are derived from B cells and are DLCL or marginal zone lymphoma, although rare cases of follicular lymphoma and other types have been reported. For reasons that remain unclear, patients with primary DLBCL of the breast are at increased risk for involvement of the CNS and must receive intrathecal chemotherapy or other chemotherapeutic prophylaxis to prevent the development of CNS disease.

LYMPHOMA OF THE TESTICLE

Most lymphomas of the testicle are high-grade lesions—DLBCL, lymphoblastic lymphoma, or Burkitt lymphoma. Involvement of the testicle with DLBCL is a risk factor for involvement of the CNS, and these patients must receive intrathecal chemotherapy or other chemotherapeutic prophylaxis to prevent the development of CNS disease. Also, because the blood-testis barrier can prevent chemotherapy from effectively penetrating

into testicular tissue, these patients often receive adjuvant irradiation to the contralateral testicle.

LYMPHOMA OF THE GASTROINTESTINAL TRACT

The GI tract is the most common site of primary extranodal lymphoma, which accounts for approximately 2% of GI neoplasms and most commonly involves the stomach followed by the small intestine and then the colon. Approximately 5% of gastric neoplasms are malignant lymphomas, the majority of which are DLBCL. They most commonly occur in middle or late adulthood, typically arising in the body of the stomach; they are often large and diffuse or may appear as nodular masses. Direct spread to the liver or spleen, as well as dissemination to other areas, occasionally occurs. Gastric lymphomas carry a better prognosis than gastric carcinomas; the 5-year survival rate is approximately 50% for all stages.

Extranodal marginal zone lymphomas of MALT account for a significant percentage of GI lymphomas and also occur in several other extranodal sites that normally contain MALT, including breast, lung, head, and neck areas, including the thyroid, and the urogenital tract. It may be low grade or high grade. Low-grade MALT lymphoma is composed of small B cells with round to irregular nuclear outlines, notable cytoplasm, associated plasma cells, and a tendency to invade epithelium, resulting in characteristic lymphoepithelial lesions. Tumor cells are immunoreactive for pan-B-cell markers (e.g., CD20) but not CD5, seen in other low-grade B-cell lymphomas, or CD10, seen in follicular center cell lymphomas. Low-grade MALT lymphomas tend not to disseminate widely, and surgical excision results in an excellent long-term prognosis. Of note, NHL (particularly low-grade MALT type) affecting the stomach but not other sites is associated with previous *H. pylori* infection (Parsonnet et al., 1994). Despite lymphoma regression with therapy for *H. pylori*, the causative role, while plausible, still remains unproven (Isaacson, 1994).

LYMPHOMA OF THE KIDNEY

Although primary renal lymphoma is rare, about 5% to 10% of patients with disseminated lymphoma show clinically detectable renal involvement and up to 50% of cases reveal renal lesions at autopsy. High-grade lymphomas are most commonly encountered, particularly Burkitt lymphoma. Occasionally patients present with renal failure due to infiltration of the kidney by lymphoma cells, with resultant bilateral enlargement.

INTRAVASCULAR LYMPHOMA

Historically also referred to as malignant angio-endotheliomatosis, this rare B- or T-cell–derived neoplastic proliferation of large pleomorphic mononuclear cells may preferentially involve the lumens of small arteries and veins, and capillaries, without significant infiltration of vessel walls or parenchymal involvement that may be seen in angioimmunoblastic T-cell lymphoma. Intravascular lymphoma typically involves multiple organs, with effects particularly notable in the CNS (with associated dementia and neurologic impairment) and skin (with plaques and nodules), and is usually rapidly fatal.

CLINICAL EVALUATION AND STAGING

The staging workup for all patients includes a detailed history and physical examination; complete blood count with differential; blood chemistries; serum protein electrophoresis; chest radiograph (now largely replaced by CT scanning); CT scan of the chest, abdomen, and pelvis; and bone marrow aspiration with biopsy. Selected patients may require the following additional studies for complete evaluation: magnetic resonance imaging (MRI; to evaluate the nervous system or bone), GI series or endoscopy, bone scan, CT scan of the head (in the presence of symptoms of lymphoma in the head and neck area), and lumbar puncture. Evaluation of the peripheral blood by a sensitive cytofluorometric technique (cell sorter) may reveal circulating monoclonal lymphocytes, especially in B-cell lymphomas. As with Hodgkin disease, PET scans have largely replaced gallium scans and have become relatively routine for the staging and therapeutic monitoring of NHL (particularly the aggressive subtypes).

The Ann Arbor staging system is used for NHLs, except that the designation of stages III_1 and III_2 as applied to Hodgkin disease is not necessary (see Fig. 16.13). This system, however, is not optimal, for it does not reflect important prognostic factors such as size, or "bulk," of the tumor, the number of extranodal sites of disease, performance status, or the lactate dehydrogenase (LDH) concentration. Separate staging classification systems have been devised for childhood lymphomas, particularly Burkitt lymphoma and lymphoblastic lymphoma.

CLINICAL MANIFESTATIONS

In contrast to Hodgkin disease, most patients with NHL present with advanced disease (stage III or IV), which is often reflected by generalized adenopathy. In addition, the disease may occur at unusual sites, such as epitrochlear or popliteal nodes, Waldeyer's ring (nasopharynx), skin, GI tract, brain, and ovaries or testes—sites rarely affected in Hodgkin disease. Patients with low-grade lymphomas have a long history of slowly progressing disease, which may temporarily regress— so-called "spontaneous" remission—in 5% to 10% of cases. High-grade and aggressive intermediate-grade lymphomas, on the other hand, usually have a more rapidly progressive course, with 40% to 50% of patients developing B symptoms. Although the presence of B symptoms has been considered an adverse prognostic factor, multivariate analysis after modern intensive chemotherapy programs reveals that B symptoms no longer affect survival.

Bone marrow involvement occurs in 10% to 40% of cases. The incidence is highest in lymphoblastic, follicular, and Burkitt and Burkitt-like lymphomas (20% to 40%) and lowest in DLBCL (10% to 15%). Such involvement is often focal and does not affect peripheral blood counts, although in some patients the marrow may be extensively infiltrated, leading to the development of pancytopenia or a leukemic phase. Immunofluorescent microscopy has revealed small numbers of monoclonal B cells in the peripheral blood in about one third of patients with low-grade lymphomas and in 15% to 20% of those with intermediate- and high-grade lymphomas.

PROGNOSTIC FACTORS

Modern combination chemotherapy programs have markedly improved the prognosis, particularly in intermediate- and high-grade lymphomas. While formerly only 10% of patients were cured, 50% to 60% are now cured with intensive multidrug regimens. As a result of the clinical, histologic, and immunobiologic heterogeneity of NHL, many prognostic factors have been identified that separate patients into various risk categories for

relapse and decreased survival. This allows for planning of lesser or greater intensity of treatment (see Table 16.2).

A prognostic index has been developed by the International Non-Hodgkin Lymphoma Prognostic Factors Project based upon patient data from 16 single institutions and cooperative groups (Shipp, 1994; Shipp et al., 1993). A total of 2031 evaluable patients with aggressive NHL (NCI categories E to H; see Fig. 16.35) were treated with doxorubicin-containing regimens between 1982 and 1987. Multiple clinical and laboratory features were analyzed to define adverse prognostic factors that were present at the time of diagnosis and predicted for relapse and death. The International Index Model, based upon age, stage, serum LDH, performance status, and number of extranodal disease sites, identified four risk groups with predicted 5-year survivals of 73%, 51%, 43%, and 26% (see Tables 16.3 and 16.4). It was found that while older patients (>60 years) had similar complete remissions (CRs) to younger patients (<60 years), they were less likely to maintain their CR than younger patients, especially low- and low- to intermediate-risk patients, with resultant shorter survival. Survival curves for the age-adjusted International Index are noted in Figure 16.36. The advantage of a prognostic index is that good-risk patients can be identified for conventional therapy while poor-risk (high-relapse) patients can be identified for new research protocols to improve the cure rate. Furthermore, treatment results among institutions and cooperative groups can be compared, since standardized prognostic factors will have been used.

Additional poor prognostic factors include long time to achieve CR, lower dose intensity and schedule, T-cell phenotype versus B-cell phenotype (data, however, are not uniformly in agreement), elevated serum β_2-microglobulin level, increased expression of adhesion molecules (CD44), increased serum level of IL-10, *BCL2-MBR* gene rearrangement, and lack of rearrangement of the *BCL6* gene (Shipp, 1994; Blay et al., 1993; Tang et al., 1994; Offit et al., 1994).

Follicular lymphoma grades I and II have a similar, generally indolent clinical course, and therefore the clinical outcome is not well predicted by the IPI. Very often patients can be observed for long periods of time without requiring any therapy. Recently a prognostic scoring system has been developed called the Follicular Lymphoma Prognostic Index that allows clinicians to estimate treatment-free intervals and overall survival based upon the patient's age, stage of disease, number of lymph node sites involved, presence or absence of anemia, and serum concentration of LDH (Solal-Celigny et al., 2004). Patients are divided into low (no or one risk factor), intermediate (two risk factors), and high (three or more risk factors) groups. The 5-year overall survivals by group were 90%, 77%, and 52%, respectively, while the 10-year overall survivals by group were 70%, 50%, and 35%, respectively. Grade III follicular lymphoma behaves like and is generally treated like the aggressive NHL DLBCL, and therefore the IPI is best used for prognostication.

A significant proportion of low-grade follicular lymphomas will eventually progress (transform) to an aggressive intermediate- or high-grade lymphoma. Specific genetic changes have recently been described that are associated with the latter, including *TP53* mutation and alterations in *c-MYC* (Sander et al., 1993; Chang et al., 1994). An understanding of the molecular mechanisms predating or coinciding with clonal evolution of malignant lymphoma may permit early detection of this event so that effective (intensive) therapy can be used when the tumor burden is minimal.

	WHO classification	
Abbreviated updated (1992) NCI working formulation equivalent	**B-cell neoplasms**	**T-cell neoplasms**
Low-grade malignant lymphoma	Precursor B-cell lymphoblastic leukemia/lymphoma	Precursor T-cell lymphoblastic leukemia/lymphoma
A Small lymphocytic (and small lymphocytic-plasmacytoid)	Mature B-cell neoplasms	Mature T-cell and natural killer cell neoplasms
B Follicular, predominantly small cleaved cell	B-cell chronic lymphocytic leukemia/small lymphocytic lymphoma	T-cell prolymphocytic leukemia
C Follicular, mixed, small cleaved, and large cell	B-cell prolymphocytic leukemia	T-cell large granular lymphocytic leukemia
	Lymphoplasmacytic lymphoma (lymphoplasmacytoid lymphoma)	Aggressive natural killer cell leukemia
II Intermediate-grade malignant lymphoma	Mantle cell lymphoma	T/natural killer cell lymphoma, nasal and nasal-type (angiocentric lymphoma)
D Follicular, predominantly large cell	Follicular lymphoma (follicle center lymphoma)	Mycosis fungoides
E Diffuse small cleaved cell		Sézary syndrome
	Cutaneous follicle center lymphoma	Angioimmunoblastic T-cell lymphoma
F Diffuse mixed, small and large cell	Marginal zone B-cell lymphoma of mucosa-associated lymphoid tissue type	Peripheral T-cell lymphoma (unspecified)
G Diffuse large cell, cleaved/noncleaved	Nodal marginal zone lymphoma =/– monocytoid B-cell	Adult T-cell leukemia/lymphoma (HTLV1 +)
III High-grade malignant lymphoma	Splenic marginal zone B-cell lymphoma	Anaplastic large-cell lymphoma (T-cell and null-cell types)
H Diffuse large cell immunoblastic	Hairy cell leukemia	Primary cutaneous CD30-positive T-cell lymphoproliferative disorders (cutaneous anaplastic large cell lymphoma)
I Lymphoblastic (convoluted/non-convoluted)	Diffuse large B-cell lymphoma	Subcutaneous panniculitis-like T-cell lymphoma
J Small noncleaved cell (Burkitt/non-Burkett types)	Mediastinal (thymic)	Enteropathy-type intestinal T-cell lymphoma
IV Miscellaneous	Intravascular	Hepatosplenic g/d T-cell lymphoma
Composite	Primary effusion lymphoma	
Mycosis fungoides	Burkitt lymphoma	
True histiocytic	Plasmacytoma	
Unclassified	Plasma cell myeloma	

FIGURE 16.35 Comparison of the updated (1992) NCI's International Working Formulation classification and the WHO classification (Harris et al., 1999) of non-Hodgkin lymphomas.

Table 16.1

Frequency of Non-Hodgkin Lymphoma (NHL) Subgroups According to the NCI Working Formula Classification, Together with Survival Range by Grade*

Category	Subgroup	Frequency (%)[†]	Survival Range (yr)
Low grade	A	14	
	B	26	5–10
	C	19	
Intermediate grade	D	4	
	E	8	
	F	7	2–5
	G	22	
High grade	H	9	
	I	5	0.5–2
	J	6	

*See Figure 16.35 for definitions. Working Formulation subgroups G and H are often called diffuse large cell lymphoma (DLCL) and treated as high-grade or poor-prognosis lymphomas. "Aggressive" lymphomas refer to subgroups E to H. "Very aggressive" lymphomas refer to subgroups I and J.
[†]Frequency in US whites.
Compiled from data in Rosenberg (1980) and Newell et al. (1987).

Table 16.2

Association between Host/Tumor Characteristics and Clinical Prognostic Features in Aggressive Non-Hodgkin Lymphoma*

Host/Tumor Characteristics	Clinical Prognostic Factors
Tumor's growth and invasive potential	Serum LDH
	Number of nodal and extranodal sites of disease
	Mass size
	Stage according to Ann Arbor classification
	BM involvement
Patient's response to the tumor	Systemic B symptoms
	Performance status
Patient's ability to tolerate intensive therapy	Age at diagnosis
	Performance status
	BM involvement

BM, bone marrow; LDH, lactate dehydrogenase.
*Aggressive lymphomas refer to NCI categories E to H; see Table 16.1.

Table 16.3

Prognostic Risk Factors for Survival in Aggressive Non-Hodgkin Lymphoma in International Index Patients

Risk Factor	Relative Risk	P Value
Patients of All Ages		
• Age (≤60 years vs >60 years)	1.96	<0.001
• LDH (≤nL vs >nL)	1.85	<0.001
• Performance status (0.1 vs 2–4)	1.80	<0.001
• Stage (I/II vs III/IV)	1.47	<0.001
• Extranodal involvement (≤1 site vs >1 site)	1.48	<0.001
Patients ≤60 Years of Age		
• Stage (I/II vs III/IV)	2.17	<0.001
• LDH (≤nL vs >nL)	1.95	<0.001
• Performance status (0, 1 vs 2–4)	1.81	<0.001

LDH, lactate dehydrogenase.
From Shipp MA: Prognostic factors in aggressive non-Hodgkin's lymphoma: who has 'high-risk' disease? *Blood* 83:1165–1173, 1994.

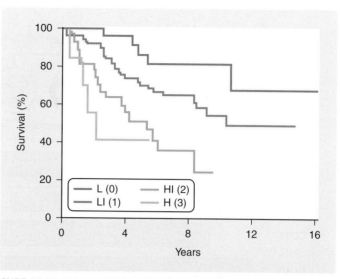

FIGURE 16.36 PROGNOSTIC FACTORS IN AGGRESSIVE NON-HODGKIN LYMPHOMA. Overall predicted survival in patients under 60 using the age-adjusted International Index. Risk groups are defined from risk factors noted in Table 16.4: low (L), low-intermediate (LI), high-intermediate (HI), and high (H). The numbers in parentheses refer to the number of risk factors. (Modified with permission from Shipp et al., 1993.)

Table 16.4

Prognostic Factors in Patients of All Ages in Aggressive Non-Hodgkin Lymphoma: The International Index

Risk Group	Risk Factors	Distribution of Cases (%)	CR Rate (%)	RFs of CRs (%) 2-Year Rate	RFs of CRs (%) 5-Year Rate	Survival (%) 2-Year Rate	Survival (%) 5-Year Rate
Low	0.1	35	87	79	70	84	73
Low-intermediate	2	27	67	66	50	66	51
High-intermediate	3	22	55	59	49	54	43
High	4.5	16	44	58	40	34	26

CR, complete response.
From Shipp MA: Prognostic factors in aggressive non-Hodgkin's lymphoma: who has 'high-risk' disease? *Blood* 83:1165–1173, 1994.

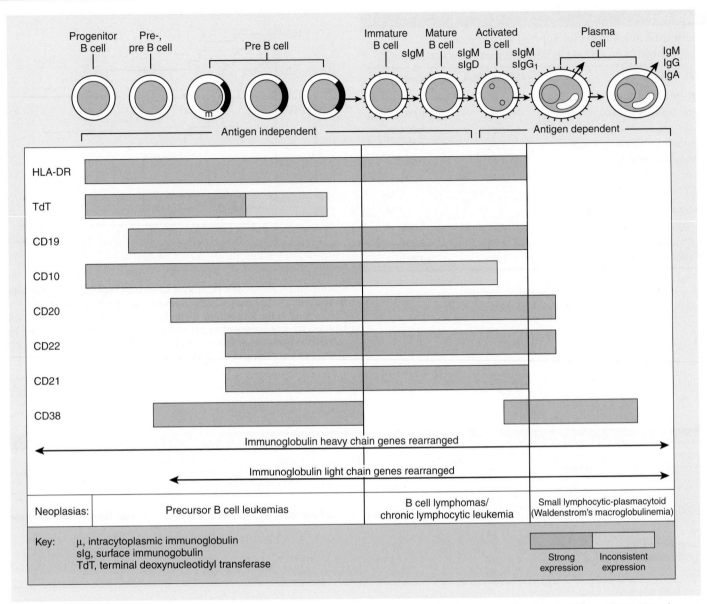

FIGURE 16.37 MAbs specific to human B-cell surface antigens can be used to detect sequential stages in B-cell maturation. The malignant lymphomas and leukemias reflect these stages of normal B-cell development. (Modified with permission from Jaffe, 1990, with additional data from Uckun, 1990.)

Table 16.5

Predominant Phenotypes of B-Cell Neoplasms*

Neoplasm	CD19	CD20	CD22	CD10	CD5	CD25	CD11c	CD21	CD38	TdT
Common ALL	+	±	±	+	−	−	−	−	+/−	+
Small non–cleaved cell Burkitt lymphoma	+	+	+	+	−	−	−	+/−	−	−
Large cell/large cell immunoblastic lymphoma	+	+	+	±	−	±	−	±	+	−
Nodular (follicular) lymphomas	+	+	+	+	−	−	−	+	+/−	−
Mantle cell lymphoma	+	+	+	−/+	+	−	−	+/−	−	−
Marginal zone lymphoma	+	+	+	−	−	+/−	+/−	−	+/−	−
Small lymphocytic/CLL	+	+	+	−	+	−	−	+/−	−	−
Small lymphocytic-plasmacytoid (Waldenstrom's macroglobulinemia)	+/−	+/−	+/−	−	+/−	+	−	−	+	−
Hairy cell leukemia	+	+	+	−	−	+	+	−	−/+	−
Myeloma	−	−	−	−	−	−	−	−	+	−

ALL, acute lymphoblastic leukemia; CLL, chronic lymphocytic leukemia; TdT, terminal deoxynucleotidyl transferase; +, nearly always positive; ±, sometimes positive; −, usually negative; +/−, more often positive than negative; −/+, more often negative than positive.
*Cluster designation (CD) groupings are noted as well as the commonly used terms.
Modified from Stetter-stevenson M, Medeiros L, Jaffe E: Immunophenotypic methods and findings in the diagnosis of lymphoproliferative disorders. In Jaffe E, editor: *Surgical pathology of the lymph nodes and related organs*, Philadelphia, 1995, Saunders, pp 22–57.

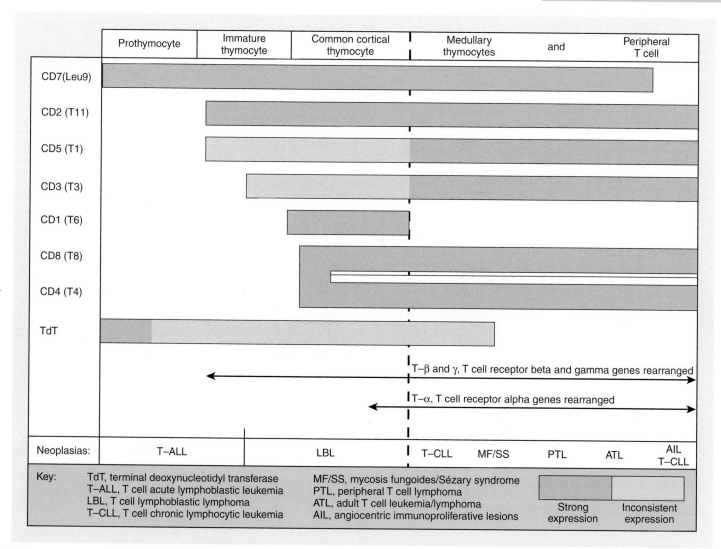

FIGURE 16.38 MAbs specific to human T-cell surface antigens can be used to detect sequential stages in T-cell development. Malignancies can be phenotypically related to stages of normal T-cell maturation. CD4 (T4) (helper/inducer) cells represent 60% to 70% of peripheral blood cells, whereas CD8 (T8) (cytotoxic/suppressor) cells constitute 30% to 40%. (Modified with permission from Jaffe, 1990.)

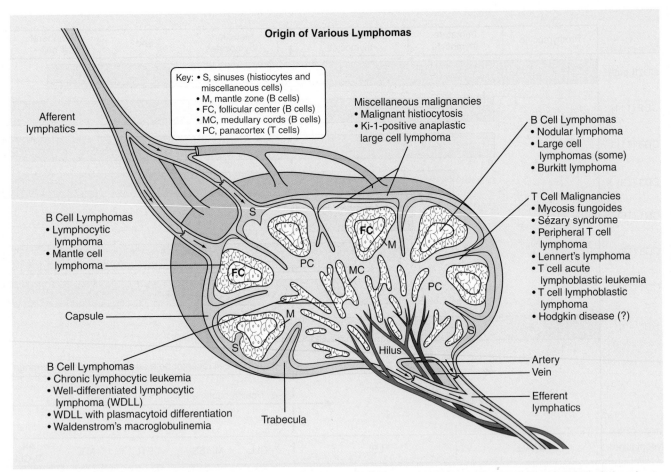

FIGURE 16.39 ORIGINS OF VARIOUS LYMPHOMAS. This diagram represents anatomic areas and functionally related compartments of a lymph node at which different lymphoid malignancies arise. For example, B-cell lymphomas arise from the follicles (mantle zone and follicular center), whereas T-cell lymphomas arise from the paracortical areas normally populated by T lymphocytes.

FIGURE 16.40 GENETIC DEFECTS IN B-CELL LYMPHOMA. The translocations t(14;18) and t(11;14), and some t(8;14) translocations, probably occur in primitive B cells in the bone marrow. Lymphomas arise after these genetically damaged B cells mature, leave the bone marrow, and acquire additional genetic lesions because of unknown secondary events (the *arrows* do not imply that lymphomas themselves arise in the bone marrow). These secondary events may include the antigen-driven proliferation of B cells. Other events in B cells carrying the t(14;18) translocation may lead directly to primary (nodal) large B-cell lymphomas. *BCL6* rearrangements at band 3q27 occur mainly in primary extranodal lymphomas (*thick blue arrows*) (Offit et al., 1994). Additional gene rearrangements occur in follicular lymphoma (*thin blue arrows*). Because nothing is known about the origin of breakpoints at 3q27 during B-cell maturation, these *arrows* have no identifiable starting point. Other oncogenic factors include the direct infection of B cells by Epstein-Barr virus in Burkitt lymphoma and the possible stimulation of MALT lymphoma cells by *H. pylori* infection. All lymphomas may subsequently spread to lymph nodes, the bone marrow, or other sites, but this process is not shown in the figure. (Modified and reprinted with permission from Kluin, 1994.)

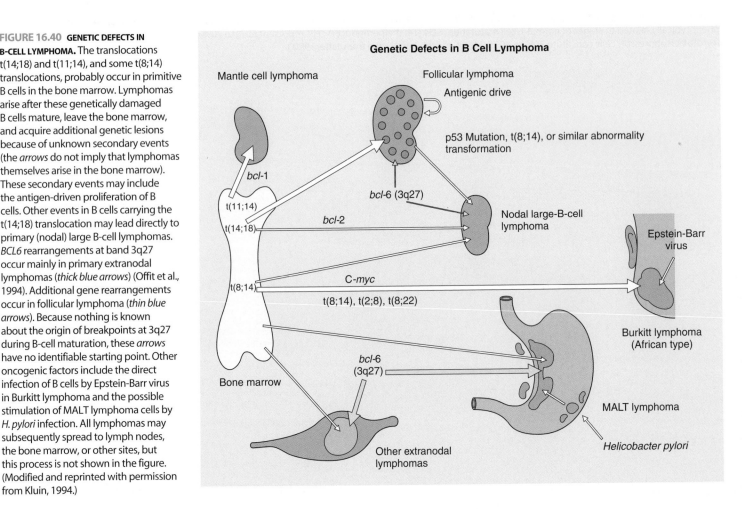

Table 16.6

Most Common Molecular Abnormalities Studied in Non-Hodgkin Lymphoma

Gene Studied	Chromosomal Site	Most Common Disease Associations
Immunoglobulin heavy-chain (*IgH*) rearrangements	14q32	B-cell neoplasms*
Immunoglobulin κ light-chain (*Igκ*) rearrangements	2p11	B-cell neoplasms
J_H/BCL1	t(11;14)(q13;q32)	Mantle cell lymphoma
J_H/BCL2	t(14;18)(q32;q21)	Follicular lymphoma, some diffuse large B-cell lymphomas
PAX5/IgH	t(9;14)(p13;q32)	Lymphoplasmacytic lymphoma
AP12/MLT	t(11;18)(q21;q21)	Extranodal marginal zone lymphoma
BCL6 translocations	t(3;n)(q27;n)	Some diffuse large B-cell lymphomas
c-MYC translocations	t(8;n)(q24;n)	Burkitt lymphoma
T-cell receptor β-chain (*TCRβ*) rearrangements	7q34	T-cell neoplasms*
T-cell receptor γ-chain (*TCRγ*) rearrangements	7q15	T-cell neoplasms*
NPM/ALK	t(2;5)(p23;q35)	Anaplastic large cell lymphoma

*Lineage infidelity may occur in some neoplasms, particularly lymphoblastic leukemias and lymphomas, which may result in detection of aberrant gene rearrangements (see text).

Adapted from Aber DA: Molecular diagnostic approach to non-Hodgkin lymphoma, *J Mol Diagn* 2:178–190, 2000.

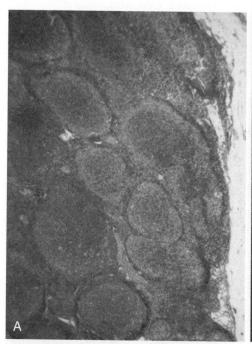

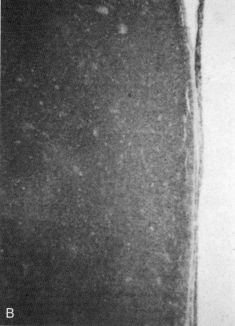

FIGURE 16.41 **NODULAR VERSUS DIFFUSE LYMPHOMAS. (A)** Low magnification of a nodular lymphoma shows many of the architectural features that are helpful in the diagnosis of follicular lymphomas. These features include complete effacement of lymph node architecture, high density of follicles with a back-to-back arrangement, infiltration of the lymph node capsule by follicles with extension into perinodal fat, and loss of a distinct boundary separating the follicles from the surrounding peripheral cuff of lymphocytes. **(B)** Low magnification of a diffuse lymphoma reveals complete effacement of the normal nodal architecture by a diffuse lymphomatous process.

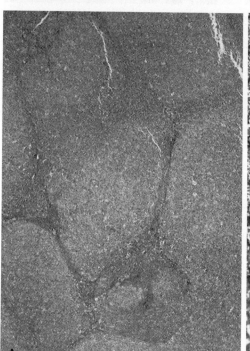

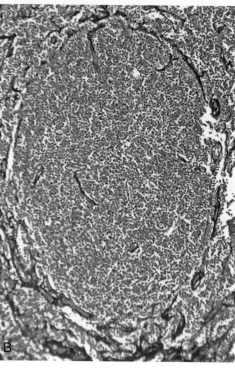

FIGURE 16.42 **NODULAR (FOLLICULAR) LYMPHOMA. (A)** The well-defined, uniform follicles seen in this low-power photomicrograph are due to compression of reticulin around the neoplastic follicles, shown **(B)** in this high-power view (reticulin stain).

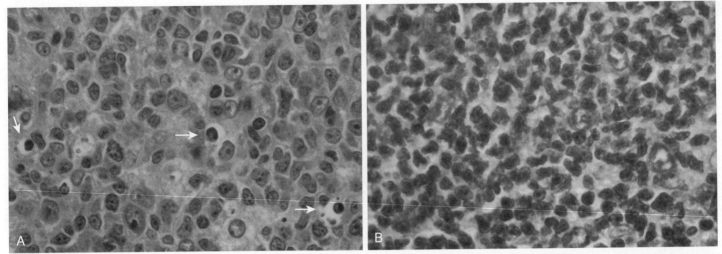

FIGURE 16.43 **(A)** Apoptosis (programmed cell death) is a normal finding in germinal centers where scattered, individual necrotic cells are readily identified (*arrows*). In contrast, the nodular infiltrates of follicular center cell–derived nodular lymphomas **(B)** have far fewer apoptotic cells. Follicular center cell lymphomas typically exhibit a t(14;18) chromosomal translocation, which results in deregulation of expression of the *BCL2* proto-oncogene on chromosome 18. This gene blocks apoptosis, and its overexpression results in prolongation of the lifespan of involved cells, contributing to the pathogenesis of lymphoma. Approximately 20% of diffuse non-Hodgkin lymphomas of follicular center cell origin exhibit the t(14;18) translocation as well.

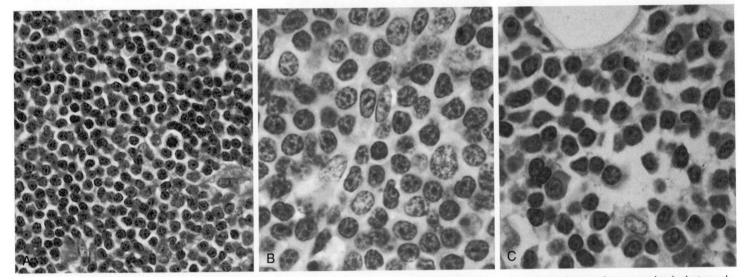

FIGURE 16.44 **CHRONIC LYMPHOCYTIC LEUKEMIA (SMALL LYMPHOCYTIC LYMPHOMA) (NCI SUBGROUP A). (A)** Sheets of small lymphocytes have completely destroyed the normal lymph node architecture. Virtually all cases show a diffuse pattern. **(B)** Such monotonous sheets of mature lymphocytes may also be seen in the lymph nodes in chronic lymphocytic leukemia. **(C)** This example shows plasmacytoid differentiation. All cases are of B-cell origin and usually show aberrant immunoreactivity for CD5, a T-cell marker.

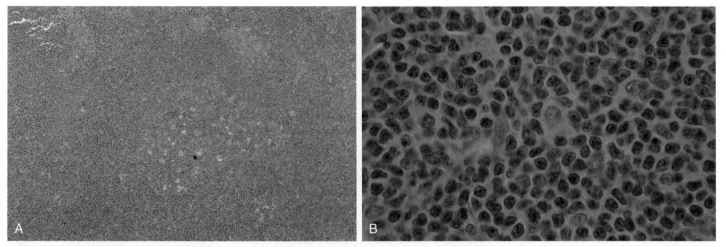

FIGURE 16.45 **MANTLE CELL LYMPHOMA. (A)** A vaguely nodular proliferation of small lymphocytes surrounds germinal centers in a mantle zone pattern, effacing normal lymph node architecture. Mantle cell lymphoma may also present with a diffuse pattern of lymph node involvement, usually with residual germinal centers present as well. **(B)** Higher power reveals uniform, small lymphoid cells with scant cytoplasm and small irregular to notched or cleaved nuclei with coarse chromatin. All cases are of B-cell origin and usually show aberrant immunoreactivity for CD5. A significant percentage of cases show a t(11;14) chromosomal translocation.

Table 16.7

Comparison of Low-Grade Lymphomas

Characteristic	Small Lymphocytic Lymphoma (SLL), Chronic Lymphocytic Leukemia (CLL)	Mantle Cell Lymphoma	Small Cleaved FCC Lymphoma	Marginal Zone Lymphoma, Monocytoid B-Cell MALT Types
Nuclear appearance	Round	Irregular	Cleaved	Round to irregular
Lymph node infiltration patterns	Diffuse	Diffuse or mantle zone	Diffuse or follicular	Sinusoid interfollicular diffuse
Immunoreactivity for CDS (T1)	+	+(−)	−	−
CD10 (CALLA)	−	−(+)	+	−
CD23	+	−	+/−	−
Surface immunoglobulin expression	IgM weak	IgM/D intermediate	IgG bright	IgM/A
Genotypic features	(*BCL1*)[†]	*BCL1*	*BCL2*	*BCL1*(−) *BCL2*(−)
Cytogenetic features	+12	t(11;14)	t(14;18)	
Median survival	5–7 years	2–5 years	Diffuse 3–4 years, follicular 7–8 years	Indolent course
Salient clinical features	Autoimmune phenomena; Richter's transformation	Splenomegaly, GI lesions	Spontaneous remission; transformation	Tend to remain localized

FCC, follicular center cell; GI, gastrointestinal; MALT, mucosa-associated lymphoid tissue.

*B-cell markers expressed (CD19, CD20, CD22). Low-grade lymphomas of T-cell lineage are not common but include T-cell CLL, peripheral T-cell lymphoma, and Sézary syndrome.

[†]t(11;14) and upregulation of *BCL1* are uncommon in CLL/SLL.

FIGURE 16.46 FOLLICULAR LYMPHOMA, GRADE I.
(A) High-power microscopic section shows small cells with nuclear irregularity including cleaves (notches) and indentations. **(B)** Touch prep of a lymph node demonstrates classic cleaved cells, some with split nuclei. Lymph node architecture may be either nodular or diffuse. All cases are of B-cell origin.

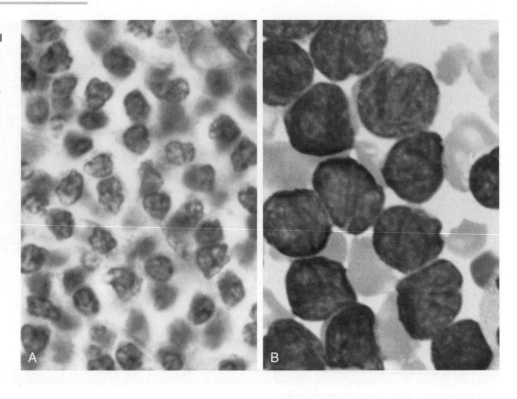

FIGURE 16.47 FOLLICULAR LYMPHOMA, GRADE II.
(A) Low- and **(B)** high-power photomicrographs demonstrate a lymphoma composed of both small lymphocytes and large lymphoid cells. Lymph node architecture may be either nodular (NCI subgroup C) or diffuse (NCI subgroup F).

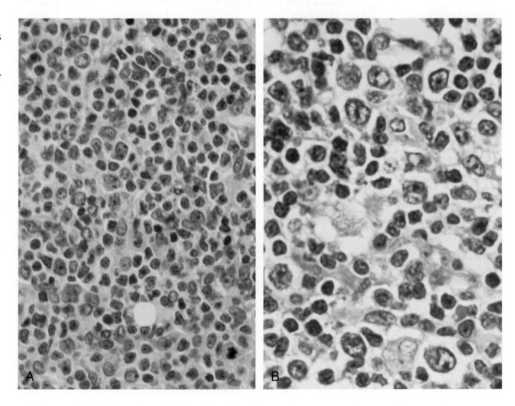

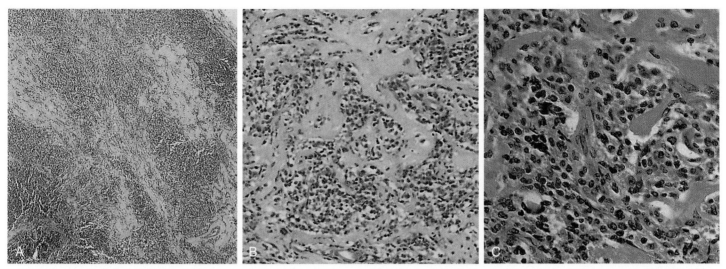

FIGURE 16.48 **FOLLICULAR LYMPHOMA, GRADE II, DIFFUSE. (A)** Low-power photomicrograph of a retroperitoneal lesion shows a sclerosing mixed lymphoma exhibiting broad birefringent bands of collagen. **(B)** In other areas the compartmentalizing bands are hyalinized. This pattern of sclerosis is also seen with diffuse large cell lymphomas, particularly in the mediastinum. **(C)** High-power view of areas compartmentalized by hyalinized collagenous bands shows that the tumor is composed of small and large cleaved follicular center cells.

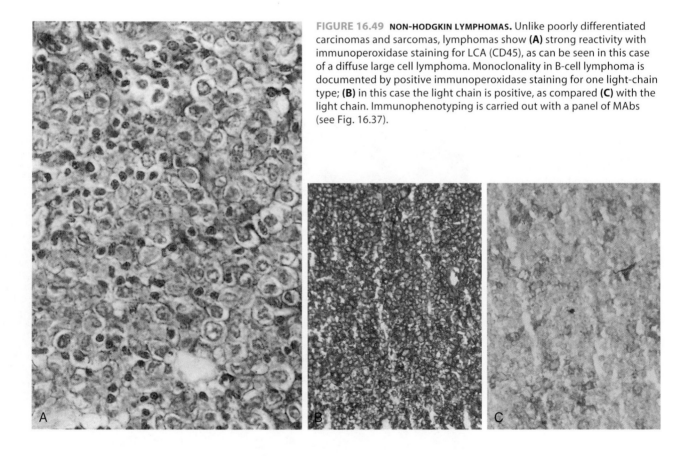

FIGURE 16.49 **NON-HODGKIN LYMPHOMAS.** Unlike poorly differentiated carcinomas and sarcomas, lymphomas show **(A)** strong reactivity with immunoperoxidase staining for LCA (CD45), as can be seen in this case of a diffuse large cell lymphoma. Monoclonality in B-cell lymphoma is documented by positive immunoperoxidase staining for one light-chain type; **(B)** in this case the light chain is positive, as compared **(C)** with the light chain. Immunophenotyping is carried out with a panel of MAbs (see Fig. 16.37).

Table 16.8

Histologic Subtypes of Diffuse Large Cell Lymphoma*

Subtype	NCI Subgroup	Cell of Origin
Large cleaved follicular center cell	G	B
Large noncleaved follicular center cell	G	B
Mixed cleaved/noncleaved follicular center cell	G	B
Large clear cell	G	B
Immunoblastic	H	B (80%), T (20%)
Multilobulated cell	–	T (90%), B (10%)
Ki-1 lymphoma	–	T (80%), B (10%)
True diffuse histiocytic lymphoma	IV	Monocyte (histiocytes)
Unclassified	IV	Undefined

*Various morphologic or descriptive types are listed with the cell of origin. Considerable heterogeneity is noted.

FIGURE 16.50 **LARGE CELL LYMPHOMA (LARGE, NONCLEAVED CELL TYPE) (NCI SUBGROUP G). (A)** High magnification reveals large cells with predominantly round nuclei, distinct nucleoli, and a moderate amount of cytoplasm. Small lymphocytes in the background allow size comparison. Note the lack of well-defined cell borders and an absence of an organoid pattern, features more commonly associated with carcinomas. **(B)** Touch prep of a lymph node shows large cells with large, prominent nucleoli and basophilic cytoplasm.

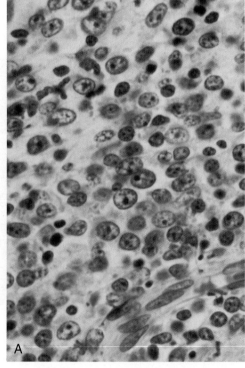
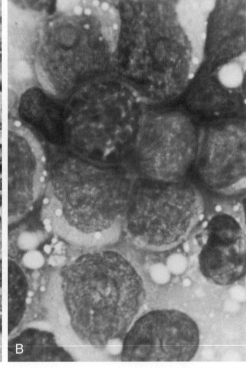

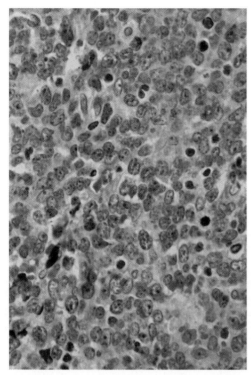

FIGURE 16.51 **LARGE CELL LYMPHOMA (LARGE, CLEAVED CELL TYPE) (NCI SUBGROUP G).** Large cells are part of a heterogeneous population composed predominantly of irregular and cleaved cells, as well as occasional round forms.

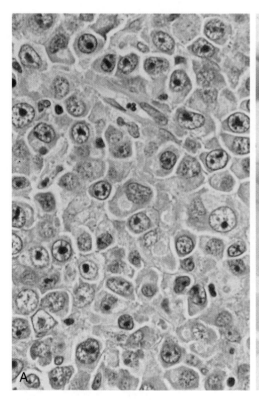

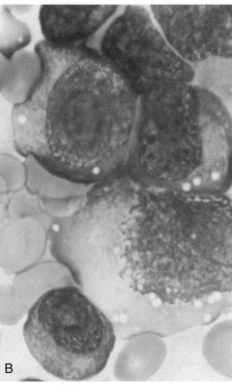

FIGURE 16.52 **LARGE CELL LYMPHOMA (B-CELL TYPE) (NCI SUBGROUP H). (A)** High-power photomicrograph shows large cells with eccentric nuclei and prominent nucleoli, abundant amphophilic cytoplasm and pale-staining perinuclear hof or halo (representing the location of the Golgi apparatus). **(B)** Cytocentrifuge prep from a pleural effusion shows large, immature cells with eccentric nuclei and basophilic cytoplasm. Note the large, prominent nucleoli.

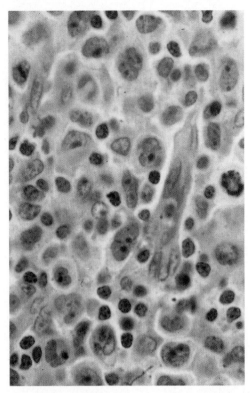

FIGURE 16.53   LARGE CELL LYMPHOMA (T-CELL TYPE) (NCI SUBGROUP H). The predominant cell population is composed of large cells with round to lobated nuclei, prominent magenta nucleoli, and abundant pale cytoplasm. Note the range of cell sizes and scattered eosinophils.

FIGURE 16.54   LARGE CELL LYMPHOMA (MULTILOBULATED CELL TYPE). (A, B) This high-grade lymphoma, most often arising from peripheral (post-thymic) T lymphocytes, is marked by large, multilobulated or multisegmented nuclei, with relatively fine chromatin and small to inconspicuous nucleoli. Under high magnification the nucleus of a typical cell has a "popcorn" shape. (Courtesy of Dr G. Pinkus, Pathology Department, Brigham and Women's Hospital, Boston, MA.)

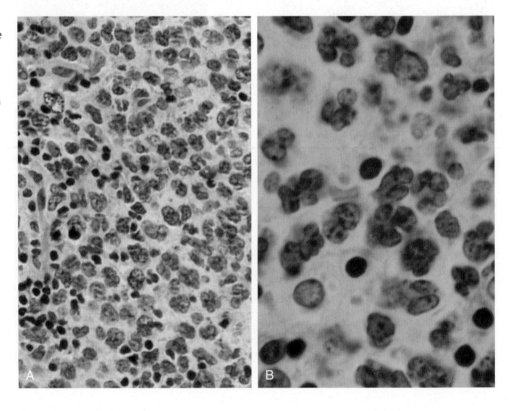

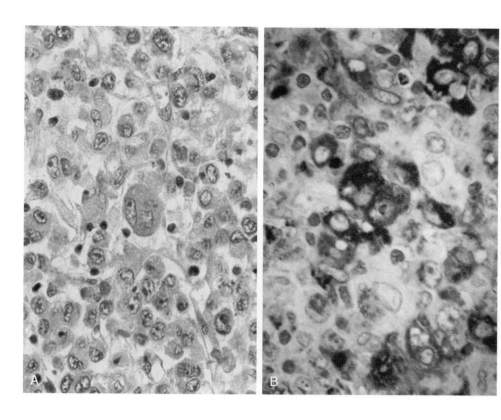

FIGURE 16.55 **LARGE CELL LYMPHOMA (TRUE HISTIOCYTIC TYPE). (A)** Large cells with membranes are present together with occasional focal erythrophagocytosis, a helpful but nonspecific indicator of this type of lymphoma. Nuclei typically show conspicuous lobulation, often appearing multinucleate. Confirmatory histochemical staining shows positivity for **(B)** α_1-antichymotrypsin and (not shown) α_1-naphthylacetate esterase (nonspecific esterase), lysozyme, and acid phosphatase in some cases. In this patient, MAbs specific to MO-1 (a monocyte marker), LCA (CD45), lysozyme, and epithelial membrane antigen were positive; B- and T-cell markers were all negative. Ultrastructural studies showed pseudopod-like projections of the plasma membrane, microfilaments, phagolysosomes, and phagocytized material.

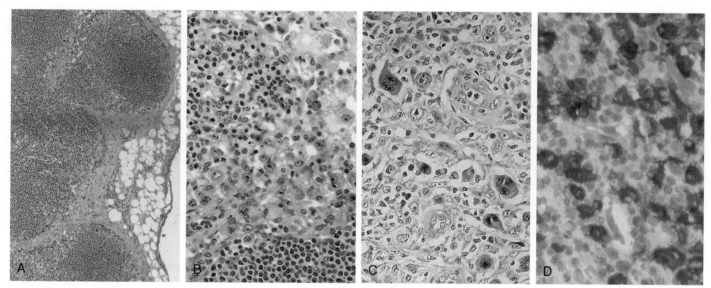

FIGURE 16.56 **ANAPLASTIC LARGE CELL LYMPHOMA (ALCL). (A)** Low-power photomicrograph demonstrates sinusoidal and paratrabecular infiltration by lymphoma cells surrounding intact, uninvolved germinal centers. **(B)** With higher magnification, the bizarre cells of the sinusoidal infiltrate can be better appreciated. The cells have irregular nuclei and prominent nucleoli. An uninvolved germinal center is seen in the lower part of the field. **(C)** Under high magnification, some of the typically large, bizarre lymphoma cells are suggestive of Reed-Sternberg cells. **(D)** Immunoperoxidase staining shows immunoreactivity for Ki-1 (CD30) antigen; there was no reactivity for CD15 (Leu-M1) antigen (not shown). This lymphoma may be misdiagnosed as Hodgkin disease or metastatic carcinoma unless appropriate studies are carried out (see Table 16.9).

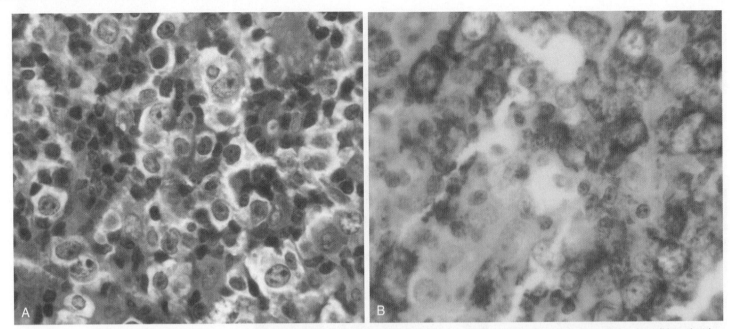

FIGURE 16.57   LARGE CELL LYMPHOMA (T-CELL–RICH B-CELL TYPE). (A) Nodal architecture is effaced by a diffuse infiltrate composed mainly of small lymphoid cells with interspersed large mononuclear cells. **(B)** Immunoperoxidase studies reveal that the small cells are reactive T cells (not shown), whereas the large cells are a clonal population of B cells, here shown to be reactive for B-cell marker CD20. Clinical features parallel those of other B-cell large cell lymphoma patients, although about 30% of patients have splenomegaly. It is important not to confuse T-cell–rich B-cell lymphoma with Hodgkin disease or cases of peripheral T-cell lymphoma that require different therapy.

Table 16.9

Monoclonal Antibodies Useful in the Diagnosis of Large Cell Lymphomas, Hodgkin Disease, and Undifferentiated Metastatic Carcinomas

Monoclonal Antibody	Hodgkin Disease*	Diffuse Large Cell Lymphoma				Undifferentiated Metastatic Carcinoma
		T Cell	B Cell	ALCL Type†	True DHL	
Ki-1 (CD30)	+	−	−	+		−
CD15 (Leu-MI)	+	−	−	−	−	±
T-cell markers	−	+	−	±	−	−
B-cell markers	−	−	+	±	−	−
LCA (CD45)	−	+	+	+	+	−
EMA	−	−	−	+	+	+

ALCL, anaplastic large cell lymphoma; DHL, diffuse histiocytic lymphoma; EMA, epithelial membrane antigen; LCA, leukocyte common antigen; +, positive; −, negative; ±, may be positive or negative.
*Reed-Sternberg cells (excluding the lymphocyte predominance type).
†A small percentage of T- and B-cell lymphomas are positive for Ki-1 (CD30) antigen.

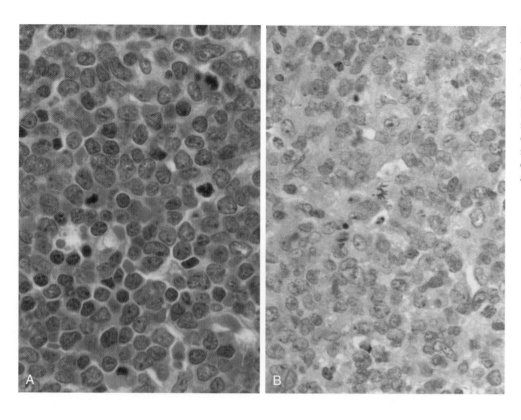

FIGURE 16.58 LYMPHOBLASTIC (PRECURSOR T-CELL) LYMPHOMA (NCI SUBGROUP I). **(A)** Malignant cells are small and light staining and have round to convoluted nuclei with delicate, evenly dispersed chromatin and indistinct nucleoli. **(B)** Most lymphoblasts show characteristic prominent nuclear convolutions or cerebriform shapes, although rare, nonconvoluted types exist. Mitoses are often seen, as well as a "starry sky" appearance. In most instances the cells are derived from immature T lymphocytes, although a B-cell phenotype can be seen in rare cases.

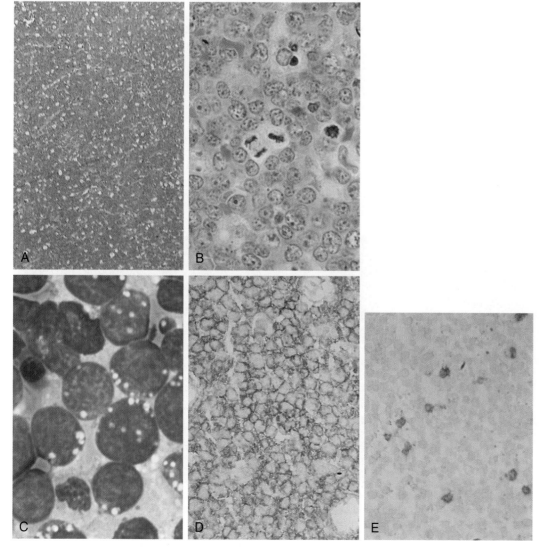

FIGURE 16.59 BURKITT LYMPHOMA (NCI SUBGROUP J). **(A)** Low-power photomicrograph reveals a "starry sky" appearance resulting from the presence of benign macrophages, which are active in the phagocytosis of necrotic cells and debris. This pattern is nonspecific and can be seen with any rapidly proliferating lymphoma. **(B)** With higher magnification, monotonous small to intermediate-sized cells can be seen; these cells have round nuclear outlines, multiple basophilic nucleoli, and abundant mitoses. **(C)** Bone marrow aspirate shows small, immature cells with deep basophilic cytoplasm containing many vacuoles. Distinct nucleoli are seen in several of the cells. **(D)** Immunoperoxidase staining demonstrates immunoreactivity for CD20 (B1) antigen; **(E)** only background, scattered benign T cells are present, which show reactivity for CD2 (T11) antigen.

FIGURE 16.60 BURKITT-LIKE LYMPHOMA (NCI SUBGROUP J). (A) Lymph node biopsy specimen shows diffuse replacement by small to intermediate-sized lymphoid cells having sparse cytoplasm, round to irregular nuclei, and distinct nucleoli. Many mitoses are evident. **(B)** Benign histiocytes are scattered in the background. Immunoperoxidase studies (not shown) demonstrated positivity for LCA (CD45), CD20 (B1), and CD22, with monotypic expression of light chains. Morphologically, non-Burkitt lymphoma differs from Burkitt lymphoma by a greater variation in cell size and shape, as well as a larger, more distinct, single central nucleolus, as shown here. Unlike Burkitt lymphoma, this subtype usually does not have c-*MYC* gene rearrangement.

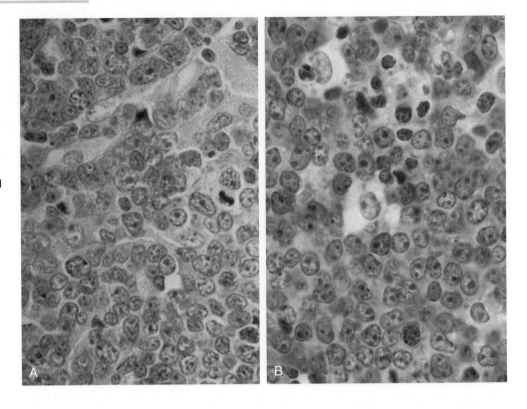

Table 16.10

Monoclonal Antibodies Useful in the Diagnosis of T-Cell Lymphomas

	Pan-T-Cell Markers			Other T-Cell Markers			Other Markers		
	CD2	CD3	CD5	CD4	CD8	CD10	CD30	ALK	TdT
T PLL	+	+	+	+/−	−/+	−	−	−	−
Cerebriform (mycosis fungoides)	+	+	+	+	−	−	−	−	−
Pleomorphic (small cell; mixed small and large cell; large cell)	+	+	+	+/−	−/+	−	−/+	−	−
Anaplastic large cell*	+/−	+/−	+/−	+/−	−/+	−	+	+	−
Precursor T-cell (lymphoblastic)*	+/−	+/−	+/−	+/−	−/+	+/−	−	−	+

ALK, ALK protein; TdT, terminal deoxynucleotidyl transferase; PLL, prolymphocytic leukemia; +, positive; −, negative; +/−, more often positive than negative; −/+, more often negative than positive.

*Some cases may express B-cell markers.

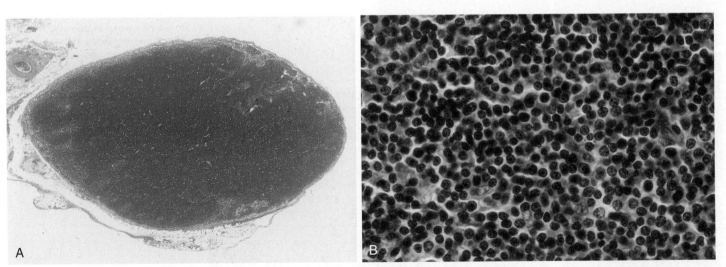

FIGURE 16.61 PERIPHERAL T-CELL NON-HODGKIN LYMPHOMA, SMALL LYMPHOCYTIC TYPE. (A, B) Nodal architecture is effaced by a uniform population of small lymphoid cells with scant cytoplasm and small nuclei with coarse chromatin and round, slightly irregular nuclear outlines. The lymphoid cells are immunoreactive for pan-T-cell markers (not shown). T-cell lymphoma of small lymphocytic type often has associated inv(14) and +8q chromosomal abnormalities.

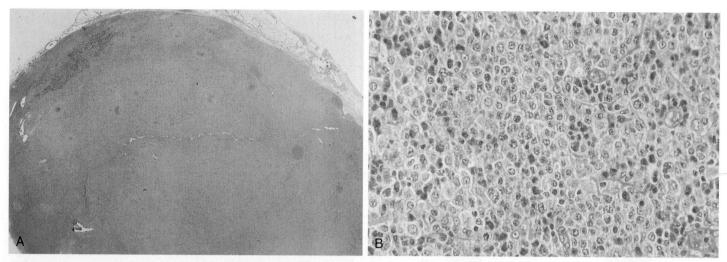

FIGURE 16.62 **PERIPHERAL T-CELL NON-HODGKIN LYMPHOMA, UNSPECIFIED. (A, B)** A cervical lymph node biopsy specimen from a 50-year-old man reveals architectural effacement by a diffuse infiltrate composed of small to large-sized cells, most with prominent nuclear irregularity, and with moderate amounts of pale cytoplasm in the larger cells. Note the presence of numerous admixed eosinophils, a finding frequently seen in T-cell lymphomas.

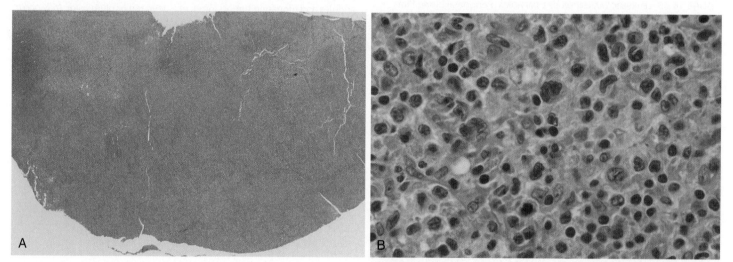

FIGURE 16.63 **PERIPHERAL T-CELL NON-HODGKIN LYMPHOMA, UNSPECIFIED. (A, B)** A 71-year-old man presented with left axillary lymphadenopathy. Biopsy revealed a diffuse infiltrate of large lymphoid cells with pale cytoplasm and large irregular to cleaved nuclei, including occasional Reed-Sternberg–like cells with pale prominent nucleoli. Tumor cells were immunoreactive for pan-T-cell markers, including CD2 and CD5, and were nonreactive for pan-T-cell marker CD7, consistent with the phenomenon of antigen deletion frequently observed in T-cell non-Hodgkin lymphomas. No immunoreactivity was evident for Leu M1 (CD15), a marker of Reed-Sternberg cells seen in Hodgkin disease.

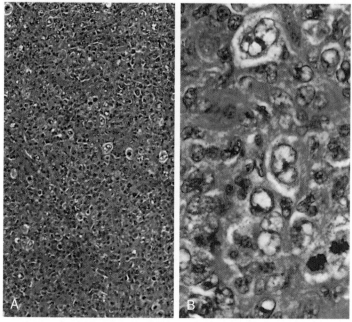

FIGURE 16.64 **ADULT T-CELL LYMPHOMA-LEUKEMIA. (A)** Low-power microscopic section of lymph node shows replacement of the normal architecture by pleomorphic lymphoid cells. **(B)** Under high magnification, occasional bizarre, polylobulated giant cells and prominent mitotic figures can be seen.

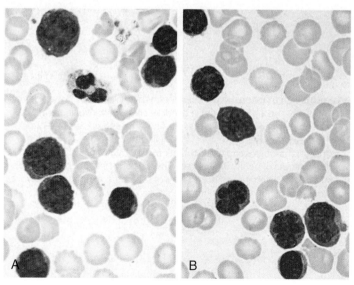

FIGURE 16.65 **ADULT T-CELL LYMPHOMA-LEUKEMIA. (A, B)** Peripheral blood films reveal characteristic abnormal lymphocytes with convoluted nuclei. (Courtesy of Dr. D. Catovsky.)

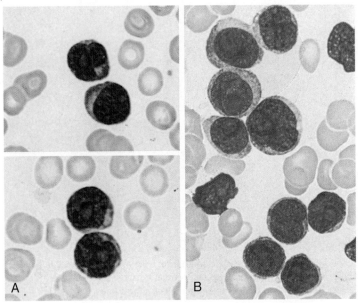

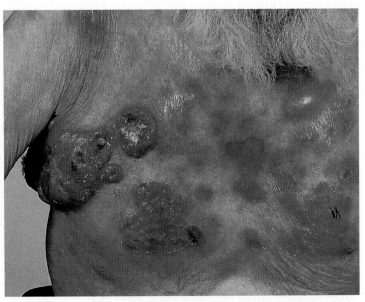

FIGURE 16.66 **LEUKEMIC TRANSITION OF LYMPHOMA.** Peripheral blood films show **(A)** lymphoid cells, two of which show prominent nuclear clefts, in a patient with nodular, poorly differentiated lymphocytic lymphoma. **(B)** In a patient with widely disseminated, terminal large cell lymphoma, abnormal large and medium-sized immature lymphoid cells are present in peripheral blood, showing abundant cytoplasm and prominent nucleoli.

FIGURE 16.67 **CUTANEOUS INVOLVEMENT IN DIFFUSE LARGE CELL LYMPHOMA.** Large nodules and fungating tumors, often of a deep red or plum color, may occur. Skin biopsy is essential for diagnosis and distinction from mycosis fungoides. Although T-cell lymphomas often involve the skin, B-cell lymphomas may also occasionally spread to the skin and subcutaneous tissues. Dissemination to other organs eventually occurs in most cases.

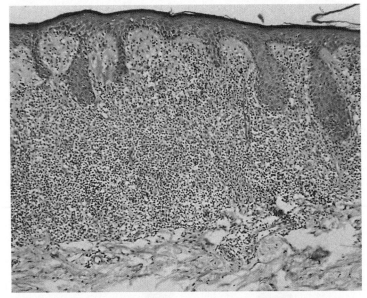

FIGURE 16.68 **CUTANEOUS INVOLVEMENT IN SYSTEMIC LYMPHOMA.** The epidermis is not affected, and a "Grenz zone" (a bandlike area of noninvolvement between epidermis and tumor) is present. The latter and the absence of Pautrier microabscesses are features that help distinguish B-cell lymphomas from mycosis fungoides and other cutaneous T-cell lymphomas. A dense bandlike infiltrate of poorly differentiated lymphocytic cells occupies the upper and mid-dermis. Infiltration of hair follicles or sebaceous glands (not shown) is a common feature of most lymphomas that secondarily involve the skin.

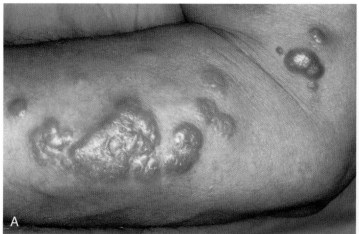

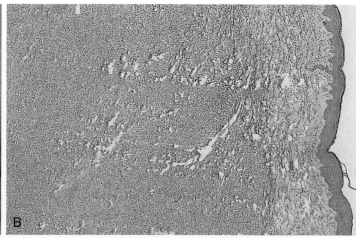

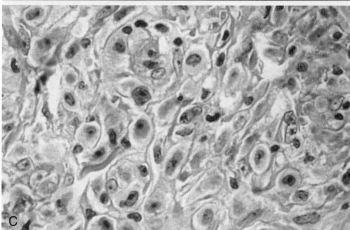

FIGURE 16.69 **CUTANEOUS ANAPLASTIC LARGE CELL LYMPHOMA (ALCL).** This 68-year-old man presented with slowly progressive cutaneous lesions, together with retroperitoneal and groin adenopathy. **(A)** Close-up view of the arm shows multiple raised, firm, irregular lesions. **(B)** Low-power microscopic section of a skin biopsy specimen reveals diffuse involvement of the reticular dermis by a blue cell infiltrate. **(C)** Higher magnification shows large cells with bizarre, hyperlobated nuclei, prominent nucleoli, and abundant cytoplasm. The cells usually express CD30, or less commonly T-cell antigens, or they may not express any lineage-specific antigens. Systemic ALCL represents about 2% of all non-Hodgkin lymphomas and has a bimodal age distribution (second and seventh decades). The ALK fusion protein is usually expressed, which carries a better prognosis than ALK$^-$ systemic disease. Primary cutaneous ALCL is CD30$^+$ ALK$^-$ but has a better prognosis than the systemic form of the disease.

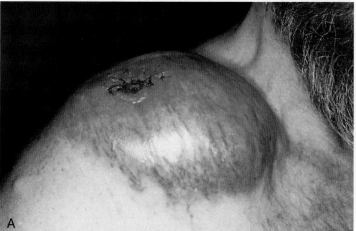

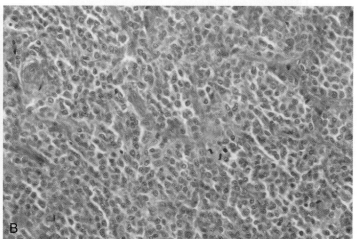

FIGURE 16.70 **CUTANEOUS INVOLVEMENT IN PERIPHERAL T-CELL LYMPHOMA, UNSPECIFIED. (A)** This 57-year-old man developed a large mass in the right shoulder, with no other lesions or adenopathy found on extensive evaluation. **(B)** Biopsy of the lesion shows intermediate- to large-sized lymphoid cells with round to irregular nuclear outlines, indistinct nucleoli, and pale eosinophilic cytoplasm. The lesion diffusely infiltrates from the dermis into the subcutaneous tissue but shows no epidermotropism. The malignant cells stained positive for LCA (CD45) and CD4 but were negative for CD5, CD3, CD1, CD8, CD2, and B-cell antigens (not shown). Primary cutaneous T-cell lymphoma is not common. The patient responded to chemotherapy followed by local radiation therapy. (Courtesy of Dr. D. Roberts, Department of Pathology, Brigham and Women's Hospital, Boston, MA.)

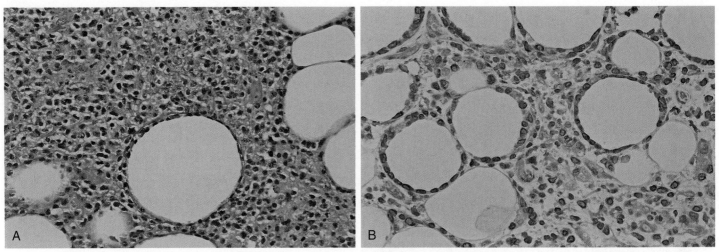

FIGURE 16.71 Subcutaneous panniculitis-like T-cell lymphoma, which occurs in young patients, typically involves the subcutaneous tissues of the extremities and may be associated with a hemophagocytic syndrome. **(A)** Intermediate-sized T-cells infiltrate subcutaneous and adipose tissues and are typically immunoreactive for **(B)** CD3, CD8, and cytotoxic markers TIA-1 and perforin.

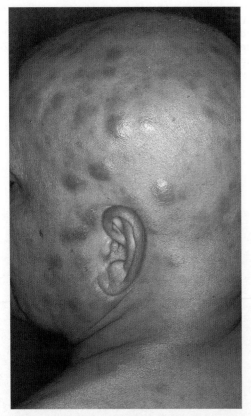

FIGURE 16.72 NK-CELL LYMPHOMA IN A 46-YEAR-OLD MAN. Numerous scalp and other cutaneous lesions are noted. The malignant cells were positive for both CD3 and CD56. He eventually developed generalized lymphadenopathy, a leukemic phase, and CNS involvement, including spread to the spinal fluid. Although initial response to chemotherapy was dramatic, progressive recurrent disease was fatal. A more indolent NK-cell lymphoma (also called large granular lymphocyte lymphoma or leukemia) is positive for CD3 but negative for CD56 antigens, and a third type is negative for CD3 and positive for CD56. (Reproduced from Lamy and Loughran, 1998, with permission.)

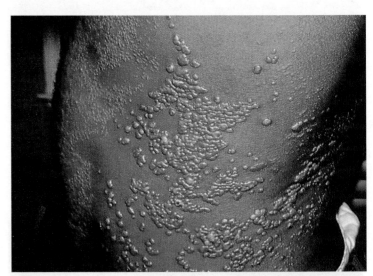

FIGURE 16.73 CUTANEOUS INVOLVEMENT IN ADULT T-CELL LYMPHOMA-LEUKEMIA. This unusual lymphoproliferative malignancy typically involves the skin, as well as lymph nodes, early in its course. Skin involvement in this case is extensive. (Courtesy of Dr. J.W. Clark.)

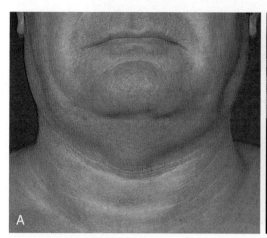
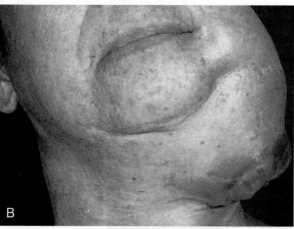

FIGURE 16.74 **CERVICAL ADENOPATHY IN NON-HODGKIN LYMPHOMA. (A)** Bilateral cervical lymphadenopathy is present in this patient with follicular lymphoma. **(B)** In another patient with diffuse large cell lymphoma, massive enlargement of lymph nodes in the left submandibular area has occurred together with extensive ulceration of the overlying skin.

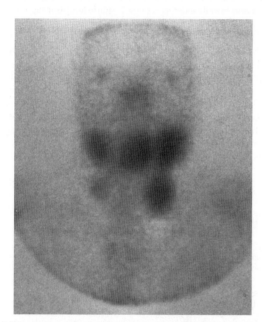

FIGURE 16.75 **CERVICAL ADENOPATHY IN DIFFUSE LARGE CELL LYMPHOMA (STAGE IIA).** Gallium-67 citrate scan in a 55-year-old man who presented with bulky lymphadenopathy involving only the neck nodes shows intense uptake in the submandibular and submental nodes and lower neck bilaterally. Gallium scan is useful in detecting sites of disease that are not palpable, as well as in following the response to therapy. PET scans are now used for staging and prognosis because of rapid results and direct comparison to CT images.

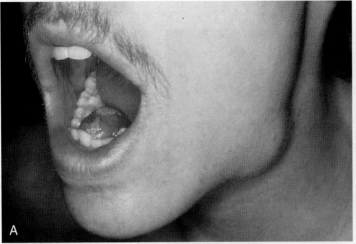

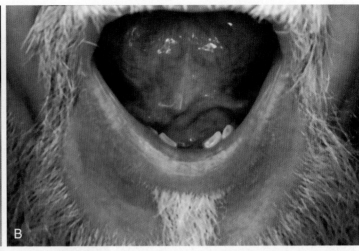

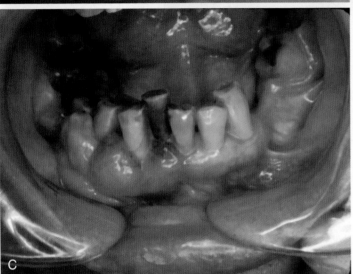

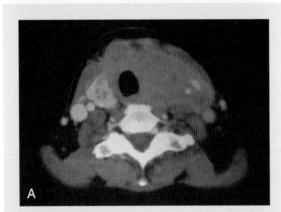

FIGURE 16.76 **MANDIBULAR AND INTRAORAL INVOLVEMENT IN BURKITT-LIKE LYMPHOMA.** **(A)** This 22-year-old man presented with a prominent tumor mass in the mandible and was found to have widespread disease. Note also the lymphomatous mass protruding through the floor of the mouth; superficial ulceration is present. Jaw lesions are particularly common in both Burkitt and Burkitt-like types of high-grade lymphomas. Intensive chemotherapy resulted in a rapid and complete remission. **(B)** A prominent tender mass at the base of the tongue was the presenting lesion in this 66-year-old man. Biopsy showed a large B-cell lymphoma. Multiple lymph node masses were found on staging evaluation, and he responded to multidrug chemotherapy. **(C)** A 56-year-old woman complained to her dentist about painful "gum lesions," seen on physical examination. Biopsy showed infiltration of the soft tissues by a follicular center cell lymphoma that was also present in the bone marrow biopsy specimen obtained. Systemic chemotherapy resulted in marked improvement with regression of symptoms and findings.

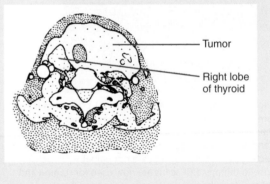

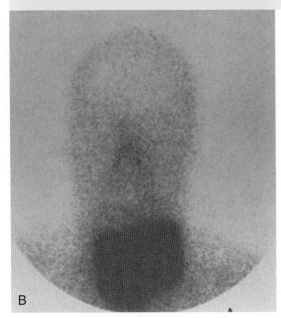

FIGURE 16.77 **THYROID INVOLVEMENT IN DIFFUSE LARGE CELL LYMPHOMA (STAGE I$_e$).** **(A)** CT scan of a 68-year-old woman who presented with a large neck mass shows extensive involvement of the anterior neck and left portion of the thyroid. The normal thyroid has a high attenuation number because of its normal iodine content. **(B)** A gallium-67 citrate scan shows uptake in the primary mass.

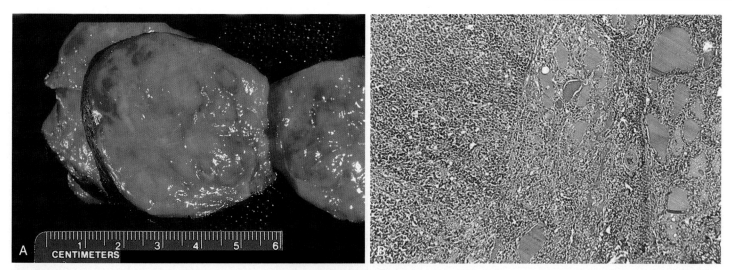

FIGURE 16.78 **THYROID INVOLVEMENT IN DIFFUSE LARGE CELL LYMPHOMA (DLCL). (A)** Diffusely enlarged, focally hemorrhagic, and necrotic thyroid involved by DLCL. **(B)** Histologic section of thyroid shows sheets of neoplastic cells on the *left* adjacent to residual colloid-filled acini on the *right*. Immunoperoxidase staining for light chains confirmed the monoclonality of the tumor cells. Although thyroid involvement is most common with large cell lymphomas, particularly B-cell immunoblastic lymphoma, occasional lymphocytic and nodular lymphomas have been reported. Most patients have evidence of coexisting Hashimoto's thyroiditis.

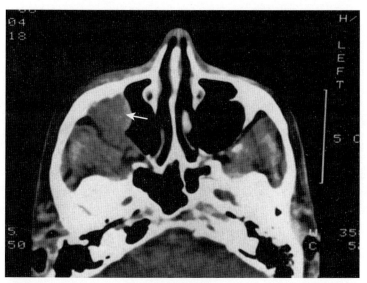

FIGURE 16.79 **NASOPHARYNGEAL INVOLVEMENT IN DIFFUSE LARGE CELL LYMPHOMA (STAGE I$_E$).** CT scan of a 34-year-old man who presented with frontal headaches and swelling around the eye reveals a tumor mass (*arrow*) primarily arising from the right maxillary sinus. He was treated successfully with surgery and radiation therapy; subsequently he developed a testicular mass and was placed on intensive combination chemotherapy.

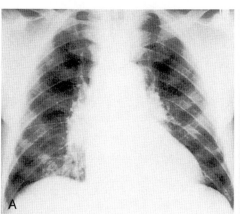
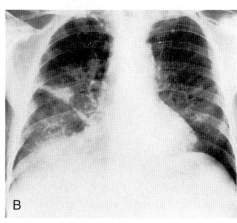

FIGURE 16.80 **MEDIASTINAL AND PULMONARY INVOLVEMENT IN FOLLICULAR LYMPHOMA.** Chest radiographs show **(A)** bilateral hilar lymph node enlargement and **(B)** interstitial and confluent shadowing, particularly in the lower and mid-zones, which biopsy showed to be due to lymphomatous infiltration.

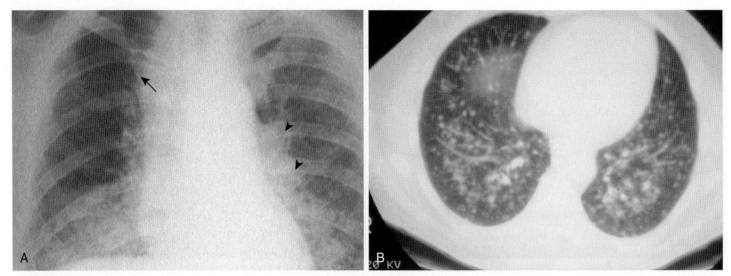

FIGURE 16.81 **MEDIASTINAL AND PULMONARY INVOLVEMENT IN DIFFUSE LARGE CELL LYMPHOMA. (A)** Frontal chest radiograph shows innumerable tiny bilateral lung nodules. The mediastinum is also widened because of adenopathy, particularly in the right paratracheal region (*black arrow*), and the left hilum is enlarged and lobular in contour (*arrowheads*). **(B)** CT image at the level of the lung bases displayed with lung windows also demonstrates the many tiny, well-defined nodules in both lungs. The patient, a 66-year-old man, had presented with a follicular lymphoma several years earlier. Transition to a large cell lymphoma occurs in over 30% of patients with low- or intermediate-grade lymphomas, particularly with long-standing disease (see Fig. 16.88).

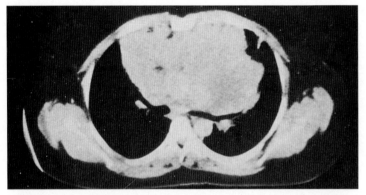

FIGURE 16.82 **MEDIASTINAL INVOLVEMENT IN PRECURSOR T-CELL LYMPHOBLASTIC LYMPHOMA.** CT scan through the midthorax shows gross enlargement of anterior mediastinal lymph nodes. This high-grade non-Hodgkin lymphoma of early T-cell lineage may arise in the mediastinum and occurs mainly in boys and adolescent males, which contrasts with mediastinal diffuse large cell lymphoma of B-cell lineage. With the latter, women outnumber men 2:1 and the median age at presentation is less than 30 years (see Fig. 16.83).

FIGURE 16.83 **MEDIASTINAL INVOLVEMENT IN DIFFUSE LARGE CELL LYMPHOMA.** Chest film shows bulky mediastinal adenopathy in an 18-year-old man with stage I before **(A)** and after **(B)** complete remission, which was achieved in only 6 weeks after the initiation of combination chemotherapy. The patient was disease-free more than 17 years later. Microscopically, primary large cell lymphoma is associated with dense sclerosis in about half of the cases. Clinically, adverse prognostic features include bulky (>7 cm) masses, extranodal disease, pleural effusion, elevated LDH or persistent gallium-67 or 2-[^{18}F]-fluoro-2-deoxy-D-glucose–PET (^{18}F-FDG-PET) avidity after treatment (Kirn et al., 1993).

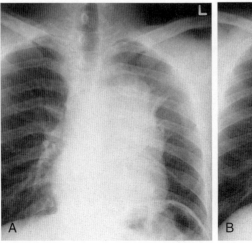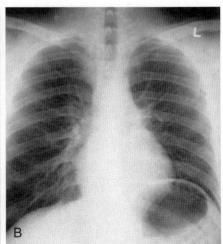

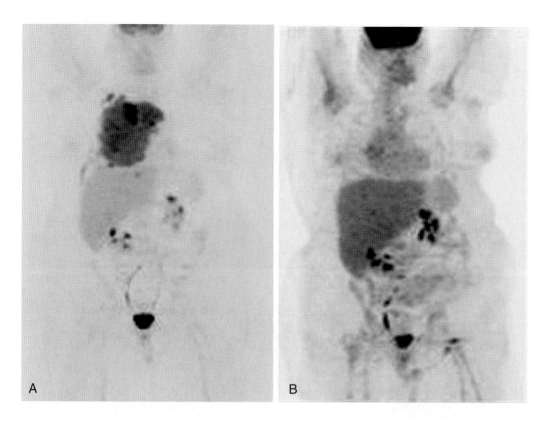

FIGURE 16.84 Pre-therapy **(A)** and follow-up post-therapy **(B)** PET scans of patient with diffuse large B-cell lymphoma with extensive ^{18}F-FDG–avid disease in the mediastinum. Follow-up scan demonstrates complete resolution of disease.

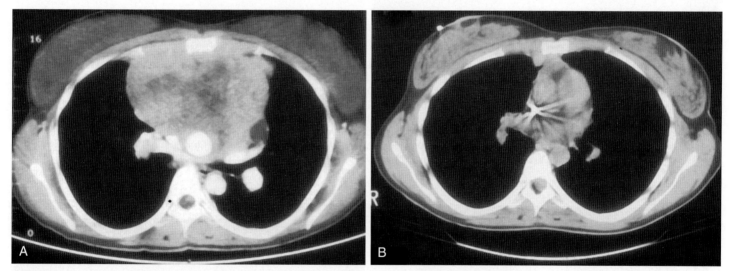

FIGURE 16.85 CT scans of a 40-year-old woman with primary large B-cell lymphoma of the mediastinum before **(A)** and after **(B)** two cycles of combination chemotherapy showing dramatic response.

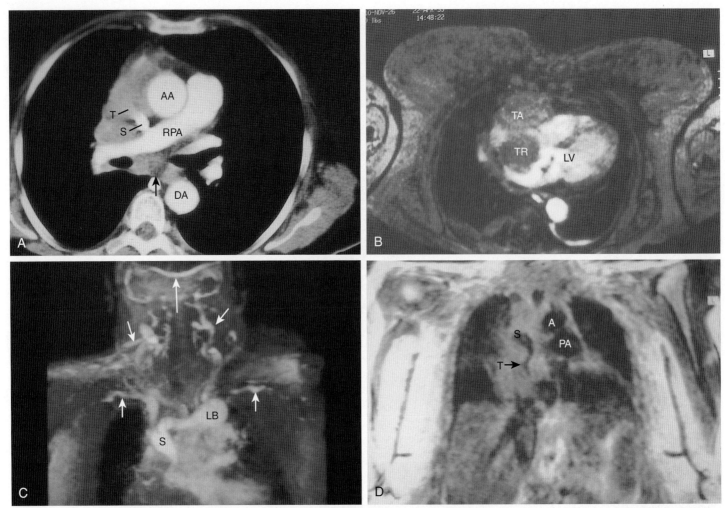

FIGURE 16.86 **SUPERIOR VENA CAVA (SVC) SYNDROME IN DIFFUSE LARGE CELL LYMPHOMA. (A)** CT image with intravenous contrast at the level of the right pulmonary artery (RPA) showing tumor (T) infiltrating into the area of the SVC (S), which is narrowed. Tumor is also present in the subcarinal space (*arrow*). AA, ascending aorta; DA, descending aorta. **(B)** MR image in the axial plane at the level of the left ventricle (LV) using a sequence that produces a high signal from flowing blood. Tumor is seen both anterior to the heart (TA) and protruding into the lumen of the right atrium (TR). A small left pleural effusion is also present. **(C)** MR image in the coronal plane at the level of the anterior neck using a sequence that produces a high signal from flowing blood. Numerous tortuous and dilated neck collateral vessels are present (*arrows*), indicating obstruction of venous return. LB, left brachiocephalic vein; S, SVC. **(D)** T_1-weighted MR image in the coronal plane through the main pulmonary artery (PA). Tumor is seen filling the right atrium (T). A markedly narrowed SVC (S) passes through the tumor, tapering to a slit inferiorly (*arrow*). A, aortic arch.

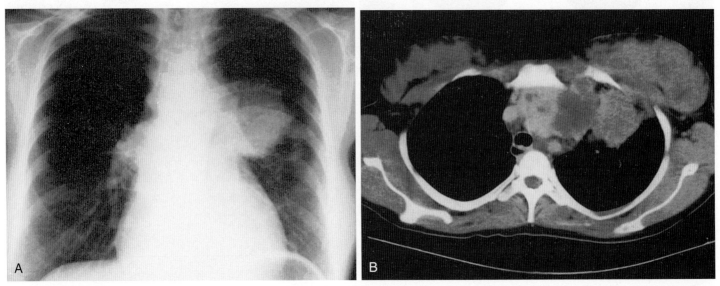

FIGURE 16.87 **MEDIASTINAL INVOLVEMENT IN DIFFUSE LARGE CELL LYMPHOMA (STAGE IVB). (A)** Chest film of a 30-year-old woman who presented with cough, fever, and weight loss shows a large upper mediastinal mass. **(B)** On CT scan the mass appears heterogeneous, a result of necrosis within the tumor. There is also a second mass extending from the mediastinum and involving the lung parenchyma. Spread of the lymphoma through the chest wall and into the pectoralis muscles and breast is evident. Biopsy showed a B-immunoblastic sarcoma subtype of large cell lymphoma. A complete remission was obtained with combination chemotherapy.

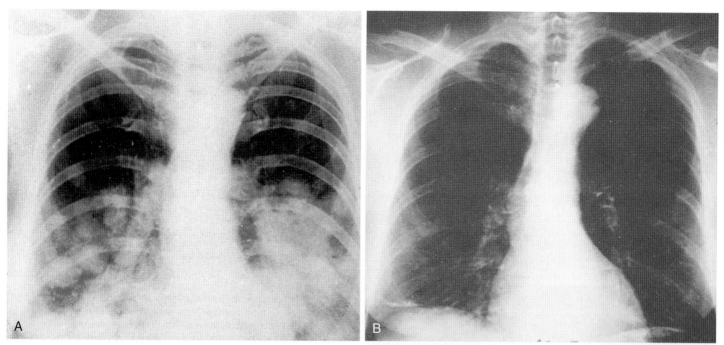

FIGURE 16.88 **PULMONARY INVOLVEMENT IN DIFFUSE LARGE CELL LYMPHOMA (STAGE IVB). (A)** A 64-year-old woman who presented with fever, weight loss, and dyspnea was found to have multiple pulmonary nodules on chest radiography. Biopsy yielded the diagnosis. **(B)** Two months after chemotherapy there is complete remission. Non-Hodgkin lymphomas in the lung show a broad spectrum of radiographic findings, ranging from purely linear or "reticular" (reticulonodular) infiltrates to the extensive large nodules seen in this case. Less commonly, a single nodule or a focal infiltrate resembling pneumonia may be seen.

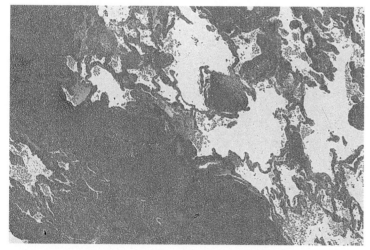

FIGURE 16.89 **PRIMARY PULMONARY LYMPHOCYTIC LYMPHOMA.** Low-power view of a lung biopsy shows sheets of neoplastic lymphocytes at the edge of the tumor infiltrating the surrounding lung along bronchovascular bundles and alveolar septa. Primary pulmonary non-Hodgkin lymphomas are uncommon, although lung involvement is frequent as part of disseminated disease, most often with diffuse large cell lymphoma. In some patients morphologic features are diagnostic of a low-grade MALT lymphoma.

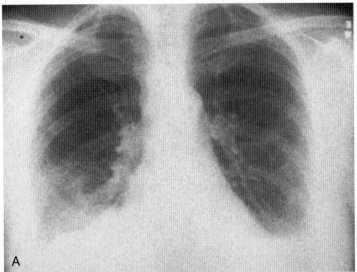

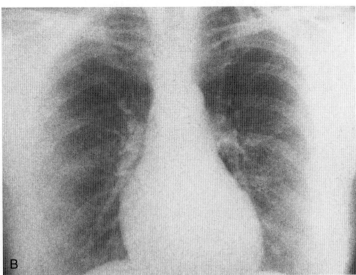

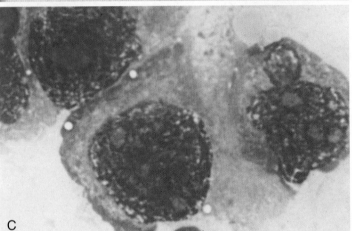

FIGURE 16.90   **MALIGNANT PLEURAL EFFUSION IN FOLLICULAR LYMPHOMA (STAGE IVA). (A)** Chest film of a 57-year-old woman who presented with increasing dyspnea and cough shows small bilateral pleural effusions. Further workup revealed retroperitoneal adenopathy with ascites. A dramatic response occurred within 3 weeks of initiation of combination chemotherapy. **(B)** Follow-up film shows complete resolution of the pleural effusions. Four years later fever and weight loss occurred, in association with pleural effusions, adenopathy, and subcutaneous nodules. **(C)** Cytocentrifuge preparation of pleural fluid shows large malignant cells with irregular nuclei containing prominent nucleoli, findings diagnostic of a large cell lymphoma. Lymph node biopsy (not shown) confirmed histologic progression to a diffuse large cell lymphoma (see Fig. 16.81).

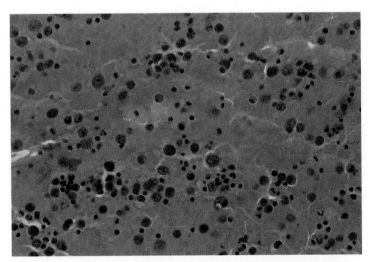

FIGURE 16.91   Primary effusion lymphoma, typically found in HIV-positive patients, presents in pleural, pericardial, or ascitic fluid without a tumor mass. It is a high-grade B-cell lymphoma with a poor prognosis (median survival <1 year). Neoplastic cells are positive for CD45, CD30, and HLA-DR, as well as being positive for Kaposi sarcoma–associated herpesvirus, human herpesvirus 8, and EBV.

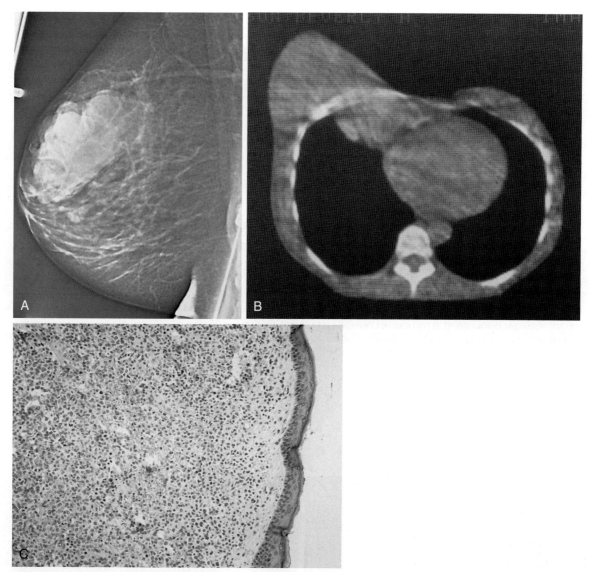

FIGURE 16.92 **LYMPHOMA OF THE BREAST (STAGE I$_E$). (A)** Mammogram of a 35-year-old woman who presented with a large upper left breast mass shows a soft tissue mass with no suspicious calcifications. The differential diagnosis included adenocarcinoma of the breast, cystosarcoma phylloides, lymphoma, and, less likely, metastases or a benign process. Biopsy was positive for a diffuse large cell lymphoma (DLCL). **(B)** Staging CT scan in another patient, who developed rapid enlargement of the right breast and axillary adenopathy, dramatically reveals how extensively the tumor has infiltrated the breast; there is also extension of the lymphoma into the internal mammary nodes. Biopsy also showed a DLCL. **(C)** Microscopic section of a breast biopsy from a woman who presented with an inflammatory breast lesion demonstrates involvement by a DLCL. Primary lymphomas of the breast represent a B-cell spectrum, varying from high-grade to low-grade follicular and MALT types (Mattia et al., 1993).

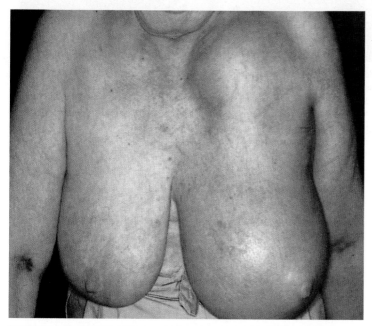

FIGURE 16.93 **INVOLVEMENT OF THE BREAST IN LYMPHOMA (STAGE IV).** This 75-year-old woman presented with advanced diffuse large cell lymphoma including involvement of lung and heart. Note the enlarged left breast with inflammatory skin changes due to lymphatic obstruction, simulating primary inflammatory breast carcinoma. A greatly enlarged left upper chest wall mass is also evident, arising from underlying adenopathy.

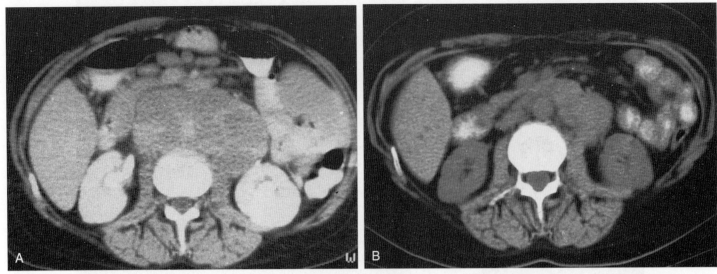

FIGURE 16.94 **RETROPERITONEAL INVOLVEMENT IN FOLLICULAR LYMPHOMA (STAGE IIIA). (A)** Staging CT scan in a 42-year-old woman who presented with generalized adenopathy shows enlarged retroperitoneal nodes that demonstrated marked uptake on gallium-67 citrate scan (not shown). **(B)** Following combination chemotherapy there is dramatic regression in the retroperitoneal nodes.

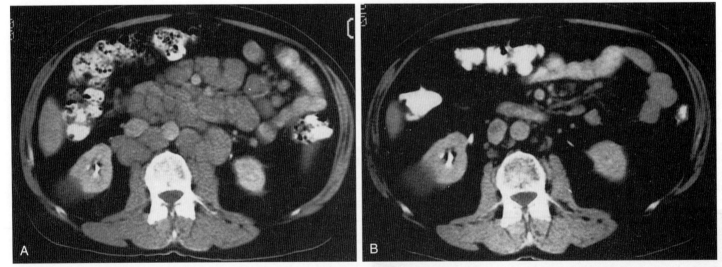

FIGURE 16.95 **MESENTERIC AND RETROPERITONEAL INVOLVEMENT IN SMALL LYMPHOCYTIC LYMPHOMA (STAGE IVA).** A 58-year-old man presented with generalized adenopathy, mild anemia, and thrombocytopenia. Bone marrow biopsy revealed infiltration by small, well-differentiated lymphocytes. Surface marker studies were consistent with a monocolonal population of B lymphocytes. **(A)** Abdominal CT scan demonstrates many enlarged mesenteric and retroperitoneal lymph nodes. **(B)** Follow-up CT scan 16 months later after intermittent chemotherapy shows regression in all nodes, confirming a complete clinical remission. As an incidental finding, note the benign renal cyst in the right kidney.

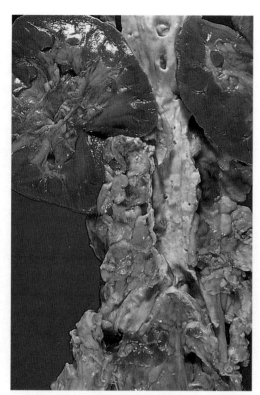

FIGURE 16.96 **RETROPERITONEAL INVOLVEMENT IN DIFFUSE LARGE CELL LYMPHOMA.**
Confluent adenopathy of retroperitoneal lymph nodes has led to bilateral
encasement and compression of the ureters by pink-tan, fleshy tumor.

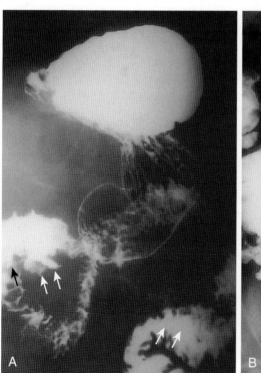

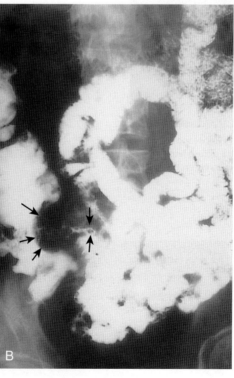

FIGURE 16.97 **MALT MARGINAL ZONE LYMPHOMA
OF THE GI TRACT. (A)** Abdominal film from upper
GI series showing thickened nodular folds in the
duodenum (*arrows*) and less prominent nodularity
of the mucosa in the jejunum (*arrows*) consistent
with infiltrative process in the small bowel mucosa.
(B) Abdominal film from a small bowel follow-
through series showing the relatively normal
appearance of the distal jejunum and proximal
ileum, but marked narrowing and irregularity of
the terminal ileum (*arrows*), with a large filling
defect in the region of the ileocecal valve (*arrows*),
consistent with markedly thickened, infiltrated
mucosa (see also Fig. 16.98).

FIGURE 16.98 **MARGINAL ZONE LYMPHOMA OF MALT OF THE STOMACH. (A, B)** The stomach wall is extensively infiltrated by small lymphoid cells with a moderate amount of cytoplasm and round to irregular nuclei, with occasional plasma cells and scattered germinal centers. **(B)** Higher power reveals scattered lymphoepithelial lesions. The lymphoid cells are positive for pan-B-cell markers and negative for CD5 and CD10. Some patients seem to respond to therapy for *H. pylori* infection, which has been implicated as an etiologic agent (Isaacson, 1994).

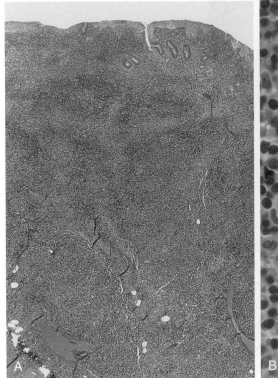
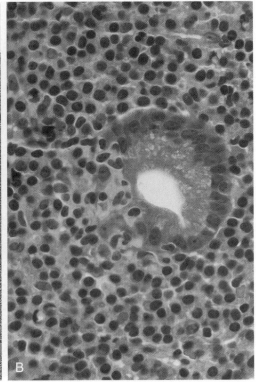

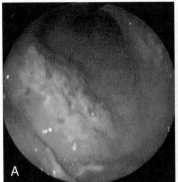
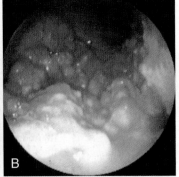

FIGURE 16.99 **LYMPHOMA OF THE STOMACH. (A, B)** These endoscopic views show diffuse nodular involvement of the gastric wall by a diffuse large cell lymphoma. This lesion was associated with a protein-losing enteropathy.

FIGURE 16.100 **LYMPHOMA OF THE STOMACH.** **(A)** Barium study shows mucosal and mural involvement of the fundus and body of the stomach. **(B)** Histologic section reveals invasion of the gastric glands, lamina propria, and deeper areas by sheets of tumor cells of a diffuse large cell lymphoma. **(A**, Courtesy of Dr. D. Nag.)

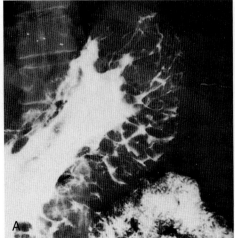
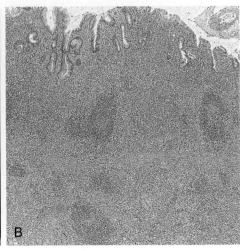

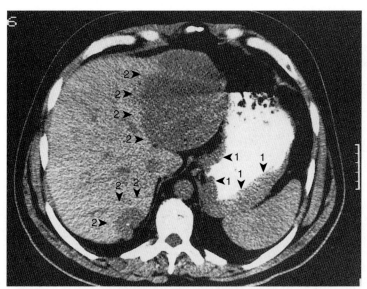

FIGURE 16.101 **LYMPHOMA OF THE STOMACH.** CT scan of a 45-year-old man who presented with weight loss and epigastric distress shows thickening of the wall of the body of the stomach (*arrowheads 1*), as well as two low-attenuation masses in the liver (*arrowheads 2*). Although these abnormalities are compatible with the diagnosis of lymphoma, there is no way to distinguish them from gastric adenocarcinoma with metastases to the liver. Endoscopic gastric biopsy showed a diffuse large cell lymphoma.

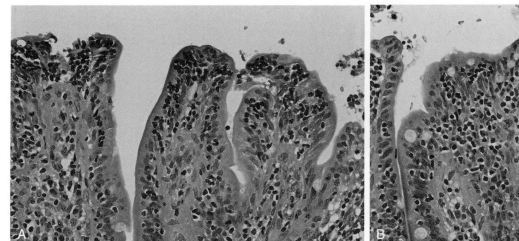
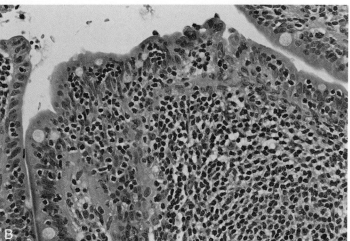

FIGURE 16.102 Enteropathy-type T-cell lymphoma occurs in older patients, many of whom have a history of celiac disease. Neoplastic T cells infiltrate segments of small bowel **(A)**, leading to villous blunting, atrophy, and malabsorption **(B)**. The neoplastic cells are immunoreactive for pan-T-cell markers such as CD3 as well as CD103.

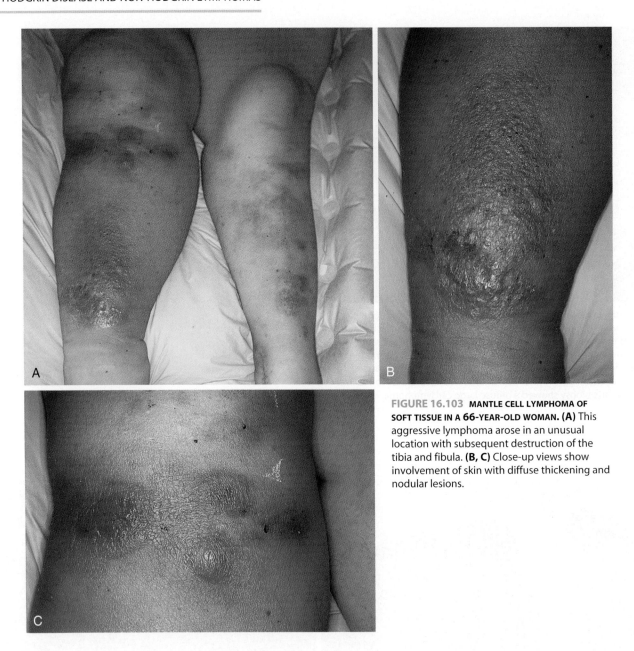

FIGURE 16.103 **MANTLE CELL LYMPHOMA OF SOFT TISSUE IN A 66-YEAR-OLD WOMAN. (A)** This aggressive lymphoma arose in an unusual location with subsequent destruction of the tibia and fibula. **(B, C)** Close-up views show involvement of skin with diffuse thickening and nodular lesions.

FIGURE 16.104 **GI INVOLVEMENT IN B-CELL LARGE CELL LYMPHOMA.** A 55-year-old man presented with abdominal complaints. On workup he was found to have mediastinal, hilar, and peripheral adenopathy, as well as **(A)** diffuse narrowing and irregularity of several loops of small bowel, consistent with involvement by lymphoma. A mass effect in the right lower quadrant can also be seen. **(B)** Combination chemotherapy resulted in complete remission, as can be seen in this follow-up barium film.

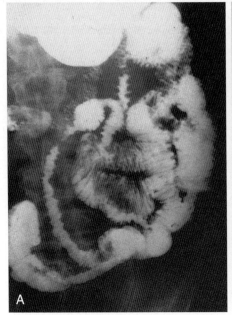

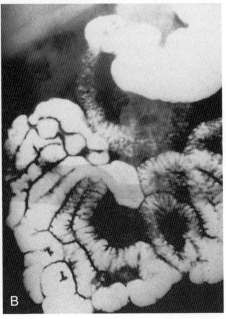

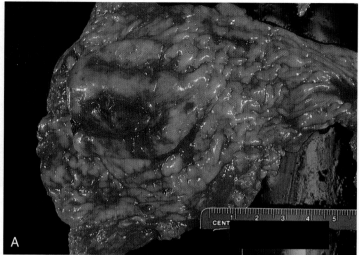

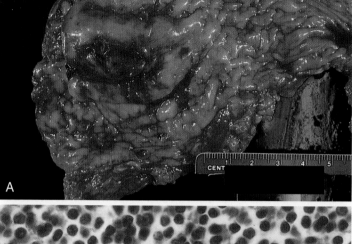

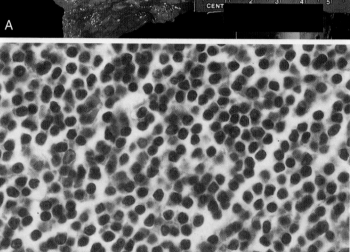

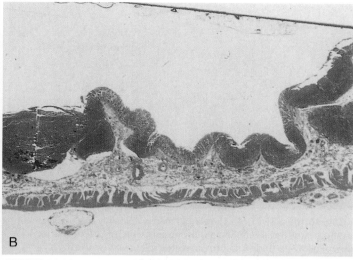

FIGURE 16.105 **MANTLE CELL LYMPHOMA OF THE COLON, PRESENTING AS MULTIPLE LYMPHOMATOUS POLYPOSIS.** A 67-year-old woman presented with GI bleeding. Biopsies and subsequent resection reveal multiple submucosal tumor masses in the right colon and ileum that focally erode the mucosa and infiltrate to lamina propria **(A, B)**. The infiltrate is composed of small lymphoid cells with irregular to cleaved nuclei **(C)**. Tumor was present in numerous pericolic lymph nodes and, at autopsy, was found to have spread extensively with the retroperitoneum and to involve lung, liver, spleen, and bone marrow. Early, wide dissemination is a characteristic feature in multiple lymphomatous polyposis. Tumor cells are positive for pan-B-cell markers and CD5.

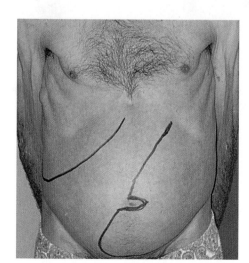

FIGURE 16.106 **SPLENIC AND LIVER INVOLVEMENT IN FOLLICULAR LYMPHOMA.** Massive enlargement of the spleen and hepatomegaly are apparent in this patient.

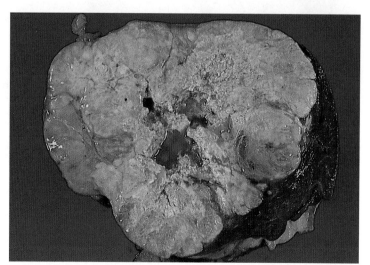

FIGURE 16.107 **SPLENIC INVOLVEMENT IN B-CELL DIFFUSE LARGE CELL LYMPHOMA.** This spleen, removed at laparotomy, has been sectioned to show widespread replacement of tissue by pale tumor with extensive areas of necrosis.

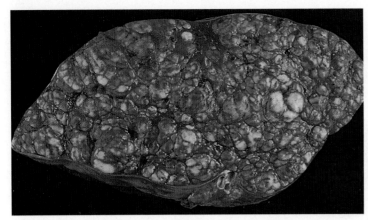

FIGURE 16.108 PET/CT of a 55-year-old man with mainly liver involvement by diffuse large B-cell lymphoma showing subtle foci of FDG uptake (A, arrow). Follow-up study 6 months later after relapse revealed extensive lymphoma lesions that were FDG-avid in the liver.

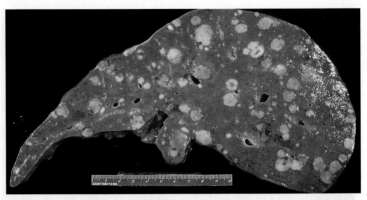

FIGURE 16.109 **HEPATIC INVOLVEMENT IN B-CELL DIFFUSE LARGE CELL LYMPHOMA.** A 64-year-old woman with a stage IV DPDL lymphoma responded to treatment at first but then relapsed with a downhill course despite further therapy. Autopsy showed widespread disease, and histologic examination revealed transition to a high-grade lymphoma. The liver may be involved in up to 50% of cases of disseminated disease. Histologic progression from a low-grade to an intermediate- or high-grade lymphoma occurs clinically in about 30% of cases, but at autopsy as many as 60% to 70% of cases show a change in histology to a higher grade (aggressive) lymphoma.

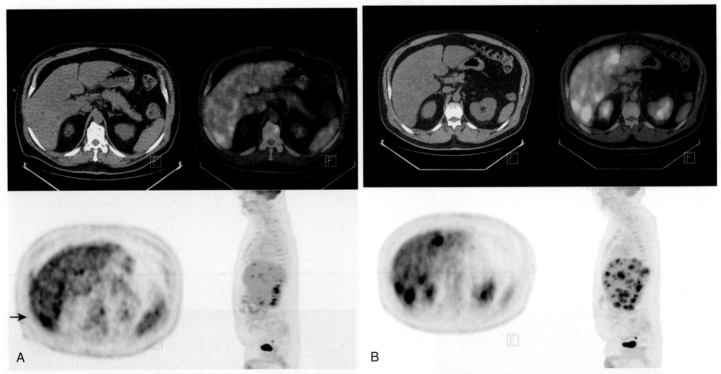

FIGURE 16.110 **HEPATIC INVOLVEMENT IN FOLLICULAR LYMPHOMA. (A)** Dark patches *(arrow)* of lymphocytic tumor cells infiltrate the liver, causing **(B)** expansion of a portal tract. This type of periportal involvement is often seen in lymphocytic lymphomas and may not be associated with very abnormal liver chemistry tests.

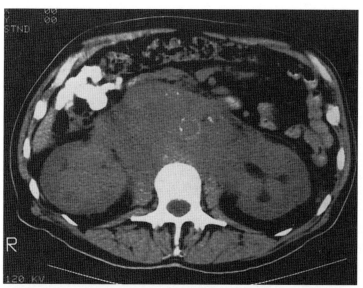

FIGURE 16.111 **RENAL INVOLVEMENT IN DIFFUSE LARGE CELL LYMPHOMA.** A 54-year-old man who had a stage III poorly differentiated lymphocytic lymphoma for 7 years suddenly developed increasing abdominal distention. This CT scan shows diffuse retroperitoneal adenopathy encasing the aorta and extending directly into the renal parenchyma bilaterally. A cauda equina syndrome developed and cerebrospinal fluid examination showed large lymphoma cells, indicating histologic conversion to an aggressive malignancy.

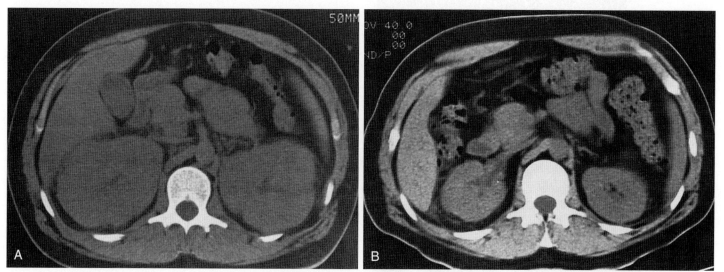

FIGURE 16.112 **RENAL INVOLVEMENT IN PRECURSOR T-CELL LYMPHOBLASTIC LYMPHOMA.** A 31-year-old man presented with weight loss, fatigue, and low back pain. Evaluation revealed acute renal failure. **(A)** Abdominal CT scan shows greatly enlarged kidneys, which on biopsy yielded the diagnosis. Bone marrow was also involved by lymphoma. Immunophenotyping of bone marrow cells showed positivity for CD2 (71%), CD5 (53%), CD3 (22%), CD8 (30%), and CD4 (8%). The patient's condition improved dramatically with intensive chemotherapy. **(B)** Follow-up CT scan 1 month later shows essentially normal kidneys.

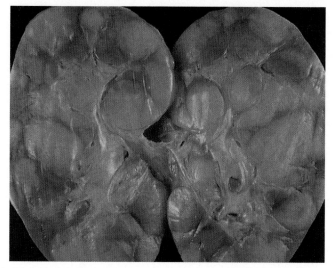

FIGURE 16.113 **RENAL INVOLVEMENT IN DIFFUSE LARGE CELL LYMPHOMA.** There is little remaining parenchyma in this specimen, which exhibits many large, gray-white nodules of tumor.

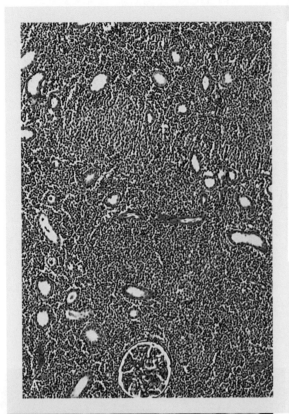

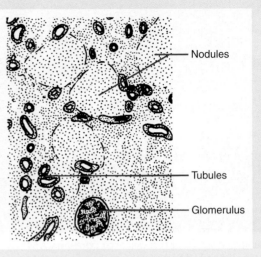

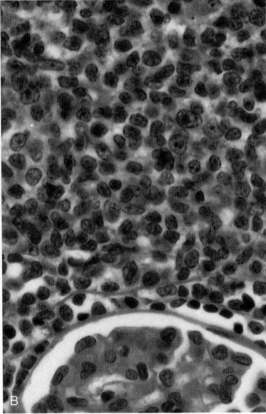

FIGURE 16.114   **RENAL INVOLVEMENT IN FOLLICULAR LYMPHOMA. (A)** The presence of nodular infiltrates in the renal cortex is consistent with involvement by a B-cell lymphoma. **(B)** Higher magnification demonstrates that the infiltrate is composed of a mixture of large and small lymphocytes, as well as scattered small, cleaved cells typical of a follicular center cell lymphoma. (Reproduced from Schumann and Weiss, 1981.)

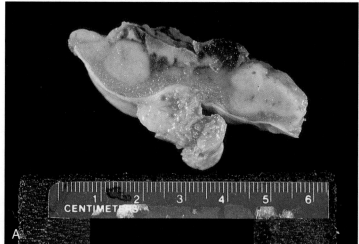

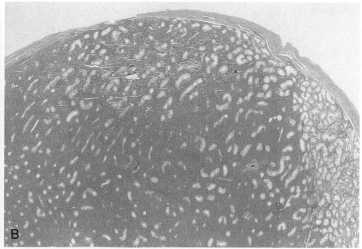

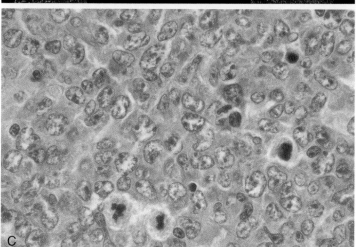

FIGURE 16.115 **TESTICULAR INVOLVEMENT BY DIFFUSE LARGE CELL LYMPHOMA (DLCL). (A)** A tan-pink tumor mass accounts for the testicular enlargement in a 51-year-old man. **(B)** Low-power view of the interstitial DLCL infiltrate that characteristically surrounds seminiferous tubules. **(C)** High-power view reveals a population of large lymphoid cells, many with irregular and cleaved nuclei. Non-Hodgkin lymphoma is the most common testicular tumor in men over 60 years of age and is most commonly a large cell type of B-cell origin, as was true in this case.

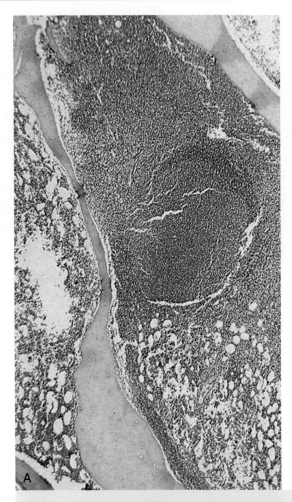

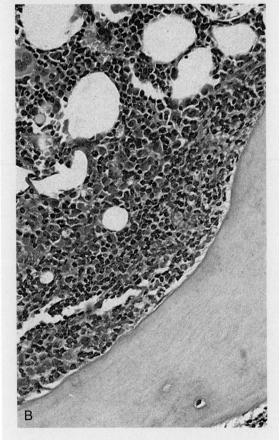

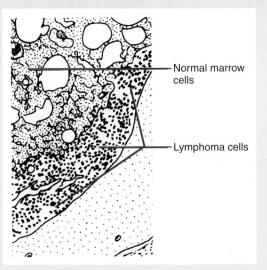

Normal marrow cells

Lymphoma cells

FIGURE 16.116   BONE MARROW INVOLVEMENT IN FOLLICULAR LYMPHOMA. (A) Low-power microscopic section of a needle biopsy specimen reveals almost complete replacement of normal hematopoietic tissue in the upper portion of the field and a paratrabecular collection of neoplastic lymphoid cells below. **(B)** Higher magnification shows the demarcation between the paratrabecular lymphoid cells and the normal hematopoietic cells and fat.

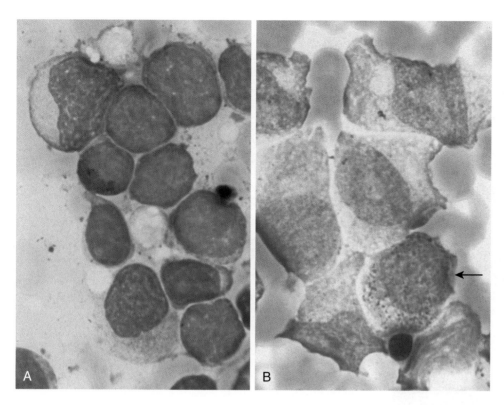

FIGURE 16.117   **BONE MARROW INVOLVEMENT IN NON-HODGKIN LYMPHOMA. (A)** Smear from a bone marrow aspiration in a patient with follicular lymphoma shows small, poorly differentiated cells with scanty cytoplasm; irregular nuclear contours are apparent, with slight indentations in some of the cells. Nuclear chromatin is fine and light staining. Nucleoli are not evident. **(B)** In this patient with a diffuse large cell lymphoma, immature cells have large, prominent nucleoli. A promyelocyte (granulated cell) is seen in the lower right field (*arrow*).

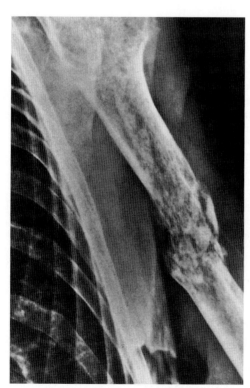

FIGURE 16.118   **BONE INVOLVEMENT IN DIFFUSE LARGE CELL LYMPHOMA (STAGE 1$_E$).** Radiograph of the left upper arm of a 45-year-old man who complained of sudden onset of pain shows a pathologic fracture through an area of permeative destruction of cortical and medullary bone. The fracture is quite recent, since there is little or no periosteal reaction either to the tumor itself or to the complicating fracture. Biopsy yielded the diagnosis.

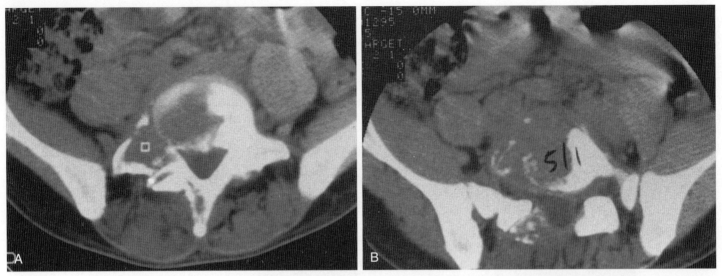

FIGURE 16.119 **BONE INVOLVEMENT IN BURKITT-LIKE LYMPHOMA (STAGE IVB). (A, B)** CT scans in an 18-year-old man who presented with weight loss and severe low back pain reveal destruction at the L5–S1 vertebrae. Further workup disclosed multiple bone lesions and retroperitoneal adenopathy.

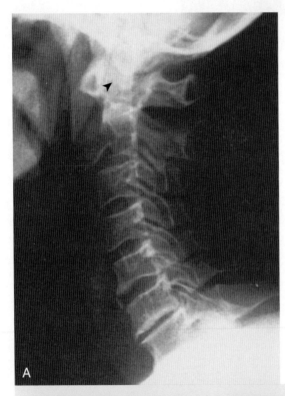

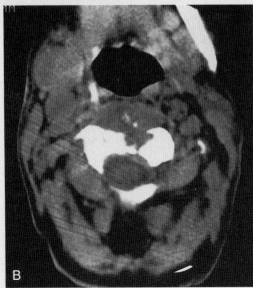

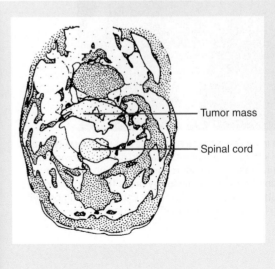

FIGURE 16.120 **BONE INVOLVEMENT IN FOLLICULAR LYMPHOMA (STAGE IV).** A 62-year-old man with a 3-year history of lymphoma, involving mainly the bone marrow and lymph nodes, showed a partial response with chemotherapy but suddenly developed severe neck pain. **(A)** Plain radiograph of the cervical spine shows lytic destruction of the body of C1 (*arrowhead*). **(B)** CT scan reveals tumor invasion of C1–C2 with extension into the spinal canal. Stabilization of the neck was achieved by a bone graft. Further workup disclosed other bone lesions and retroperitoneal adenopathy.

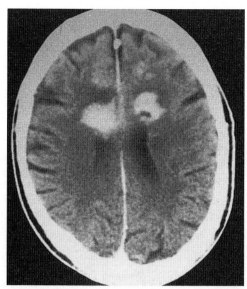

FIGURE 16.121 CNS INVOLVEMENT IN DIFFUSE LARGE CELL LYMPHOMA.
A 62-year-old man who was diagnosed 3 years earlier with a stage IIA
lymphoma involving the mediastinum achieved complete remission with
chemotherapy. Subsequently a testicular mass developed, followed by
headaches. This CT scan shows several enhancing periventricular lesions
consistent with CNS involvement by lymphoma.

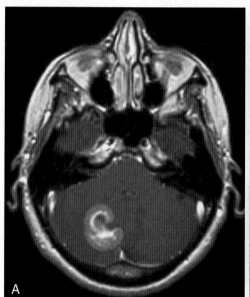
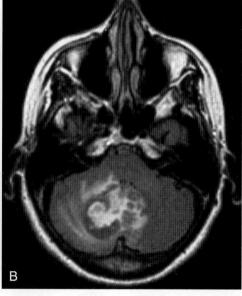

FIGURE 16.122 A 57-year old woman
developed vertigo, headaches, nausea,
vomiting and diplopia with subsequent
speech difficulties. A brain MRI with contrast
showed a heterogeneous cystic-appearing
mass with surrounding vasogenic edema
and near obliteration of the lateral and third
ventricle with some midbrain compressions
(A,B). Resection showed a diffuse large B-cell
lymphoma that was CD20⁺, MUM⁺, BCL2⁺,
CD10⁻, EBER⁻, and Ki-67 = 90%. Staging showed
no other sites of disease. She was treated for
primary CNS lymphoma with subsequent high-
dose methotrexate and continues in complete
remission at more than 2 years. (Courtesy of Dr.
Julia Gold and Dr. Alexi Wright.) Recent data
show that BCL6 expression in patients with
primary CNS lymphoma is associated with a
better prognosis (Levy et al., 2008).

FIGURE 16.123 CNS INVOLVEMENT IN DIFFUSE LARGE CELL LYMPHOMA. A 70-year-old woman with a lymphoma in remission developed blindness and diffuse weakness of all extremities. This MR scan shows evidence of meningeal involvement. Cerebrospinal fluid examination revealed increased protein, low sugar, and many large, immature lymphoma cells.

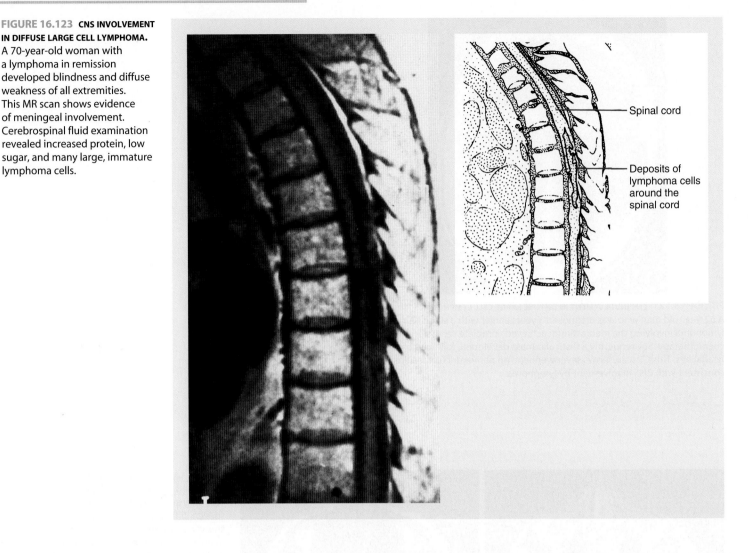

Spinal cord

Deposits of lymphoma cells around the spinal cord

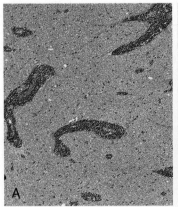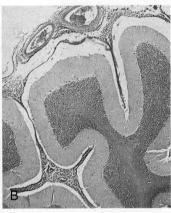

FIGURE 16.124 CNS INVOLVEMENT IN PRECURSOR T-CELL LYMPHOBLASTIC LYMPHOMA. (A) Invasion has occurred along perivascular spaces, and **(B)** the meninges are extensively involved. A similar pattern occurs in primary lymphoma of the brain, which in most cases is an undifferentiated or large cell lymphoma. Primary lymphoma of the brain is an AIDS-defining illness and the second most frequent extranodal disease site after the GI tract. Almost all cases are of B-cell type. EBV is thought to have a role in the pathogenesis of CNS lymphomas in immunocompromised patients, including AIDS patients (see Chapter 19).

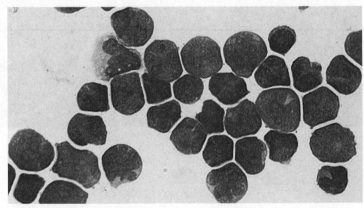

FIGURE 16.125 CNS INVOLVEMENT IN PRECURSOR T-CELL LYMPHOBLASTIC LYMPHOMA. High-power view of a cytospin preparation of cerebrospinal fluid shows typical T lymphoblasts. The nucleus in many of the cells has a convoluted or cloverleaf appearance. Another high-grade lymphoma, small non–cleaved cell lymphoma, Burkitt-type, also has a predilection for involvement of the meninges.

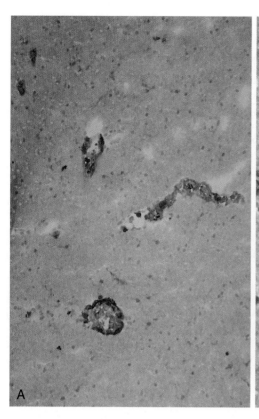
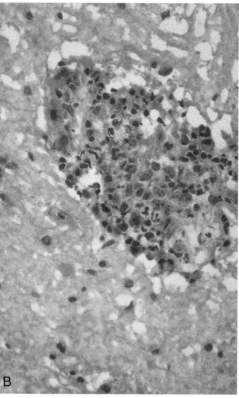

FIGURE 16.126 **CNS INVOLVEMENT IN INTRAVASCULAR LYMPHOMATOSIS (IVL). (A)** Low-power view of the brain shows several intravascular foci of lymphoma cells in a 43-year-old man who presented with confusion and other neurologic features (immunoperoxidase stain for LCA). **(B)** Higher-power view shows cluster of large lymphoid cells within a vessel. Immunophenotyping revealed monoclonal B lymphocytes (not shown). The patient had widespread involvement of the CNS as well as of the blood vessels of the lungs. IVL is an unusual aggressive lymphoma with a variety of CNS, cutaneous, and pulmonary manifestations (Demirer et al., 1994). Few cases are diagnosed before death. The mechanisms for trapping of neoplastic lymphocytes within small vessels of diffuse organs remain unexplained. (Courtesy of Dr. M. Kilo.)

References and Suggested Readings

Abramson J, Shipp MA: Advances in the biology of diffuse large B-cell lymphoma: moving toward a molecularly targeted approach, *Blood* 106:1164–1174, 2005.

Amin HM, Lai R: Pathobiology of ALK+ anaplastic large-cell lymphoma, *Blood* 110:2259–2267, 2007.

Arber DA: Molecular diagnostic approach to non-Hodgkin's lymphoma, *J Mol Diagn* 2:178–190, 2000.

Armitage JO, Bierman PJ, Bociek RG, et al: Lymphoma 2006: classification and treatment, *Oncology* 20:231–249, 2006.

Arnold A, Cossman J, Bakhshi A, et al: Immunoglobulin-gene rearrangements as unique clonal markers in human lymphoid neoplasms, *N Engl J Med* 309:1593–1599, 1983.

Baddoura F, Chan W, Masih A, et al: T-cell-rich B-cell lymphoma, *Am J Clin Pathol* 103:65–75, 1995.

Bea S, Zettl A, Wright G, et al: Diffuse large B-cell lymphoma subgroups have distinct genetic profiles that influence tumor biology and improve gene-expression-based survival prediction, *Blood* 106: 3183–3190, 2005.

Carey JL, Hanson CA: Flow cytometric analysis of leukemia and lymphoma. In Keren DF, Hanson CA, Hurtubise PE, editors: *Flow cytometry and clinical diagnosis*, Chicago, 1994, American Society of Clinical Pathologists, pp 197–308.

Chan JKC, Banks PM, Clearly ML, et al: A revised European-American classification of lymphoid neoplasms proposed by the International Lymphoma Study Group, *Am J Clin Pathol* 103:543–560, 1995.

Chang H, Benchimol S, Minden MD, et al: Alterations of p53 and c-myc in the clonal evolution of malignant lymphoma, *Blood* 83(2):452–459, 1994.

Chen YB, Rahemtullah A, Hochberg E: Primary effusion lymphoma, *Oncologist* 12:569–576, 2007.

Clarke C, Glaser SL: Changing incidence of non-Hodgkin lymphomas in the United States, *Cancer* 94:2015–2023, 2002.

Cordier JF, Chailleux E, Lauque D, et al: Primary pumonary lymphomas: a clinical study of 70 cases in nonimmunocompromised patients, *Chest* 103:201–208, 1993.

Dabbs DJ, Moul-Manager L, Mignon F, et al: Glomerular lesions in lymphomas and leukemias, *Am J Med* 80:63–70, 1986.

Dave SS, Fu K, Wright GW, et al: Molecular diagnosis of Burkitt's lymphoma, *N Engl J Med* 354:2431–2442, 2006.

DeFalco G, Leucci E, Lenze D, et al: Gene-expression analysis identifies novel RBL2/p130 target genes in endemic Burkitt lymphoma cell lines and primary tumors, *Blood* 110:1301–1307, 2007.

Del Giudice I, Morilla A, Osuji N, et al: Zeta-chain associated protein 70 and CD38 combined predict the time to first treatment in patients with chronic lymphocytic leukemia, *Cancer* 104:2124–2132, 2005.

Diepstra A, van Imhoff GW, Henrike E, et al: HLA Class II expression by Hodgkin Reed-Sternberg cells is an independent prognostic factor in classical Hodgkin's lymphoma, *J Clin Oncol* 25:3101–3108, 2007.

Ferry JA: Burkitt's lymphoma: clinicopathologic features and differential diagnosis, *Oncologist* 11:375–383, 2006.

Fisher R, Dahlberg S, Hathwani B, et al: A clinical analysis of two indolent lymphoma entities: mantle cell lymphoma and marginal zone lymphoma (including the mucosa-associated lymphoid tissue and monocytoid B-cell subcategories): a Southwest Oncology Group study, *Blood* 85:1075–1082, 1995.

Freedman AS, Nadler LM: Cell surface markers in hematologic malignancies, *Semin Oncol* 14:193–212, 1987.

Harris NL, Horning SJ: Burkitt's lymphoma—the message from microarrays, *N Engl J Med* 354:2495–2498, 2006.

Harris NL, Jaffe ES, Diebold J, et al: World Health Organization classification of neoplastic diseases of the hematopoietic and lymphoid tissues: report of the clinical advisory committee meeting, Airlie House, Virginia, November 1997, *J Clin Oncol* 17:3835–3849, 1999.

Harris NL, Jaffe ES, Stein H, et al: A revised European-American classification of lymphoid neoplasms: a proposal from the International Lymphoma Study Group, *Blood* 84:1361–1392, 1994.

Hecht JL, Aster JC: Molecular biology of Burkitt's lymphoma, *J Clin Oncol* 18:3707–3721, 2000.

Hodgson DC, Gilbert ES, Dores GM, et al: Long-term solid cancer risk among 5-year survivors of Hodgkin's lymphoma, *J Clin Oncol* 25:1489–1497, 2007.

Hoster E, Dreyling M, Klapper W, et al: A new prognostic index (MIPI) for patients with advanced-stage mantle cell lymphoma, *Blood* 111:558–565, 2008.

Hummel M, Bentink S, Berger H, et al: A biologic definition of Burkitt's lymphoma from transcriptional and genomic profiling, *N Engl J Med* 354:2419–2430, 2006.

Iqbal J, Neppalli VT, Wright G, et al: BCL2 expression is a prognostic marker for the activated B-cell-like type of diffuse large B-cell lymphoma, *J Clin Oncol* 24:961–968.

Isaacson PG: Gastric lymphoma and *Helicobacter pylori*, *N Engl J Med* 350(18):1310–1311, 1994.

Jacobsen E: Anaplastic large-cell lymphoma, T-/null-cell type, *Oncologist* 11:831–840, 2006.

Jaffe ES: The role of immunophenotypic markers in the classification of non-Hodgkin's lymphomas, *Semin Oncol* 17:11–19, 1990.

Kadin ME: Ki-1/CD30+ (anaplastic) large-cell lymphoma: maturation of a clinicopathologic entity with prospects of effective therapy, *J Clin Oncol* 12(5):884–887, 1994.

Kaleem Z, White G, Vollmer RT: Critical analysis and diagnostic usefulness of limited immunophenotyping of B-cell non-Hodgkin lymphomas by flow cytometry, *Am J Clin Pathol* 115:136–142, 2000.

Kienle D, Katzenberger T, Ott G, et al: Quantitative gene expression deregulation in mantle-cell lymphoma: correlation with clinical and biologic factors, *J Clin Oncol* 25:2770–2777, 2007.

Kirn D, Mauch P, Shaffer K, et al: Large cell and immunoblastic lymphoma of the mediastinum: prognostic features and treatment outcome in 57 patients, *J Clin Oncol* 11:1336, 1993.

Kluin P: BCL-6 in lymphoma: sorting out a wastebasket? *N Engl J Med* 331:116–118, 1994.

Kutok JL, Aster JC: Molecular biology of anaplastic lymphoma kinase-positive anaplastic large-cell lymphoma, *J Clin Oncol* 3691–3702, 2002.

Kwee TC, Kwee RM, Nievelstein AJ: Imaging in staging of malignant lymphoma: a systemic review, *Blood* 111:504–516, 2008.

Lamy T, Loughran TP Jr: Large granular lymphocyte leukemia, *Cancer Control* 5:25, 1998.

Lenz G, Wright G, Dave SS, et al: Stromal gene signatures in large- B-cell lymphomas, *N Engl J Med* 359:2313–2323, 2008.

Levy O, DeAngelis LM, Filippa, et al: BCL-6 predicts improved prognosis in primary central nervous system lymphoma, *Cancer* 112:151–156, 2008.

Lossos IS, Morgensztern: Prognostic biomarkers in diffuse large B-cell lymphoma, *J Clin Oncol* 24:995–1007, 2006.

Mattia AR, Ferry JA, Harris NL: Breast lymphoma: a B-cell spectrum including the low grade B-cell lymphoma of mucosa associated lymphoid tissue, *Am J Surg Pathol* 17:574–587, 1993.

Morice WG, Kurtin PJ, Hodnefield JM, et al: Predictive value of blood and bone marrow flow cytometry in B-cell lymphoma classification: comparative analysis of flow cytometry and tissue biopsy in 252 patients, *Mayo Clin Proc* 83:776–785, 2008.

Muslimani AA, Spiro TP, Daw HA, et al: Neurolymphomatosis: the challenge of diagnosis and treatment, *Commun Oncol* 5:339–341, 2008.

Nathwani BN, Mohrmann RL, Brynes RK, et al: Monocytoid B-cell lymphomas: an assessment of diagnostic criteria and a perspective on histogenesis, *Hum Pathol* 23:1061–1071, 1992.

Newell GR, Cabanillas FG, Hagemeister FJ, et al: Incidence of lymphoma in the US classified by the working formulation, *Cancer* 59:857–861, 1987.

Non-Hodgkin's Lymphoma Classification Project: A clinical evaluation of the international study group classification of non-Hodgkin's lymphoma, *Blood* 89:3909–3918, 1997.

Offit K, Lo Coco F, Louie DC, et al: Rearrangement of the BCL-6 gene as a prognostic marker in diffuse large-cell lymphoma, *N Engl J Med* 331:74–80, 1994.

Oscier DG, Gardiner AC, Mould SJ, et al: Multivariate analysis of prognostic factors in CLL: clinical stage, IGVH gene mutational status, and loss or mutation of the p53 gene are independent prognostic factors, *Blood* 100:1177–1184, 2002.

Parsonnet J, Hansen S, Kodriguez L, et al: *Helicobacter pylori* infection and gastric lymphoma, *N Engl J Med* 330:1267–1271, 1994.

Penny RJ, Blaustein JC, Longtime JA, et al: Ki-1-positive large cell lymphomas, a heterogeneous group of neoplasms: morphologic, immunophenotypic, genotypic, and clinical features of 24 cases, *Cancer* 68:362–373, 1991.

Pinkus GS, Lones M, Shintaku IP, Said JW: Immunohistochemical detection of Epstein-Barr virus-encoded latent membrane protein in Reed-Sternberg cells and variants of Hodgkin's disease, *Mod Pathol* 7:454–461, 1994.

Pinkus GS, O'Hara CJ, Said JW: Peripheral/post-thymic T-cell lymphomas: a spectrum of disease, *Cancer* 65:971–998, 1990.

Ravandi F, Kantarjian H, Jones D, et al: *Cancer* 104:1808–1818, 2005.

Re D, Thomas RK, Behringer K, et al: From Hodgkin disease to Hodgkin lymphoma: biologic insights and therapeutic potential, *Blood* 105:4553–4560, 2005.

Rizvi MA, Evens AM, Tallman MS: T-cell non-Hodgkin lymphoma, *Blood* 107:1255–1264, 2006.

Rosenberg SA: National Cancer Institute sponsored study of classifications of non-Hodgkin's lymphomas: summary and description of a working formulation for clinical usage, *Cancer* 45:2188–2193, 1980.

Sanchez J, Aventin A: Detection of chromosomal abnormalities in chronic lymphocytic leukemia increased by interphase fluorescence in situ hybridization in tetradecanoylphorbol acetate-stimulated peripheral blood cells, *Cancer Genet Cytogenet* 175:57–60, 2007.

Savage KJ: Primary mediastinal large B-cell lymphoma, *Oncologist* 11:488–495, 2006.

Savage KJ, Harris NL, Vose JM, et al: ALK-anaplastic large-cell lymphoma is clinically and immunophenotypically different from both ALK + ALCL and peripheral T-cell lymphoma, not otherwise specified: report from the International Peripheral T-Cell Lymphoma Project, *Blood* 111:5496–5504, 2008.

Seam P, Juweid ME, Cheson BD: The role of FDG-PET scans in patients with lymphoma, *Blood* 110:3507–3516, 2007.

Sehn LH, Berry B, Chhanabhai M, et al: The revised International Prognostic Index (R-IPI) is a better predictor of outcome than the standard IPI for patients with diffuse large B-cell lymphoma treated with R-CHOP, *Blood* 109:1857–1861, 2007.

Senff NJ, Hoefnagel JJ, Jansen PM, et al: Reclassification of 300 primary cutaneous B-cell lymphomas according to the new WHO-EORTC classification for cutaneous lymphomas: comparison with previous classifications and identification of prognostic markers, *J Clin Oncol* 25:1581–1587, 2007.

Shipp MA: Prognostic factors in aggressive non-Hodgkin's lymphoma: who has "high-risk" disease? *Blood* 83:1165–1173, 1994.

Shipp MA, Harrington DP, Anderson JR, et al: Development of a predictive model for aggressive lymphoma: the International Non-Hodgkin's Lymphoma Prognostic Factors Project, *N Engl J Med* 329:987–994, 1993.

Shivdasani RA, Hess JL, Skarin AT, et al: Intermediate lymphocytic lymphoma: clinical and pathologic features of a recently characterized subtype of non-Hodgkin's lymphoma, *J Clin Oncol* 11(4):802–811, 1993.

Siebert JD, Harvey LAC, Fishkin PAS, et al: Comparison of lymphoid neoplasm classification, *Am J Clin Pathol* 115:650–655, 2001.

Siebert JD, Mulvaney DA, Potter KL, et al: Relative frequencies and sites of presentation of lymphoid neoplasms in a community hospital according to the revised European-American classification, *Am J Clin Pathol* 111:379–386, 1999.

Skarin AT: Non-Hodgkin's lymphoma. In Stollerman GH, Harrington WJ, La Mont JT, et al, editors: *Annals of internal medicine*, Chicago, 1989, Year Book Medical Publishers, pp 209–242.

Solal-Celigny P, Roy P, Colombat P, et al: Follicular lymphoma international prognostic index, *Blood* 108:1258–1265, 2004.

Staudt LM: The molecular and cellular origins of Hodgkin's disease, *J Exp Med* 191:207–212, 2000.

Stetter-Stevenson M, Medeiros L, Jaffe E: Immunophenotypic methods and findings in the diagnosis of lymphoproliferative disorders. In Jaffe E, editor: *Surgical pathology of the lymph nodes and related organs*, Philadelphia, 1995, Saunders, pp 22–57.

Tsimberidou AM, O'Brien S, Khouri I, et al: Clinical outcomes and prognostic factors in patients with Richter's syndrome treated with chemotherapy or chemoimmunotherapy with or without stem-cell transplantation, *J Clin Oncol* 24:2343–2351, 2006.

Tun HW, Baskerville KA, Menke DM, et al: Pathway analysis of primary central nervous system lymphoma, *Blood* 111:3200–3210, 2008.

Uckun FM: Regulation of human B-cell ontogeny, *Blood* 76:1908–1923, 1990.

Van Besien K, Kelta M, Bahaguna P: Primary mediastinal B-cell lymphoma: a review of pathology and management, *J Clin Oncol* 19:1855–1864, 2001.

Weiss R, Mitrou P, Arasteh K, et al: Acquired immunodeficiency syndrome-related lymphoma, *Cancer* 106:1560–1568, 2006.

Went P, Agostinelli C, Gallamini A, et al: Marker expression in peripheral T-cell lymphoma: a proposed clinical-pathologic prognostic score, *J Clin Oncol* 24:2472–2479, 2006.

Whang-Peng J, Knutsen T, Jaffe ES, et al: Sequential analysis of 43 patients with non-Hodgkin's lymphoma: clinical correlations with cytogenetic, histologic, immunophenotyping, and molecular studies, *Blood* 85:203–216, 1995.

Willemze R, Jaffe ES, Burg G, et al: WHO-EORTC classification for cutaneous lymphomas, *Blood* 105:3768–3785, 2005.

Yee KWL, O'Brien SM, Giles FJ: Richter's syndrome: biology and therapy, *Cancer J* 11:161–174, 2005.

Zinzani PL, Quaglino P, Pimpinelli N, et al: Prognostic factors in primary cutaneous B-cell lymphoma: the Italian Study Group for cutaneous lymphomas, *J Clin Oncol* 24:1376–1382, 2006.

Zuckerman D, Seliem R, Hochberg E: Intravascular lymphoma: the oncologist's "great imitator," *Oncologist* 11:496–502, 2006.

Figure Credits

The following books published by Gower Medical Publishing are sources of figures in the present chapter. The figure numbers given in the listing are those of the figures in the present chapter. The page numbers given in parentheses are those of the original publication.

Bullough PG, Boachie-Adjei O: *Atlas of spinal diseases*. Philadelphia/New York, 1988, Lippincott/Gower Medical Publishing: Fig. 16.30 (p. 203).

Bullough PG, Vigorita VJ: *Atlas of orthopedic pathology*. Baltimore/New York, 1984, University Park Press/Gower Medical Publishing: Figs. 16.7 (p. 13.8), 16.31 (p. 13.8), 16.118 (p.13.6).

Cawson RA, Eveson JW: *Oral pathology and diagnosis*. London, 1987, Heinemann Medical Books/Gower Medical Publishing: Figs. 16.5 (p. 18.15), 16.11 (p. 18.15), 16.42 (p. 18.10), 16.44A (p. 18.10), 16.44B, C (p. 18.12).

du Bois RM, Clarke SW: *Fibreoptic bronchoscopy in diagnosis and management*. Philadelphia/London, 1987, Lippincott/Gower Medical Publishing: Fig. 16.16 (p. 3.17).

du Vivier A: *Atlas of clinical dermatology*. Edinburgh/London, 1986, Churchill Livingstone/Gower Medical Publishing: Figs. 16.67 (p. 8.14), 16.68 (p. 8.15).

Fletcher CDM, McKee PH: *An atlas of gross pathology*. London, 1987, Edward Arnold/Gower Medical Publishing: Figs. 16.25B (p. 52), 16.108 (p. 52).

Hewitt PE: *Blood diseases (pocket picture guides)*. London, 1985, Gower Medical Publishing: Fig. 16.18 (p. 43).

Hoffbrand AV, Pettit JE: *Clinical haematology illustrated*. Edinburgh/London, 1987, Churchill Livingstone/Gower Medical Publishing: Figs. 16.1 (p. 10.4), 16.3A (p. 10.4), 16.9 (p. 10.5), 16.10 (p. 10.5), 16.12 (p. 10.6), 16.13 (p. 10.6), 16.21 (p. 10.2), 16.25A (p. 10.3), 16.27 (p. 10.2), 16.28 (p. 10.2), 16.34 (p. 10.3), 16.64 (p. 10.18), 16.65 (p. 10.18), 16.66 (p. 10.13), 16.73 (p. 10.18), 16.74 (p. 10.8), 16.78 (p. 10.15), 16.80 (p. 10.14), 16.81 (p. 10.14), 16.89 (p. 10.15), 16.100 (p. 10.15), 16.106 (p. 10.9), 16.107 (p. 10.9), 16.116 (p. 10.13), 16.124 (p10.15), 16.125 (p. 10.16).

Kassner EG, editor: *Atlas of radiopathic imaging*. Philadelphia/New York, 1989, Lippincott/Gower Medical Publishing: Fig. 16.22 (p. 8.39).

Schumann GB, Weiss MA: *Atlas of renal and urinary tract cytology and its histopathologic bases*. Philadelphia, 1981, Lippincott: Fig. 16.114.

Silverstein FE, Tytgat GNJ: *Atlas of gastrointestinal endoscopy*. Philadelphia/New York, 1987, Saunders/Gower Medical Publishing: Fig. 16.99 (p. 6.11).

Weiss MA, Mills SE: *Atlas of genitourinary tract disorders*. Philadelphia/New York, 1988, Lippincott/Gower Medical Publishing: Figs. 16.47A, B (p. 8.25), 16.96 (p. 8.24), 16.113 (p. 11.58).

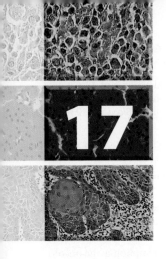

17

Multiple Myeloma and Plasma Cell Dyscrasias

NOOPUR RAJE • KENNETH C. ANDERSON • DAVID M. DORFMAN • ARTHUR T. SKARIN

Multiple myeloma and related disorders compose a spectrum of diseases that are characterized by the autonomous proliferation of differentiated lymphoid cells and plasma cells whose physiologic function is to secrete immunoglobulins. Plasma cell dyscrasias account for 1% of all cancers in the United States, and approximately 10% of hematologic malignancies. Multiple myeloma is the most common of the dyscrasias, representing about 75% of cases and affecting approximately 15,000 individuals each year. Waldenstrom's macroglobulinemia accounts for about 20% of cases, with the remainder consisting of other types of heavy-chain disease.

Multiple Myeloma

Multiple myeloma (MM) is a malignancy of clonal plasma cells involving primarily the bone and bone marrow (BM). The median age at diagnosis is approximately 65 years, and fewer than 3% of patients are younger than 40 years. MM remains incurable, with a median survival of approximately 3.5 years. In 2009 an estimated 20,580 patients will be diagnosed, and 10,580 patients will die from the disease (Jemal et al., 2009).

DISEASE BIOLOGY

The available evidence suggests that the clonal precursor cell in MM is a B cell that has undergone somatic hypermutation and passed through the germinal center. Within the lymph node illegitimate immunoglobulin (Ig) class switching occurs, resulting in chromosome 14q32 translocations and the dysregulation of a number of oncogenes (*FGFR3/MMSET*, cyclin D1, *c-MAF*) (Avet-Loiseau et al., 1999). Chemokines then mediate homing of the immortalized MM cells from the lymph node to the BM, where binding of MM cells to BM stromal cells (BMSCs) occurs, localizing the MM cells within the BM microenvironment. Adhesion of MM cells results in an increase in the transcription and secretion of a number of cytokines involved in MM cell growth and survival, including interleukin-6, insulin-like growth factor-1, vascular endothelial growth factor, stromal cell–derived growth factor-1α, tumor necrosis factor-α, transforming growth factor-β, and B-cell activating factor, which augment MM cell growth, survival, drug resistance, and migration in the BM milieu. Besides localizing tumor cells in the BM microenvironment, our studies demonstrate that adhesion of MM cells to

BMSCs also triggers the paracrine nuclear factor-κB-dependent transcription and secretion in BMSCs of interleukin-6, the major cytokine mediating MM cell growth, survival, and resistance to drug (dexamethasone)-induced apoptosis via mitogen-activated protein kinase and phosphoinositide 3-kinase/Akt, Jak/signal transduction and transcription activator, and phosphoinositide 3-kinase/Akt signaling cascades, respectively. Most importantly, adhesion of MM cells to the BM induces changes in gene profile—that is, upregulation of growth, survival, and drug resistance genes in tumor cells; upregulation of adhesion molecules on MM cells and BMSCs; and changes in cytokines in BMSCs both in vitro and in our in vivo models of human MM in mice. Interaction of MM cells with BMSCs activates Notch signaling, which induces melphalan resistance. Others have shown that MM cell adhesion to fibronectin confers cell adhesion–mediated drug resistance to conventional chemotherapy, with induction of p27 and G1 growth arrest. Excitingly, novel agents including thalidomide and derivatives including lenalidomide, as well as proteasome inhibitor bortezomib (Velcade; PS-341, Millenium Takeda Oncology) can target both the tumor cell and its BM microenvironment, thereby overcoming cell adhesion–mediated drug resistance. Induction of proteasome activity when MM cells bind to BMSCs may sensitize them to therapy. Other cytokines are produced that promote bone resorption, tumor migration, and invasion, including matrix metalloproteinase-1, interleukin-1β, and vascular endothelial growth factor (Hideshima et al., 2007). As disease progresses, the development of plasma cell leukemia (PCL) is characterized by increasing genetic instability of the MM cell associated with a high frequency of *RAS*, *TP53*, and *c-MYC* mutations (Corradini et al., 1993; Davies et al., 2003). This is accompanied by a decreased expression of certain adhesion molecules, which facilitates tumor cell mobilization into the peripheral blood. The acquisition of other adhesion molecules on the MM cell surface leads to the metastasis of MM cells to sites outside the BM and the development of extramedullary plasmacytoma.

DIAGNOSIS AND MORPHOLOGY

The Durie and Salmon major and minor diagnostic criteria have been conventionally used for the diagnosis of MM. These include the presence of excess monotypic marrow plasma cells, monoclonal Ig in either the serum or urine, decreased normal Ig levels, and lytic bone lesions (Durie and Salmon, 1975). These diagnostic criteria are now being replaced by the International Myeloma Working Group criteria (2003; Durie et al., 2006). They help in distinguishing active MM from other disorders characterized by monoclonal gammopathies, both malignant and otherwise, in particular monoclonal gammopathy of undetermined significance (MGUS) and smoldering MM. Other conditions such as Waldenstrom's macroglobulinemia, non-Hodgkin lymphoma, light-chain amyloid, idiopathic cold agglutinin disease, essential cryoglobulinemia, and heavy-chain disease should also be differentiated from MM.

The morphology of plasma cells in MM varies from typical small, mature cells that appear normal to larger cells with immature nuclei containing prominent clear nucleoli, little or no perinuclear clear area (hof), and a rim of basophilic cytoplasm. In between these extremes are medium-sized cells, often characterized by an eccentric nucleus with one or several small nucleoli, a diffuse chromatin pattern, perinuclear hof, and a variable amount of blue cytoplasm. On biopsy normal BM architecture is lost, and the plasma cells are found as single cells or small clusters between adipocytes. As the disease progresses, diffuse marrow replacement occurs, resulting in a packed marrow.

The diagnosis of MM can be confirmed by immunoperoxidase staining that demonstrates the presence of monoclonal cytoplasmic-staining light chains (κ or λ) or monoclonal heavy chains (IgG, IgA, or IgD). Since plasma cells are terminally differentiated B cells, they express a number of B-cell antigens as well as myeloma-associated antigens including CD38, CD138 (syndecan-1), Muc-1, and PCA-1. They lack CD10, CD20, CD23, CD34, and CD45RO.

STAGING OF MULTIPLE MYELOMA

The Durie-Salmon staging system was conventionally used to separate patients into prognostic groups using laboratory measurements. These stages are now being replaced by the International Staging System (Greipp et al., 2005). This is simple and correlates well with survival. It relies on serum albumin and β_2-microglobulin (β2m) levels at diagnosis. In addition to a full physical examination, a complete blood count with blood smear, and blood chemistries including renal studies, are required. Serum electrophoresis with quantification of protein, as well as a 24-hour urine electrophoresis and quantification of Bence-Jones protein (light chains), should also be performed. The serum-free light-chain assay is a new test that allows diagnosis of patients with light-chain disease. BM aspirate and biopsy are indicated. An estimation of the extent of bone disease using a skeletal bone survey is advisable, although in many centers this has now been superceded by magnetic resonance imaging.

CLINICAL MANIFESTATIONS

The clinical picture of MM involves a combination of bone destruction leading to pain or fracture with hypercalcemia; infection due to immune deficiency; BM failure leading to anemia and, less commonly, thrombocytopenia; and renal failure due to hypercalcemia, direct damage from paraprotein, or precipitation of light chain in renal tubules. A hyperviscosity syndrome may occur in some patients, and neurologic complications such as spinal cord compression and peripheral neuropathy may be seen.

A number of studies have evaluated various parameters for prognostic significance. β2m, a polypeptide that forms the extracellular portion of the light chain of the class I major histocompatibility complex, is the single most important variable. Levels correlate with a high tumor burden and decreasing renal function. The extent and type of BM infiltration are also important: patients with a plasmablastic morphology have a much shorter median survival compared with patients with other morphologic subtypes (Greipp et al., 1998). Measures of tumor cell proliferation such as the plasma cell labeling index (PCLI) are also useful; a high PCLI correlates with a shorter survival time independent of tumor cell mass. The presence of certain cytogenetic abnormalities also has prognostic significance: patients with partial or complete deletions of chromosome 13 or abnormalities of 11q have an adverse outcome.

Three recent prognostic staging systems have been proposed to better predict patient outcome. First, an international staging system based upon serum β2m and albumin has provided a new three-stage International Staging System (Greipp et al., 2005). Second, cyclin D dysregulation has been identified as an early and unifying event in MM. Using gene expression profiling to identify five recurrent translocations, specific trisomies, and expression of cyclin D2 genes, MM can prognostically be divided into eight translocation/cyclin D groups (Bergsagel and Kuehl, 2005). Additional molecular classifications have been proposed, with high-risk myeloma defined by deregulated expression of genes mapping to chromosome 1. Most recently, the first DNA-based classification scheme has been proposed to predict outcome to high-dose therapy (Carrasco et al., 2006).

THERAPY

Treatment for MM has evolved significantly in the last 3–4 years. Although the use of conventional low-dose chemotherapy or high-dose chemotherapy with autologous or allogeneic stem cell transplantation is able to reduce tumor burden, complete molecular remission of disease is rare, and all patients eventually relapse. Novel pharmacologic agents including thalidomide, lenalidomide, and proteasome inhibitors like bortezomib are now approved by the U.S. Food and Drug Administration for the treatment of MM (Raje et al., 2006; Richardson et al., 2007). These agents have been used, either alone or in combination with conventional and high-dose chemotherapy, to improve response and outcome.

Other novel single agents of great promise include new proteasome inhibitors NPI-0052 and PR-171, fibroblast growth factor receptor-3 (FGFR3) inhibitors, humanized antibodies to CD40, antibody to CS1, mitogen-activated protein/extracellular signal–regulated kinase kinase (MEK) inhibitor AZD6244, cyclin-dependent kinase inhibitor P276.00, Hsp90 inhibitors, and histone deacetylase (HDAC) inhibitors. NPI-0052 and PR-171 are next-generation proteasome inhibitors that are active against bortezomib-resistant MM, are nontoxic in preclinical models, and are already in clinical trials in relapsed MM. FGFR3 inhibitors specifically target those 15% to 20% of patients with t(4;14) translocation. CD40 humanized antibodies have demonstrated early activity against MM, and Hsp90 inhibitors as single agents can achieve responses in relapsed refractory MM. HDAC inhibitors block aggresomal breakdown of ubiquinated proteins; combined with proteasome inhibitors to inhibit proteasomal degradation of ubiquinated proteins, they mediate significant toxicity. Clinical testing of the HDAC inhibitor panobinostat (LBH589; Novartis) is ongoing, with a combination LBH and bortezomib trial soon to follow. Immunologic-based treatment approaches (e.g., vaccination, antibody therapy) are also being actively evaluated (Hideshima et al., 2005, 2007).

Plasma Cell Leukemia

PCL is characterized by the presence of more than 2×10^9 plasma cells per liter within the peripheral blood, which constitutes 20% of all circulating cells. The majority (60%) of cases are de novo or primary, in which a leukemic picture develops in the absence of documented preceding myeloma, whereas 40% of cases are secondary and occur in 1% of myeloma patients with advanced myeloma that is refractory to treatment (Garcia-Sanz et al., 1999). The symptoms of primary disease are similar to myeloma, although the disease course is often more aggressive with symptoms relating to extramedullary disease (plasmacytomas and hepatosplenomegaly) and BM failure (anemia, infections, and bleeding).

Monoclonal Gammopathy of Undetermined Significance

MGUS describes a condition characterized by the presence of a low level of paraprotein in the absence of other clinical features of MM, Waldenstrom's macroglobulinemia, or other B-cell lymphoproliferative disorders. MGUS is present in 3.2% of persons 50 years of age or older and 5.3% of persons 70 years of age or older. Independent prognostic factors associated with MGUS transformation to MM include (1) more than 5% BM plasmacytosis, (2) Bence-Jones proteinuria, (3) decrease in polyclonal serum Ig, and (4) an elevated erythrocyte sedimentation rate. More recently, risk factors for progression include an abnormal serum κ/λ free light-chain ratio, a high serum monoclonal protein level, and non IgG MM. The risk of progression from smoldering MM to symptomatic disease is related to the proportion of BM plasma cells and serum monoclonal protein level at diagnosis (Kyle and Rajkumar, 2003, 2006; Kyle et al., 2007; Rajkumar et al., 2007). The previous term "benign monoclonal gammopathy" is a misleading description of the disease, since approximately 25% of patients will go on to develop an overt plasma cell disorder.

Waldenstrom's Macroglobulinemia

Waldenstrom's macroglobulinemia (WM) is a chronic B-cell lymphoproliferative disorder in which most of the clinical manifestations are due to the presence of a high level of serum IgM paraprotein (Dimopoulos et al., 2005). It is predominantly a disease of the elderly, with a median age at presentation of 65 years, and remains incurable with a median survival of 5 years. The disorder is characterized by BM infiltration with small lymphocytes, plasma cells, and characteristic lymphoplasmacytoid cells, which have the nucleus of a lymphocyte and cytoplasm of a plasma cell. The immunophenotype of WM cells is between that of well-differentiated small lymphocytes and plasma cells, since cells express monoclonal surface and cytoplasmic IgM pan-B-cell markers CD19, CD20, and CD22, and late B-cell differentiation markers such as CD38 and FMC7, but lack CD5, CD10, and CD23. Most patients develop symptoms due to tumor cell infiltration of BM resulting in anemia, increased infections, and bleeding. Splenomegaly, hepatomegaly, and lymphadenopathy are common. Many patients present with hyperviscosity syndrome accompanied by headache, confusion, and blurred vision. Cryoglobulinemia, cold agglutinin disease, and neurologic manifestations may also occur. In contrast to other plasma cell disorders, there is an absence of bony changes and lytic lesions.

LIGHT CHAIN–ASSOCIATED AMYLOIDOSIS

Light-chain amyloid, previously called primary amyloid, is characterized by the extracellular deposition of fibrillar protein derived from monoclonal light chains (Falk et al., 1997). The fragments form β-pleated sheets, which become insoluble and resistant to degradation following the deposition of glycosaminoglycans and the normal protein serum amyloid P component. The clinical features depend on the spectrum of organ involvement, with the most commonly affected organs being the heart, kidneys, and peripheral nerves. Other features include macroglossia (infrequent but pathognomonic), gastrointestinal malabsorption, hepatosplenomegaly, and skin involvement including papular and nodular lesions and characteristic purpura around the eyes. A monoclonal component is usually present in the serum or urine, although immunofixation is often required to demonstrate its presence, since the peak may be small. Amyloid may occur as a long-term complication of most clonal B-cell disorders, especially myeloma and, less commonly, WM.

Heavy-Chain Disorders

This group of rare plasma cell disorders is characterized by the production of a monoclonal Ig that is formed from truncated heavy chains with no associated light chains (Fermand and Brouet, 1999). α-Heavy-chain disease, a subtype of immunoproliferative small intestine disease, is diagnosed by the identification of monoclonal Ig α-heavy-chain fragments in the plasma or urine. The pathologic process consists of a lymphoma-like proliferation of lymphoid cells and plasma cells in the lamina propria of the small intestine and in mesenteric nodes, accompanied by diarrhea and malabsorption. Occasionally the disease may present with respiratory symptoms due to infiltration in the respiratory tract. It was previously referred to as Mediterranean abdominal lymphoma, but it may also be identified in patients of non-Mediterranean ancestry.

Acknowledgments

We are extremely grateful to Dr. Andrew Jack (Haematological Malignancy Diagnostic Service, Leeds General Infirmary, Leeds, UK) and Professor Gareth Morgan and Dr. Faith Davies (Royal Marsden Hospital, Sutton, UK) for allowing us to use some of their figures.

Table 17.1

Diseases Associated with the Production of Paraprotein

Stable Production	Uncontrolled Production
MGUS	MGUS
Idiopathic cold agglutinin disease	Smoldering myeloma
Essential cryoglobulinemia	Multiple myeloma
Transient M proteins	Light-chain amyloidosis
Occasionally metastatic carcinoma, connective tissue disorders, and skin disorders	Waldenstrom's macroglobulinemia
	Heavy-chain disease
	Non-Hodgkin lymphoma

MGUS, monoclonal gammopathy of undetermined significance.

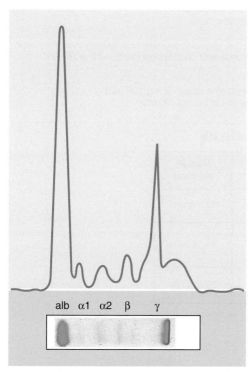

FIGURE 17.1. BENIGN MONOCLONAL GAMMOPATHY. Serum protein electrophoresis shows M-protein in the γ region. Unlike the pattern in multiple myeloma, there is no reduction in the background normal β- and γ-globulins. In about 25% of cases, multiple myeloma or a lymphoproliferative disorder will develop within 10 years. For the remaining 75%, no significant illness may become apparent within that time interval.

Criteria for the diagnosis of multiple myeloma

Major criteria

1. Plasmacytoma on tissue biopsy
2. Bone marrow plasmacytosis (>30% plasma cells)
3. Monoclonal immunoglobulin spike on serum electrophoresis IgG >3.5 g/dL or IgA >2 g/dL; K or l light chain excretion >1 g/day on 24-hour urine electrophoresis

Minor criteria

a. Bone marrow plasmacytosis (10%–30% plasma cells)
b. Monoclonal immunoglobulin spike present but of lesser magnitude than above
c. Lytic bone lesions
d. Normal IgM <50 mg/dL, IgA <100 mg/dL or IgG <600 mg/dL

Any of the following criteria will confirm the diagnosis:
Any two major criteria
Major criterion 1 plus minor criterion b, c, or d
Major criterion 3 plus minor criterion a or c
A Minor criteria a, b, and c or a, b, and d

**International Myeloma Working Group
diagnostic criteria for multiple myeloma**

1. Monoclonal plasma cells in the bone marrow >10% and/or presence of a biopsy-proven plasmacytoma
2. Monoclonal protein present in the serum and/or urine*
3. Myeloma-related organ dysfunction (1 or more)[†]
   • [C] Calcium elevation in the blood S. Calcium >11.5 mg/L or upper limit of normal
   • [R] Renal insufficiency S. Creatinine >2 mg/dL
   • [A] Anemia hemoglobin <10 g/dL or 2 g < normal[‡]
   • [B] Lytic bone lesions or osteopenia

* In patients with no detectable M-component, an abnormal serum FLC ratio on the serum FLC assay can substitute and satisfy this criterion. For patients with no serum or urine M-component and normal serum FLC ratio, the baseline bone marrow must have ≥10% clonal plasma cells; these patients are referred to as having "nonsecretory myeloma." Patients with biopsy-proven amyloidosis and/or systemic light chain deposition disease (LCDD) should be classified as "myeloma with documented amyloidosis" or "myeloma with documented LCDD," respectively, if they have ≥30% plasma cells and/or myeloma-related bone disease.

[†] Must be attributable to the underlying plasma cell disorder.

B [‡] *Note*: Hemoglobin of 10 g/dL is 12.5 mmol/L [or 100 g/L].

FIGURE 17.2 (A) Diagnostic criteria for multiple myeloma. **(B)** International Myeloma Working Group Diagnostic Criteria for Multiple Myeloma. (Adapted from Durie BG, Harousseau JL, Miguel JS, et al: International uniform response criteria for multiple myeloma, *Leukemia* 20(9):1467–1473, 2006.)

FIGURE 17.3 **(A)** Staging system for multiple myeloma. **(B)** New International Staging System for Multiple Myeloma. **(A**, Modified from Durie BG, Salmon SE: A clinical staging system for multiple myeloma. Correlation of measured myeloma cell mass with presenting clinical features, response to treatment, and survival. *Cancer* 36:842–854, 1975; **B**, adapted from Greipp PR, San Miguel J, Durie BG, et al: International staging system for multiple myeloma, *J Clin Oncol* 23:3412–3420, 2005.)

	Criteria	Measured myeloma cell mass (cells × 10^{12}/m^2)

Stage I	All of the following:
	
	1. Hemoglobin value >10 g/100 mL
	2. Serum calcium value normal (<12 mg/100 mL)
	3. On radiograph, normal bone structure (scale 0) or solitary bone plasmacytoma only
	4. Low M-component production rates
	  A. IgG value <5 g/100 mL
	  B. IgA value <3 g/100 mL
	  C. Urine light chain M-component on electrophoresis <4 g/24 h
		<0.6 (low)

Stage II	Fitting neither stage I nor stage III	0.6–1.20 (intermediate)

Stage III	One or more of the following:
	
	1. Hemoglobin value <8.5 g/100 mL
	2. Serum calcium value >12 mg/100 mL
	3. Advanced lytic bone lesions (scale 3)
	4. High M-component production rates
	  A. IgG value >7 g/mL
	  B. IgA value >5 g/mL
	  C. Urine light chain M-component on electrophoresis >12 g/24 h
		>1.20 (high)

Subclassifications
A = relatively normal renal function (serum creatinine value <2 mg/100 mL)
B = abnormal renal function (serum creatinine value ≥2 mg/100 mL)

A

New International Staging System for MM

Stage	Serum β2 microglobulin	Serum albumin	Median survival
I	<3.5 mg/L	≥3.5 g/dL	62 months
II	<3.5 mg/L 3.5–5.5 mg/L	<3.5 mg/L regardless of albumin	44 months
III	≥5.5 mg/L		29 months

B

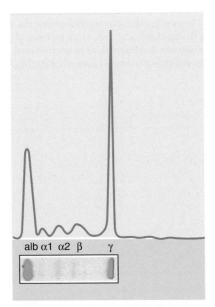

FIGURE 17.4 **MULTIPLE MYELOMA.** Serum protein electrophoresis demonstrates an M-protein in the γ-globulin region and a reduced level of background γ-globulin. This "spike" and deficiency pattern is typical of patients with myeloma.

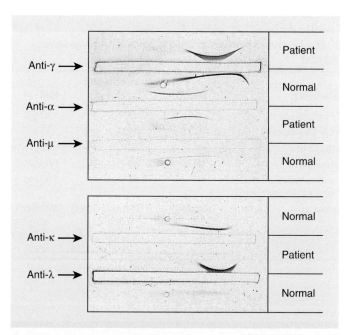

FIGURE 17.5 MULTIPLE MYELOMA (IgG-λTYPE). Normal protein is recognized by characteristic arc patterns on immunoelectrophoresis. In the reactions against anti-γ and anti-λ, the IgG-λ M-protein maintains its electrophoretic position but appears as a "bow" or thickened arc with a smaller than usual radius. Reduced levels of IgA and IgM are reflected in small or absent arcs in the reactions with anti-α and anti-μ.

Table 17.2

Frequency of M-Protein Types in Multiple Myeloma

Types	Frequency (%)
IgG	52
IgA	22
κ only	9
λ only	7
IgD	2
Biclonal	1
IgM*	0.5
Negative	6.5

*IgM rarely occurs, since it usually indicates Waldenstrom's monoglobulinemia. Light-chain disease is defined by circulating light chains only with Bence-Jones proteinuria and hypogammaglobulinemia. As the result of imbalanced immunoglobulin production, most patients with an M component also have monoclonal light chains that vary from barely detectable levels to grams per day.
Data from 984 patients with multiple myeloma at the Mayo Clinic (1982–1994).

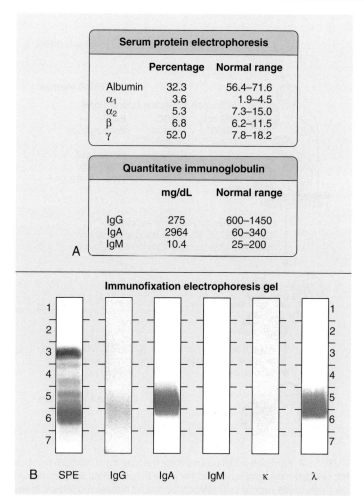

Serum protein electrophoresis

	Percentage	Normal range
Albumin	32.3	56.4–71.6
α₁	3.6	1.9–4.5
α₂	5.3	7.3–15.0
β	6.8	6.2–11.5
γ	52.0	7.8–18.2

Quantitative immunoglobulin

	mg/dL	Normal range
IgG	275	600–1450
IgA	2964	60–340
IgM	10.4	25–200

FIGURE 17.6 MULTIPLE MYELOMA (IgA-λTYPE). Immunoelectropherogram shows an excess of γ-globulin, which is overwhelmingly IgA-λ. SPE, serum protein electrophoresis.

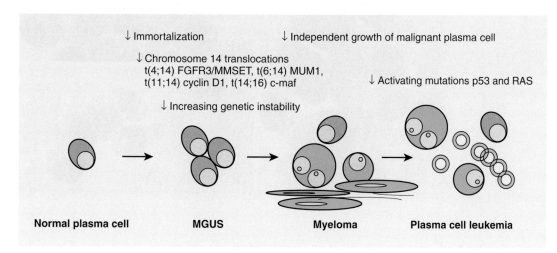

FIGURE 17.7 It is thought that the transformation from monoclonal gammopathy of undetermined significance (MGUS) to multiple myeloma and plasma cell leukemia (PCL) occurs in an orderly fashion, although not all stages are present within the individual patient. One of the initial events involves the translocation of chromosome 14q32 with oncogene dysregulation during immunoglobulin class switching. This results in genetic instability and later independent cell growth. A high frequency of chromosomal abnormalities including *RAS*, *TP53*, and c-*MYC* mutations characterizes PCL.

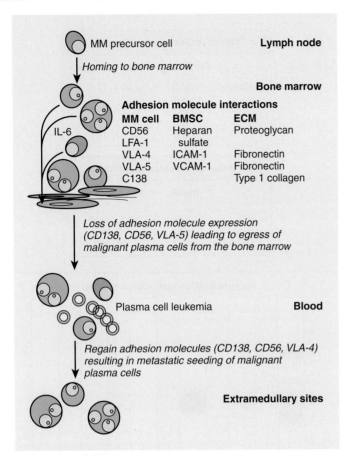

FIGURE 17.8 Adhesion molecules mediate the homing of multiple myeloma (MM) cells from the lymph node to the bone marrow (BM), where binding of MM cells to BM stromal cells (BMSCs) occurs. As disease progresses, there is a decreased expression of some adhesion molecules, which facilitates tumor cell mobilization into the peripheral blood. The acquisition of other adhesion molecules on the MM cell surface leads to the metastasis of MM cells to sites outside the BM. ECM, extracellular matrix.

Table 17.3

Criteria for the Diagnosis of MGUS, Smoldering Myeloma, and MM

Parameter	MGUS	Smoldering myeloma	MM
M component	<30 g/L	>30 g/L	>30 g/L
% BM plasma cells	<10%	>10%, <30%	>30%
Symptoms	Nil	Nil	Yes
Bone lesions	Nil	Nil	Present
Anemia, hypercalcemia, or renal impairment	Nil	Nil	Present
Follow-up	Stable	Stable initially, once progressed similar to MM	Median survival 3.5 years

BM, bone marrow; MGUS, monoclonal gammopathy of undetermined significance.

Table 17.4

Cytokines Involved in (MM) Disease Biology

Cytokine	Role
(IL-6)	Proliferation and survival of MM cells
Vascular endothelial growth factor	Proliferation and migration of MM cells; angiogenesis
Tumor necrosis factor-α	Upregulation of adhesion molecules on MM cell surface; osteoclast activation
Transforming growth factor-β	Increased IL-6 secretion by BM stromal cells; inhibition of T-cell proliferation
IGF	Proliferation and survival of MM cells
IL-1β	Osteoclast activation; induction of IL-6 secretion by osteoblasts; increased expression of adhesion molecules on MM cell surface
Lymphotoxin	Osteoclast activation
TRANCE/RANKL	Differentiation and maturation of osteoclast progenitors
(IL-11)	Stimulation of osteoclastogenesis and inhibition of bone formation
Hepatocyte growth factor	Induction of IL-11 secretion by osteoblasts

BM, bone marrow; IL, interleukin; mm, multiple myeloma.

FIGURE 17.9 **MULTIPLE MYELOMA.** These bone marrow aspirates demonstrate the morphology of abnormal plasma cells. **(A)** Some myeloma cells are binuclear, with nucleoli; one mitotic figure can be seen. **(B)** The nuclei of a single binucleate cell vary greatly in size. **(C)** Abnormal cytoplasmic and nuclear vacuolation can also be encountered.

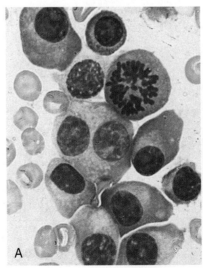

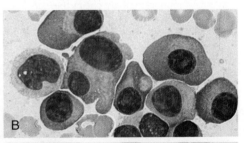

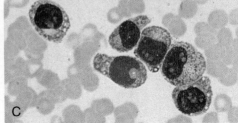

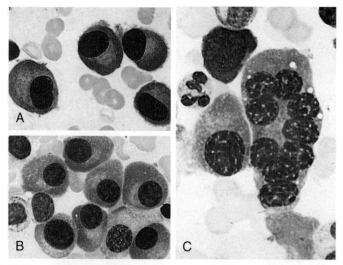

FIGURE 17.10 **MULTIPLE MYELOMA. (A, B)** Considerable variation in nuclear size and cytoplasmic volume of abnormal plasma cells can be seen in these bone marrow aspirates. **(C)** One of the myeloma cells is multinucleate.

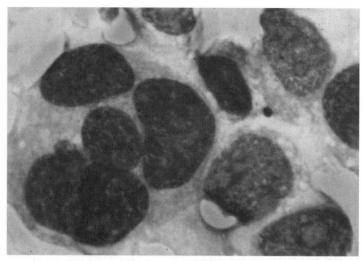

FIGURE 17.12 Bone marrow aspirate from a patient with rapidly progressive disease shows large bizarre multinucleate plasmablasts. Plasmablasts have a fine reticular chromatin pattern, large nucleoli, and less abundant cytoplasm (less than half of the nuclear area). This morphologic subset is associated with a high plasma cell labeling index, more advanced and aggressive disease, and a worse prognosis. Histologically it may be mistaken for metastatic carcinoma or large cell lymphoma; however, immunophenotyping is diagnostic for a monoclonal population of malignant plasma cells. It was formerly called "anaplastic" myeloma.

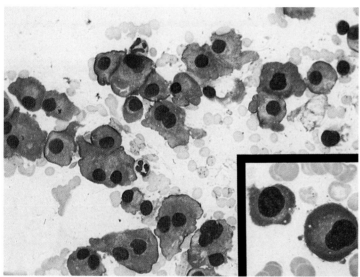

FIGURE 17.11 Numerous thesaurocytes—large plasma cells with small, sometimes pyknotic, nuclei and expanded fibrillary cytoplasm that also shows "flaming" of the cell rim *(inset)*—are evident in this bone marrow aspirate. Although "flaming cells" occur most frequently with IgA production, they may also be seen with M protein of other classes. The red color results from the high carbohydrate content of IgA protein.

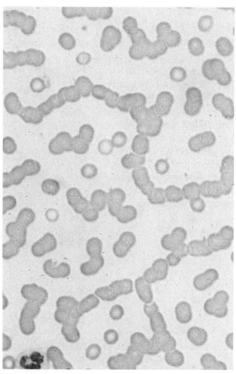

FIGURE 17.13 **MULTIPLE MYELOMA.** Peripheral blood film demonstrates marked rouleaux formation of red cells and increased background staining due to the high protein level.

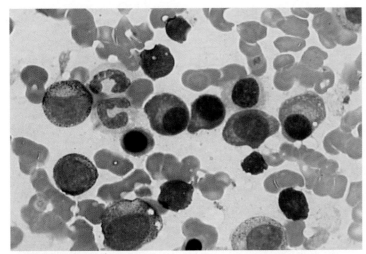

FIGURE 17.14 The peripheral blood is characterized by the presence of a large number of circulating plasma cells, which may be morphologically normal or have blastic features. Anemia is invariably present, and both neutropenia and thrombocytopenia are common. Rouleaux formation is usually also present with a high nonspecific background staining, especially in secondary plasma cell lymphoma cases where the level of paraprotein is often high. (From Wickramasinghe SN, McCullough J: *Blood and bone marrow pathology.* © 2003 Churchill Livingstone.)

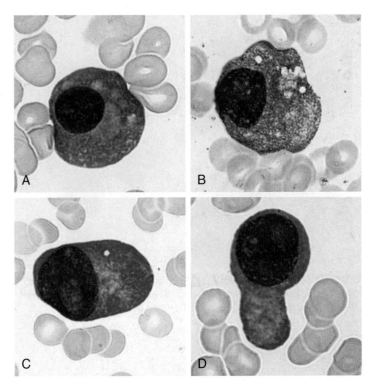

FIGURE 17.15 **MULTIPLE MYELOMA. (A to D)** Isolated myeloma cells are visible in peripheral blood smears from two patients. Plasma cell leukemia is rare, occurring in 2% to 5% of patients. It may be the presenting feature or may occur as a terminal event. Most cases exhibit rapidly progressive disease, with prominent bone symptoms, marked anemia, azotemia, and infiltration of organs and tissues.

FIGURE 17.16 **MULTIPLE MYELOMA. (A)** Low-power view of a bone marrow core biopsy specimen shows diffuse replacement of marrow by a monoclonal population of plasma cells. Plasma cells stain positive for antibodies to κ-light chain **(B)** but not antibodies to λ-light chain **(C)** with the immunoperoxidase technique. **(D)** At high power, plasma cells are characterized by clumped "clock face" chromatin, eccentric nuclei, and perinuclear hof (halo).

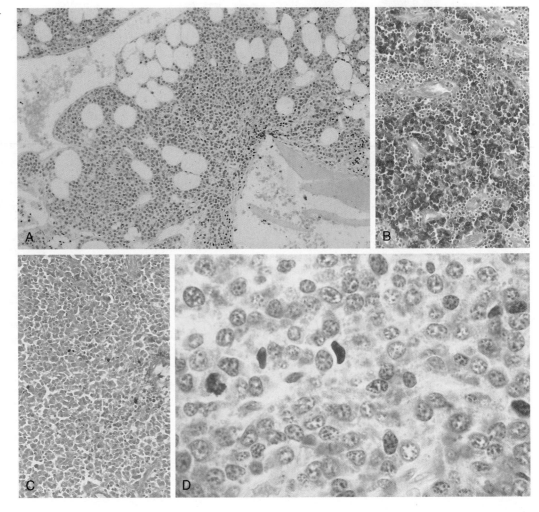

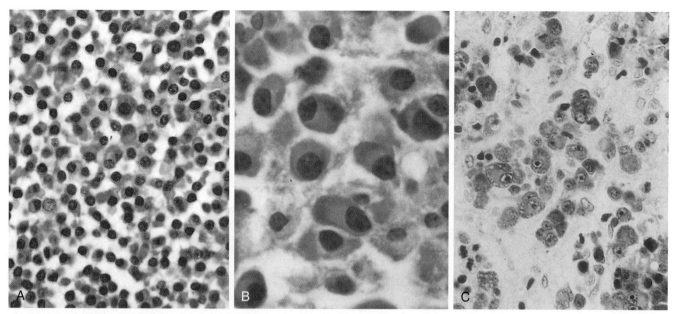

FIGURE 17.17 **MULTIPLE MYELOMA. (A)** In this well-differentiated tumor, the deposits consist of plasma cells. **(B)** At higher power, the typically eccentric nuclei, relatively large areas of basophilic or amphophilic cytoplasm, and perinuclear hof can be appreciated. **(C)** High-power view of a poorly differentiated myeloma tumor containing plasma cells with prominent nucleoli and multinucleate cells.

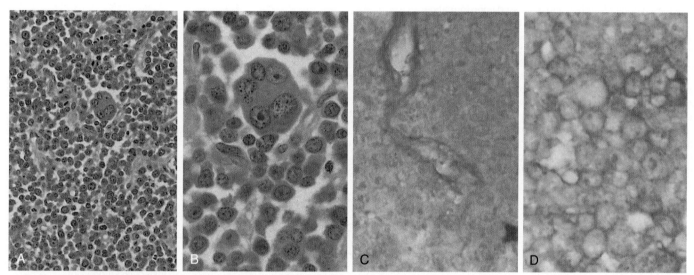

FIGURE 17.18 **EXTRAMEDULLARY PLASMACYTOMA. (A)** This anterior chest wall lesion exhibits scant, delicate connective tissue stroma and a relatively monomorphous population of cells, unlike the findings in plasma cell granuloma. **(B)** Plasma cells have eccentric nuclei with a "clock face" chromatin pattern and amphophilic cytoplasm. This tumor contains many immature forms and occasional multinucleate cells. **(C, D)** Demonstration of a single light-chain class by immunoperoxidase staining confirms the presence of a monoclonal (neoplastic) population of plasma cells **(C**, κ negative; **D,** λ positive). (Courtesy of S. Swerdlow, MD, Cincinnati, OH.)

FIGURE 17.19 Although the exact mechanism of action of thalidomide and lenalidomide in myeloma is unclear, it can be postulated that their pharmacologic effects may be mediated via a number of pathways involving both the tumor cell and the bone marrow microenvironment: a direct effect on tumor or bone marrow stromal cells, an alteration in the adhesion profile between myeloma and bone marrow stromal cells, an inhibition of cytokine release from bone marrow stromal cells, an antiangiogenic effect, or an immunomodulatory effect. bFGF, basic fibroblast growth factor; IFNγ, interferon-γ; IL-2 etc., interleukins; NK, natural killer; TNFα, tumor necrosis factor-α; VEGF, vascular endothelial growth factor.

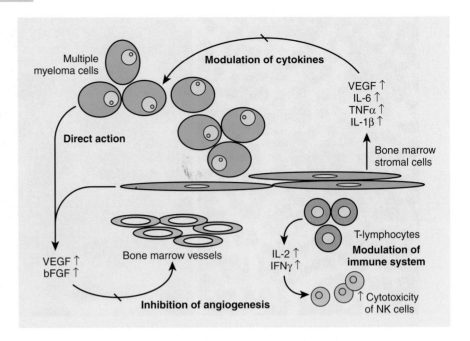

FIGURE 17.20 There is an uncoupling of normal bone remodeling with increased bone resorption and decreased bone formation. When multiple myeloma (MM) cells bind to bone marrow stroma, cytokines are produced that stimulate bone marrow stromal cells and osteoblasts to produce tumor necrosis factor–related activation-induced cytokine (TRANCE), which leads to the differentiation and maturation of osteoclast progenitors. Osteoprotegrin (OPG) directly regulates osteoclast activity by acting as an alternative receptor for TRANCE. However, syndecan produced by MM cells traps OPG, leading to an excess of TRANCE. The increased osteoclast activity results in bone resorption and secretion of cytokines, further stimulating MM cell growth. FGF, fibroblast growth factor; IGF, insulin-like growth factor; IL-1β, etc., interleukins; TGFβ, transforming growth factor-β.

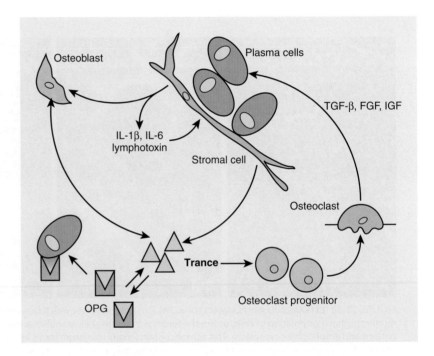

FIGURE 17.21 Variants in the radiographic presentation of myeloma.

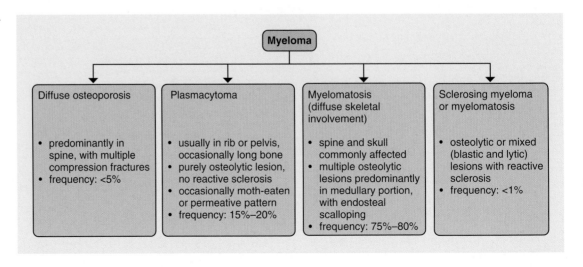

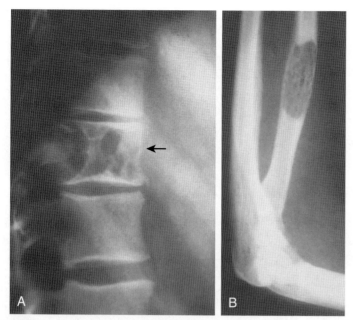

FIGURE 17.22   MULTIPLE MYELOMA. (A) Plain film of the thoracic spine shows multiple radiolucencies in the body of T12 (*arrow*). **(B)** In another patient a deposit of myeloma is apparent in the midshaft of the radius.

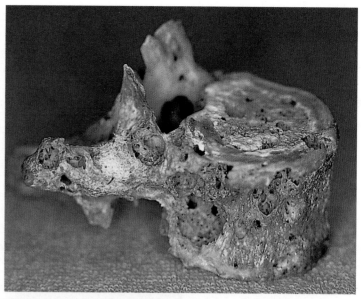

FIGURE 17.24   MULTIPLE MYELOMA. A macerated vertebral body exhibits many destructive round defects throughout the bone. (Specimen from the collection of the Smithsonian Institution; courtesy of Dr. Donald J. Ortner.)

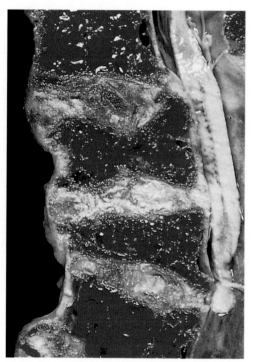

FIGURE 17.23   MULTIPLE MYELOMA. This segment of the lower thoracic spine has been sectioned to show extensive replacement of the bone and marrow by gelatinous red tissue. The resultant osteoporosis has caused multiple compression fractures. (Courtesy of Howard Dorfman, MD.)

FIGURE 17.25 PLASMACYTOMA.
(A) Anteroposterior view of the lumbosacral spine in a 68-year-old man who presented with lower back pain shows a large lytic lesion (*arrowheads*) in the right side of the sacrum adjacent to the sacroiliac joint. **(B)** Computed tomography (CT) scan demonstrates an adjacent soft tissue mass (*arrowheads*). On the basis of these findings a solitary plasmacytoma, a metastatic lesion, malignant fibrous histiocytoma, and fibrosarcoma were considered in the differential diagnosis. A fluoroscopy-guided biopsy yielded the diagnosis.

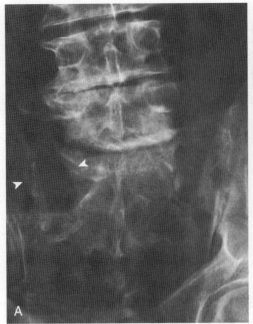
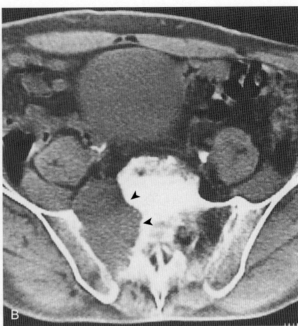

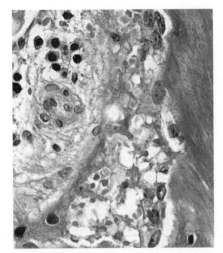

FIGURE 17.26 MULTIPLE MYELOMA. Although plasma cells are seen in the *upper left* of this bone biopsy specimen, osteoclasts (the multinucleate cells at the bone–intertrabecular tissue interface) are the cells responsible for the bone absorption around the osteolytic lesion.

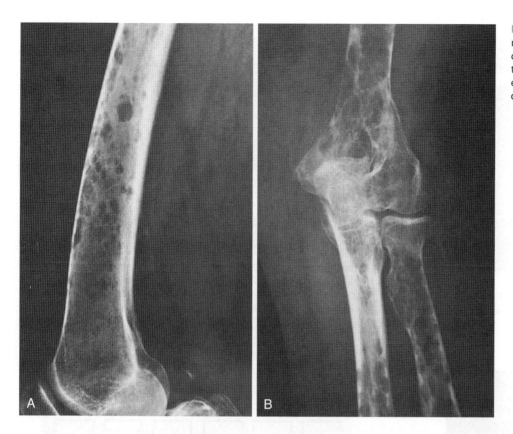

FIGURE 17.27 **MULTIPLE MYELOMA. (A)** Lateral radiograph of the distal femur shows numerous classic punched-out lytic lesions. **(B)** Plain film of the elbow in a 65-year-old woman demonstrates endosteal scalloping of the cortex, typical of diffuse myelomatosis.

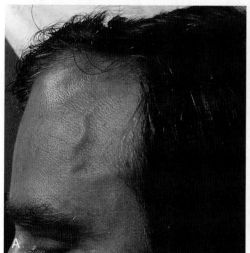

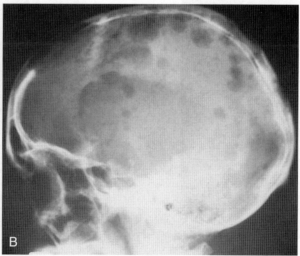

FIGURE 17.28 **MULTIPLE MYELOMA.**
(A) A 35-year-old man developed multiple osseous lesions; in this instance, a plasmacytoma involves the forehead. **(B)** Skull radiograph reveals other osteolytic areas in addition to the large frontal lesion. Bone marrow aspirations were normal. A small amount of Bence-Jones protein was detected in concentrated urine by immunoelectrophoresis.

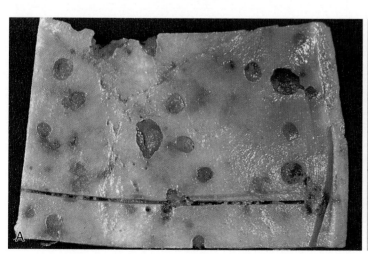

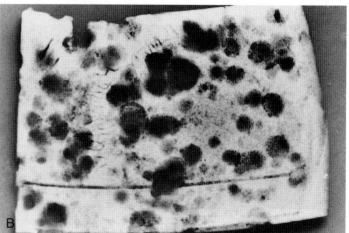

FIGURE 17.29 **MULTIPLE MYELOMA. (A)** A portion of the skull removed from a patient with multiple myeloma shows many round defects filled with pinkish gray tissue. **(B)** Specimen radiograph of the portion of skull demonstrates the clearly demarcated lytic lesions.

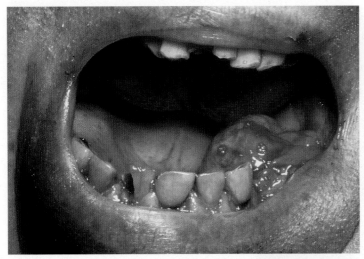

FIGURE 17.30 PLASMACYTOMA. This 60-year-old man with IgD multiple myeloma presented with a lesion of the lower mandible, with soft tissue extension into the floor of the mouth. He also had severe anemia and uremia.

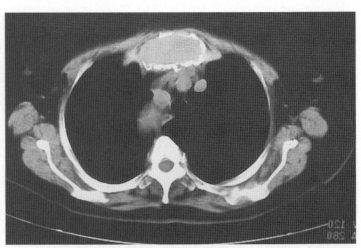

FIGURE 17.32 Computed tomography scan shows a destructive, expansile mass of the manubrium. Biopsy was diagnostic of a plasmacytoma composed of monoclonal IgG_κ plasma cells. Of note, iliac crest bone marrow biopsy showed 5% involvement by IgG_L plasma cells.

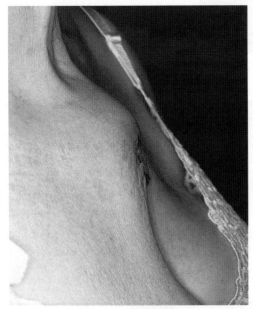

FIGURE 17.31 PLASMACYTOMA. This 78-year-old woman presented with a painful slowly enlarging mass protruding from her upper sternum.

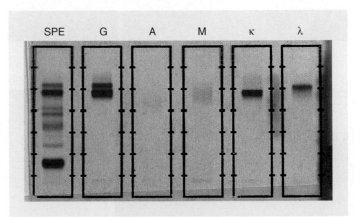

FIGURE 17.33 Serum protein electrophoresis demonstrates a "biclonal gammopathy" with two IgG M components in the γ-globulin region. Biclonal gammopathies are unusual, seen in only about 1% of cases of multiple myeloma. Of note, 6 months later, the patient's 42-year-old son presented with a pathologic lumbar spine fracture and was found to have stage IIIB myeloma. Familial multiple myeloma is not common but is occasionally reported. SPE, serum protein electrophoresis.

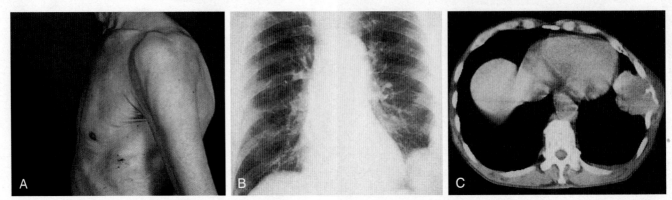

FIGURE 17.34 SOLITARY OSSEOUS PLASMACYTOMA. (A) A firm, ovoid mass, measuring 9 cm in diameter, is visible over the lower lateral aspect of the left chest wall. Protein studies, complete blood count, and bone marrow were normal. No other skeletal lesions were detected. **(B)** Chest film shows a well-defined mass, approximately 5 cm in diameter, in the lower left chest; the mass is pleural in position and arises from the ninth rib. **(C)** On CT scan, erosion of the rib is apparent, together with a soft tissue mass extending both into the pleural space and outward.

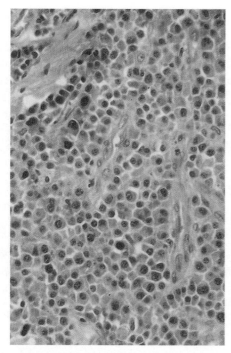

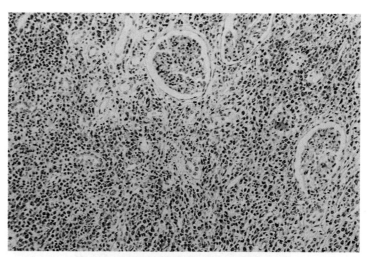

FIGURE 17.36 MULTIPLE MYELOMA (RENAL INVOLVEMENT). Photomicrograph of renal tissue from a patient who died from advanced multiple myeloma shows replacement of the majority of the stroma by tumor cells; several glomeruli and tubules are spared. Both kidneys were diffusely infiltrated by plasma cells, which led to renal failure.

FIGURE 17.35 SOLITARY OSSEOUS PLASMACYTOMA. Bone biopsy specimen reveals dense collections of plasma cells supported by a vascular stroma.

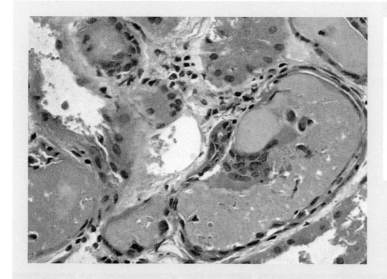

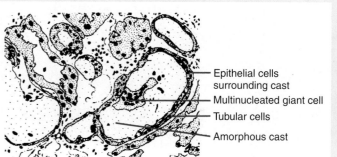

Epithelial cells surrounding cast
Multinucleated giant cell
Tubular cells
Amorphous cast

FIGURE 17.37 MULTIPLE MYELOMA (RENAL INVOLVEMENT). Histologic section of kidney shows a cast lined by epithelial cells within a dilated renal tubule. There is also a giant cell reaction to the proteinaceous material within the cast. "Myeloma kidney" refers to a variety of findings, like those shown here, including tubular atrophy and the presence of chronic inflammatory cells. The tubular, often laminated proteinaceous material consists of Bence-Jones protein, albumin, and often fibrinogen.

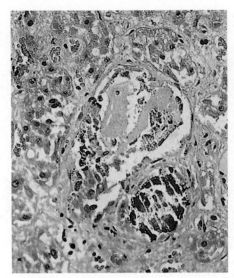

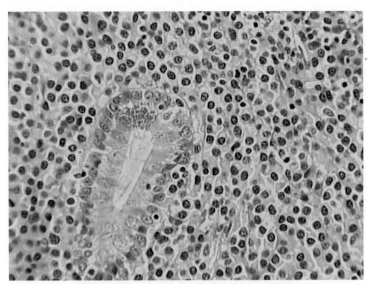

FIGURE 17.38 **MULTIPLE MYELOMA (NEPHROCALCINOSIS).** Irregular fractured hematoxylinophilic deposits of calcium are seen in this fibrotic renal tissue.

FIGURE 17.40 Plasma cells are deposited throughout the gut in this unusual presentation of IgA extramedullary disease. (From Wickramasinghe SN, McCullough J: *Blood and bone marrow pathology.* © 2003 Churchill Livingstone.)

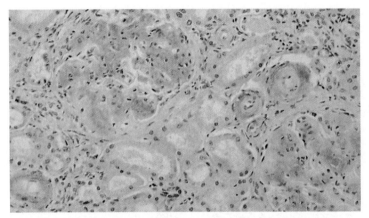

FIGURE 17.39 **MULTIPLE MYELOMA (RENAL AMYLOID DISEASE).** Microscopic section of renal tissue reveals extensive amyloid deposition in the glomeruli and associated arterioles.

FIGURE 17.41 **AMYLOID. (A)** Exceptionally large amounts of amyloid are evident in this microscopic section as homogeneous masses staining positive with Congo red. **(B)** Under polarized light these areas show brilliant apple-green birefringence. Amyloidosis is a well-recognized complication in about 20% of cases of multiple myeloma, in which circumstance the characteristic β-pleated sheets of fibrillary protein are composed of abnormal Ig light chains. Most often there is diffuse deposition in the kidneys, heart, vessels, skin, and gastrointestinal tract. Nodular, tumor-like deposition, as seen here, is extremely unusual.

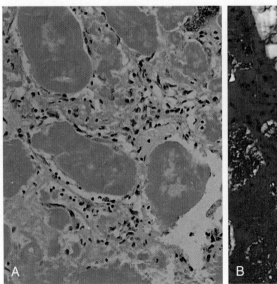
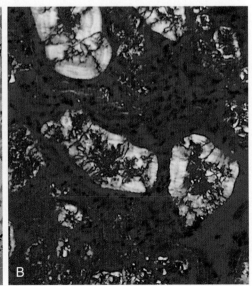

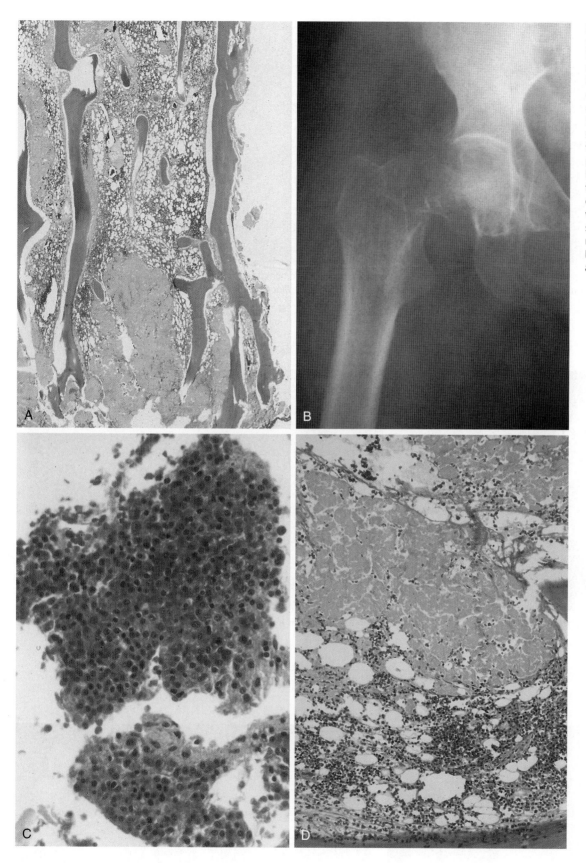

FIGURE 17.42 **AMYLOID. (A)** Low-power photomicrograph of a bone marrow (BM) biopsy from a patient with multiple myeloma involving BM as well as extensive deposits of myeloma-associated amyloid within marrow, and also involving the joint space and surrounding soft tissue. **(B)** Hip film revealing the presence of a pathologic fracture of the right hip and lytic lesions within the femur, as well as radiolucent deposits consistent with amyloid within the joint and surrounding soft tissue. **(C)** Homogeneous nodule of plasma cells within the BM. **(D)** Amorphous eosinophilic amyloid deposit within BM.

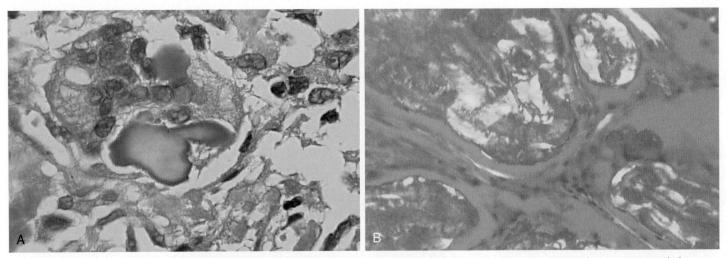

FIGURE 17.43   An unusual presentation of light-chain amyloid within the postnasal space. **(A)** On hematoxylin-eosin staining there are scattered plasma cells. **(B)** Fibrils stain apple green under polarized light. (From Wickramasinghe SN, McCullough J: *Blood and bone marrow pathology*. © 2003 Churchill Livingstone.)

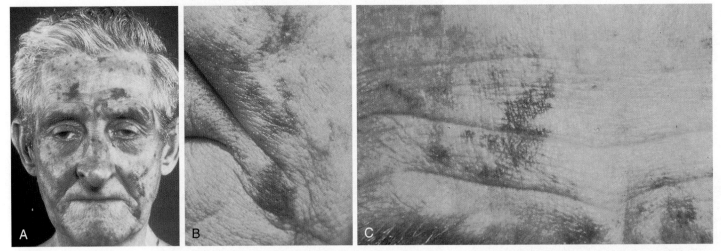

FIGURE 17.44   **AMYLOID SKIN DEPOSITS. (A to C)** The purpuric skin lesions visible on the face of this man can be ascribed to the deposition of amyloid in cutaneous blood vessels.

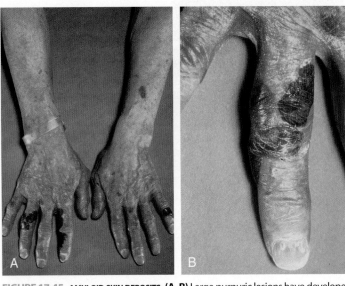

FIGURE 17.45   **AMYLOID SKIN DEPOSITS. (A, B)** Large purpuric lesions have developed on the hands and fingers, exacerbated by minimal friction and pressure.

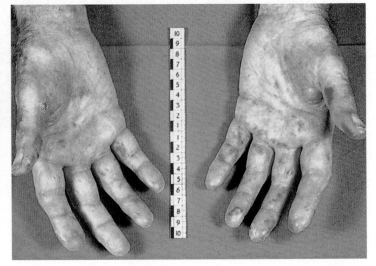

FIGURE 17.46   **AMYLOID SKIN DEPOSITS.** Purpuric skin lesions with characteristic smooth, yellowish deposits can be seen in this patient with multiple myeloma. The skin is hard, dense, and waxy.

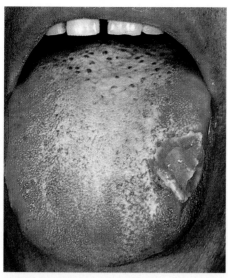

FIGURE 17.47 **AMYLOID.** The tongue exhibits macroglossia and a deep ulcer on the upper and anterolateral surfaces. The floor of the ulcer has the waxy appearance typical of amyloid deposition.

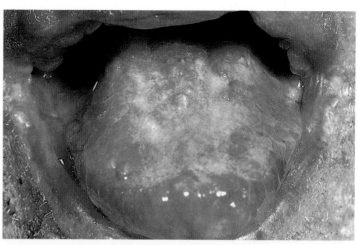

FIGURE 17.49 **AMYLOID DISEASE.** These nodular deposits of amyloid contrast with the diffuse enlargement shown in Figure 17.47. Similar nodules are also evident on the lips. Changes in taste sensation may occur.

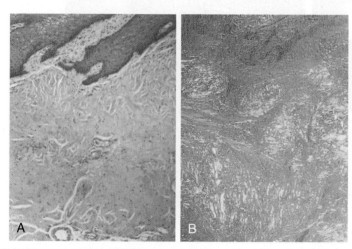

FIGURE 17.48 **AMYLOID. (A)** Photomicroscopic section of the ulcer seen in Figure 17.47 shows extensive deposition of pale-staining acidophilic material. **(B)** Stained with Congo red, this material shows the characteristic green birefringence of amyloid.

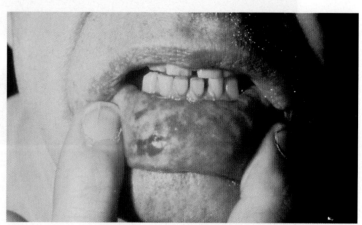

FIGURE 17.50 **MULTIPLE MYELOMA (ECCHYMOSES).** Abnormal bleeding is noted in 10% to 20% of patients at presentation. Cutaneous hemorrhages and epistaxis are the most common bleeding manifestations. This patient had recurrent "blood blisters" in the mouth, combined with periorbital hematomas and subconjunctival hemorrhages. The pathogenesis is complex but probably involves interference with platelet-capillary interaction and/or with clotting factors by the paraprotein. Uremia and thrombocytopenia may contribute.

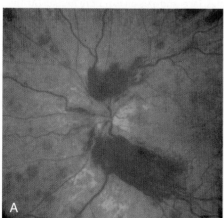
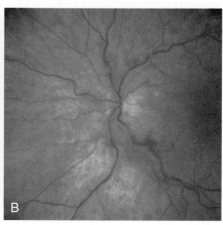

FIGURE 17.51 **MULTIPLE MYELOMA (HYPERVISCOSITY SYNDROME). (A)** Distention of retinal veins and widespread hemorrhage accompany the hyperviscosity syndrome. The patient presented with some loss of vision and headache. **(B)** Two months after plasmapheresis and chemotherapy, the vessels are normal and almost all hemorrhage has cleared. (Courtesy of Prof. J.C. Parr.)

Table 17.5

Causes of the Hyperviscosity Syndrome

Causes*	Diseases
M proteins	Waldenstrom's macroglobulinemia Multiple myeloma
Polycythemia	Polycythemia vera Severe secondary polycythemia
Leukostasis	Chronic myelogenous leukemia Acute nonlymphocytic leukemias with white cell counts 100,000 cells/mm³
Hyperfibrinogenemia	Following factor VIII replacement therapy with large amounts of cryoprecipitate

*M proteins are the dominant cause, but others of importance are polycythemia, leukostasis, and hyperfibrinogenemia.

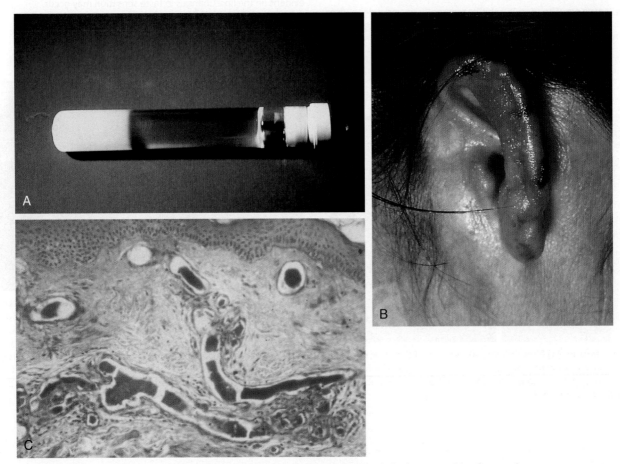

FIGURE 17.52   MULTIPLE MYELOMA (IgG CRYOGLOBULINEMIA). This patient experienced severe pain in the extremities, face, and ears on exposure to cold. **(A)** The concentration of cryoglobulin (6 g/100 mL) was vividly demonstrated by keeping the plasma in a refrigerator overnight, resulting in precipitation. **(B)** Crusted hemorrhagic lesions are present on the ears. **(C)** Skin biopsy reveals precipitation of cryoglobulin in small cutaneous vessels.

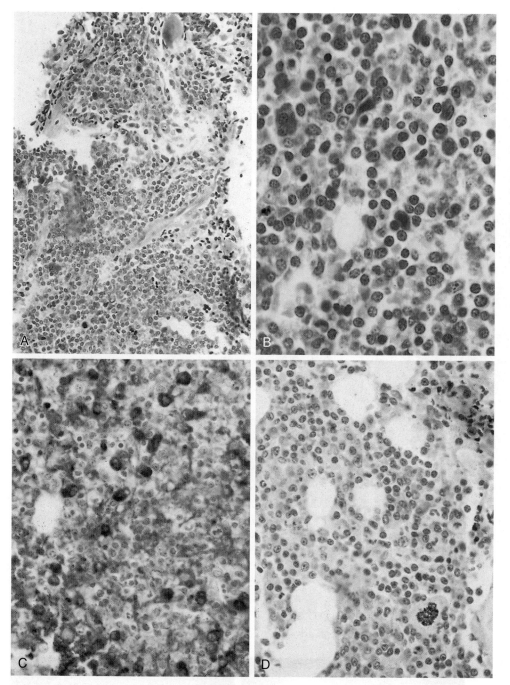

FIGURE 17.53 **WALDENSTROM'S MACROGLOBULINEMIA. (A)** Low-power photomicrograph of a bone marrow core biopsy specimen shows marked hypercellularity with loss of the normal 50:50 fat-to-cell ratio due to infiltration by tumor cells. **(B)** High magnification reveals lymphocytes, plasma, cells, and lymphoplasmacytoid cells typical of Waldenstrom's macroglobulinemia. The presence of mast cells, with their distinctive granules that stain purple with Giemsa, is sometimes a helpful diagnostic feature because of their association with this disease. Immunoperoxidase studies reveal that the plasmacytoid cells are **(C)** strongly immunoreactive for IgM heavy chains but **(D)** negative for IgG. The cells were also positive for κ-light chains but negative for λ-light chains (not shown).

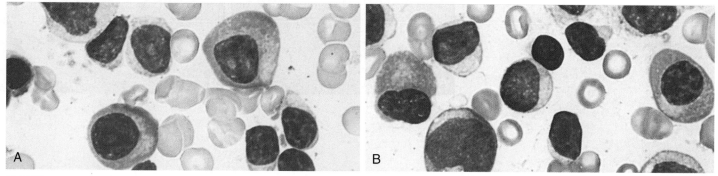

FIGURE 17.54 **WALDENSTROM'S MACROGLOBULINEMIA. (A, B)** Characteristically, the cells have features combining those of classic lymphocytes with those of plasma cells. For example, some cells have the nuclear appearance of a lymphocyte and the cytoplasmic features of a plasma cell. The chromatin patterns in the larger nuclei are more open and primitive.

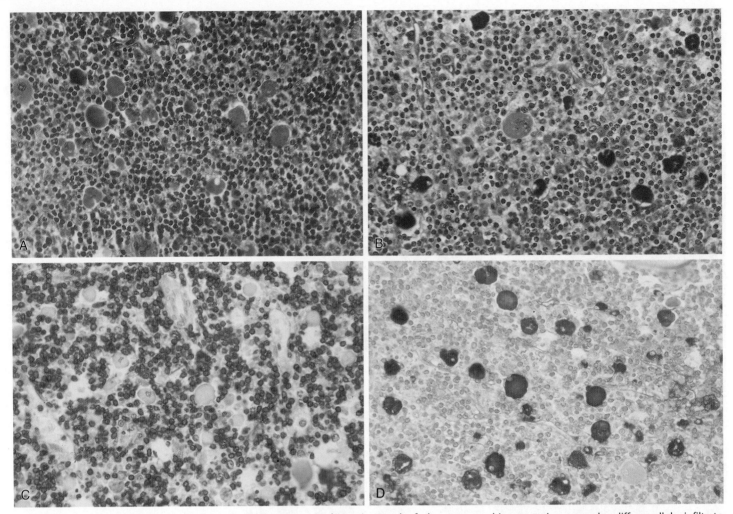

FIGURE 17.55 WALDENSTROM'S MACROGLOBULINEMIA. (A) Low-power photomicrograph of a bone marrow biopsy specimen reveals a diffuse cellular infiltrate composed of small lymphocytes as well as lymphoplasmacytoid cells and plasma cells, many of which contain prominent intracytoplasmic Ig inclusions, which are periodic acid–Schiff positive **(B)**. The small lymphocytes are immunoreactive for B-cell marker CD74 **(C)**, and Ig inclusions exhibit positive staining for IgM **(D)**.

FIGURE 17.56 **WALDENSTROM'S MACROGLOBULINEMIA (HYPERVISCOSITY SYNDROME). (A)** The retina of a patient who presented with blurred vision, headache, and dizziness shows gross distention of vessels, particularly the veins, which show bulging and constriction (the "linked sausage" effect), as well as areas of hemorrhage. **(B)** After plasmapheresis the vascular diameters are normal and the hemorrhagic areas have cleared.

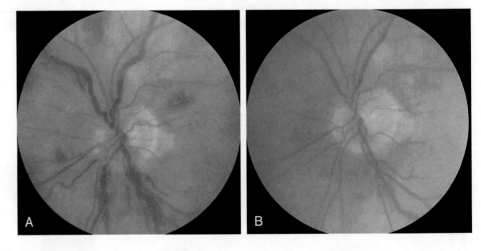

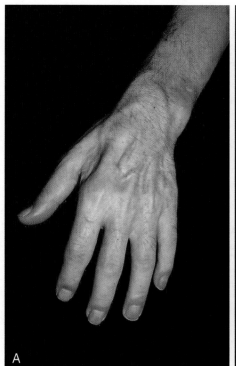

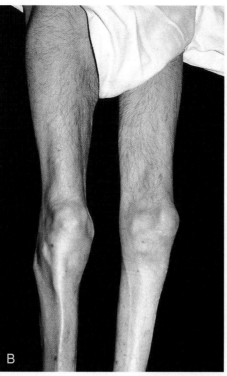

FIGURE 17.57 **WALDENSTROM'S MACROGLOBULINEMIA (NEUROPATHY).** This 75-year-old man developed severe hand and leg weakness due to peripheral neuropathy. **(A)** Evaluation of the hand shows marked atrophy of the interosseous muscles. **(B)** The legs show marked muscle atrophy. These features are mainly the result of amyloid deposition in small vessels supplying nerves.

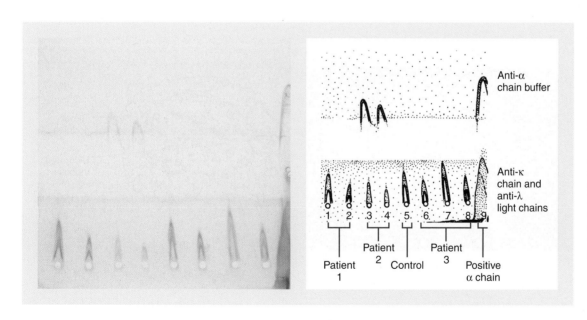

FIGURE 17.58 α-**HEAVY CHAIN DISEASE.** Gel electrophoresis results are shown for a case of α-chain disease (patient 2) with accompanying positive control (9). Patients 1 and 3 are negative. The numbered wells contain the sera to be tested. When they migrate across the plate under the influence of an electrophoretic current, the light chains are precipitated in the proximal one-third of their course by the anti-κ and anti-λ in the gel. Any serum containing heavy chains is precipitated in the distal third of the gel by anti-α chain. (Courtesy of Dr. A. Howard.)

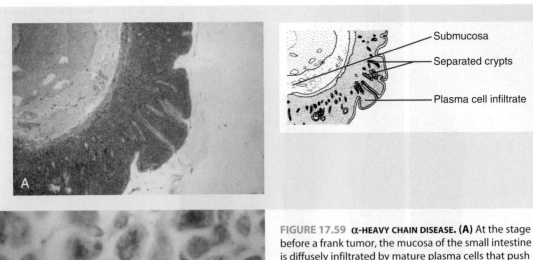

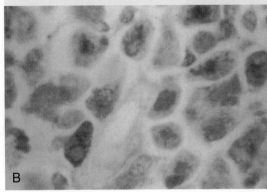

FIGURE 17.59 α-HEAVY CHAIN DISEASE. (A) At the stage before a frank tumor, the mucosa of the small intestine is diffusely infiltrated by mature plasma cells that push the crypts apart. (B) The immunoperoxidase technique demonstrates only IgA (staining brown) in the plasma cells and no light chain.

FIGURE 17.60 α-HEAVY CHAIN DISEASE. This surgical specimen of ileum shows frank tumor nodules clearly visible in the mesentery, ulcerating the ileal mucosa. (Courtesy of Dr. F. Asselah.)

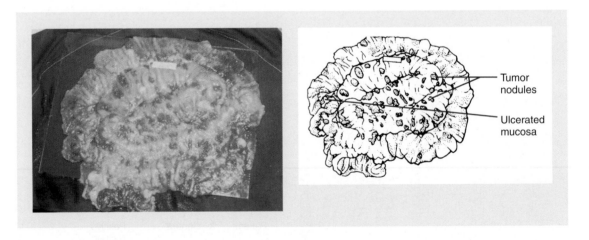

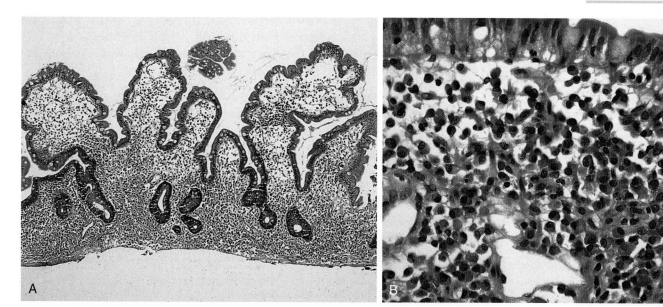

FIGURE 17.61 α-HEAVY CHAIN DISEASE. A 25-year-old Algerian man presented with malabsorption syndrome consisting of weight loss, chronic diarrhea, steatorrhea, and hypocalcemia, which responded to broad-spectrum antibiotics. **(A)** Biopsy specimen of small intestine shows diffuse infiltration of the lamina propria by **(B)** a mixture of lymphocytes, plasma cells, and plasmacytoid cells. Immunocytochemical staining showed that the vast majority of these cells contained α-heavy chains without κ- or λ-light chains. Serum and urine samples revealed a broad band in the α2 region, which precipitated with an anti-IgA antiserum but showed no reactivity to anti-κ or anti-α. (Courtesy of Dr. J.E. McLaughlin.)

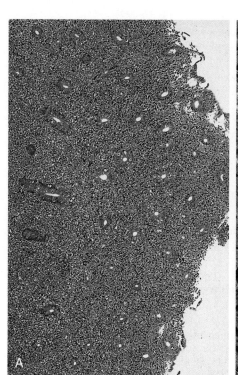
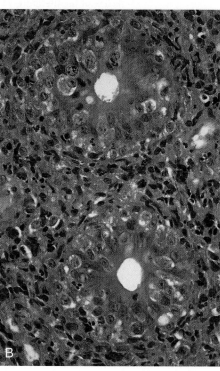

FIGURE 17.62 α-HEAVY CHAIN DISEASE. Two years after presentation, the same patient as presented in Figure 17.61 developed small intestinal obstruction. After resection the small bowel was found to be heavily infiltrated by a large cell immunoblastic lymphoma, with an additional mixed infiltrate of neutrophils, plasma cells, and macrophages. Despite intensive chemotherapy, the tumor relapsed, involving the large and small bowel and intra-abdominal lymph nodes, which showed similar histologic findings. The rectal mucosa seen at **(A)** low power and **(B)** high power shows complete loss of normal architecture; remaining crypt cells are surrounded by a diffuse infiltrate composed of large malignant cells and mixed inflammatory cells. The α-heavy chain could still be detected in serum but not in urine at this relapse. (Courtesy of Dr. J.E. McLaughlin.)

References and Suggested Readings

Avet-Loiseau H, Brigaudeau C, Morineau N, et al: High incidence of cryptic translocations involving the Ig heavy chain gene in multiple myeloma, as shown by fluorescence in situ hybridization, *Genes Chromosomes Cancer* 24:9–15, 1999.

Bergsagel PL, Kuehl WM: Molecular pathogenesis and a consequent classification of multiple myeloma, *J Clin Oncol* 23:6333–6338, 2005.

Carrasco DR, Tonon G, Huang Y, et al: High-resolution genomic profiles define distinct clinico-pathogenetic subgroups of multiple myeloma patients, *Cancer Cell* 9:313–325, 2006.

Corradini P, Ladetto M, Voena C, et al: Mutational activation of N- and K-ras oncogenes in plasma cell dyscrasias, *Blood* 81:2708–2713, 1993.

Davies FE, Dring AM, Li C, et al: Insights into the multistep transformation of MGUS to myeloma using microarray expression analysis, *Blood* 102:4504–4511, 2003.

Dimopoulos MA, Kyle RA, Anagnostopoulos A, et al: Diagnosis and management of Waldenström's macroglobulinemia, *J Clin Oncol* 23:1564–1577, 2005.

Durie BG, Harousseau JL, Miguel JS, et al: International uniform response criteria for multiple myeloma, *Leukemia* 20:2220, 2006.

Durie BG, Salmon SE: A clinical staging system for multiple myeloma: correlation of measured myeloma cell mass with presenting clinical features, response to treatment, and survival, *Cancer* 36:842–854, 1975.

Falk RH, Comenzo RL, Skinner M: The systemic amyloidoses, *N Engl J Med* 337:898–909, 1997.

Fermand JP, Brouet JC: Heavy-chain diseases, *Hematol Oncol Clin North Am* 13:1281–1294, 1999.

Garcia-Sanz R, Orfao A, Gonzalez M, et al: Primary plasma cell leukemia: clinical, immunophenotypic, DNA ploidy, and cytogenetic characteristics, *Blood* 93:1032–1037, 1999.

Gonzáles D, van der Burg M, García-Sanz R, et al: Immunoglobulin gene rearrangements and the pathogenesis of multiple myeloma, *Blood* 110:3112–3121, 2007.

Greipp PR, Leong T, Bennett JM, et al: Plasmablastic morphology—an independent prognostic factor with clinical and laboratory correlates: Eastern Cooperative Oncology Group (ECOG) myeloma trial E9486 report by the ECOG Myeloma Laboratory Group, *Blood* 91:2501–2507, 1998.

Greipp PR, San Miguel J, Durie BG, et al: International staging system for multiple myeloma, *J Clin Oncol* 23:3412–3420, 2005.

Hideshima T, Chauhan D, Richardson P, et al: Identification and validation of novel therapeutic targets for multiple myeloma, *J Clin Oncol* 23:6345–6350, 2005.

Hideshima T, Mitsiades C, Tonon G, et al: Understanding multiple myeloma pathogenesis in the bone marrow to identify new therapeutic targets, *Nat Rev Cancer* 7:585–598, 2007.

International Myeloma Working Group: Criteria for the classification of monoclonal gammopathies, multiple myeloma and related disorders: a report of the International Myeloma Working Group, *Br J Haematol* 121:749–757, 2003.

Jagannath S: Value of serum free light chain testing for the diagnosis and monitoring of monoclonal gammopathies in hematology, *Clin Lymphoma Myeloma* 7:518–523, 2007.

Jemal A, Siegel R, Ward E, et al: Cancer statistics, 2009, *CA Cancer J Clin* 59:225–249, 2009.

Kyle RA, Rajkumar SV: Monoclonal gammopathies of undetermined significance: a review, *Immunol Rev* 194:112–139, 2003.

Kyle RA, Rajkumar SV: Monoclonal gammopathy of undetermined significance, *Br J Haematol* 134:573–589, 2006.

Kyle RA, Rajkumar SV: Multiple myeloma, *Blood* 111:2962–2972, 2008.

Kyle RA, Remstein ED, Therneau TM, et al: Clinical course and prognosis of smoldering (asymptomatic) multiple myeloma, *N Engl J Med* 356:2582–2590, 2007.

Lynch HT, Ferrara K, Barlogie B, et al: Familial myeloma, *N Engl J Med* 359:152–157, 2008.

Munshi NC: Monoclonal gammopathy of undetermined significance: genetic vs environmental etiologies, *Mayo Clin Proc* 82:1457–1459, 2007.

Nieuwenhuizen L, Biesma DH: Central nervous system myelomatosis: review of the literature, *Eur J Haematol* 80:1–9, 2007.

Raje N, Hideshima T, Anderson KC: Therapeutic use of immunomodulatory drugs in the treatment of multiple myeloma, *Expert Rev Anticancer Ther* 6:1239–1247, 2006.

Rajkumar SV, Lacy MQ, Kyle RA: Monoclonal gammopathy of undetermined significance and smoldering multiple myeloma, *Blood Rev* 21:255–265, 2007.

Richardson PG, Mitsiades C, Schlossman R, et al: New drugs for myeloma, *Oncologist* 12:664–689, 2007.

Figure Credits

The following books published by Gower Medical Publishing are sources of figures in the present chapter. The figure numbers given in the listing are those of the figures in the present chapter. The page numbers given in parentheses are those of the original publication.

Asscher AW, Moffat DB, Sanders E: *Nephrology illustrated.* Oxford/London, 1982, Pergamon Medical Publications/Gower Medical Publishing: Fig. 17.37 (p. 8.15).

Bullough PG, Boachie-Adjei O: *Atlas of spinal diseases.* Philadelphia/New York, 1988, Lippincott/Gower Medical Publishing: Figs. 17.6 (p. 191); 17.23 (p. 192); 17.24 (p. 192).

Bullough PG, Vigorita VJ: *Atlas of orthopaedic pathology.* Baltimore/New York, 1984, University Park Press/Gower Medical Publishing: Figs. 17.29A (p. 13.9); 17.29B (p. 13.9).

Cawson RA, Eveson JW: *Oral pathology and diagnosis.* London, 1987, Heinemann Medical Books/Gower Medical Publishing: Figs. 17.17 (p. 18.18); 17.41 (p. 18.20).

Dieppe PA, Bacon PA, et al: *Atlas of clinical rheumatology.* Philadelphia/London, 1986, Lea and Febiger/Gower Medical Publishing: Fig. 17.22 (p. 21.6).

Greenspan A: *Orthopedic radiology.* Philadelphia/New York, 1988, Lippincott/Gower Medical Publishing: Figs. 17.21 (p. 16.20); 17.25 (p. 16.22); 17.27 (p. 16.20).

Hewitt PE: *Blood diseases* (Pocket Picture Guides). London, 1985, Gower Medical Publishing: Figs. 17.28 (p. 48); 17.45 (p. 49); 17.50 (p. 48).

Hoffbrand AV, Pettit JE: *Clinical haematology illustrated.* Edinburgh/London, 1987, Churchill Livingstone/Gower Medical Publishing: Figs. 17.1 (p. 11.10); 17.4 (p. 11.3); 17.85 (p. 11.3); 17.9 (p. 11.2); 17.10 (p. 11.2); 17.11 (p 11.2); 17.13 (p. 11.3); 17.15 (p. 11.4); 17.26 (p. 11.5); 17.31 (p. 11.8); 17.34B (p. 11.8); 17.34C (p. 11.8); 17.38 (p. 11.6); 17.39 (p. 11.6); 17.46 (p. 13.5); 17.47 (p. 11.6); 17.43 (p. 11.7); 17.49 (p. 11.7); 17.51 (p. 11.10); 17.54 (p. 11.9); 17.56 (p. 11. 9); 17.61 (p. 11.11); 17.62 (p. 11.12); Table 17.1 (p. 11.10); Table 17.5 (p. 11.10).

Misiewicz JJ, Bartram CI, Cotton PB, et al: *Atlas of clinical gastroenterology.* London, 1985, Gower Medical Publishing: Figs. 17.58 (p. 6.13); 17.54 (p. 6.14); 17.60 (p. 6.14).

Weiss MA, Mills SE: *Atlas of genitourinary tract disorders.* Philadelphia/New York, 1988, Lippincott/Gower Medical Publishing: Fig. 17.18 (p. 11.45).

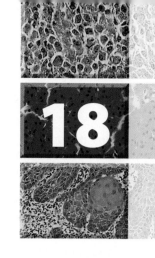

Solid Tumors in Childhood

STEPHAN D. VOSS • ANTONIO PEREZ-ATAYDE • FREDRIC A. HOFFER • HOLCOMBE E. GRIER

The incidence of cancer in childhood is quite rare compared with the incidence in adults; approximately 6500 new cases are diagnosed in the United States each year. Nevertheless, cancer remains the second most common cause of death during childhood. The common childhood cancers and their frequency are shown in Table 18.1. It is important to note that the relative incidence of tumors is not constant through childhood. The median age for neuroblastoma, for instance, is 1–2 years, and the tumor is unusual after 5 years of age. In contrast, the incidence of Hodgkin disease peaks in adolescence and is rare in children younger than 5 years of age.

Childhood cancers have provided insights into the biology and treatment of neoplasia in general. The identification of recessive oncogenes, for example, as well as the advantage of multimodal therapy on cure rates were first described in the context of childhood malignancies such as Wilms' tumor, retinoblastoma, and other solid tumors of childhood.

Several malignancies seen in adults and children are covered in other chapters and will not be reviewed here. Brain tumors and germ cell tumors are discussed in Chapters 8 and 14, acute leukemias in Chapter 15, and lymphomas in Chapter 16.

Table 18.1

Common Malignant Tumors in Childhood and Their Relative Frequency*

Malignant Tumor	Frequency (%)
Leukemia (mostly ALL, some AML)	30
Brain tumors	19
Lymphomas (Hodgkin and non-Hodgkin)	13
Neuroblastoma	8
Kidney (mostly Wilms' tumor)	6
Soft tissue sarcoma (rhabdomyosarcoma most common)	7
Retinoblastoma	3
Bone	5
Liver	1
Other	8

ALL, acute lymphoblastic leukemia; AML, acute myeloid leukemia
*<15 years of age.
Compiled from SEER data, National Cancer Institute.

Retinoblastoma

Retinoblastoma is a malignancy of early childhood that arises in the retina. It is often present at birth and is rarely diagnosed later than 6 years of age. The disease is hereditary in 60% of cases. The hereditary type may be transmitted as an autosomal-dominant trait from an affected parent or may occur as a spontaneous mutation. This type of retinoblastoma, which is passed on to 50% of subsequent offspring, is diagnosed earlier than the nonhereditary form and is usually multifocal at presentation. It is associated with the somatic loss of a recessive oncogene, the retinoblastoma (*RB1*) gene, from chromosome 13. Loss of both *RB1* genes leads to the tumor, thus explaining why multiple tumors occur in patients lacking one of the *RB1* genes (the first "hit" of the two-hit process has occurred in all the cells). Patients are at high risk for secondary sarcomas, both at previous irradiation sites and elsewhere. A staging system developed by Reese and Ellsworth predicts the likelihood of tumor control and preservation of vision, based on the location of the tumor for disease confined to the orbit (intraocular retinoblastoma).

In contrast to the hereditary form, nonhereditary retinoblastoma is always unilateral and does not have a high risk of second tumors except in the irradiated field. Up to 10% of unilateral tumors may be hereditary, and genetic counseling along with molecular analysis of the germline *RB1* genes is necessary for all patients even with unilateral presentation.

Patients with retinoblastoma most commonly present with leukokoria, a whitish reflex from a mass behind the lens. In the United States the disease is usually confined to the globe at diagnosis, although it may grow along the optic tract or extend through the globe and invade bone. Microscopically, retinoblastoma cells have hyperchromatic nuclei with scanty cytoplasm. The vast majority of patients with retinoblastoma are cured with a combination of surgery and/or radiation therapy. Chemotherapy is used only for the very rare patient with extraocular disease or distant metastases.

The size and extent of retinoblastoma can be measured by many means including direct ophthalmoscopy, computed tomography (CT), magnetic resonance imaging (MRI), and sonography. Fluorescein angiography (not illustrated) will detect small vascular lesions. It is performed by intravenous injection of a fluorane dye and direct photography of the retina illuminated by an ultraviolet light.

Wilms' Tumor

Wilms' tumor is the most common tumor of the kidney in childhood; other rarer, malignant renal tumors of childhood include clear cell sarcoma and rhabdoid tumor. The median age at diagnosis of Wilms' tumor is between 2 and 3 years. The tumor is uncommon after 8 years of age. The classic histologic appearance of Wilms' tumor is triphasic, comprising blastemal, epithelial (tubules and glomeruloid structures), and mesenchymal elements, although many tumors exhibit only one or two of these elements. The presence of anaplasia is associated with a poorer prognosis.

Most patients with Wilms' tumor present with an abdominal mass, usually first palpated by the parents. Less common presentations include hematuria and hypertension; systemic symptoms are rare. Bilateral tumors are found at presentation in 4% to 7% of cases. In 5% of cases Wilms' tumor is associated with other abnormalities of the genitourinary (GU) system and, more rarely, with hemihypertrophy, the Beckwith-Wiedemann syndrome (macroglossia, somatic gigantism, abdominal wall defects, and hypoglycemia), Drash syndrome (pseudohermaphroditism and nephropathy), and aniridia. The latter syndrome led to the discovery of an association in some patients between Wilms' tumor and loss of the *WT1* gene on the long arm of chromosome 11. This gene is a zinc-finger DNA-binding protein that is expressed in the developing kidney.

The grouping system developed by the National Wilms' Tumor Study is shown in Figure 18.7. The workup for Wilms' tumor includes urinalysis, chest radiography, and abdominal and chest CT scan. The lung is the most common site of metastases. MRI of the abdomen may also be useful and may substitute for abdominal CT. MRI may help differentiate nephrogenic rests from bilateral Wilms' tumor. Either MRI or ultrasonography of the abdomen should be done preoperatively to visualize tumor within the inferior vena cava (IVC).

Neuroblastoma

Neuroblastoma is the most common extracranial solid tumor in childhood and the most common cancer in infants. The median age at diagnosis is 2 years, although neuroblastoma occasionally occurs in adults. The tumor, originating in neural crest cells, can occur anywhere along the sympathetic nerve chain. By far the most common location for a primary tumor is the adrenal gland. In its most primitive form, the histology of neuroblastoma is marked by poorly differentiated small, round blue cells. At an intermediate stage of maturation, there is differentiation toward ganglion cells. Tumors composed of a mixture of neuroblasts and mature ganglion cells are classified as ganglioneuroblastomas. At the most differentiated end of the spectrum is ganglioneuroma, a benign tumor composed entirely of mature ganglion cells, neuritis, and Schwann cells.

The International Neuroblastoma Staging System (INSS) is shown in Table 18.2.

Stage 4S neuroblastoma is an unusual malignancy that has a high likelihood of spontaneous resolution despite the existence of extensive, generalized metastases at the time of presentation. The most common fatal complication in stage 4S disease is respiratory compromise secondary to massive enlargement of the liver. For other patients with neuroblastoma, the prognosis overall is stage- and age-related, with a markedly improved survival rate for patients who present before the age of 1 year.

The presenting signs and symptoms of neuroblastoma depend on the location of the primary tumor. An abdominal mass associated with an adrenal tumor is the most common presentation. Paraspinal tumors may present with cord compression, and thoracic tumors are occasionally associated with Horner syndrome. Patients with metastatic disease frequently present with proptosis and periorbital ecchymosis. Metastases occur to lymph nodes, bone, bone marrow, liver, and skin. Patients frequently show systemic symptoms of irritability and poor food intake, probably occasioned by pain from extensive bone involvement. Urinary excretion of catecholamines is increased in 85% to 90% of patients with neuroblastoma; in fact, the diagnosis can be made on the basis of increased urinary catecholamines associated with typical neuroblastoma cells in the bone marrow. Workup should also include a bone scan and MR or CT imaging of the primary; many centers are doing MIBG scanning, utilizing the tumor uptake of the radiolabeled catecholamine precursor meta-iodobenzylguanidine. Rarely, patients present with diarrhea from secretion of vasoactive intestinal polypeptide or with the syndrome of opsoclonus-myoclonus; the latter syndrome may be an autoimmune phenomenon and may not regress even with successful treatment of the tumor.

Table 18.2

International Neuroblastoma Staging System Criteria

Stage	Definition
1	Localized tumor with complete gross excision, with or without microscopic residual disease; representative ipsilateral nonadherent* lymph nodes negative for tumor microscopically
2A	Localized tumor with incomplete gross excision; representative ipsilateral nonadherent lymph nodes negative for tumor microscopically
2B	Localized tumor with or without complete gross excision, with ipsilateral, nonadherent lymph nodes positive for tumor. Enlarged contralateral lymph nodes must be negative microscopically.
3	Unresectable unilateral tumor infiltrating across the midline,† with or without regional lymph node involvement or Localized unilateral tumor with contralateral regional lymph node involvement or Midline tumor with bilateral extension by infiltration (unresectable) or by lymph node involvement
4	Any primary tumor with dissemination to distant lymph nodes, bone marrow, liver, skin, and/or other organs (except as defined for stage 4S)
4S	Localized primary tumor (as defined for stages 1, 2A, or 2B), with dissemination limited to skin, liver, and/or bone marrow‡ (limited to infants <1 year of age)

*Lymph nodes attached to and removed with the primary tumor.
†The midline is defined as the vertebral column. Tumors originating on one side and crossing the midline must infiltrate to or beyond the opposite side of the vertebral column.
‡Marrow involvement in stage 4S should be minimal (i.e., <10% of total nucleated cells identified as malignant on bone marrow biopsy or on marrow aspirate). More extensive marrow involvement would be considered to be stage 4. The MIBG scan, if performed, should be negative in the marrow.

Neuroblastoma is one of the first tumors noted in some cases to involve amplification of a dominant oncogene. Cytogenetic studies of cell lines and fresh tumor specimens may show double minutes or homogeneous staining regions representing multiple copies of the *MYCN* oncogene. Amplification of this gene conveys a less favorable prognosis. Several other biologic variables predict outcome in neuroblastoma. The International Neuroblastoma Risk Groups Committee is attempting to define patient subsets based on these variables.

Hepatic Tumors

The most common primary malignant tumors of the liver in childhood are hepatoblastoma and hepatoma (hepatocellular carcinoma). (See also text and illustrations on "Hepatoma" in Chapter 7.) The distinguishing clinical characteristics of hepatoblastoma and hepatoma are shown in Table 18.3.

Hepatoblastoma is a rare, embryonal malignant neoplasm that typically presents in infancy, showing a predilection for males. It may be associated with a variety of congenital anomalies and with the syndrome of familial polyposis coli (FPC). Children with hepatoblastoma and FPC may exhibit congenital hypertrophy of the retinal pigment epithelium (CHRPE), which is sometimes seen with FPC. There is an increased incidence of hepatoblastoma in low-birth-weight infants; the cause for this association is not known. Most children with hepatoblastoma present with an asymptomatic abdominal mass, which grossly appears tan and lobulated. Workup includes measurement of α-fetoprotein, which is elevated in nearly all patients. CT scan of the lung, the most common site of metastasis, is part of patient workup, as well as abdominal MRI, ultrasonography, and, finally, angiography of the liver if the potential for resection is unclear. Complete resection of the primary tumor is of utmost importance for cure in hepatoblastoma.

Adjuvant chemotherapy improves outcome in completely resected cases, and neoadjuvant chemotherapy may convert some patients' tumors from being unresectable to resectable; this approach has considerably increased the cure rate in hepatoblastoma.

Rhabdomyosarcoma

Rhabdomyosarcoma, a malignancy that differentiates toward striated muscle cells, is the most common soft tissue sarcoma of childhood. (See also text and illustrations on "Rhabdomyosarcoma" in Chapter 12.) Pathologic sections occasionally show cross-striations, but their presence is not necessary to establish the diagnosis. Antibodies against muscle-specific proteins (especially myogenin and Myod1) and electron microscopy showing bundles of actin and myosin filaments can be extremely helpful in distinguishing rhabdomyosarcoma from other tumors. Two histologic patterns have been identified: embryonal and alveolar. Cytogenetics is an important tool in the diagnosis of rhabdomyosarcoma. The vast majority of tumors with alveolar characteristics have a translocation between the *FKHR* (now *FOXO1*) gene (one of the forkhead transcription factor genes) on chromosome 13 and the *PAX3* gene on chromosome 2 (or, less commonly, the *PAX7* gene on chromosome 1).

The median age at presentation for childhood rhabdomyosarcoma is 2–3 years for GU tumors and 6 years for tumors of the head and neck (see Table 18.4). Patients with rhabdomyosarcoma are assigned both a stage and a group. The stage is determined by factors at presentation. The system used is a TNM system but also incorporates the site of the tumor, since this is highly prognostic. Grouping is a surgical staging system and helps determine local control methods and dosing of radiation therapy. It is also prognostic when added to stage (see Table 18.5 and Figure 18.25), although in recent years there has been greater use of a TNM system. Proper staging requires MRI of the primary, CT of the lungs, and bone marrow aspirates and biopsies. As with other childhood sarcomas, FDG-PET imaging is being used increasingly for staging and post-treatment evaluation.

Table 18.3

Comparison of the Clinical Characteristics of Hepatoblastoma and Hepatoma

Characteristic	Hepatoblastoma	Hepatoma
Age	0–3 years	5–18+ years
Previous liver disease	Uncommon	Common
Pain	Uncommon	Common
Jaundice	Uncommon	¼ of cases
Elevated α-fetoprotein	⅔ of cases	½ of cases

Table 18.4

Patterns of Clinical Presentation in Rhabdomyosarcoma

Location	Relative Frequency (%)	Median Age (years)	Histology
Head and neck	40	6	Embryonal > alveolar
Genitourinary	20	2–3	Embryonal
Extremity, trunk	30	12–20	Alveolar > embryonal

Table 18.5

Intergroup Rhabdomyosarcoma Study Group Presurgical Staging Classification

Stage	Sites	Tumor (T)*	Size	Node (N)†	Metastasis (M)‡	
I	Orbit, head, and neck (excluding parameningeal) GU: Nonbladder/nonprostate	T_1 or T_2	a or b	N_0, N_1, or b	N_x	M_0
II	Bladder/prostate, extremity, cranial, parameningeal, other (includes trunk, retroperitoneum, etc.)	T_1 or T_2	a	N_0 or N_x	M_0	
III	Bladder/prostate, extremity, cranial parameningeal, other (includes trunk, retroperitoneum, etc.)	T_1 or T_2	a b	N_1 N_0, N_1, or N_x	M_0	
IV	All	T_1 or T_2	a or b	N_0 or N_1	M_1	

GU, genitourinary.
*T_1, confined to anatomic site of origin; T_2, extension and/or fixative to surrounding tissue; a, ≤ 5 cm in diameter in size; b, >5 cm in diameter in size.
†Regional nodes: N_0, regional nodes not clinically involved; N_1, regional nodes clinically involved by neoplasm; N_x, clinical status of regional nodes unknown.
‡Metastasis: M_0, no distant metastasis; M_1, metastasis present.

Surgery, radiation therapy, and chemotherapy are all important for long-term survival. Prognosis depends on the site of origin of the tumor and its histology: orbital, paratesticular, and most GU primary tumors have a more favorable prognosis than those of the extremities, trunk, and head and neck with extensive bone destruction; the alveolar histologic variant carries a less favorable prognosis than the embryonal variant.

The Ewing Family of Tumors

EWING SARCOMA AND PERIPHERAL PRIMITIVE NEUROECTODERMAL TUMOR OF BONE AND SOFT TISSUE

Ewing sarcoma is the second most common malignant bone tumor in children and adolescents. (See also text and illustrations on "Ewing Sarcoma" in Chapter 12.) Although its cell of origin is unclear, its histology is marked by small, round blue cells, classically often containing periodic acid–Schiff-positive material. Ewing sarcoma of bone and soft tissue has a continuum of differentiation, with the most differentiated form frequently termed primitive neuroectodermal tumor (PNET). The pathogenesis and cytogenetics of PNET are clearly different from the group of central nervous system tumors (central PNET) that unfortunately carry the same name. PNETs exhibit neuroectodermal differentiation as demonstrated on electron microscopy or by positivity with neuronal markers such as neuron-specific enolase. The clinical importance of this variation in differentiation is unclear. PNET and Ewing sarcoma cells both stain positively to antibodies to CD99, the protein product of the *MIC2* (now *CD99*) gene. Ewing sarcoma and PNET have a high incidence of a clonal abnormality, a translocation between chromosomes 11 and 22. This translocation creates a novel chimeric protein consisting of parts of two genes: *FLI1* (an ETS-like oncogene) and *EWS* (now *EWSR1*), a gene encoding an RNA-binding protein. This information can often be obtained by needle aspiration, using polymerase chain reaction or fluorescence in situ hybridization techniques. These tumors have a peak occurrence in the early second decade but can occur in patients as young as infants or as old as 30 years of age. The disease is extremely rare in blacks and Asians.

For patients with bone primaries, the most common symptom is a painful mass. For both soft tissue and bone primaries, fever may be a symptom at presentation in about one third of patients and occurs more commonly with large tumors or tumors with metastases. The most common bone site is the pelvis, followed closely by the femur, although the tumor can occur in virtually any bone. When a long bone is the site of the primary tumor, the midshaft of the femur is the most commonly involved area. Soft tissues in nearly every region of the body can develop PNETs, including the extremities, pelvis, or retroperitoneum. Most common sites include the paraspinal and thoracopulmonary regions. The paraspinal masses often impinge on the spinal cord. The thoracopulmonary tumor is commonly referred to as the Askin tumor of the chest wall.

The workup of a patient with Ewing sarcoma/PNET should include plain films and MR scanning of the primary tumor. In addition, CT scan of the lungs, bone scan, bone marrow aspiration and biopsy, and determination of lactate dehydrogenase concentration are part of the patient workup. There is also an increasing role for FDG-PET imaging, both for staging and post-treatment evaluation. The most common site of metastases is the lung, followed by bone and bone marrow. Poor prognostic factors for patients with bone primaries, in order of importance, are the presence of metastases, large size of the primary tumor, and location of the primary. Pelvic involvement carries a worse prognosis than involvement of the femur or humerus, which in turn has a worse prognosis than involvement distal to the knee and elbow. Treatment includes systemic chemotherapy for control of micrometatastic disease, which is present in more than 90% of patients, as indicated by the cure rate achieved with amputation alone. Radiation therapy can control the primary lesion in the majority of patients; it is unclear whether or not surgical excision of the primary tumor improves local control or overall disease-free survival.

Osteosarcoma

Osteosarcoma (osteogenic sarcoma) is the most common malignant tumor of bone in children and adolescents. (See also text and illustrations on "Osteosarcoma" in Chapter 12.) Derived from primitive mesenchymal bone-forming cells, osteosarcoma is defined histologically by malignant sarcomatous cells that form osteoid. The tumor most commonly arises in the second decade of life, with peak occurrence during the adolescent growth spurt. Most adolescents present with pain, often in conjunction with a soft tissue mass. Osteosarcoma is primarily a disease that affects the metaphysis of long bones. The distal femur is the most common primary site, followed by the proximal tibia and the proximal humerus.

Workup of a patient with presumed osteosarcoma should include plain films and MR scan of the primary lesion, as well as CT scan of the lung, bone scan, and determination of lactate dehydrogenase concentration. Metastases at the time of presentation are associated with a poor prognosis. Successful treatment of patients with nonmetastatic osteosarcoma requires complete surgical excision of the primary tumor and adjuvant chemotherapy. It is not clear at present whether preoperative chemotherapy improves the overall survival rate.

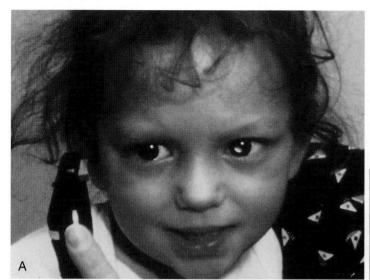

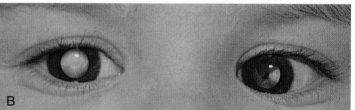

FIGURE 18.1 **RETINOBLASTOMA. (A)** Frequently, families first note leukokoria by a white reflex in the retina seen in photographs of their child. A retinal tumor is responsible for loss of the normal red reflex. **(B)** This 1-year-old child shows gross ocular involvement. A convergent squint is also present. (**A**, Courtesy of Nancy Tarbell, MD, Children's Hospital, Boston, MA.)

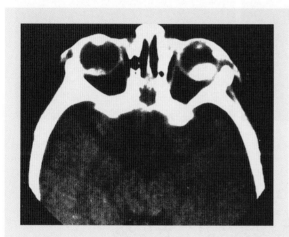

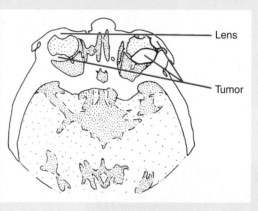

FIGURE 18.2 **RETINOBLASTOMA.** CT scan in a child with hereditary disease shows several tumor foci involving the orbits bilaterally. (Courtesy of Roy Strand, MD, Children's Hospital, Boston, MA.)

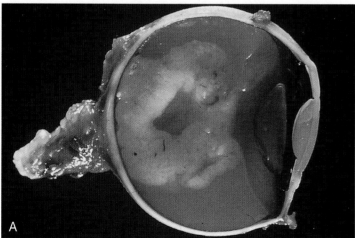

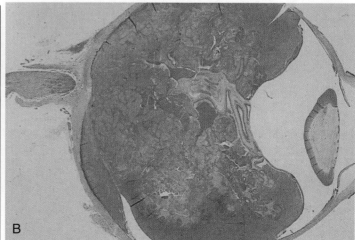

FIGURE 18.3 **RETINOBLASTOMA. (A)** Cross-section of an eye shows a tumor growing into the vitreous humor from its origin along the posterior wall of the retina. **(B)** Whole-mount section of an eye demonstrates a similar retinoblastoma invading the vitreous body and extending into the optic nerve.

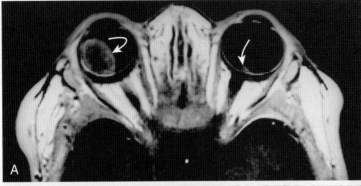

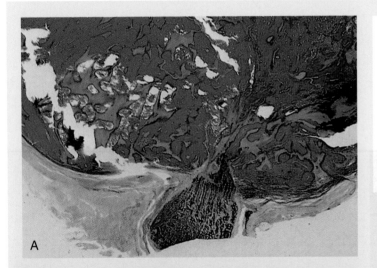

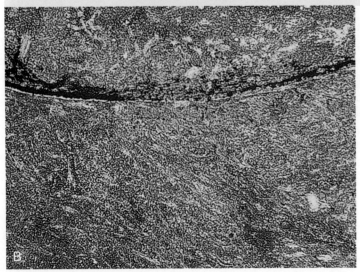

FIGURE 18.4 This 3-month-old girl has bilateral retinoblastoma. **(A)** Post-contrast T$_1$-weighted axial MRI demonstrates the larger right and smaller left retinal masses (*curved arrows*). **(B)** Longitudinal transorbital high-resolution (13 MHz) ultrasound shows the 1.4-cm–diameter right globe mass (cross-hatches) nearly filling the globe. **(C)** A more medial ultrasound section demonstrates the retinal detachment (*curved arrow*) not seen by MR or CT. **(D)** The left retinal mass (cross-hatches) measured 5 mm on this ultrasound.

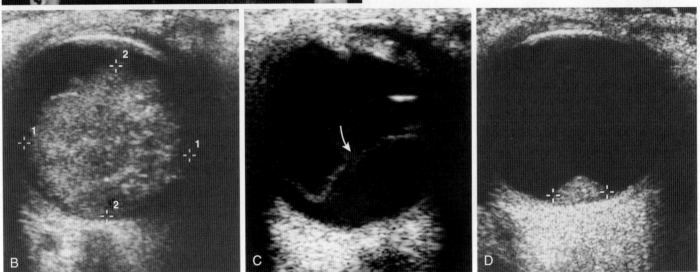

Necrotic tumor
filling globe

Tumor invasion
of optic nerve

FIGURE 18.5 **RETINOBLASTOMA.** **(A)** Tumor completely fills the vitreal cavity and extends into the optic nerve in this microscopic section. **(B)** Photomicroscopy in another case reveals direct extension into the underlying choroid.

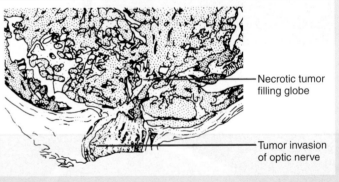

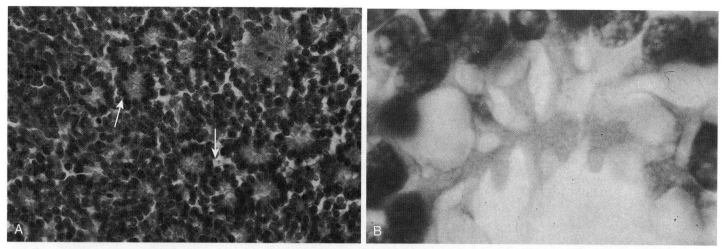

FIGURE 18.6 RETINOBLASTOMA. (A) Small cells with round, hyperchromatic nuclei are arranged in well-developed Flexner-Wintersteiner rosettes (*arrows*), which are interpreted as a primitive attempt at photoreceptor differentiation. **(B)** With high magnification, careful inspection reveals apical intraluminal protrusions indicating photoreceptor differentiation.

Group 1
- Tumor limited to kidney and completely excised
- Surface of renal capsule intact
- No tumor rupture before or during removal
- No residual tumor apparent beyond margins of excision

Group II
- Tumor extending beyond kidney but completely excised
- Regional extension of tumor (i.e., penetration through outer surface of renal capsule into perirenal soft tissues)
- Vessels outside kidney substance infiltrated or contain tumor thrombus
- Tumor may have been biopsied, or local spillage of tumor confined to flank
- No residual tumor apparent at or beyond margins of excision

Group III
- Residual nonhematogenous tumor confined to abdomen, with any of the following:
- Lymph nodes (hilar, periaortic, or beyond) found on biopsy to be involved
- Diffuse peritoneal contamination by tumor (e.g., by spillage of tumor beyond flank before or during surgery or by tumor growth through peritoneal surface)
- Implants found on peritoneal surface
- Tumor extending beyond surgical margins (microscopically or grossly)
- Tumor not completely resectable due to local infiltration into vital structures

Group IV
- Hematogenous metastases
- Deposits beyond stage III (i.e., lung, liver, bone, brain)

Group V
- Bilateral renal involvement at diagnosis

FIGURE 18.7 National Wilms' Tumor Study grouping system.

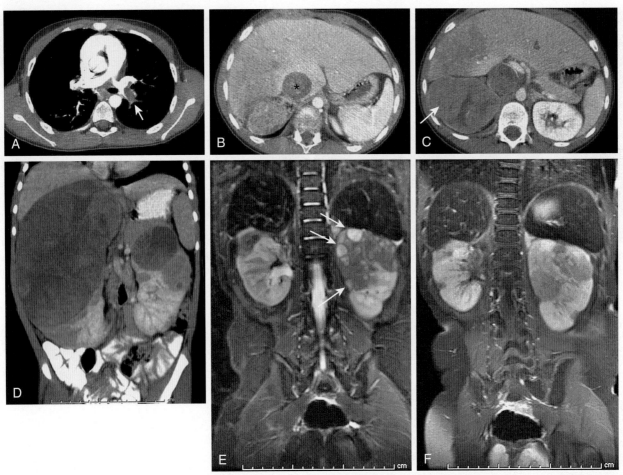

FIGURE 18.8 **WILMS' TUMOR.** An 11-year-old patient who presented with shortness of breath. **(A)** A CT angiogram demonstrated multiple pulmonary emboli and a large saddle embolus in the left main pulmonary artery (*arrow*). Contrast-enhanced CT of the abdomen shows a solid right renal mass with extension into the inferior vena cava (IVC; *). **(B, C)** Ill-defined low density throughout the right lobe of the liver was due to obstruction of hepatic venous drainage secondary to the tumor thrombus in the IVC. The study emphasizes the importance of evaluating the IVC, right atrium, and pulmonary vessels for intravascular extension of Wilms' tumor. Ultrasound is usually the first modality of choice in imaging Wilms' tumor and is effective at demonstrating vascular invasion. As shown here; both contrast-enhanced CT with multiplanar reconstructions and MRI can be used for this evaluation, and also allow assessment for extent of disease spread and presence of retroperitoneal lymph nodes. Subsequent chemotherapy treatment resulted in tumor shrinkage and gradual recanalization of the IVC. However the extent of hematogenous spread led to multiple intracranial metastases and a poor outcome. **(D)** Contrast-enhanced CT should always include multiplanar reconstructions, as shown in this 3-year-old patient with bilateral Wilms' tumor. MRI is superior at demonstrating small nephrogenic rests **(E, F).** The patient shown in **D** underwent right upper pole nephrectomy and chemotherapy. Following gadolinium enhancement, the heterogeneous signal intensity nephrogenic rests seen on the T_2-weighted MRI images (*arrows*) do not show any enhancement relative to the normal renal parenchyma, arguing against degeneration into Wilms' tumor. MRI has been advocated as a superior modality for monitoring degeneration of nephrogenic rests into Wilms' tumor, and should be considered in the monitoring of patients with nephroblastomatosis.

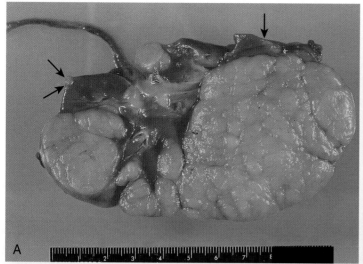

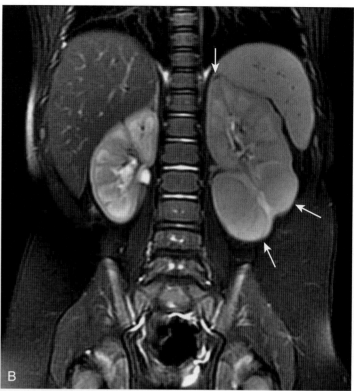

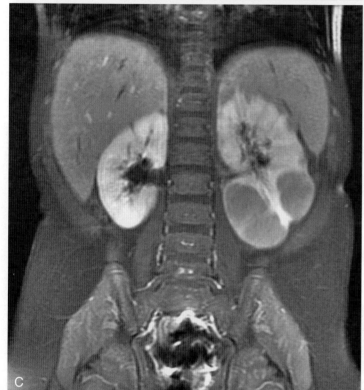

FIGURE 18.9 **(A)** Wilms' tumor with nephroblastomatosis. Bisected nephrectomy specimen shows multicentric Wilms' tumors. Multicentric tumors are usually associated with nephroblastomatosis, sometimes bilateral. Nephroblastomatosis is seen as small cortical nodules (*arrows*). **(B, C)** A 15-month-old patient who presented with palpable renal masses. Ultrasound showed extensive bilateral perilobar nephroblastomatosis. As shown here, MRI depicts the perilobar nephrogenic rests (*arrows*), characterized as isointense to renal cortex on T_2-weighted images **(B)**. These benign hyperplastic perilobar lesions do not show enhancement following gadolinium infusion **(C)** and typically spontaneously regress, in contrast to the intralobar nephrogenic rests seen in the setting of Wilms' tumor.

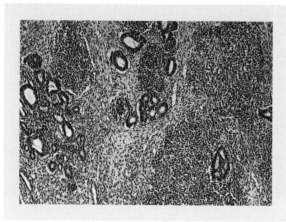

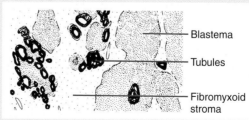

FIGURE 18.10 **WILMS' TUMOR.** Its classic triphasic pattern is marked by circumscribed nodules of blastema showing variable epithelial differentiation and tubule formation, surrounded by a fibromyxoid stroma. (Reproduced with permission from Schumann and Weiss, 1981.)

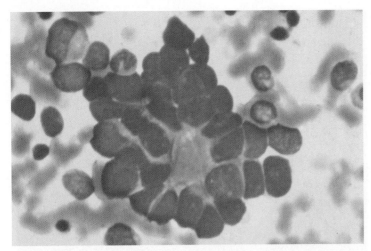

FIGURE 18.11 NEUROBLASTOMA. This bone marrow aspirate shows a clump of tumor cells in a rosette formation with central fibrillar material. The individual cells, resembling lymphoblasts, are small and have scanty cytoplasm.

FIGURE 18.12 NEUROBLASTOMA. A 5-month-old child presented with left periorbital bruising and anemia. Unenhanced CT of the brain shows left proptosis and a left periorbital mass (*arrow*) with associated bone destruction **(A)**. Contrast-enhanced abdominal CT shows the associated retroperitoneal/left adrenal mass with punctate calcifications throughout **(B)**, characteristic of neuroblastoma. The axial and coronal contrast-enhanced T$_1$-weighted MRI images of the brain emphasize the additional value of MRI in demonstrating the extensive bilateral periorbital soft tissue masses **(C)**, as well as the extension into the skull base and the spread of disease along the dura (*arrows*) **(D)**.

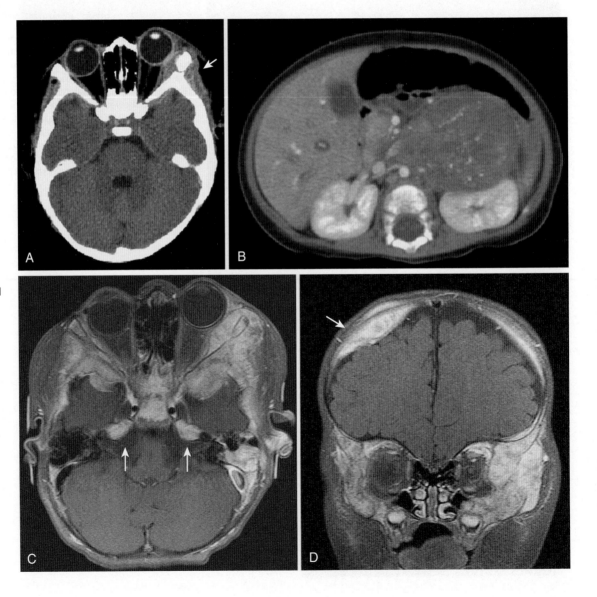

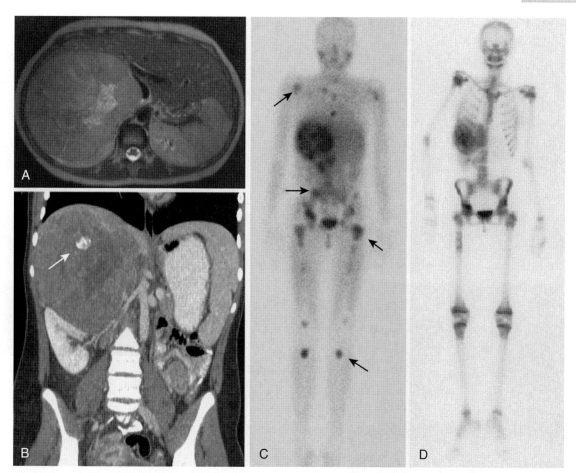

FIGURE 18.13   NEUROBLASTOMA. A 13-year-old patient presented with a palpable abdominal mass. This series of images demonstrates the multimodality approach to imaging that is often necessary in evaluating patients with neuroblastoma. An initial ultrasonogram documented a solid right upper quadrant mass that was difficult to separate from the kidney (not shown). Axial T_2-weighted MRI image shows a heterogeneous solid mass **(A)**, with primary differential considerations in a patient this age, including Wilms' tumor and other renal masses. Contrast-enhanced CT demonstrated calcifications within the solid mass (*arrow*), and the coronal images clearly demonstrate the suprarenal nature of the lesion **(B)**, making neuroblastoma the most likely diagnosis. ^{123}I-MIBG scintigraphy shows extensive foci of MIBG uptake **(C)**, in the primary mass, as well as at multiple sites of intramedullary bone marrow involvement (*arrows* indicate some of the multiple sites). Only a subset of the MIBG-avid sites show accumulation of radiotracer on the technetium-99m–methylene diphosphonate bone scan **(D)**, demonstrating the distinction between cortical bone involvement shown by bone scintigraphy and the intramedullary marrow involvement shown by MIBG. Each of these imaging studies played a complementary role in evaluating and properly staging this patient with stage IV disease.

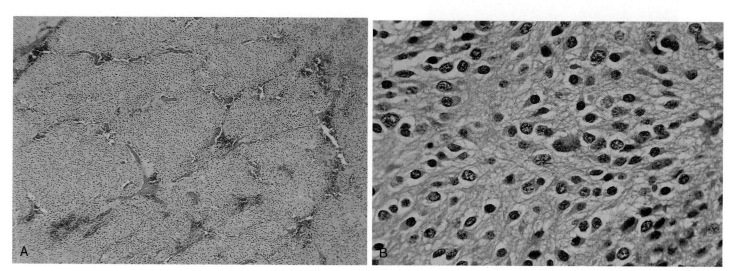

FIGURE 18.14   NEUROBLASTOMA. (A) This low-power view shows the characteristic lobular pattern of neuroblastoma with discrete, large nests of tumor cells surrounded by a delicate fibrovascular stroma. **(B)** A higher-power view of the same tumor reveals that small, round tumor cells are separated by an abundant, pink fibrillary network (neuropile). The neuropile represents cytoplasmic processes (neurites). The tumor cells at the center of this photograph show signs of maturation as evidenced by the abundant cytoplasm, resembling immature ganglion cells.

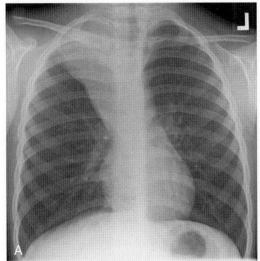

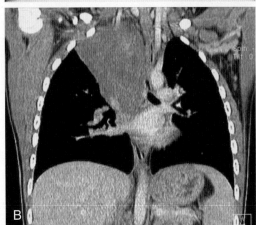

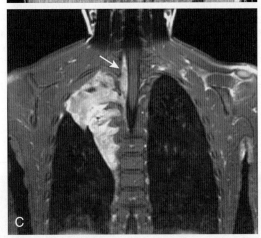

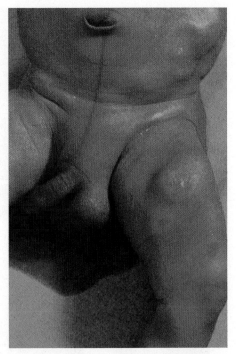

FIGURE 18.16 **SKIN AND SUBCUTANEOUS METASTASES.** Skin lesions can vary in size and are frequently smaller than those seen in this infant with stage 4S neuroblastoma.

FIGURE 18.15 **POSTERIOR MEDIASTINAL GANGLIONEUROBLASTOMA.** A 5-year-old patient who initially presented with upper respiratory symptoms. **(A)** Chest radiograph showed right upper lobe opacity, interpreted as lung consolidation, possibly with partial collapse. When this failed to resolve, a contrast-enhanced CT showed a solid right upper lobe/posterior mediastinal mass **(B)**, which had mass effect on midline structures and appeared to extend into the spinal canal. **(C)** The contrast-enhanced fat-suppressed coronal T_1-weighted MRI clearly demonstrates the multiple levels of extension into neural foramina, as well as the extensive intraspinal extension of the patient's tumor (*arrow*). MRI is superior to CT at determining the extent of intraspinal involvement, as well as evaluating the spinal cord for any evidence of edema/cord compression. In this case, the patient first underwent a decompression laminectomy and resection of the intraspinal portion of his tumor, followed by resection of the extraspinal posterior mediastinal/intrathoracic component of the mass. It is frequently not possible to completely resect all foci of disease in these patients, and residual post-operative abnormalities must be followed to ensure stability. The choice of imaging depends on the modality best suited to the patient's sites of disease involvement; in this case the patient has been followed by MRI.

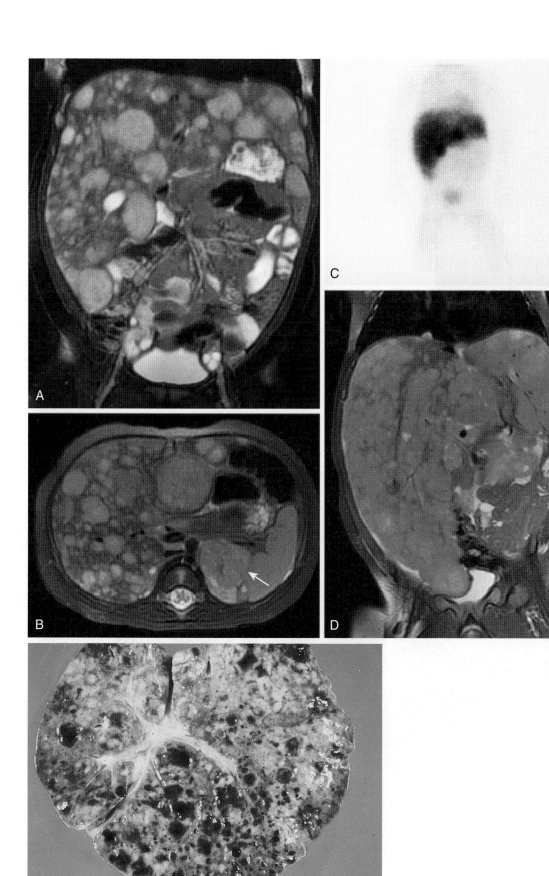

FIGURE 18.17 STAGE 4S NEUROBLASTOMA. A 3-month-old child who developed skin lesions and on subsequent evaluation was found to have a palpable abdominal mass. Ultrasonography showed extensive liver involvement and a left adrenal mass (not shown). As shown here, coronal **(A)** and axial **(B)** T_2-weighted fat-suppressed MRI images demonstrate multiple foci of hepatic involvement throughout the entire liver, as well as the primary left adrenal mass (*arrow*). Staging evaluation showed minimal marrow involvement. ^{123}I-MIBG scintigraphy **(C)** showed disease limited to the liver and the left adrenal mass. This patient's tumor was therefore classified, based on INSS staging, as stage 4S, with the primary tumor localized to the left adrenal and metastatic lesions limited to liver, skin, and bone marrow, with less than 10% bone marrow involvement. Although there is a high rate of spontaneous regression in patients with stage 4S neuroblastoma, as shown here **(D)** a significant percentage of patients will require intensive chemotherapy as a result of disease progression and the associated morbidity and increased mortality from the high disease burden. **(E)** Similar to the clinical story above, this patient had progressive enlargement of his liver despite chemotherapy and radiation therapy and eventually died of respiratory failure from mechanical compression. Autopsy specimen shows virtual replacement of the liver by metastases, many of which were hemorrhagic. The liver weighed 2374 g.

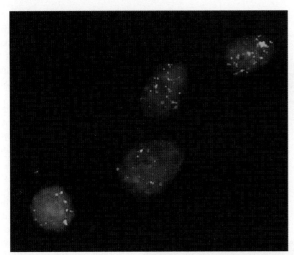

FIGURE 18.18 NEUROBLASTOMA. Utilizing the fluorescence in situ hybridization technique, these neuroblastoma cells show the multiple copies of *MYCN* characteristic of high-risk, high-stage neuroblastoma. On karyotypes the amplification may show up as double minutes or homogeneous staining regions. *MYCN* amplification predicts a poorer outcome independent of stage. (Courtesy of Lisa Moreau and Rani George, Dana-Farber Cancer Institute, Boston, MA.)

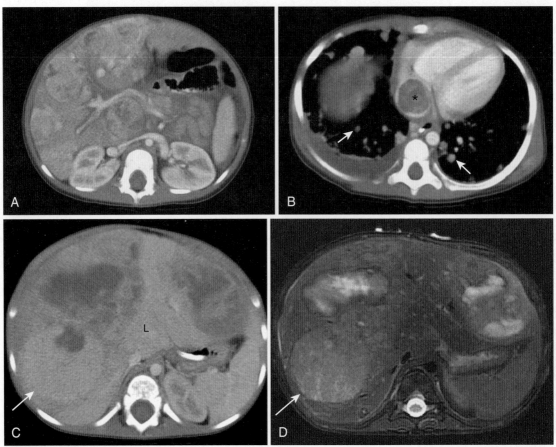

FIGURE 18.19 HEPATOBLASTOMA. This 15-month-old child presented with a palpable liver mass. Contrast-enhanced CT demonstrates extensive liver involvement with masses seen throughout the liver **(A)**. **(B)** There is also extension of the mass into the IVC and right atrium (*) as well as multiple pulmonary metastases (*arrows* indicate representative lesions). As with Wilms' tumor, evaluation of patients with suspected hepatoblastoma must be rigorous with respect to assessing for intravascular extension. Ultrasound, CT, and/or MRI are all effective modalities at assessing for intravascular extension of tumor. CT, reviewed under lung windows (not shown), is superior at visualizing the lung nodules detected on review of the soft tissue windows **(B)**; MRI may be better at delineating the heterogeneous foci of disease characteristic of hepatoblastoma **(C, D)**. In particular, lesions that are isointense to the liver on CT **(C,** *arrow*) are clearly shown as distinct sites of tumor involvement by MRI **(D)**, and MRI may be superior at delineating the extent of intrahepatic involvement.

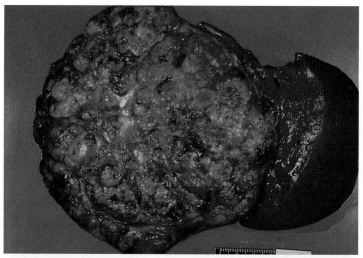

FIGURE 18.20 **HEPATOBLASTOMA.** Typical hepatoblastoma: a single, round, well-demarcated lobulated mass with variegated appearance and areas of necrosis and hemorrhage. Normal liver included in the resection specimen is seen at the *right*.

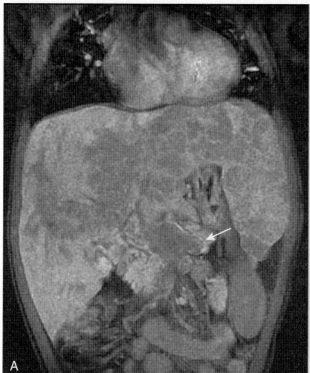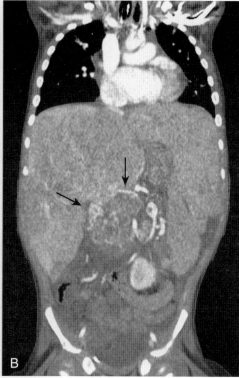

FIGURE 18.21 **PORTAL VEIN THROMBOSIS AND CAVERNOUS TRANSFORMATION IN HEPATOBLASTOMA.** Coronal MRI **(A)** in a 2-year-old patient with extensive hepatoblastoma shows widespread liver involvement and demonstrates extension of disease into periportal lymph nodes and into the portal vein, back to its confluence with the superior mesenteric vein (*white arrow*). Multiphase contrast-enhanced CT **(B)** clearly demonstrates cavernous transformation of the portal vein, with multiple collateral vessels that have arisen (*black arrows*) as a result of tumor thrombus extending into and occluding the main portal vein. Evaluating for the presence of tumor thrombus in the portal vein is essential in the imaging assessment of patients with hepatoblastoma and may influence surgical decision making and eligibility for liver transplantation.

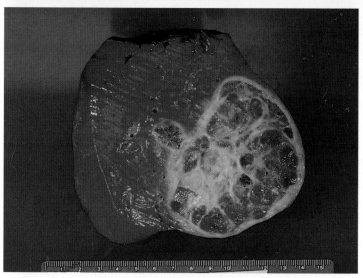

FIGURE 18.22 **HEPATOBLASTOMA RESECTED AFTER THREE CYCLES OF INDUCTION CHEMOTHERAPY.** The tumor is markedly reduced in size (as compared with pretreatment MRI scans, not shown) and displays central scarring and necrosis along with a thick fibrous capsule. The dark, fleshy tumor seen between the central scarring and the periphery is made up of granulation tissue with hemosiderosis and scattered residual tumor cells. Normal liver is included with the specimen (*on the left side*).

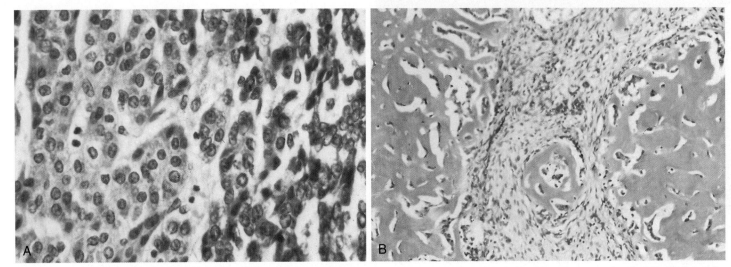

FIGURE 18.23 HEPATOBLASTOMA. (A) This tumor exhibits a mixture of the embryonal type (*on the right*) with the fetal histologic type (*on the left*). **(B)** Osteoid (pinkish areas) is often observed.

FIGURE 18.24 HEPATOBLASTOMA. Congenital hypertrophy of the retinal pigment epithelium (CHRPE) is sometimes seen in patients with hepatoblastoma associated with familial polyposis coli. **(A)** The CHRPE is seen as discoloration. **(B)** In another patient the discoloration is more rounded. (Courtesy of Dr. J. Garber, MD, Dana-Farber Cancer Institute, Boston, MA.)

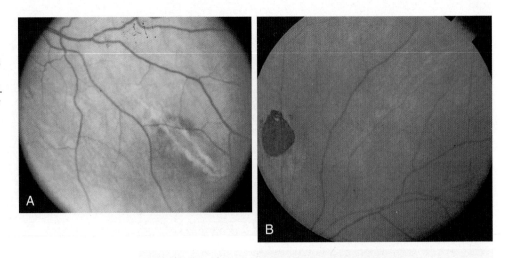

FIGURE 18.25 Intergroup Rhabdomyo-sarcoma Study Group post-surgical group classification.

IRSG Post-Surgical Groups Classification	
Group 1	Localized disease, completely excised, no microscopic residual
A	Confined to site of origin, completely resected
B	Infiltrating beyond site of origin, completely resected
Group 2	Total gross resection
A	Gross resection with evidence of microscopic local residual
B	Regional disease with involved lymph nodes, completely resected with no microscopic residual
C	Microscopic local and/or nodal residual
Group 3	Incomplete resection or biopsy with gross residual
Group 4	Distant metastases

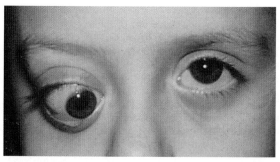

FIGURE 18.26 ORBITAL RHABDOMYOSARCOMA. This patient presented with unilateral proptosis of very recent onset. Often rhabdomyosarcoma develops rapidly and causes lid redness. It may be mistaken for orbital inflammation.

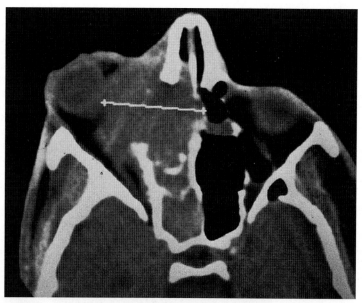

FIGURE 18.27 ORBITAL RHABDOMYOSARCOMA. CT scan at the level of the orbits in a patient who presented with marked unilateral proptosis shows extensive bone destruction with involvement of the ethmoid sinus.

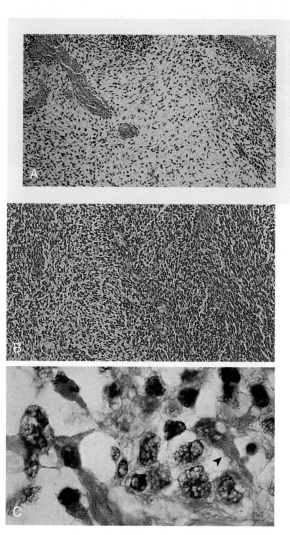

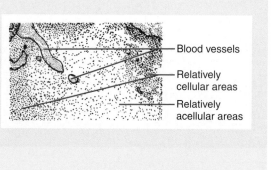

Blood vessels

Relatively cellular areas

Relatively acellular areas

FIGURE 18.28 EMBRYONAL RHABDOMYOSARCOMA.
(A) Microscopy shows an embryonic cellular pattern. **(B)** Higher magnification reveals the primitive nature of the rhabdomyoblasts, which tend to cluster in groups, separated by relatively acellular areas. **(C)** Some rhabdomyoblasts exhibit characteristic cross-striations (*arrowhead*) in their cytoplasm.

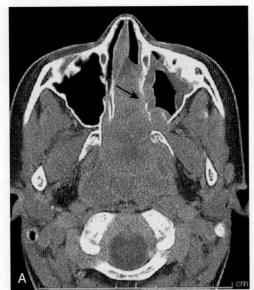

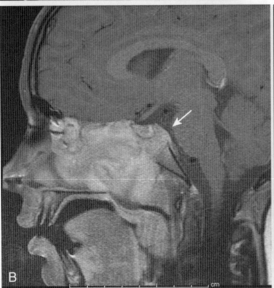

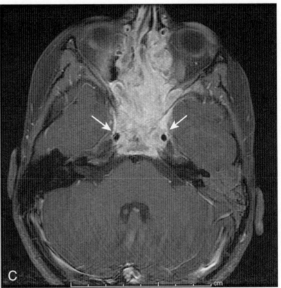

FIGURE 18.29 **RHABDOMYOSARCOMA.** A 7-year-old with a history of nasal congestion, nosebleeds, and headaches. Unenhanced CT of the paranasal sinuses **(A)** shows a soft tissue mass filling much of the left maxillary sinus, with extension into the nasal cavity and posteriorly into the nasopharynx. CT also demonstrates deviation of the nasal septum and bone destruction along the medial left maxillary sinus wall (*arrow*). Sagittal **(B)** and axial **(C)** fat-suppressed T_1-weighted images obtained after gadolinium enhancement show the extent of tumor involvement in the nasopharynx and sinuses, with improved delineation of the degree of skull base extension **(B)** and extension into the cavernous sinus **(C)**.

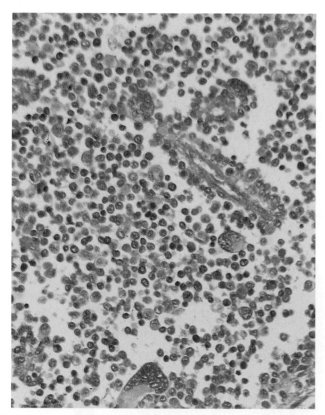

FIGURE 18.30 **ALVEOLAR RHABDOMYOSARCOMA.** Characteristically, tumor cells are loosely attached to trabeculae or lie free within alveolar spaces. Occasional multinucleate giant cells are seen in this photograph and are a helpful diagnostic feature. Cross-striations are rare in this type of rhabdomyosarcoma.

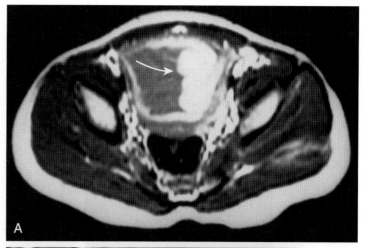

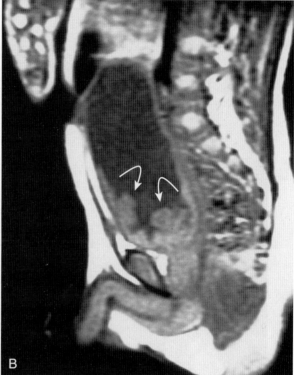

FIGURE 18.31 **RHABDOMYOSARCOMA (SARCOMA BOTRYOIDES).** Axial **(A)** and sagittal **(B)** MR scans of a 2-year-old patient who presented with urinary obstruction. The tumor can be seen in the bladder with ball-like projections into the bladder space (*arrows*) as well as extension along the bladder wall. This extension usually occurs in the anatomic plane between the mucosa and the muscularis. The tumor was biopsied transurethrally during cystoscopy.

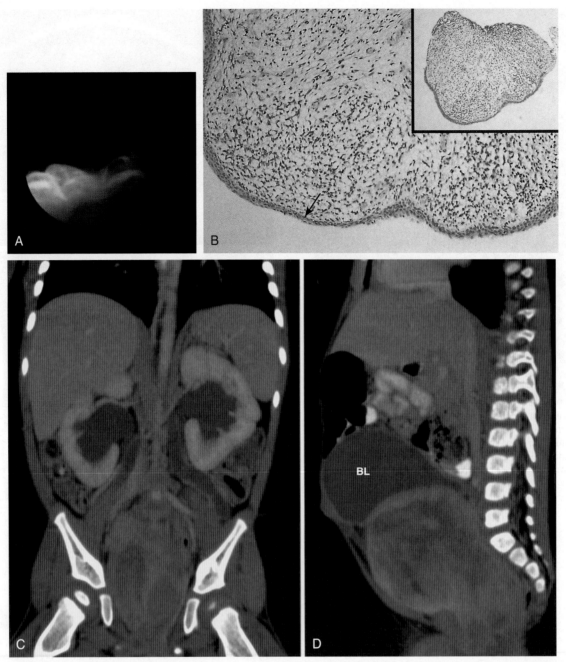

FIGURE 18.32   RHABDOMYOSARCOMA (SARCOMA BOTRYOIDES). Cystoscopy **(A)** reveals the delicate, grapelike projections of tumor from the bladder wall. The pathologic section **(B)** further illustrates this process: the tumor cells push out from the bladder wall and are covered with a layer of normal mucosa (*arrow*). The most common site for botryoid sarcoma is the GU tract, but occasionally it presents in the gallbladder or bile duct. **(C, D)** Rhabdomyosarcomas arising from the base of the bladder or prostate frequently compress the distal ureters, resulting in hydroureteronephrosis, as shown here. Contrast-enhanced CT scanning of the abdomen in this 1-year-old, who presented with difficulty voiding and urinary obstruction, demonstrates a large soft tissue mass, shown to be rhabdomyosarcoma of the prostate. Presenting symptoms may differ in these patients, depending on whether tumor extends into the bladder or displaces/obstructs the bladder (as is the case here; BL, bladder) and lower urinary tract. Nonetheless, there is no evidence that clinical outcome is significantly different for these different groups of patients.

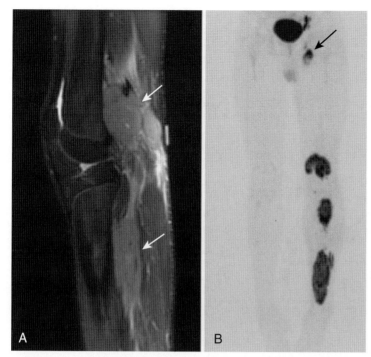

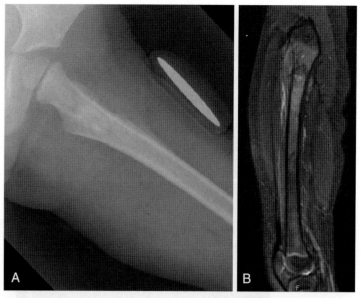

FIGURE 18.33 **RHABDOMYOSARCOMA.** A 16-year-old patient with a palpable left leg mass initially underwent MRI evaluation of the knee. Sagittal fat-suppressed T_2-weighted image shows solid masses in the popliteal fossa as well as posterior to the tibia **(A)** (*arrows*). 2-[^{18}F]-fluoro-2-deoxy-D-glucose–positron emission tomography (^{18}F-FDG-PET) scanning, obtained to further stage this patient, demonstrates additional masses posterior to the distal tibia that were not seen on the initial MRI, which was limited to the knee joint. **(B)** ^{18}F-FDG PET also demonstrated left inguinal lymph node involvement (*arrow*) that would not have been detected on the MRI examinations done to stage the patient's local disease. Biopsy showed alveolar rhabdomyosarcoma. Most patients with primary-extremity rhabdomyosarcomas are teenagers. Rhabdomyosarcomas at this location, as well as the trunk, carry a poorer prognosis than GU, orbital, and head and neck tumors without extensive bone destruction.

FIGURE 18.34 **EWING SARCOMA/PRIMITIVE NEUROECTODERMAL TUMOR (PNET).** **(A)** The midshaft of long bones is a common site of occurrence, as illustrated here in the left femur of a 4-year-old boy. Almost any bone in the body may be affected. Ewing sarcoma's classic radiographic appearance is marked by the permeative bone destruction and a lamellated ("onion skinning") periosteal reaction shown here. As shown in the accompanying MRI of the left lower extremity **(B)**, MRI imaging is superior at delineating the extent of intramedullary involvement typical of Ewing sarcoma, and is also superior at better defining the size of the soft tissue component of disease and the extent of extramedullary disease involvement. Though not shown here, pulmonary metastases frequently occur in the setting of Ewing sarcoma, and all patients should receive a chest CT for staging of their disease.

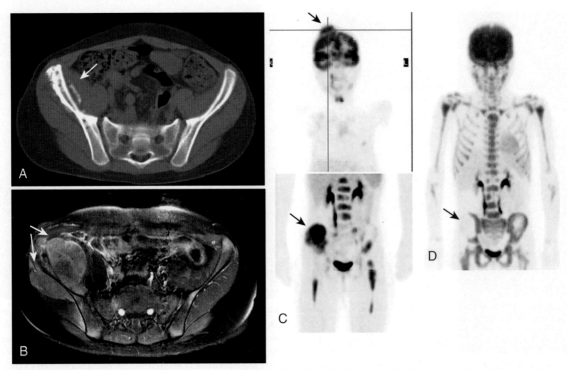

FIGURE 18.35 EWING SARCOMA/PNET. This 8-year-old girl presented with right-sided hip pain. Radiographs showed a mixed lytic and sclerotic process involving the right iliac bone. CT scan **(A)** shows a soft tissue mass and extensive bone destruction, common findings with pelvic Ewing sarcoma. MRI is superior at delineating an associated soft tissue mass and showing the extent of soft tissue involvement and local spread of disease. The fat-suppressed T_2-weighted image shown here **(B)** demonstrates the large soft tissue mass surrounding the right iliac bone seen on the corresponding CT **(A)** and shows the soft tissue mass predominating relative to the degree of bone involvement, as is typical of pelvic Ewing sarcoma. ^{18}F-FDG-PET imaging is becoming more widely used both in staging patients with Ewing sarcoma and in response assessment. Pretreatment ^{18}F-FDG-PET imaging shows intense uptake in the right iliac mass, as well as extensive bone marrow disease and metastatic disease to the skull **(C,** *arrows***).** Following treatment, there is a photopenic area in the right hemipelvis corresponding to the loss of metabolic activity at the primary site of disease, demonstrating an excellent response to therapy **(D).** Residual MRI findings (not shown) probably relate to residual necrotic tumor rather than active disease, given the absence of significant metabolic activity. The skull lesion also shows no residual ^{18}F-FDG uptake following therapy.

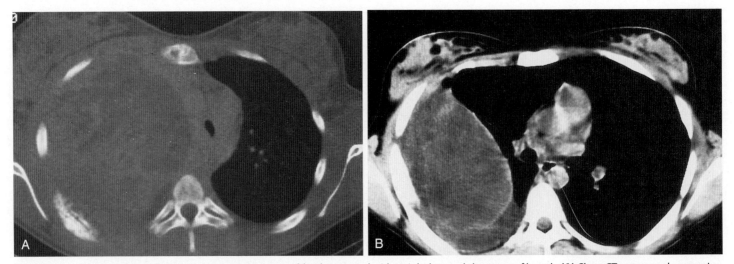

FIGURE 18.36 EWING SARCOMA/PNET (ASKIN TUMOR). A 17-year-old girl presented with weight loss and shortness of breath. **(A)** Chest CT scan reveals a massive tumor filling the right hemithorax and deviating the mediastinum to the left. Rib erosion can be seen posteriorly. **(B)** After two courses of chemotherapy there was a dramatic response. After further shrinkage with drug therapy, the tumor was removed. The majority of the specimen showed necrosis, with only rare scattered areas of tumor remaining.

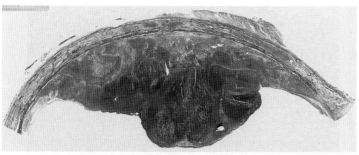

FIGURE 18.37 **EWING SARCOMA/PNET.** This giant histologic section shows another typical Ewing family tumor adjacent to a rib. These lesions are commonly referred to as Askin tumors. The bone may not be involved at all or only focally by the tumor. The tumor protrudes into the pleural cavity and may be associated with pleural fluid or pleural studding with metastases.

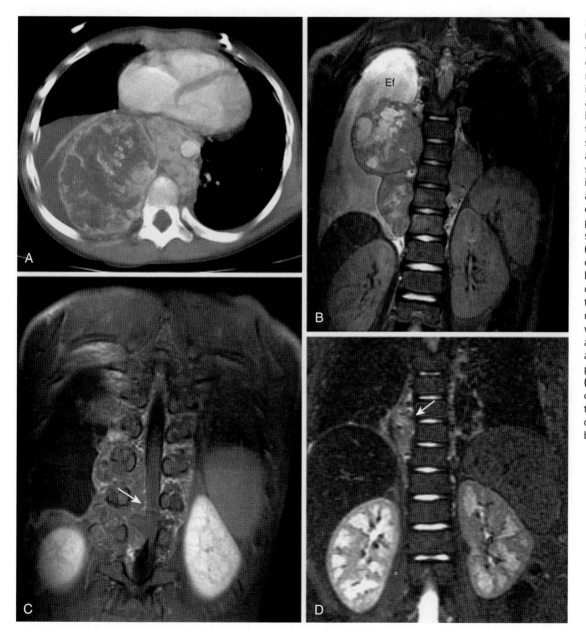

FIGURE 18.38 **EWING SARCOMA/ PNET.** A 4-year-old who presented with right hip pain. Evaluation of the abdomen revealed a retroperitoneal mass extending into the thorax. Chest CT shows a massive tumor filling the right hemithorax and displacing the heart anteriorly **(A)**. Fat-suppressed T_2-weighted **(B)** and post-gadolinium fat-suppressed T_1-weighted **(C)** MRI imaging demonstrate the large accompanying right pleural effusion (Ef), and the lobulated paraspinal mass abutting both sides of the vertebral column **(B)**, with extension into the spinal canal and compression of the lower spinal cord **(C, *arrow*)**. As is often seen in patients with this tumor, there was an excellent response to chemotherapy, with the MRI obtained 4 months after diagnosis showing only a small amount of residual paraspinal disease remaining **(D, *arrow*)**. Following successful chemotherapy reduction, these tumors, which are frequently quite large at diagnosis, can often be surgically resected.

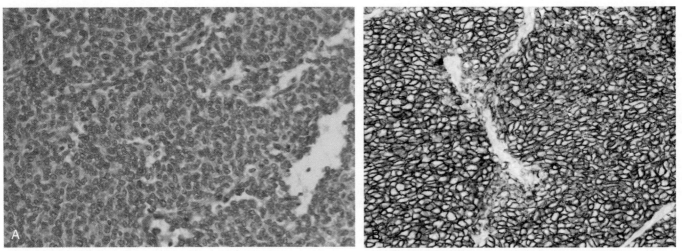

FIGURE 18.39 EWING SARCOMA/PNET. (A) This tumor is marked by small, round blue cells. A capillary network gives a lobular pattern to the tumor. Poorly formed rosettes can be seen as in this slide. **(B)** The tumor frequently stains with stains to CD99, the protein product of the *MIC2* (now *CD99*) gene. The staining in Ewing sarcoma is membranous, as shown here.

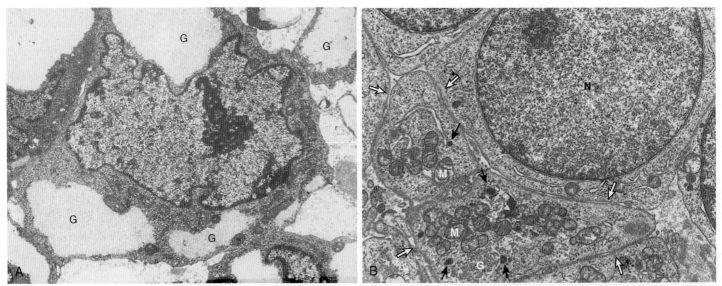

FIGURE 18.40 EWING SARCOMA/PNET. (A) Electron micrograph of a "typical" Ewing tumor shows large pools of cytoplasmic glycogen (G). **(B)** In contrast, the PNET variant tends toward neural differentiation. Neuritic processes (*open arrows*) contain mitochondria (M), dense-core granules (*smaller arrows*), and looser areas of glycogen (G). N, nucleus.

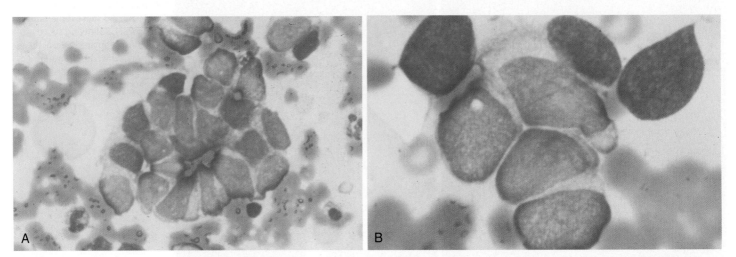

FIGURE 18.41 BONE MARROW METASTASES. (A) Low-power view of a bone marrow aspirate shows a clump of undifferentiated malignant cells. **(B)** Higher magnification reveals small blue cells with scanty cytoplasm and indistinct nucleoli. Unlike osteosarcoma, Ewing sarcoma frequently spreads to bone marrow.

11 der(11) 22 der(22)

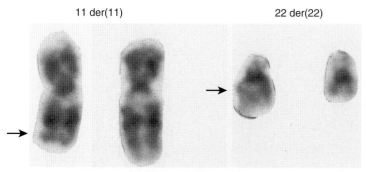

FIGURE 18.42 **PNET.** This partial karyotype demonstrates the t(11;22) abnormally (*arrows*) seen in almost all cases of PNET and Ewing sarcoma (see also Figs. 12.20–12.22). (Courtesy of Jonathan Fletcher, MD, Dana-Farber Cancer Institute, Boston, MA.)

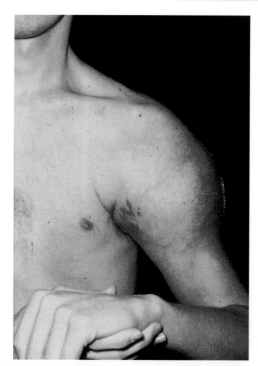

FIGURE 18.43 **OSTEOSARCOMA.** This 21-year-old man presented with a prominent soft tissue mass at the left proximal humerus. He first noted pain while at basic training, and the mass followed a few weeks later. Proximal humoral malignancies can usually be treated with a limb-sparing operation. In this patient, however, chest wall involvement required a forequarter amputation. (Courtesy of Mark Gebhardt, MD, Children's Hospital, Boston, MA.)

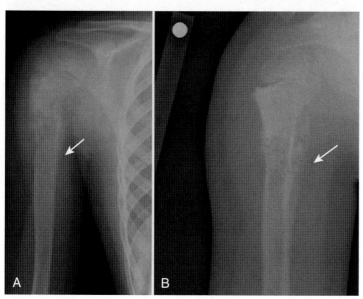

FIGURE 18.44 **OSTEOSARCOMA.** Anteroposterior (**A**) and lateral (**B**) radiographs of the right humerus in a 6-year-old boy show the typical lytic and sclerotic lesion with extensive bone destruction, osteoblastic activity, and periosteal reaction characteristically seen in osteosarcoma. A Codman triangle is present (*arrow*), indicating the ongoing bone remodeling at the sites of bone destruction. Although there is usually a prominent associated soft tissue mass, as is shown here, the soft tissue component of the lesion, relative to the degree of bone involvement, may be relatively small. The distal femur is the most common site of occurrence, followed by the proximal tibia and proximal humerus.

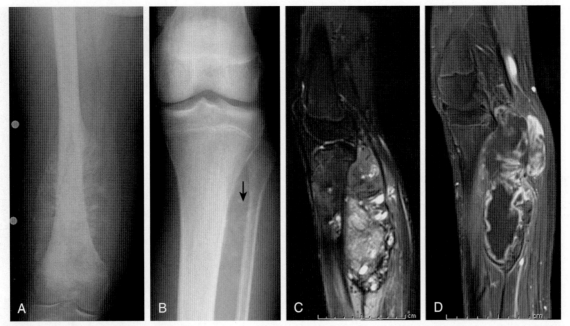

FIGURE 18.45 **OSTEOSARCOMA.** Anteroposterior radiographs in 13-year-old **(A)** and 16-year-old **(B)** patients with osteogenic sarcoma of right femur **(A)** and left tibia **(B)** show the sunburst periosteal reaction that is typically seen in patients with osteogenic sarcoma **(A)**, with an associated Codman triangle along the upper margin of the lesion. In contrast to the distal femoral lesion, where the osteoblastic activity is quite prominent, the proximal tibial lesion **(B)** has only very subtle soft tissue calcifications (*arrow*). However, T_2-weighted **(C)** and post-gadolinium–enhanced fat-suppressed T_1-weighted **(D)** MRI imaging of the left lower extremity shows the large associated soft tissue mass, as well as the extensive necrosis **(D)** that occurred following therapy. The use of MRI to document the extent of local disease spread and the relationship of the tumor to the neurovascular bundle, as well as to monitor tumor response following therapy is now fairly standard in most major centers and is important in determining resectability of the tumor and may be of value in determining the extent of tumor necrosis occurring after therapy.

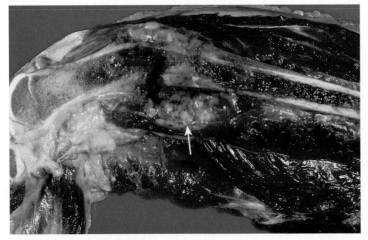

FIGURE 18.46 **OSTEOSARCOMA.** Sagittal section through the thigh shows a large metaphyseal mass with soft tissue extension (*arrow*). Note the pathologic fracture.

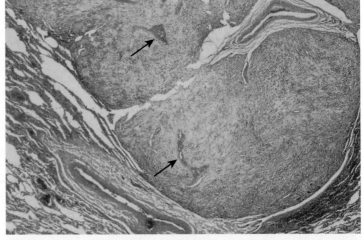

FIGURE 18.47 **LUNG METASTASES.** A photomicrograph of a pulmonary metastatic nodule compressing the lung parenchyma (periphery). Osteoid formation (*arrows*) is present within a sarcomatous stroma.

References and Suggested Readings

Retinoblastoma

Chintagumpala M, Chevez-Barrios P, Paysse EA, et al: Retinoblastoma: review of current management, *Oncologist* 12:1237–1246, 2007.

Eng C, Li FP, Abramson DH, et al: Mortality from second tumors among long-term survivors of retinoblastoma, *J Natl Cancer Inst* 85:1121–1128, 1993.

Friend SH, Bernards R, Rogelj S, et al: A human DNA segment with properties of the gene that predisposes to retinoblastoma and osteosarcoma, *Nature* 323:643–646, 1986.

Garber JE, Diller L: Screening children at genetic risk of cancer, *Curr Opin Pediatr* 5:712–715, 1989.

Wetzig P: Fluorescein photography in the differential diagnosis of retinoblastoma, *Am J Ophthalmol* 61:341–343, 1966.

Yandell DW, Campbell TA, Dayton SH, et al: Oncogenic point mutations in the human retinoblastoma gene: their application to genetic counseling, *N Engl J Med* 321:1689–1695, 1989.

Wilms' Tumor

Bonadio JF, Storer B, Norkool P, et al: Anaplastic Wilms' tumor: clinical and pathologic studies, *J Clin Oncol* 3:513–520, 1985.

Cotton CA, Peterson S, Norkool PA, et al: Early and late mortality after diagnosis of Wilms tumor, *J Clin Oncol* 27:1304–1309, 2009.

Fischbach BV, Trout KL, Lewis J, et al: WAGR syndrome: a clinical review of 54 cases, *Pediatrics* 116:984–988, 2005.

Friedman GK, Castleberry RP: Changing trends of research and treatment in infant neuroblastoma, *Pediatr Blood Cancer* 49:1060–1065, 2007.

Grundy PE, Breslow NE, Li S, et al: Loss of heterozygosity for chromosomes 1p and 16q is an adverse prognostic factor in favorable-histology Wilms tumor: a report from the National Wilms Tumor Study Group, *J Clin Oncol* 23:7312–7321, 2005.

Metzger ML, Dome JS: Current therapy for Wilms' tumor, *Oncologist* 10:815–826, 2005.

Pritchard-Jones K: Controversies and advances in the management of Wilms' tumour, *Arch Dis Child* 87:241–244, 2002.

Shamberger RC, Guthrie KA, Ritchey ML, et al: Surgery-related factors and local recurrence of Wilms tumor in National Wilms Tumor Study 4, *Ann Surg* 229(2):292–297, 1999.

Schumann GB, Weiss MA: Atlas of Renal and Urinary Tract Cytology and its Histopathologic Basis, Philadelphia, J. B. Lippincott Co., 1981.

Weirich A, Ludwig R, Graf N, et al: Survival in nephroblastoma treated according to the trial and study SIOP-9/GPOH with respect to relapse and morbidity, *Ann Oncol* 15:808–820, 2004.

Neuroblastoma

Attiyeh EF, London WB, Mossé YP, et al: Chromosome 1p and 11q deletions and outcome in neuroblastoma, *N Engl J Med* 353:2243–2253, 2005.

Castleberry R, Pritchard J, Ambros P, et al: The International Neuroblastoma Risk Group (INRG): a preliminary report, *Eur J Cancer* 33:2113–2116, 1997.

Janoueix-Lerosey I, Schleiermacher G, Michels E, et al: Overall genomic pattern is a predictor of outcome in neuroblastoma, *J Clin Oncol* 27:1026–1033, 2009.

Kusher BH, Kramer K, Modak S, Cheung N-KV: Sensitivity of surveillance studies for detecting asymptomatic and unsuspected relapse of high-risk neuroblastoma, *J Clin Oncol* 27:1041–1046, 2009.

London WB, Castleberry RP, Matthay KK, et al: Evidence for an age cutoff greater than 365 days for neuroblastoma risk group stratification in the Children's Oncology Group, *J Clin Oncol* 23:6459–6465, 2005.

Maris JM, Hogarty MD, Bagatell R, et al: Neuroblastoma, *Lancet* 369(9579):2106–2120, 2007.

Matthay KK, Villablanca JG, Seeger RC, et al: Treatment of high-risk neuroblastoma with intensive chemotherapy, radiotherapy, autologous bone marrow transplantation, and 13-cis-retinoic acid. Children's Cancer Group, *N Engl J Med* 341:1165–1173, 1999.

Nitschke R, Smith EI, Shochat S, et al: Localized neuroblastoma treated by surgery: a Pediatric Oncology Group study, *J Clin Oncol* 6:1271–1279, 1988.

Seeger RC, Brodeur GM, Sather H, et al: Association of multiple copies of the N-*myc* oncogene with rapid progression of neuroblastomas, *N Engl J Med* 313:1111–1116, 1985.

Hepatoblastoma

McLaughlin CC, Baptiste MS, Schymura MJ, et al: Maternal and infant birth characteristics and hepatoblastoma, *Am J Epidemiol* 163:818–828, 2006.

Ortega JA, Douglass EC, Feusner JH, et al: Randomized comparison of cisplatin/vincristine/fluorouracil and cisplatin/continuous infusion doxorubicin for treatment of pediatric hepatoblastoma: a report from the Children's Cancer Group and the Pediatric Oncology Group, *J Clin Oncol* 18:2665–2675, 2000.

Otte JB, Pritchard J: Liver Transplantation for Hepatoblastoma: results From the International Society of Pediatric Oncology (SIOP) Study SIOPEL-1 and review of the world experience, *Pediatr Blood Cancer* 42:74–83, 2004.

Hepatic Tumors

Haliloglu M, Hoffer F, Gronemeyer S, et al: 3D gadolinium-enhanced MRA: evaluation of hepatic vasculature in children with hepatoblastoma, *J Magn Reson Imaging* 11:65–68, 2000.

Ikeda H, Matsuyama S, Tanimura M: Association between hepatoblastoma and very low birth weight: a trend or a chance? *J Pediatr* 130:557–560, 1997.

Rhabdomyosarcoma

Arndt CA, Crist WM: Common musculoskeletal tumors of childhood and adolescence, *N Engl J Med* 341:342–352, 1999.

Breitfeld PP, Meyer WH: Rhabdomyosarcoma: new windows of opportunity, *Oncologist* 10:518–527, 2005.

Crist WM, Anderson JR, Meza JL, et al: Intergroup rhabdomyosarcoma study-IV: results for patients with nonmetastatic disease, *J Clin Oncol* 19:3091–3102, 2001.

Mercado GE, Barr FG: Fusions involving PAX and FOX genes in the molecular pathogenesis of alveolar rhabdomyosarcoma: recent advances, *Curr Mol Med* 7(1):47–61, 2007.

Pappo AS, Shapiro DN, Crist WM, et al: Biology and therapy of pediatric rhabdomyosarcoma, *J Clin Oncol* 13:2123–2139, 1995.

Pizzo PA, Triche TJ: Clinical staging in rhabdomyosarcoma: current limitations and future prospects (editorial), *J Clin Oncol* 5:8–9, 1987.

Sung L, Anderson JR, Donaldson SS, et al: Late events occurring five years or more after successful therapy for childhood rhabdomyosarcoma: a report from the Soft Tissue Sarcoma Committee of the Children's Oncology Group, *Eur J Cancer* 40:1878–1885, 2004.

Ewing Family of Tumors: Ewing Sarcoma and PNET

Delattre O, Zucman J, Melot T, et al: The Ewing family of tumors—a subgroup of small round cell tumors defined by specific chimeric transcripts, *N Engl J Med* 331:294–299, 1994.

Leavey PJ, Mascarenhas L, et al: Prognostic factors for patients with Ewing sarcoma (EWS) at first recurrence following multi-modality therapy: a report from the Children's Oncology Group, *Pediatr Blood Cancer* 51:334–338, 2008.

McAllister NR, Lessnick SL: The potential for molecular therapeutic targets in Ewing's sarcoma, *Curr Treat Options Oncol* 6:461–471, 2005.

Meyer JS, Nadel HR, et al: Imaging guidelines for children with Ewing sarcoma and osteosarcoma: a report from the Children's Oncology Group Bone Tumor Committee, *Pediatr Blood Cancer* 51:163–170, 2008.

Pearlman E, Dickman PS, Askin FB, et al: Ewing's sarcoma: routine diagnostic utilization of MIC2 analysis, *Hum Pathol* 25:304–307, 1994.

Osteosarcoma

Chou AJ, Merola PR, Wexler LH, et al: Treatment of osteosarcoma at first recurrence after contemporary therapy: the Memorial Sloan-Kettering Cancer Center experience, *Cancer* 104:2214–2221, 2005.

Hayashida Y, Yakushiji T, Awai K, et al: Monitoring therapeutic responses of primary bone tumors by diffusion-weighted image: initial results, *Eur Radiol* 16(12):2637–2643, 2006.

Link MP, Goorin AM, Miser AW, et al: The effect of adjuvant chemotherapy on relapse-free survival in patients with osteosarcoma of the extremity, *N Engl J Med* 314:1600–1606, 1986.

Meyer JS, Nadel HR, Marina N, et al: Imaging guidelines for children with Ewing sarcoma and osteosarcoma: a report from the Children's Oncology Group Bone Tumor Committee, *Pediatr Blood Cancer* 51:163–170, 2008.

Whelan J, Seddon B, Perisoglou M: Management of osteosarcoma, *Curr Treat Options Oncol* 7:444–455, 2006.

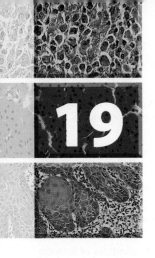

19

AIDS-Associated Malignancies

JEREMY S. ABRAMSON • DAVID T. SCADDEN

The acquired immunodeficiency syndrome (AIDS) epidemic is in its third decade, and the number of people infected with the human immunodeficiency virus-1 (HIV) in the United States is approaching 1 million, with nearly 40 million individuals infected worldwide. Since early in the HIV epidemic it has been recognized that certain tumors occur with increased frequency in the setting of HIV-induced immunosuppression. These include most prominently Kaposi sarcoma (KS), B-cell non-Hodgkin lymphoma (NHL), and anogenital neoplasia. Less common, but also of increased frequency compared with the general population, are Hodgkin lymphomas and, in children, leiomyosarcomas. The advent of highly active antiretroviral therapy (HAART) has markedly reduced the morbidity and mortality of HIV-infected individuals with access to such medications. Oncologic complications are among those markedly reduced in the era of better viral control, although the impact has not been uniform across neoplasms.

Pathogenesis of AIDS-Related Neoplasms

Several possible contributing pathophysiologic mechanisms probably participate in the predisposition to neoplasms in the setting of HIV infection, including altered immune activation, impaired innate tumor surveillance, dysregulated cytokine production, and inadequate control of oncogenic pathogens. Such issues are not unique to HIV-related immunosuppression and are analogous in certain respects to malignancy in patients with congenital or therapeutic immune deficiency states, although there are clear differences among these entities.

Organ transplant data indicate that the risk of post-transplant lymphoproliferative disease increases proportionately with the depth and duration of therapeutic immunosuppression (see Table 19.1). There are also data suggesting that immune activation may contribute to the emergence of lymphoid neoplasms. There is an increased incidence of lymphomas in the setting of autoimmune diseases such as Sjögren syndrome, systemic lupus erythematosus, rheumatoid arthritis, and celiac disease. Similarly, immune activation may be directly driven by an infectious agent. Inadequate host immunologic responses to infectious agents may result in tumor development due to a combination of impaired immunity and viral oncogenesis. The geographic clustering of KS and its association with specific sexual practices strongly suggested an association with a

Table 19.1	
Incidence of Post-transplant Lymphoproliferative Disorders Based on Data Using Historic Immunosuppression Regimens	
Transplant Type	**Incidence (%)***
Renal	1.0
Heart	1.8
Liver	2.2
Heart and lung	5.0
Bone marrow (BM)	<1.0
T cell–depleted BM	12.0
Mismatched, T cell–depleted BM	24.0

*Incidence figures would be expected to be lower using current protocols.

secondary infectious process, a process subsequently identified as human herpesvirus-8 (HHV-8) or KS herpesvirus, a member of the γ-herpesvirus family. The common association between KS and the polyclonal lymphoproliferative disorder multicentric Castleman disease led to the identification of HHV-8 as the driving pathogen of that disorder, and it has subsequently been implicated in the pathogenesis of primary effusion lymphoma, as well. The role for immune control of HHV-8 and Epstein-Barr virus (EBV) in oncogenesis is now strongly supported by evidence that improved immune function with HAART markedly reduces HHV-8- and EBV-related tumors. Notably, however, data regarding the impact of HAART on human papillomavirus (HPV)-related tumors are less clear, and it is not yet known to what extent improved immune function will affect anogenital neoplasia. What is clear is that HIV itself does not play a direct role in tumor generation. Other than in very rare cases of T-cell lymphoma, HIV is not detectable in HIV-related malignancies. HIV provides the immunologic dysfunction permissive of tumor emergence. These tumors may be regarded as opportunistic neoplasms in much the same way as specific infections are regarded as opportunistic in the immunocompromised host.

Perturbations in the tissue cytokine milieu may provide the specific signals altering the control of cellular proliferation in tumors of immune suppression. KS serves as an example of this, in that KS cells, unlike normal mesenchymal cells, both secrete interleukin-6 (IL-6) and have a proliferative response to IL-6 in an autocrine fashion. Similarly, some AIDS-lymphoma cells appear to produce IL-10, and their growth rate is affected by it. These events may not be sufficient for tumor generation but provide the proliferative background against which transforming events may occur.

Kaposi Sarcoma

KS has been the most common HIV-related neoplasm, although the incidence has declined significantly since the introduction of HAART. It is believed to arise from mesodermally derived cells, the exact nature of which remains controversial. Histologically these lesions are composed of multiple cell types, including smooth muscle, endothelial, and immune cells. The histologic picture raises the unanswered question of whether this disease represents a true malignancy or is the result of dysregulated proliferation of otherwise normal cells in response to an abnormal signal. Efforts to define clonality in lesions have conflicting results, showing that clonal disease may evolve, but polyclonality is common. The abnormal drive for cell proliferation may be due to products of KS herpesvirus itself such as a constitutively active G protein–coupled receptor the virus encodes. In addition, the HIV gene product, *tat*, may induce the lytic phase of HHV-8, resulting in increased viral transcripts, IL-6 production, and stimulation of the JAK/STAT proliferation pathway, which may account for the extraordinary predilection for KS seen in HIV-infected individuals above that of other immunosuppressed populations. The epidemiology of KS is outlined in Figures 19.1 and 19.2.

KS lesions occur clinically in the skin, on mucosal surfaces, in lymph nodes, and in solid organs, most commonly the lung and gastrointestinal (GI) tract. Cutaneous manifestations vary from erythematous, macular lesions to raised, nodular masses with a violaceous hue. Large, plaquelike lesions may develop when clusters of tumors coalesce, and central necrosis can occur. KS tends to appear at multiple sites concurrently, with no ordered pattern of spread. An important differential diagnosis is bacillary angiomatosis, which is an infectious disease occurring in HIV patients caused by *Bartonella* organisms. Cutaneous *Pneumocystis carinii* infection has also been reported to cause an erythematous lesion resembling KS. Early KS lesions may also be mistaken for benign skin lesions such as dermatofibromas or angiomas. Thus, biopsy of clinically suspected KS lesions is recommended at the time of first clinical presentation.

Mucosal involvement by KS may occur in the oral cavity, conjunctiva, or more rarely the urethral meatus and may result in local discomfort. Cutaneous lesions, however, are mostly of cosmetic significance, and their successful treatment can overcome a major source of distress in affected patients. Approximately one half of patients with mucocutaneous disease will also have KS involving other organs. While skin disease usually accompanies organ involvement, up to 15% of patients have been reported to have lymph node, GI, or lung KS without skin manifestations.

Pulmonary KS may involve the large airways, interstitium, alveoli, or pleural surfaces, and the clinical features vary accordingly. Patients may complain of dyspnea, cough, hemoptysis, or wheezing, but the disease is often asymptomatic. When parenchymal involvement is extensive it may be life-threatening, prompting most clinicians to aggressively treat patients in whom infiltrates on chest radiography are thought to be due to KS. GI tract lesions are generally asymptomatic but may result in nonspecific symptoms such as abdominal pain and bloating. These lesions may be the cause of minor chronic blood loss, but massive hemorrhage is uncommon.

Finally, KS can involve lymph nodes and local lymphatics, causing marked local edema. This is exacerbated by the increased permeability of the vascular component of KS and by a permeability factor elaborated by KS cells, vascular endothelial

Table 19.2

Staging System (TIS) for HIV-Associated Kaposi Sarcoma (KS)

	Good Risk (All of the Following)	Poor Risk (Any of the Following)
Tumor (T)	Confined to skin and/or lymph nodes and/or minimal oral disease	Tumor-associated edema or ulceration Extensive KS Gastrointestinal disease Other visceral involvement
Immune system (I)	CD4 > 200 cells/μL	CD4 <200 cells/μL
Systemic illness (S)	No opportunistic infections or thrush (*Candida*) No "B" symptoms Karnofsky score >70%	History of or current opportunistic infection or thrush "B" symptoms Karnofsky score <70% Other HIV-related illness (CMV, PCP, MAI, PML)

"B" symptoms, significant weight loss, fevers, and drenching night sweats. CMV, cytomegalovirus; MAI; *Mycobacterium avium-intracellulare*; PCP, *Pneumocystis carinii*; PML, progressive multifocal leukoencephalopathy.

growth factor. Edema is commonly seen in the groin, distal lower extremities, or head and neck regions, and is a major cause of morbidity. It is the most common cause of symptoms from KS and is generally regarded by us as an indication to proceed with a more aggressive treatment approach. A system for clinically staging KS is outlined in Table 19.2.

KS is not curable with standard therapies, and so goals of treatment are to prevent deleterious consequences of the disease, including organ dysfunction from extracutaneous involvement as well as discomfort or cosmetics associated with skin lesions. Initiation of HAART often results in regression of KS lesions, and so antiretroviral therapy should be considered in all patients. It should be noted, however, that rarely, rapid progression of KS has been reported after HAART initiation as a component of the immune reconstitution inflammatory syndrome. For local control, topical approaches include topical retinoids, local radiation therapy, cryotherapy, laser therapy, and direct intralesional injections of chemotherapy. Treatment of advanced disease most commonly consists of single-agent chemotherapy, with liposomal doxorubicin, paclitaxel, vinca alkaloids, or etoposide. Novel treatments that have shown early promise and are the subject of ongoing clinical trials include angiogenesis inhibitors, mTOR inhibitors, and the tyrosine kinase inhibitor imatinib mesylate, among others.

Non-Hodgkin Lymphoma

The increased incidence of NHL in AIDS patients was first noted in 1984; NHL became recognized as an AIDS-defining illness in 1987. The estimated incidence of NHL in patients ranges from 1.6% to 2.0% per year, with patients from all HIV risk groups being susceptible to the disease. AIDS-related NHLs are a heterogeneous group in terms of pathogenesis, histologic appearance, clinical behavior, and treatment. Diffuse large B-cell lymphoma (DLBCL) is the most common, particularly the immunoblastic variant. DLBCL may be limited to the brain and leptomeninges, in which case it is referred to as the distinct entity of primary central nervous system (CNS) lymphoma. Burkitt lymphoma is the second most common systemic HIV-related lymphoma and is the only AIDS-related NHL that customarily occurs with CD4 counts over 200, and thus, not surprisingly, is the only AIDS-related NHL not to see a decrease in incidence since the introduction of HAART. Rare AIDS-related lymphomas occurring only at very low CD4 counts are plasmablastic lymphoma and primary effusion lymphoma, also known as body cavity lymphoma.

The pathogenesis of AIDS-related lymphoma is related to underlying immune dysfunction, stimulation of B cells by abnormally produced cytokines, and co-infecting oncogenic organisms such as EBV and HHV-8. DLBCLs are associated with EBV in up to 75% of cases and in virtually all primary CNS lymphomas, while Burkitt lymphomas are EBV-associated in only 20% to 35%. Interestingly, the endemic form of Burkitt lymphoma, traditionally presenting as jaw tumors in African children, is uniformly EBV-positive, while traditional nonendemic Burkitt lymphomas in non-HIV-infected patients are uniformly EBV-negative. The pattern of EBV expression in AIDS-related lymphomas differs from that seen in post-transplant lymphoproliferative disease. In systemic AIDS lymphomas a unique combination of Epstein-Barr nuclear antigen-1 and latent membrane protein-1 expression occurs. In post-transplant patients and primary CNS AIDS lymphomas, Epstein-Barr nuclear antigen-2 through -5 are expressed along with latent membrane protein-1 and -2. Transplant-related neoplasms may regress upon withdrawal of administered immunosuppressive agents or occasionally with antiviral therapy. However, this is not the case in AIDS, where tumor regression is rare even in the face of improved immune function with HAART.

Several genetic abnormalities have been found in AIDS-related NHL. Rearrangements of the c-MYC proto-oncogene located on chromosome 8 with the immunoglobulin genes situated on chromosomes 14 and 2 are the most common mutations noted, with a frequency of 23% to 79%. The rearrangement occurs in the mature B cell, in which immunoglobulin gene rearrangement has already occurred. The resultant juxtaposition of the c-MYC and immunoglobulin genes may play a central role in the transformation of cells bearing this molecular translocation. Other oncogene mutations that occur less frequently than that involving c-MYC include abnormalities of the TP53 tumor suppressor gene and the RAS oncogene. EBV is implicated in the pathogenesis of virtually all cases of plasmablastic lymphoma, a highly aggressive B-cell lymphoma often presenting in the oral cavity. HHV-8 underlies the rare cases of primary effusion lymphoma, which occurs without accompanying nodal disease in serosal sites such as the peritoneum, pleura, and pericardium. EBV co-infection is also common. Plasmablastic and primary effusion lymphomas predominantly occur with CD4 counts less than 50.

Histologically, AIDS-related NHLs are high-grade B-cell malignancies demonstrating aggressive clinical behavior. Rarely, T-cell malignancies such as large granular lymphoproliferative disease, Sézary syndrome, or angioimmunoblastic T-cell lymphoma are encountered in HIV-infected patients. In some cases these rare T-cell malignancies have been demonstrated to harbor HIV, some of which have integrated into the host genome resulting in a transforming mutation.

The clinical features of AIDS-related NHL are similar to those of aggressive lymphomas in general. Patients with AIDS-related lymphomas are, however, more likely to present with advanced-stage disease and involvement of multiple extranodal sites, as compared with their HIV-negative counterparts. There is also a

Table 19.3

Primary CNS and Systemic HIV Lymphoma

	Primary CNS	**Systemic**
CD4 (cells/μL)	~30	~189
Prior AIDS	~73%	~37%
Immunoblastic histology	~100%	18% to 43%
EBV genome detected	~100%	38% to 68%
Median survival	2–18 months	43 months

CNS, central nervous system; EBV, Epstein-Barr virus.

high proportion of patients with systemic "B" symptoms of significant weight loss, fevers, and drenching night sweats (see Fig. 19.3). Patients presenting with such symptoms should have a thorough microbiologic evaluation to exclude bacterial, mycobacterial, viral, fungal, or parasitic disease. HHV-8–associated multicentric Castleman disease should also be considered in the differential diagnosis of AIDS-related lymphoma, because it presents similarly with diffuse adenopathy and profound "B" symptoms and often precedes the development of, or presents concurrently with, AIDS-related lymphoma.

Prognosis is closely linked to the status of the immunodeficiency (as indicated by CD4 count and prior AIDS diagnosis) as well as tumor-related factors. Prognosis has improved significantly since the introduction of HAART, with the median survival in AIDS-related DLBCL increasing from 8 months to 43 months (see Fig. 19.4). High-risk international prognostic index score is a poor prognostic factor in AIDS-related lymphoma, as it is in non-AIDS-related lymphoma. Other poor prognostic factors include Burkitt, plasmablastic, or primary effusion histologies, CD4 count less than 100 cells/μL, and failure to achieve a complete remission to initial therapy. When one is treating patients with AIDS-related lymphoma, the status of the HIV disease itself must always be kept in mind, since prognosis and tolerance of therapy are different for patients with advanced AIDS failing antiretrovirals compared with those tolerating and benefiting from HAART.

Primary CNS lymphoma is an important subgroup of HIV-associated lymphoma and composes 15% to 20% of all AIDS NHLs. It tends to occur in patients with more advanced immunosuppression; one study demonstrated a mean CD4 count of 30 cells/mm³ in primary CNS lymphoma versus 190 cells/mm³ in patients with systemic NHL. Primary CNS lymphoma in AIDS resembles transplant lymphoma in that it is of immunoblastic histology and is virtually always associated with the EBV genome (see Table 19.3). This is in contrast to systemic HIV lymphoma, which differs from lymphoma developing in patients who are immunocompromised for other reasons (see Table 19.4). This subset of HIV-associated lymphomas has substantially declined in the era of HAART. The improved immune function associated with more effective control of HIV probably

Table 19.4

Features of Lymphoma in Immunosuppressed Patients

Feature	**Organ Transplantation Patients**	**AIDS Patients**
EBV genome	~100%	38% to 68%
Burkitt histology	~1%	36%
MYC translocation	Not reported	30% to 80%

EBV, Epstein-Barr virus.

accounts for the decrease in patients with this devastating complication. Clinical presentation is with neurologic symptoms which may be as vague as subtle personality changes with a CNS mass lesion found by radiographic imaging studies. In AIDS patients, lymphoma must be distinguished from *Toxoplasma* or other infectious brain abscesses, as well as progressive multifocal leukoencephalopathy. Certain radiologic criteria are useful in differentiating lymphoma from *Toxoplasma* lesions: NHL is typically located centrally, is often larger than 2 cm, and may cross the midline, while converse features may suggest toxoplasmosis. Brain biopsy is required to establish a definitive diagnosis, but the presence of EBV by cerebrospinal fluid (CSF) polymerase chain reaction strongly supports a lymphoma diagnosis and has a sensitivity and specificity of greater than 90% in patients with a negative *Toxoplasma* titer who have been on trimethoprim-sulfamethoxazole prophylaxis. Analysis of the CSF for a clonal IgH gene rearrangement by polymerase chain reaction is also highly suggestive of CNS lymphoma, while routine cytologic evaluation and flow cytometry are much less sensitive as a result of the paucity of circulating cells. For those in whom ambiguity remains, a therapeutic trial of antitoxoplasmosis therapy may be useful, since a majority of patients with *Toxoplasma* infection will respond within 2 weeks.

Certain aspects of the management of systemic AIDS-related lymphoma require special consideration. First, the CNS should be examined carefully with radiologic scanning and cytologic analysis of the CSF due to the high incidence of CNS involvement by these lymphomas. Many centers administer intrathecal chemotherapy to prevent CNS relapse even if there is no evidence of disease in the CSF initially. The presence of EBV in the primary tumor is highly associated with CNS involvement and may be useful in discriminating those patients who most benefit from prophylactic chemotherapy to the CNS. Patients with B symptoms must be evaluated to exclude coincident HIV-related infections, which can cause symptoms such as fever and weight loss and that would require a different treatment approach. In general, patients should receive prophylaxis for *P. carinii* infection while undergoing chemotherapy, regardless of the pretreatment CD4 count. Patients with very low CD4 counts before treatment are also candidates for prophylaxis against *Toxoplasma* and atypical mycobacteria. During treatment of lymphoma in the HIV population the physician should be particularly wary of the myelotoxic effects of chemotherapy, since these may be compounded by the concomitant administration of drugs for *P. carinii* prophylaxis (trimethoprim-sulfamethoxazole) as well as by certain antiretroviral agents. Granulocyte colony–stimulating factors (filgrastim, pegfilgrastim, or sargramostim) have been useful in mitigating neutropenia in this setting and should be used prophylactically in all patients.

Treatment of systemic disease is usually with combination chemotherapy regimens such as CHOP (cyclophosphamide, doxorubicin, vincristine, and prednisone) or the infusional regimen of dose-adjusted EPOCH (etoposide, prednisone, vincristine, cyclophosphamide, and doxorubicin), which have yielded overall response rates of 50% to 70% and 87%, respectively. Bolus and infusional strategies have not yet been compared head to head, and so there is no evidence yet on the superiority of one over the other. Lower-dose regimens have been tested in comparison to full-dose regimens with comparably poor results in the pre-HAART era, but have not been well studied since the introduction of HAART, where response rates and survival have all significantly improved, and so low-dose regimens should be reserved for those patients with advanced

AIDS who have failed antiretroviral therapy. The introduction of the CD20-directed monoclonal antibody rituximab has revolutionized the treatment of non-HIV–related B-cell lymphomas, where it provides a broad benefit in response and survival with minimal additional toxicity. Trials assessing the benefit of rituximab-containing therapy in AIDS-related NHLs have not been as compelling. A randomized trial of CHOP versus CHOP plus rituximab (R-CHOP) in AIDS-related B-cell lymphoma found similar complete response rates and event-free survivals; however, the rituximab-treated patients had an increased rate of infectious-related death (14% vs. 2%). On subset analysis, most deaths were limited to patients with CD4 counts less than 100, with 60% of deaths occurring in patients with CD4 counts less than 50. Furthermore, there was a 3-month maintenance rituximab period following R-CHOP, during which time 40% of infectious-related deaths occurred. While rituximab may be safe and effective in certain settings, these data suggest that the additional immune suppression may markedly increase risk in HIV-infected patients and should be used cautiously. An ongoing randomized trial is asking whether sequential rituximab administration will offer benefit while minimizing infectious-related toxicity. Burkitt lymphoma is a highly aggressive lymphoma that may be treated with more intensive therapy than DLBCL. Since the introduction of HAART, evidence suggests that HIV-infected patients can tolerate highly aggressive chemotherapy with outcomes that rival those of their non–HIV-infected counterparts.

For those individuals with AIDS-related NHL failing initial therapy, a standard salvage regimen has not been defined. High-dose chemotherapy with autologous stem cell support may successfully salvage a proportion of relapsed or refractory patients, although stem cell transplantation in these patients should probably be performed at centers with particular expertise in treating this high-risk patient population.

Treatment of CNS lymphoma is generally limited to radiation therapy and corticosteroids, often with inclusion of high-dose methotrexate. Combination chemotherapy and radiation therapy seems to add little beyond toxicity. The overall prognosis in this group of patients is grim, with survival estimated to be 2–5 months limited approximately equally by recurrent lymphoma and other complications of AIDS.

Hodgkin Lymphoma

Hodgkin lymphoma occurs more frequently in AIDS patients than in the general population but of a magnitude less pronounced than NHL (an approximately fivefold increase compared with a 60-fold increase for NHL). Unlike most AIDS-related lymphomas, the incidence of Hodgkin lymphoma has not declined since the introduction of HAART. This may be related to the observation that Hodgkin lymphoma is more likely to occur at moderately decreased CD4 counts than in the setting of severe immunodeficiency. The cause of this is speculative, but it may be due to the critical role played by the host inflammatory microenvironment in the pathogenesis of classical Hodgkin lymphoma. Partial immune reconstitution with antiviral therapy may sufficiently allow necessary signaling from infiltrating host lymphocytes but still leave the patient at risk for infection and transformation by EBV, which is present in virtually all cases of HIV-related Hodgkin lymphomas.

The histologic subtypes of this disease also differ in the context of HIV infection, with the mixed-cellularity subtype seen most commonly, compared to nodular sclerosis Hodgkin lymphoma in patients without concomitant HIV infection. Presentation is usually with advanced-stage disease, with 82% of patients having stage III or IV disease at diagnosis. There is a propensity for extranodal and bone marrow involvement with 67% and 48%, respectively, in one series. Treatment consists of standard Hodgkin lymphoma approaches based on stage, with durable remissions well documented. Patients with advanced-stage Hodgkin lymphoma treated with standard ABVD (doxorubicin, bleomycin, vinblastine, and dacarbazine) along with concurrent HAART are reported to have a complete-response rate of 87%, and event-free and overall survival at 5 years of 71% and 76%, respectively. As with the care of any malignancy in HIV disease, the vigor with which a curative strategy is pursued should be tempered by the status of the HIV infection itself. Individuals with end-stage AIDS for whom all available antiretroviral therapies have failed may be better approached with a palliative intent. Chemotherapy regimens such as ABVD may require additional supportive measures and attention must be paid to the prevention and treatment of opportunistic infections.

Squamous Epithelial Lesions

Anal intraepithelial neoplasia and invasive squamous cell cancer are increased among men who have sex with men. The additional risk imposed by HIV infection is substantial for dysplasia, although the impact on frank invasive cancer is more ambiguous. Similarly, dysplasia of the uterine cervix is increased in HIV-infected women, although a substantial increase in invasive cervical cancer has not been detected in most studies. The incidence of preinvasive and frankly invasive squamous neoplasms has not declined since the introduction of HAART, and so as patients with AIDS live longer, the incidence and impact of these malignancies may increase without effective screening techniques. Anogenital squamous cell neoplasia in the setting of HIV disease is highly linked to HPV infection with known oncogenic serotypes. The ability to intervene to eradicate HPV is extremely limited at this time, although screening strategies may prevent the development of frank invasive cancer. It is not clear whether the newly US Food and Drug Administration–approved HPV vaccine will prove to be a valuable prophylactic tool against HPV-related neoplasms in HIV-infected patients given that the prevalence of HPV infection is already high in these patients at the time of HIV diagnosis. There are no clinical trials published thus far in this high-risk population. For women the guidelines for treating cervical dysplasia and cancer outside the context of HIV disease are those generally applied. Additional vigilance in screening and following women with HIV infection for the presence of high-grade dysplasia, recurrent dysplasia, or frank cancer is warranted. For anal and perianal dysplasia in men who have sex with men, cytologic screening will detect anal intraepithelial neoplasms in a high proportion of at-risk individuals, and those lesions may benefit from local therapy. Lesions of the anal verge may benefit from topical therapy with agents such as imiquimod and lesions in the anal canal from local therapies with cryosurgery or laser surgery. For patients with invasive anal cancer, the combination of chemotherapy and radiation therapy is recommended and can result in long-term elimination of the disease.

Occurring in the Mediterranean basin—generally elderly males often with immunologic abnormalities

Occurring in Central Africa—male predominance, antedated the HIV epidemic

Post-transplant on immunosuppressive drugs

HIV-related—20,000-fold increased incidence over the general population

FIGURE 19.1 Epidemiology of Kaposi sarcoma.

Predominantly in homosexual/bisexual risk group for HIV

Incidence in HIV-positive homosexual males is 15%–20% (decreased from 48% in 1981 pre-HAART*; much reduced (<5% on HAART)

Associated with infection by human herpesvirus 8 (HHV-8), also known as Kaposi sarcoma herpesvirus (KSHV)

*HAART, highly active antiretroviral therapy

FIGURE 19.2 HIV-associated Kaposi sarcoma.

Histology	
Small noncleaved cell (Burkitt-like)	(36%)
Immunoblastic	(21%)
Diffuse large cell	(24%)
Other type	(9%)
Stage at presentation	
I, II	(27%)
III, IV	(73%)
Extranodal sites	
CNS	(23%)
Bone marrow	(23%)
GI tract	(21%)
Liver	(18%)

FIGURE 19.3 HIV-associated non-Hodgkin lymphoma.

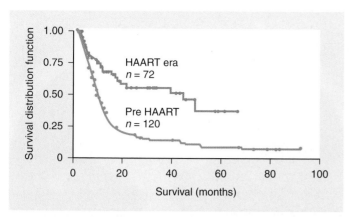

FIGURE 19.4 Survival of patients with HIV-related DLBCL treated with curative intent: pre-HAART era versus HAART era. (Figure used with permission: Lim ST, Karim R, Tulpule A, et al: Prognostic factors in HIV-related diffuse large-cell lymphoma: before versus after highly active antiretroviral therapy, *J Clin Oncol* 23:8477–8482, 2005.)

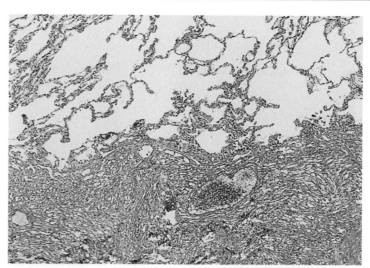

FIGURE 19.6 **PULMONARY KAPOSI SARCOMA (KS).** A 27-year-old graduate student with a history of asthma presented with progressive dyspnea on exertion unresponsive to antiasthma medications and a declining diffusing capacity of the lung for carbon monoxide. Chest radiography revealed patchy areas of consolidation (not shown). Thoracoscopic biopsy revealed KS adjacent to normal lung parenchyma. Low-power microscopic view shows infiltration of the lung by a spindle cell neoplasm with large and small thin-walled vascular spaces. With ongoing chemotherapy the patient became oxygen-independent with no respiratory symptoms 1 year following diagnosis. He had no mucocutaneous KS when he initially presented, a situation that may occur in up to 20% of patients with pulmonary KS. (Courtesy of Dr. Bradford Sherburne.)

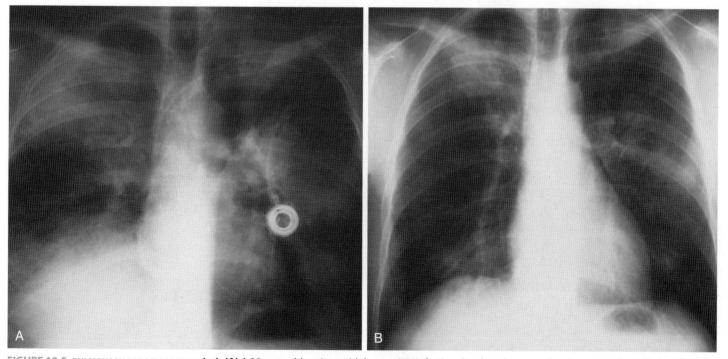

FIGURE 19.5 **PULMONARY KAPOSI SARCOMA (KS). (A)** A 28-year-old patient with known HIV infection developed progressive shortness of breath, cough, and hemoptysis. Evaluation for an infectious etiology as the basis for the multiple infiltrates was negative. Bronchoscopy revealed multiple endobronchial KS lesions, and a gallium-67 citrate scan was negative (characteristic of KS but not infection). Treatment with chemotherapy initially resulted in resolution of his respiratory symptoms and improvement of his chest radiograph. **(B)** However, 6 months later new infections interrupted his KS therapy. He developed progressive respiratory compromise, worsening of the KS infiltrates, and new pleural effusions.

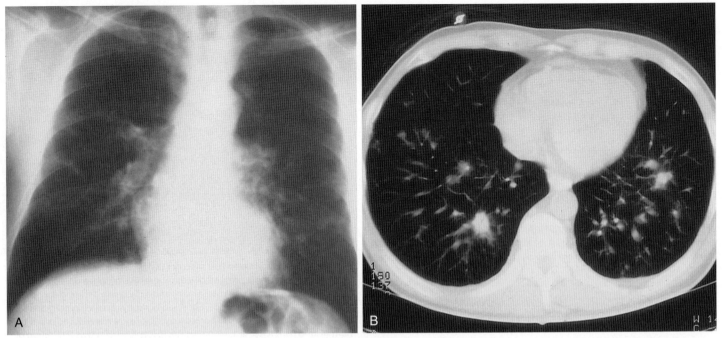

FIGURE 19.7 **PULMONARY KAPOSI SARCOMA.** A 41-year-old man previously diagnosed with cutaneous KS developed persistent cough without fever. Chest radiography revealed hilar fullness and parenchymal nodules **(A)** more clearly defined on chest computed tomography scan **(B)**. This radiographic appearance is common for pulmonary KS.

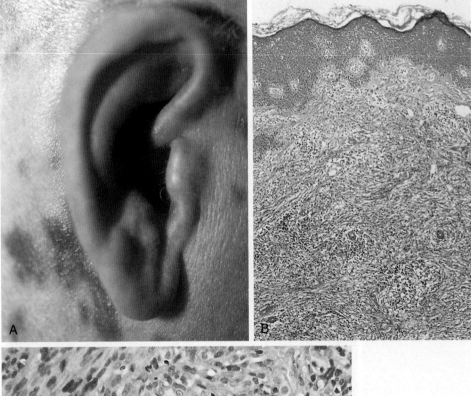

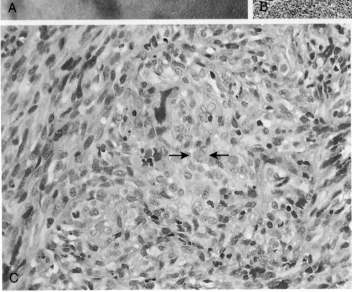

FIGURE 19.8 **CUTANEOUS KAPOSI SARCOMA.** **(A)** Typical appearance of cutaneous KS with irregularly shaped, macular papular lesions of erythematous or violaceous hue. There is often a surrounding halo of pigment representing the breakdown of heme pigments from red cells that diapedese into KS lesions. **(B)** Skin punch biopsy from an erythematous macule reveals a dermal infiltrate of spindle cells forming vascular arrays expanding the reticular dermis (×40). This is a characteristic appearance of KS in the skin. **(C)** A higher-magnification view (×100) of the biopsy specimen in **B** reveals spindle cell vascular channels with enlarged "boxcar nuclei" in parallel bundles arranged haphazardly. These are interspersed between scattered mononuclear inflammatory cell infiltrates. In the center there are eosinophilic cytoplasmic droplets characteristic of KS (*arrows*). (Courtesy of Dr. Steven Tahan.)

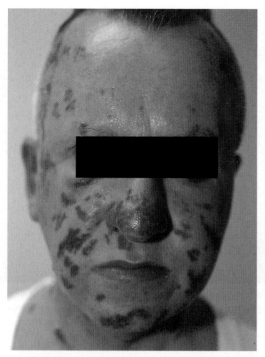

FIGURE 19.9 **CUTANEOUS KAPOSI SARCOMA.** The marked disfigurement evident in this photograph demonstrates why patients with only cutaneous involvement may seek aggressive therapy. This 32-year-old clerk also has evidence of early periorbital edema.

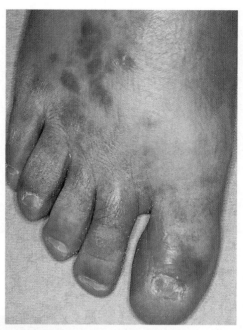

FIGURE 19.11 **CUTANEOUS KAPOSI SARCOMA.** Involvement of the skin can often result in local edema. In this patient, painful swelling of the first two digits occurred from cutaneous involvement.

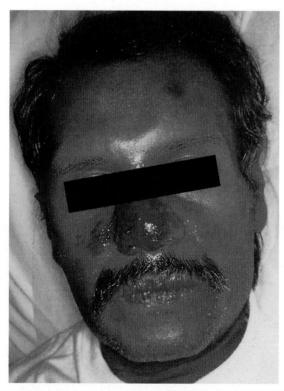

FIGURE 19.10 **CUTANEOUS KAPOSI SARCOMA.** Facial KS often has a predilection for the nose. In this 26-year-old male this resulted in marked edema of the nose and eventual sloughing of the overlying skin. The latter is a rare complication.

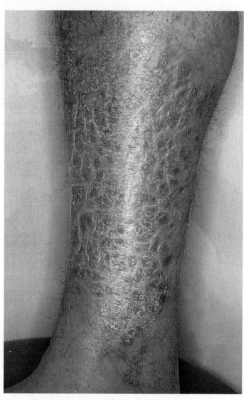

FIGURE 19.12 **CUTANEOUS KAPOSI SARCOMA.** Extensive KS can become consolidated and can result in marked local edema. This is particularly true in the lower extremity—as evident in this photograph—often resulting in joint stiffness and discomfort limiting mobility.

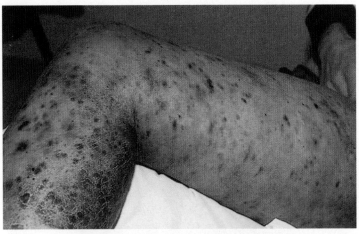

FIGURE 19.13 **CUTANEOUS KAPOSI SARCOMA.** Massive edema from presumed lymph node involvement can accompany local skin involvement. This 28-year-old male developed complete immobility of his right lower extremity that confined him to bed despite aggressive treatment.

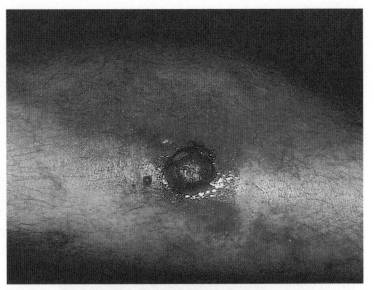

FIGURE 19.15 **CUTANEOUS KAPOSI SARCOMA.** Extensive KS can occasionally ulcerate as in this 54-year-old woman. The ulcer occurred in the setting of extensive local edema and radiation therapy. The resulting ulcer and surrounding cellulitis slowly responded to antibiotics and fastidious wound care.

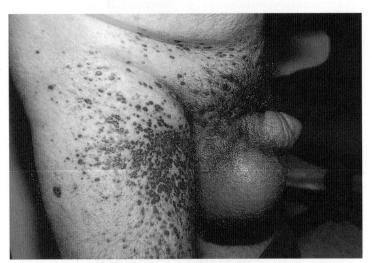

FIGURE 19.14 **CUTANEOUS KAPOSI SARCOMA.** Edema of the lower extremities, peripubic area, genitalia, and face is common in advanced KS. This can often result in extreme discomfort and immobility. This patient had complete resolution of genital and peripubic edema with systemic chemotherapy. Remaining woody edema of the upper thigh did not compromise the mobility of his leg function, and he was able to continue his career for 9 months after beginning chemotherapy.

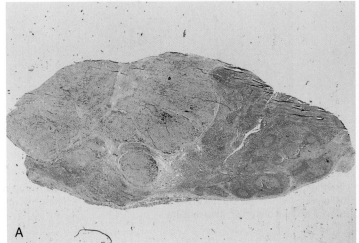
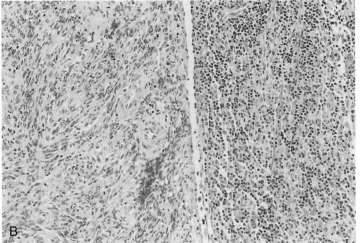

FIGURE 19.16 **CUTANEOUS KAPOSI SARCOMA: LYMPHADENOPATHY.** A 23-year-old patient, seropositive for HIV and previously diagnosed with KS of the extremities and hard palate, developed unilateral inguinal adenopathy and woody edema of the thigh. **(A)** A lymph node biopsy revealed KS disrupting the normal architecture of the node (×2.5). **(B)** Higher power shows lymphoid tissue on right with reactive changes (increase in macrophages, small lymphocytes, and endothelial cells, as well as venules) with sharp transition to Kaposi infiltrate consisting of spindle cells and frequent extravasated red blood cells (×50). No infectious organisms or lymphomas were noted. The patient improved on systemic chemotherapy but did not have resolution of the edema and died of an opportunistic infection 6 months later. (Courtesy of Dr. Bradford Sherburne.)

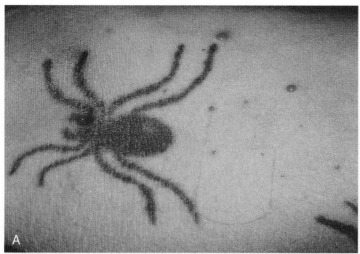

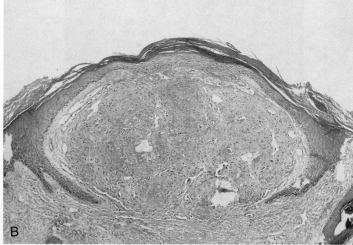

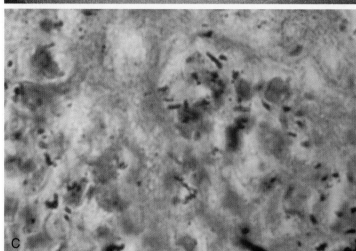

FIGURE 19.17 **CUTANEOUS LESIONS: BACILLARY ANGIOMATOSIS.** An important differential diagnosis in pigmented skin lesions in HIV-infected patients is bacillary angiomatosis. **(A)** Seen here on the tattooed forearm of a 26-year-old male, these lesions may be mistaken for KS and have very different implications for therapy. **(B)** A characteristic collar of epidermis around a dermal papule is seen (×40) on skin punch biopsy of one of the lesions shown in **A**. This appearance is classic for bacillary angiomatosis. **(C)** Warthin-Starry silver stain reveals organisms consistent with *Bartonella*, confirming the diagnosis of bacillary angiomatosis. (**A**, Courtesy of Dr. Richard Johnson; **B, C**, courtesy of Dr. Steven Tahan.)

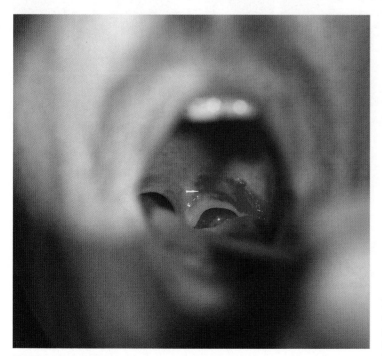

FIGURE 19.18 **MUCOSAL KAPOSI SARCOMA.** Typical appearance of oral KS visualized here on the soft palate of a 44-year-old man. Note the erythematous, patchy, raised lesions.

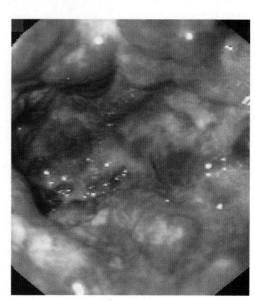

FIGURE 19.19 **MUCOSAL KAPOSI SARCOMA.** Mucosal involvement by KS is common. Note the red, violaceous, raised colonic nodules. It is often noted as an asymptomatic finding on either bronchoscopy or GI endoscopy. The colonoscopic findings depicted above were thought to be a potentially contributory factor, but unlikely to be the primary cause, of intractable, watery diarrhea. (Courtesy of Dr. Harry Anastopoulos.)

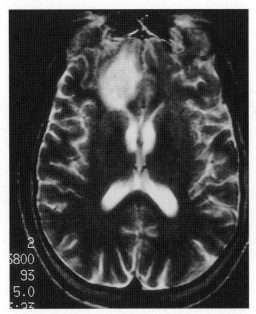

FIGURE 19.20 **CENTRAL NERVOUS SYSTEM LESIONS: CYTOMEGALOVIRUS.** A 20-year-old male with a history of *Pneumocystis carinii* pneumonia and cytomegalovirus retinitis developed headache, lethargy, and irritability. Magnetic resonance imaging (MRI) revealed a space-occupying lesion in the frontal lobe that enhanced with gadolinium and on T$_2$-weighted image. He transiently responded to therapy but relapsed and died of intractable seizures 3 months later.

FIGURE 19.21 **CENTRAL NERVOUS SYSTEM LESION: TOXOPLASMOSIS.** A 26-year-old female with multiple prior opportunistic infections developed left-sided motor and sensory deficits. MRI scan revealed multiple focal effects on T$_1$-weighted imaging **(A)** that enhanced with gadolinium **(B)**. The patient failed to respond to empiric anti-*Toxoplasma* therapy, but on stereotactic biopsy had a histologically confirmed *Toxoplasma* abscess to which she rapidly succumbed.

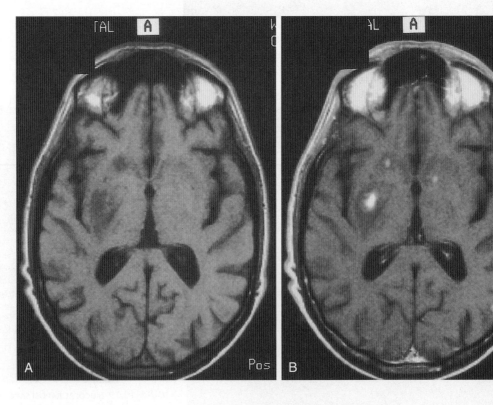

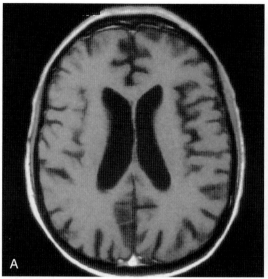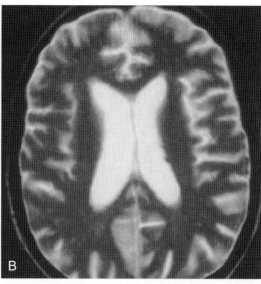

FIGURE 19.22 **CENTRAL NERVOUS SYSTEM LESION: PROGRESSIVE MULTIFOCAL LEUKOENCEPHALOPATHY.** A 44-year-old man who had been HIV-seropositive for 10 years had three episodes of *Pneumocystis carinii* pneumonia. He developed profound wasting, recurrent fevers, generalized weakness, and ataxia. MRI revealed a low-signal intensity T_1-weighted lesion **(A)**, high-signal intensity T_2-weighted lesion **(B)** that did not enhance or show mass effect, which was consistent with localized demyelination. The presumptive diagnosis was progressive multifocal leukoencephalopathy. The patient had progressive neurologic deterioration and generalized wasting, and died from pneumonia 4 weeks later.

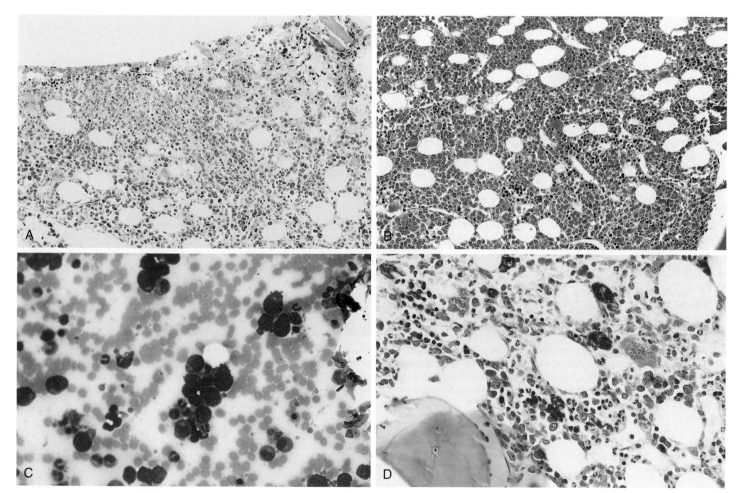

FIGURE 19.23 **BONE MARROW FINDINGS IN HIV DISEASE.** Bone marrow morphology of patients with HIV disease is often abnormal. Typically cellularity will be normal or increased and mild dysplastic changes will be noted, often accompanied by increased plasma cells, eosinophils, and reticulin. Atypical lymphoid aggregates are often noted **(A)**. These are to be distinguished from the infiltrating involvement by lymphoma seen in approximately 23% of patients with AIDS-related lymphoma **(B)**. The small non-cleaved cell lymphoma seen in **B** was further evident in the accompanying bone marrow aspirate **(C)**. Whenever evaluating patients with cytopenia and fever in AIDS, it is particularly important to exclude lymphoma or infiltrating infectious diseases such as those caused by mycobacteria and fungi. Abundant acid-fast organisms are noted in bone marrow **(D)** from a patient presenting with fever and cytopenia, splenomegaly, and retroperitoneal adenopathy. (Courtesy of Dr. Bradford Sherburne.)

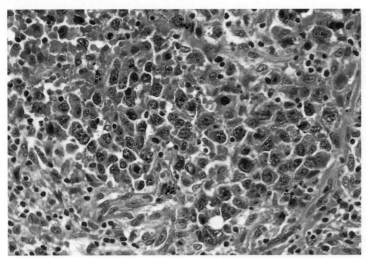

FIGURE 19.24 AIDS-ASSOCIATED LYMPHOMAS. A 54-year-old male developed idiopathic thrombocytopenic purpura (ITP) and was found to be HIV-seropositive. His thrombocytopenia responded to zidovudine. However, 2 years later he developed a scalp nodule that on biopsy revealed high-grade anaplastic large B-cell lymphoma (×100). He is currently without evidence of disease in his second remission 12 months after diagnosis. (Courtesy of Dr. Bradford Sherburne.)

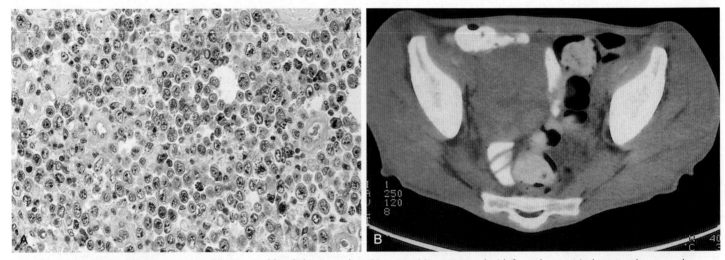

FIGURE 19.25 AIDS-ASSOCIATED LYMPHOMAS. A 41-year-old male known to be HIV-seropositive presented with fever, hematuria, hepatosplenomegaly, and inguinal adenopathy. Cystoscopic and inguinal lymph node biopsy revealed diffuse large B-cell lymphoma with immunoblastic histology **(A)** (×100). The patient failed to respond to chemotherapy and developed hepatosplenomegaly and a lower abdominal mass **(B)**. On autopsy, he was found to have a large pelvic tumor mass as well as extensive lymphomatous involvement of the right ventricle of the heart, liver, spleen, and bladder. ((**A**), Courtesy of Dr Bradford Sherburne.)

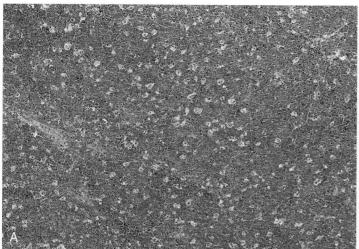

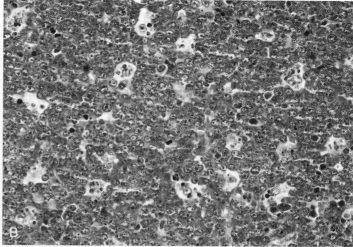

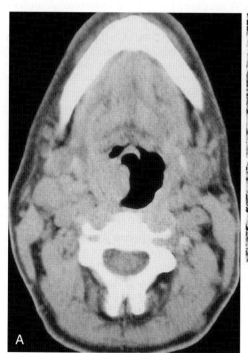

FIGURE 19.26 **AIDS-ASSOCIATED LYMPHOMAS. (A, B)** A 26-year-old male noted a swelling in the left axilla. He was otherwise well and had no prior knowledge of HIV infection. A lymph node biopsy revealed a small non-cleaved cell lymphoma (**A**, ×25; **B**, ×100), and a serologic test for HIV was positive. Note the "starry-sky" appearance of the lymph node due to the presence of light-staining benign histiocytes among a diffuse population of Burkitt-like undifferentiated lymphoma cells. He initially responded to chemotherapy. However, he developed perioral numbness and radicular back pain 6 months after his original diagnosis. He was found to have CSF involvement with relapsed lymphoma that was refractory to therapy (**C**). (**A, B**, Courtesy of Dr. Bradford Sherburne.)

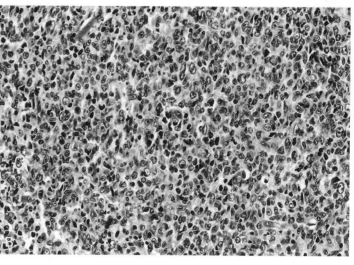

FIGURE 19.27 **AIDS-ASSOCIATED LYMPHOMAS.** A 38-year-old male with a remote history of intravenous drug use presented with persistent hoarseness and dysphagia. The patient was found to have extensive involvement of the tonsil, piriform fossa, cervical nodes, and associated soft tissue (**A**). Excisional biopsy of the tonsil revealed diffuse large cell lymphoma (**B**, ×100). He received chemotherapy and is disease-free with an excellent performance status and CD4 count of 350 cells/mm³ 18 months after diagnosis. (**B**, Courtesy of Dr. Bradford Sherburne.)

References and Suggested Readings

Epidemiology

Besson C, Goubar A, Gabarre J, et al: Changes in AIDS-related lymphoma since the era of highly active antiretroviral therapy, *Blood* 98(8):2339–2344, 2001.

Biggar RJ, Chaturvedi AK, Goedert JJ, Engels EA: AIDS-related cancer and severity of immunosuppression in persons with AIDS, *J Natl Cancer Inst* 99(12):962–972, 2007.

Navarro WH, Kaplan LD: AIDS-related lymphoproliferative disease, *Blood* 107:13–20, 2006.

Sierra del Rio M, Rousseau A, Soussain C, et al: Primary CNS lymphoma in immunocompetent patients, *Oncologist* 14:526–539, 2009.

Spano J-P, Costagliola D, Katlama C, et al: AIDS-related malignancies: state of the art and therapeutic challenges, *J Clin Oncol* 26:4834–4842, 2008.

Kaposi Sarcoma

Chang Y, Cesarman E, Pessin MS, et al: Identification of herpesvirus-like DNA sequences in AIDS-associated Kaposi's sarcoma, *Science* 266:1865–1869, 1994.

Gill P, Tulpule A, Espina B, et al: Paclitaxel is safe and effective in the treatment of advanced AIDS-related Kaposi's sarcoma, *J Clin Oncol* 17:1876–1883, 1999.

Gill PS, Wernz J, Scadden DT, et al: Randomized phase III trial of liposomal daunorubicin versus doxorubicin, bleomycin, and vincristine in AIDS-related Kaposi's sarcoma, *J Clin Oncol* 14:2353–2364, 1996.

Karcher DS, Alkan S: Human herpesvirus-8-associated body cavity-based lymphoma in human immunodeficiency virus-infected patients: a unique B-cell neoplasm, *Hum Pathol* 28:801–805, 1997.

Martin JN, Ganem DE, Osmond DH, et al: Sexual transmission and the natural history of human herpesvirus 8 infection, *N Engl J Med* 338:948–954, 1998.

Northfelt DW, Dezube BJ, Thommes JA, et al: Efficacy of pegylated-liposomal doxorubicin in the treatment of AIDS-related Kaposi's sarcoma after failure of standard chemotherapy, *J Clin Oncol* 15:653–659, 1997.

Sgadari C, Barillari G, Toschi E, et al: HIV protease inhibitors are potent anti-angiogenic molecules and promote regression of Kaposi sarcoma, *Nat Med* 8(3):225–232, 2002.

Whitby D, Boshoff C: Kaposi's sarcoma herpesvirus as a new paradigm for virus-induced oncogenesis, *Curr Opin Oncol* 10:405–412, 1998.

Zeng Y, Zhang X, Huang Z, et al: Intracellular Tat of Human Immunodeficiency Virus Type 1 Activates Lytic Cycle Replication of Kaposi's Sarcoma-Associated Herpesvirus: Role of JAK/STAT Signaling, *J Virol* 81:2401–2417, 2007.

Non-Hodgkin Lymphoma

Antinori A, Ammassari A, De Luca A, et al: Diagnosis of AIDS-related focal brain lesions: a decision-making analysis based on clinical and neuroradiologic characteristics combined with polymerase chain reaction assays in CSF, *Neurology* 48:687–694, 1997.

Cingolani A, Gastaldi R, Fassone L, et al: Epstein-Barr virus infection is predictive of CNS involvement in systemic AIDS-related non-Hodgkin's lymphomas, *J Clin Oncol* 18:3325–3330, 2000.

Hoffmann C, Tabrizian S, Wolf E, et al: Survival of AIDS patients with primary central nervous system lymphoma is dramatically improved by HAART-induced immune recovery, *AIDS* 15:2119–2127, 2001.

Jacomet C, Girard PM, Lebrette MG, et al: Intravenous methotrexate for primary central nervous system non-Hodgkin's lymphoma in AIDS [see comments], *AIDS* 11:1725–1730, 1997.

Kaplan LD, Lee JY, Ambinder RF, et al: Rituximab does not improve clinical outcome in a randomized phase 3 trial of CHOP with or without rituximab in patients with HIV-associated non-Hodgkin lymphoma: AIDS-Malignancies Consortium Trial 010, *Blood* 106:1538–1543, 2005.

Kaplan LD, Straus DJ, Testa MA, et al: Low-dose compared with standard-dose m-BACOD chemotherapy for non Hodgkin's lymphoma associated with human immunodeficiency virus infection, *N Engl J Med* 336:1641–1648, 1997.

Kirk O, Pederson C, Cozzi-Lepri A, et al: Non-Hodgkin lymphoma in HIV-infected patients in the era of highly active antiretroviral therapy, *Blood* 98(12):3406–3412, 2001.

Krishnan A, Molina A, Zaia J, et al: Durable remissions with autologous stem cell transplantation for high-risk HIV-associated lymphomas, *Blood* 105:874–878, 2005.

Lim ST, Karim R, Nathwani BN, et al: AIDS-related Burkitt's lymphoma versus diffuse large-cell lymphoma in the pre-highly active antiretroviral therapy (HAART) and HAART eras: significant differences in survival with standard chemotherapy, *J Clin Oncol* 23:4430–4438, 2005.

Lim ST, Karim R, Tulpule A, et al: Prognostic factors in HIV-related diffuse large-cell lymphoma: before versus after highly active antiretroviral therapy, *J Clin Oncol* 23:8477–8482, 2005.

Little RF, Butierrez M, Jaffe ES, et al: HIV-associated non-Hodgkin's lymphoma: incidence, presentation, and prognosis, *J Am Med Assoc* 285(14):1880–1885, 2001.

Rabkin CS, Yang Q, Goedert JJ, et al: Chemokine and chemokine receptor gene variants and risk of non-Hodgkin's lymphoma in human immunodeficiency virus-1-infected individuals, *Blood* 93:1838–1842, 1999.

Ratner L, Lee J, Shengui T, et al: Chemotherapy for HIV-associated non-Hodgkin's lymphoma in combination with highly active antiretroviral therapy, *J Clin Oncol* 19:2171–2178, 2001.

Straus DJ, Huang J, Testa MA, et al: Prognostic factors in the treatment of human immunodeficiency virus associated non-Hodgkin's lymphoma: analysis of AIDS Clinical Trials Group protocol 142—low-dose versus standard-dose m-BACOD plus granulocyte-macrophage colony-stimulating factor. National Institute of Allergy and Infectious Diseases, *J Clin Oncol* 16:3601–3606, 1998.

Wang ES, Straus DJ, Teruya-Feldstein J, et al: Intensive chemotherapy with cyclophosphamide, doxorubicin, high-dose methotrexate/ifosfamide, etoposide, and high-dose cytarabine (CODOX-M/IVAC) for human immunodeficiency virus-associated Burkitt lymphoma, *Cancer* 98:1196–1205, 2003.

Hodgkin Lymphoma

Biggar RJ, Jaffe ES, Goedert JJ, et al: Hodgkin lymphoma and immunodeficiency in persons with HIV/AIDS, *Blood* 108:3786–3791, 2006.

Levine AM: HIV-associated Hodgkin's disease: biologic and clinical aspects, *Hematol Oncol Clin North Am* 10:1135–1148, 1996.

Re A, Casari S, Cattaneo C, et al: Hodgkin disease developing in patients infected by human immunodeficiency virus results in clinical features and a prognosis similar to those in patients with human immunodeficiency virus-related non-Hodgkin lymphoma, *Cancer* 92(11):2739–2745, 2001.

Xicoy B, Ribera JM, Miralles P, et al: Results of treatment with doxorubicin, bleomycin, vinblastine and dacarbazine and highly active antiretroviral therapy in advanced stage, human immunodeficiency virus-related Hodgkin's lymphoma, *Haematologica* 92:191–198, 2007.

Squamous Epithelial Lesions

Cranston RD, Hart SD, Gornbein JA, et al: The prevalence, and predictive value, of abnormal anal cytology to diagnose anal dysplasia in a population of HIV-positive men who have sex with men, *Int J STD AIDS* 18:77–80, 2007.

Frisch M, Biggar RJ, Goedert JJ: Human papillomavirus-associated cancers in patients with human immunodeficiency virus infection and acquired immunodeficiency syndrome, *J Natl Cancer Inst* 92(18):1500–1510, 2000.

Palefsky JM, Holly EA, Efirdc JT, et al: Anal intraepithelial neoplasia in the highly active antiretroviral therapy era among HIV-positive men who have sex with men, *AIDS* 19:1407–1414, 2005.

Peddada AV, Smith DE, Rao AR, et al: Chemotherapy and low-dose radiotherapy in the treatment of HIV-infected patients with carcinoma of the anal canal, *Int J Radiat Oncol Biol Phys* 37:1101–1105, 1997.

Sun XW, Kuhn L, Ellerbrock TV, et al: Human papillomavirus infection in women infected with the human immunodeficiency virus [see comments], *N Engl J Med* 337:1343–1349, 1997.

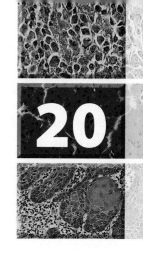

Complications of Cancer

NADINE JACKSON McCLEARY • ARTHUR T. SKARIN

Cancer affects all body systems, potentially leading to metabolic derangements, structural changes, and infection. Most individuals diagnosed with cancer will experience a complication at some time during their illness (Halfdanarson et al., 2006). Clinicians need to be able to recognize such complications so as to rapidly diagnose, treat, and prevent chronic sequelae. Complications of cancer include acute or subacute changes, sometimes also referred to as oncologic emergencies, and chronic changes. These may be categorized by the systems affected—infectious, structural, metabolic, hematologic, vascular, and neurologic (Table 20.1). Key complications and their pictorial descriptions are reviewed in this chapter.

Table 20.1
Complications of Cancer
Metabolic
Hypercalcemia
Hyponatremia
Tumor lysis syndrome
Lactic acidosis
Adrenal insufficiency
Infectious
Neutropenic fever
Typhlitis (cecitis)
Hematologic
Hyperviscosity syndrome
Hyperleukocystosis
Hypercoagulable states
Nonbacterial thrombotic endocarditis
Pulmonary embolism
Deep venous thrombosis
Trousseau's syndrome
Antiphospholipid syndrome
Sweet's syndrome
Vascular/Structural
Superior vena cava syndrome
Malignant pericardial effusion
Hemorrhagic cystitis
Malignant effusions
Pleural effusion
Pericardial effusion
Peritoneal effusion (ascites)
Neurologic
Spinal cord compression
Intracranial metastases
Leptomeningeal carcinomatosis
Paraneoplastic Syndromes (see Chapter 5, Table 5.7)

Infectious Complications

NEUTROPENIC FEVER

Infections in cancer account for a significant portion of morbidity and mortality, particularly in patients receiving chemotherapy. Neutropenic fever is defined as an oral temperature of 38°C (100.4°F) or greater in the setting of an absolute neutrophil count less than 1×10^9 per liter. It is more likely to occur with longer duration and depth of neutrophil nadir. Although the causative agents often elude diagnosis, enteric gram-negative bacilli are the most common organisms recovered from blood cultures. Factors favoring a lower risk of serious infection in the setting of neutropenic fever include absolute monocyte count of 1×10^9 per liter or more, normal chest radiograph, duration of neutropenia less than 7 days, no intravenous catheter site infection, and malignancy in remission (Table 20.2). Some studies support the use of white blood cell growth factors to prevent or reduce the occurrence of neutropenic fever. Patients may present with symptoms supporting infection, although some patients are asymptomatic with the exception of a fever. Management comprises obtaining cultures of blood, urine, wounds, and cerebrospinal fluid (CSF) if applicable, as well as initiating broad-spectrum antibiotics. A fungal blood culture and antifungal medications are added if the patient does not defervesce within

Table 20.2
Factors That Favor Low Risk for Severe Infection in Patients with Neutropenic Fever
Absolute neutrophil count $\geq 1.0 \times 10^9$ cells/L
Absolute monocyte count $\geq 1.0 \times 10^9$ cells/L
Normal chest radiograph
Normal or only minimally abnormal renal and liver chemical test results
Duration of neutropenia <7 days
Resolution of neutropenia expected in <10 days
No intravenous catheter-site infection
Early evidence of bone marrow recovery
Malignancy in remission
Peak temperature of <39°C
No mental or neurologic changes
No appearance of illness
No abdominal pain
No comorbidity complications (e.g., shock, hypoxia, pneumonia, deep-organ infection, vomiting, or diarrhea)

From Halfdanarson TR, Hogan WJ, Moynihan TJ: Oncologic emergencies: diagnosis and treatment, *Mayo Clin Proc* 81(6): 835–848, 2006.

Table 20.3

Multinational Association for Supportive Care in Cancer Scoring System for Patients with Neutropenic Fever*

Characteristic	Score
Burden of illness: no or mild symptoms	5
No hypotension	5
No chronic obstructive pulmonary disease	4
Solid tumor or no previous fungal infection	4
No dehydration	3
Burden of illness: moderate symptoms	3
Outpatient status	3
Age <60 years	2

*Patients with a total score of ≥21 have a low risk of having serious medical complications. Points attributed to the variable "burden of illness" are not cumulative. Therefore, the maximum theoretical score is 26.
From Halfdanarson TR, Hogan WJ, Moynihan TJ: Oncologic emergencies: diagnosis and treatment, *Mayo Clin Proc* 81(6): 835–848, 2006.

24 hours of presentation. Patients with a total score of 21 or more on the Multinational Association for Supportive Care Cancer Scoring System have a low risk of serious complications from neutropenic fever (Table 20.3).

Metabolic Complications

HYPERCALCEMIA

Hypercalcemia occurs in up to 30% of patients during the course of their malignancy. Hypercalcemia is one of the complications of malignancy with skeletal involvement (Table 20.4). Although it occurs predominantly in lung, breast, and multiple myeloma cancer, any malignancy can be associated with high levels of serum calcium (Coleman, 1997). Hypercalcemia is mediated by ectopic parathyroid hormone production (parathyroid hormone–related protein), generation of vitamin D analogues, or cytokine-induced local bone destruction. Parathyroid hormone–related protein, usually detected in cases of hypercalcemia associated with small cell lung cancer, mimics the action of parathyroid hormone, leading to bone resorption and distal tubular calcium resorption. In contrast, hypercalcemia associated with lymphoma is mediated by the generation of vitamin D analogues, such as calcitriol. The sequelae of hypercalcemia include constipation, psychosis, lethargy, excessive thirst and urination, hypovolemia, and renal failure. Treatment includes aggressive intravenous hydration and bisphosphonates to block osteoclastic bone resorption. Dialysis may also be required.

HYPONATREMIA

Hyponatremia may occur due to the syndrome of inappropriate antidiuretic hormone secretion (SIADH) or salt-wasting

Table 20.4

Frequency of Major Complications of Skeletal Involvement*

Complication	No. (%) of Patients
Hypercalcemia of malignancy	70 (19%)
Pathologic feature of a long bone	68 (19%)
Spinal cord compression	36 (10%)
Bone marrow failure/leukoerythroblastic anemia	33 (9%)

*Data from Coleman et al. (1997).

nephropathy. SIADH is due to ectopic vasopressin production by tumor leading to renal retention of water and reduced aldosterone secretion associated with sodium loss in the urine and consequent reduced serum osmolarity. Chemotherapy, particularly high-dose cyclophosphamide and cisplatin, can also contribute to SIADH. Patients may present with euvolemia or hypovolemia. In hypovolemic states, oliguria and low urine sodium levels characterize SIADH. In contrast, nonoliguria and high urine sodium levels in the setting of hypovolemia characterize salt-wasting nephropathy. Salt-wasting nephropathy can occur as a result of chemotherapy, adrenal insufficiency, or cerebral salt wasting after intracranial surgery or subarachnoid hemorrhage. Treatment of hyponatremia includes water and salt restriction, hypertonic saline to slowly correct serum sodium levels, and administration of vasopressin receptor antagonists as indicated (Spinazze and Schrijvers, 2006).

TUMOR LYSIS SYNDROME

Tumor lysis syndrome occurs when intracellular materials are released from rapidly dying tumor cells leading to excess serum levels of uric acid, potassium, phosphorus, and reduced levels of calcium. The Cairo-Bishop definition of tumor lysis syndrome includes criteria for laboratory evaluation (Table 20.5) and a grading classification (Table 20.6). These metabolic derangements often occur within 5 days of chemotherapy or irradiation and can lead to hypovolemia, renal failure, seizures, and cardiac arrhythmias. Treatment involves frequent monitoring of serum laboratory values, aggressive intravenous hydration, alkalinization of the urine, and uric acid sequestrants (allopurinol or rasburicase).

ADRENAL INSUFFICIENCY

Adrenal insufficiency results when mineralocorticoids and glucocorticoids stores are reduced in the adrenal gland (see Chapter 5). Secondary or tertiary adrenal insufficiency is the most common manifestation of adrenal failure. Primary adrenal failure (Addison's disease) is uncommon, requiring over 90% of the adrenal gland to be replaced by tumor (Spinazze and Schrijvers 2006). Megestrol acetate administration is the most frequent cause of secondary adrenal failure associated with cancer while chronic corticosteroid administration is frequently the cause of tertiary adrenal failure. Patients present with symptoms of decreased appetite, weight loss, fatigue, and nausea and vomiting, and signs of hyperpigmentation and postural hypotension. Adrenal insufficiency should be suspected in patients receiving

Table 20.5

Cairo-Bishop Definition of Laboratory Tumor Lysis Syndrome and Clinical Tumor Lysis Syndrome

Laboratory tumor lysis syndrome
  Uric acid ≥8 mg/dL (≥476 μmol/L) or 25% increase from baseline
  Potassium ≥6.0 mEq/L (≥6 mmol/L) or 25% increase from baseline
  Phosphorus ≥6.5 mg/dL (≥2.1 mmol/L) or 25% increase from baseline
  Calcium ≤7 mg/dL (≤1.75 mmol/L) or 25% decrease from baseline
Clinical tumor lysis syndrome
  Creatinine ≥1.5 times upper limit of normal
  Cardiac arrhythmia or sudden death
  Seizure

From Halfdanarson TR, Hogan WJ, Moynihan TJ: Oncologic emergencies: diagnosis and treatment, *Mayo Clin Proc* 81(6): 835–848, 2006; adapted from *Br J Haematol*, with permission from Blackwell Publishing Group. Copyright © 2004. All rights reserved.

Table 20.6

Cairo-Bishop Grading Classification of Tumor Lysis Syndrome

	Grade 0*	Grade I	Grade II	Grade III	Grade IV	Grade V
LTLS	No	Yes	Yes	Yes	Yes	Yes
Creatinine[†]	≤1.5 × ULN	1.5 × ULN	>1.5–3.0 × ULN	>3.0–6.0 × ULN	>6 × ULN	Death[‡]
Cardiac arrhythmia[†]	None	Intervention not needed	Nonurgent intervention needed	Symptomatic and incompletely controlled medically or controlled with a device	Life-threatening (e.g., arrhythmia associated with CHF, hypotension, or shock)	Death[‡]
Seizures[†]	None	None	One brief, generalized seizure, seizures controlled with anticonvulsant drugs, or infrequent motor seizures	Seizures with impaired consciousness, poorly controlled seizures, generalized seizures despite medical interventions	Status epilepticus	Death[‡]

CHF, congestive heart failure; LTLS, laboratory tumor lysis syndrome; ULN, institutional upper limit of normal adjusted for age and sex.
*Not LTLS.
[†]Not attributable to a therapeutic drug or an intervention.
[‡]Attributable probably or definitively to clinical tumor lysis syndrome.
From Halfdanarson TR, Hogan WJ, Moynihan TJ: Oncologic emergencies: diagnosis and treatment, *Mayo Clin Proc* 81(6): 835–848, 2006; adapted from *Br J Haematol*, with permission from Blackwell Publishing Group. Copyright © 2004. All rights reserved.

megestrol acetate or chronic corticosteroid therapy, or in patients with documented metastatic disease to the adrenal glands. It can be diagnosed using a low-dose adrenocorticotrophic hormone stimulation test. Treatment is based on repletion of depleted mineralocorticoid and glucocorticoid stores.

LACTIC ACIDOSIS

Lactic acidosis is defined as accumulation of serum lactate in the setting of metabolic acidosis (serum pH <7.37). It occurs as a result of hypoperfusion or ischemic states as well as in association with predisposing diseases, including cancer. Patients present with signs and symptoms of poor organ perfusion (e.g., confusion, decreased urine output, hypotension, tachycardia). Treatment includes targeted therapy for the underlying disease (chemotherapy in the case of cancer) and volume replacement.

Hematologic Complications

HYPERVISCOSITY SYNDROME

Excess production of abnormal proteins occurring in leukemia, Waldenstrom's macroglobulinemia, and multiple myeloma can lead to increased blood viscosity. This is particularly prominent in Waldenstrom's macroglobulinemia as a result of excess production of immunoglobulin M (IgM) or in other IgG, IgD, IgE, or IgA myeloma. IgA can polymerize to form larger molecules. Symptoms of hyperviscosity due to impaired perfusion of organs (brain, kidney, eyes) occur at serum visocity levels of greater than 4 centipoise or with serum IgM levels of greater than 4 g/L. Management includes intravenous fluid hydration, avoiding blood product transfusions that can exacerbate hyperviscosity, treatment of the underlying disease with chemotherapy, and plasmapheresis.

LEUKOSTASIS

Hyperleukocytosis, generally defined as white blood cell count greater than 100,000 cells/μL, occurs in acute leukemia, particularly in acute myeloid leukemia because of the larger size of myeloblasts contributing to leukostasis at lower cell counts than lymphoid leukemias. Symptoms of leukostasis are similar to those of hyperviscosity syndrome given increased blood viscosity leading to poor perfusion of organs. Additionally, dyspnea due to pulmonary infiltrates of leukocytes is common, as are thrombocytopenia and coagulopathy (see Fig. 15.107). Similar to hyperviscosity syndrome, which can also be caused by leukostasis, reduction of the viscous state is imperative to prevent complications of viscosity. This is achieved with treatment of the underlying disease, intravenous fluid hydration, and leukapheresis once the leukocyte count exceeds 1×10^9 per liter.

HYPERCOAGULABLE STATES

Overall 15% of cancer patients suffer a thrombotic event during the course of their illness; up to 50% of patients are noted to have thromboses at autopsy (el-Shami et al., 2007). Patients with cancer are thought to be more susceptible to thromboembolic disease due to alterations in the procoagulant cascade and increased host inflammatory response both favoring coagulation (Horton, 2005a). Cancer-associated thrombophilia presents as a range of disease including venous thromboembolism (pulmonary embolism, deep venous thrombosis), migratory thrombophlebitis (Trousseau's syndrome), arterial thrombosis, disseminated intravascular coagulation, thrombotic microangiopathy, or nonbacterial thrombotic endocarditis (marantic endocarditis; NBTE) (Bell et al., 1985; el-Shami et al., 2007; Varki, 2007).

NONBACTERIAL THROMBOTIC ENDOCARDITIS

The average incidence of NBTE is 42% (el-Shami et al., 2007). It is associated with 25% of ischemic cerebrovascular strokes in cancer patients (Newton, 1999). It is due to sterile vegetations of collections of degenerating platelets interwoven with fibrin on previously undamaged cardiac valves in the absence of bacterial infection often called marantic endocarditis (NBTE; Newton, 1999; el-Shami et al., 2007). The aortic and mitral valves are primarily affected, although any cardiac valve is susceptible to involvement. Patients present with organ embolic phenomena, particularly in the central nervous system and coronary arteries. Symptoms are due to systemic emboli and not to valvular dysfunction (Horton, 2005b). NBTE should be suspected in cancer patients with sudden-onset neurologic deficit. It is best diagnosed with transesophageal echocardiography as well as diffusion-weighted magnetic resonance imaging (MRI) as indicated. Treatment involves indefinite anticoagulation.

ANTIPHOSPHOLIPID SYNDROME

Antiphospholipid syndrome usually occurs secondary to another disease, such as autoimmune disorders or malignancy. It is characterized by recurrent vascular thrombosis, thrombocytopenia, prolongation of activated partial thromboplastin time or prothrombin time, marantic endocarditis, or pregnancy loss due to increased levels of antiphospholipid antibodies (Miesbach et al., 2006). Antiphospholipid syndrome may precede the diagnosis of cancer in some patients and is therefore considered a paraneoplastic phenomenon due to an autoimmune-mediated thrombophilic state. Diagnosis is based on detection of phospholipid antibodies (anticardiolipin antibodies, anti-β_2-glycoprotein I, and lupus anticoagulant). Anticoagulation is the mainstay of treatment.

Vascular Complications

SUPERIOR VENA CAVA SYNDROME

Compression of the superior vena cava (SVC) is a characteristic presentation of lung cancer and lymphoma. It occurs as a result of extrinsic compression of the SVC by tumor but can also occur as a result of intraluminal extension of tumor or in association with indwelling central venous catheters. Patients typically present with bilateral facial swelling and shortness of breath worsened with forward position further limiting venous return. Additionally, patients may have prominent superficial collateral vessels evident on the neck, chest, and upper extremities. Management entails diagnosis of malignancy, radiation therapy to reduce tumor bulk, and SVC stenting if necessary (Higdon and Higdon, 2006) (see Fig. 5.55).

Neurologic Complications

As many as 20% of cancer patients suffer neurologic complications during their illness (Newton, 1999).

SPINAL CORD COMPRESSION

As many as 5% to 14% of patients with malignancy experience spinal cord compression during the duration of their illness, with breast, lung, and prostate cancer accounting for two thirds of these cases (Newton, 1999). In fact, spinal cord compression is the first manifestation of cancer in a quarter of patients. The patient's neurologic status and duration of symptoms at presentation are predictive of neurologic outcome. Initial compression of the spinal cord by extension of neoplastic disease from the vertebral bodies into the spinal canal can lead to spinal cord edema and then spinal cord ischemia with irreversible neurologic injury. The majority of patients present with back pain with varying degrees of motor weakness, bowel or bladder dysfunction,

and gait disturbance. Diagnosis of spinal cord compression is best done using MRI of the spine, although plain radiographs can be used to detect some symptomatic spinal cord metastases with sensitivity of 85% to 90%. Management consists of rapid recognition, steroid administration to reduce spinal cord edema, radiation therapy, and neurosurgical evaluation for possible surgical intervention. Of patients who are ambulatory at presentation, 80% remain so after treatment in comparison to only 5% to 10% of patients who are paraplegic at presentation.

INTRACRANIAL METASTASES

Intracranial metastases occur in 20% to 40% of adult patients with cancer (Newton, 1999). Although many malignant conditions are associated with intracranial metastasis, presentation with neurologic disease warrants rapid evaluation given concern for increased intracranial pressure, seizures, and possible hemorrhagic stroke. Intracranial metastases occur most often in advanced disease and portend a poor prognosis. The primary sites in order of frequency are lung (50% to 60%), breast (15% to 20%), melanoma (5% to 10%), gastrointestinal (4% to 6%), genitourinary (3% to 5%), unknown (4% to 8%), other (3% to 5%). Treatment involves steroids to reduce edema, anticonvulsants to prevent seizures, and radiation therapy or surgical resection as appropriate.

LEPTOMENINGEAL CARCINOMATOSIS

Leptomeningeal carcinomatosis, also known as carcinomatosis meningitis, occurs in up to 8% of cancers as a late complication of progressive neoplastic disease (Pavlidis, 2004). It is most often seen in breast malignancies (5%), lung malignancies (9% to 25%), and melanoma (23%), but is also known to occur in hematologic malignancies as well (see Figs. 5.75, 10.67, 14.91, 16.120, 16.122). Leptomeningeal carcinomatosis occurs when tumor cells spread into the CSF of the subarachnoid space separating the arachnoid membrane from the pia mater. Tumor cells spread via hematogenous or lymphatic routes, via direct extension from a primary brain tumor, or via seeding during surgical resection. The spine is primarily affected in 75% to 80% of cases; the brain is additionally affected in up to 50% of cases. Symptoms and signs of leptomeningeal carcinomatosis include cranial nerve palsies, cerebral signs, headache, spinal nerve disorder, altered mental status, weakness, gait disturbance, and seizure. Diagnosis is based on lumbar puncture results; cerebrospinal protein elevation (sensitivity 75%), increased opening pressure (sensitivity 50% to 70%), decreased glucose (sensitivity 40%), and pleocytosis are characteristic. Gadolinium-enhanced MRI has a sensitivity of 70% in comparison to computed tomography (CT) scans (sensitivity 30%) for leptomeningeal carcinomatosis. Treatment often consists of intrathecal chemotherapy and sometimes radiation therapy.

PARANEOPLASTIC SYNDROMES

Cancer causes dysfunction of both nerve and muscle due to tumor infiltration, compression, or direct extension. This occurs in the form of cranial neuropathies, brachial and lumbosacral plexopathy, chemotherapy-induced neuropathy, paraneoplastic neuropathy, paraneoplastic disorders (e.g., inflammatory myopathies, Lambert-Eaton syndrome) (Newton, 1999). Lumbosacral or brachial plexopathy is often associated with an apical lung mass (Pancoast tumor). Paraneoplastic syndromes encompass all body systems and usually precede cancer diagnosis. Paraneoplastic neurologic disorders occur via an immune response to ectopic expression of neuronal antigens by tumor with pathology showing loss of neurons in affected areas with inflammatory infiltration by CD4+ T-helper cells, CD8+ T cells, and B cells (Table 21.7). Incidence varies with tumor type. Immunotherapy is usually not helpful in reversing the disorder, although rapid diagnosis of the underlying malignancy and subsequent treatment may reverse or stabilize the paraneoplastic disorder.

Subacute Cerebellar Degeneration

Subacute cerebellar degeneration occurs in the acute or subacute setting, stabilizing over months, and is the most commonly occurring paraneoplastic neurologic disorder. Patients present with nausea, vomiting, ataxia, weakness, diplopia, nystagmus,

mental status change, and dysarthria. MRI and CT imaging may reveal cerebellar atrophy later in the course of the disease. Anti-Yo, anti-Tr, and anti-mGluR1 are the antineuronal antibodies most frequently associated with cerebellar degeneration.

Limbic Encephalitis

Limbic encephalitis is a rare, subacute process involving the limbic system and hypothalamus. At least half of patients presenting with limbic encephalitis are later diagnosed with a malignancy. This most often occurs in the setting of lung disease, specifically small cell lung cancer, (with anti-Hu antibodies) and testicular germ cell (with anti-Ma2 antibodies) cancer. Another group of patients present without any associated antineuronal antibody. All present with memory impairment, confusion, seizures, hyperthermia, and endocrine abnormalities (de Beukelaar

Table 20.7

Paraneoplastic Neurologic Syndromes and Their Response to Treatment

Clinical Syndrome	Autoantibody	Response to Immunotherapy	Response to Tumor Therapy	Comments
Encephalomyelitis	Hu (ANNA-1)	No established effect	Stabilizes the patient in better condition	Spontaneous improvement very rarely described
Limbic encephalitis	Hu (ANNA-1), Ma2	Some patients respond	May improve	Partial improvement may occur spontaneously
Subacute cerebellar degeneration	Yo (PCA-1)	No established effect	No effect on neurologic outcome	
	Tr (PCA-Tr), mGluR1	May improve	May improve	Subacute cerebellar degeneration associated with Hodgkin disease may also improve spontaneously
Opsoclonus-myoclonus (adults)	Ri (ANNA-2)	May improve	Partial neurologic recovery	Thiamin, baclofen, and clonazepam may be effective
Opsoclonus-myoclonus (pediatric)	No antibody	Two thirds improve	Partial neurologic recovery	
Stiff-person syndrome	Amphiphysin	May improve	May improve	Responds to baclofen, diazepam, valproate, vigabatrine, and carbamazepine; painful spasms may require opioids
Cancer-associated retinopathy	Recoverin	Vision may slightly improve	No established effect	
Melanoma-associated retinopathy	Anti-bipolar cells	Anecdotal vision improvement	Anecdotal vision improvement	
Paraneoplastic optic neuropathy	CV2/CRMP5	Anecdotal vision improvement	Anecdotal vision improvement	
Subacute sensory neuronopathy	Hu (ANNA-1)	No established effect; rare partial responses	Stabilizes the patient in better condition	Treatment of neuropathic pain with tricyclic antidepressants and antiepileptic drugs
Chronic sensorimotor neuropathy with M protein	MAG (IgM)	May improve	May improve	
Chronic sensorimotor neuropathy with osteosclerotic myeloma	No antibody	No established effect	Often responds	Radiation therapy, chemotherapy, and surgery effective
Subacute autonomic neuropathy	Hu	No established effect	No established effect	Symptomatic treatment of orthostatic hypotension; neostigmine in pseudo-obstruction
Paraneoplastic peripheral nerve vasculitis	Hu	May improve	May improve	
Lambert-Eaton myasthenic syndrome	P/Q-type VGCC	Often responds	Often responds	2,3-diaminopyridine; cholinesterase inhibitors may be tried (efficacy unclear)
Myasthenia gravis	AChR	Often responds	Often responds	Cholinesterase inhibitors
Neuromyotonia	VGKC	May respond	Not known	Antiepileptic drugs (carbamazepine, phenytoin)
Dermatomyositis	Mi-2	Usually responds	May respond	

AChR, acetylcholine receptor; ANNA, antineuronal nuclear antibody; MAG, myelin-associated glycoprotein; mGluR1, metabotropic glutamate receptor type 1; PCA, Purkinje cytoplasmic antibody; VGCC, voltage-gated calcium channels; VGKC, voltage-gated potassium channel.
Data from de Beukelaar JW, Sillevis Smitt PA: Managing paraneoplastic neurological disorders, *Oncologist* 11(3):292–305, 2006.

and Sillevis Smitt, 2006). MRI studies may be diagnostic in up to 80% of patients, as is lumbar puncture with CSF showing pleocytosis, protein elevation, and the presence of IgG or oligoclonal bands.

Lambert-Eaton Myasthenic Syndrome

Lambert-Eaton myasthenic syndrome occurs most frequently in the setting of small cell lung cancer. Patients present with proximal weakness of the lower extremities, muscle fatigue on repeated stimulation, and decreased or absent deep tendon reflexes of the lower extremities, and they later develop autonomic dysfunction. Approximately 20% of patients present with anti-MysB antibodies. Electromyographic testing is diagnostic with a classic pattern of muscle potential variation with levels of repetitive stimulation.

Dermatologic Complications

Patients presenting with a heliotrope rash characteristic of dermatomyositis are at a sixfold increased risk for malignant disease. The rash often precedes proximal muscle weakness that also occurs in this disease. Patients present with anti-Mi2 antibodies in one third of cases. A biopsy of muscle or involved skin is diagnostic. Other dermatologic paraneoplastic syndromes include acanthosis nigricans, acquired ichthyosis, paraneoplastic pemphigus, pyoderma gangrenosum, and Sweet syndrome (see Fig. 15.45) (Chung et al., 2006).

Structural Complications

MALIGNANT EFFUSIONS

Body cavity effusion in the setting of cancer portends a poor prognosis, because it indicates spread of the disease beyond the primary site and heralds disease progression (Davidson, 2004; Haas et al., 2007). Effusions typically occur in pleural, peritoneal, and pericardial spaces. In women, effusions occur in the setting of breast or ovarian adenocarcinoma. In fact, peritoneal effusions (ascites) are present in 66% of ovarian cancer patients at diagnosis (Davidson, 2004). In both genders, effusions occur most often in the setting of lung cancer or malignant mesothelioma. Diagnosis is made based on morphologic examination of cytology as well as immunocytochemistry, and genetic analysis using fluorescent in-situ hybridization and reverse transcription–polymerase chain reaction.

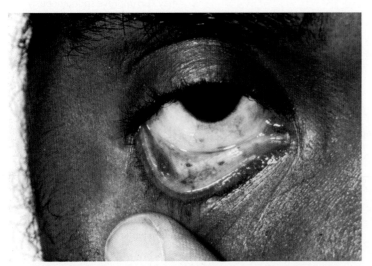

FIGURE 20.1 **JANEWAY LESIONS OF ENDOCARDITIS IN A MAN WITH LUNG CANCER.** These conjunctival lesions represent thromboembolic phenomena associated with endocarditis and occlusion of end vessels. Presentation with these phenomena should prompt rapid evaluation for thromboembolic disease and associated diseases, in this case, lung cancer.

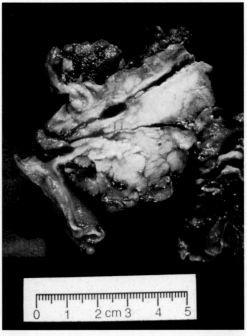

FIGURE 20.2 Pancreatic cancer with tumor infiltration causing external compression of the pancreatic duct. Patients may present with obstructive symptoms, including jaundice, nausea, vomiting, and possibly abdominal pain in the epigastric or right upper quadrant regions. Evaluation includes laboratory evaluation as well as imaging with CT scan, endoscopic retrograde cholangiopancreatography, or MR cholangiopancreatography.

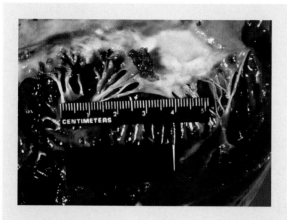
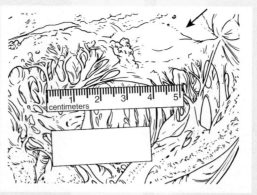

FIGURE 20.3 **MARANTIC ENDOCARDITIS IN A PATIENT WITH METASTATIC COLON CANCER AT AUTOPSY.** Thrombi shown are noninfectious but can lead to serious complications inclusive of myocardial infarction, cerebrovascular accident, or even death. If detected rapidly, indefinite anticoagulation is warranted.

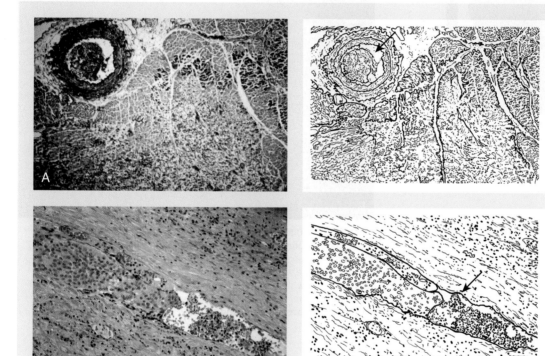

FIGURE 20.4. Pathologic picture denoting partial **(A)** and complete **(B)** arterial occlusion by thrombus associated with a tissue infarct.

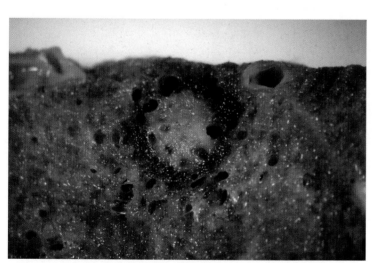

FIGURE 20.5 Pulmonary *Aspergillus* infection with characteristic gross targetoid appearance. Pulmonary infections are common in the setting of neutropenic fever. Severe infections are associated with the duration of neutropenia, the depth of the nadir, and the status of the malignancy.

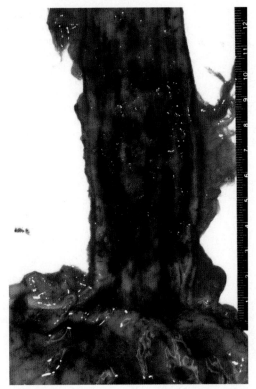

FIGURE 20.6 Candidal esophagitis is one of the most common infectious etiologies in malignancy. It is associated with neutropenia, malnutrition, mucositis, and steroid use.

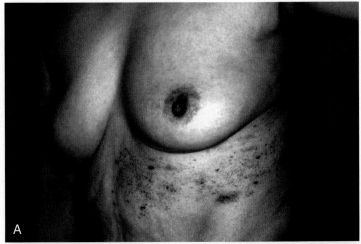

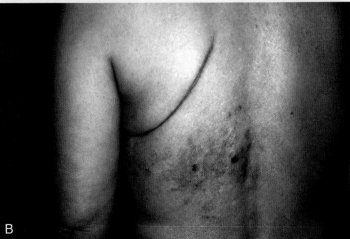

FIGURE 20.7 **HERPES ZOSTER, LEFT CHEST WALL.** This 50-year-old woman with recent thoracotomy for lung cancer has two reasons for left chest pain: post-thoracotomy pain syndrome and the pain associated with herpes zoster. In this patient there seems to be no connection between the two problems. **(A)** Anterior view shows the dermatome distribution of the zoster. **(B)** Lateral view shows the recent healing thoracotomy site. Note that the dermatome involvement by zoster ends at the midline.

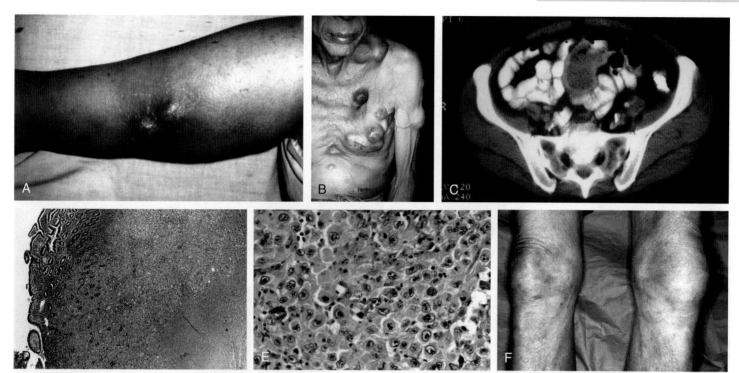

FIGURE 20.8 **METASTATIC CANCER SITES.** Virtually any tissue or organ can be involved by disseminated disease. **(A)** Skin metastases are very common, as noted in this patient with colon cancer presenting with a cluster of upper arm lesions. **(B)** Multiple skin as well as nodal metastases occurred in the 65-year-old man with small cell lung cancer. Most skin metastases are symptomatic, but some cause considerable local pain. Other cancers that commonly spread to the skin include malignant melanoma, breast, pancreas, and lymphoma. **(C)** Gastrointestinal involvement. In this 63-year-old patient with previously resected non–small cell lung cancer, sudden abdominal pain and small bowel obstruction heralded isolated metastases as diagnosed on this CT scan. **(D)** Successful resection of a bowel segment was carried out on the patient shown in **C**. Histologic section shows low-power view of bowel wall with metastatic poorly differentiated adenocarcinoma. **(E)** Higher-power view shows the malignant cells. The patient was evaluated, and no other sites of disease were found. Most patients, however, are found to have other metastases requiring treatment. **(F)** Knee metastases from lung cancer occurred in this man with involvement of only the left patella, an unusual event. Spread to distal bone sites, called acrometastases, is uncommon.

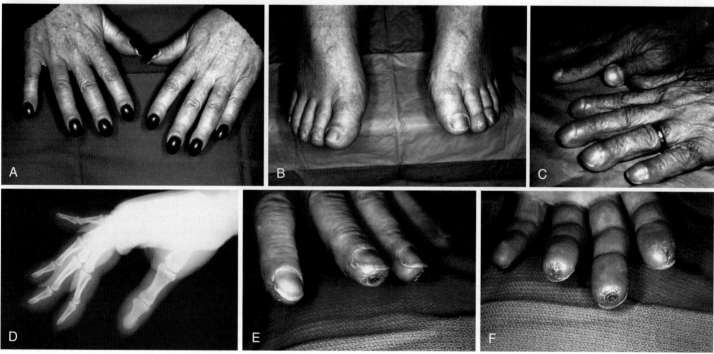

FIGURE 20.9 **DIGITAL CLUBBING (HYPERTROPHIC PULMONARY OSTEOARTHROPATHY, HPO).** **(A)** This 47-year-old woman presented with gradual asymptomatic thickening of her distal fingers. She was referred to an arthritis specialist who astutely carried out a chest radiograph to diagnose early lung cancer. **(B)** Her toes also show clubbing. **(C)** This 65-year-old man presented with dramatic HPO of gradual onset but associated with digital pain. A resectable non–small cell lung cancer was diagnosed. His pain regressed after thoracotomy with successful resection. **(D)** Digital radiographs show soft tissue swelling along with a slight digital flair, especially in the distal thumb. Bone scan abnormalities with periosteal elevation in the tibia can occur in HPO associated with leg edema and pain, often misdiagnosed as congestive heart failure, cellulitis, or arthritis. **(E, F)** HPO and skin necrosis. This 48-year-old man who smoked three to four packs of cigarettes per day presented with digital clubbing but also had very painful ulcers and necrosis of skin at the fingertips. Stage IIIB non–small cell lung cancer was diagnosed along with Buerger disease of the fingertips (thromboangiitis obliterans) related to the heavy cigarette smoking. His lung cancer regressed after treatment with chemotherapy and radiation therapy, but his Buerger disease responded only to complete discontinuation of smoking cigarettes.

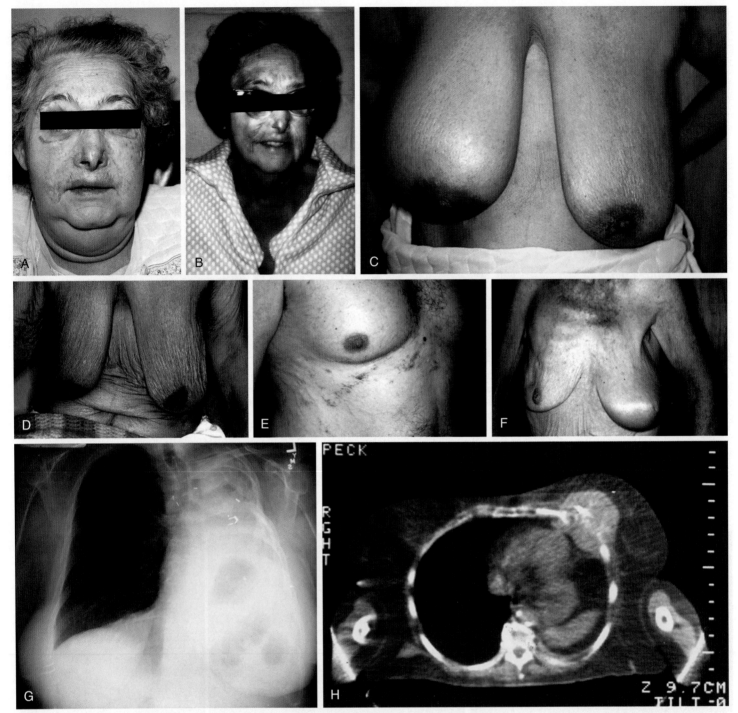

FIGURE 20.10 SVC syndrome usually occurs in the setting of advanced lung cancer or lymphoma, but almost any malignancy can cause it by external compression of the SVC or direct intraluminal tumor extension. It may be complicated by clot formation requiring anticoagulation or placement of a stent in chronic cases. Rarely, benign diseases like infection or fibrosis from a variety of etiologies can be causative, and thus an intensive workup is recommended. (See Fig. 5.55.) **(A)** This 68-year-old woman had an unusual breast cancer relapse with a solitary tumor mass surrounding the SVC with resultant face and neck edema. **(B)** Dramatic regression of the SVC syndrome 2 months later after localized radiation therapy to the tumor site. **(C)** SVC syndrome may sometimes present with gradual breast enlargement due to edema as occurred in this 74-year-old woman with metastatic sarcoma to the mediastinum. **(D)** Dramatic improvement occurred 2½ months later after radiation therapy. **(E)** SVC syndrome results in development of collateral circulation around the obstructed site with dilated skin veins and capillaries both on the chest and abdomen. This 50-year-old man had underlying advanced lung cancer. **(F)** Unilateral breast edema. This unusual problem occurred in a 74-year-old woman with locally advanced non–small cell lung cancer that invaded the chest wall and left breast causing lymphatic obstruction, simulating an early SVC syndrome. **(G)** Chest radiograph of the patient shown in **F** showing a left lung cancer with adenopathy and atelectasis and enlarged left breast. **(H)** CT scan of a patient showing invasion of the lung cancer through the chest wall into the left breast. In some cases, the opposite occurs, with primary breast cancer invading the lungs directly with or without parenchymal, pleural, and nodal metastases.

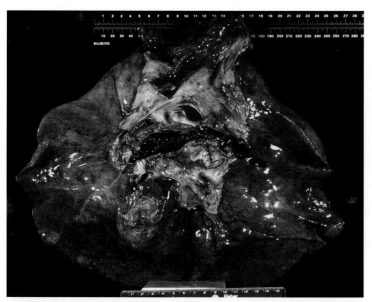

FIGURE 20-11 PULMONARY EMBOLI This gross specimen of the central thorax dramatically illustrated a large fatal "saddle embolism" to both the right and left pulmonary arteries in a 60-year-old patient with lung cancer. Increasing clotting occurs commonly in cancer patients (see text) and can lead to Trousseau's syndrome, which is characterized by migratory thrombophlebitis. Early diagnosis is important for use of heparin and new heparin-related drugs to reverse these vascular complications.

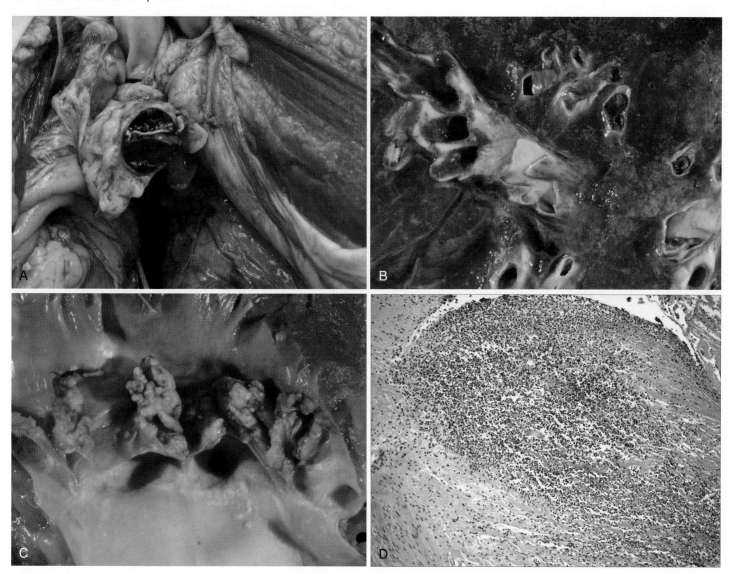

FIGURE 20.12 Clotting problems and acute bacterial endocarditis resulted in the demise of a 39-year-old man with advanced metastatic adenocarcinoma of the esophagus. **(A)** Inferior vena cava thrombus is noted, related to an underlying hypercoagulable state. **(B)** The lung shows multiple pulmonary vessels with emboli. **(C)** Acute bacterial endocarditis is evident on the mitral valve. **(D)** Microscopic view of acute bacterial endocarditis due to gram-positive cocci. The patient also had acute bronchopneumonia with sepsis, myocarditis, and glomerulonephritis. (Images courtesy of Drs. Stefan Kraft and Betsy Steensma, Department of Pathology, Brigham and Women's Hospital, Boston, MA.)

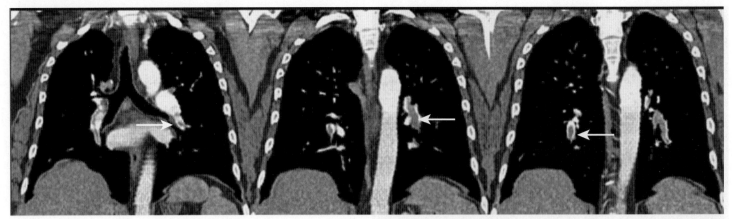

FIGURE 20.13 Early diagnosis of a pulmonary embolism can be made by a CT scan with contrast as noted in this image from a 55-year-old man with sudden chest pain and shortness of breath (see *arrow* indicating clots in right and left pulmonary arteries). (Images courtesy of Dr. Ciaran Johnston, Department of Radiology, Dana-Farber Cancer Institute, Boston, MA.)

References and Suggested Readings

Bell WR, et al: Trousseau's syndrome: devastating coagulopathy in the absence of heparin, *Am J Med* 79(4):423–430, 1985.

de Beukelaar JW, Sillevis Smitt PA: Managing paraneoplastic neurological disorders, *Oncologist* 11(3):292–305, 2006.

Cho S, Ra YJ, Lee C-T, et al: Difficulties in diagnosis and management of ectopic Cushing syndrome, *J Thorac Oncol*, 3:444–446, 2008.

Chung VQ, et al: Clinical and pathologic findings of paraneoplastic dermatoses, *J Am Acad Dermatol* 54(5):745–762, 2006; quiz 763–766.

Coleman RE: Skeletal complications of malignancy, *Cancer* 80(Suppl 8):1588–1594, 1997.

Davidson B: Malignant effusions: from diagnosis to biology, *Diagn Cytopathol* 31(4):246–254, 2004.

el-Shami K, Griffiths E, Streiff M: Nonbacterial thrombotic endocarditis in cancer patients: pathogenesis, diagnosis, and treatment, *Oncologist* 12(5):518–523, 2007.

Haas AR, Sterman DH, Musani AI: Malignant pleural effusions: management options with consideration of coding, billing, and a decision approach, *Chest* 132(3):1036–1041, 2007.

Halfdanarson TR, Hogan WJ, Moynihan TJ: Oncologic emergencies: diagnosis and treatment, *Mayo Clin Proc* 81(6):835–848, 2006.

Higdon ML, Higdon JA: Treatment of oncologic emergencies, *Am Fam Physician* 74(11):1873–1880, 2006.

Horton J: Venous thromboembolism and cancer: current issues and treatment updates, *Cancer Control* 12(Suppl 1):3–4, 2005b; quiz 38–40.

Horton J: Venous thrombotic events in cancer: the bottom line, *Cancer Control* 12(Suppl 1):31–37, 2005a.

Lyman GH, Khorana AA, Falanga A, et al: American society of clinical oncology guideline: recommendations for venous thromboembolism prophylaxis and treatment in patients with cancer, *J Clin Oncol* 25:5490–5505, 2007.

Miesbach W, Scharrer I, Asherson R: Thrombotic manifestations of the antiphospholipid syndrome in patients with malignancies, *Clin Rheumatol* 25(6):840–844, 2006.

Newton HB: Neurologic complications of systemic cancer, *Am Fam Physician* 59(4):878–886, 1999.

Pavlidis N: The diagnostic and therapeutic management of leptomeningeal carcinomatosis, *Ann Oncol* 15(Suppl 4):iv285–iv291, 2004.

Spinazze S, Schrijvers D: Metabolic emergencies, *Crit Rev Oncol Hematol* 58(1):79–89, 2006.

Varki A: Trousseau's syndrome: multiple definitions and multiple mechanisms, *Blood* 110(6):1723–1729, 2007.

Yu JB, Wilson LD, Detterbeck FC: Superior vena cava syndrome—a proposed classification system and algorithm for management, *J Thorac Oncol* 3:811, 2008.

Systemic and Mucocutaneous Reactions to Chemotherapy

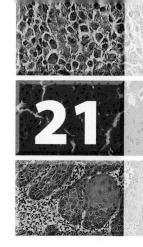

21

JOSEPH P. EDER • ARTHUR T. SKARIN

Cancer chemotherapy is a major component of cancer therapy, along with surgery and irradiation. Classical cancer chemotherapy agents differ from most drugs in that they are intentionally cytotoxic to human cells. This aspect of cancer chemotherapeutic agents produces a narrow therapeutic index (desired vs. undesired) for most, but not all, agents in this class. The target of classical cancer chemotherapeutic agents is the proliferating cancer cell. While many normal tissues are nonproliferating, others are, and toxicity of this class tends to preferentially overlap proliferating tissues—hematopoietic, gastrointestinal mucosa, and skin. In addition, each agent often has specific organ toxicity related to its chemical class or unique mechanism of action.

The major groups of classical cancer chemotherapeutic agents are the direct-acting alkylating agents, the indirect-acting anthracyclines and topoisomerase inhibitors, the antimetabolites, the tubulin-binding agents, hormones, receptor-targeted agents, and a class of miscellaneous agents. Despite the disparate nature of this broad class of agents, some generalizations about the effects of chemotherapy are still possible.

Molecularly targeted cancer chemotherapeutic agents have become the standard of care in an increasing number of cancers. Molecularly targeted agents may be monoclonal antibodies or small-molecule competitive adenosine triphosphate kinase inhibitors. Monoclonal antibodies may be directed at ligands (i.e., bevacizumab) or receptors (i.e., trastuzumab). Toxicities are related either to the mechanism of action or, if the antibody is not fully human, to allergic reactions. Despite the best efforts of medicinal chemists, no small molecule is exclusively selective for its intended targets, and off-target as well as mechanistic toxicities occur. For more information readers are referred to detailed reports (Weiss, 2006; Crawford et al., 2006).

Acute Hypersensitivity Reactions

Acute hypersensitivity can occur with any drug. However, several cancer chemotherapeutic agents are derived from hydrophobic plant chemicals and must be solubilized with agents with a marked propensity for causing acute hypersensitivity reactions, especially histamine-mediated anaphylactic reactions, such as the polyethoxylated castor oil (Cremophor EL; BASF Corp., Mt. Olive, NJ) used with paclitaxel. Docetaxel has a lower incidence of this complication. The incidence of severe hypersensitivity reactions with paclitaxel may be up to 25% without ancillary measures.

With antihistamine H1 and H2 blockade and corticosteroids the incidence falls to 2% to 3%. Hypersensitivity reactions occur in up to 40% of patients receiving single-agent L-asparaginase but only 20% when administered in combination therapy with glucocorticoids and 6-mercaptopurine, perhaps as a result of immunosuppression. The hypersensitivity usually occurs after several doses and in successive cycles. The reaction may be only urticaria (see Fig. 21.1) but may be severe with laryngospasm or, rarely, serum sickness. Fatal reactions occur less than 1% of the time. Changing the source of enzyme is the appropriate initial step. Two other proteins in clinical use, rituximab and trastuzumab, have a similar incidence of hypersensitivity reactions.

Certain drugs such as etoposide are associated with a greater incidence of reactions, but most are not true hypersensitivity reactions. The polysorbate 80 (Tween 80; ICI Americas, Inc., Bridgewater, N.J.) diluent in the clinical etoposide formulation produces hypotension, rash, and back pain. The platinum compounds carboplatin and cisplatin are associated with hypersensitivity reactions, particularly on subsequent cycles; most of these reactions are severe (75%). Hypersensitivity to platinum and related compounds is actually quite frequent, up to 14% in industrial workers, so such reactions in patients receiving these agents parenterally should not be surprising; they are often unappreciated in combination chemotherapy regimens, as with taxanes, and may be equally suppressed by the prophylactic regimens used. Liposomal-encapsulated anthracyclines are associated with an increased incidence of hypersensitivity compared with the parent drugs. Like the reaction to polyethoxylated castor oil and radiocontrast agents, the reaction is a "complement activation pseudoallergy." Up to 45% of cancer patients show activation of the classical or alternative complement pathway, or both, although the incidence of clinical reactions is about 20%.

Monoclonal antibodies such as trastuzumab, rituximab, bevacizumab, and cetuximab have had enormous impact on cancer therapeutics. Monoclonal antibodies may be chimeric (a murine Fab binding site but human amino acid sequences elsewhere) or fully human. Allergic or hypersensitivity reactions are more frequent with chimeric proteins such as cetuximab (1% to 5% clinically significant) and are treated with antihistamines and steroids plus slowing of the infusion.

L-Asparaginase is a bacterial protein that frequently results in hypersensitivity reactions. These reactions are more frequent with interrupted schedules and with subsequent rechallenge. Changing the source from *Escherichia coli* to *Erwinia* is one accepted strategy if immunosuppression does not work.

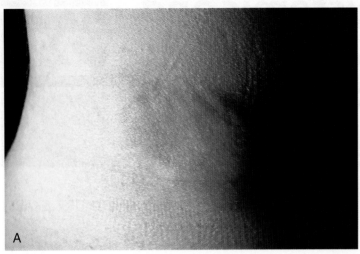
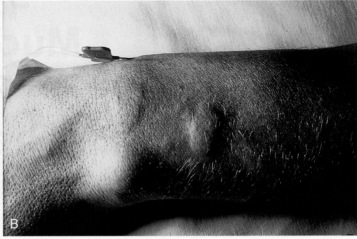

FIGURE 21.1 **ACUTE HYPERSENSITIVITY REACTIONS.** Urticaria, with giant localized hives, occurred **(A)** in a 40-year-old man within a few minutes of receiving intravenous 5-FU and **(B)** in the lower arm of a 50-year-old man after receiving adriamycin. The urticaria was self-limiting in both patients.

Alopecia

Many antineoplastic drugs can produce marked hair loss (see Fig. 21.2). This includes not only scalp hair but also facial, axillary, pubic, and all body hair. The germinating hair follicle has an approximately 24-hour doubling time. Cancer chemotherapy agents preferentially affect actively growing (anagen) hairs. The interruption of mitosis produces a structurally weakened hair prone to fracture easily from minimal trauma such as brushing. Since 80% to 90% of scalp hairs are in anagen phase, the degree of hair loss can be substantial. Hair loss, while often emotionally difficult for patients, is reversible, although hair may regrow more curly and of a slightly different color.

FIGURE 21.2 **ALOPECIA. (A)** Near-total alopecia in a 38-year-old woman receiving cyclophosphamide and adriamycin. Note the loss of eyebrow and eyelid hair. **(B)** Total alopecia developed in this 64-year-old woman due to chemotherapy and cranial irradiation for brain metastases. The duration of alopecia after both treatment modalities may be many months or even permanent in some patients. In this woman the scalp edema and erythema are related to an allergic cutaneous reaction from diphenylhydantoin.

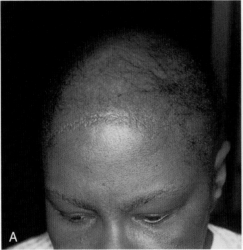
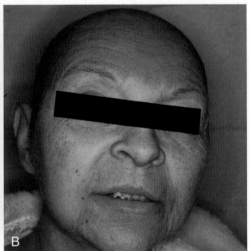

Stomatitis/Mucositis

The oral complications of cancer chemotherapy are many and frequently severe. The disruption of the protective mucosal barrier serves as a portal of entry for pathogens, which, especially when combined with chemotherapy-induced neutropenia, predisposes to local infection and systemic sepsis. Once established, these infections may be difficult to eradicate in immunocompromised patients. The most common infectious organisms are *Candida albicans*, herpes simplex virus, β-hemolytic streptococci, staphylococci, opportunistic gram-negative bacteria, and mouth anaerobes.

Several agents of the antimetabolite class of cancer chemotherapeutic agents, especially those that target pyrimidine biosynthesis such as methotrexate, 5-fluorouracil (5-FU), and cytosine arabinoside, and the anthracycline agents, such as doxorubicin and daunorubicin, are particularly toxic to the mucosal epithelium (see Fig. 21.3). These agents have a marked capacity to produce more severe injury in irradiated tissues, even if the irradiation is temporally remote. These agents produce marked ulceration and erosion of the mucosa. These lesions occur initially on those mucosal surfaces that abrade the teeth and gums, such as the sides of the tongue, the vermilion border of the lower lip, and the buccal mucosa. More advanced mucosal injury may occur on the hard and soft palate and the posterior oropharynx. These ulcerations cannot often be distinguished from those caused by infectious organisms. Appropriate tests must be performed to exclude viral, fungal, and bacterial causes or superinfection.

In addition to the risk of infection, the resultant pain makes patients unable to maintain adequate nutrition and hydration. This may compromise the capacity to complete a course of chemotherapy and require prolonged administration of parenteral fluids and even parenteral nutrition.

Stomatitis occurs with several kinase inhibitors, including sunitinib, erlotinib, and sorafenib. The incidence is 15% to 25% and is usually mild in severity.

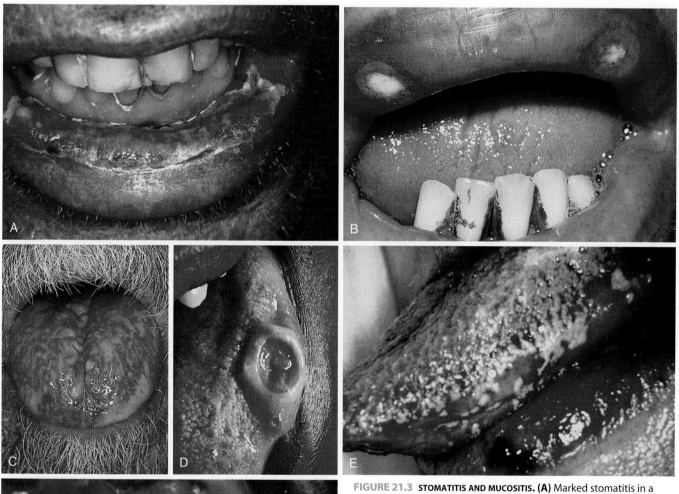

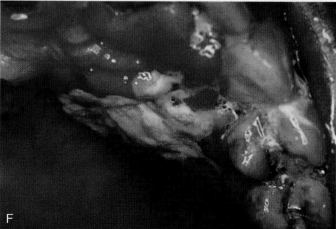

FIGURE 21.3 STOMATITIS AND MUCOSITIS. (A) Marked stomatitis in a patient receiving methotrexate. **(B)** Aphthous stomatitis related to severe granulocytopenia after chemotherapy. The ulcers may be due to herpes simplex or other infection. **(C)** Mucositis in a patient receiving combination chemotherapy for head and neck cancer. **(D)** Marked ulcer of the tongue in a 32-year-old man receiving induction chemotherapy for acute leukemia. **(E)** Mucositis of the tongue due to *Monilia* infection (thrush) in a patient receiving corticosteroids for brain metastases. **(F)** Marked oral mucositis due to mixed infection in a patient receiving chemotherapy for acute leukemia.

Dermatitis, Skin Rashes, and Hyperpigmentation

Superficial manifestations of cancer chemotherapy agents are noted frequently by patients, although they are considered significant much less often by clinicians. The cosmetic changes may be disturbing to patients without requiring discontinuation of therapy.

Of the direct-acting alkylating agents, busulfan has been associated with a wide variety of specific and nonspecific cutaneous changes. Diffuse hyperpigmentation has been noted (see Fig. 21.4), which resolves with discontinuation of therapy. Systemic mechlorethamine (nitrogen mustard) has no cutaneous toxicity. However, when applied topically for cutaneous T-cell lymphomas, telangiectasias, hyperpigmentation, and allergic contact dermatitis may occur. The development of more effective, safer alternative agents has made busulfan and mechlorethamine of essentially historical interest only or for narrow indications (busulfan in allogeneic bone marrow transplant for hematologic malignancies). Cyclophosphamide, ifosfamide, and melphalan produce hyperpigmentation of nails, teeth, gingiva, and skin. The antimetabolites methotrexate and 5-FU are frequently associated with cutaneous reactions. In contrast, the purine antimetabolites 6-mercaptopurine, 6-thioguanine, cladribine, fludarabine, and pentostatin are devoid of cutaneous toxicity. Methotrexate, a folate antagonist, may cause reactivation of ultraviolet burns when given in close proximity to previous sun exposure. This is not prevented by leucovorin, a reduced folate that prevents the myelosuppression and stomatitis of high doses of methotrexate. Methotrexate should be given more than a week after a significant solar burn. It may cause stomatitis and cutaneous ulcerations at high dose, despite the use of leucovorin. Extensive epidermal necrolysis may occur and be fatal. Multiple areas of vesiculation and erosion over pressure areas have been noticed.

5-FU is an antimetabolite with steric properties similar to uracil. Like methotrexate, 5-FU produces increased sensitivity to ultraviolet-induced toxic reactions in a large number of patients, over 35% in one study. Enhanced sunburn erythema and increased posterythema hyperpigmentation characterize these reactions. A hyperpigmentation reaction over the veins in which the drug is administered may occur. This is probably hyperpigmentation secondary to chemical phlebitis due to chemotherapeutic agents in the superficial venous system. Nail and generalized skin hyperpigmentation have been reported with 5-FU. Occasionally, acute inflammation of existing actinic keratosis is seen in patients receiving 5-FU. This differs from a drug reaction in that it occurs in discrete inflamed regions only in sun-exposed areas, not in a generalized distribution. The end result is usually the disappearance of the actinic keratosis as a result of an inflammatory infiltration into the atypical epidermis and resultant removal of atypical cells. High doses of cytosine arabinoside may produce ocular toxicity through an ulcerating keratoconjunctivitis. This may be prevented by the prophylactic administration of steroid eyedrops. Excessive lacrimation may be noted with 5-FU therapy due to lacrimal duct stenosis. This is corrected by surgical dilatation of the duct.

The indirect-acting anticancer drugs may produce superficial cutaneous toxicity. The anthracyclines doxorubicin, daunorubicin, epirubicin, and idarubicin produce complete alopecia. Radiation recall reactions are frequent, even when the two modalities are separated by years. Skin, nail, and mucous membrane hyperpigmentation may be striking; these may be localized or general. Hyperpigmentation of the hands, feet, and face may occur in patients of African descent. Liposomal anthracyclines, such as Doxil (doxorubicin) and Daunosome (daunorubicin), may produce a severe erythromayalagia with palmar and plantar erythema and desquamation similar to 5-FU. Actinomycin D produces a characteristic skin eruption in many patients. Beginning 3–5 days after drug administration, patients develop facial erythema followed by papules, pustules, and plugged follicles similar to the open comedones of acne. This eruption is benign, self-limited, and not a reason to stop therapy. A similar acneiform skin rash occurs in patients taking the new oral epidermal growth factor receptor inhibitors such as gefitinib and erlotinib (see Fig. 21.4). In most patients the rash is mild and may regress with continued treatment. When severe the skin lesions will rapidly regress with discontinuation of the drug. Topical steroids and antibiotics may be indicated.

Bleomycin is actually a mixture of peptides isolated from *Streptomyces verticullus*. Its most common toxic effects involve the lungs and skin because of high concentrations in these organs due to the deficiency of the catabolic enzyme bleomycin hydrolase in these tissues. Cutaneous toxicity occurs in the majority of patients treated with bleomycin doses in excess of 200 mg. Bleomycin causes a morbilliform eruption 30 minutes to 3 hours after administration in approximately 10% of patients (see Fig. 21.4). It most likely represents a transient hypersensitivity response (it may be accompanied by fever). Linear or "flagellate" hyperpigmentation may occur on the trunk. This may likewise represent postinflammatory hyperpigmentation. Bleomycin may cause a scleroderma-like eruption of the skin. Infiltrative plaques, nodules, and linear bands of the hands have been described. Pathologic findings include dermal sclerosis and appendage entrapment similar to that seen in scleroderma. These changes are reversible when the drug is stopped.

Etoposide has relatively few cutaneous manifestations at standard doses ($<600 \, mg/m^2$). At higher doses ($1800–4200 \, mg/m^2$) a generalized pruritic, erythematous, maculopapular rash occurs in approximately 25% of patients. The most severe toxicity occurs at the highest doses. In these patients an intense, well-defined palmar erythema develops. Affected areas become edematous, red, and painful. Bullous formation and desquamation follow. The severity of the reaction is related to the dose. A short course (3–5 days) of corticosteroids controls the symptoms.

Cutaneous rashes are the most common toxicities encountered with gefitinib and erlotinib. The chimeric monoclonal antibodies cetuximab and panitumumab are associated with dermatologic toxicity. The severity and extent of the skin changes, including dry skin, desquamation, erythema, nail changes, and acneiform eruptions, vary from report to report, and no consistent grading system for incidence and severity is universally agreed upon. There is neutrophil and macrophage infiltration of the dermis and hair follicles, with thinning of the epidermis and stratum corneum. The incidence and severity is dose-dependent. Certain epidermal growth factor receptor polymorphisms increase the incidence of developing a rash. For erlotinib, cetuximab, and panitumumab, several studies support a positive correlation between development of a rash and response, and rash and survival (Ando et al., 2006). Management is usually supportive with creams, including 1% clindamycin, 5% benzoyl peroxide, and systemic antibiotics when there is evidence of infection, including tetracycline and amoxicillin/clavulanate. These should be used only when necessary.

Sunitinib causes a yellowing of the skin in 10% of patients. This is not due to deposition of bilirubin in the skin, since there is no scleral icterus and there are no changes in serum bilirubin. Between 10% and 20% of patients experience loss of hair pigmentation in 2–3 weeks, which resolves in the same period of time after discontinuation of the drug (Kerr et al., 2007).

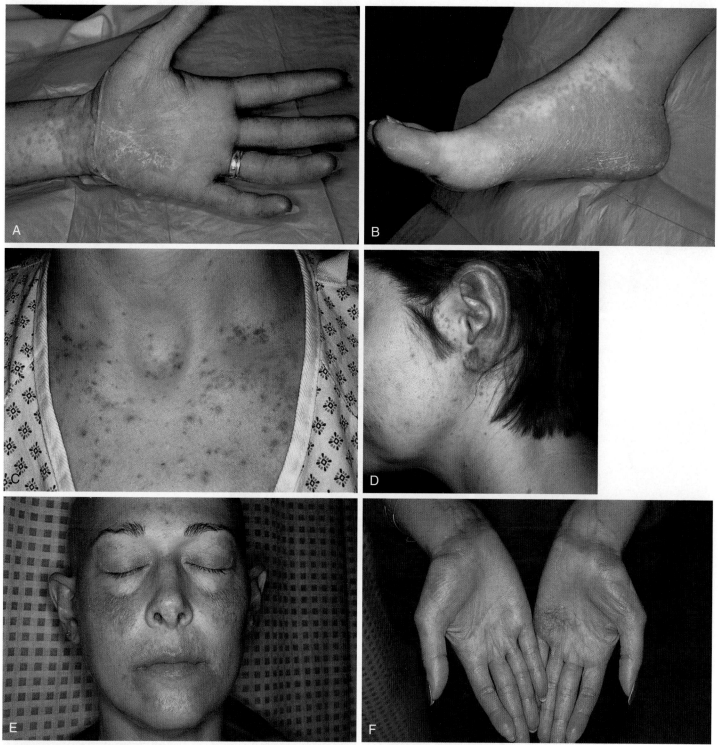

FIGURE 21.4 **(A, B)** Dermatitis, skin rashes, and hyperpigmentation: hand-foot syndrome related to 5-FU chemotherapy in metastatic colon cancer. Note the erythema, edema, rash, and early skin desquamation. Severe pain is associated with this toxic reaction. **(C, D)** Skin reaction to Ara-C (also known as cytosine arabinoside and cytarabine). Note the erythematous macular rash on the chest and diffuse erythema and edema of the ears in this 22-year-old woman receiving Ara-C for acute leukemia. **(E, F)** Skin reaction to docetaxel. Note periorbital and malar flush along with erythema and edema of the palms in this patient. **(G, H)** Cutaneous reactions to bleomycin include raised, erythematous, and pruritic lesions around pressure points, especially the elbows **(G)**, as well as desquamation of skin **(H)**. **(I, J)** Acneiform skin lesions occur in patients taking gefitinib, especially on the face **(I)**, chest, and back **(J)**. These rashes may regress when the drug is temporarily withheld or the dose is lowered. Similar skin reactions occur after actinomycin D and corticosteroids. **(K)** Hyperpigmentation of the skin along veins occurs after the use of many chemotherapeutic agents, including vinorelbine (Navelbine; Glaxo Wellcome), actinomycin D, and 5-FU infusion, as in this patient. In many cases the veins become sclerotic because of thrombophlebitis. **(L–N)** Hyperpigmentation of the skin after 5-FU **(L)**. Hyperpigmentation of the skin occurs after adriamycin and other drugs **(M)**, while increased pigment in the mucous membranes **(N)** and nails **(M)** is mainly related to adriamycin.

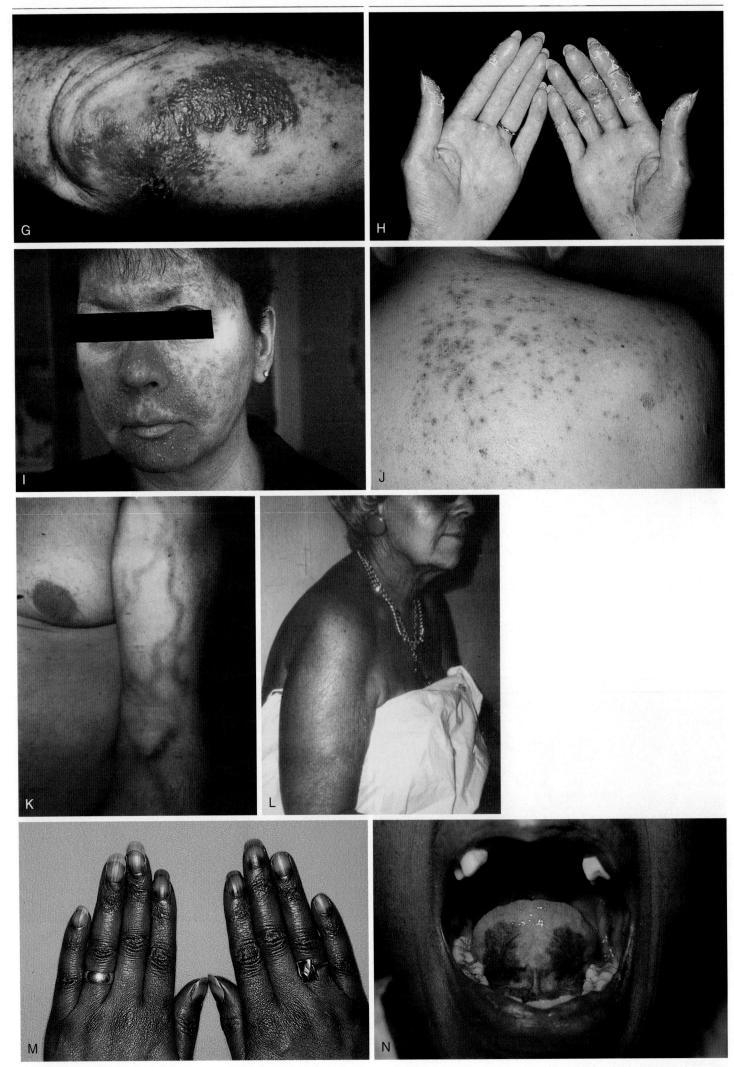

FIGURE 21.4—CONT'D

Skin Ulceration and Extravasation

Vesicant reactions from extravasated cancer chemotherapeutic agents are one of the most debilitating complications seen with cancer therapy (see Fig. 21.5). The anthracyclines, especially doxorubicin, are particularly noted for an intense inflammatory chemical cellulitis caused by subcutaneous extravasation. This results in ulceration and necrosis of affected tissue. No local measures have proven unequivocally helpful once the accident has occurred. Doxorubicin should be stopped immediately but the intravenous line left in place. Dilution of doxorubicin with sodium bicarbonate and the local instillation of steroids before catheter withdrawal are standard measures, but their efficacy is uncertain. Rest and warm compresses are recommended. If healing does not proceed well, excision of the affected area and surgical grafting are recommended to avoid excess morbidity. Other agents with vesicant properties include the vinca alkaloids (vincristine, vinblastine, vinorelbine) and actinomycin. General recommendations for the administration of vesicant drugs include the use of veins as far away from the hands and joints as possible and placement of the intravenous line so that infusion occurs at a rapid rate and blood return is good. The use of venous access devices is accepted as appropriate in this situation unless contraindicated on specific clinical grounds.

Generalized skin ulceration is an infrequent, albeit dramatic, occurrence. Mucocutaneous ulcerations are frequently noted with bleomycin. These begin as edema and erythema over pressure points such as the elbows, knees, and fingertips and in intertriginous areas such as the groin and axillae. These areas then proceed to shallow ulcerations. These ulcerations may also occur in the oral cavity. Biopsy shows epidermal degeneration and necrosis with dermal edema. Total epidermal necrosis can even be found without any dermal changes. This suggests that the epidermal toxicity is the primary event.

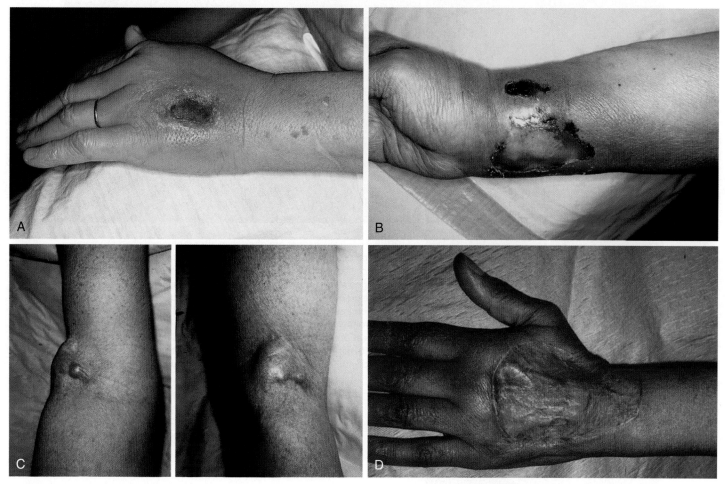

FIGURE 21.5 Extravasation of drugs and skin ulcers occurs with vesicant drugs. Acute changes with adriamycin **(A, B)**. **(C)** Chronic healed scarring with adriamycin and **(D)** mitomycin-C. Other vesicant drugs include actinomycin D, vincristine, and vinorelbine. Immediate medical attention is necessary, and sometimes skin grafts are required (see text).

Nail Changes

Banding of the nails is the appearance of linear horizontal depressions in the nails that occur as a result of growth interruptions in the nail germinal cell layer by a cytostatic effect from the administration of cancer chemotherapy agents. These occur in other disease settings and are called Beau's lines (see Fig. 21.6). The direct-acting alkylating agents cyclophosphamide, ifosfamide and melphalan may also produce hyperpigmentation of nails. The nails may show linear or transverse banding or hyperpigmentation. These changes begin proximally and progress distally and clear, proximally to distally, when the agents are discontinued. Similar effects are seen with the indirect-acting anthracyclines, such as doxorubicin, and bleomycin. The anthracyclines may cause hyperpigmentation of the hyponychia (the soft layer of skin beneath the nail), especially in dark-skinned persons.

Onycholysis is separation of the nail plate from the nail bed (see Fig. 21.6). Anthracyclines, anthracenediones, and taxanes are the drugs most frequently associated with onycholysis. The combination of these agents is most frequently reported with onycholysis. Most of the reports are associated with docetaxel, administered either weekly or every 3 weeks. These changes occur after hyperpigmentation of the hyponychia, often with hyperkeratosis and splinter hemorrhages. Ultraviolet light may be a facilitating factor. Onycholysis can occur within weeks or months of the initiation of therapy.

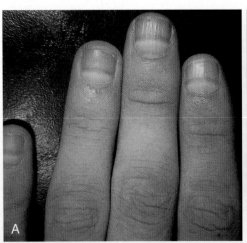
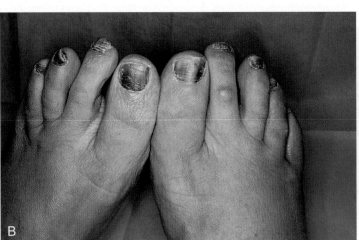
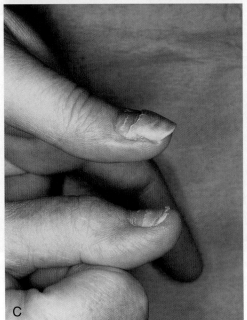

FIGURE 21.6 Nail changes are often seen after prolonged chemotherapy. **(A)** Banding of the nails results from growth interruptions in the nail germinal cell layer by the cytostatic effect of chemotherapy. These white bands (called Mee's lines) will grow outward eventually. Beau's lines are transverse grooves across the nail plate due to temporary nail matrix malfunction, seen with chemotherapy or associated with other illnesses (acute coronary or severe febrile episodes). Nail hyperpigmentation occurs occasionally after prolonged use of adriamycin **(B)**, especially in people with dark skin. Onycholysis or separation of the nail from its bed is associated with use of adriamycin **(C)**, cyclophosphamide, and taxanes.

Radiation Recall

Radiation recall dermatitis is a cutaneous toxicity that develops in patients with prior exposure to therapeutic doses of radiation and subsequent treatment with a cancer chemotherapeutic agent (see Fig. 21.7). These reactions occur in the previously irradiated field and not elsewhere. A previous cutaneous reaction at the time of irradiation is not a prerequisite. The onset of symptoms is days to weeks after drug treatment and can occur any time after irradiation, even years later. Cutaneous manifestations include erythema with maculopapular eruptions, vesiculation, and desquamation. The intensity of the cutaneous response can vary from a mild rash to skin necrosis. Radiation recall reactions in other organs can produce gastrointestinal mucosal inflammation (stomatitis, esophagitis, enteritis, proctitis), pneumonitis, and myocarditis.

An extensive number of anticancer agents have been implicated in radiation recall reactions. The anthracyclines (doxorubicin as an example), bleomycin, dactinomycin, etoposide, taxanes, vinca alkaloids, and antimetabolites (hydroxycarbamide, 5-FU, methotrexate, gemcitabine) are the most commonly implicated in cutaneous toxicity. In addition, these skin reactions have been seen in association with targeted therapy with drugs such as gefitinib.

Methotrexate and dactinomycin are reported to cause radiation enhancement in the central nervous system (CNS). The antimetabolites doxorubicin, dactinomycin, and bleomycin enhance gastrointestinal toxicity from irradiation. Cyclophosphamide, taxanes, hydroxycarbamide, doxorubicin, dactinomycin, gemcitabine (2′,2′-difluoro-2′-deoxycytidine), cytosine arabinoside, and, most importantly, bleomycin exacerbate pulmonary irradiation toxicity. Optic toxicity is increased by treatment with 5-FU and cytosine arabinoside. Irradiation lowers the dose of doxorubicin that produces cardiomyopathy.

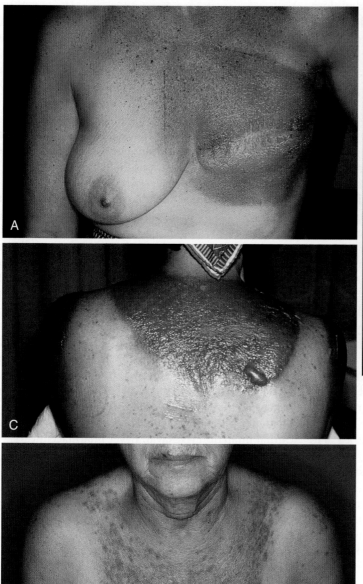

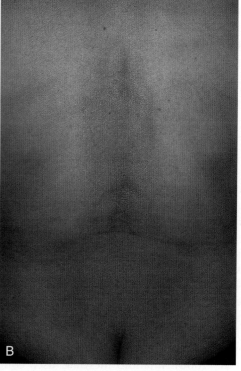

FIGURE 21.7 Radiation recall dermatitis may occur in a radiation therapy field after systemic chemotherapy, with development of hyperemia and then hyperpigmentation in the healing phase **(A)**. The patient in **A** received adjuvant Alkeran (melphalan) 1 month after postoperative irradiation to the chest wall. **(B)** This patient had radiation therapy to the lower spine for bone metastases from breast cancer and developed recall dermatitis 6 months later, when gemcitabine was administered. **(C)** Chemotherapy can also sensitize the skin to adverse reactions to solar radiation. This young woman developed severe dermatitis in a sun-exposed area while taking methotrexate. **(D)** This patient also developed acute dermatitis in a sun-exposed area while receiving 5-FU.

Hand-Foot Syndrome/ Erythromelalgia

When 5-FU is given by intravenous continuous infusion, the most common dose-limiting toxicity is erythromelalgia, the so-called hand-foot syndrome (see Fig. 21.4). The hands and feet become red, edematous, and often painful. The skin often peels afterward. The nails become dry and brittle and develop linear cracks. This may occur at doses lower than those that produce the hand-foot syndrome. A similar reaction occurs with 5-FU or 5-FU prodrugs administered orally on a daily schedule. Capecitabine, an oral prodrug that is eventually converted to 5-FU intracellularly, produces erythromelalgia as its most common toxicity. Interestingly, oral 5-FU does not produce this syndrome when combined with enyluracil, an irreversible inhibitor of dihydropyrimidine dehydrogenase, the major enzyme in 5-FU catabolism.

Sorafenib and a related drug, sunitinib malate, are oral multitargeted receptor tyrosine kinase inhibitors that block signal transduction through the *RAF* kinases, vascular endothelial growth factor receptor 2 (VEGFR2), and the platelet-derived growth factor receptors. At the recommended dose there is a 33% incidence of skin rashes or desquamation, 27% incidence of hand-foot syndrome, and 22% incidence of alopecia (all grades of severity) (Escudier et al., 2005).

Organ Toxicity

CARDIAC AND CARDIOVASCULAR TOXICITY

Cardiotoxicity is a well-recognized consequence of anthracycline use, especially doxorubicin because of its wide spectrum of antineoplastic therapy. This peculiar and potentially lethal problem can be classified as acute or chronic. The acute toxicity is usually asymptomatic arrhythmias, including heart block. Acute myopericarditis occurs at low total doses in an idiosyncratic fashion or at high single doses (>110–120 mg/m²). Fever, pericarditis, and congestive heart failure (CHF) are the clinical manifestations. Chronic cardiomyopathy is characterized by progressive myofibrillar damage with each dose, dilatation of sarcoplasmic reticulum, loss of myofibrils, and myocardial necrosis/fibrosis. Various syndromes of cardiac toxicity related to antineoplastic agents have been recently reviewed in detail (Kerkela et al., 2006). Imatinib mesylate, used commonly in chronic myelogenous leukemia and gastrointestinal stromal tumors, has been associated with a low incidence of cardiomyopathy syndrome (Floyd et al., 2006).

A doxorubicin total dose lower than 550 mg/m² has a 1% to 10% occurrence of CHF (daunorubicin 900–1000 mg/m²) and a 40% incidence at 800 mg/m² of doxorubicin; the incidence of CHF approaches 100% at 1 g/m² of doxorubicin. Cardiac function is tested using noninvasive techniques to measure the resting and exercise ejection fraction, including radionuclide ventriculograms and echocardiograms, or invasively by cardiac biopsy. Factors that increase the risk of developing CHF include preexisting heart disease, hypertension, and cardiac radiation therapy. Concomitant dosing with trastuzumab increases the cardiac toxicity of doxorubicin. Cardiac toxicity is a function of *peak* dose level, so continuous infusions or weekly dosing decrease the risk. Dexrazoxane, an iron chelator, decreases cardiotoxicity and is approved for use.

Biochemical mechanisms implicated include calcium-mediated damage to the sarcoplasmic reticulum, which increases calcium ion (Ca²⁺) release with increased Ca²⁺ uptake in mitochondria in preference to adenosine triphosphate. Lipid peroxidations of the sarcoplasmic reticulum, which decrease high Ca²⁺ binding sites, and lipid peroxidation due to drug •Fe³⁺ complexes with hydroxyl radical (•OH) generation may contribute to cardiotoxicity. The heart has no catalase, and anthracyclines decrease glutathione peroxidase activity, which increases the sensitivity of the myocardium to oxidative damage.

Idarubicin and epirubicin have less cardiotoxicity but are still capable of causing cardiotoxicity. High-dose cyclophosphamide, at doses higher than 60 mg/kg as used in bone marrow transplantation, can cause a hemorrhagic cardiomyopathy. Paclitaxel produces clinically insignificant atrial arrhythmias. Agents that can produce arterial smooth muscle spasm may produce ischemic myocardial infarction in the absence of fixed coronary vascular disease. These agents include 5-FU, vincristine, and vinblastine. Combination chemotherapy in colorectal cancer with bevacizumab has been associated with an incidence (1% to 3%) of ischemic cardiac events above that observed with conventional therapy alone. This increase in cardiovascular events, while of low overall incidence, nonetheless represents about a threefold increase (Kerr et al., 2007).

Cardiomyopathy has been increasingly observed with newer molecularly targeted agents. Decreases in left ventricular ejection fraction to below the lower limits of normal occur in 10% to 20% of patients treated with sunitinib. Sunitinib has a 10% incidence of usually reversible clinical cardiomyopathy. Patients can often be treated with lower doses if and when symptoms resolve (Kerkela et al., 2006). Imatinib produces clinical cardiomyopathy in 1% of patients. This incidence comes from unmonitored trials, so the true incidence is unknown. Molecular studies confirm this due to c-ABL inhibition, and the pathologic findings are similar to other cardiomyopathies (Kerkela et al., 2006).

Hypertension has been recognized as a class effect for agents that target VEGFR2. Hypertension is so common that it serves as a pharmacodynamic end point in the early development of agents of this class. Hypertension of a moderate degree (grade 2, recurrent or persistent, symptomatic increase of diastolic blood pressure to >200 mm Hg systolic or to >100 mm Hg diastolic or requiring monotherapy) or severe degree (grade 3, requiring more than one agent or more intensive therapy) occurs in 10% to 25% of patients receiving bevacizumab, sorafenib, or sunitinib. Patients with preexisting or borderline hypertension are more susceptible. No specific treatment algorithm has yet been applied to the management of these patients.

Ischemic cardiovascular events have been reported with increasing frequency with VEGF-targeted agents. Sorafenib has an incidence of 2.9% of acute coronary syndrome, including myocardial infarction (Nexavar; Bayer Pharmaceuticals) (Force et al., 2007). In pooling data from five randomized, controlled, clinical trials involving over 1500 patients, the overall incidence of cardiovascular events was increased to 4.4% among the patients treated with bevacizumab in combination with chemotherapy as compared to 1.9% in patients treated with chemotherapy only. Fatal events occurred in 0.7% of patients treated with bevacizumab and combination chemotherapy, compared to 0.4% in chemotherapy-only patients. The incidences of both cerebrovascular arterial events (1.9% vs. 0.5%) and cardiovascular arterial events (2.1% vs. 1.0%) were increased in patients receiving bevacizumab (Avastin; Genentech Pharmaceuticals, 2004). There was a correlation between increasing age (65 years and over) and increased risk of arterial thromboembolic events.

PULMONARY TOXICITY

Bleomycin produces pulmonary toxicity, which is the major problem with subacute or chronic interstitial pneumonitis complicated by late-stage fibrosis (see Fig. 21.8). The incidence is 3% to 5% with doses of less than $450 U/m^2$, in patients over 70, with emphysema, and after high single doses ($>25 U/m^2$). The incidence rises to 10% at doses higher than $450 mg/m^2$, but can occur at cumulative doses of less than 100 mg. Pulmonary injury can occur during high FiO_2 and volume overload during surgery for many years after exposure.

Toxicity results from free radicals produced by an intercalated $Fe_{(II)}$-bleomycin-O^2 complex between DNA strands. Intercalation of drug into the DNA is the first step; then $Fe_{(II)}$ is oxidized and O^2 is reduced to oxygen ($\bullet O^{2-}$) or hydroxyl radicals $\bullet OH$. DNA cleavage occurs after the activated bleomycin complex is assembled. Strand breakage absolutely requires O^2, which is converted to O^{2-} and $\bullet OH$, and peroxidation products of DNA (and protein) are formed. Free-radical scavengers and superoxide dismutase inhibit DNA breakage. Bleomycin is hydrolyzed by bleomycin hydrolase, a cysteine present in normal and malignant cells but decreased in lung and skin.

Busulfan, mitomycin C, and carmustine are direct-acting alkylating agents that can cause chronic interstitial pneumonitis and fibrosing alveolitis. This chronic fibrosis produces the clinical picture of progressive, often fatal, restrictive lung disease. The symptoms occur insidiously, often after prolonged therapy. The chronic use of busulfan for the treatment of chronic myelogenous leukemia is now a historical footnote, but carmustine remains the mainstay of treatment for glioblastoma and anaplastic astrocytomas. Cyclophosphamide has been implicated in chronic pulmonary toxicity but rarely as a single agent and more often after irradiation.

The antimetabolite methotrexate may produce an acute eosinophilic pneumonitis, which represents an allergic reaction. Cytosine arabinoside and gemcitabine may also cause an acute pneumonitis, which may be fatal if unrecognized. In these circumstances, withdrawal of the offending agent, supportive care, and corticosteroids may prevent a fatal outcome. Some of the reported pulmonary syndromes associated with chemotherapy drugs are noted in Table 21.1.

Both erlotinib and gefitinib, new oral agents targeted at the epidermal growth factor receptor 1, both have a low (<1%) but real incidence of interstitial pneumonitis that resolves if the agent is stopped. The highest incidence is in Asian patients, where 3.5% of patients may develop interstitial disease also referred to as ground-glass opacities, which carries a mortality rate of 1.6% (Ando et al., 2006).

HEPATOTOXICITY

The liver is a frequent organ for toxicity with cancer chemotherapeutic agents. Centrilobular hepatocyte injury is the frequent histologic finding and elevated transaminases the biochemical manifestation. Antimetabolite drugs such as cytosine arabinoside, methotrexate, hydroxycarbamide, and 6-mercaptopurine are all associated with hepatic injury. 6-Mercaptopurine produces a cholestatic picture, with an elevated alkaline phosphatase and bilirubin. L-Asparaginase and carmustine cause hepatotoxicity as well. The injury reverses with discontinuation of the drug. Chronic methotrexate administration, as in the treatment of autoimmune diseases, is associated with irreversible fibrosis and cirrhosis.

Hepatic vascular injury is another type of injury to the liver associated with cancer chemotherapeutic agents. Hepatic venoocclusive disease may occur in up to 20% of patients receiving high-dose chemotherapy in conjunction with bone marrow transplantation, with a mortality rate of up to 50%. Jaundice, ascites, and hepatomegaly are the full manifestations of venoocclusive disease, but right upper quadrant pain and weight gain occur more frequently. Obliteration of the central hepatic venules and resulting pressure necrosis of the hepatocytes is seen at autopsy. Many regimens and many individual drugs have been implicated. With busulfan, adjustment of the plasma concentration–time profile may reduce the risk. Dacarbazine, a monofunctional alkylating agent, may produce an eosinophilic centrilobular injury with hepatic vein thromboses.

GASTROINTESTINAL TOXICITY

Chemotherapy-induced diarrhea has been described with several drugs including the fluoropyrimidines (particularly 5-FU), irinotecan, methotrexate, and cisplatin. However, it is the major toxicity of regimens containing a fluoropyrimidine and/or irinotecan that can be dose-limiting. Both 5-FU and irinotecan cause acute damage to the intestinal mucosa, leading to loss of epithelium. 5-FU causes a mitotic arrest of crypt cells, leading to an increase in the ratio of immature secretory crypt cells to mature villous enterocytes. The increased volume of fluid that leaves the small bowel exceeds the absorptive capacity of the colon, leading to clinically significant diarrhea.

In patients treated with irinotecan, early-onset diarrhea, which occurs during or within several hours of drug infusion in 45% to

Table 21.1	
Pulmonary Syndromes Associated with Specific Cancer Chemotherapy Drugs	
Syndrome	**Associated Cancer Chemotherapy Drugs**
Pulmonary capillary leak	IL-2, recombinant TNF-α, cytarabine, mitomycin
Asthma	IL-2, vinca alkaloids plus mitomycin
Bronchiolitis obliterans organizing pneumonia	Bleomycin, cyclophosphamide, methotrexate, mitomycin
Hypersensitivity pneumonitis	Busulfan, bleomycin, etoposide, methotrexate, mitomycin, procarbazine
Interstitial pneumonia/fibrosis	Bleomycin, busulfan, chlorambucil, cyclophosphamide, melphalan, methotrexate, nitrosureas, procarbazine, vinca alkaloids (with mitomycin), gefitinib, erlotinib
Pleural effusion	Bleomycin, busulfan, IL-2, methotrexate, mitomycin, procarbazine
Pulmonary vascular injury	Busulfan, nitrosureas

IL-2, interleukin 2; TNF-α, tumor necrosis factor.
Adapted with permission from Belknap SM, Kuzel TM, Yarnold PR, et al: Clinical features and correlates of gemcitabine-associated lung injury. *Cancer* 106: 2051–2057, 2006.

50% of patients, is cholinergically mediated. This effect is thought to be due to structural similarity with acetylcholine. In contrast, late irinotecan-associated diarrhea is not cholinergically mediated. The pathophysiology of late diarrhea seems to be multifactorial with contributions from dysmotility and secretory factors as well as a direct toxic effect of the drug on the intestinal mucosa.

Irinotecan produces mucosal changes associated with apoptosis, such as epithelial vacuolization, and goblet cell hyperplasia, suggestive of mucin hypersecretion. These changes seem to be related to the accumulation of the active metabolite of irinotecan, SN-38, in the intestinal mucosa. SN-38 is glucuronidated in the liver and is then excreted in the bile. The conjugated metabolite SN-38G does not seem to cause diarrhea. However, SN-38G can be deconjugated in the intestines by β-glucuronidase present in intestinal bacteria. A direct correlation has been noted between mucosal damage and either low glucuronidation rates or increased intestinal β-glucuronidase activity. Severe toxicity has been described following irinotecan therapy in patients with Gilbert's syndrome, who have defective hepatic glucuronidation. Experimental studies have shown that inhibition of intestinal β-glucuronidase activity with antibiotics protects against mucosal injury and ameliorates the diarrhea. Several recently approved receptor tyrosine kinase inhibitors have diarrhea associated with use, including sorafenib, sunitinib, erlotinib, and gefitinib. The frequency varies from 30% to 40% with less than 5% grade 3 (severe) (Niko et al., 2006). Also, rare cases of gastrointestinal perforation have been reported using new agents with several mechanisms of action, including inhibitors of tumor vasculature (Ratain et al., 2006). Hypertension and rare strokes are also side effects that have been reported.

NEUROTOXICITY

Neurotoxicity from cancer chemotherapeutic agents is an increasingly recognized consequence of cancer treatment. The toxicities observed may affect the brain and spinal cord (CNS), peripheral nerves, or supporting neurologic tissues such as the meninges. Neurotoxicity from cancer therapeutic drugs must be distinguished from the effects of space-occupying metastatic lesions, toxic metabolic effects from disorders of blood chemistry, adjunctive drugs (such as opiate narcotics), and paraneoplastic syndromes. Toxicity may be acute, subacute, or chronic, reversible, or irreversible.

The direct-acting alkylating agents ifosfamide and carmustine cause somnolence, confusion, and coma at high doses. The toxicity of ifosfamide is secondary to accumulation of a metabolite, chlorethyl aldehyde, in cerebrospinal fluid. Renal dysfunction may cause CNS toxicity at low doses when acidosis results in increased chlorethyl aldehyde levels.

Damage from the antimetabolite methotrexate occurs in three forms and is worse when the drug given intrathecally with radiation therapy. Chemical arachnoiditis, characterized by headache, fever, and nuchal rigidity, is the most common and most acute toxicity. This may be due to additives in the diluent (benzoic acid in sterile water). Subacute toxicity is delayed for 2–3 weeks after administration and is characterized by extremity motor paralysis, cranial nerve palsy seizures, and coma. This is due to prolonged exposure to high doses of methotrexate. Chronic demyelinating encephalitis produces dementia and spasticity. There is cortical thinning with enlarged ventricles and cerebral calcifications. Types 2 and 3 may be increased after irradiation, especially if concomitant systemic therapy with high (or intermediate) doses is used.

Cytosine arabinoside, when given at high doses, produces cerebral and cerebellar dysfunction due to Purkinje cell necrosis and damage. At standard doses, leukoencephalopathy occurs rarely. When given intrathecally, cytosine arabinoside can produce transverse myelitis with resulting paralysis. 5-FU may produce acute cerebellar toxicity due to inhibition of aconitase, an enzyme in the cerebellar Krebs cycle. The purine adenine deaminase inhibitors pentostatin and fludarabine may produce several types of neurotoxicity. Pentostatin produces somnolence and coma at high doses. Fludarabine may cause delayed-onset coma or cortical blindness at high doses and peripheral neuropathy at low doses. Peripheral neuropathy is a frequent toxicity encountered with many cancer chemotherapeutic agents of many classes. Cisplatin and oxaliplatin, the vinca alkaloids, and the taxanes all produce peripheral neuropathy in a cumulative dose-dependent manner.

Posterior reversible leukoencephalopathy syndrome (PRES) or reversible posterior leukoencephalopathy syndrome (RPLS) is a neurologic syndrome defined by clinical and radiologic features. Typically patients present with headache, confusion, visual loss, and seizures. PRES/RPLS most often occurs in the setting of hypertensive crisis, of preeclampsia, or with cytotoxic immunosuppressive therapy. PRES/RPLS has been reported with classical chemotherapy agents for many years as an extremely rare event. Case reports of PRES/RPLS in cancer patients treated with bevacizumab, sorafenib, and sunitinib have appeared in recent years. In this clinical context, the diagnosis is confirmed by radiologic imaging. Typical magnetic resonance imaging findings are consistent with vasogenic edema and are predominantly localized to the posterior cerebral hemispheres. Diffusion-weighted images can be helpful in distinguishing RPLS from stroke. In the setting of hypertension, treatment is focused on lowering blood pressure, removing the offending agent, and antiseizure prophylaxis. Most patients recover without sequelae, though not all do (Neill et al., 2007; Rajasekhar and George, 2007).

NEPHROTOXICITY

One of the most serious side effects of chemotherapeutic agents is nephrotoxicity. Any part of the kidney structure (e.g., the glomerulus, the tubules, the interstitium, or the renal microvasculature) could be vulnerable to damage. The clinical manifestations of nephrotoxicity can range from an asymptomatic elevation of serum creatinine to acute renal failure requiring dialysis. Intravascular volume depletion secondary to ascites, edema, or external losses, concomitant use of nephrotoxic drugs, urinary tract obstruction secondary to the underlying malignancy, tumor infiltration of the kidney, and intrinsic renal disease can potentiate renal dysfunction in the cancer patient.

Platinum compounds are the agents most associated with renal toxicity. Cisplatin is one of the most commonly used and effective chemotherapeutic agents available and also the best-studied antineoplastic nephrotoxic drug. It is a potent tubular toxin, particularly in a low-chloride environment, such as the interior of cells. Cell death results via apoptosis or necrosis as DNA-damaged cells enter the cell cycle. Approximately 25% to 35% of patients will develop a mild and partially reversible decline in renal function after the first course of therapy. The incidence and severity of renal failure increase with subsequent courses, eventually becoming in part irreversible. As a result, discontinuing therapy is generally indicated in those patients who develop a progressive rise in plasma creatinine concentration. In addition to this rise, potentially irreversible hypomagnesemia due to urinary magnesium wasting may occur in over one half of cases.

There is suggestive evidence that the nephrotoxicity of cisplatin can be diminished by vigorous hydration and perhaps by giving the drug in a hypertonic solution. A high chloride concentration may minimize both the formation of the highly reactive platinum compounds described above and the uptake of cisplatin by the renal tubular cells. Amifostine, an organic thiophosphate, seems to diminish cisplatin-induced toxicity by donating a protective thiol group, an effect that is highly selective for normal, but not malignant, tissue. Discontinuation of platinum therapy once the plasma creatinine concentration begins to rise should prevent progressive renal failure.

Carboplatin has been synthesized as a non-nephrotoxic platinum analogue, but even though it is less nephrotoxic, it is not free of potential for renal injury. Hypomagnesemia seems to be the most common manifestation of nephrotoxicity. Other, less common renal side effects include recurrent salt wasting. No significant clinical nephrotoxicity due to oxaliplatin has yet been reported. Limited data have shown no exacerbation of preexisting mild renal impairment. Studies of oxaliplatin in patients with progressive degrees of renal failure are in progress.

Cyclophosphamide may produce significant side effects involving the urinary bladder (hemorrhagic cystitis). The primary renal effect of this agent is hyponatremia, which is due to impairment of the ability of the kidney to excrete water. The mechanism seems to be due to a direct effect of cyclophosphamide on the distal tubule and not to increased levels of antidiuretic hormone. Hyponatremia usually occurs acutely and resolves upon discontinuation of the drug (approximately 24 hours). It is recommended that isotonic saline be infused before cyclophosphamide administration to ameliorate this effect.

Ifosfamide nephrotoxicity has a primary renal effect to produce tubular renal toxicity. The damage produced by ifosfamide is concentrated in the proximal renal tubule, and a Fanconi syndrome has been observed after therapy. Other clinical syndromes that have been associated with ifosfamide include nephrogenic diabetes insipidus, renal tubular acidosis, and rickets. Preexisting renal disease is an important risk factor for ifosfamide nephrotoxicity.

Carmustine, lomustine, and semustine are lipid-soluble nitrosureas, which have been used against brain tumors. The exact mechanism of nephrotoxicity, however, is incompletely understood. High doses of semustine in children and adults have been associated with progressive renal dysfunction to marked renal insufficiency 3–5 years after therapy. The characteristic histologic changes include glomerular sclerosis without immune deposits and interstitial fibrosis. The incidence of nephrotoxicity was reported at 26% in patients with malignant melanoma treated with methyl CCNU (also known as lomustine) in the adjuvant setting. Nephrotoxicity has been reported in 65% to 75% of patients treated with streptozotocin for prolonged periods of time. Proteinuria is often the first sign of renal damage. This is followed by signs of proximal tubular damage, such as phosphaturia, glycosuria, aminoaciduria, uricosuria, and bicarbonaturia. Renal toxicity lasts approximately 2–3 weeks after discontinuing the drug.

The most common form of nephrotoxicity associated with mitomycin C is hemolytic uremic syndrome. It has been reported in patients who were treated with total doses of mitomycin C in excess of $60\,mg/m^2$. The renal damage caused by this antineoplastic agent seems to be direct endothelial damage. The incidence of

this syndrome ranges from 4% to 6% of patients who receive this drug alone or in combination.

Low or standard doses of methotrexate are usually not associated with renal toxicity, unless patients have underlying renal dysfunction. High doses $(1-15\,g/m^2)$ are associated with a 47% incidence of renal toxicity, accompanied by methotrexate crystals in the urine. The mechanism for methotrexate-induced nephrotoxicity is explained in part by its limited solubility at an acid pH, which leads to intratubular precipitation. Patients who are volume-depleted and excrete an acidic urine are at higher risk for nephrotoxicity. With aggressive hydration and urine alkalinization, the incidence of renal failure with high doses of methotrexate can be decreased. The clinical picture of methotrexate-induced renal failure is that of a nonoliguric renal failure. Preventive measures when using high doses of methotrexate include aggressive intravenous hydration with saline and urine alkalinization with sodium bicarbonate to maintain a urine pH around 7.0. If renal failure develops, methotrexate levels will increase and the risk of systemic toxicity will also be enhanced. In addition to supportive measures, patients should be started on folinic acid rescue, until levels of methotrexate fall below $0.5\,\mu M$.

VEGF- or VEGFR2-targeted agents produce albuminuria in 10% to 25% of patients, sometimes to nephrotic range. The exact mechanism has not been elucidated, but studies in mice with conditional expression of VEGF in the podocytes confirms a major role for VEGF in endothelial development and maintenance of a fenestrated endothelium (Arriaga et al., 2006). Like hypertension, this seems to be a class effect, but the factors associated with occurrence and severity are unknown. If clinically significant, decreasing the dose or discontinuation of drug are the only current approaches.

Late Complications of Cancer Chemotherapy

As cancer therapy has become increasingly effective and more patients live longer, late complications have become apparent separate from the direct toxic effects on organ system function described above. Gonadal dysfunction is one. In males, the primary lesion is depletion of germinal epithelium of seminiferous tubules with marked decrease in testicular volume, oligospermia or azoospermia, and infertility. There is an increase in follicle-stimulating hormone (FSH) and occasionally in luteinizing hormone (LH). No change is seen in serum testosterone. Alkylating agents (and irradiation) are the most damaging, and toxicity is dose-related. About 80% of males with Hodgkin disease treated with MOPP (mechlorethamine/vincristine/procarbazine/prednisone) are oligoazoospermic. About half recover in up to 4 years. Procarbazine is a major offender. Anthracyclines also cause azoospermia in a dose-related fashion. In females the primary lesion is ovarian fibrosis and follicle destruction. Amenorrhea ensues, with increase in FSH and LH and a decrease in estradiol leading to vaginal atrophy and endometrial hypoplasia. Onset and duration are dose- and age-related. Alkylating agents (and irradiation) again are the worst offenders.

In children the prepubertal effects may be less profound and reversible in males, although the pubertal effects may be more severe with often irreversible azoospermia, decreased testosterone, and increased FSH and LH. Less is known about females, but young girls seem quite resistant to alkylating agents.

No more tragic toxicity is seen with cancer chemotherapeutic agents than the induction of a second, treatment-related cancer in a patient cured of one cancer (Bhatia and Landier, 2005; Hudson et al., 2004). Of the wide variety of environmental and chemical agents causing cancer, there is one common thread in their mode of action—interaction with DNA. Clinical studies detailing this consequence of therapy have many problems, including the inherent bias of reporting index cases, the retrospective nature of many reports, the lack of reliable information on drug dosage, the total amount of drug given and duration of therapy, and the underlying incidence of a second malignancy. The direct-acting alkylating agents are most often implicated, and chronic, low-dose administration is a greater risk factor. Acute nonlymphocytic leukemia or myelodysplasia is the best described. The indirect-acting topoisomerase II agents produce a specific 11q23 translocation.

Osteonecrosis of the jaw has been seen with increasing frequency during the past few years, related in part to chronic use of intravenous bisphosphonates for advanced cancer. The incidence has been estimated at 1% to 10% of patients receiving these medications (Badros et al., 2006). The pathogenesis and optimal management for osteonecrosis of the jaw are poorly understood, with multiple risk factors and various treatments involved (Ruggerio et al., 2006).

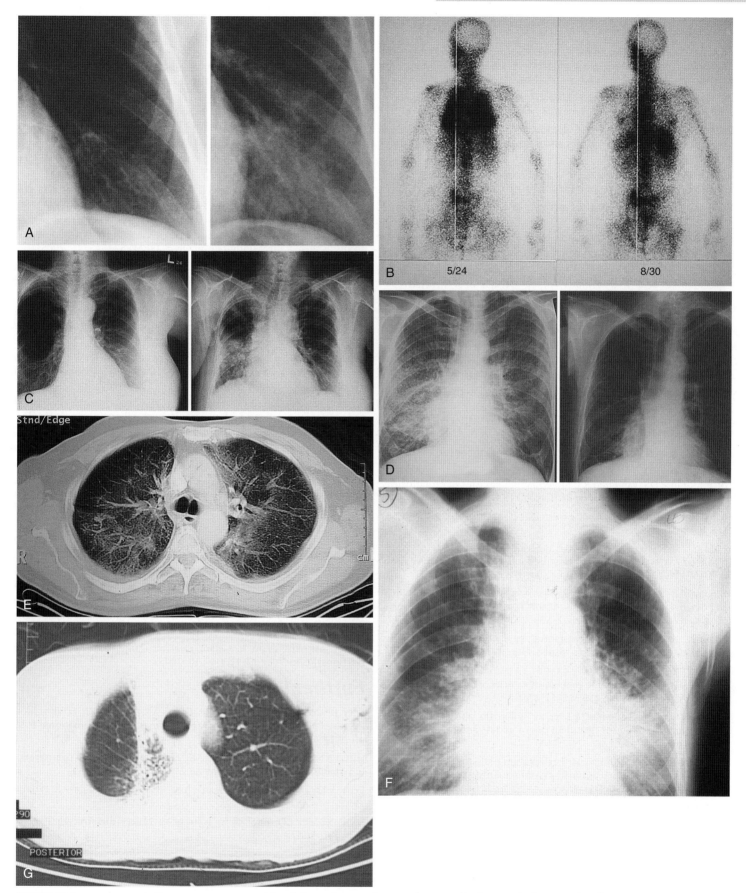

FIGURE 21.8 **ORGAN TOXICITY.** Nonmucocutaneous toxicity of chemotherapeutic agents is covered in the text. The lung may be affected by several agents including bleomycin. **(A)** The earliest radiographic changes are linear infiltrates in the lower lung fields. **(B)** Gallium-67 uptake is quite striking but is reversible, as this serial study demonstrates. **(C)** While usually dose-related, progressive changes may occur resulting in fibrosis and pulmonary insufficiency. Other drugs such as alkylating agents and high-dose methotrexate may result in diffuse infiltrates **(D)**, which were reversible 4 months later. **(E)** In this patient several courses of gemcitabine resulted in acute dyspnea and decreased oxygen saturation. Evaluation with lung biopsy and other studies showed no evidence of infection, pulmonary emboli, or other diagnosable disease. Use of prednisone led to rapid improvement and regression of the interstitial infiltrates. **(F)** Acute radiation pneumonitis in a 58-year-old man who received palliative mediastinal radiation therapy for regional lung cancer nodal metastases. Prednisone was prescribed for significant cough and dyspnea, which gradually regressed over several weeks. A higher dose (>3000 cGy) and large radiation therapy fields increase this lung toxicity, as does concomitant use of some chemotherapeutic drugs and irradiation. **(G)** Chronic radiation pneumonitis in a 64-year-old man due to previous therapeutic radiation therapy for unilateral right hilar adenopathy from lung cancer. The acute effects were subclinical, but chronic fibrosis and reduced lung volumes are quite common and may slowly progress over months and years. These problems can be reduced by use of modern three-dimensional conformal radiation therapy.

References and Selected Readings

Ando M, Okamoto I, Yamamoto N, et al: Predictive factors for interstitial lung disease, antitumor response, and survival in non-small-cell lung cancer patients treated with gefitinib, *J Clin Oncol* 24:2549–2556, 2006.

Arriaga Y, Becerra: Adverse effects of bevacizumab and their management in solid tumors, *Supportive Cancer Therapy* 3:247–250, 2006.

Badros A, Weikel D, Salama A, et al: Osteonecrosis of the jaw in multiple myeloma patients: clinical features and risk factors, *J Clin Oncol* 24:945–952, 2006.

Belknap SM, Kuzel TM, Yarnold PR, et al: Clinical features and correlates of gemcitabine-associated lung injury, *Cancer* 106:2051–2057, 2006.

Bhatia S, Landier W: Evaluating survivors of pediatric cancer, *Cancer J* 11:340–354, 2005.

Crawford J, Cella D, Sonis ST: Managing chemotherapy-related side effects: trends in the use of cytokines and other growth factors, *Oncology* 20(Suppl):2006.

Cristaaudo A, Sera F, Severino V, et al: Occupational hypersensitivity to metal salts, including platinum, in the secondary industry, *Allergy* 60(2):138–139, 2005.

Drake MT, Clarke BL, Khosla S: Bisphosphonates: mechanism of action and role in clinical practice, *Mayo Clin Proc* 83:1032–1045, 2008.

Erimina V, Quaggin SE: The role of VEGF-A in glomerular development and function, *Curr Opin Nephrol Hypertens* 13:9–15, 2004.

Escudier B, Szczylik C, Eisen T, et al: Randomized phase III trial of the Raf kinase and VEGFR inhibitor sorafenib (BAY 43–9006) in patients with advanced renal cell carcinoma (RCC), *J Clin Oncol* 23(Suppl 18), 2005. abstract 4510.

Floyd JD, Nguyen DT, Lobins RL, et al: Cardiotoxicity of cancer therapy, *J Clin Oncol* 23:7685–7696, 2005.

Force T, Krause DS, Van Etten RA: Molecular mechanisms of cardiotoxicity of tyrosine kinase inhibition, *Nat Rev Cancer* 7(5):332–334, 2007.

Genetech Pharmaceuticals: *Avastin prescribing information*, 2004, Physicians Desk Reference@pdr.net.

Hudson MM, Mertens AC, Yasui Y, et al: Health status in adults treated for childhood cancer: a report from the childhood survivor study, *Am J Oncol Rev* 3:165–170, 2004.

Hurwitz H: Integrating the anti-VEGF—a humanized monoclonal antibody bevacizumab with chemotherapy in advanced colorectal cancer, *Clin Colorectal Cancer* 4(Suppl 2):S62–S68, 2004.

Ibrahim T, Barbanti F, Giorgio–Marrano G, et al: Osteonecrosis of the jaw in patients with bone metastases treated with bisphosphonates: a restrospective study, *Oncologist* 13:330–336, 2008.

Kerkela R, Grazette L, Yacobi R, et al: Cardiotoxicity of the cancer therapeutic agent imatinib mesylate, *Nat Med* 12(8):908–916, 2006.

Kerr DJ, Dunn JA, Langman MJ, et al: Rofecoxib and cardiovascular adverse events in adjuvant treatment of colorectal cancer, *N Engl J Med* 357:360–369, 2007.

Kirshner JJ, Hickok J, Hofman M: Pegfilgrastim-induced bone pain: incidence, risk factors, and management in a community practice, *Community Oncology* 4:455–458, 2007.

Lai SE, Kuzel T, Lacouture ME: Hand-foot and stump syndrome to sorafenib, *J Clin Oncol* 25:341–346, 2007.

Letter to the editor: Bisphosphonate-induced osteonecrosis of the jaw: long-term outcomes, *J Support Oncol* 7:9–10, 2009.

Lorusso P, Karmanos BA: Toward evidence-based management of the dermatologic effects of EFGR inhibitors, *Oncology* 23:186–198, 2009.

Motzer RJ, Hutson TE, Tomczak P, et al: Phase III randomized trial of sunitinib malate (SU11248) versus interferon alfa as first line systemic therapy for patients with metastatic renal cell carcinoma, *J Clin Oncol* 24(Suppl 18):930s, 2006. abstract LBA3.

Moy B, Goss PE: Lapatinib-associated toxicity and practical management recommendations, *Oncologist* 12:756–765, 2007.

Nalluri SR, Chu D, Keresztes R, et al: Risk of venous thromboembolism with the angiogenesis inhibitor be vacizumab in cancer patients, *JAMA* 300:2277–2285, 2008.

Niho S, Kubota K, Goto K, et al: First-line single agent treatment with gefitinib in patients with advanced non-small cell lung cancer: a phase II study, *J Clin Oncol* 24(1):64–69, 2006.

Perez-Solar R, Saltz L: Cutaneous adverse effects with HER1/EGFR-targeted agents: is there a silver lining? *J Clin Oncol* 23(24):5235–5246, 2005.

Ratain MJ, Eisen T, Stadler WM, et al: Phase II placebo-controlled randomized discontinuation trial of sorafenib in patients with metastatic renal cell carcinoma, *J Clin Oncol* 24:2505–2512, 2006.

Rajasekhar A, George TJ: Gemcitabine-induced reversible posterior leukoencephalopathy syndrome: a case report and review of the literature, *Oncologist* 12:1332–1335, 2007.

Ruggiero S, Gralow J, Marx RE, et al: Practical guidelines for the prevention, diagnosis and treatment of osteonecrosis of the jaw in patients with cancer, *J Oncol Pract* 2:7–14, 2006.

Schmidinger M, Zielinski CC, Vogl UM, et al: Cardiac toxicity of sunitinib and sorafenib in patients with metastatic renal cell carcinoma, *J Clin Oncol* 26:5204–5212, 2008.

Strevel EL, Ing DJ, Siu LL: Molecularly targeted oncology therapeutics and prolongation of the QT interval, *J Clin Oncol* 25:3362–3371, 2007.

Strumberg D, Clark JW, Awada A, et al: Safety, pharmacokinetics, and preliminary antitumor activity of sorafenib: a review of four phase I trials in patients with advanced refractory solid tumors, *Oncologist* 12:426–437, 2007.

Szebeni J: Complement activation-related pseudoallergy: a new class of drug-induced acute immune toxicity, *Toxicology* 216:106–121, 2005.

Telli ML, Hunt SA, Carlson RW, et al: Trastuzumab-related cardiotoxicity: calling into question the concept of reversibility, *J Clin Oncol* 25:3525–3533, 2007.

Weiss RB: Toxicity of chemotherapy—the last decade, *Semin Oncol* 33:1, 2006.

Zorzou MP, Efstathiou E, Galani E, et al: Carboplatin hypersensitivity reactions, *J Chemother* 17(1):104–110, 2005.

Further Reading

Eder JP: Neoplasms. In Page CP, Curtis MJ, Sutter MC, et al, editors: *Integrated pharmacology*, London, Mosby–Times Mirror International,1997, pp. 501–522.

Hussain S, Anderson DN, Salvatti ME, et al: Onycholysis as a complication of systemic chemotherapy, *Cancer* 88:2367–2371, 2000.

Perry MD: *The chemotherapy source book*, Baltimore, Williams & Wilkins, 1992.

Sonis ST, Fey EG: Oral complications of cancer therapy, *Oncology* 16: 680–691, 2002.

Index

Notes: Page numbers suffixed with 'f' indicate figures: page numbers suffixed with 't' indicate tables: page numbers suffixed with 'b' indicate boxes

A

Abdomen
  plain film radiographs of, 8
    marginal zone lymphoma in, 623f
  ultrasonography of, 12
Ablation
  tumor, 26
  ultrasound, 12
ABVD regimen, for Hodgkin disease, 697–698
Acidophilic adenoma, pituitary, 392f
Acidosis, lactic, cancer-associated, 711
Acinic cell carcinoma, of salivary glands, 61t, 73f
Acoustic neuroma (schwannoma), 508, 508f, 509f
Acquired immunodeficiency syndrome (AIDS), 694
  malignancies associated with. *See* AIDS-associated malignancy(ies).
Acquired sideroblastic anemia, MDS type II, 551f
Acromegaly, colorectal cancer associated with, 213
Actinomycin
  skin eruptions due to, 724
  skin ulceration/extravasation due to, 727
Acute febrile neutrophilic dermatoses (Sweet's syndrome), 546f
Acute leukemia, 529–550
  clinical manifestations of, 529–550
  definition of, 529
  mixed-cell type, 541f
  morphology and biology of, 529
  myelofibrosis transformed to, 553f, 554f
  WHO classification of, 530t
Acute lymphoblastic leukemia
  clinical manifestations of, 529–550
    cutaneous, 543f
    mediastinal involvement in, 542f
    meningeal infiltration in, 542f
  CNS metastasis in, 523–527, 526f
  complications of, 549f
    therapy-induced, 549f
  immunologic classification of, 531t
  in adults, 529
  in children, 529
  L1 subtype, 531f, 533f, 534f
  L2 subtype, 534f
  L3 subtype, 535f
Acute megakaryocytic leukemia, M7 subtype, 541f
Acute monocytic leukemia
  M5A subtype, 539f, 540f
  M5B subtype, 539f
Acute myeloblastic leukemia
  CNS metastasis in, 523–527, 526f
  M0 subtype, 536f
  M1 subtype, 536f, 537f
  M2 subtype, 537f, 538f

Acute myeloid leukemia
  classification of, 532t
  clinical manifestations of, 529–550
    acute febrile neutrophilic dermatoses (Sweet's syndrome), 546f
    cutaneous, 543f, 544f
    intraoral, 544f, 545f
    myeloblastoma, 545f, 546f
    ophthalmic infiltration in, 547f
    renal infiltration in, 547f
    vertebral infiltration in, 547f
  complications of, 548f
Acute myelomonocytic leukemia, M4 subtype, 539f
Acute promyelocytic leukemia, M3 subtype, 538f, 539f
Adamantinoma, 420f
Adamantinomatous craniopharyngioma, 520–522
Addison's disease, 710–711
Adenocarcinoma
  ampulla of Vater, 195–203, 202f, 203f
  bladder, 234–235, 258f, 259f
  cecal, 224f, 225f
  colonic, 226f
    in ascending colon, 225f
    in sigmoid colon, 225f
  differential diagnosis of, antibody panel in, 1, 2t
  endometrial, 298f, 295
  esophageal, 169, 175f, 176f
  gallbladder, 200f, 201f
  gastric, 177, 178f, 179f, 180f
    diffuse type, 177, 182f, 183f
    fungating type, 177, 181f, 182f
    polypoid type, 177, 181f
    scirrhous pattern of, 177
    superficial type of, 177
    ulcerative variant of, 177, 180f
  lung, 99, 111f, 112f
    stage I, 127f
    stage II, 129f
    stage IIA, 129f
    stage IIIB, 133f, 134f, 135f, 138f, 139f, 140f
  pancreatic, 185, 191f
  parotid gland, 95f
  prostatic, 233, 239f, 241f, 242f, 243f, 245f, 246f
  rectal, 227f
  salivary gland, 61t, 72f
  small bowel, 203
    of appendix, 207f
    of ileum, 206f
    of jejunum, 205f
  thyroid
    follicular, 365t, 366, 372f, 373f
    papillary, 365–366, 365t, 369f, 370f
      metastatic, 369f

Adenoid cystic adenoma, 120f
Adenoid cystic carcinoma, salivary gland, 61t, 72f, 73f
Adenoma
  adenoid cystic, 120f
  adrenocortical, 380f, 381f
  colorectal
    tubular, 216f, 217f
    tubulovillous, 217f, 218f
    villous, 218f, 219f
      sessile, 218f
  lactating, 326, 329f
  pituitary, 389, 392f
    chromophobe, 391f
  pleomorphic
    of parotid gland, 93f, 94f
    of salivary glands, 61, 70f
    of submandibular gland, carcinoma arising in, 95f
  renal cortical, 261f
  thyroid, follicular, 371f, 372f
Adenomatosis, diffuse, in familial adenomatous polyposis, 205f
Adenosis, sclerosing, of breast, 326, 330f
Adhesion molecules, in multiple myeloma, 640, 646f
Adrenal gland tumor(s), 377–382
  cortical
    adenoma, 380f, 381f
    carcinoid tumor, 380f
    carcinoma, 380f, 381f, 382f
      metastatic, 381f, 382f
    clinical manifestations of, 378, 378t
    incidence of, 377–378
    lymphoma, 382f
    molecular biology of, 378–382
    morphology of, 378
    myelolipoma, 381f
  medullary
    ganglioneuroma, 388f
    paraganglioma, 383–388. *See also* Paraganglioma.
    pheochromocytoma, 382–383, 384f, 385f
Adrenal insufficiency, cancer-associated, 710–711
Adrenal metastasis, from lung cancer, 143f, 382f
Adrenocortical adenoma, 380f, 381f
  in Conn's syndrome, 380f
Adrenocortical hyperplasia, in Cushing's syndrome, 379f
Adrenocorticotrophic hormone (ACTH), 388t
  in Cushing's syndrome, 378
  overproduction of, pituitary and ectopic, clinical features of, 388, 388t
Adriamycin, skin ulceration/extravasation due to, 727f
Adult T-cell lymphoma-leukemia, 590, 609f
  cutaneous involvement in, 612f

Gorlin syndrome (basal cell nevus syndrome), 452, 460f
  medullablastoma associated with, 484–485
Graft-versus-host disease, after bone marrow transplantation, 549f
Granulocytic sarcoma (myeloblastoma), in acute myeloid leukemia, 545f, 546f
Granuloma, midline lethal nonhealing, of head and neck, 62
Granulosa cell tumor, ovarian, 278t, 279–295, 284f, 285f, 293f
Growth factor(s), abnormal, in small cell lung cancer, 103
Growth hormone (GH), 388t
Gums
  hypertrophy of, in acute myeloid leukemia, 545f
  leukemic infiltration of, 544f
Gynecologic tumor(s), 278–324. *See also under anatomy or specific malignancy for details.*
  cervical, 307–313
  clinical manifestations of, cervical, 307–313
  endometrial, 295–307
  fallopian tube, 313
  gestational trophoblastic neoplasia, 314–323
  ovarian, 278–295
  peritoneal, 313–314
  vaginal, 313
  vulvar, 313
Gynecomastia, associated with diethylstilbestrol therapy, for prostate cancer, 250f

H

Hair loss, chemotherapy-induced, 722–723, 722f
Hairy cell leukemia, 556, 563f, 564f, 565f
  splenic involvement in, 564f, 565f
Halstead theory, of breast cancer spread, 327, 335f
Hamartoma, bronchial, 119f
Hamartomatous polyp, in Peutz-Jeghers syndrome, 205f
Hand-foot syndrome, chemotherapy-induced, 725f, 730
Head and neck cancer, 60–97. *See also under anatomy or malignancy for details.*
  clinical manifestations of, 74
  FDG-PET scan of, 37, 40f
  histology of, 60–61
  hypopharyneal, 75, 76f, 80f
  laryngeal, 75, 76f, 86f
  less frequent lesions in, 61–62
  lip, 74, 76f
  molecular biology of, 62–73
  nasal cavity, 75
  nasopharyngeal, 74–75, 74t, 77f, 80f
  nodal and metastatic categories for, 76f
  oral cavity, 74, 78f
  oropharyngeal, 75, 76f, 80f
  paranasal sinuses, 75, 76f, 88f
  risk factors for, 60
  salivary glands, 61, 61t, 76f
    major and minor, 75–96
  staging of, 73–74, 73t
  tumor categories for, 76f
  tumor type in, classification of, 61, 61t
Heart, tumors of. *See* Cardiac tumor(s).
Heavy-chain disease, 642, 663f, 664f, 665f
Helicobacter pylori
  extranodal marginal zone lymphoma associated with, 588
  gastric cancer associated with, 177
Heliotrope rash, in dermatomyositis, 714
Hemangioblastoma, capillary, 511–518, 515f, 516f
Hemangiopericytoma (angioblastic meningioma), 426, 511
Hematologic complications, of malignancy, 709t, 711–712

Hematologic diseases, leukemic transformation in, 550–554
Hemochromatosis, hepatocellular carcinoma in, 195, 197f
Hemolytic anemia, autoimmune, chronic lymphocytic leukemia with, 557f
Hemorrhagic cystitis, 254f
Hemothorax, in mesothelioma, 161, 162f
Hepatic. *See also* Liver *entries.*
Hepatic angiosarcoma, 198f, 199f, 433f
Hepatic vascular tumors, vinyl chloride exposure associated with, 199f
Hepatic vein, obstruction of (Budd-Chiari syndrome), 195
Hepatobiliary cancer, 195–203. *See also* Biliary cancer; Liver cancer.
Hepatoblastoma, 669, 680f, 681f, 682f
  vs. hepatoma, 669t
Hepatocellular carcinoma, 195
  cirrhotic liver and, 195, 196f
  metastatic, 195, 198f
  multifocal, 197f
  staging of, 195, 197f
  uninodular, 197f
  with esophageal varices, 196f
Hepatoma, 195, 196f, 669
  malignant. *See* Hepatocellular carcinoma
  vs. hepatoblastoma, 669t
Hepatomegaly, follicular lymphoma and, 627f
Hepatosplenic gamma delta T-cell lymphoma, 589–590
Hepatotoxicity, chemotherapy-induced, 731
HER family receptors, 333f
HER2 gene, in breast cancer, 3–5
HER2/neu status, determination of, 328, 362f
Hereditary nonpolyposis colon cancer, 212
Hermatite pneumoconiosis, 111f
Herpes zoster infection, 716f
  in chronic lymphocytic leukemia, 560f
  in Hodgkin disease, 586f
Highly active antiretroviral therapy (HART)
  for Hodgkin disease, 697–698
  for Kaposi sarcoma, 695
  for non-Hodgkin lymphoma, 696
Histone deacetylase (HDAC) inhibitor, for multiple myeloma, 641–642
Hodgkin disease, 571–586
  AIDS-related, 697–698, 705f, 706f, 707f
  Ann Arbor staging of, 571–572, 576f
    stage IA, 577f
    stage II, 580f
    stage IIA, 578f, 579f
    stage III, 583f
    stage IIIA, 581f, 582f
    stage IIIB, 581f
    stage IV, 583f, 584f, 585f
    stage IVB, 584f
  clinical evaluation and staging of, 571–572
  clinical manifestations of, 572–586
  diagnosis of, monoclonal antibodies in, 606t
  gallium-67 scan of, 46, 50f, 51f
  histologic classification of, 571, 572f
  immunobiology of, 571
  lymphocyte-predominant, 572–586, 572f
  metastatic, involving central nervous system, 523
  mixed-cellularity type, 575f
  nephrotic syndrome in, 585f
  nodular-sclerosis type, 573f, 574f
  PET scan of, 571
  Reed-Sternberg cells in, 571, 572f, 573f, 574f, 575f
  relapse of, 586f
  splenic involvement in, 583f
  thymic, 577f
Hormonal therapy, for breast cancer, 328
Horn pattern, cutaneous, in premalignant lesions, 450f

Horner's syndrome, in lung cancer, 104, 131f
HRAS gene, in non-small cell lung cancer, 101
Human herpesvirus-8 (HHV-8), in AIDS-related neoplasms, 694, 696
Human papillomavirus (HPV)
  in cervical cancer, 307, 698–708
  in head and neck cancer, 60, 62–73
  warty carcinoma associated with, 462f
Human T-cell lymphoma-leukemia virus 1 (HTLV-1) infection, 586–587
Humerus
  chondrosarcoma of, 418f
  giant cell tumor of, 419f, 420f
  osteosarcoma of, 691f
Hürthle cells, in follicular thyroid adenocarcinoma, 373f
Hydatidiform mole, 324
  complete, 321f
  invasive, 322f
  partial, 321f
Hydroxycarbamide
  hepatotoxicity of, 731
  radiation recall reactions due to, 729–730
Hypercalcemia, cancer-associated, 710, 710t
Hypercoagulable states, cancer-associated, 711
Hyperleukocytosis, definition of, 711
Hyperpigmentation, chemotherapy-induced, 724–727, 725f
Hyperpigmented plaques, in Kaposi sarcoma, 434f
Hypersensitivity reactions
  chemotherapy-induced, 721–722, 722f
  in chronic lymphocytic leukemia, 560f
Hypertrophic osteoarthropathy
  bone scan of, 32, 35f
  pulmonary, 149f, 150f, 717f
Hyperviscosity syndrome
  cancer-associated, 711
  causes of, 660t
  in multiple myeloma, 659f
  in Waldenström's macroglobulinemia, 662f, 711
Hyponatremia, cancer-associated, 710
Hypopharyngeal cancer, 75, 76f, 80f
  squamous cell carcinoma, 85f
  tumor categories for, 80f
Hypoxia-induible factor (HIF), 235

I

Idarubicin, cardiac toxicity due to, 730
Ifosfamide
  nail changes due to, 728
  nephrotoxicity of, 733
  neurotoxicity of, 732
  skin hyperpigmentation due to, 724
Ileal metastasis, from malignant melanoma, 211f
Ileum
  adenocarcinoma of, 203, 206f
  carcinoid tumor of, 208f, 394f
Image-guided biopsy, 26
Image-guided therapy, 26–27
  response to, 27–28, 28f
Imaging coils, in magnetic resonance imaging, 25
Imaging studies, 6–29
  computed tomographic, 12–19, 13f, 14f. *See also* Computed tomography (CT).
  contrast agents in
    gastrointestinal, 9
    intravenous, 9
  cost and radiation dose comparison in, 8t
  digital radiographs in, 7
  goals of, 6–7, 7f
  image-guided biopsy in, 26
  magnetic resonance, 22–26, 23f, 24f. *See also* Magnetic resonance imaging (MRI).
  mammographic, 9–11. *See also* Mammography.